CORNEAL TRANSPLANTATION

VIDEO CONTENTS

Scan QR code to access the videos

CORNEAL TRANSPLANTATION

Third Edition

Editors

Namrata Sharma
MD FRCOphth FRCSEd
Professor of Ophthalmology
Cataract, Cornea and Refractive Surgery Services
Dr Rajendra Prasad Centre for Ophthalmic Sciences
All India Institute of Medical Sciences
New Delhi, India

Ritu Nagpal
MD FLVPEI (Cornea)
Senior Research Associate
Cataract, Cornea and Refractive Surgery Services
Dr Rajendra Prasad Centre for Ophthalmic Sciences
All India Institute of Medical Sciences
New Delhi, India

Rasik B Vajpayee
MS FRCSEd FRANZCO
Professor of Ophthalmology
Cornea, Cataract and Refractive Surgery Services
Vision Eye Institute, Melbourne
Royal Victorian Eye and Ear Hospital
University of Melbourne
Melbourne, Australia

Forewords

Hugh R Taylor
Mark J Mannis
Jorge L Alió

JAYPEE

JAYPEE BROTHERS MEDICAL PUBLISHERS
The Health Sciences Publisher
New Delhi | London

Jaypee Brothers Medical Publishers (P) Ltd

Headquarters
Jaypee Brothers Medical Publishers (P) Ltd
EMCA House, 23/23-B
Ansari Road, Daryaganj
New Delhi 110 002, India
Landline: +91-11-23272143, +91-11-23272703
+91-11-23282021, +91-11-23245672
Email: jaypee@jaypeebrothers.com

Corporate Office
Jaypee Brothers Medical Publishers (P) Ltd
4838/24, Ansari Road, Daryaganj
New Delhi 110 002, India
Phone: +91-11-43574357
Fax: +91-11-43574314
Email: jaypee@jaypeebrothers.com

Overseas Office
JP Medical Ltd.
83 Victoria Street, London
SW1H 0HW (UK)
Phone: +44 20 3170 8910
Fax: +44 (0)20 3008 6180
Email: info@jpmedpub.com

Website: www.jaypeebrothers.com
Website: www.jaypeedigital.com

Corneal Transplantation

First Edition: 2002
Second Edition: 2010
Third Edition: **2023**

ISBN: 978-93-89587-22-7

Printed at Replika Press Pvt. Ltd.

Dedication

To my respectable parents, Dr Ramesh C Sharma and Mrs Maitreyi Pushpa, my husband, Dr Subhash Chandra and my beloved daughter, Vasavdatta

–Namrata Sharma

To my mentors, who taught me the art of corneal transplantation and my ever supportive family

–Ritu Nagpal

To my wife, Madhu and my dearly loved children, Mihika and Shubhankar

–Rasik B Vajpayee

Contributors

Ahmad Kheirkhah MD
Assistant Professor
Department of Ophthalmology
Long School of Medicine
University of Texas Health San Antonio
San Antonio, TX, USA

Amar Agarwal MS FRCS FRCOphth
Chairman
Dr Agarwal's Group of Eye Hospitals
Chennai, Tamil Nadu, India

Anahita Kate MS
Consultant
The Cornea Institute, KVC Campus
LV Prasad Eye Institute
Vijayawada, Andhra Pradesh, India

Angeli Christy Yu MD
Doctoral Student
University of Ferrara
Department of Translational Medicine
Ferrara, Italy
Ospedali Privati Forlì "Villa Igea"
Department of Ophthalmology
Forlì, Italy
Istituto Internazionale per la Ricerca e Formazione in Oftalmologia
Forlì, Italy

Ankita B Dube MS
Consultant Ophthalmologist
Chandra Nursing home
Dewas, Madhya Pradesh, India

Antonio Moramarco MD
Consultant
Ophthalmology Unit, DIMES
Alma Mater Studiorum
University of Bologna and S Orsola–Malpighi Teaching Hospital
Bologna, Italy

Asaf Friehmann MD
Head, Cornea Services
Meir Medical Center
Kfar Saba, Israel
Ospedali Privati Forlì "Villa Igea"
Department of Ophthalmology
Forlì, Italy
Istituto Internazionale per la Ricerca e Formazione in Oftalmologia
Forlì, Italy

Ben Connell BMBS FRANZCO MPH
Consultant, Cornea Unit
Royal Victorian Eye and Ear Hospital
32 Gisborne St, East Melbourne VIC 3002
Australia

Bhaskar Srinivasan MS
Senior Consultant
Cornea and Refractive Surgery Services
Sankara Nethralaya
Chennai, Tamil Nadu, India

Bhavana Sharma MS MAMS
Professor and Head
Department of Ophthalmology
All India Institute of Medical Sciences
Bhopal, Madhya Pradesh, India

Bruce D Allan MD FRCOphth
Consultant
Cornea and External Disease Service
Moorfields Eye Hospital
London, UK

C Banu Cosar MD
Professor of Ophthalmology
Director
Department of Ophthalmology
Acibadem Mehmet Ali Aydinlar University
Istanbul, Turkey

C Maya Tong BSc MD
Cornea and Anterior Segment Fellow
Vancouver, British Columbia, Canada
Netherlands Institute for Innovative Ocular Surgery and
Department of Ophthalmology
University of Montreal Health Centre
Montreal, Canada

Chandrashekhar Kumar MD
Consultant Ophthalmologist
Cornea and Refractive Surgeon
Shekhar Eye Care and Laser Centre
Patna, Bihar, India

Christopher J Rapuano MD
Chief, Cornea Services
Wills Eye Hospital
840 Walnut Street, Suite 920
Philadelphia, PA 19107

Collin Ross CEBT MPM
Vice President—Global Development
Eversight
Ann Arbor, Michigan, USA

David S Rootman MD
Medical Director
Department of Ophthalmology and Vision Sciences
University of Toronto, Toronto
Ontario, Canada

Denisse Pinkus MD FICO
Cornea and Refractive Surgery Specialist
CODET Vision Institute
Blvd Padre Kino No 10159
Zona Urbana Río Tijuan, 22010
Tijuana BC, México

Elsie Chan MBBS (Hon) MPH FRANZCO
Consultant Ophthalmologist
Royal Victorian Eye and Ear Hospital
University of Melbourne
Melbourne, Australia

Eric Donnenfeld MD
Cornea, Laser Cataract and Refractive Surgeon
Ophthalmic Consultants of Long Island
Rockville Centre
New York, USA

Francis W Price Jr MD
Founder and CEO
Price Vision Group, 9002
N. Meridian St, Suite 100
Indianapolis, IN 46260, USA

Geetha Iyer MS
Senior Consultant
Dr G Sitalakshmi Memorial Clinic for Ocular Surface Disorders
Sankara Nethralaya
Chennai, Tamil Nadu, India

Gerald W Zaidman MD
Professor
Department of Ophthalmology
Westchester Medical Center
New York Medical College
Valhalla, New York, USA

Gerrit RJ Melles MD PhD
Director
Netherlands Institute for Innovative Ocular Surgery
Melles Cornea Clinic, Rotterdam
Amnitrans Eye Bank
Rotterdam, Netherlands

Giuseppe Giannaccare MD PhD
Professor
Department of Ophthalmology
University of Magna Graecia
Catanzaro, Italy

Graeme A Pollock
BSc (Hons) GCUT MPH PhD OAM
Director
Lions Eye Donation Service
Centre for Eye Research, Australia
The University of Melbourne
Melbourne, Australia

Gurnarinder Singh MD
Consultant
Prabodh Chander Eye Hospital
Gurdaspur, Punjab, India

Haitham Al-Mahrouqi
BMedSc (Hons) MBChB OMSB ABO
Fellow in Cornea and Anterior Segment
The University of Auckland
Auckland, New Zealand

Harsha Saxena
Department of Ophthalmology
All India Institute of Medical Sciences
Bhopal, Madhya Pradesh, India

Hassan Mansoor
Assistant Professor/Consultant Eye Surgeon
Department of Cornea and Refractive Surgery
Al-Shifa Trust Eye Hospital
Punjab, Pakistan

Heather Machin
Senior Project Manager and Lions Fellow (LEDS-Eye Bank/CERA-Biobank/Corneal Research Unit)
Centre for Eye Research Australia (CERA)
Project Consultant
The Fred Hollows Foundation, NZ

Hiren Matai
Sankara Nethralaya
Medical Research Foundation
Chennai, Tamil Nadu, India

Hugh R Taylor AC LLD (Hon) MD
FAHMS FRANZCO
Professor
Past President
The International Council of Ophthalmology
Melbourne Laureate Professor and Harold Mitchell Chair of Indigenous Eye Health
Melbourne School of Population and Global Health, University of Melbourne
Melbourne, Australia

James Chodosh MD MPH
Professor
Department of Ophthalmology
Harvard Medical School
Boston, MA, USA

Jeewan S Titiyal MD
Professor and Head
Department of Ophthalmology
Cataract, Cornea and Refractive Surgery Services
Dr Rajendra Prasad Centre for Ophthalmic Sciences
All India Institute of Medical Sciences
New Delhi, India

Jodhbir S Mehta MBBS FRCOphth
FRCS (Ed) FAMS PhD (UK)
Head
Corneal and External Eye Disease Service
Senior Consultant Refractive Service
Singapore
National Eye Centre
Deputy Executive Director, Head Tissue Engineering and Stem Cells Group
Singapore Eye Research Institute
Deputy Vice Chair (Research) of Ophthalmology and Visual Sciences
Academic Clinical Programme
SingHealth Duke-NUS Academic Medical Centre (AMC)
Professor, Duke-NUS Graduate Medical School
Adjunct Professor
School of Material Science and Engineering and School of Mechanical and Aerospace Engineering
Nanyang Technological University
Adjunct Professor
Yong Loo Lin School of Medicine
Department of Ophthalmology
National University of Singapore

Jonathan G Crowston MD
Professor of Ophthalmology
Center for Eye Research
Melbourne University
Melbourne, Australia

Jorge L Alió MD PhD FEBO
Professor and Chairman of Ophthalmology
University Miguel Hernandez de Elche
Alicante, Spain

Jorge L Alió del Barrio MD PhD FEBOS-CR
Consultant and Surgeon in Ophthalmology Cornea, Cataract and Refractive Surgery Unit
Vissum Instituto Oftalmológico de Alicante
Associate Professor, Universidad Miguel Hernández, Alicante (Spain)

Karl Anders Knutsson
Consultant Ophthalmologist
Cornea and Ocular Surface Unit
San Raffaele Scientific Institute
Milan, Italy

Karl David Brown BSc MPhil PhD
Research Scientist
Centre for Eye Research Australia and Department of Ophthalmology
University of Melbourne
Melbourne, Australia

Keamela Vasanthananthan MD
Consultant
Netherlands Institute for Innovative Ocular Surgery
Melles Cornea Clinic
Rotterdam, Netherlands

Louis J Stevenson MD PhD
Head of Department
Royal Victorian Eye and Ear Hospital
Melbourne, Australia

Luigi Fontana MD PhD
Head of Department
Ophthalmology Unit
DIMES, Alma Mater Studiorum
University of Bologna and S Orsola—Malpighi Teaching Hospital
Bologna, Italy

Mark J Mannis MD FACS
Professor and Chair
Department of Ophthalmology and Vision Science
University of California, Davis
California, USA

M Vanathi MD
Professor of Ophthalmology
Cataract, Cornea and Refractive Surgery Services
Dr Rajendra Prasad Centre for Ophthalmic Sciences
All India Institute of Medical Sciences
New Delhi, India

Manotosh Ray MBBS MD (AIIMS) FRCSEd
Senior Consultant and Head
Cornea and Refractive Service
Department of Ophthalmology
National University Health System
Associate Professor and UG Education Director
Yong Loo Lin School of Medicine
National University of Singapore
Singapore

Marianne O Price PhD MBA
Executive Director
Cornea Research Foundation of America, 9002
N Meridian St, Suite 212
Indianapolis, IN 46260, USA

Massimo Busin MD
Professor
University of Ferrara
Department of Translational Medicine
Ferrara, Italy
Ospedali Privati Forlì "Villa Igea"
Department of Ophthalmology, Forlì, Italy
Istituto Internazionale per la Ricerca e Formazione in Oftalmologia Forlì, Italy

Michael S Loughnan MBBS PhD FRANZCO
Senior Consultant, Cornea Services
Royal Victorian Eye and Ear Hospital
32 Gisborne St, East Melbourne VIC 3002
Australia

Mohamed Ibrahime Asif MD DNB
Consultant
Cornea and Refractive Surgery Services
Eye7 Hospital
New Delhi, India

Mohammed Ziaei MBChB (Hons) MD CertLRS FRCOphth FRANZCO
Department of Ophthalmology
University of Auckland
Auckland, New Zealand

Monica Chaudhry MSc PhD
Consultant Optometrist and Educator
Founder Learn Beyond Vision
Former Director (Health Sciences)
Sushant University
Gurugram, Haryana, India

Mukesh Taneja MS
Consultant, Cornea and Refractive Surgery Services
Tetravue Super Speciality Eye Centre
New Delhi, India

Nagib Du Toit
Consultant
University of Cape Town
Cape Town, 7700, South Africa

Namrata Sharma MD FRCOphth FRCSEd
Professor of Ophthalmology
Cataract, Cornea and Refractive Surgery Services
Dr Rajendra Prasad Centre for Ophthalmic Sciences
All India Institute of Medical Sciences
New Delhi, India

Nandyala Sushma MSc PhD Scholar
Junior Research Fellow
Dr Rajendra Prasad Centre for Ophthalmic Sciences
All India Institute of Medical Sciences
New Delhi, India

Nicholas York
Consultant Ophthalmologist
St George's Hospital
Port Elizabeth Area, South Africa
Royal Victorian Eye and Ear Hospital
Melbourne, Australia

Nikhil S Gokhale MD
Consultant, Cornea Services
Gokhale Eye Hospital
Mumbai, Maharashtra, India

Nir Sorkin MD
Assistant
Professor of Ophthalmology
Director of Research, Cornea and Anterior Segment
Department of Ophthalmology
Tel Aviv Medical Center and the Tel Aviv University
Tel Aviv, Israel

Olena Al-Shymali
Ophthalmology and Research Fellow
Research and Development
Department Vissum Innovation
Alicante, Spain

Olivia Mead
R&D Department, TissueTech Inc.
Miami, Florida, USA

Paolo Rama
Director
Ophthalmology—Cornea and Ocular Surface Unit
San Raffaele Scientific Institute—Cornea and Ocular Surface Unit
Milan, Italy

Peter R Laibson
Consultant
Department of Ophthalmology Buyukdere Cad. No: 40
Maslak 34457
Acibadem Mehmet Ali Aydınlar University
Istanbul, Turkey

Prabhakar Singh MD
Senior Resident
Department of Ophthalmology
All India Institute of Medical Sciences
Patna, Bihar, India

Prafulla K Maharana MD DNB
Associate Professor of Ophthalmology
Cataract, Cornea and Refractive Surgery Services
Dr Rajendra Prasad Centre for Ophthalmic Sciences
All India Institute of Medical Sciences
New Delhi, India

Prakash Chand Agarwal MD Contributors
Consultant
Prakash Eyecare and Laser Centre
Bhopal, Madhya Pradesh, India

Prakhyat Roop MD
Senior Resident
Dr Rajendra Prasad Centre for Ophthalmic Sciences
All India Institute of Medical Sciences
New Delhi, India

Pranita Sahay MD FRCS (Glasgow) DNB FICO (Cornea) FAICO (Ref. Sx.)
Associate Consultant
Cataract, Cornea and Refractive Surgery Services
Centre for Sight
New Delhi, India

Prashant Garg MS
Incoming Executive Chair
Paul Dubord Chair of Cornea
LV Prasad Eye Institute (LVPEI)
Kallam Anji Reddy Campus
Hyderabad, Telangana, India

Prerna Agarwal MS
Associate Professor
Saraswati Institute of Medical Sciences
Ghaziabad, Uttar Pradesh, India

Priyadarshini K MD
Senior Resident
Dr Rajendra Prasad Centre for Ophthalmic Sciences
All India Institute of Medical Sciences
New Delhi, India

Rahul Kumar Bafna MD
Senior Resident
Dr Rajendra Prasad Centre for Ophthalmic Sciences
All India Institute of Medical Sciences
New Delhi, India

Raj Maini MD FRCSC
Consultant
Uptown Eye Specialist
Concord, ON L4K 2Z5, Canada
Department of Ophthalmology and Visual Science University of Toronto
Toronto, Canada

Rajesh Fogla FRCS FACS MMED
Consultant
Cornea and Refractive Surgery Services
Concord, ON L4K 2Z5, Canada
Apollo Hospitals
Hyderabad, Telangana, India

Rajesh Sinha MD DNB FRCS
Professor of Ophthalmology
Cataract, Cornea and
Refractive Surgery Services
Dr Rajendra Prasad Centre for
Ophthalmic Sciences
All India Institute of Medical Sciences
New Delhi, India

Rakesh Ahuja MBBS (AIIMS) MD (AIIMS)
UBC Fellowship (Canada) Harvard MEEI Fellowship (Boston MA, USA)
Attending Physician
Overlook Medical Center, Summit NJ (USA)

Rakhi Nathawat
Consultant
Eye Bank Association of India
Head of Programmes, South Asia
Motivation India

Rashmi Deshmukh MS
Consultant
The Cornea Institute
LV Prasad Eye Institute
Kallam Anji Reddy Campus
Hyderabad, Telangana, India

Rasik B Vajpayee MS FRCSEd FRANZCO
Professor of Ophthalmology
Cornea, Cataract and
Refractive Surgery Services
Vision Eye Institute, Melbourne
Royal Victorian Eye and Ear Hospital
University of Melbourne
Melbourne, Australia

Rinky Agarwal MD
Associate Professor
Lady Hardinge Medical College
New Delhi, India

Rishi Swarup MBBS DOMS Fellowship in Cornea FRCS (General Surgery) FICO (UK)
Consultant
Swarup Eye Centre
Hyderabad, Telangana, India

Ritika Sachdev MS
Director–Medical Services
Centre for Sight, Eye Hospital
Safdarjung Enclave, New Delhi, India

Ritu Arora
Director
Guru Nanak Eye Center
New Delhi, India

Ritu Nagpal MD FLVPEI (Cornea)
Senior Research Associate
Cataract, Cornea and
Refractive Surgery Services
Dr Rajendra Prasad Centre for
Ophthalmic Sciences
All India Institute of Medical Sciences
New Delhi, India

Robin G Abell MBBS MMed FRANZCO
Consultant, Cornea, Cataract and
Refractive Surgery Services
Royal Victorian Eye and Ear Hospital
32 Gisborne St
East Melbourne VIC 3002, Australia

Samar K Basak MD DNB FRCS
Consultant
Disha Eye Hospitals
Kolkata, West Bengal, India

Sameer Kaushal MD DNB
Head of Ophthalmology
Artemis Hospital
Gurugram, Haryana, India

Sarath S MD
Senior Resident
Dr Rajendra Prasad Centre for
Ophthalmic Sciences
All India Institute of Medical Sciences
New Delhi, India

Sayan Basu MS
Consultant
The Cornea Institute, Professor Brien
Holden Eye Research Centre (BHERC)
LV Prasad Eye Institute
Hyderabad, Telangana, India

Scheffer CG Tseng MD
Director
R&D Department, TissueTech Inc.
Miami, Florida, USA
Ocular Surface Center and
Ocular Surface Research Education
Foundation
Miami, FL, USA

Sean Tighe PhD
Research Scientist
R&D Department, TissueTech Inc.
Miami, Florida, USA
Department of Ophthalmology
Herbert Wertheim College of Medicine
Florida International University
Miami, Florida, USA
Department of Biochemistry and
Molecular Biology
Miller School of Medicine
University of Miami
Miami, FL, USA

Shaunak K Bakshi MD
Research Fellow, Ophthalmology
Harvard Medical School
Boston, Massachusetts, USA

Shikha Gupta MD
Associate Professor
Department of Ophthalmology
Dr Rajendra Prasad Centre for
Ophthalmic Sciences
All India Institute of Medical Sciences
New Delhi, India

Shipra Sarda MS
Senior Resident
Department of Ophthalmology
Guru Nanak Eye Center
New Delhi, India

Shokufeh Tavassoli BSc (Hons) MBChB (Hons) CertLRS FRCOpht
Consultant
Department of Ophthalmology
Royal United Hospitals, Bath, UK

Shreya Thatte MS
Professor and Head
Department of Ophthalmology
Sri Aurobindo Medical College
and Postgradaute Institute
Indore, Madhya Pradesh, India

Shweta Agarwal MBBS DO
Consultant
Dr G Sitalakshmi Memorial Clinic for
Ocular Surface Disorders
Sankara Nethralaya
Chennai, Tamil Nadu, India

Smrutirekha Priyadarshini MS
Consultant, Cornea and
Anterior Segment Services
LV Prasad Eye Institute
Bhubaneshwar, Odisha, India

Soham Basak MS DNB
Consultant
Disha Eye Hospitals
Kolkata, West Bengal, India

Sohini Mandal MD
Senior Resident
Dr Rajendra Prasad Centre for
Ophthalmic Sciences
All India Institute of Medical Sciences
New Delhi, India

Somasheila I Murthy MS
Consultant, Cornea Services
The Cornea Institute
LV Prasad Eye Institute
Hyderabad, Telangana, India

Sridevi Nair MD
Senior Resident
Dr Rajendra Prasad Centre for Ophthalmic Sciences
All India Institute of Medical Sciences
New Delhi, India

Sri Vatsa Sehra MD
Assistant Commissioner of Income Tax
Indian Revenue Services

Sujata Das MS FRCS (Glasg) AMPH DSc
Consultant (Cornea and Anterior Segment Service)
Medical Director
Drushti Daan Eye Bank
LV Prasad Eye Institute
Bhubaneshwar, Odisha, India

Suman Lata MD DNB
Senior Resident
Dr Rajendra Prasad Centre for Ophthalmic Sciences
All India Institute of Medical Sciences
New Delhi, India

Swapna S Shanbhag MS
Consultant
The Cornea Institute
LV Prasad Eye Institute
Hyderabad, Telangana, India

Trupti Dubey
Fellow
Gomabai Netralaya
Neemuch, Madhya Pradesh, India

Tushar Agarwal MD
Professor of Ophthalmology
Cataract, Cornea and Refractive Surgery Services
Dr Rajendra Prasad Centre for Ophthalmic Science
All India Institute of Medical Sciences
New Delhi, India

Urmimala Ghatak MD
Consultant
Department of Ophthalmology
Dr Joseph's Polyclinic
Dubai, UAE

Usha Gopinathan
Former Associate Executive Director
LV Prasad Eye Institute
Technical and Scientific Director, RIEB
Hyderabad, Telangana, India

Verónica Vargas MD
Fellow
Cornea, Cataract and Refractive Surgery Unit
Vissum Corporación
Alicante, Spain

Vincenzo Scorcia
Professor
Department of Ophthalmology
University of Magna Graecia
Catanzaro, Italy

Viney Gupta MD
Professor
Department of Ophthalmology
Dr Rajendra Prasad Centre for Ophthalmic Sciences
All India Institute of Medical Sciences
New Delhi, India

Vishal Gupta MD
Dr Rajendra Prasad Centre for Ophthalmic Sciences
All India Institute of Medical Sciences
New Delhi, India

Vishal Jhanji
MD FRCS (Glasgow) FRCOphth FARVO
Professor of Ophthalmology
Cornea, Cataract and External Disease Services
Refractive Surgery Service
Clinical Co-Director of the Funderburgh Corneal Regeneration Project
University of Pittsburgh
School of Medicine
Pittsburgh, Pennsylvania, USA

Foreword

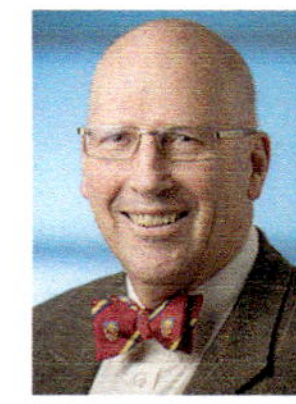

What an exciting book? It has been written by a range of surgeons who really enjoy what they do, they do it so well, and they love sharing their skills and experiences. They are all leaders globally and in their own specific subspecialty areas.

The book is totally comprehensive. Sections start with the instruments you need for a particular procedure. Then the procedure is clearly laid out with many figures and excellent photographs. If complications do occur, their management is also clearly described and discussed. The expertise and the experience that has been captured in these chapters is truly remarkable.

The first edition of this book was written in 2002 and the second edition in 2010. As so clearly shown in the book, corneal transplantation surgery has undergone a remarkable evolution over the last few decades. Previous corneal transplantation predominantly consisted of penetrating keratoplasty, lamellar keratoplasty was an unusual procedure. How different things are today? In addition to the wonderful and detailed chapters on penetrating keratoplasty, this book describes in detail some 21 different lamellar transplantation surgical techniques with clear descriptions and explanations of particular benefits of the different variations.

The book also covers the whole range of corneal transplantation surgeries and treatment options. Other areas include limbal stem cell and buccal mucosal grafts, keratoprosthesis, and prosthetic contact lenses. Of course, it also covers eye banking, the basis for all transplantation surgeries. What a treasure trove and an educational experience this book provides.

A foreword does not need to be lengthy, but I hope that I have been able to convey the breadth, authority and comprehensiveness of the coverage of this rapidly progressing area. This is a must-have book for those learning about corneal transplantation. But also for those who are already corneal surgeons who can refine and improve their own surgery with the wonderful, clear and up-to-date descriptions given by this amazing group of world experts.

Hugh R Taylor
AC LLD (Hon) MD FAHMS FRANZCO
Past President
The International Council of Ophthalmology
Melbourne Laureate Professor and
Harold Mitchell Chair of Indigenous Eye Health
Melbourne School of Population and Global Health
University of Melbourne
Melbourne, Australia

Foreword

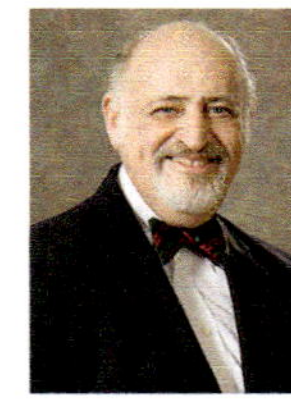

The last three decades have witnessed a dramatic evolution in corneal transplantation. This evolution—indeed, a *revolution* in the surgical approaches to corneal diseases—has occurred based on an enhanced understanding of corneal structure, biology, and immunology. Our increased understanding of how the cornea works has led to a panoply of procedural approaches that are layer- and disease entity-specific. These focused surgical approaches provide a new repertoire of surgical procedures for the contemporary corneal surgeon.

In this volume, the editors have collected a wealth of knowledge and experience to provide the modern corneal surgeon with clinically pragmatic information in virtually every aspect of keratoplasty.

The text begins appropriately at the beginning—with the critical role of eye banking to the practice of keratoplasty. Unique in ophthalmology, the cornea subspecialty relies on the eye-banking system for its surgical success. The ever increasing and essential role of the eye bank in corneal surgery is outlined in detail.

The editors then move through the details of penetrating keratoplasty in all of its manifestations: indications, techniques, follow-up, and complication management. From there, the book concentrates on selective, layer-based keratoplasty in all its surgical variations. Tectonic and therapeutic keratoplasty, disease-specific surgical approaches, shaped keratoplasty, contact lens applications, prosthokeratoplasty and keratopigmentation techniques are all discussed in practical detail.

There are few texts of this scope in the modern ophthalmic library, and this very comprehensive text will serve as a distinctly useful tool for residents, fellows, and practitioners at every stage of their careers. It is a truly comprehensive manual on keratoplasty, and I am confident that this volume will serve the rapidly evolving field of keratoplasty for decades to come.

Mark J Mannis
MD FACS
Professor and Chair
Department of Ophthalmology and Vision Science
University of California
Davis, California, USA

Foreword

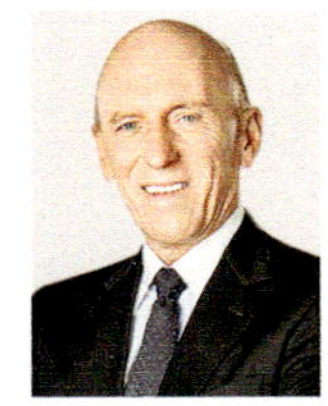

Jorge L Alió

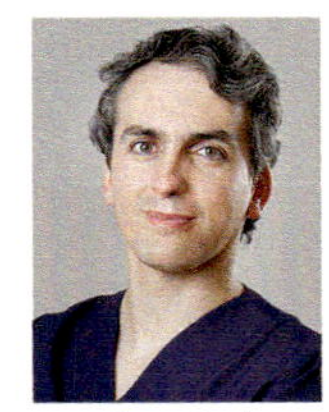

Jorge Alio del Barrio

Corneal transplantation has evolved in the last decades into a sophisticated series of surgical techniques aiming to solve the different causes of corneal blindness. Cornea, as an ophthalmic subspecialty, has evolved accordingly requiring higher skills and a longer and deeper level of study and training, which are included in the cornea fellowship programs. However, the cornea specialist is frequently involved in other areas of Ophthalmology, but corneal surgery is the main motivation behind all of them. Even though we might also dedicate part of our practice to other fields such as refractive surgery, cataract or glaucoma, it is when we face a challenging cornea case that our medical spirit really awakens and we stretch our brains to solve the most challenging cases, requiring both experience and also sometimes "art" and inspiration to improvise a solution for those cases whose characteristics make them unique. To achieve this, the first thing a surgeon needs is knowledge, acquired from intense study that always involves the first step of any learning curve: study, observe, and finally practice. This book aims to provide the necessary material for this first step of learning curve, a reference book the reader can use as baseline knowledge to start their training in corneal transplantation.

This subspecialized area of ophthalmology has seen incredible progress in the last two decades with the introduction of lamellar keratoplasty techniques, thanks to the outstanding work of some colleagues who will be remembered in the history of ophthalmology and are also the authors in this book. The introduction of lamellar keratoplasty techniques has allowed us to significantly and progressively improve our visual outcomes and graft survival with progressively less invasive techniques. However, we should remember that there is still space for the old keratoplasty techniques, and classical surgeries (such as penetrating keratoplasty or limbal autografts among others) which must not be forgotten, since we still need to use them regularly in our practice. In this scenario, with the current book the reader will be able to have access to the old (but still valid) knowledge and the new techniques, learning from the classical keratoplasty techniques, including something as basic and critical as graft suturing, ending with an overview of the most modern lamellar keratoplasty techniques.

Despite the fact that in the last few years, with the advent of DMEK we have reached a new threshold, exciting years are still ahead with the standardization and introduction of new cellular therapies and regenerative medicine techniques in real clinical practice, that are expected to change the field of corneal grafting in the next two decades.

But we do expect even larger advances in the future, as topics such as genomics and regenerating procedures and new technologies will further widen the broad spectrum of surgical techniques and corneal therapies for the benefit of the patients affected by corneal diseases. The Cornea Specialist faces an exciting future that will be in part announced in the pages of this book.

We congratulate the Editors and Co-Authors of the splendid book for their dedication and success in providing medical education in this area.

Jorge L Alió MD PhD FEBO
Jorge Alio del Barrio MD PhD FEBOS-CR
Cornea, Cataract and Refractive Surgery Unit
Vissum Corporación, Alicante, Spain
Division of Ophthalmology
School of Medicine, Universidad Miguel Hernández
Alicante, Spain

Preface to the Third Edition

The journey of *"Corneal Transplantation"* book started in late 1990s with the joint efforts of corneal surgeons, including Professors Rasik B Vajpayee, Namrata Sharma, Geoffrey C Tabin, and Hugh R Taylor. The conceptualization of developing a practical handbook of corneal surgeries was aimed to cater to the needs of both a surgeon practicing in a rural area as well as a fellowship trained surgeon. First edition of this book was brought out in the year 2002, followed by a second edition in 2010.

The previous decade has witnessed significant popularization in terms of expanding indications of various techniques of corneal grafting such as the techniques of anterior as well as posterior lamellar keratoplasty, use of femtosecond laser for assisting various steps of corneal transplantation and limbal stem cell transplantation. This updated version "the third edition" is a conglomeration of 74 chapters, including the updated versions as well as the new ones.

New highlights of this edition include many innovative techniques of corneal transplantation such as Superficial Anterior Lamellar Keratoplasty, Diamond Knife-assisted Deep Anterior Lamellar Keratoplasty (Dia-DALK), Cannula Assisted DALK, Groove and Peel DALK, Thin Lenticule Descemet's Stripping Automated Endothelial Keratoplasty, Pre-Descemet's Endothelial Keratoplasty, Shaped Keratoplasty, Non-circular Corneal Grafts, Hemi-automated Lamellar Keratoplasty and Bowman's Layer Transplantation. A separate section on indication specific techniques of corneal transplantation has been included, consisting of a detailed description of several clinical conditions.

Providing cutting-edge information from experts all over the world, has been the primary focus of this book, since its inception. The aim is to help the corneal surgeons understand the intricacies of various techniques of corneal transplantation including the novel as well as the established ones. Relevant clinical photographs, sketch diagrams and surgical videos have been incorporated to further provide a lucid understanding of the facts.

Future treatment options for the management of corneal pathologies include use of tissue-engineered cornea, mesenchymal stem cell and cultured corneal endothelial cell therapy, use of ROCK inhibitors and gene therapy. These modalities are still in their initial phase of use, with limited number of patients being enrolled in certain parts of the world. End of this decade, will further determine their feasibility and effectiveness for the management of different types of corneal pathologies.

We are thankful to all our authors for sharing their expertise, their patience and cooperation and investing their precious time in writing the chapters in a reader-friendly and well-structured manner.

Namrata Sharma
Ritu Nagpal
Rasik B Vajpayee

Preface to the First Edition

Corneal Transplantation Surgery has undergone tremendous advancements over the last few decades. Innovative minds have been contributing novel and original concepts in an ongoing pursuit, aimed towards achieving optimal long-term success of this craft. My journey in the field of corneal grafting surgery began during my residency at Gandhi Medical College, Bhopal, Madhya Pradesh, India. In those formative years, it was thrilling to observe surgeons replace diseased and scarred corneas with healthy donor tissue. After a formal training in corneal surgery at Dr Rajendra Prasad Centre for Ophthalmic Sciences, I learnt the finer points of this craft at the Cornea Service of Melbourne University Department of Ophthalmology in Australia. I would like to express my heartfelt gratitude to my teachers Professor Santokh Singh, Professor MK Rathore, Dr Salil Kumar, Professor Madan Mohan, Professor VK Dada, Professor Hugh R Taylor and Professor Peter R Laibson. These luminaries have helped me to shape my skills as an ophthalmologist and a corneal surgeon and have been a source of inspiration in my academic endeavors including this book.

This book was conceived in Australia, when Dr Geoff Tabin and myself were working as corneal fellows with Professor Hugh R Taylor. Our interactions with him made us realize that the profile of corneal diseases and their management modalities in the developing world differ somewhat from those of the developed nations. We felt that there was a need for a concise, user-friendly and practical book on corneal grafting surgery. The book was planned as an amalgamation of knowledge about the newer technological advances of the developed world and the simpler alternatives appropriate and optimal for the developing countries. Another principal purpose of this venture is to generate interest amongst ophthalmic surgeons of the developing countries in the field of corneal grafting surgery, as corneal blindness is a major health issue here.

Bringing out a book on a subject such as corneal transplantation is a kind of mammoth exercise and it is clear that work of such enormity is the congregation of efforts of many individuals. I am grateful for the esprit de corps, collaboration, education and altruism that my Australian, American and other International and Indian colleagues have bestowed on me over the years. Many of them are contributing authors to this book. I am obliged to all the contributing authors for the time and effort they have put in to share their expertise and knowledge with the readers. I am indebted to my co-editors Dr Namrata Sharma, Dr Geoff Tabin and Professor Hugh R Taylor for their invaluable help and guidance at every step. I would also like to acknowledge my residents, and my assistants Mr Rajkumar and Ms Meena Verma for providing useful inputs and assistance. And finally, I would like to thank my wife Madhu and children Mihika and Shubhankar for their patience in allowing me to spend time to accomplish this work.

This book has been designed as a practical guide to the various aspects of corneal grafting surgery. It elucidates the basic aspects in preoperative evaluation, investigations, established surgical procedures and the advanced techniques in special situations as well as the newer technology in corneal grafting. Theoretical as well as research aspects of corneal grafting have been dealt in a practical manner. An extensive and well-illustrated section provides up-to-date knowledge of complications in corneal transplantation and their management. This should be of particular assistance to ophthalmologists practicing in remote areas and involved in the postoperative care of the grafted patients.

Overall our book provides students, surgeons and practitioners a concise treatise on corneal transplantation that contains essential information intended to help a beginner and can be consulted by the experienced corneal transplantation surgeons to acquaint themselves with the state-of-the-art techniques in corneal grafting surgery.

Rasik B Vajpayee

Preface to the First Edition

In the early 1990s Rasik B Vajpayee and I were corneal fellows together under the guidance of Professor Hugh R Taylor at the Royal Victorian Eye and Ear Hospital in Melbourne, Australia. Dr Vajpayee had come from the busy corneal unit at the All India Institute of Medical Sciences in New Delhi and he was concerned about the difficulties of corneal surgery in the developing world. I trained at Harvard Medical School and Brown University's Department of Ophthalmology in the United States of America and arrived with a bias towards modern technology and no holds barred best possible care for every individual patient. Professor Taylor's superb corneal fellowship provided us with both a state-of-the-art corneal fellowship experience and the opportunity to discuss wider global issues surrounding the delivery of medical care both in the developed and developing world.

Dr Vajpayee returned to India where he quickly became one of the busiest and most influential corneal surgeons in the world. He has an enormous surgical volume and innovative mind. He has developed numerous new techniques and has advanced the art of corneal surgery in a myriad of areas. Along with his publications, he experienced a meteoric rise through the academic ranks. Dr Vajpayee is now a full Professor at the All India Institute of Medical Sciences and Director of Cornea Services. In addition to being involved with many aspects of cutting edge research and technology, he has continued to be concerned about the difficulties of delivering high quality corneal care in the developing world.

Dr Vajpayee and I spoke at the American Academy of Ophthalmology meeting one year ago. He felt that there was a need for a practical book on modern corneal surgery that would transcend the boundaries of modern technology and the developing world. He noted that there was no single book that would allow a rural surgeon in India to quickly learn what he needs to treat a specific difficult corneal pathology that also provides in depth discussions and insights for the western fellowship trained corneal surgeon. Professor Vajpayee's enthusiasm was infectious. We discussed ideas and possible formats and drew up a list of topics. We then discussed who in the world was currently at the absolute cutting edge in dealing with those specific problems. We enlisted the help of Professor Taylor from Australia and Dr Namrata Sharma from India as co-editors and approached an all star cast of corneal specialists from around the world.

We asked the authors to write succinct practical chapters geared towards patient care while still including sufficient academic support for their views. In each chapter, the authors delivered an excellent treatise on their topic of specific corneal expertise. We hope this book will be a valuable resource for general ophthalmologists who are faced with a corneal crisis, residents and corneal specialists alike. As we enter a new millennium, corneal disease and injury remains the second leading cause of blindness in the world. We hope this book will provide a practical, yet comprehensive, guide to surgical corneal care.

I am indebted to all of our chapter authors and to my co-editors for their hard work. I am particularly grateful to Rasik B Vajpayee for having the vision of this book and the enthusiasm to make it a reality. Happy reading!

Geoffrey C Tabin

Preface to the First Edition

I was very pleased when Rasik B Vajpayee first raised the possibility of writing a book on corneal transplantation. Dr Vajpayee, in addition to being an expert surgeon is also one of the most industrious and productive members of a new generation of corneal surgeons and is rapidly becoming a world leader.

He has assembled a most distinguished group of leading corneal surgeons from around the world to contribute to this very important and impressive book.

There have been many significant and exciting developments in the technical aspects of corneal transplantation over recent years and these have been beautifully set out in the chapters that follow. The precision and beauty of corneal transplantation still amazes me after thirty years. With the large numbers of cases done around the world each year and the high success rate, corneal transplantation must be without doubt the most successful example of transplantation in the whole of medicine. Although exquisite surgical skill and attention to detail throughout the operation are extremely important in determining the successful outcome of corneal transplantation, they are only part of the story.

Data from the Australian Corneal Transplant Registry show that the single most important factor affecting the long-term survival of corneal grafts is the surgeon. This does not relate to the surgical skill and dexterity as much as it relates to meticulous postoperative management. The key to the successful postoperative management of a corneal transplant is not how many patients are seen, or whether they are seen exactly at the time of their appointment without having to wait, or whether they are first examined by an ophthalmic assistant, the key is the meticulous attention to detail in the postoperative management especially the recognition of early stages of low-grade rejection and its appropriate management. Attention to detail is a key to success in ophthalmology, and in no area is this more true than the postoperative management of corneal transplantation.

One of the great strengths of this book is the wide range of experience and opinion that is presented here. This book does not give a simplistic cookbook recipe for the management of these sometimes complex and difficult cases, rather it gives the distilled experience of the world's leaders in this field in which they outline their approach and their justification for the decisions they have taken. I trust you will find this book as interesting and as informative as I have and sustain the excitement I first felt when this book was first discussed.

Hugh R Taylor

Contents

SECTION 4: Lamellar Keratoplasty

A: Anterior Lamellar Keratoplasty Techniques

B: Endothelial Keratoplasty Techniques

SECTION 5: Specific Techniques in Corneal Transplantation

Synopsis

The first edition of "*Corneal Transplantation*" was published in the year 2002 by the combined effort of various experts in corneal transplantation across the globe. It was Professor Rasik B Vajpayee's idea to have a single book which would guide the corneal surgeons, as to how to address a specific corneal pathology. In quest of better postoperative outcomes and improved survival rates for corneal grafts, corneal surgeons continue to refine the techniques of corneal transplantation. We have moved from transplanting full thickness donor corneal tissues to transplantation of selective tissue layers such as Bowman layer transplantation, automated lamellar therapeutic keratoplasty (ALTK) and Descemet stripping automated endothelial keratoplasty (DSAEK) and Descemet membrane endothelial keratoplasty. The understanding as well as the management of various corneal pathologies has undergone tremendous changes in the past few years. The third edition of this book amalgamates the most recent advances in corneal transplantation techniques with newer concepts of various corneal pathologies, the upgradation of previously described surgical techniques and introduction to the novel techniques in component surgery of cornea.

SECTION 1

Evolution, Preoperative Considerations, and Eye Banking

1 Evolution of Corneal Grafting Surgery

Namrata Sharma, Prabhakar Singh, Chandrashekhar Kumar

INTRODUCTION: HISTORY OF CORNEAL TRANSPLANTATION

Today, corneal transplantation is considered the most widely performed successful organ transplantation surgery worldwide. It has gradually evolved since the 19th century, when the suggestion of replacing an opaque cornea of one animal with the clear cornea of another was put forth by *K Himly* of Germany (1813). However, the idea to replace opaque human cornea with a transparent one of an animal was suggested by *F Reisinger* in 1824. The term "keratoplasty" was also coined by him. The first successful penetrating allograft was performed by *Samuel Bigger* in animals. The experimental work of *Henry Power*, on animals and humans was reported in 1872.[1] His work was the first of its kind to shed light upon the need for proper graft placement, nullifying risk of infection, using fresh donor graft and minimizing trauma to the endothelium. The first lamellar corneal grafting was reported by *Von Hippel* in 1886.[2] Nearly a century ago in 1906, *Edward Konrad Zirm* performed the first successful penetrating keratoplasty (**Fig. 1**) on a patient, who had presented with alkali burns.[3] The donor was harvested from an 11-year-old boy who had sustained penetrating scleral injury with retained intraocular foreign body and hence had to undergo enucleation of his eyeball.

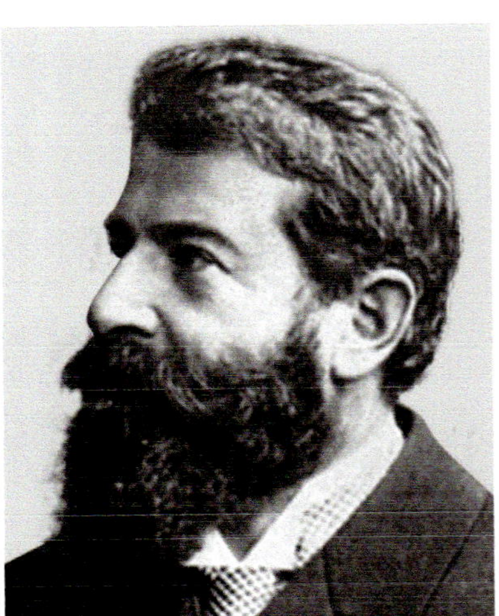

Fig. 1: Edward Konrad Zirm.

For the succeeding 30 years, enucleated eyes of living donors were used for corneal grafting. In 1908, the first autokeratoplasty was performed by *Plange*, where the transparent cornea of the patient's blind eye was used to replace the scarred cornea of his other eye.

VP Filatov is a Russian ophthalmologist, who is lauded as the father of modern eye banking.[4,5] He fixated the graft using an egg membrane, which later became widely popular. He made use of a cadaver cornea as the donor graft, insisted on the importance of safeguarding the intraocular tissues during trephination of the host tissue and implemented direct suturing. In 1940s, the availability of a range of antibiotics and introduction of steroids played a major role in the evolution of corneal transplant surgery.

In late 1950s, *Paufique* and *Charleux* introduced limbal and eccentric grafts and popularized lamellar corneal grafting. It was around this time that small fine needles were introduced for suturing. In the past 30 years, great advances have taken place in the arena of corneal transplant surgery, though its evolution began in the 1st half of 20th century. The success rates of corneal transplant surgery increased with gradual understanding of corneal anatomy and physiology, evolution of microsurgical techniques and corneal preservation methods, interpretation of corneal immunology, and use of anti-inflammatory and immunosuppressive drugs.

Edward Maumenee identified corneal graft rejection to be the greatest limiting factor with respect to graft survival. *Khododoust* designed the experimental models and gave the classic scientific description for the same.

The world's first successful human keratoplasty was performed by *Ramon Castroviejo* (**Fig. 2**). He has also designed numerous instruments, such as Castroviejo calipers, corneal scissors, forceps, cyclodialysis spatula, corneoscleral punch, needle holder, tying, and suturing forceps. He also pioneered various surgical techniques in corneal transplant surgery. He demonstrated the use of continuous external silk suture along a square graft in his

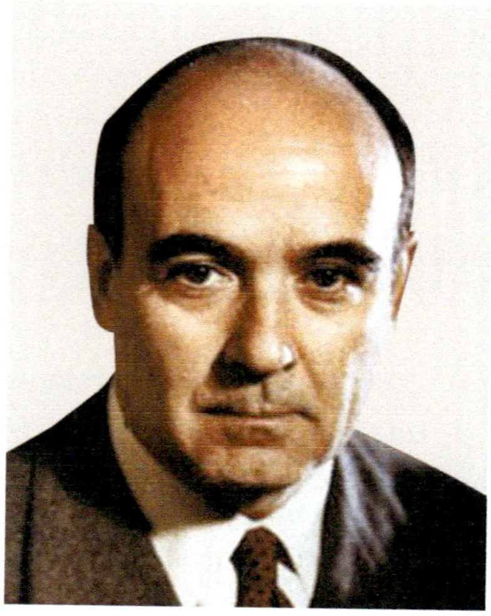

Fig. 2: Ramon Castroviejo.

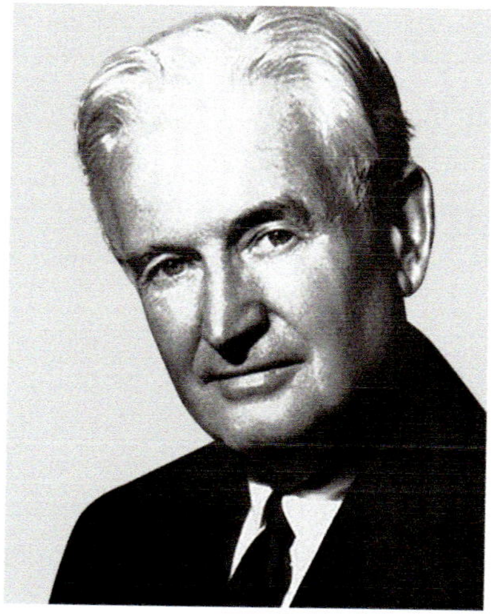

Fig. 3: Townley Paton.

original suturing technique, which held the graft in place with the aid of intraocular pressure holding the graft against the suture. Most of his square grafts had a good survival providing good visual acuity for a long period.

The surgical microscope and many other microsurgical instruments were designed by *Richard Troutman*.[6] He circumvented astigmatism by the invention of surgical keratometer and his innovative technique of wedge resection.

The first eye bank was setup in 1959 by *Townley Paton* (**Fig. 3**) in New York. In 1961, it paved way to the setting up of Eye Bank Association of America, by which the standards for obtaining, preservation, storage, and usage of donor corneal tissue was laid down. *Maurice* invented the specular microscope which aids in studying the endothelium of host and donor corneas, which plays a key role in the success of corneal transplantation.

The outcome of keratoplasty is greatly influenced by the preservation of donor cornea. A preservation technique should ideally enable safe transportation of the corneal tissue increasing its duration of storage and ensuring endothelial viability, thus enhancing efficient use of harvested cornea. In 1954, *Eastcott* reported the first successful use of cryopreserved donor cornea in keratoplasty. In 1965, the basic method of cryopreservation was described by *Capella* and *Kaufman*.[7,8] *McCarey* and *Kaufman (MK)*, in 1974, introduced the MK medium which assured storage of donor cornea for at least 3–4 days, enabling elective planning of keratoplasty procedures.[9]

KERATOPLASTY: TECHNOLOGICAL DEVELOPMENTS

In the last two decades, with the improvement in surgical techniques and instrumentation lamellar keratoplasty has undergone a revolution. The various types of lamellar keratoplasty include anterior and posterior lamellar keratoplasty (PLK) depending on the level of pathology. With the advent of the microkeratomes, automated lamellar therapeutic keratoplasty (ALTK) has given way to manual lamellar keratoplasty.

Deep lamellar keratoplasty was introduced to improve the postoperative visual performance in cases with corneal pathology involving the stromal layers of the cornea. It provides all the advantages of lamellar keratoplasty such as extraocular technique, less stringent criteria for donor tissue, less graft rejection and intraocular complications and yet offers a better visual acuity in terms of contrast sensitivity. In 1974, *Anwar* described the use of a big air bubble to dissect the plane between the Descemet's membrane (DM) and stromal layers under direct visualization.[10] *Archilla* in 1980s was first to use intrastromal air injection and spatula dissection to facilitate access to DM without perforating it.[11] *Sugita* also described hydrodelamination of the stroma from DM.[12] *Melles* described the technique of deep anterior lamellar keratoplasty (DALK) in which deeper dissection was done with the help of viscoelastic injection through the lamellar stromal pocket.[13] In 2002, *Anwar* and *Teichmann* in their "big bubble" technique described the dissection of DM from the overlying stroma with injection of air.[14]

Endothelial keratoplasty (EK) is an alternative to penetrating keratoplasty in cases where corneal endothelium is diseased alone. In 1998, *Dr Gerrit Melles* described a technique for PLK,[15] and a year later, he successfully implemented the technique for pseudophakic corneal edema. A deep stromal pocket was created which was subsequently dissected out and replaced by donor cornea comprising similar layers. The unfolded posterior lamellar graft was introduced through a 9 mm incision in the early days, however, later *Melles* modified the technique by folding the graft. This resulted in decrease in incision size from 9 to 5 mm. In 2001, a similar procedure was described by *Terry and Ousley*, called deep lamellar endothelial keratoplasty (DLEK) in which some slight modifications like stabilizing the anterior chamber using viscoelastic substance were added.[16] *Price and Price* made the EK technique more popular and easier by eliminating the need to dissect stroma. In this procedure, only diseased endothelium and DM were stripped off from the host cornea and this technique was called as Descemet's stripping endothelial keratoplasty (DSEK).[17] In 2006, *Gorovoy* described the technique of Descemet's stripping automated endothelial keratoplasty (DSAEK) in which the manual stromal dissection was replaced by the more reproducible microkeratome dissection.[18] This results in a smoother interface. Smoother interface results in a comparatively faster visual recovery; however, the hyperopic shift due to graft thickness[19] and presence of interface still pose a hindrance to unaided visual clarity.

In 2006, *Tappin* described the clinical transplantation of 7.5 mm diameter DM through an 8.0 mm scleral incision using a flat carrier device.[20] In the same year *Melles* described the first clinical results of only DM and endothelium transplantation through a self-sealing corneal incision and referred it to as Descemet's membrane endothelial keratoplasty (DMEK) (**Table 1**).[21] Further modifications like DMAEK and DMEK-S with a frill of stromal rim in a DMEK graft were deviced.[22]

The experimental studies are on to make cultured human endothelial cell transplantation successful. Promising results were seen when cultured human corneal endothelial cells were transplanted with a collagen sheet in a rabbit model.[23] This was further substantiated by the report of Perisamy P et al., wherein they transplanted the human corneal endothelial cell using nanocomposite gel in eyes with bullous keratopathy.[24] The visual acuity and symptoms improved following this procedure. However, the procedure needs further validation.

In 2015, another paper published by Agarwal A et al., introduced a newer technique of EK and termed it pre-Descemet's endothelial keratoplasty (PDEK). Here, donor endothelial graft was created using pneumatic dissection and attaining type 1 bubble. The grafts so obtained had a mean thickness of 28 + 5.6 μm with good postoperative outcome.[25]

An observation of corneal clearing without attachment of grafts in some patients led to the evolvement of a new technique termed as Descemetorhexis without endothelial keratoplasty (DWEK) by Kaufman et al.[26]

Table 1: Major contributions in the field of corneal transplantation.

S. No.	*Year*	*Name*	*Contribution*
1.	1813	K Himly	Suggested replacing opaque cornea in one animal with clear cornea from another animal
2.	1824	F Reisinger	Suggested replacing opaque human cornea with clear animal cornea • Coined the term *keratoplasty*
3.	1837	Samuel Bigger	Successfully performed corneal allograft in animals
4.	1872	Henry Power	Experimental corneal grafting
5.	1880	Von Hippel	• Introduced *lamellar keratoplasty* • Invented circular trephine
6.	1906	Edward Konrad Zirm	Reported *first successful penetrating keratoplasty in a human*
7.	1908	Plange	Autokeratoplasty
8.	1910–1950	VP Filatov	• *Father of keratoplasty* • Performed systematic study of keratoplasty • Suggested using cadaver corneas as donor tissues • Devised numerous instruments and surgical innovations
9.	1930–1950	R Castroviejo	Devised numerous instruments for microsurgery
10.	1950s	Paufique and Charleux	• *Lamellar keratoplasty* • *Limbal and eccentric grafts*
11.	1944	RT Paton	Founded the first Eye Bank in USA
12.	1954	Eastcott	Transplantation using cryopreserved cornea
13.	1960	E Maumenee	Recognition of "graft rejection" as a clinical entity
14.	1965	Troutman	Surgical microscope and surgical keratometer
15.	1965	Capella and Kaufman	*Cryopreservation*
16.	1968	D Maurice	Developed *specular microscope*
17.	1974	B McCarey and H Kaufman	Developed *corneal storage media*
18.	1985	Archila EA	*Deep anterior lamellar keratoplasty (DALK)* with air assisted dissection
19.	1998	Melles GR	• Deep anterior lamellar keratoplasty • Posterior lamellar keratoplasty
20.	2001	Mark Terry	Deep lamellar endothelial keratoplasty (DLEK)
21.	2006	Price and Gorovoy	Descemet's stripping endothelial keratoplasty (DSEK) and Descemet's stripping automated endothelial keratoplasty (DSAEK)
22.	2006	Melles GR	Descemet's membrane endothelial keratoplasty (DMEK)

The femtosecond laser-assisted DSEK (FS-DSEK) came into vogue with more promising outcome; however, visual outcome appeared limited when compared to DSAEK or PK.[27,28] Femtosecond and excimer laser-assisted EK (FELEK) is another technique in which combined thin graft dissection followed by smoothening of graft with excimer laser is being done.[29] Another promising technique using femtolaser is femtosecond laser-enabled descemetorhexis DMEK (F-DMEK) and the outcomes seem to be better with lesser rates of graft detachment.[30-32]

Over time, diseased individual layers of cornea are being replaced and Bowman's layer transplantation is being practiced for management of postlaser surface complications and keratoconus.[33,34]

REFERENCES

1. Power H. Report of the Fourth International Ophthalmological Congress. London: Savill Edwards and Co; 1872. p. 172.
2. Von Hippel A. Albrecht von Graefes Arch Ophthalmol. 1888; 34:108-30.
3. Zirm EK. Eine erfolgreiche totale keratoplastik. Von Graefes Arch Ophthalmol. 1906;64:580-93.
4. Filatov VP. Transplantation of the cornea. Arch Ophthalmol. 1935;13:321-47.
5. Filatov VP, Bajenova MA. Culture of dried corneal tissue. Arch Ophthalmol. Rev Gen Ophthalmol. 1937;1:385.
6. Troutman RC. The operating microscope in ophthalmic surgery. Trans Am Ophthalmol Soc. 1965;63:335-48.
7. Capella JA, Kaufman HE, Robbins JE. Preservation of viable corneal tissue. Arch Ophthalmol. 1965;74:669-73.
8. McCarey BE, Kaufman HE. Improved corneal storage. Invest Ophthalmol. 1974;13:165-73.
9. Lindstrom RL. Advances in corneal preservation. Trans Am Ophthalmol Soc. 1990;88:555-648.
10. Anwar M. Dissection technique in lamellar keratoplasty. Br J Ophthalmol. 1972;56(9):711-3.
11. Archila EA. Deep lamellar keratoplasty dissection of host tissue with intrastromal air injection. Cornea. 1984-1985;3(3):217-8.
12. Sugita J, Kondo J. Deep anterior lamellar keratoplasty with complete removal of pathological stroma for vision improvement. Br J Ophthalmol. 1997;81:184-8.
13. Melles GR, Lander F, Rietveld FJ, Remeijer L, Beekhuis WH, Binder PS. A new surgical technique for deep stromal, anterior lamellar keratoplasty. Br J Ophthalmol. 1999;83(3):327-33.
14. Anwar M, Teichmann KD. Big-bubble technique to bare Descemet's membrane in anterior lamellar keratoplasty. J Cataract Refract Surg. 2002;28(3):398-403.
15. Melles GR, Eggink FA, Lander F, Pels E, Rietveld FJ, Beekhuis WH, et al. A surgical technique for posterior lamellar keratoplasty. Cornea. 1998;17:618-26.
16. Terry MA, Ousley PJ. Deep lamellar endothelial keratoplasty in the first United States patients: early clinical results. Cornea. 2001;20:239-43.
17. Price FW Jr, Price MO. Descemet's stripping with endothelial keratoplasty in 50 eyes: a refractive neutral corneal transplant. J Refract Surg. 2005;21:339-45.
18. Gorovoy MS. Descemet's stripping and automated endothelial keratoplasty. Cornea. 2006;25:886-9.
19. Ham L, Dapena I, Moutsouris K, Balachandran C, Frank LE, van Dijk K, et al. Refractive change and stability after Descemet membrane endothelial keratoplasty. Effect of corneal dehydration-induced hyperopic shift on intraocular lens power calculation. J Cataract Refract Surg. 2011;37(8):1455-64.
20. Tappin M. A method for true endothelial cell (Tencell) transplantion using a custom made cannula for the treatment of endothelial cell failure. Eye. 2007;21:775-9.
21. Melles GR, Ong TS, Ververs B, van der Wees J. Descemet's membrane endothelial keratoplasty (DMEK). Cornea. 2006; 25:987-90.
22. Price MO, Giebel AW, Fairchild KM, Price FW Jr. Descemet's membrane endothelial keratoplasty: prospective multicenter study of visual and refractive outcomes and endothelial survival. Ophthalmology. 2009;116(12):2361-8.
23. Mimura T, Yamagami S, Yokoo S, Usui T, Tanaka K, Hattori S, et al. Cultured human corneal endothelial cell transplantation with a collagen sheet in a rabbit model. Invest Ophthalmol Vis Sci. 2004;45(9):2992-7.
24. Parikumar P, Haraguchi K, Senthilkumar R, Abraham SJ. Human corneal endothelial cell transplantation using nanocomposite gel sheet in bullous keratopathy. Am J Stem Cells. 2018;7(1):18-24.
25. Agarwal A, Dua HS, Narang P, Kumar DA, Agarwal A, Jacob S, et al. Pre-Descemet's endothelial keratoplasty (PDEK). Br J Ophthalmol. 2014;98(9):1181-5.
26. Kaufman AR, Nosé RM, Pineda R. Descemetorhexis without endothelial keratoplasty (DWEK): Proposal for nomenclature standardization. Cornea. 2018;37(4):e20-e21.
27. Chen H, Tian L, Le Q, Zhao F, Zhao Y, Chen Y, et al. Femtosecond laser-assisted Descemet's stripping endothelial keratoplasty: a prospective study of 6-month visual outcomes, corneal thickness and endothelial cell loss. Int Ophthalmol. 2020;40(8):2065-75.
28. Cheng YY, van den Berg TJ, Schouten JS, Pels E, Wijdh RJ, van Cleynenbreugel H, et al. Quality of vision after femtosecond laser-assisted descemet stripping endothelial keratoplasty and penetrating keratoplasty: a randomized, multicenter clinical trial. Am J Ophthalmol. 2011;152(4):556-66.e1.
29. Trinh L, Saubaméa B, Auclin F, Denoyer A, Lai-Kuen R, El Hamdaoui M, et al. Femtosecond and excimer laser-assisted endothelial keratoplasty (FELEK): a new technique of endothelial transplantation. J Fr Ophthalmol. 2014;37(3):211-9.
30. Einan-Lifshitz A, Sorkin N, Boutin T, Showail M, Borovik A, Alobthani M, et al. Comparison of femtosecond laser-enabled descemetorhexis and manual descemetorhexis in Descemet membrane endothelial keratoplasty. Cornea. 2017;36(7):767-70.
31. Pilger D, von Sonnleithner C, Bertelmann E, Maier AB, Joussen AM, Torun N. Exploring the precision of femtosecond laser-assisted descemetorhexis in Descemet membrane endothelial keratoplasty. BMJ Open Ophthalmol. 2018;3(1):e000148.
32. Sorkin N, Mednick Z, Einan-Lifshitz A, Trinh T, Santaella G, Telli A, et al. Three-year outcome comparison between femtosecond laser-assisted and manual Descemet membrane endothelial keratoplasty. Cornea. 2019;38(7):812-6.
33. Lie J, Droutsas K, Ham L, Dapena I, Ververs B, Otten H, et al. Isolated Bowman layer transplantation to manage persistent subepithelial haze after excimer laser surface ablation. J Cataract Refract Surg. 2010;36(6):1036-41.
34. Parker JS, van Dijk K, Melles GR. Treatment options for advanced keratoconus: A review. Surv Ophthalmol. 2015;60(5):459-80.

2 Indications and Outcomes of Penetrating Keratoplasty

Urmimala Ghatak, Sridevi Nair, Ritu Nagpal, Namrata Sharma

INTRODUCTION

Corneal transplantation surgery is performed for a wide variety of reasons, the major indication being improvement in visual acuity. Improvement of two or more lines of Snellen's visual acuity chart is taken as a significant improvement in vision after corneal grafting. This may encompass one or more of the following:

- Attainment of acceptable optical correction
- Restoration of binocularity
- Elimination of corneal disease
- Improvement in function and lifestyle
- Improvement in pain

INDICATIONS OF PENETRATING KERATOPLASTY

In today's date penetrating keratoplasty (PK) is performed for a wide variety of conditions (**Box 1**). These may be unilateral or bilateral. The indications can be divided into four categories:[1-9]

1. Optical
2. Tectonic
3. Therapeutic
4. Cosmetic

Box 1: Clinical indications of penetrating keratoplasty.

- *Pseudophakic corneal edema*
- *Aphakic corneal edema*
- *Stromal corneal dystrophies*:
  - Granular dystrophy
  - Lattice dystrophy
  - Macular dystrophy
  - Central crystalline dystrophy of Schnyder
  - Central cloudy dystrophy of François
- *Endothelial dystrophies*:
  - Fuchs' endothelial dystrophy
  - Congenital hereditary endothelial dystrophy
  - Posterior polymorphous dystrophy
  - Iridocorneal endothelial syndrome
  - Chandler's syndrome
- *Ectasias/thinning*:
  - Anterior keratoconus
  - Keratoglobus
  - Posterior keratoconus
- *Congenital opacities*:
  - Peters anomaly
  - Sclerocornea
  - Congenital glaucoma/buphthalmos
  - Aniridia
- *Viral/post-viral keratitis*:
  - Herpes simplex virus
  - Varicella zoster virus
  - Adenovirus—epidemic keratoconjunctivitis
- *Microbial/post-microbial keratitis*:
  - Bacterial
  - Infectious crystalline keratopathy
  - Fungal
  - Chlamydial keratitis
  - Trachoma
  - Parasitic
  - Acanthamoeba keratitis
- *Nutritional deficiencies*: Keratomalacia
- *Noninfectious ulcerative keratitis*:
  - Keratoconjunctivitis sicca
  - Sjögren's syndrome
  - Neuroparalytic/neurotrophic keratopathy
  - Exposure keratitis
  - Mooren's ulcer
- *Corneal degenerations*:
  - Terrien's marginal degeneration
  - Calcific band keratopathy
- *Chemical injuries*:
  - Alkaline
  - Acid
- *Mechanical trauma, nonsurgical*: Traumatic opacity/irregular astigmatism
- *Regraft related to allograft rejection*
- *Regraft unrelated to allograft rejection*:
  - Primary tissue failure
  - Pseudophakic corneal edema
  - Vitreocorneal touch
  - Recurrent stromal dystrophy
  - Trauma/rupture
  - Glaucoma
- *Other causes of corneal opacification/distortion*:
  - Uveitis
  - Detached Descemet's membrane
  - Failed epikeratoplasty
  - Post-laser/postrefractive surgery
  - Silicone oil keratopathy
  - Epithelial downgrowth

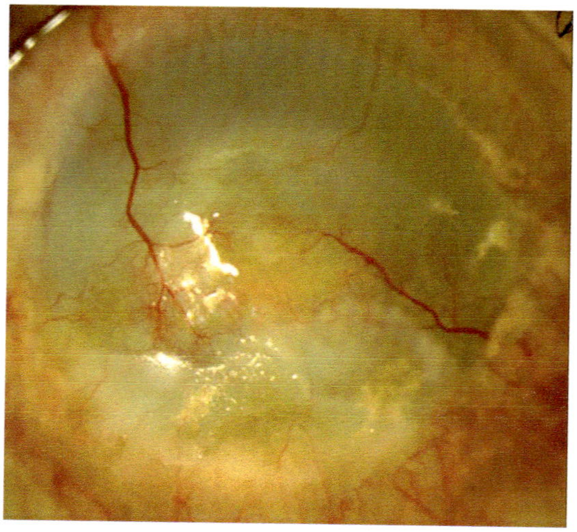

Fig. 1: Diffuse leucomatous corneal scarring in an eye with vascularization and lipid deposition following an episode of infectious keratitis.

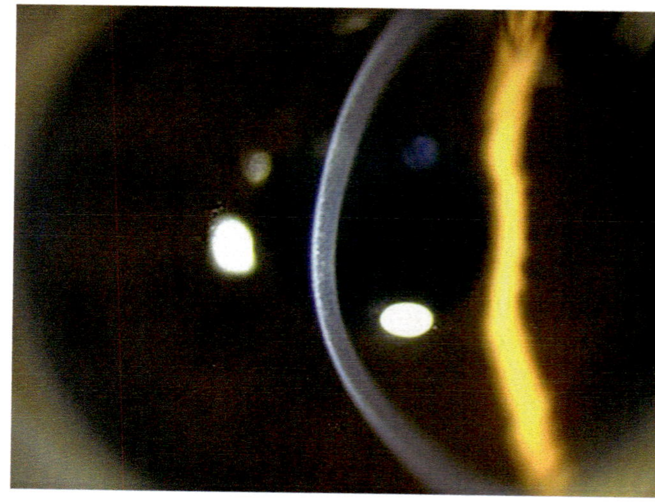

Fig. 2: Slit lamp biomicroscopic photograph of the right eye of a patient with keratoconus having paracentral corneal ectasia and corresponding thinning.

Another indication is deep anterior lamellar keratoplasty (DALK) with intraoperative Descemet membrane (DM) macroperforation necessitating conversion to a PK. The incidence of intraoperative DM perforation in DALK ranges 1.3–54.5%, and about 0.3–20.7% of cases require conversion to full-thickness keratoplasty due to such perforations.[10,11]

Optical Keratoplasty

Optical keratoplasty is performed with the primary purpose of improving visual acuity. This is the most common indication of PK and comprises >90% of the total penetrating keratoplasties performed in the developed world.[3] The indication of keratoplasty depends on the visual requirement and the expected long-term benefits arising out of surgery. A corneal pathology causing reduction in visual acuity to below 6/18 on Snellen's visual acuity chart is an acceptable norm for performing a full-thickness graft. Common indications of optical keratoplasty include aphakic bullous keratopathy and pseudophakic bullous keratopathy, corneal opacities following infectious keratitis (**Fig. 1**), trauma, graft failure, aphakic and pseudophakic bullous keratopathy with deep stromal scarring, corneal stromal dystrophies, corneal degenerations and congenital corneal opacities.[4] With the increasing adoption of component corneal surgeries, there has been a tremendous shift in the management of pathologies limited to specific layers of the cornea such as anterior lamellar keratoplasty for keratoconus and posterior lamellar keratoplasty for endothelial pathologies. Overall, keratoconus (**Fig. 2**), pseudophakic bullous keratopathy (**Fig. 3**) and Fuchs' dystrophy are the most common indications for an optical keratoplasty in the western world.[12,13]

In developing countries, post infectious corneal scarring, corneal opacification following trauma, malnutrition, previously failed graft and stromal scarring as a sequelae of long standing corneal edema.[14-16]

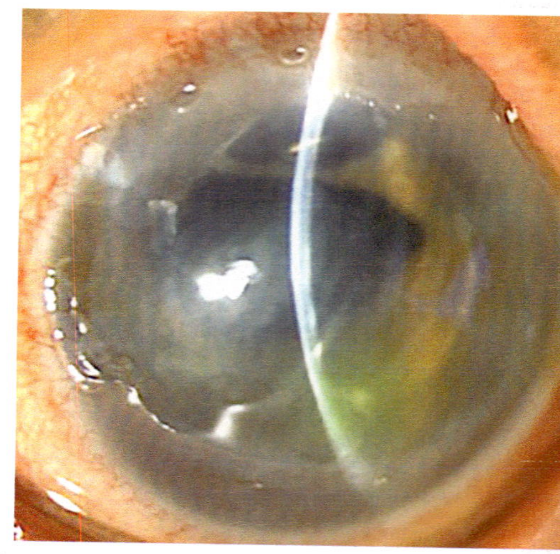

Fig. 3: Slit-lamp biomicroscopic photograph of the right eye of a patient with pseudophakic bullous keratopathy showing corneal stromal edema and Descement membrane folds. The iris architecture is distorted with dialysis in the superior part and a fixed and dilated pupil.

With the advent of intraocular lenses, there has been a rapid rise in the numbers of cataract surgery.[9] This resulted in plenty of cases of pseudophakic bullous keratopathy throughout the world. Presently, the incidence of pseudophakic bullous keratopathy appears to be decreasing, presumably because of improved intraocular implant design and almost universal use of posterior chamber intraocular lens (PC-IOL). The last two decades has also seen a rise in the popularity of posterior lamellar keratoplasty techniques such as Descemet stripping endothelial keratoplasty (DSEK) and Descemet membrane endothelial keratoplasty (DMEK) over PK for the treatment of endothelial pathologies all over the world.[17]

Tectonic/Reconstructive Keratoplasty

The prime purpose of tectonic/reconstructive keratoplasty is to restore the altered corneal anatomy. Although improved

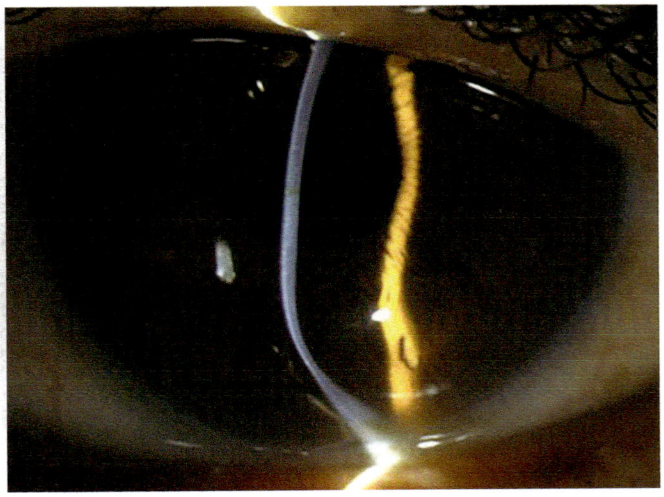

Fig. 4: Slit-lamp biomicroscopic view of a patient with pellucid marginal degeneration having a characteristic "beer belly appearance". The area of corneal protrusion can be clearly located above the area of thinning which is situated 1-2 mm inner to the limbus. There is no vascularization or scarring of the involved cornea.

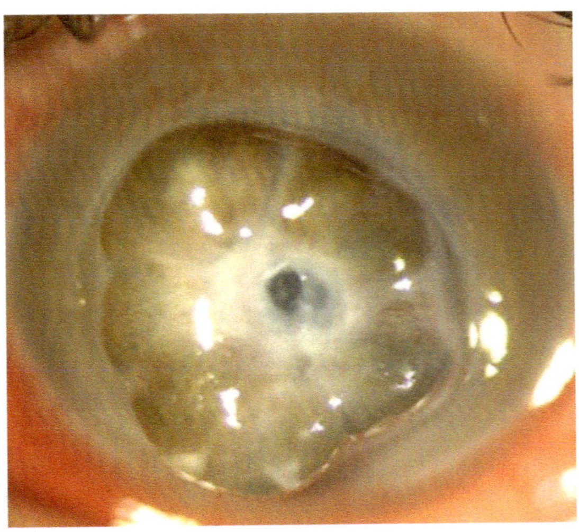

Fig. 5: Slit-lamp biomicroscopic photograph showing post infectious severe corneal stromal melting with iris tissue prolapse and pseudomembrane formation, necessitating a tectonic corneal graft.

visual acuity remains a relevant consideration, restoration or at least preservation of ocular anatomy and physiology are the principal indications for tectonic corneal grafts. This is required in eyes with cornea thinning or ectasia such as keratoconus, pellucid marginal degeneration (**Fig. 4**) and keratoglobus, corneal perforation or loss of corneal tissue, corneal melting associated with autoimmune disorders and in eyes with a corneal fistula and post infectious stromal melts (**Fig. 5**).[18,19] A reconstructive graft may also improve the patient's visual function and the option for future optical graft remains viable.

Therapeutic Keratoplasty

Therapeutic keratoplasty is indicated in cases with infectious keratitis unresponsive to specific antimicrobial therapy (**Fig. 6**).[20] In these cases, corneal transplantation

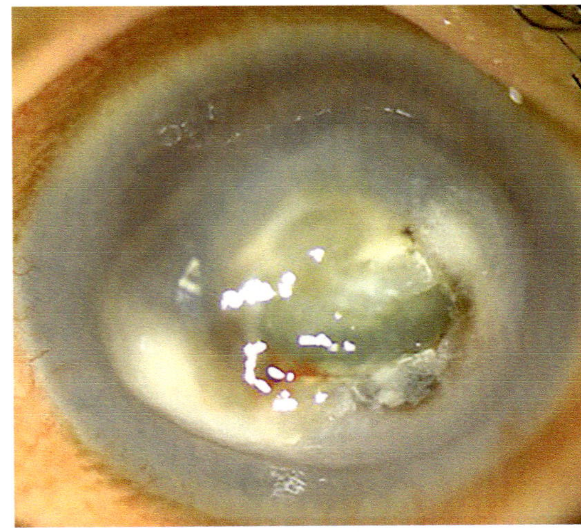

Fig. 6: Slit-lamp biomicroscopic photograph of a patient with long standing infectious keratitis with stromal thinning, non-responding to medical therapy requiring a therapeutic graft.

provides a form of surgical therapy as actively diseased tissue is removed. Transplants that are done to preserve the globe therapeutically often have the added advantage of improving visual clarity. Therapeutic keratoplasty performed for microbial keratitis still accounts for a major share of PKs performed in the developing countries.[12,21] Other therapeutic indications include long standing, non-resolving corneal edema, corneal scarring and deposits. Pain may be a significant factor in advanced corneal swelling with bullous epithelial changes. Penetrating keratoplasty is effective in reducing, and usually eliminating the pain of bullous keratopathy. Sometimes, therapeutic keratoplasty is necessitated for visualization of fundus to perform retinal procedure, such as pars plana vitrectomy, photocoagulation or repair of complicated retinal detachment. Therapeutic keratoplasty is usually considered when all other treatment modalities have failed; therefore, alternative treatments should always be tried, wherever applicable. Conjunctival flaps can be a successful alternative in cases with nonhealing corneal ulcers. Small perforations can be treated effectively with cyanoacrylate glue application and placement of a soft bandage contact lens.

Cosmetic Keratoplasty

The primary purpose of a cosmetic keratoplasty is to restore the normal appearance of the eye, which has limited or no visual potential.

This is usually performed in cases of unsightly corneal scars or corneal deposits. Patients should be informed prior about the possibility of graft opacification and the need for long-term medications similar to grafts performed for optical reasons. With the availability of painted soft contact lenses, corneal tattooing, enucleation or evisceration with a skillfully prepared prosthesis or cosmetic shields, cosmetic keratoplasty has become a rare procedure.

REGIONAL DIFFERENCES AND CHANGING INDICATIONS OF PENETRATING KERATOPLASTY

The leading indications of PK in developing countries include corneal scarring including adherent leukoma, active infectious keratitis, and previously failed graft.[14,15,21] In a study by Sony et al., in India, leading indications for PK were corneal scarring (38.03%) followed by acute infectious keratitis (28.38%), regrafting (11.5%), aphakic bullous keratopathy (7.27%), pseudophakic bullous keratopathy (6.18%), and corneal dystrophy (3.85%).[16] More recently Arya et al. reported previously failed graft (29.7%) followed by healed keratitis (15.8%) and pseudophakic or aphakic bullous keratopathy (14.8%) to be the most common indications for performing optical PK in a tertiary eye care center in northern India.[15] This is unlike developed countries where indications such as keratoconus, pseudophakic bullous keratopathy, and Fuchs' endothelial dystrophy are more common.[12,13]

Some interesting trends in the clinical indications for PK have been observed in the developed countries over the last two decades.[19] Before 1980, keratoconus and aphakic corneal edema were the most common indications and pseudophakic corneal edema was just emerging.[4,7,8,22,23] The emergence of pseudophakic corneal edema as the most common indication correlated with the overwhelming increase in the number of the cataract surgeries and lens implantations since mid-1970s.

Pseudophakic bullous keratopathy remains the leading indication for corneal transplantation in the United States.[12,22] Cosar et al. reported increase in percentage of pseudophakic bullous keratopathy cases associated with PC-IOLs have as compared to the anterior chamber intraocular lens (AC-IOLs). Relative number of regrafts increased with the increasing number of keratoplasties performed in the population and comprise the second most common indication for performing PK in the United States.[12,13,22,24] Keratoconus is the leading indication for PK in Europe, New Zealand, Australia, and the Middle East.[12,25,26]

PENETRATING KERATOPLASTY IN THE FELLOW EYE

An optimal visual recovery after corneal grafting surgery usually takes 4–8 months. Prior to this, vision may in fact be worse than before surgery in some of the cases. Considering this fact, it is wise to wait for at least 6 months after corneal grafting surgery in one eye before performing corneal transplantation in the fellow eye.[27] Following a corneal transplant in the second eye, the risk of rejection, to both eyes, has been found to be lower, if the time between two transplantation procedures is longer, with best survival if there was no rejection for 3 years in the first eye prior to surgery on the second.[28]

Box 2: Expected outcomes after penetrating keratoplasty.

Category 1 (Excellent prognosis >90% success rate):
- Keratoconus
- Lattice dystrophy
- Granular dystrophy
- Early Fuchs' dystrophy

Category 2 (Very good prognosis: 80–90% success rate):
- Pseudophakic bullous keratopathy
- Aphakic bullous keratopathy
- Fuchs' dystrophy
- Herpetic keratitis
- Iridocorneal endothelial syndromes
- Interstitial keratitis
- Macular dystrophy

Category 3 (Fair prognosis: 50–80% success rate):
- Keratoglobus
- Pellucid marginal degeneration
- Congenital hereditary endothelial dystrophy
- Corneal opacities in the pediatric group
- Chemical injury (mild)
- Dry eye (mild)
- Corneal perforations
- Active keratitis

Category 4 (Poor prognosis: <50% success rate):
- Ocular pemphigoid
- Stevens–Johnson syndrome
- Congenital glaucoma
- Anterior chamber cleavage syndrome
- Neuroparalytic/neurotrophic disease
- Multiple graft failures

EXPECTED OUTCOMES OF PENETRATING KERATOPLASTY

A successful outcome of corneal grafting surgery depends on many variables, indication of surgery being the most important one. There are certain indications of PK, which carry a relatively better prognosis. The definition of success includes presence of a clear graft along with improvement of two or more lines on a Snellen's visual acuity chart. This also implies visual rehabilitation with glasses instead of contact lenses, attainment of binocularity, decreased glare, and lesser pain. Expected outcomes of corneal graft surgery may be classified into four major categories based on the groups described by Buxton et al. (**Box 2**).[2]

Category 1 (Excellent Prognosis)

This group consists of corneas with central corneal disease and normal peripheral architecture. The limbal anatomy, corneal sensations and the microenvironment of the eyelids, as well as the tear film is healthy. Examples include keratoconus, lattice or granular stromal dystrophies, and early central Fuchs' dystrophy or other inactive central or paracentral scars. Prognosis in this group is excellent with over 90% success rate. The best reported rates of keratoplasty success have been reported in keratoconic eyes. Keates and Falkenstein[29] reported 100% graft success and 81% patients acheiving 20/40 or better visual acuity. Studies comparing the outcomes of DALK versus PK in keratoconic eyes report better or comparable visual outcomes with PK as opposed to DALK, albeit with a higher associated rate of long-term complications and graft rejection.[30-32] Kirkness et al. reported 97% graft clarity in cases of keratoconus at 4 years follow-up.[33] Studies reporting the extended long-term outcomes of PK in keratoconus patients have reported a decrease in graft survival and increase in disease recurrence rates after 20 years of surgery.[34,35]

Category 2 (Very Good Prognosis)

This group includes corneal lesions which involve either a part or entire corneal periphery with minimal vascularization (stromal vascularization in <2 quadrants). Examples include pseudophakic bullous keratopathy, aphakic bullous keratopathy, diffuse Fuchs' dystrophy, inactive herpetic keratitis, iridocorneal endothelial syndromes, interstitial keratitis, and macular stromal dystrophy. Prognosis in this group is very good with 80–90% success rates. Polack[36] et al. reported 78% of clear grafts performed for aphakic bullous keratopathy at 1 year and Olson[37] reported 89% of clear aphakic grafts. Pineros et al. reported[38] results in Fuchs' dystrophy with 89% graft clarity and visual acuity of 20/40 or better in 64% of cases after 8 years of follow-up.

Tanaka et al. reported outcomes of PK in patients with herpes zoster ophthalmicus (HZO)-associated complications.[39] They found a graft survival rate of 75% at 5 year and observed that preoperative corneal neovascularization and postoperative acyclovir did not impact the graft survival. Meanwhile, a longer quiescent period between active episode and PK was found to be associated with better graft survival.[39,40]

Category 3 (Fair Prognosis)

Corneas in this group are characterized by extremes of corneal thickness, involving a large part of the recipient zone adjacent to the limbus and Langerhans' cells, e.g., keratoglobus, pellucid marginal degeneration, congenital hereditary endothelial dystrophy, keratoplasty in young children, mild chemical injury, and mild dry eye. This may also include certain active infectious or inflammatory disease, corneal perforations, peripheral descemetoceles, and active bacterial, fungal, and herpetic keratitis. Prognosis in this group is fair with a success rate varying from 50 to 80%. The reported success rate of cornea in pediatric PK for congenital opacities is about 60% at 1 year.[41,42] The graft survival rates in pediatric PKs performed for congenital and acquired corneal opacities are reported to be comparable.[41,43] Lin et al. reported outcomes of PK for congenital corneal opacities in children <7 years of age. They found 55% of the grafts remaining clear during the follow-up period (6–82 months). While patients with sclerocornea were found to have the worst outcomes with only 12% achieving ambulatory vision, cases with minimal or no anterior segment involvement such as dermoid tumors, opacities without iridocorneal adhesions, and congenital hereditary endothelial dystrophy were found to associated with much better outcomes. Primary grafts were associated with better visual outcome than regraft cases (79% vs. 55% patients achieved ambulatory vision).[44]

The most frequent indication for pediatric keratoplasty may vary depending on the geographical location; infectious keratitis is the most frequent indication in developing countries while corneal dystrophies and congenital corneal opacities are the more common indications in the developed world.[14,45]

Category 4 (Poor Prognosis)

In this group, there is absence of normal limbal stem cells and normal maturation of corneal epithelium. These cases include ocular pemphigoid (**Fig. 7**), Stevens-Johnson syndrome (**Fig. 8**), congenital glaucoma, anterior chamber

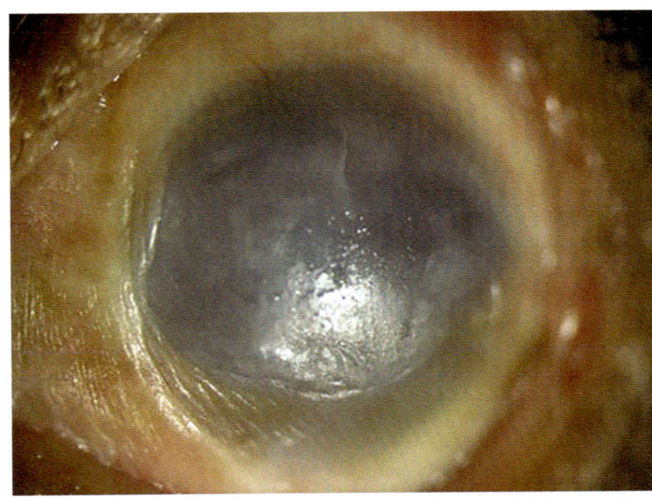

Fig. 7: Slit-lamp image of a patient with ocular cicatricial pemphigoid showing conjunctival scarring, symblepharon formation and corneal opacification with keratinization.

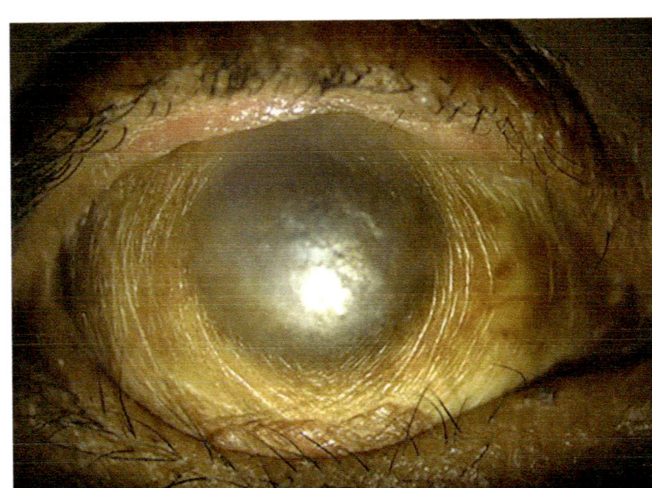

Fig. 8: Slit-lamp image of a patient with ocular Stevens–Johnson syndrome sequelae showing lower lid entropion with trichiasis and a completely dry and keratinized ocular surface.

cleavage syndromes, neuroparalytic or neurotrophic disease, and multiple graft failures. Prognosis in this group is very poor with a success rate of less than 50%. Full-thickness graft the preferred therapeutic option in this group; however, surgery may be undertaken with guarded prognosis when the disease is bilateral or involves the patient's only seeing eye. In chemical injury patients, simple or cultivated limbal stem cell transplantation (LSCT) followed by a sequential PK has been reported to provide better outcomes compared to PK alone or PK performed simultaneously with LSCT.[46,47] Gupta et al. reported an 85% graft survival rate at 6 months in patients undergoing a two-stage simple limbal epithelial cell transplantation (SLET) followed by PK in unilateral chemical injury patients.[47]

Various studies have evaluated different risk factors for graft survival after PK. The Collaborative Corneal Transplant Study, identified various high-risk factors affecting graft survival including:[48]

- Indication for the graft (keratoconus showed the best survival)
- Number of grafts performed in the ipsilateral eye
- Corneal vascularization at the time of the graft
- Presence of anterior synechiae during surgery
- History of raised intraocular pressure
- Presence of aphakia or pseudophakia
- History of previous intraocular surgery
- Recipient age <40 years
- Graft size <8 mm
- Time to preservation of donor cornea >6 hours
- Blood group ABO incompatibility

Williams et al. examined graft survival and visual outcome after full-thickness corneal transplantation in the Australian corneal graft registry. Probability of corneal graft survival was 0.87, 0.73, 0.60, and 0.46 at 1, 5, 10, and 15 years, respectively. Reasons for graft failure included irreversible rejection (34%), corneal endothelial cell failure including cases of glaucoma (24%), and infection (14%). Variables predicting graft failure in multivariate analysis included transplant center (centers performing >20 grafts per year showed increased survival), location, and volume of surgeon's case-load, graft era, indication for graft, number of previous ipsilateral grafts, lens status, corneal neovascularization at transplantation, a history of ocular inflammation or raised intraocular pressure, graft diameter (a graft size of >8.5 mm in diameter or a graft disparity of >0.5 mm showing poorer prognosis), and postoperative events including graft neovascularization and rejection. Best-corrected Snellen acuity of 6/12 or better was achieved by 45%, and of <6/60 by 26%, of grafted eyes at last follow-up. Most penetrating grafts were performed for visual improvement.[49]

The UK Transplant Study noted the following to be statistically significant risk factors for graft failure: Recipient diagnosis other than keratoconus or other central corneal disease, large grafts (trephine size = 14.5 mm), combined running and interrupted sutures.[50]

In the study done by Dandona et al.,[23] 5-year survival rate was highest if the corneal transplant was done for keratoconus and lowest if carried out for previous transplant failure. The relative risk of transplant failure was higher if the preoperative diagnosis was previous transplant failure, aphakic bullous keratopathy, corneal clouding due to congenital conditions, and glaucoma. Patients with lower socioeconomic status and patients <10 years of age also had higher risk of transplant failure. This was also associated with vascularization of the host cornea before transplantation and the use of fair quality donor cornea for transplantation compared with excellent, very good or good quality donor cornea.

The New Zealand National eye bank study published 1-year outcome of the PKs performed in a 10-year period between 1994 and 2003. They observed that while the donor characteristics did not significantly affect graft survival, various other factors such as previous episodes of reversible rejection, active anterior chamber inflammation at the time of surgery, preexisting corneal vascularization, intraoperative complications, small graft size (<7.25 mm), large graft size (>8.5 mm), preoperative glaucoma, and cases of regraft or past trauma adversely affected the graft survival. Keratoconus and Fuchs' cases were found to have the best outcomes in accordance with the previous reports, while bullous keratopathy, noninfective keratitis, and preoperative trauma cases were found to have a poorer visual outcome.[51]

Hassan et al. attempted to determine how donor health status affects the risk of infection after corneal transplant.[52] Postkeratoplasty endophthalmitis was associated with recent hospitalization and fatal cancer among donors. Endophthalmitis appeared more likely with tissues transplanted longer than 5 days after donation. The prevalence of concordant microbial isolates from donors and recipients was greater among fungal endophthalmitis than among bacterial endophthalmitis. In a separate study,[53] Hassan et al. tracked the relative frequency and explored possible risk factors of fungal compared with bacterial endophthalmitis after corneal transplantation. They noted that concordant cultures of the residual donor corneoscleral rim or preservation medium occurred significantly more often with fungal than bacterial endophthalmitis. After the introduction of Optisol-GS, the odds of bacterial relative to fungal endophthalmitis decreased by 77%. After adjustment for the preservation method and other eye-banking variables, the odds of fungal endophthalmitis were 3.4 times that of bacterial endophthalmitis, when donor corneal preservation was 4 days or longer.

In poor prognostic category such as aniridia, postoperative complications include whorl keratopathy, persistent epithelial defects, central subepithelial scarring, peripheral vascularization with pannus, and graft rejection. In a study by Kremer et al., glaucoma was well-controlled medically but five of nine patients (56%) with preexisting glaucoma needed an increase in medication for intraocular pressure control. Graft rejection occurred in seven of 11 eyes (64%) and three of these eyes required repeat transplantation.[54]

ALTERNATIVES AND CONTRAINDICATIONS TO PENETRATING KERATOPLASTY

While there are no absolute contraindications for PK except for the presence of no light perception, there are certain conditions of corneal opacification in which the morphological and functional outcome is so poor that most surgeons would not prefer to perform a corneal grafting surgery in such cases. These eyes as such should not be operated but surgery may be undertaken, especially, if the disease is bilateral or involves patient's only eye. Patients who are satisfied with their present level of vision and whose lifestyles are not compromised should not be operated. In developing countries like India, because of very high chances of graft failure, patient who have ambulatory vision in the eye with better vision and seem incapable of abiding by the postoperative care regimen should not have surgery. In cases of advanced dry eye, grade IV chemical burns, anterior staphyloma and severe cases of Stevens–Johnson syndrome, ocular cicatricial pemphigoid, with no tear film, and bad ocular surface may jeopardize a successful PK. Keratoprosthesis may be a better option for these patients.[37] Multiple graft failure is a relative contraindication for PK.

Cases of patients with inaccurate projection of rays and underlying retinal detachment are also relative contraindications for surgery. Patients with central corneal opacities and clear paracentral areas may obtain useful ambulatory vision with optical iridectomy alone.[38] Keratoplasty may also be deferred in patients who have severely scarred corneas with anterior segment distortion due to trauma or infection in one eye and the fellow eye has a visual acuity of 20/20. This topic is covered in details in section VI.

REFERENCES

1. Paytar D, Jones DB. Penetrating keratoplasty. Outcome monograph. Alcon monograph series 1(1). Texas: Alcon laboratories Fort Worth; 1976.
2. Buxton JN. Corneal surgery. In: Collins JF (Ed). Handbook of Clinical Ophthalmology. New York: Masson Publishers; 1982.
3. Williams KA, Muehlberg SM, Lewis RF, Coster DJ. How successful is corneal transplantation? A report from the Australian Corneal Graft Register. Eye (Lond). 1995;9(Pt 2):219-27.
4. Hyman L, Wittpenn J, Yang C. Indications and techniques of penetrating keratoplasties, 1985-1988. Cornea. 1992;11(6):573-6.
5. Mamalis N, Anderson CW, Kreisler KR, Lundergan MK, Olson RJ. Changing trends in the indications for penetrating keratoplasty. Arch Ophthalmol. 1992;110(10):1409-11.
6. The Australian Corneal Graft Registry. 1990 to 1992 report. Aust N Z J Ophthalmol. 1993;21(2 Suppl):1-48.
7. Sharif KW, Casey TA. Changing indications for penetrating keratoplasty, 1971-1990. Eye (Lond). 1993;7(Pt 4):485-8.
8. Haamann P, Jensen OM, Schmidt P. Changing indications for penetrating keratoplasty. Acta Ophthalmol (Copenh). 1994;72(4):443-6.
9. Robin JB, Gindi JJ, Koh K, Schanzlin DJ, Rao NA, York KK, et al. An update of the indications for penetrating keratoplasty, 1979 through 1983. Arch Ophthalmol. 1986;104(1):87-9.
10. Huang OS, Htoon HM, Chan AM, Tan D, Mehta JS. Incidence and outcomes of intraoperative Descemet membrane perforations during deep anterior lamellar keratoplasty. Am J Ophthalmol. 2019;199:9-18.
11. Gadhvi KA, Romano V, Fernández-Vega Cueto L, Aiello F, Day AC, Allan BD. Deep anterior lamellar keratoplasty for keratoconus: multisurgeon results. Am J Ophthalmol. 2019;201:54-62.
12. Matthaei M, Sandhaeger H, Hermel M, Adler W, Jun AS, Cursiefen C, et al. Changing indications in penetrating keratoplasty: A systematic review of 34 years of global reporting. Transplantation. 2017;101(6):1387-99.
13. Patel NP, Kim T, Rapuano CJ, Cohen EJ, Laibson PR. Indications for and outcomes of repeat penetrating keratoplasty, 1989-1995. Ophthalmology. 2000;107(4):719-24.
14. Sharma N, Prakash G, Titiyal JS, Tandon R, Vajpayee RB. Pediatric keratoplasty in India: indications and outcomes. Cornea. 2007;26(7):810-3.
15. Arya SK, Raj A, Bamotra RK, Bhatti A, Deswal J, Sindhu M. Indications and graft survival analysis in optical penetrating keratoplasty in a tertiary care center in North India: a 5-year study. Int Ophthalmol. 2018;38(4):1669-79.
16. Sony P, Sharma N, Sen S, Vajpayee RB. Indications of penetrating keratoplasty in northern India. Cornea. 2005;24(8):989-91.
17. Zhang AQ, Rubenstein D, Price AJ, Côté E, Levitt M, Sharpen L, et al. Evolving surgical techniques of and indications for corneal transplantation in Ontario: 2000-2012. Can J Ophthalmol. 2013;48(3):153-9.
18. Soong HK, Farjo AA, Katz D, Meyer RF, Sugar A. Lamellar corneal patch grafts in the management of corneal melting. Cornea. 2000;19(2):126-34.
19. Taylor DM, Stern AL. Reconstructive keratoplasty in the management of conditions leading to corneal destruction. Ophthalmology. 1980;87(9):892-904.
20. Nurözler AB, Salvarli S, Budak K, Onat M, Duman S. Results of therapeutic penetrating keratoplasty. Jpn J Ophthalmol. 2004;48(4):368-71.
21. Sharma N, Arora T, Singhal D, Maharana PK, Garg P, Nagpal R, et al. Procurement, storage and utilization trends of eye banks in India. Indian J Ophthalmol. 2019;67(7):1056-9.
22. Cosar CB, Sridhar MS, Cohen EJ, Held EL, Alvim P de TS, Rapuano CJ, et al. Indications for penetrating keratoplasty and associated procedures, 1996-2000. Cornea. 2002;21(2):148-51.
23. Dandona L, Ragu K, Janarthanan M, Naduvilath TJ, Shenoy R, Rao GN. Indications for penetrating keratoplasty in India. Indian J Ophthalmol. 1997;45(3):163-8.
24. Sheldon CA, McCarthy JM, White VA. Correlation of clinical and pathologic diagnoses of corneal disease in penetrating keratoplasties in Vancouver: a 10-year review. Can J Ophthalmol. 2012;47(1):5-10.
25. Cunningham WJ, Brookes NH, Twohill HC, Moffatt SL, Pendergrast DG, Stewart JM, et al. Trends in the distribution of donor corneal tissue and indications for corneal transplantation: the New Zealand National Eye Bank Study 2000-2009. Clin Exp Ophthalmol. 2012;40(2):141-7.
26. Edwards M, Clover GM, Brookes N, Pendergrast D, Chaulk J, McGhee CN. Indications for corneal transplantation in New Zealand: 1991-1999. Cornea. 2002;21(2):152-5.
27. Buxton JN, Schuman M, Pecego J. Graft reactions after unilateral and bilateral keratoplasty for keratoconus. Ophthalmology. 1981;88(8):771-3.

28. Tuft SJ, Gregory WM, Davison CR. Bilateral penetrating keratoplasty for keratoconus. Ophthalmology. 1995;102(3):462-8.
29. Keates RH, Falkenstein S. Keratoplasty in keratoconus. Am J Ophthalmol. 1972;74(3):442-4.
30. Henein C, Nanavaty MA. Systematic review comparing penetrating keratoplasty and deep anterior lamellar keratoplasty for management of keratoconus. Cont Lens Anterior Eye. 2017;40(1):3-14.
31. Keane M, Coster D, Ziaei M, Williams K. Deep anterior lamellar keratoplasty versus penetrating keratoplasty for treating keratoconus. Cochrane Database Syst Rev. 2014;(7):CD009700.
32. Khattak A, Nakhli FR, Al-Arfaj KM, Cheema AA. Comparison of outcomes and complications of deep anterior lamellar keratoplasty and penetrating keratoplasty performed in a large group of patients with keratoconus. Int Ophthalmol. 2018;38(3):985-92.
33. Kirkness CM, Ficker LA, Steele AD, Rice NS. The success of penetrating keratoplasty for keratoconus. Eye (Lond). 1990;4(Pt 5): 673-88.
34. Pramanik S, Musch DC, Sutphin JE, Farjo AA. Extended long-term outcomes of penetrating keratoplasty for keratoconus. Ophthalmology. 2006;113(9):1633-8.
35. Jensen LB, Hjortdal J, Ehlers N. Long-term follow-up of penetrating keratoplasty for keratoconus. Acta Ophthalmol. 2010;88(3):347-51.
36. Polack FM. Keratoplasty in aphakic eyes with corneal edema: results in 100 cases with 10-year follow-up. Ophthalmic Surg. 1980;11(10):701-7.
37. Olson RJ, Mattingly TP, Waltman SR, Kaufman HE. Aphakic keratoplasty: visual acuity and optical errors. Ophthalmology. 1980;87(7):680-6.
38. Pineros O, Cohen EJ, Rapuano CJ, Laibson PR. Long-term results after penetrating keratoplasty for Fuchs' endothelial dystrophy. Arch Ophthalmol. 1996;114(1):15-8.
39. Tanaka TS, Hood CT, Kriegel MF, Niziol L, Soong HK. Long-term outcomes of penetrating keratoplasty for corneal complications of herpes zoster ophthalmicus. Br J Ophthalmol. 2019;103(12):1710-5.
40. Kosker M, Duman F, Suri K, Hammersmith KM, Nagra PK, Rapuano CJ. Long-term results of keratoplasty in patients with herpes zoster ophthalmicus. Cornea. 2013;32(7):982-6.
41. Huang C, O'Hara M, Mannis MJ. Primary pediatric keratoplasty: indications and outcomes. Cornea. 2009;28(9):1003-8.
42. Stulting RD, Sumers KD, Cavanagh HD, Waring GO, Gammon JA. Penetrating keratoplasty in children. Ophthalmology. 1984; 91(10):1222-30.
43. Xavier Dos Santos Araújo ME, Santos NC, Souza LB, Sato EH, de Freitas D. Primary pediatric keratoplasty: Etiology, graft survival, and visual outcome. Am J Ophthalmol. 2020;212:162-8.
44. Lin Q, Shi W, Miao S, Zhang Y, Li L, Pan Z. Visual outcomes and prognostic factors of successful penetrating keratoplasty in 0- to 7-year-old children with congenital corneal opacities. Cornea. 2018;37(10):1237-42.
45. Majander A, Kivelä TT, Krootila K. Indications and outcomes of keratoplasties in children during a 40-year period. Acta Ophthalmol. 2016;94(6):618-24.
46. Basu S, Mohamed A, Chaurasia S, Sejpal K, Vemuganti GK, Sangwan VS. Clinical outcomes of penetrating keratoplasty after autologous cultivated limbal epithelial transplantation for ocular surface burns. Am J Ophthalmol. 2011;152(6):917-924.e1.
47. Gupta N, Farooqui JH, Patel N, Mathur U. Early results of penetrating keratoplasty in patients with unilateral chemical injury after simple limbal epithelial transplantation. Cornea. 2018; 37(10):1249-54.
48. Maguire MG, Stark WJ, Gottsch JD, Stulting RD, Sugar A, Fink NE, et al. Risk factors for corneal graft failure and rejection in the collaborative corneal transplantation studies. Collaborative Corneal Transplantation Studies Research Group. Ophthalmology. 1994;101(9):1536-47.
49. Williams KA, Lowe M, Bartlett C, Kelly TL, Coster DJ; All Contributors. Risk factors for human corneal graft failure within the Australian corneal graft registry. Transplantation. 2008;86(12):1720-4.
50. Bradley BA, Vail A, Gore SM, Rogers CA, Armitage WJ, Nicholls SM, et al. Penetrating keratoplasty in the United Kingdom: an interim analysis of the corneal transplant follow-up study. Clin Transpl. 1993;293-315.
51. Patel HY, Ormonde S, Brookes NH, Moffatt SL, Sherwin T, Pendergrast DG, et al. The New Zealand National Eye Bank: survival and visual outcome 1 year after penetrating keratoplasty. Cornea. 2011;30(7):760-4.
52. Hassan SS, Wilhelmus KR, Dahl P, Davis GC, Roberts RT, Ross KW, et al. Infectious disease risk factors of corneal graft donors. Arch Ophthalmol. 2008;126(2):235-9.
53. Hassan SS, Wilhelmus KR; Medical Review Subcommittee of the Eye Bank Association of America. Eye-banking risk factors for fungal endophthalmitis compared with bacterial endophthalmitis after corneal transplantation. Am J Ophthalmol. 2005;139(4):685-90.
54. Kremer I, Rajpal RK, Rapuano CJ, Cohen EJ, Laibson PR. Results of penetrating keratoplasty in aniridia. Am J Ophthalmol. 1993;115(3):317-20.

3

Preoperative Evaluation

Namrata Sharma, Sridevi Nair, Ritika Sachdev, Manotosh Ray

INTRODUCTION

The principal objective of preoperative evaluation is to identify the underlying corneal disease, to anticipate potential intraoperative and postoperative problems and to prognosticate a case of keratoplasty. It is imperative that a correct etiological diagnosis of corneal pathology and associated disorder, if any, is established. An attempt must be made to cure all associated conditions that can complicate a desired result of corneal transplantation surgery. Any active corneal disease must be identified preoperatively and if required, effective measures should be taken to prevent its adverse influence on a successfully performed corneal grafting surgery. A proper patient selection and comprehensive preoperative evaluation enhance the potential for a favorable outcome.

OCULAR HISTORY

A detailed history is taken to identify the related local or systemic conditions. Patients should be carefully screened for ocular injury, infectious keratitis, nutritional deficiencies, history of previous surgery, and for systemic diseases such as collagen vascular disease and Stevens–Johnson syndrome.[1-3]

Prognosis for successful outcome may be related to the knowledge of patient's preoperative history. Corneal grafts for herpetic scars develop recurrence of the disease postoperatively and may require long-term systemic acyclovir therapy.

A history of good visual acuity prior to the development of corneal opacity in the affected eye suggests chances of a better functional outcome, postoperatively. A meticulous evaluation to rule out presence of amblyopia in cases with long standing corneal opacities, anisometropia, and strabismus is crucial. A patient with childhood onset of opacity presenting later during adulthood might have coexisting amblyopia. Information should be obtained pertaining to the onset of visual disturbance, whether a prior intraocular surgery or infection preceded it, or whether it simply deteriorated over time. Previous retinal and macular pahologies may result in poor visual gain despite a clear graft.

History-taking should also document the use of antiglaucoma medications. Poor control of intraocular pressure after keratoplasty reduce the chances of graft survival. Chronic elevation of intraocular pressure may lead to decreased endothelial cell counts.[4,5]

Changes in the quality of vision, as the day progresses should also be ascertained; for example, in Fuchs' dystrophy, vision is often worse immediately upon awakening with gradual improvement as the day progresses. When available, old records should be looked into. These can caution the physician regarding the possibility of occurrence of intra- and postoperative problems and confirm important information such as prior best-corrected visual acuity (BCVA), intraocular pressure control, and previous intraocular lens (IOL) powers used. A history should be sought about prior ophthalmic surgical procedures such as cataract extraction, filtering procedures or neodymium-doped yttrium aluminum garnet (Nd:YAG) laser for posterior capsular opacification. A candidate for regrafting carries a high-risk of rejection.

GENERAL HISTORY

The main question when obtaining the patient's history relates to the ability of the patient to undergo proposed operative procedure. In considering for local anesthesia, for example, the ability of the patient to lie flat during the procedure could be compromised by pulmonary or cardiac abnormalities and severe arthritis.[6] Preexisting medical problems such as hypertension and diabetes should be stabilized. Allergies to medications such as antibiotics, systemic medications, and anesthetics should be noted and reviewed to avoid subsequent complications.

Medication history especially pertaining to the intake of anticoagulant or antiplatelet drugs should be elicited. Conclusive evidence associating an increased risk of intraoperative hemorrhage in keratoplasty patients receiving antithrombotics is lacking. Furthermore, discontinuation of these drugs may lead to serious arterial or venous thromboembolic events. Continuation of drugs such as aspirin, clopidrogel, vitamin K antagonists, and heparin during the perioperative period may be considered depending on the indication for anti-thrombotic agent and risk of thromboembolic events provided, the anticoagulation level remains within the therapeutic range. Discontinuation of more potent and newer antiplatelet agents such as ticagrelor and direct oral anticoagulants should be considered prior to surgery while using an appropriate bridge therapy. A multidisciplinary approach including the eye surgeon, cardiologist, and anesthetist is warranted in these patients.[7]

Patient's social and family support system also needs to be reviewed. Because consistent follow-up and proper use of postoperative medications is required, patient's compliance is important for the ultimate success of the graft.

OCULAR EXAMINATION

Visual Acuity

Assessment of visual acuity is extremely important before the patient is taken up for a penetrating keratoplasty. This should include recording of both uncorrected as well as corrected distance visual acuity (UDVA and CDVA). Standard Snellen's chart is commonly used to record visual acuity. Contact lens corrected visual acuity should be recorded in cases of irregular astigmatism.[8]

In cases with poor visual acuity, it must be documented as counting fingers, hand movements or light perception. One of the most important acuity factors involves the careful documentation of projection of rays, as this is an important indication of retinal and optic nerve function. In eyes with corneal edema, instilling topical glycerin after anesthesia and waiting 20–30 minutes for corneal clearing may improve acuity and facilitate retinal examinations. Pinhole visual acuity, potential acuity meter, and glare testing may have limited value in predicting best visual acuity due to severe light scattering from corneal pathology. In cases of small central scars stenopic slit visual acuity should be recorded after complete pupillary dilatation. It is possible that some of these patients may significantly benefit from a simple optical iridectomy and hence a penetrating keratoplasty may be deferred.[9]

Quantifying visual function in children is important to prognosticate the case. Occlusion of one eye, which is strongly objected by the child, can indicate a poorer acuity in the uncovered eye. Preferential looking test can also be performed to assess visual acuity in children, which is based on the fact that infants prefer to fixate on a pattern rather than a homogeneous stimulus. The infant is exposed to stimulus and the examiner observes the eye for fixation movements using Teller acuity cards or Cardiff acuity cards. In children >2 years multiple picture test or Sheridan–Gardiner test can be performed which is based on matching prototypes.

Gross Ocular Examination

Eyes are examined with an emphasis on external ocular disorders. The lids are evaluated for ectropion, entropion, lagophthalmos, and trichiasis. Surgical correction of these conditions prior to keratoplasty is advised. Because normal tear production is crucial to graft re-epithelialization, one should note any kind of tear film abnormalities if present, during preoperative examination. Any evidence of blepharitis should be looked for and must be treated aggressively. The status of the lacrimal sac and punctal position is examined to rule out any lacrimal system disorder. These anomalies must be corrected before the patient is taken up for keratoplasty. If significant dryness is present, partial or complete punctal occlusion should be performed either preoperatively or intraoperatively, sometimes in combination with medial or lateral tarsorrhaphy particularly, if exposure keratitis is present.

Slit-lamp Biomicroscopy

Conjunctiva and Cornea

The tear film should be evaluated under slit lamp to look for any signs of dry eye such as decreased tear meniscus height and presence of debris in the tear film. Palpebral and tarsal conjunctiva should be examined to look for any evidence of scarring or, symblepharon suggestive of presence of an ocular surface pathology such as Stevens–Johnson syndrome, ocular cicatricial pemphigoid or chemical burns. These patients are at increased risk of for developing, nonhealing epithelial defects, and postoperative infections as the normal external immune defense mechanisms are compromised.

Slit-lamp examination is also performed to assess the size, shape, extent and severity of corneal opacity, degree, and extent of vascularization. The corneal sensations are checked using the fine tip of a cotton wisp 7 (**Fig. 1**).

Consideration must be given to the condition of the host graft bed, its corneal thickness especially in the peripheral area, particularly in cases of regrafts. The presence of corneal vascularization may dictate the type of suturing technique to be used in a particular case. The underlying pathology and the diameter of the host cornea guide the diameter of host trephination and corresponding disparity in the size of donor button. In cases with postinfectious scarring with thinning and vascularization or corneal ectasias such as pellucid marginal degeneration, sizing, and placement of the graft may require some decentering. Interrupted sutures may be preferred in corneas with excessive vascularization or in pediatric eyes due to their faster healing response seen after keratoplasty.

Anterior Segment and Iris

The anterior chamber must be evaluated for any evidence of any active inflammation. A transplant is best performed

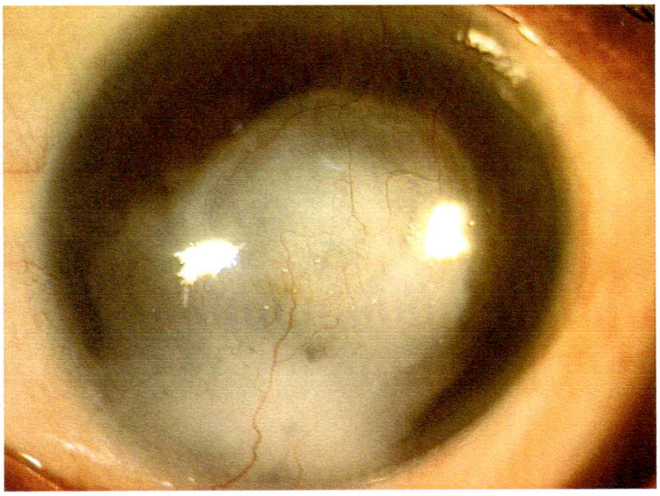

Fig. 1: Postinfectious corneal scarring with vascularization.

in an uninflamed and a quiet eye. Presence of ciliary flush, keratic precipitates, anterior synechia, and iridocorneal adhesions are signs of past or present inflammation. Iris should be examined for the presence of iridocorneal synechiae, rubeosis, and also fibrovascular membranes obscuring the pupillary area and location of peripheral iridectomies. Presence of extensive anterior synechiae may warrant use of special techniques like corneal debulking[10] and use of oversized grafts.[11] The pupil should be examined for size, shape, and relative afferent pupillary defect.

Lens

The lens status must be determined for the presence of cataract, aphakia, and pseudophakia. Slit-lamp microscopy is performed after dilatation of pupil to detect lenticular opacities. The lens may have weakened zonules and exhibit phakodonesis. Preexisting early cataract progresses very rapidly after penetrating keratoplasty. Moreover, coexistent cataract and corneal opacities are common, especially when the patient is older than 50 years. Therefore, it may be mandatory to remove cataract at the time of keratoplasty, even if it is minimal.[12] This can avoid the risk of endothelial damage during subsequent cataract surgery.

If the eye is aphakic, status of the anterior hyaloid, presence and extent of iris coloboma, and pupillary status must be evaluated. Such eyes may additionally require anterior segment reconstruction including coreoplasty, anterior vitrectomy, and an anterior chamber or scleral fixated posterior chamber IOL implantation.

If pseudophakos is present, the type of IOL should be identified. If an anterior chamber IOL is present, it must be identified as either an open looped or a closed loop lens. Iris supported closed loop anterior chamber lenses and open-looped anterior chamber lens should be replaced especially if any pseudophakodonesis is suspected.

Intraocular Pressure

Intraocular pressure should be measured preoperatively. Applanation tonometry may not be possible in corneas with opacities and scarring. A MacKay–Marg, pneumotonometer, scleral tonometer or Tono-Pen may be required for more accurate assessment in these patients. The use of rebound tonometer and ocular response analyzer (cornea compensated intraocular pressure) has been found to be more accurate in cases of corneal clouding due to mucopolysaccharidosis.[13] Raised intraocular pressure must be controlled either medically or surgically, before the patient is planned for keratoplasty. Intraocular pressure should not be higher than the low twenties on no more than two medications. If it is not, primary filtering or combined filtering and penetrating keratoplasty should be considered.[4] Since, all keratoplasty patients require intraoperative viscoelastics to coat the endothelium, control of bleeding, and help prevent synechiae formation, eyes with preexisting glaucoma should be screened out. Further, the use of long-term topical steroids to prevent graft rejection may lead to steroid-induced glaucoma.[4,5]

Fundus Evaluation

If possible, a thorough evaluation of retina and vitreous should be performed to ensure that the decreased vision is secondary to corneal pathology only. Eyes with macular pathology, e.g., macular holes, macular degeneration, and cystoid macular edema are unlikely to improve after penetrating keratoplasty despite a successful graft. This may be of particular significance in cases of aphakic and pseudophakic bullous keratopathy with a history of intraoperative vitreous disturbance and postoperative iridocylitis. Knowledge of such conditions helps to explain the prognosis to the patients. Direct and indirect ophthalmoscopy should be done under mydriasis and fundus evaluation is performed from relatively clear areas, wherever possible.

Preoperative Evaluation in Endothelial Keratoplasty

Appropriate patient selection is the key to achieving good outcomes after endothelial keratoplasty. In addition to what has been described above, certain important aspects should be considered while planning a patient for endothelial keratoplasty. Presence of corneal stromal scarring or fibrosis must be documented because such cases are less suited for Descemet stripping endothelial keratoplasty (DSEK) or Descemet membrane endothelial keratoplasty (DMEK). The stromal scar or haze may persist after surgery and hinder with optimal visual rehabilitation after surgery. An intact iris-lens diaphragm improves the chances of retaining an air bubble within the anterior chamber during the early postoperative period following endothelial keratoplasty (EK). Graft unfolding is more difficult in DMEK, making it technically challenging in patients with large iris defects, extensive peripheral anterior synechiae, anterior chamber intraocular lens, glaucoma drainage devices in situ, previously operated trabeculectomy or aphakia. Post vitrectomized eye often have deep anterior chambers which could make the unfolding and attachment of a DMEK graft difficult in these cases. With increasing surgeon experience, however, DMEK has been shown to have good outcomes even in these difficult scenarios.[14] Unfolding the DMEK graft and determining the graft correct orientation can be challenging in cases with poor corneal visibility due to inadequate intraoperative visualization.[15]

INVESTIGATIONS

Refraction

An accurate refraction under mydriasis is mandatory for all cases, wherever possible. In cases such as keratoconus, where retinoscopy is impossible, keratometry may be checked and patient refracted.

Tear Film Status

The use of fluorescein and/or rose bengal dye for ocular surface evaluation and Schirmer testing provide the ophthalmologist an indication of the extent of dryness and epitheliopathy.

Keratometry

Keratometry may be warranted in cases of corneal ectasias such as keratoconus, pellucid marginal degeneration, and keratoglobus.

Gonioscopy

Gonioscopy may be performed to examine iridocorneal adhesions, peripheral iridectomies, and to locate the position of the lens haptics if an anterior chamber lens is present.

Pachymetry

Pachymetry should be performed to quantify corneal thickness using ultrasonic pachymeter or sonogage, especially in cases of corneal thinning disorders such as keratoconus, keratoglobus, and pellucid marginal degeneration. Not only central but also paracentral and peripheral readings should be obtained in each of the four meridians. Pachymetry is also mandatory in cases where, automated therapeutic lamellar keratectomy is contemplated for proper selection of the microkeratome head to be used. Michieletto et al. have reported a very high-risk of perforation of the Descemet's membrane while performing big-bubble technique of deep anterior lamellar keratoplasty (DALK) in cases with preoperative pachymetry <250 µm.[16] They hypothesized that the weakening of the Descemet's membrane is related to end-stage keratoconus corneal thinning and this ultrastructurally weakened Descemet's membrane is more likely to rupture during the DALK procedure.

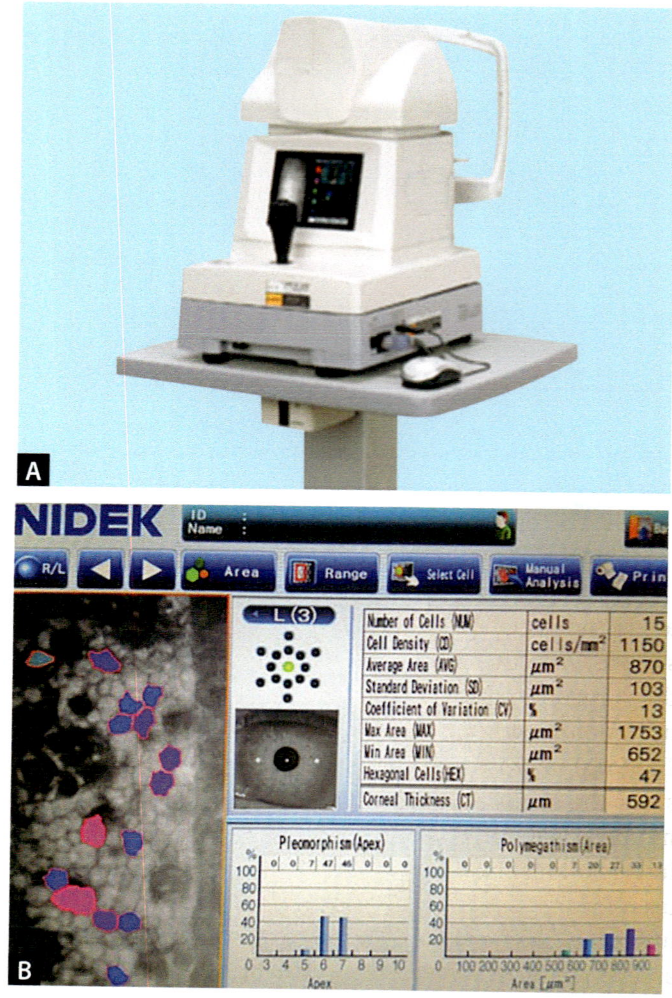

Figs. 2A and B: (A) Specular microscope; (B) Specular microscopic features of Fuchs' dystrophy: extensive guttae are visible.

In patients planned for endothelial keratoplasty corneal pachymetry helps to determine the severity of disease. While there is no single cutoff value for corneal edema which helps ascertain the need for surgery, a stromal thickness greater that 650 microns or progressive worsening of stromal edema are considered to be the indications for surgical intervention.[14]

Specular Microscopy, Confocal Microscopy and Straylight Meter

Specular microscopy and confocal microscopy may be undertaken, wherever possible. Specular microscopic features help to diagnose cases of Fuchs' endothelial corneal (**Figs. 2A and B**) and also help to differentiate various other pathologies such as posterior polymorphous dystrophy and iridocorneal endothelial syndromes. Endothelial cell counts and morphology may also be relevant in cases of superficial opacities where lamellar grafts are contemplated and a normal endothelial reserve is essential. Quantitative assessment of corneal endothelial guttae may be performed using multifocal specular microscopy. The area ratio of corneal guttae measured has been found to adversely

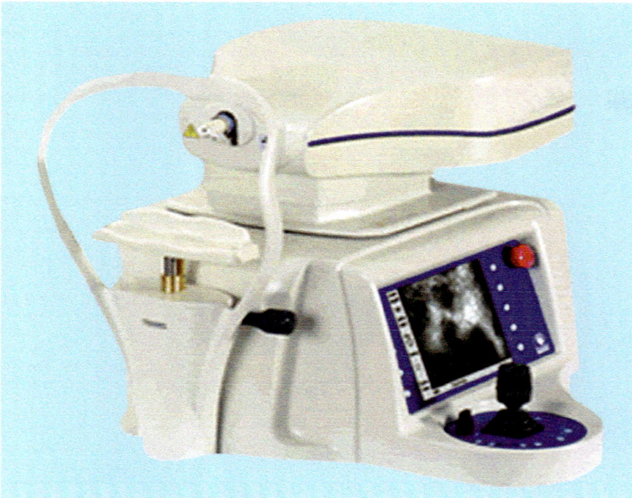

Fig. 3: Confocal microscopy.

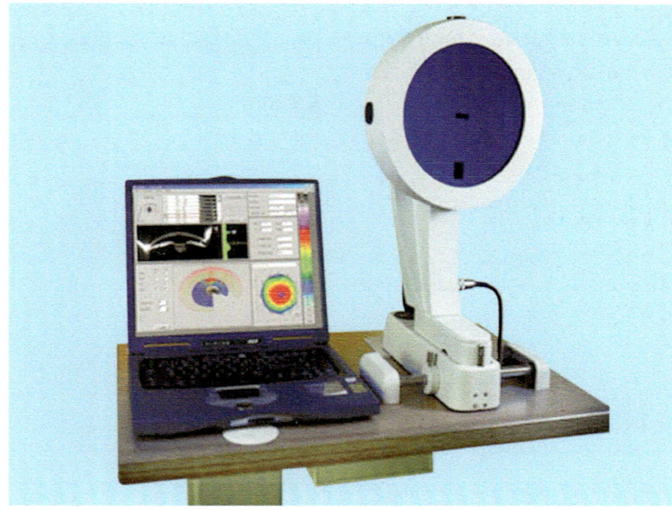

Fig. 4: Pentacam: The Scheimpflug imaging system

affect the visual quality and cause increased corneal light scatter. Objective assessment of this parameter may guide the surgeon in deciding on whether to intervene surgically in patients without clinically evident stromal edema.[17,18] Confocal microscopy, a more recent research tool helps to study the status of the epithelium as well as keratocytes. It noninvasively resolves the structural as well as functional interrelationships (**Fig. 3**). Confocal microscopy has been used for the detection and management of pathologic and infectious conditions, corneal dystrophies and ectasias, and assessment of the depth of corneal scarring prior to lamellar keratoplasty. Abnormalities in anterior corneal cellular and architectural features such as increased anterior corneal backscatter, reduced anterior stromal cell density and abnormal subepithelial cells have been observed on confocal images of patients with early Fuchs endothelial corneal dystrophy.[19] Straylight meter is used to assess the functional forward light scatter and is beneficial in the assessment of FECD patients.[20,21] The Oculus C-Quant straylight meter (Oculus GmbH, Wetzlar, Germany) is one such device which reports forward light scatter as the logarithm of the straylight parameter. Straylight is a psychophysical measurement that is proportional to forward light scatter; a higher value of forward light scatter indicates more straylight (more sensitivity to glare). Meulen et al. reported that younger patients with Fuchs' dystrophy can have symptoms of increased straylight despite having good visual acuity and that endothelial keratoplasty may improve their symptoms. They proposed preoperative straylight as a useful clinical metric to predict postoperative improvement, especially in cases where preoperative visual acuity approximates 20/20 on a Snellen chart.[21]

Laser Interferometry

More sophisticated testing with potential acuity meters and laser interferometers may be helpful for evaluation of prognosis of a transplant surgery in patients with corneal opacities.

Scheimpflug Imaging

Slit scanning (Orbscan) and Scheimpflug (Pentacam) evaluation of the anterior and posterior corneal surface as well as the corneal thickness may be useful in ectatic disorders of the cornea (**Figs. 4 and 5**). Their role is however limited in opaque corneas and ultrasonic evaluation may be more useful in these cases. Yamaguchi T et al. demonstrated that postoperative BCVA following Descemet stripping automated endothelial keratoplasty (DSAEK) correlated with irregularity of the anterior surface but not the posterior surface as evaluated using the Scheimpflug imaging system.[22] Riss et al. reported Pentacam-pachymetry based big-bubble DALK using a 90% intended depth of initial lamellar trephination to be a safe and effective procedure for disorders such as keratoconus.[23] More recently, Pentacam has been employed to detect subclinical stromal edema in patients with Fuchs' endothelial corneal dystrophy without clinically apparent corneal edema. The following tomographic features, namely, loss of parallel isopachs, displacement of the thinnest point of the cornea, and focal posterior corneal surface depression, were found to characterize the presence of subclinical edema independent of pachymetry.[24] Staging of FECD based on the above tomographic features was also found to be highly repeatable by the authors.[25] The authors reported that loss of regular isopachs and displacement of thinnest point were the most important clinical risk factors for progression and potential need for intervention. The risk of FECD progression and intervention, including that following uncomplicated cataract surgery, was found to increase in accordance with the number of parameters present. The cumulative probability of disease progression or intervention over 5 years increased from 7% when none of the patterns were present to 89% when all were present. They also reported central corneal thickness was a weak predictor of prognosis as compared to the pachymetry map and posterior elevation map parameters.[26]

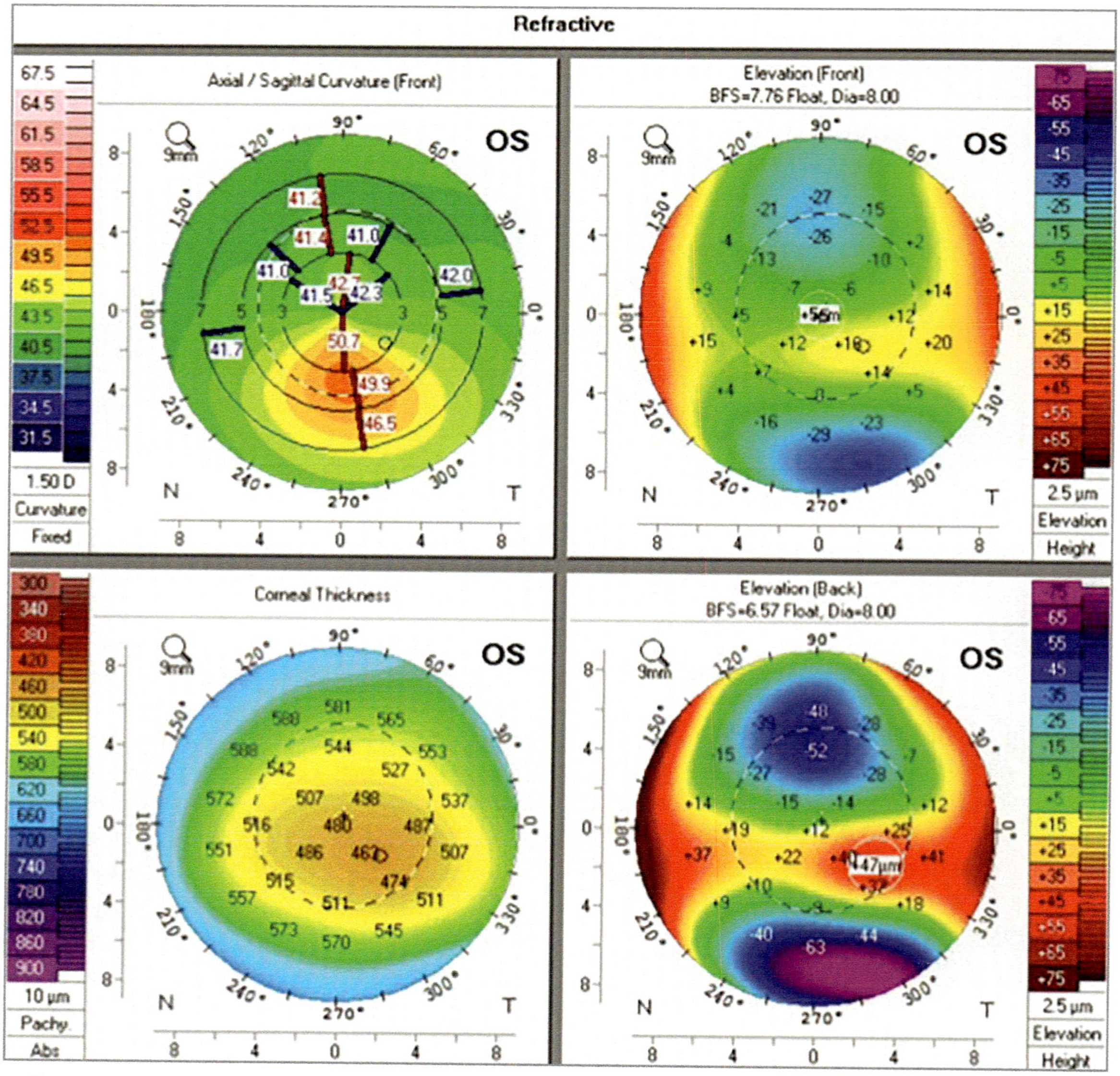

Fig. 5: Four quadrant refractive map of a patient with Keratoconus showing inferior corneal steepening and thinning.

Ultrasound Biomicroscopy

The original ultrasound biomicroscope (UBM) developed by Pavlin, Sherar, and Foster is based on 50–100 MHz transducer, incorporated into the B-mode clinical scanner. High frequency transducers permit increased resolution, but only at the expense of decreased tissue penetration depth. The commercially available UBM is most often configured with a 50 MHz transducer, which provides a tissue resolution of approximately 50 μm and a penetration depth of 4–5 mm. This permits visualization of the anterior segment. The presence of a corneoiridic scar may necessitate an ultrasound biomicroscopy to assess the angle and ciliary body (**Figs. 6 and 7**). While performing keratoplasty, corneal debulking by sequential lamellar separation[9] and subsequent anterior segment reconstruction may be undertaken in such cases. Ultrasound biomicroscopic evaluation can be used to determine the presence and extent of peripheral anterior synechiae (PAS), the status of the lens or the intraocular implant, and the capsular status in aphakes. Madhavan et al. have reported its role as a useful adjunct in preoperative planning and prognostication of patients requiring penetrating

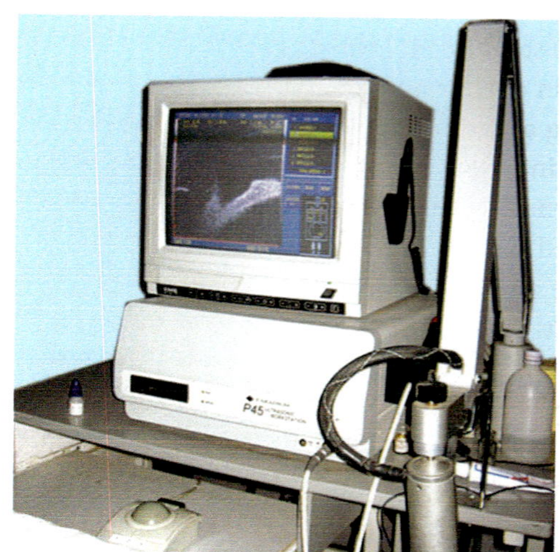

Fig. 6: Ultrasound biomicroscopy.

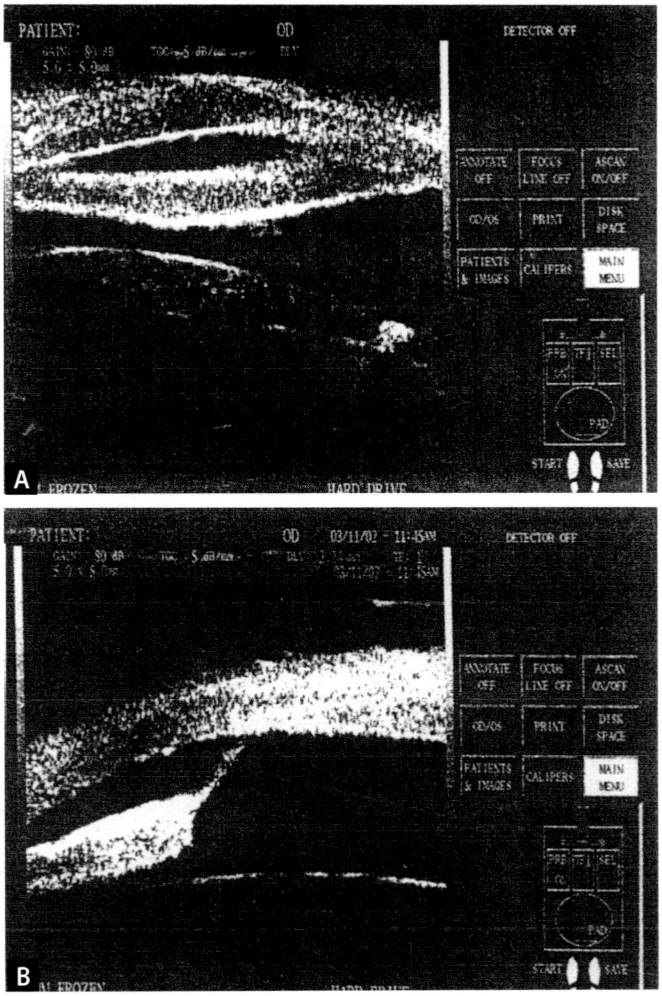

Figs. 7A and B: Ultrasound biomicroscopy of corneoiridic scar.

keratoplasty.[27] Lanzl et al. demonstrated the role of UBM in surgical planning of limbal dermoids. UBM is able to assess the depth of involvement of opaque corneal lesions such as limbal dermoids as it distinguishes the normal cornea from the more sonolucent lesion.[28]

Rutnin et al. evaluated the role of UBM as a method for assessing anterior chamber IOL haptics before combined penetrating keratoplasty and IOL exchange in eyes with poor corneal clarity resulting from pseudophakic bullous keratopathy.[29] They concluded that UBM can evaluate the presence and extent of fibrotic encasement of the haptics in cases with an opaque cornea and the extent of fibrotic encasement was found to be predictive of the surgical difficulty encountered while removing the intraocular implant. UBM plays a vital role in preoperative evaluation of patients with congenital corneal opacities and anterior segment dysgenesis such as Peter's anomaly. It helps in characterizing corneal pathology, anterior chamber angle details, lens status, and keratolenticular or iridocorneal adhesions. This information is crucial for establishing a diagnosis, preoperative decision-making, and planning additional procedures such as lens extraction and IOL implantation.[30] Nischal et al. reported that UBM findings based diagnosis matched the histopathological diagnosis in 100% of their patients, and, helped change the clinical diagnosis in 38% of their cases.[31]

Anterior Segment Optical Coherence Tomography

Anterior segment optical coherence tomography (ASOCT) is a noncontact imaging system that allows cross-sectional visualization of the anterior segment. It enables qualitative and quantitative analysis of the corneal and anterior chamber details. It differs from UBM in three important aspects; it is a noncontact procedure, employs an infrared light source and produces higher resolution images. Two major OCT platforms are currently available: time domain (TD-OCT) and spectral domain (SD-OCT). The TD-OCT includes Visante OCT (Carl Zeiss Meditec, Oberkochen, Germany) and slit-Lamp OCT (Heidelberg Engineering GmbH, Heidelberg, Germany). These devices use a long wavelength (1,310 nm) light which allows deeper penetration with 15–20 μm resolution and a wider area of capture in a single image. The SD-OCT devices include the Spectralis (Heidelberg Engineering GmbH, Heidelberg, Germany), RTVue (Optovue, Inc., CA, USA), and Cirrus OCT (Carl Zeiss Meditec, Oberkochen, Germany). They employ shorter wavelengths (830 nm) and have better axial resolution of about 4–7 μm. SD-OCT devices, however, have the disadvantage of a smaller horizontal scan width and shorter scan depth as compared to TD-OCT.[32] ASOCT plays a crucial role in preoperative evaluation of patients undergoing a full-thickness or lamellar keratoplasty. It aids in the assessment of corneal thickness, the depth and extent of corneal lesions or scarring, anterior chamber depth, presence of PAS or corneoiridic scars, and lens status. The information regarding the nature, depth and extent of corneal pathology is crucial both for establishing a correct diagnosis as well as for deciding the type of keratoplasty (**Fig. 8A**).[33] ASOCT aids in decision-making of patients planned for DALK or anterior lamellar keratoplasty. The measured depth of corneal pathology guides the depth of the initial trephination during surgery. ASOCT also provides corneal pachymetry across the various zones of cornea including central, midperipheral, and peripheral areas, and helps to detect any areas of thinning or scarring. This helps the surgeon to decide whether to proceed with a big-bubble DALK or manual dissection. The presence of a corneal scar or excessive corneal thinning detected on ASOCT may alert the surgeon regarding the increased risk of intraoperative Descemet membrane (DM) perforation on attempting a big-bubble procedure.[34] In patients planned for endothelial keratoplasty (EK), preoperative ASOCT imaging helps the surgeon to objectively quantify the corneal thickness and document its progression on serial follow-up (**Fig. 8B**). It helps in detection of epithelial hyperplasia, subepithelial fibrosis and stromal haze. An excessively thick cornea and presence of subepithelial fibrosis are suggestive of a chronic

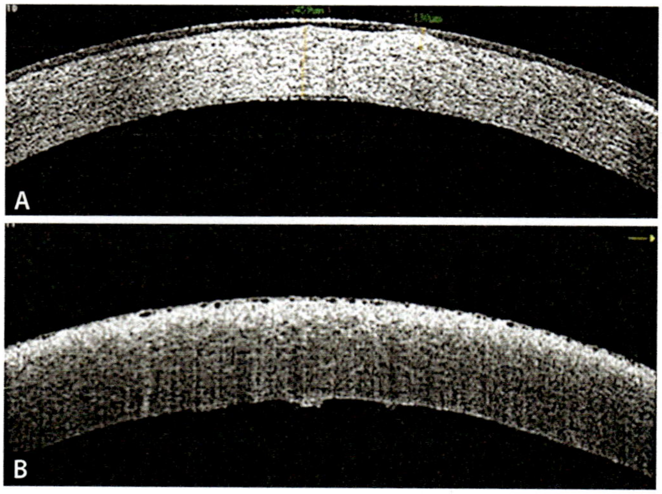

Figs. 8A and B: (A) An anterior segment optical coherence tomography image of a macular corneal dystrophy patient depicting corneal thickness and the extent of pathology; (B) An anterior segment optical coherence tomography image of a Fuchs' endothelial corneal dystrophy patient depicting stromal edema and epithelial bullae without a significant stromal scarring or fibrosis.

long-standing edema predictive of suboptimal visual outcome after surgery.[35] Wertheimer et al. graded corneal stromal opacity using optical density measurements by spectral domain ASOCT. They reported increased optical densities in FECD corneas which correlated well with other parameters such as corneal pachymetry and visual acuity. Being an objectively quantifiable parameter it has been proposed as a potentially useful tool for identifying disease progression as well for deciding on the need for surgical intervention in these patients.[36] The role of artificial intelligence in the diagnosis of ocular pathologies is being studied increasingly over the past few years. Deep learning enables computers to execute direct classification from images rather than through features recognized by human experts. Recently, Eleiwa et al. demonstrated the successful application of a deep learning algorithm using high definition ASOCT to diagnose both early and late FECD cases as well as distinguish these from non-diseased patients with a very high sensitivity and specificity.[37] In patients with failed EK, ASOCT imaging helps to detect the presence of DM remnants in the graft-host interface. In patients with a previously failed full-thickness graft ASOCT helps in the assessment of posterior graft host junction. This is especially crucial while planning to an EK in these patients. ASOCT can give crucial details about the lens status, especially in cases where corneal haze precludes adequate visibility. Also, the presence of significant PAS or corneoiridic scars are suggestive of an increased risk of postoperative glaucoma.

Ultrasonography

A and B-scan ultrasonography should be performed in all eyes with corneal opacity to rule out any coexistent posterior segment pathology such as old retinal detachment wherein a keratoplasty may not be undertaken due to poor prognosis. Determination of axial length using A-scan biometry is critical for IOL power calculation while planning triple procedure.

Electrophysiological Tests

Use of electrophysiologic methods is helpful for assessment of retinal functions in eyes dense corneal opacities. Bright-flash electroretinogram (ERG) is able to elicit a response despite most media opacities. However, ERG only measures the gross retinal function. Visual evoked response (VER) is a better indicator of optic nerve function. Pattern stimuli give a relatively precise measurement of visual function when the media is clear, however flash stimuli are used for opaque corneas. A decreased amplitude and prolonged latency in VER indicates poor visual prognosis.

Once, the evaluation is over, one must establish a diagnosis and prognosticate the case carefully. Several factors including age of patient, status of the other eye, compliance of the patient, and need of binocularity play a role in decision-making. The procedure should be clearly explained to the patient and relatives. The risks of the procedure specifically regarding long follow-up time, chances of rejection, long-term use of medications should be discussed. The patient should have a realistic expectation regarding visual gain after the surgical procedure.

REFERENCES

1. Williams KA, Roder D, Esterman A, Muehlberg SM, Coster DJ. Factors predictive of corneal graft survival. Report from the Australian Corneal Graft Registry. Ophthalmology. 1992; 99(3):403-14.
2. Price FW, Whitson WE, Johns S, Gonzales JS. Risk factors for corneal graft failure. J Refract Surg. 1996;12(1):134-43; discussion 143-7.
3. Chang SD, Pecego JG, Zadnik K, Danneffel MB, Mutti DO, Mannis MJ. Factors influencing graft clarity. Cornea. 1996;15(6):577-81.
4. Charlin R, Polack FM. The effect of elevated intraocular pressure on the endothelium of corneal grafts. Cornea. 1982;1(3):241-50.
5. Sekhar GC, Vyas P, Nagarajan R, Mandal AK, Gupta S. Post-penetrating keratoplasty glaucoma. Indian J Ophthalmol. 1993;41(4):181-4.
6. Altman AJ, Albert DM, Fournier GA. Cocaine's use in ophthalmology: Our 100-year heritage. Surv Ophthalmol. 1985; 29(4):300-6.
7. Bonhomme F, Hafezi F, Boehlen F, Habre W. Management of antithrombotic therapies in patients scheduled for eye surgery. Eur J Anaesthesiol. 2013;30(8):449-54.
8. Vail A, Gore SM, Bradley BA, Easty DL, Rogers CA, Armitate WJ. Clinical and surgical factors influencing corneal graft survival, visual acuity, and astigmatism. Corneal Transplant Follow-up Study Collaborators. Ophthalmology. 1996;103(1):41-9.
9. Vajpayee RB, Sharma N, Dada T, Pushker N. Optical sector iridectomy in corneal opacities. Cornea. 1999;18(3):262-4.
10. Vajpayee RB, Angra SK, Honavar SG, Taherian K. Protection of the iris by lamellar dissection of corneal layers. A technique in penetrating keratoplasty. Cornea. 1994;13(1):16-9.
11. Vajpayee RB, Dada T, Ray M, Tandon R, Sethi A, Turaka K. Oversized corneal grafts for corneal opacities with iridocorneal adhesions. Ophthalmology. 2001;108(11):2026-8.

12. Flowers CW, McLeod SD, McDonnell PJ, Irvine JA, Smith RE. Evaluation of intraocular lens power calculation formulas in the triple procedure. J Cataract Refract Surg. 1996;22(1):116-22.
13. Wasielica-Poslednik J, Butsch C, Lampe C, Elflein H, Lamparter J, Weyer V, et al. Comparison of rebound tonometry, Perkins applanation tonometry and ocular response analyser in mucopolysaccharidosis patients. PLoS One. 2015;10(8):e0133586.
14. Trindade BLC, Eliazar GC. Descemet membrane endothelial keratoplasty (DMEK): an update on safety, efficacy and patient selection. Clin Ophthalmol. 2019;13:1549-57.
15. Sharma N, Sahay P, Maharana PK, Kumar P, Ahsan S, Titiyal JS. Microscope integrated intraoperative optical coherence tomography-guided DMEK in corneas with poor visualization. Clin Ophthalmol. 2020;14:643-51.
16. Michieletto P, Balestrazzi A, Balestrazzi A, Mazzotta C, Occhipinti I, Rossi T. Factors predicting unsuccessful big bubble deep lamellar anterior keratoplasty. Ophthalmologica. 2006;220(6):379-82.
17. Oie Y, Watanabe S, Nishida K. Evaluation of visual quality in patients with Fuchs' endothelial corneal dystrophy. Cornea. 2016;35 (Suppl 1):S55-8.
18. Watanabe S, Oie Y, Fujimoto H, Soma T, Koh S, Tsujikawa M, et al. Relationship between corneal guttae and quality of vision in patients with mild Fuchs' endothelial corneal dystrophy. Ophthalmology. 2015;122(10):2103-9.
19. Amin SR, Baratz KH, McLaren JW, Patel SV. Corneal abnormalities early in the course of Fuchs' endothelial dystrophy. Ophthalmology. 2014;121(12):2325-33.
20. Patel SV, McLaren JW, Hodge DO, Baratz KH. Scattered light and visual function in a randomized trial of deep lamellar endothelial keratoplasty and penetrating keratoplasty. Am J Ophthalmol. 2008;145(1):97-105.
21. van der Meulen IJE, Patel SV, Lapid-Gortzak R, Nieuwendaal CP, McLaren JW, van den Berg TJTP. Quality of vision in patients with Fuchs' endothelial dystrophy and after Descemet stripping endothelial keratoplasty. Arch Ophthalmol. 2011; 129(12):1537-42.
22. Yamaguchi T, Negishi K, Yamaguchi K, Murat D, Uchino Y, Shimmura S, et al. Effect of anterior and posterior corneal surface irregularity on vision after Descemet-stripping endothelial keratoplasty. J Cataract Refract Surg. 2009;35(4):688-94.
23. Riss S, Heindl LM, Bachmann BO, Kruse FE, Cursiefen C. Pentacam-based big bubble deep anterior lamellar keratoplasty in patients with keratoconus. Cornea. 2012;31(6):627-32.
24. Sun SY, Wacker K, Baratz KH, Patel SV. Determining subclinical edema in Fuchs' endothelial corneal dystrophy: Revised classification using Scheimpflug tomography for preoperative assessment. Ophthalmology. 2019;126(2):195-204.
25. Patel SV, Hodge DO, Treichel EJ, Spiegel MR, Baratz KH. Repeatability of Scheimpflug tomography for assessing Fuchs' endothelial corneal dystrophy. Am J Ophthalmol. 2020;215:91-103.
26. Patel SV, Hodge DO, Treichel EJ, Spiegel MR, Baratz KH. Predicting the prognosis of Fuchs' endothelial corneal dystrophy by using Scheimpflug tomography. Ophthalmology. 2020;127(3):315-23.
27. Madhavan C, Basti S, Naduvilath TJ, Sangwan VS. Use of ultrasound biomicroscopic evaluation in preoperative planning of penetrating keratoplasty. Cornea. 2000;19(1):17-21.
28. Lanzl IM, Augsburger JJ, Hertle RW, Rapuano C, Correa-Melling Z, Santa Cruz C. The role of ultrasound biomicroscopy in surgical planning for limbal dermoids. Cornea. 1998;17(6):604-6.
29. Rutnin SS, Pavlin CJ, Slomovic AR, Kwartz J, Rootman DS. Preoperative ultrasound biomicroscopy to assess ease of haptic removal before penetrating keratoplasty combined with lens exchange. J Cataract Refract Surg. 1997;23(2):239-43.
30. Alexander JL, Wei L, Palmer J, Darras A, Levin MR, Berry JL, et al. A systematic review of ultrasound biomicroscopy use in pediatric ophthalmology. Eye (Lond). 2021;35(1):265-76.
31. Nischal KK, Naor J, Jay V, MacKeen LD, Rootman DS. Clinicopathological correlation of congenital corneal opacification using ultrasound biomicroscopy. Br J Ophthalmol. 2002;86(1):62-9.
32. Han SB, Liu YC, Noriega KM, Mehta JS. Applications of Anterior Segment Optical Coherence Tomography in Cornea and Ocular Surface Diseases. J Ophthalmol. 2016;2016:4971572.
33. Yenerel NM, Kucumen RB, Gorgun E. The complementary benefit of anterior segment optical coherence tomography in penetrating keratoplasty. Clin Ophthalmol. 2013;7:1515-23.
34. Nanavaty MA, Daya SM. Outcomes of deep anterior lamellar keratoplasty in keratoconic eyes with previous hydrops. Br J Ophthalmol. 2012;96(10):1304-9.
35. Agarwal A, Narang P, Kumar DA, Agarwal A. Young donor-graft assisted endothelial keratoplasty (PDEK/DMEK) with epithelial debridement for chronic pseudophakic bullous keratopathy. Can J Ophthalmol. 2017;52(5):519-26.
36. Wertheimer CM, Elhardt C, Wartak A, Luft N, Kassumeh S, Dirisamer M, et al. Corneal optical density in Fuchs endothelial dystrophy determined by anterior segment optical coherence tomography. Eur J Ophthalmol. 2020;22:1120672120944796.
37. Eleiwa T, Elsawy A, Özcan E, Abou Shousha M. Automated diagnosis and staging of Fuchs' endothelial cell corneal dystrophy using deep learning. Eye Vis (Lond). 2020;7:44.

4 Eye Banking for Corneal Transplantation

Graeme A Pollock

INTRODUCTION

The process of corneal transplantation begins with eye donation. Corneal transplantation is not possible without the provision of a viable, disease-free donor cornea. Eye banks and effective eye banking practices are central to providing this essential service.

Since the establishment of the Eye-Bank for Sight Restoration in New York in 1944, eye banking has evolved in both professional practice and scope and moved far beyond the concept of a simple storage and supply unit for the purposes of full-thickness penetrating keratoplasty (PK). The professional practice of eye banking can be defined as encompassing two interdependent processes: (1) the coordination, identification, consent, and surgical donation of eyes from recently deceased persons (eye donation) and (2) the evaluation, processing, preservation, and equitable allocation of safe and efficacious allograft tissue for transplantation (eye banking in the technical sense). In the past decade and a half, these services have extended into customized tissue preparations to accommodate the different forms of corneal transplantation.

While the scope of activity undertaken by an individual eye bank may be determined by jurisdiction, regulation, nation, or health system in which it operates, the cornerstone of eye banking and corneal transplantation is the availability and donation of eyes from recently deceased persons. While this chapter does not deal directly with this issue, it is incumbent that any eye bank recognizes the importance of advocacy for eye donation within their health system to ensure policy, regulation, legislation, and ethical practice provide for sustainability and growth in eye donation as the demand for transplantation increases. In this respect, eye banks need to engage with, or directly provide hospital development and professional in-service programs designed to maximize the appropriate identification of suitable donors and referral to the eye bank.

The continued development, complexity, professionalism, and evolution of the services provided by eye banks has been accompanied by the development of robust quality management systems. These incorporate peer reviewed evidence-based standards with an emphasis on risk assessment and mitigation. In many nations, government regulations have mandated such standards within a framework of current of good tissue practice (cGTP) or good manufacturing practice (cGMP). As such, eye banking now not only includes the classical areas of donor selection/eligibility, retrieval/recovery, preservation and storage, and tissue evaluation, but importantly must now also address quality in traceability, personnel and training, documentation, facilities and equipment, materials, packaging and labeling, and notification and recall systems.

Increasing globalization of eye banking, transnational movement of corneas between sovereign states and new business practices employed by some organizations, has highlighted that all aspects of eye banking needs to be conducted within an acceptable ethical framework. Importantly, this now not only includes issues relevant to the donation of human ocular tissue, but also to its allocation and use. Guidance is provided by the Barcelona Principles[1] and the World Health Organization (WHO).[2]

DONOR SELECTION

While the technical aspects of eye banking must be robust to ensure the provision of safe tissue, it is in the careful selection or exclusion of potential donors that is of utmost importance in preventing the transmission of disease to the recipient. In addition, donor selection must also consider matters regarding the quality, or potential efficacy for purpose, of the tissue.

Many of the standards that have been adopted by eye banks worldwide were initially developed by the Eye Bank Association of America (EBAA)[3] who produced their first set of medical standards in 1980. A rigorous review process has ensured that these medical standards continue to evolve as new knowledge, insights, and challenges develop. These standards are supported by the EBAA procedures manual which provides valuable guidelines and rationale toward implementing the standards. Other eye banking organizations, such as the European Eye Bank Association,[4] have also developed minimum standards that are reviewed each year. The European Directorate for the Quality of Medicines and Healthcare publish a comprehensive guide to the quality and safety of tissues and cells for human application which covers general principles involved in the quality management of the technical aspects of eye and tissue banking, as well as a specific chapter on ocular tissue requirements and ocular tissue monologues.[5]

It is important however when developing medical standards that each jurisdiction analyses their own unique situation to ensure assessment of potential risk in the donor is balanced against benefit of the transplant. The balance will vary by disease prevalence in the local donor pool, the consequences of transmission of disease, available local resources available in pathology and testing, and other risk mitigation strategies. The degree of acceptable risk will therefore vary by jurisdiction. Each eye bank jurisdiction should consider their contraindications accordingly.

Contraindications for the Use of Donor Tissue

The Eye Bank Association of Australia and New Zealand (EBAANZ) contraindications for the use of donor tissue are available at www.ebaanz.org/medical-standards-and-quality.[6] These contraindications are designed to reduce the potential for (1) viral transmission of disease; (2) transmission of bacterial or fungal infections; (3) transmission of malignant disease; (4) transplantation of corneal disorders, or of those corneas which pose a risk to the success of the surgery. These standards are supported by EBAANZ guidelines for the selection of ocular tissue donors.[7]

To successfully implement these standards eye banks must have consistent policies for the examination and documentation of a prospective donor's available medical records, medical history or investigation of cause of death. Donor history gathering should be to an extent to which it is possible to make an acceptable judgment on donor risk. Sources of information may include but not be limited to:

- Medical record or hospital charts
- Donor risk assessment interview with the donor's family member or friend who can answer questions about the donor's medical and lifestyle history.
- Physical assessment of the donor to identify risk factors for potential infection with transmissible diseases (the extent of which is in keeping with the overall risk profile of the donor).
- Death certificate
- Coroner or pathologist's report on the physical assessment of death
- Treating physician or general practitioner interview/report.

In deciding on donor eligibility, all evidence should be examined together within the circumstances of the donor rather than in isolation, considering objective and subjective evidence and the validity of each piece of evidence. An individual who is qualified either by profession, education, or training to perform all the above tasks, and familiar with the potential surgical uses of the tissue should perform donor screening.

Disease Transmission from Donor Corneas

Fortunately, iatrogenic transmission of serious or fatal systemic disease from corneal transplantation is a rare event. A review of the world literature reveals only 13 reports of disease transmission since 1939 (excepting bacterial and fungal contamination and transmission).

Diseases that could potentially be transmitted by corneal transplantation fall into three categories:

1. Prion disease [Creutzfeldt–Jakob disease (CJD) and associated variants]
2. Infections (bacterial, fungal, and viral)
3. Malignancies

A good understanding of these cases and an understanding of the underlying pathogens is instructive when considering the degree of risk of transmission that each of these diseases pose.

Prion Disease

Duffy et al.[8] reported the possible transmission of CJD in 1974 and during the 1990s two further possible cases were reported.[9,10] However, the evidence for transmission in these later two cases is limited. In 1999, Hogan et al.[11] reviewed known cases of transmission of CJD by tissues and concluded that the risk of transmission was very low. In addition, they suggested that the review of a potential donor's available medical information for any evidence of a diagnosis or family history of CJD or evidence that human pituitary hormone had been administered was enough to guard against the extremely low potential risk of disease transmission.

Initial concern about the presence of variant CJD (vCJD) in the United Kingdom and the theoretical possibility of human-to-human transmission has tempered in recent years. Those nations that have excluded from donation those people who have visited or resided in the United Kingdom for a cumulative period of 6 months (some 3 months) or more between 1980 and 1996, based on increased risk of vCJD transmission from such donors, are now reviewing these policies. In 2010, Garske and Ghani[12] predicted a peak global annual incidence of vCJD around 11 cases, but with a 95% credibility interval between one and 65 cases. Notably, UK surveillance data after the 2010 modeling records a total of 10 cases from 2010 to November 2020, with no cases since 2016.[13] Variant CJD has a very different epidemiology and presentation than sporadic (classical) CJD (sCJD), and vCJD has behaved differently from sCJD with respect to transmission. Unlike blood transfusion, ocular tissues have not been implicated in any case of vCJD transmission.[14]

Interestingly, data on CJD and vCJD suggests the disease-related prion protein (PrP^{Sc}) may not be widely distributed in human eye tissue. In three cases of sporadic (or classical) CJD, no PrP^{Sc} was detected in proximal optic nerve, sclera, retina, vitreous humor, lens, aqueous humor, iris or cornea. In the one case of vCJD, investigated PrP^{Sc} in the eye was restricted to the optic nerve and retina.[15] In addition, in a widely reported case of transplantation of ocular tissues from a donor subsequently determined to have sporadic CJD (where subsequently tissues were explanted with no known transmission) there was no evidence of PrP^{Sc} in the cornea.[16] These findings, together with only one case of CJD being plausibly attributed to corneal transplants among millions of recipients, have led to cornea now being categorized as a lower-risk tissue by the WHO and the Australian Government Department of Health.[17,18]

Infections—Viral

During the history of eye banking corneas have transmitted three types of virus that have the potential for harm to the recipient or the outcome of the transplant—hepatitis B, herpes simplex, and rabies.

Nine cases of rabies transmission from six donors resulting in eight deaths have been documented between 1979 and 1996.[19-24] In all cases, rabies was not identified in the donor until transmission had occurred. In only one case, rabies in the donor was detected promptly and subsequent intensive immunotherapy for the recipient prevented their death.[25] The problem arises that diagnosis in a potential donor can be difficult if the rabies does not present with its classical picture of hydrophobia and hyperesthesia (furious rabies). In the Iran case, the donor is described as presenting only the prodromal symptoms of fever, malaise, headache, and gastrointestinal infections prior to death. However, even in the less common paralytic or dumb rabies, flaccid paralysis develops and the exclusion criteria of "death from central nervous system disease of unestablished diagnosis" would today exclude such potential donors from becoming actual donors.

The possibility of iatrogenic transmission of hepatitis B virus (HBV) has long been recognized. Two cases of transmission from 1984 and 1985 were reported by Hoft et al.[25] Both these cases took place before routine serological screening of donors for hepatitis B surface antigen (HBsAg). There have been no further reports of transmission since.

Hepatitis C virus has been detected in corneas[26] and in the media of organ-cultured corneas of seropositive donors[27] although at the very low concentration of virus detected, it remains arguable whether transmission via corneal transplantation is likely. In one case of a donor being anti-HCV-negative but HCV ribonucleic acid (RNA)-positive, HCV infection occurred in eight of 30 recipients of organ and tissues but not in the single recipient of a corneal transplant.[28] These negative reports suggest that the transmission of HCV through corneal transplantation is highly unlikely, and of course has not been reported.

Similarly, the human immunodeficiency virus (HIV) has been shown to be present in a human cornea[29] but such a presence may not lead to transmission of the disease by corneal transplantation. There are three reports in the literature of HIV-infected donors where the corneal recipients have not seroconverted.[30-32] Again, all these negative reports suggest that the transmission of HIV through corneal transplantation is highly unlikely, and of course has not been reported.

The recent corona virus SARS-CoV-2 global pandemic has created great concern about the possibility of transmission through corneal transplantation, and indeed the transmissibility of many other virus-types that may potentially be the causative agent of an epidemic. In one publication, the authors demonstrated a small but noteworthy prevalence of SARS-CoV-2 viral RNA and antigens in the corneas from coronavirus disease 2019 (COVID-19) donors, although they indicated further studies were necessary to explore the possibility of transmission via ocular tissues.[33] Fortunately, there is no evidence to suggest that any coronavirus [including severe acute respiratory syndrome (SARS-CoV) and Middle East respiratory syndrome coronavirus (MERS-CoV)], nor any influenza virus, has been transmitted by cell, tissue or organ transplantation or by blood. However, the degree of risk that a pathogen presents to eye banking is not only a factor of the likelihood of transmission via transplantation but also the degree of consequence to the recipient if a transmission should take place. The degree and type of risk mitigation measures must then consider the prevalence of the causative agent in the donor population, the consequences of transmission, the availability of validated testing for the agent, and any interventions that may inactivate the agent. This has been the approach to COVID-19 as a contraindication. Donors suspect of having coronavirus are excluded from donation while povidone-iodine readily inactivates coronavirus (SARS-CoV and MERS-CoV) infectivity.[34] The need for postmortem COVID-19 testing has been debated due to the high false positive rate, the nonvalidated nature of the test, availability of the test and its cost-effectiveness in areas of low prevalence. All of these are precautionary measures considering the low risk of transmission.

There is also a group of diseases listed as contraindications that are diseases of possible but unproved viral etiology. This includes subacute sclerosing panencephalitis, progressive multifocal leukoencephalopathy, Reyes syndrome, acute leukemia, and active disseminated lymphomas such as Hodgkin's disease. Hematological malignancies, with decreased immunological defense mechanisms, may also mask opportunistic viral or bacterial infections.

Infections—Bacterial and Fungal

Septicemia is a contraindication in a prospective corneal donor because of the risk of pathogenic organisms being harbored in the conjunctiva, surviving the antibiotics used throughout the retrieval and buttoning process, and eventually leading to an endophthalmitis in the recipient's eye. The only exception to this is if the corneas are to be placed in organ culture for preservation. The microbiological surveillance during organ culture allows the exclusion prior to transplantation of those corneas that may be harboring organisms and therefore reduces the risk of transmission to the recipient.

A search of the Project Notify library, the global vigilance, and surveillance database for medical products of human origin[35] list 25 case reports of harm to a recipient due to transmission of bacteria or fungus from the donor tissue where the imputability level has been assessed as possible, probable or certain. Several publications have also reported the incidence of endophthalmitis following PK ranging from 0.11 to 1.05% but whether donor tissue contamination was considered as causative is not defined.[36-39] A systemic review published in 2005 estimated an overall post-PK endophthalmitis rate of 0.382%.[40] All these reports are prior to widespread endothelial keratoplasty (EK) being adopted.

Importantly regarding EK, the EBAA medical review subcommittee on adverse reactions reported an increasing trend in the rate of endophthalmitis and keratitis from 2007 to 2014. This was disproportionately associated with EK and Candida species.[41] The surge in fungal infections [associated primarily with hypothermic storage and Descemet's stripping automated endothelial keratoplasty (DSAEK)] has somewhat abated since a peak in 2017 (7.6/10,000) to 5.0 and 2.3/10,000 in 2018 and 2019. This may be attributed to more efficient decontamination protocols at the time of recovery, combined with reducing warming times during donor tissue EK preparation. The role of supplementation of hypothermic media with antifungal preparations is less clear.[42]

Of note is that all reports, where the cause of infection may be attributable to donor tissue contamination, suggest that the contamination originated with the donor and was not introduced during any processing undertaken within the eye bank. This emphasizes the importance of effective epithelial donor tissue decontamination prior to corneal storage in reducing the (uncommon) instances of post-transplant keratitis or endophthalmitis.

Malignancies

There are two cases reported where a malignancy has been transmitted through corneal transplantation. In the first case, a retinoblastoma was transplanted from the donor eye to the recipient eye.[43] There is also a report of transmission of a disseminated adenocarcinoma from donor to the recipient's iris with confirmation of tumor markers with polymerase chain reaction (PCR).[44] It would be incorrect however to consider malignancies in the donor as being high risk for transmission of disease. Nonhematological malignancy is not an exclusion for donation, and a substantial percentage of the hundreds of thousands of corneal transplants performed have used corneas from donors with malignancies without any evidence of transmission. However, the two isolated cases reported above, both relating to malignancies in the donor eye, demonstrate the importance of a careful examination, including the posterior pole of the eye, to exclude the possibility of malignancy or other pathology in the donated eye.

A third report is that of patient who developed an ocular melanoma after she had limbal stem cell transplantation from a donor with history of melanoma.[45] Following this report, the EBAA amended its medical standards to exclude for transplantation, corneas from donors with known metastatic melanoma.

Although leukemia and lymphoproliferative disorders pose the greatest theoretical risk of transmission, due to a possible viral etiology, no cases of transmission have been reported. However, these latter disorders remain as a contraindication.

Intrinsic Eye Disease or Anterior Segment Surgery

Local corneal disorders or surgery may pose a risk to the success of corneal transplant surgery. Keratoconus in its early stages or corneal dystrophies may go undetected. Incisional surgery to correct myopia is detected through the appearance of radial and arcuate lines upon slit-lamp examination but detecting past photorefractive surgery in a donor cornea is difficult and can easily go undetected, particularly in organ-cultured corneas.[46] This type of surgery is best detected through interview with the donors next of kin although multiple modalities such as topography, pachymetry, specular microscopy, and optical coherence tomography have demonstrated some effectiveness in identifying these eyes.[47] Modern cataract extraction by phacoemulsification and the replacement of the host lens by an intraocular lens is not an absolute contraindication to donation. However, in these cases, microscopy of the endothelium is required to exclude those corneas showing low cell density or abnormal morphology.

Donor corneas with prior refractive surgery are unsuitable for PK, anterior lamellar keratoplasty, epikeratoplasty, or tectonic corneal grafting surgeries. However, donor tissue with a history of keratorefractive surgery retains endothelial integrity and has been used with good outcomes in DSAEK and Descemet's membrane endothelial keratoplasty (DMEK).[47]

Donor Age and Endothelial Cell Density

Evidence from the multicenter outcome registries of the United Kingdom[48] and Australia[49] and the controlled clinical trial of the Cornea Donor Study[50] shows that there is no influence of donor age on corneal transplant outcome after PK. Graft survival is equivalent across all donor age groups at all-time intervals post-transplant. Similarly, these outcome registries,[48,49] Cornea Donor Study[50] and its ancillary Specular Microscopy Ancillary Study,[51] have shown no association between preoperative endothelial cell density (ECD) (which decline with donor age) and graft survival (preoperative ECDs being above the lower limits acceptable by eye banks—generally between 1,800 and 2,200 cells/mm^2).

The influence of donor age on graft survival following DSAEK surgery is less clear and appears to have as confounding variable the experience of the operating surgeon in the relevant procedure. Data from the 2018 Report of Australian Corneal Graft Registry (ACGR) indicated a significant difference across groups with survival for grafts performed with tissue from donors aged under 40 years being better than those aged 40–69 years, and 70 years or older. Similarly, corneas with cell counts under 2,500 cells/mm^2 had significantly poorer survival than donor corneas with higher ECD. However, the Registry notes that differences in rates of follow-up across subgroups was likely to have affected survival calculations for these factors.[49] In contrast, the Swedish Cornea Transplant Registry reported that higher age or low ECD was not detrimental to graft survival following DSAEK.[52]

For DMEK the situation is more nuanced. The ACGR reports that DMEK with survival for grafts performed with tissue from donors aged *under* 50 years significantly poorer than those aged 60–69 years and 70–79 years.[49] This result is thought to be associated with the surgical difficulties and complications of handling a "tighter scroll" of DMEK tissue in donors below 50 years.[53] Price[54] has recommended that new surgeons use older donor tissue, particularly that between 60 and 75 years old. Others have reported that with surgeon experience donor characteristics such as younger donor age, higher donor age, lower preoperative ECD (<2,500) and donor diabetes did not affect outcome at 1 year.[55,56]

Lower Donor Age

There is no clearly defined lower age limit for corneal donation. The Eye Bank Association of Australia and New Zealand list the minimum age as 2 years. Problems relate to both the technical difficulties in using infant tissue and the complication of postoperative myopia. The extreme thinness of the infant cornea means that it is likely to fold upon itself during handling. This, combined with the small diameter of the cornea, creates problems during the donation surgery, trephining, and during placement and suturing in the host bed. Koenig provides a review of these problems.[57] The myopic shift after keratoplasty with infant donor corneas has been related to the steep curvature of these corneas.[58]

Key Points—Donor Selection

- Careful selection or exclusion of donors is of prime importance in preventing transmission of disease to the recipient and ensuring suitability for transplantation.
- Medical standards are available from eye banking associations but should be reviewed by local jurisdictions for their own risk versus benefit balance. Transmission of disease through corneal transplantation is rare. Corneas have transmitted rabies, hepatitis B, and possibly classical CJD.
- The risk of transmission of bacteria or fungi from donor to recipient can be mitigated by effective epithelial donor decontamination at the time of retrieval.
- Nonhematological malignancy is not an exclusion to donation.
- There is no influence of donor age on graft outcome for PK or DSAEK. In experienced surgical hands, there is no influence on graft outcome for DMEK, but over 50 years of age donors are preferred.

DONATION OF EYE TISSUE

Eye Donor Coordination

Arguably, an Eye Bank's most important work is done during consent, the interaction with bereaved family members and with the process of gathering of accurate medical histories. All of this involves multiple interactions with a variety of sources such as relatives, medical and nursing staff, pathologists, and general practitioners. The skill is in the collection, assimilation, and analysis of all this information while ensuring that the donor family is cared for and is fully informed of their choices and the processes that donation entails. All of this must be done within an ethical and professional framework to reduce the risk of harm to the donor family and to the prospective recipients of donated tissue.

The form of the consent, or authority to proceed with the donation, will of course vary depending on the jurisdiction's legislation and social culture, but regardless of this the donor coordinator should ensure that all parties that need to be fully informed are fully informed. The extent of the donation (whole globe or just cornea, transplant and research purposes) needs to be identified and recorded. The investigations about assessing medical risk or donor suitability must be conducted in a thorough and professional and considered manner that is relative to the risk being assessed. These responsibilities extend to those instances where workplace partners have been primarily involved in the consent and donor screening process (e.g., multiple tissue or organ donation); the eye donor coordinator must still cross-check and ensure that these processes have been suitably performed.

Medical and Social History Review

It is important to review all available records on each donor to an extent to which it is possible to make an acceptable judgment on donor risk (in relation to donor contraindications and safety, and likely efficacy of the tissue for purpose). This should be performed by an individual(s) who is qualified by profession, education, or training to do so. Final review of the relevant donor history should also be undertaken by individuals (the medical director of the eye bank or their delegates) who are both familiar with the intended use of the tissue and deemed competent to undertake the review.

Depending on the circumstances and the location of the donor's death sources of information may include but not be limited to:

- Medical record or hospital chart
- Donor risk assessment interview
- Physical assessment of the donor to identify risk factors for potential infection with transmissible diseases, the extent of which is in keeping with the overall risk profile of the donor.
- Death certificate
- Coroner or pathologist's report on the physical assessment of death
- Treating physician or general practitioner interview/report.

In particular, the following details should be recorded:

- Data to unambiguously identify the donor (as a minimum, name of patient and date of birth).
- Cause of death and contributing factors
- Current and past medical history
- The time of irreversible cessation of the circulation of the blood—the important point here being a record of the beginning of the ischemic period for the corneas.
- In the instance of intended hypothermic storage of corneas, a review and interpretation of laboratory results (blood cultures, temperature trends, and white blood cell counts) must be performed to exclude or bacteremia or fungemia in the donor at the time of death. Discussion with the treating physician and gaining an insight into their clinical impressions is often critical in deciding on bacteremic status. However, bacteremia can be considered suitable if organ culture storage of corneas is performed where significant infection of corneal tissue will become evident as contamination in the storage medium.

When a formal donor risk assessment interview (DRAI) can be conducted, it should be with donor next of kin and/or most knowledgeable historian within the context of the donation. Its intent is to determine risks in the donor that may not be discovered through usual medical history pathways and processes described above. Formal interview templates developed by and standardized across organ, tissue and eye sectors are available for this purpose—The North American Uniform DRAI and its direct adaptation, the AUS-DRAI.[59] However, it is important to review such templates for the applicability to the region/nation in which the eye bank operates. Abbreviated versions of the DRAI when eye-only donation is undertaken are also used by the EBAA and EBAANZ member banks.

Communicable Disease Testing

As a minimum, the donor must be tested for the HIV, HBV, and hepatitis C virus. Depending on the jurisdiction and regulators, additional tests [e.g., syphilis and human T-lymphotropic virus (HTLV)] may be mandated. Best practice is now considered to be nucleic acid testing (NAT) for these viruses, validated for cadaveric blood (NAT testing decreases the "window" period from infection to detection of these viruses over serologic testing, thus reducing risk. It also allows for a reduction in deferral times for donors considered to be at higher epidemiological risk to these viruses). However, as for any pathology test there needs to be a consideration of efficiency, sensitivity, specificity, reliability, and of course availability. In many jurisdictions, *validated cadaveric* NAT testing is not readily available, and depending on the jurisdiction the risk reduction the NAT offers over serological testing is not significant.

In cases where *the donor has undergone significant blood loss,* or the donor is <12 years of age, *and* there has been significant transfusion/infusion of fluids, there exists a possibility that plasma dilution may affect the validity of any serology conducted postinfusion. In these instances, when reviewing the donor's history, it is important to record the amount and time of any transfusion or infusions (blood, colloid, and crystalloid). When no adequate pretransfusion/infusion sample is available for communicable disease testing (CDT), then a calculation should be used to determine that there has not been plasma dilution sufficient to affect test results. Examples of appropriate algorithms to follow (including relevant calculations) are available from Food and Drug Administration (FDA)[60] guidelines.

Eye Donation Surgery

As with all surgery, there are many different possible approaches to donor surgery and donor eye preparation/dissection and therefore this chapter will only deal with some of the salient points. The Procedures Manual of the Eye Bank Association of America does cover specific procedures written broadly enough to provide a framework for the development of an Eye Bank's own procedures, yet specific enough to establish accepted baseline standards.[61] In addition, an excellent introductory handbook and atlas has also been published which provides good illustrated step-by-step guides to eye bank surgical and evaluation techniques.[62]

The person performing the donor surgery must use their professional judgment and satisfy themselves that all-reasonable steps and normal surgical precautions have been taken to minimize contamination or damage to the tissue. Ideally, the area should be one of restricted access as a first step toward aseptic technique, has appropriate lighting, sharps, and biohazard waste containers, and generally be clean and organized. Personnel must be trained in the procedures or in general surgical procedures. Importantly, retrieval personnel must be equipped and wear appropriate personal protective equipment (PPE).

Preparation of the Donor—Eye Decontamination

If an enucleation is to be performed many eye banks may forego extensive donor preparation opting instead to decontaminate the globe within the eye bank laboratory prior to the removal of the cornea. This is usually performed in the laboratory by rinsing the globe in a dilute povidone-iodine (PVP) solution (a 1–5% concentration resulting in 0.1–0.5% available iodine) for 1–2 minutes. The PVP solution must not contain any detergents as this could harm the corneal epithelium, and this should be checked beforehand. The PVP is then followed by a thorough rinse with a balanced saline solution. This is a very effective means of decontamination[63] if performed with appropriate concentrations of PVP over a short period.[64] The efficacy of the combined use of 0.02% chlorhexidine and 0.5% povidone-iodine has also been demonstrated while retaining corneal viability.[65]

Of great importance are more recent reports of an increasing trend in the rate of postkeratoplasty fungal infections and a reversal in the previously documented predominance of bacterial over fungal infections, with a disproportionate incidence of fungal infections after EK compared with PK.[66] It has been hypothesized that the additional time that lamellar tissue is exposed to warmer temperatures during tissue processing, results in prolonged exposure to a permissive environment for fungi to grow. In response the EBAA mandated double povidone-iodine soaks at the time of recovery to address contamination at an early stage of proliferation when the fungal population is most vulnerable. This, combined with reducing warming times that limits the fungi's subsequent growth, appears to have lowered risk with the EBAA reporting 2019 postkeratoplasty infection rates at their lowest in over a decade.[42]

For those eye banks that perform in situ excision of corneas, similar solutions can be used to minimize ocular flora and reduce contamination. This procedure is appropriate for donor preparation prior to both enucleation and excision. Here the delivery of the solutions is also important as the eyes should first be rinsed in a strong stream of balanced saline to remove all debris, mucus and foreign matter from the cornea and conjunctival sac. This alone will reduce microbial contamination. A strong vigorous stream may also play a role in the mechanical disruption of fungal biofilms, allowing for better removal of any fungal contaminants through mechanical means and through removal of the protective barrier to allow decontamination through PVP or chlorhexidine. A good stream of balanced saline is also required after a period of PVP application to ensure good removal of the PVP from the eye. The lids and the surrounding area can then be disinfected by a surgical skin preparation of PVP.

Enucleation, In Situ Excision and Corneoscleral Rim Sectioning

Enucleation or in situ excision can be performed in an operating theater, a morgue, hospital room or funeral home. Prime considerations are to minimize manipulation of tissues surrounding the eye to preserve donor appearance, to prevent touching or distortion of the cornea and thus minimize any cell loss (epithelial and endothelial), and to reduce bacterial contamination from both exogenous sources and from ocular flora. For in situ excision one must be especially aware of the bacteriologic considerations, as no further decontamination of the tissue is possible.

Corneoscleral rim excision after an enucleation is a similar process to the in situ excision. Ideally the procedure is performed in a biological safety cabinet which provides a clean area for the excision and at the same time protects the operator from exposure to possible pathogens residing on the eye itself. The dissection needs to be made through into and along the suprachoroidal space. Perforation of the choroid would cause vitreous leakage, which may cause the collapse of the globe and anterior chamber and compromise the cornea. In addition, the operator must be careful not to exert too much pressure on the globe, as this will increase the potential for the scissors to cut or catch on the choroid. During the procedure it is most important that as little stress as possible is placed on the cornea as any stretching of the endothelial cell layer can critically damage it.

Key Points—Donation of Eye Tissue

- Donor history gathering should be to an extent to which it is possible to make an acceptable judgment on donor risk.
- History gathering includes review of medical records/hospital chart, risk assessment interview with knowledgeable donor historian and physical assessment of the donor.
- As a minimum the donor must be tested for HIV, HBV, and HCV.
- In situ excision of corneas or enucleation of the whole globe provides equal outcomes but each has its own benefits and disadvantages (**Table 1**).
- Techniques in eye retrieval are available at www.cybersight.org/portfolio/introduction-to-eye-banking-a-handbook-and-atlas/
- Effective and careful eye decontamination through the use of PVP or equivalent solutions, and aseptic handling and processing are of great importance in mitigating the risk of fungal or bacterial transmission to the recipient.

Table 1: Tissue retrieval considerations.

	In situ excision	*Enucleation*
Legal and regulatory	Tissue removal	Organ removal
Operative procedure	More difficult	
Staff	More training	
Time	Marginally longer	
Risk	Less invasive	Risk of hemorrhage
Postretrieval processing and time	Less	
Decontamination	At donor	At donor and repeated in laboratory
Eye bank facility	Not necessary	Laboratory
Contamination rate	Similar	Similar
Inspection anterior chamber	Pen light	Slit lamp
Tissue viability	Similar or better due to shorter death to preservation times	

CORNEAL EVALUATION

Except for tissue that would be potentially hazardous because of possible transmission of disease, there are no absolutely defined criteria for the acceptance or rejection of a cornea. The final decision regarding use rests with the surgeon for each individual and unique case of donor to recipient transplantation and the transplant procedure to be undertaken. However, in reaching a decision on acceptance or rejection of tissue for clinical use the ophthalmologist must rely on the eye bank's careful evaluation of the cornea and its classification of fitness for purpose for a specific procedure.

Good corneal evaluation by each corneal layer is now central in determining the fitness for purpose for a cornea. For PK, the cornea needs to be free of refractive corneal procedures (including photoablation surgery), superficial disorders of the conjunctiva (such as pterygia) that may affect the central optical zone, scars affecting the central optical zone, infiltrates (both infectious and noninfectious), and a good endothelium that passes the eye bank's standards. Donors for anterior lamellar keratoplasty procedures, tectonic grafts, and patch grafts such as for glaucoma drainage devices need to meet the same criteria as PK except that the state of the endothelium is not important. Conversely, donors for EK procedures noninfectious anterior pathology that does not affect the posterior stroma and endothelium is acceptable if the endothelial layer is acceptable.

Gross in situ Evaluation

Corneal evaluation begins with a gross examination of the corneas in situ. A simple penlight examination can reveal epithelial defects (drying, erosion, sloughing), corneal edema with associated haze and striations due to folding of Descemet's membrane, abnormal corneal shape, blood or cloudiness in the anterior chamber, corneal scars or infiltrates, arcus senilis, and any signs of conjunctivitis and discharge.

For in situ corneoscleral rim excisions a careful in situ examination is especially important. This is the only opportunity (other than a good medical history) to determine if there has been previous anterior segment surgery or if there is any pathology of the eye not identified through the donor screening process.

Slit-lamp Evaluation

The slit lamp enables a more accurate observation of the cornea, revealing earlier stages of pathology that are visible grossly. Whole eyes can be examined by the slit lamp within the container used in retrieval, or excised corneas can be examined through the bottom of the storage vial once the cornea and vial are manipulated so that the cornea is endothelial side down. The eye or cornea should be allowed to reach room temperature which makes the endothelium easier to visualize and more normal in appearance.

The cornea should be methodically examined to ensure each layer of the cornea is adequately assessed. The surrounding limbal/scleral area should also be checked for evidence of surgical incisions (these may also be at the periphery of the clear cornea) and for any sutures.

The epithelium is inspected for integrity and overall condition specifically clarity, exposure, sloughing, defects, trauma, foreign bodies, and infiltrates. Haze is often localized and coincides with ante- and postmortem exposure across the interpalpebral area. Swelling of the epithelium may cause some layers to detach (termed sloughing). Epithelial defects appear as clear depressed areas within an otherwise hazy epithelium. The extent and position (central or peripheral) of any of these findings needs to be considered in any assessment of the suitability of the cornea for transplantation.

The stroma is examined for overall clarity, amount of edema, and stromal folding. Major opacities are usually detected by the preceding gross examination but using higher magnification and a thin slit can better identify the opacity as scarring (generally a smooth gray appearance) or inflammatory infiltrates (generally whitish appearance with discrete borders). Stromal folding and haze are associated with corneal edema. The amount of corneal edema, and thus the severity and number of folds and the amount of haze will depend on time since donor death, temperature, integrity of the epithelium, and the postmortem integrity and function of the endothelium. The thickest folds are a good indicator of the overall severity of the edema. Striae, identifiable as fine gray/white lines, may also be in the stroma and are probably indicative of very localized disruptions of the stromal lamellae.

Any detachment of Descemet's membrane can be observed as a separate membrane that seems to come from and be continuous with the endothelial side of the cornea. This finding alone is usually enough to consider the cornea unsuitable for any transplantation procedure requiring an intact endothelium.

A specular reflection of endothelial layer can be observed in a small area of the endothelial reflex. At high power magnification an impression of cell density and the degree of cell uniformity in size and shape can be obtained. Guttae-like bodies (areas where no cells can be seen) may be observed in the specular reflection. The exact nature of these areas is difficult to determine. They may be guttae (bumps or excrescences of Descemet's membrane), vacuolated cells, or stress fractures (sometimes referred to as pseudoguttae) due to trauma during the donation process. Regardless of their nature these conditions should be regarded as a degenerative condition of the endothelium. The suitability of the cornea for PK would depend on the relative number and location of these bodies. (*Note*: the term "pseudoguttae" is sometimes also used to refer to guttae that appear at hypothermic storage temperatures but disappear at room temperature).

Anterior Chamber Optical Coherence Tomography

Anterior segment optical coherence tomography (AS-OCT) (adapted for eye bank use) is now being used for characterizing and evaluating donor tissues. Primarily, it was introduced for the examination of precut DSAEK tissue with advantages of improved accuracy when compared to ultrasound pachymetry measurements of thickness with the added benefit of providing a thickness profile of the whole cut posterior lenticule.[67] It is now also finding use supporting the slit-lamp examination in characterizing and measuring depth stromal opacities or lesions which is important in determining if the cornea can still be used for EK.[68] Some banks are also routinely using OCT to assist in the detection of unreported corneal ectasias or refractive surgery in donor tissue.[69]

Endothelial Microscopy

The condition of the corneal endothelium is central to evaluating the suitability of corneal tissue for both PK and EK, as it is primarily the layer responsible for the maintenance of corneal turgor and transparency. Endothelial microscopy, whether it is through the technique of specular microscopy or transmitted light/phase microscopy, allows for a reasonable determination of ECD, cell pleomorphism and polymegathism, and the identification of corneal guttae. These changes reflect the current well-being of the endothelium as well as being indicative of its functional reserve.[70]

Such objective information and has allowed the wide use of older corneal tissue based on endothelial appearance rather than arbitrarily excluding such tissue solely based on donor age (see section on donor age). In addition, endothelial microscopy has allowed for the use of corneas from donors that have had anterior segment surgery. In both cases, if the corneas have passed the endothelial microscopy criteria and slit-lamp criteria, they should be considered for penetrating or EK (with the receiving ophthalmologist being fully informed).

A low cell density may indicate that the cornea is unlikely to be able to withstand the rigors of transplantation. Bourne and O'Fallon[71] elegantly showed that there was a loss of 23% of the transplanted endothelial cells within the first week of transplantation and others have demonstrated that this cell loss may continue for up to at least 4 years.[44] The critical ECD below which any cornea undergoes decompensation is speculative although many clinicians estimate it to be 300–500 cell/mm^2. Based on the evidence of cell loss in the postoperative period and the estimated lower limit of a functional cell density, eye banks generally have a cutoff of between 1,500 and 2,200 cells/mm^2 (depending on the bank) below which they will no longer issue a cornea for penetrating or EK. In these instances, the cornea may still be suitable for anterior lamellar keratoplasty.

In addition to a low cell density an abnormal endothelial appearance may indicate that the cornea is compromised or functionally deficient. Corneas with considerable polymegathism or pleomorphism have been reported to have a decreased functional reserve[72] and an increased incidence of postoperative decompensation.[73] Corneal guttae have also been reported to reduce endothelial function.[74,75] Inflammatory cells and bacteria can also be easily seen with endothelial microscopy and their presence would lead to the exclusion of such corneas for transplantation.

Specular Microscopy

Specular microscopy is mostly used by those eye banks using hypothermic storage of corneoscleral buttons. A limitation with specular microscopy is that the area of the central corneal endothelium is much larger than can be sampled by the specular microscope even with multiple field examinations. Therefore, the information gained from specular microscopy should be interpreted within the context of the slit-lamp evaluation.

For the best observation of the corneal endothelium, the cornea must be at room temperature. Thus, the most convenient time to perform specular microscopy is after the placement of the cornea in storage media, allowing sufficient time for the media to equilibrate with room temperature and for deturgescence of the cornea. Corneas can also be observed after a period of 4°C storage and subsequent warming to room temperature. The cycle of cooling, warming and recooling of a donor cornea has been shown to have no adverse effects on the metabolic or morphometric status of the donor cornea.[76] However, it becomes more difficult to adequately visualize the endothelium with specular microscopy after a period of storage. The Corneal Donor Study Group has demonstrated that the accuracy and interpretation of ECD measurements are directly related to factors that may affect image quality, and that variability in both endothelial image quality and ECD exists with multiple eye banks and readers. Because of this variability eye banks should standardize their approach ECD determination, set internal standards on ECD density, and consider that fair images are more likely to have a larger margin of error in determining ECDs. Thus, eye banks should provide a margin of safety when the cell count nears the lower limit established by the eye bank.[77]

Light Microscopy

Eye banks using normothermic (organ culture) storage methods use phase contrast microscopy and/or transmitted light microscopy often accompanied by intravital staining of the endothelial layer. This type of endothelial microscopy has the advantages of being able to assess the endothelium after storage and close to the time of transplantation and enables visualization of a larger area of the central cornea compared to specular microscopy. Intravital staining, usually with trypan blue, also provides some information on number of endothelial cells still functioning. Sucrose or balanced salt solutions are often added which cause the intracellular space to swell, making the cell borders easier to discern for ease of cell counting. The original technique is described by Sperling.[78] Such techniques can also be applied to corneas that are hypothermically stored.

Key Points—Corneal Evaluation

- In reaching a decision on acceptance or rejection of tissue for clinical use, the ophthalmologist must rely on the eye bank's careful evaluation of each layer of the cornea.
- Slit-lamp examination can provide information on the depth, width, and position of large to small abnormalities as well as pinpointing the depth of the pathology.
- AS-OCT is being used as an adjunct to slit lamp, and in screening for ectasias, and refractive surgery. Its use in examination of precut lamellae for DSAEK is well established.
- Specular microscopy and/or light microscopy is central to evaluating the suitability of the endothelium for PK and EK surgery.
- Accuracy of ECD is dependent on good image quality. Eye banks should set internal standards on ECD measurement and use cutoff limits as benchmarks not standards.

STORAGE

Unlike tissues such as bone or heart valves that may be extensively processed and altered from their natural state, corneas must be transplanted as a viable living tissue. Thus, the aim of all corneal storage techniques is simply to maintain this living viable state while holding the cornea for the period between donation and transplantation. This is the same aim as for solid organ transplantation such as kidney transplantation. However, while reliable kidney preservation time is still restricted to around 24 hours ischemic time, techniques developed over the past 30 years have enabled the extension of reliable corneal storage times to approximately 1 month.

Hypothermic Corneal Storage

McCarey and Kaufman modified an existing tissue culture medium, TC 199, by adding dextran as an osmotic agent to compensate for the inactivity of the cornea's normal water removal mechanism at 4°C. This extended reliable storage time is 2–3 days at 4°C and the media, MK medium, quickly became the storage system of choice for eye banks. Over the years the MK formulation has been improved by the addition of the more stable HEPES buffer and the replacement of the penicillin-streptomycin antibiotics to gentamicin which has a greater spectrum against gram-negative bacteria.[79] It remains a cheap, easy, simple and reliable form of corneal preservation.

In the mid-80s 2.5% chondroitin sulfate began being added to existing tissue culture media formulations which successfully extended corneoscleral storage times to 7–10 days. This was further modified by the addition of dextran which overcame the problem of the cornea absorbing smaller molecular weight moieties (such as chondroitin sulfate) which otherwise caused the osmotic flow of water into the cornea causing it to swell. Optisol, the widest available storage medium, is based on these formulation and actions,[80] as are other commercially available hypothermic solutions.

While the original publications suggested that Optisol was suitable for up to 14 days storage, in practice the maximum storage time most ophthalmologists feel happy with is 7–10 days with storage between 2° and 6°C. There is also data that shows Optisol is also able to preserve endothelial morphologic characteristics at 26°C for limited periods. While not recommended for storage, enhanced viability for short periods at room temperature provides a margin of safety when cold storage cannot be maintained.[81]

Commercially available hypothermic corneal storage solutions are supplemented with antibiotics (often gentamicin and streptomycin) to give broad antimicrobial coverage.[82] Concerns surrounding increasing trends in the rate of postkeratoplasty fungal infections[66] have seen renewed interest in the addition of antifungals, either by manufacturers[83] or by eye banks themselves[42,84] upon the direction of the transplanting ophthalmologist. However, the efficacy, safety, science, and cost-effectiveness of various supplementation regimes have been questioned.[42] There is preliminary data on the safety and efficacy of antifungal supplementation, but many questions remain unanswered, and many argue that larger scale validation studies must be done before for changing current standard procedures.[84] Improved eye decontamination protocols appear to have a greater role in reducing postkeratoplasty fungal infections.

Organ Culture (Normothermic) Storage

Organ-cultured corneas are incubated in nutrient medium at physiological temperature. They retain active cell metabolism and corneas stored in this way can be reliably preserved for up to 30 days. Organ culture storage has not been adopted in North America but has become the preferred storage method in the UK,[85] Europe,[86-88] New Zealand,[89] and Australia.[90] It has several advantages over hypothermic storage including fewer positive rim cultures[88] and its association with postkeratoplasty infection rates, and the expansion of the potential donor pool[90] (due to acceptance of bacteremic donors and extended death to recovery and preservation times).

In the most common method, excised corneoscleral disks from decontaminated eyes are suspended in glass bottles containing 100 mL of MEM medium with Earle's salts supplemented with 2–5% fetal bovine serum, L-glutamine and the antimicrobial agents penicillin, streptomycin, and amphotericin. Culture bottles are closed and incubated in a dry (non-CO_2) environment at a temperature between 28 and 37°C.[88] Many studies have shown that corneal ultrastructure, endothelial cell morphology, density and viability are well-maintained in organ-cultured corneas up to 48 days of storage[91,92] although in practice most are distributed between 10 and 28 days (average 16 days).[93]

Tissue swells during the culture period, becoming thickened and edematous (from 0.5 to 1 mm), but this is reversed during a period of days in dextran-containing thinning medium prior to distribution.[94] Various studies have confirmed that there is a dramatically lower incidence of endothelial cell death compared to cold-stored corneas and that despite 10–15% endothelial loss during culture, the endothelium is able to eliminate dying cells and repair itself.[95] The surface epithelial layers shed into the medium during increasing time in culture, which are quickly replaced by host cells postoperatively,[91] however, fresher tissue may be indicated for recipients with preoperative persistent epithelial defects.

Organ culture provides an inbuilt microbiological surveillance system, since any culture containing microorganisms not controlled by decontamination and antibiotics will become contaminated, and the cornea not used for transplant.[96] One study showed that 98.9% of corneoscleral rims are sterile after organ culture.[97] Contamination in culture is normally visually obvious by turbidity and pH change, however, corneal cultures are quarantined until a sample of the medium taken at 3–7 days of storage is tested and reported to show no growth of bacteria or fungi. Reported bacterial isolates are most commonly ocular flora such as *Staphylococcus* species,[96,98,99] while fungal growth most commonly is *Candida* species. Strikingly, in recent studies, *Candida* has become the most common contaminant seen in during organ culture.[96] This may reflect the changing epidemiological landscape of nosocomial fungal infections.[100] Notably, contamination during organ culture related directly to systemic infection in the donor is rare, and so with this method the donor pool can be expanded to include those with bacterial septicemia, a common reason for donor exclusion when hypothermic storage is performed.

After the incubation period, corneas cleared for serology and microbiology are evaluated by direct light microscopy of the endothelium before being transferred into thinning/transport medium containing 5% dextran prior to transplantation. Prolonged presence of dextran in culture is thought to be toxic to the cornea, therefore, the maximum recommended time in thinning medium is 2–4 days.[101,102] Since endothelial evaluation is performed at the end of the storage period near to transplantation, the quality and likely efficacy of the tissue can be determined with greater assurance. This allows for reliable use of corneas from older donors and extended death-to-preservation time, with no significant impact on graft survival when compared with younger or fresher tissue.

Compared to hypothermic storage, the organ culture technique is more complex, requiring additional equipment, testing, and greater technical expertise. Although the set-up and testing costs can make it a more expensive method, efficiency benefits can be gained by increased certainty of cornea provision and elimination of potentially unsafe tissue. It is a method best suited to an established eye bank with skilled technical staff, and where donor rates are variable, or distribution is required over wide geographical area. In addition to improved microbiological screening, the increased storage time allows the ability to provide ABO- or HLA-matched corneas for patients with high risk of rejection, and for optimizing allocation of corneas to specific patients. It more easily enables the operation of fully-scheduled transplant booking systems,[90] rather than those organized at short notice, and enables transport over long distances without the need for refrigerated conditions.

Key Points—Corneal Storage

- The benefits and disadvantages of hypothermic and organ culture storage are listed in **Table 2**.
- Both systems are equivalent in graft outcomes.
- Corneas for PK and EK must be transplanted as a viable living tissue and in this respect, corneas have more in common with organ transplantation than other tissue transplantation.

Table 2: Storage procedures for the corneoscleral disk.

	Hypothermic	*Organ culture*
Technique	Simple and fast	More complex
Storage time	Up to 14 days	Up to 4–7 weeks
Tissue available immediately	Yes	No
Maintenance of hydration/thickness	Yes	No
		Second step reversal of swelling necessary
Epithelial and endothelial wound healing	No	Yes
	Stricter concerning donor supply	More tolerant for donor conditions affecting endothelial viability, e.g., time and temperature
Endothelial evaluation	Beginning of storage	End of storage
	Noninvasive specular microscopy	Invasive light microscopy with viability assay
	Small central area	Entire surface
Graft survival	Similar	
Microbiological tests	Not required	Mandatory
		Quarantine period
Bacteremic donors	No	Acceptable
Risk of postoperative endophthalmitis	0.1–2%	0–0.1%

EYE BANK PROCESSING FOR DESCEMET'S STRIPPING AUTOMATED ENDOTHELIAL KERATOPLASTY AND DESCEMET'S MEMBRANE ENDOTHELIAL KERATOPLASTY

The emergence of DSAEK and DMEK presents new opportunities for eye banking in the preparation of donor tissue. In addition, eye banks needed to revise their acceptance criteria for eye donation and the analysis of possible anterior or posterior corneal pathologies regarding specific transplant procedures.

Precut Descemet's Stripping Automated Endothelial Keratoplasty

Studies continue to demonstrate safety and efficacy of tissue prepared, cut, and processed by technicians compared to surgeons[103-105] and some studies indicate lower rates of postoperative infections for eye bank prepared tissue.[41] Additionally, DSAEK tissue prepared by the eye bank can save between 13 and 21 minutes per procedure leading to immense cost savings.[103]

Several studies have investigated the influence of donor factors on DSAEK outcome for both organ-cultured and hypothermically preserved corneas. Donor age and preoperative endothelial cell count were found to have no correlation with graft survival.[52,106-108] Interestingly, tissue from donors with diabetes were associated with increased risk for primary or early failure but the reasons for this remain unclear.[108]

Based on a hypothesis that thicker grafts impair best-corrected visual acuity after DSAEK, some corneal surgeons request thinner grafts from eye banks or prepare "ultrathin" corneal grafts, which, in some cases, can increase the cost of care or result in donor wastage. However, a 2016 systematic review and meta-analysis[109] examining the effect of DSAEK graft thickness on visual acuity agreed with Terry and associates[110] that "graft thickness may have a small effect on visual outcomes in the extremes of thickness, but not in the common range of 100–200 μm" and that "donor thickness has a tenuous relationship with visual outcomes". Nevertheless, with time, eye banks have pursued cutting thinner and thinner DSAEK preparations as surgeons have gained experience with the transplant procedure, and preparations <100 μm are now routine.

Interestingly, for hypothermically stored corneas, a large multicenter trial has now shown that thicker prelamellar-dissection donor tissue is associated with a higher graft dislocation rate. The risk was three times higher for tissues >600 μm compared with tissues ≤ 600 μm,[111] however, the thicker tissue (for hypothermically stored tissue) could simply be a marker for reduced endothelial function before dissection rather than an inherent issue with deep dissections.

Prestripped and Preloaded Descemet's Membrane Endothelial Keratoplasty

The challenge of preparing the delicate donor graft material for DMEK has been reported by individual surgeons as a key barrier in the uptake of DMEK surgery. It has been noted that the manual preparation of the donor tissue is difficult and incurs increased risks, including donor tissue loss, associated financial loss, and cancellation of the surgery.[112,113] Conversely, a facilitator of DMEK uptake has been the preparation of the graft undertaken by the eye bank, and several studies have noted that eye bank prepared DMEK tissues demonstrated outcomes comparable to surgeon prepared tissue in terms of visual acuity, graft failure rate, and endothelial cell loss.[114,115]

Descemet's membrane endothelial keratoplasty preparation techniques include those based on manual peeling, and those based on pneumatic or hydrodissection between the Descemet's membrane and posterior stroma. Current techniques trend toward a no-touch approach in which there is no direct physical graft handling to minimize endothelial cell loss. Melles' group have noted that DMEK graft dissection techniques are diverse and feature different strengths and weaknesses and use the best technique for each specific user.[113]

More recently preloaded DMEK tissue, prepared by the eye bank, has been introduced. Many reports have now demonstrated that tissue that is trephinated, stained, and loaded into an injector by the eye bank and then shipped to the surgeon is equivalent in safety, quality, and effectiveness to surgeon-loaded DMEK, and has no difference in clinical outcomes.[116-118] Preloaded tissue has several advantages, including decreased operating room time, reduced risk of tissue damage or loss in preparation and concomitant decreased risk for case cancellation, better quality control of the tissue and substantial cost savings.

Eye banks should have a heightened awareness related to an increased risk of tissue loss during DMEK preparation associated with a donor's history of diabetes or intraocular surgery.[119,120] In addition, during donor selection they need to account in for the surgical difficulties and complications of handling a "tighter scroll" of DMEK tissue in donors below 50 years and its association with poorer graft outcomes. Ultimately, these are important parameters for eye banks to consider when evaluating quality of tissue for DMEK preparation.

Key Points—Prepared DSAEK and DMEK

- Eye bank preparation of DSAEK and DMEK tissue provides equivalent graft outcomes to surgeon prepared tissue.
- For DSAEK, donor tissue thickness has a tenuous relationship with visual outcomes.
- For DSAEK donor age and preoperative ECD has no correlation with graft survival.
- For DMEK, donors over 50 are preferred. Diabetes and previous ocular surgery are risk factors for complications in donor tissue preparation.

CONCLUSION

Established more than 70 years ago, eye banking continues to develop in complexity and professionalism and has remained vital to the success of corneal transplantation by providing new innovations and patient services. Eye banking benefits from having well-established medical standards which are continually evaluated, reviewed, and internationally promulgated, improved corneal storage techniques, and comprehensive corneal evaluation through the combined use of slit-lamp and specular microscopy and OCT. Preparation of corneas for DSAEK and DMEK has further expanded the role of eye banking and facilitates the uptake of these surgeries while maintaining efficiency, safety, and cost-effectiveness. These activities are increasingly embraced by robust quality management systems.

Importantly, the cornerstone of eye banking and corneal transplantation remains the availability and donation of eyes from recently deceased persons. Eye banks must continue to provide a service that ensures the safety and efficacy of donor tissue and ensures fair and equitable distribution of transplantable tissue. This must always be achieved by following ethical principles[1]—maintaining the dignity of the donor, the dignity of the donor's family and the dignity of the prospective recipient.

REFERENCES

1. The Barcelona Principles: An Agreement on the Use of Human Donated Tissue for Ocular Transplantation, Research, and Future Technologies®. Cornea. 2018;37(10):1213-7.
2. World Health Organization. WHO guiding principles on human cell, tissue and organ transplantation. Transplantation. 2010;90(3):229-33.
3. Eye Bank Association of America: Frequently updated Manuals available from Eye Bank Association of America, 1051 18th Street NW, Suite 1010, Washington D.C. 20036. http://www.restoresight.org.
4. European Eye Bank Association: c/o Fondazione Banca degli Occhi del Veneto, via Felisati 109, Venezia Mestre 30174, Italy. http://www.europeaneyebanks.org.
5. European Directorate for the Quality of Medicines & Healthcare (EDQM). The Guide to the quality and safety of tissues and cells for human application, 4th edition, France; Council of Europe; 2019.
6. Eye Bank Association of Australia and New Zealand. (2016). Section 8 Donor Suitability Assessment and Contraindications. EBAANZ Medical and Quality Standards 2.2. [online]. Available from: https://ebaanz.org/policies-guidelines/ [Last accessed November, 2021].
7. Eye Bank Association of Australia and New Zealand. (2019). Guidelines for the Medical Selection of Ocular Tissue Donors, 3rd edition. [online]. Available from: https://ebaanz.org/policies-guidelines/ [Last accessed November, 2021].
8. Duffy P, Wolf J, Collins G, DeVoe AG, Streeten B, Cowen D. Possible person-to-person transmission of Creutzfeldt-Jakob disease. N Engl J Med. 1974;290:692-3.
9. Heckmann JG, Lang CJ, Petruch F, Druschky A, Erb C, Brown P, et al. Transmission of Creutzfeldt-Jakob disease via a corneal transplant. J Neurol Neurosurg Psychiatry. 1997;63:388-90.
10. Uchiyama K, Ischida C, Yago S, Kuramaya H, Kitmoto T. An autopsy case of Creutzfeldt-Jakob disease associated with corneal transplantation. Dementia. 1994;8:466-73.
11. Hogan RN, Heck E, Cavanagh HD. Risk of prion disease transmission from ocular donor tissue transplantation. Cornea. 1999;18:2-11.
12. Garske T, Ghani AC. Uncertainty in the tail of the variant Creutzfeldt-Jakob disease epidemic in the UK. PLoS One. 2010;5:e15626.
13. The University of Edinburgh. The National CJD Research and Surveillance Unit (NCJDRSU). Creutzfeldt-Jakob Disease in

the U.K. [online]. Available from: http://www.cjd.ed.ac.uk/surveillance [Last accessed October, 2021].

14. Seed CR, Hewitt PE, Dodd RY, Houston F, Cervenakova L. Creutzfeldt-Jakob disease and blood transfusion safety. Vox Sang. 2018;113:220-31.
15. Wadsworth JD, Joiner S, Hill AF, Campbell TA, Desbruslais M, Luthert PJ, et al. Tissue distribution of protease resistant prion protein in variant Creutzfeldt-Jakob disease using a highly sensitive immunoblotting assay. Lancet. 2001;358:171-80.
16. Tullo AB, Buckley RJ, Kelly T, Head MW, Bennett P, Armitage WJ, et al. Transplantation of ocular tissue from a donor with sporadic Creutzfeldt-Jakob disease. Clin Exp Ophthalmol. 2006;34:645-9.
17. World Health Organization. WHO guidelines on tissue infectivity distribution in transmissible spongiform encephalopathies. Geneva: World Health Organization; 2006.
18. Australian Government Department of Health. (2013). Infection Control Guidelines—Creutzfelt-Jakob Disease. [online]. Available from: https://www1.health.gov.au/internet/main/publishing.nsf/content/icg-guidelines-index.htm [Last accessed October, 2021].
19. Houff SA, Burton RC, Wilson RW, Henson TE, London WT, Baer GM, et al. Human-to-human transmission of rabies virus by corneal transplant. N Engl J Med. 1979;300:603-4.
20. Centers for Disease Control. Human-to-human transmission of rabies via a corneal transplant. France. MMWR. 1980;29:25-6.
21. Centers for Disease Control. Human-to-human transmission of rabies via corneal transplant—Thailand. MMWR. 1981;30:473-4.
22. Gode GR, Bhide NK. Two rabies deaths after corneal grafts from one donor. Lancet. 1988;2(8614):791.
23. Javadi MA, Fayaz A, Mirdehghan SA, Ainollahi B. Transmission of rabies by corneal graft. Cornea. 1996;15:431-3.
24. Sureau P, Portnoi D, Rollin P, Lapresle C, Lapresle C, Chaouni-Berbich A. Prevention of inter-human rabies transmission after corneal graft. C R Seances Acad Sci III. 1981;293:689-92.
25. Hoft RH, Pflugfelder SC, Forster RK, Ullman S, Polack FM, Schiff ER. Clinical evidence for hepatitis B transmission resulting from corneal transplantation. Cornea. 1997;16:132-7.
26. Lee HM, Naor J, Alhindi R, Chinfook T, Krajden M, Mazzulli T, et al. Detection of hepatitis C virus in the corneas of seropositive donors. Cornea. 2001;20:37-40.
27. Sengler U, Reinhard J, Adams O, Gerlich W, Sundmacher R. Testing of corneoscleral discs and their culture media for seropositive donors for hepatitis B and C virus genomes. Graefes Arch Clin Exp Ophthalmol. 2001;239:783-7.
28. Tugwell BD, Patel PR, Williams IT, Hedberg K, Chai F, Nainan OV, et al. Transmission of hepatitis C virus to several organ and tissue recipients from an antibody-negative donor. Ann Intern Med. 2005;143:648-54.
29. Salahuddin SZ, Palestine AG, Heck E, Ablashi D, Luckenbach M, McCulley JP, et al. Isolation of the human T-cell leukemia/lymphotropic virus type III from the cornea. Am J Ophthalmol. 1986;101:149-52.
30. Pepose JS, MacRae S, Quinn TC, Ward JW. Serological markers after the transplantation of corneas from donors infected with human immunodeficiency virus. Am J Ophthalmol. 1987;106:798-801.
31. Schwartz A, Hoffman F, L'age-Stehr J, Tegzess AM, Offermann G. Human immunodeficiency virus transmission by organ donation. Outcome in cornea and kidney recipients. Transplantation. 1987;44:21-4.
32. Simonds RJ, Holmberg SD, Hurwitz RL, Coleman TR, Bottenfield S, Conley LJ, et al. Transmission of human immunodeficiency virus type 1 from a seronegative organ and tissue donor. N Engl J Med. 1992;326:726-32.
33. Sawant OB, Singh S, Wright RE III, Jones KM, Titus MS, Dennis E, et al. Prevalence of SARS-CoV-2 in human post-mortem ocular tissues. Ocul Surf. 2021;19:322-9.
34. Kampf G, Todt D, Pfaender S, Steinmann E. Persistence of coronaviruses on inanimate surfaces and their inactivation with biocidal agents. J Hosp Infect. 2020;104(3):246-51.
35. Project Notify Library. The global vigilance and surveillance database for medical products of human origin. [online]. Available from: http://notifylibrary.org [Last accessed October, 2021].
36. Alharbi SS, Alrajhi A, Alkahtani E. Endophthalmitis following keratoplasty: incidence, microbial profile, visual and structural outcomes. Ocul Immunol Inflamm. 2014;22:218-23.
37. Chen JY, Jones MN, Srinivasan S, Neal TJ, Armitage WJ, Kaye SB, et al. Endophthalmitis after penetrating keratoplasty. Ophthalmology. 2015;122:25-30.
38. Du DT, Wagoner A, Barone SB, Zinderman CE, Kelman JA, MaCurdy TE, et al. Incidence of endophthalmitis after corneal transplant or cataract surgery in a medicare population. Ophthalmology. 2014;121:290-8.
39. Hassan SS, Wilhelmus KR, Dahl P, Davis GC, Roberts RT, Ross KW, et al. Infectious disease risk factors of corneal graft donors. Arch Ophthalmol. 2008;126:235-9.
40. Taban M, Behrens A, Newcomb RL, Nobe MY, McDonnell PJ. Incidence of acute endophthalmitis following penetrating keratoplasty: a systematic review. Arch Ophthalmol. 2005;123:605-9.
41. Edelstein SL, DeMatteo J, Stoeger, CG, Macsai MS, Wang CH. Report of the Eye Bank Association of America Medical Review Subcommittee on Adverse Reactions Reported From 2007 to 2014. Cornea. 2016;35:917-26.
42. Tu EY. The Rush to Supplement: The Current Case Against Anti-Fungal Supplementation of Hypothermic Corneal Storage Media. Cornea. 2021;40(9):1091-2.
43. Hata B. The development of glioma in the eye to which the cornea of a patient, who suffered from glioma, was transplanted. Nippon Ganka Gakkai Zasshi. 1939;43:1763-7.
44. McGeorge AJ, Vote BJ, Elliot DA, Polkinghorne PJ. Papillary adenocarcinoma of the iris transmitted by corneal transplantation. Arch Ophthalmol. 2002;120:1379-83.
45. Alsara A, Raf M. Donor-transmitted melanoma after limbal stem cell transplantation. Avicenna J Med. 2017;7:75-7.
46. Bourgol SA, Ninotta S, Garcin T, Cognasse F, Trone MC, Forest F, et al. Detection of refractive photokeratectomy traces during eye banking: Impossible with organ culture but possible with an active storage machine: case report. Cell Tissue Bank. 2021;22(3):479-86.
47. Fargione RA, Channa P. Cornea donors who have had prior refractive surgery: Data from the Eye Bank Association of America. Curr Opin Ophthalmol. 2016;27:323-6.
48. Wakefield MJ, Armitage WJ, Jones MN, Kaye SB, Larkin DF, Tole D, et al. The impact of donor age and endothelial cell density on graft survival following penetrating keratoplasty. Br J Ophthalmol. 2016;100(7):986-9.
49. Flinders University. (2018). Australian Corneal Graft Registry 2018 Report. [online]. Available from: https://dspace.flinders.edu.au/xmlui/handle/2328/37917 [Last accessed October, 2021].
50. Cornea Donor Study Investigator Group. The effect of donor age on corneal transplantation outcome. Ophthalmology. 2008;115:620-6.
51. Writing Committee for the Cornea Donor Study Research Group, Lass JH, Benetz BA, Gal RL, Kollman C, Raghinaru D, et al. Donor age and factors related to endothelial cell loss 10 years after penetrating keratoplasty: Specular Microscopy Ancillary Study. Ophthalmology. 2013;120:2428-35.
52. Potapenko IO, Samolov B, Armitage MC, Byström B, Hjortdal J. Donor endothelial cell count does not correlate with Descemet's Stripping Automated Endothelial Keratoplasty transplant survival after 2 years of follow-up. Cornea. 2017;36:649-54.

53. Dapena I, Moutsouris K, Droutsas K, Ham L, van Dijk K, Melles GR. Standardized "no-touch" technique for descemet's membrane endothelial keratoplasty. Arch Ophthalmol. 2011;129:88-94.
54. Price FW Jr, Price MO. Evolution of endothelial keratoplasty. Cornea. 2013;32 Suppl 1:S28-32.
55. Schaub F, Enders P, Zachewicz J, Heindl LM, Stanzel TP, Cursiefen C, et al. Impact of donor age on Descemet's membrane endothelial keratoplasty outcome: Evaluation of donors aged 17–55 years. Am J Ophthalmol. 2016;170:119-27.
56. Straiko MD, Bauer AJ, Straiko MMW, Potts LB, Chen SY, Tran KD, et al. Donor DMEK tissue characteristics: Association with rebubble rate and 6-month endothelial cell loss. Cornea. 2020;39(10):1267-73.
57. Koenig SB. Donor age. In: Brightbill FS (Ed). Corneal Surgery: Theory, Technique and Tissue, 2nd edition. St Louis: Mosby-Year Book; 1993. pp. 555-62.
58. Wood TO, Nissenkom I. Infant donor corneas for penetrating keratoplasty. Ophthalmic Surg. 1981;12:500-2.
59. Uniform Donor Risk Assessment Interview (DRAI). [online]. Available from: https://www.aatb.org/guidance-documents [Last accessed November, 2021].
60. FDA. (2007). Guidance for Industry: Donor Eligibility Determination for Donors of Human Cells, Tissues, and Cellular and Tissue-Based Products (HCT/Ps). Appendix 1 and 2. [online]. Available from: http://www.fda.gov/downloads/BiologicsBloodVaccines/GuidanceComplianceRegulatoryInformation/Guidances/Tissue/ucm091345.pdf [Last accessed October, 2021].
61. Eye Bank Association of America. Procedures Manual. Washington DC: Eye Bank Association of America. Frequently revised. [online]. Available from https://restoresight.org/what-we-do/publications/medical-standards-procedures-manual/ [Last accessed November, 2021].
62. Cybersight. (2003). Introduction to Eye Banking: A Handbook and Manual. [online]. https://cybersight.org/portfolio/introduction-to-eye-banking-a-handbook-and-atlas/ Available from: [Last accessed October, 2021].
63. Badenoch PR, Alfrich SJ, Wedding TR, Coster DJ. Effectiveness of a decontamination method for donor corneas. Br J Ophthalmol. 1988;72:225-7.
64. Pels E, Vrensen GF. Microbial decontamination of human donor eyes with povidone-iodine: penetration, toxicity and effectiveness. Br J Ophthalmol. 1999;83:1019-26.
65. van Luijk CM, Bruinsma M, van der Wees J, Lie JT, Ham L, Melles GR. Combined chlorhexidine and PVP-I decontamination of human donor eyes prior to corneal preservation. Cell Tissue Bank. 2012;13:333-9.
66. Aldave AJ, DeMatteo J, Glasser DB, Tu EY, Iliakis B, Nordlund ML, et al. Report of the eye bank association of America medical Advisory board Subcommittee on fungal infection after corneal transplantation. Cornea. 2013;32:149-54.
67. Amato D, Lombardo M, Oddone F, Nubile M, Colabelli Gisoldi RA, et al. Evaluation of a new method for the measurement of corneal thickness in eye bank posterior corneal lenticules using Anterior Segment Optical Coherence Tomography. Br J Ophthalmol. 2011;95:580-4.
68. Hsu ST, Perry I, Botsay S, Ko N, Stinnett SS, Kuo AN, et al. Characterization of corneal donor tissue lesions by anterior segment optical coherence tomography compared with eye bank technician slit-lamp examination. Cornea. 2018;37:1318-23.
69. Janunts E, Langenbucher A, Seitz B. In vitro corneal tomography of donor cornea using anterior segment OCT. Cornea. 2016;35:647-53.
70. Armitage WJ, Dick AD, Bourne WM. Predicting endothelial cell loss and long-term corneal graft survival. Invest Ophthalmol Vis Sci. 2003;44(8):3326-31.
71. Bourne WM, O'Fallon WM. Endothelial cell loss during penetrating keratoplasty. Am J Ophthalmol. 1978;85:760-6.
72. Yee RW, Geroski DH, Matsuda M, Champeau EJ, Meyer LA, Edelhauser HF. Correlation of corneal endothelial pump site density, barrier function, and morphology in wound repair. Invest Ophthalmol Vis Sci. 1985;26:1191-201.
73. Rao GN, Shaw EL, Arthur EJ, Aquavella JV. Endothelial cell morphology and corneal deturgescence. Ann Ophthalmol. 1979;11:885-99.
74. Bigar F, Schimmelpfennig B, Hurlzeler R. Cornea guttata in donor material. Arch Ophthalmol. 1978;96:653-5.
75. Burns RR, Bourne WM, Brubaker RF. Endothelial function in patients with corneal guttata. Invest Ophthalmol Vis Sci. 1981;20:77-85.
76. Oak SS, Laing RA, Chiba HM, Tsubata K. Thermal cycling effects on the stored cornea. Invest Ophthalmol Vis Sci. 1989; 30:1584-7.
77. Cornea Donor Study Group. An evaluation of image quality and accuracy of eye bank measurement of donor cornea endothelial cell density in the Specular Microscopy Ancillary Study. Ophthalmology. 2005;112:431-40.
78. Sperling S. Early morphological changes in organ cultured human corneal endothelium. Acta Ophthalmol. 1978;56:785-92.
79. Waltman SR, Palmberg PF. Human penetrating keratoplasty using modified M-K Medium. Ophthalmic Surg. 1978;9:48-50.
80. Lindstrom RL, Kaufman HE, Skelnik DL, Laing RA, Lass JH, Musch DC, et al. Optisol corneal storage medium. Am J Ophthalmol. 1992; 114:345-56.
81. Kaufman HE, Beuerman RW, Steinemann TL, Thompson HW, Varnell ED. Optisol Corneal Storage Medium. Arch Ophthalmol. 1991;109(6):864-8.
82. Smith TM, Popplewell J, Nakamura T, Trousdale MD. Efficacy and safety of gentamicin and streptomycin in Optisol-GS, a preservation medium for donor corneas. Cornea. 1995; 14:49-55.
83. Perry I, Peterson K, Tóthová JD, Tramber M, Botsay S, Tremblay D. Performance of new hypothermic corneal storage media with an antimycotic tablet in comparison to traditional hypothermic media during simulated eye bank processing. Cornea. 2020; 39(8):1031-9.
84. Thareja T, Kowalski R, Kamyar R, Dhaliwal D, Jeng BH, Tu E, et al. Fungal infection after keratoplasty and the role of antifungal supplementation to storage solution: a review. Br J Ophthalmol. 2020;104:1036.
85. Tullo AB, Armitage WJ. Ocular tissue for transplantation—fresh, chilled, warmed, frozen or pickled? Eye (Lond). 2004;18:865-6.
86. Pels E, Schuchard Y. Organ culture preservation of human corneas. Doc Ophthalmol. 1983;56:147-53.
87. Ehlers N. Corneal banking and grafting. The background to the Danish Eye Bank System, where corneas await their patients. Acta Ophthalmol Scand. 2002;80:572-8.
88. Pels E, Pollock GA. Storage of door cornea for penetrating and lamellar transplantation. In: Reinhard T, Larkin F (Eds). Corneal Disease. Heidelberg; Springer; 2013. pp. 91-106.
89. Patel HY, Brookes NH, Moffatt LS, Sherwin T, Ormonde S, Clover GM, et al. The New Zealand National Eye Bank Study 1991-2003: A Review of the Source and Management of Corneal Tissue. Cornea. 2005;24(5):576-82.
90. Devasahayam R. Georges P, Hodge C, Treloggen J, Cooper S, Petsoglou C, et al. Implementation of Organ Culture storage of donor corneas: a 3 year study of its impact on the corneal transplant wait list at the Lions New South Wales Eye Bank. Cell Tissue Bank. 2016;17:377-85.
91. Crewe JM, Armitage WJ. Integrity of epithelium and endothelium in organ-cultured human corneas. Invest Ophthalmol Vis Sci. 2001;42(8):1757-61.

92. Borderie VM, Kantelip B, Delbosc B. Morphology, histology and ultrastructure of human 31°C organ-cultured corneas. Cornea. 1995;14:300-10.
93. European Eye Bank Association Directory. (2016). European Eye Association. [online]. Available from: http://www.eeba.eu [Last accessed October, 2021].
94. Pels E, Schuchard Y. The effects of high molecular weight dextran on the preservation of human corneas. Cornea. 1985;3:219-27.
95. Doughman DJ, Van Horn DL, Rodman W, Byrnes P, Lindstrom RL. Human corneal endothelial layer repair during organ culture. Arch Ophthalmol. 1976;94:1791-6.
96. Ling LH, Wells M, Petsoglou C, Luo K, Georges P, Devasahayam R, et al. Factors affecting corneal organ culture contamination: A 6-year study at the New South Wales Tissue Bank. Cornea. 2019;38:829-35.
97. Borderie VM, Lopez M, Laroche L. Donor corneo-scleral rim cultures after organ culture. Br J Ophthalmol. 1997;81:516.
98. Albon J, Armstrong M, Tullo A. Bacterial contamination of human organ-cultured corneas. Cornea. 2001;20:260-3.
99. Zanetti E, Bruni A, Mucignat G, Camposampiero D. Bacterial contamination of human organ-cultured corneas. Cornea. 2005;24:603-7.
100. Doshi H, Pabon S, Price MO, Feng MT, Price FW Jr. Overview of systemic Candida infections in hospital settings and report of Candida after DMEK successfully treated with antifungals and partial graft excision. Cornea. 2018;37:1071-4.
101. Van der Want HJL, Pels E, Schuchard Y, Oleson B, Sperling S. Electron microscopy of cultured human corneas. Osmotic dehydration and the use of a dextran fraction (dextran T500) in organ culture. Arch Ophthalmol. 1983;101:1920-6.
102. Borderie V, Baudrimont M, Lopez M, Carvajual S, Laroche L. Evaluation of the deswelling period in dextran-containing medium after corneal organ culture. Cornea. 1997;16:215-23.
103. Kitzmann AS, Goins KM, Reed C, Padnick-Silver L, Macsai MS, Sutphin JE. Eye bank survey of surgeons using precut donor tissue for Descemet's stripping automated endothelial keratoplasty. Cornea. 2008;27(6):634-9.
104. Katzman LR, Hoover CK, Khalifa YM, Jeng BH. Assessment of the accuracy and cut-failure rates of eye bank-cut corneas for use in endothelial keratoplasty: a comparison of outcomes between 2010 and 2013. Cornea. 2015;34(11):1365-8.
105. Price MO, Baig KM, Brubaker JW, Price FW Jr. Randomized, prospective comparison of precut vs surgeon dissected grafts for Descemet's stripping automated endothelial keratoplasty. Am J Ophthalmol. 2008;146:36-41.
106. Rosenwasser GO, Szczotka-Flynn LB, Ayala AR, Liang W, Aldave AJ, Dunn SP, et al. Effect of cornea preservation time on success of Descemet's stripping automated endothelial keratoplasty: A randomized clinical trial. JAMA Ophthalmol. 2017;135:1401-9.
107. Patel SV, Lass JH, Benetz BA, Szczotka-Flynn LB, Cohen NJ, Ayala AR, et al. Postoperative endothelial cell density is associated with late endothelial graft failure after Descemet's Stripping Automated Endothelial Keratoplasty. Ophthalmology. 2019;126:1076-83.
108. Terry MA, Aldave AJ, Szczotka-Flynn LB, Liang W, Ayala AR, Maguire MG, et al. Donor, recipient, and operative factors associated with graft success in the Cornea Preservation Time Study. Ophthalmology. 2018;125:1700-9.
109. Wacker K, Bourne WM, Patal SV. Effect of Graft Thickness on Visual Acuity After Descemet's Stripping Endothelial Keratoplasty: A Systematic Review and Meta-Analysis. Am J Ophthalmol. 2016;163:18-28.
110. Terry MA, Straiko MD, Goshe JM, Li JY, Davis-Boozer D. Descemet's stripping automated Endothelial Keratoplasty: The tenuous relationship between donor thickness and postoperative vision. Ophthalmology. 2012;119:1988-96.
111. Ross KW, Stoeger CG, Rosenwasser GOD, O'Brien RC, Szczotka-Flynn LB, Ayala AR, et al. Prelamellar dissection donor corneal thickness is associated with Descemet's Stripping Automated Endothelial Keratoplasty operative complications in the Cornea Preservation Time Study. Cornea. 2019;38(9):1069-76.
112. Terry MA. Endothelial keratoplasty: Why aren't we all doing Descemet's Membrane Endothelial Keratoplasty? Cornea. 2012;31(5):469-71.
113. Birbal RS, Sikder S, Lie JT, Groeneveld-van Beek EA, Oellerich S, Melles GRJ. Donor tissue preparation for Descemet's Membrane Endothelial Keratoplasty: An Updated Review. Cornea. 2018; 37:128-35.
114. Guerra FP, Anshu A, Price MO, Giebel AW, Price FW. Descemet's membrane endothelial keratoplasty: Prospective study of 1-year visual outcomes, graft survival, and endothelial cell loss. Ophthalmology. 2011;118(12):2368-73.
115. Ham L, Dapena I, van Luijk C, van der Wees J, Melles GR. Descemet's membrane endothelial keratoplasty (DMEK) for Fuchs endothelial dystrophy: Review of the first 50 consecutive cases. Eye (Lond). 2009;23(10):1990-8.
116. Potts LB, Bauer AJ, Xu DN, Chen SY, Alqudah AA, Sanchez PJ, et al. The last 200 surgeon-loaded Descemet's Membrane Endothelial Keratoplasty tissue versus the first 200 preloaded Descemet's Membrane Endothelial Keratoplasty Tissue. Cornea. 2020;39:1261-6.
117. Böhm MS, Wylegala A, Leon P, Ong Tone S, Ciolino JB, Jurkunas UV. One-year clinical outcomes of preloaded Descemet's membrane endothelial keratoplasty versus non-preloaded Descemet's membrane endothelial keratoplasty. Cornea. 2021;40:311-9.
118. Català P, Vermeulen W, Rademakers T, van den Bogaerdt A, Kruijt PJ, Nuijts RMMA, et al. Transport and preservation comparison of preloaded and prestripped-only DMEK grafts. Cornea. 2020;39:1407-14.
119. Greiner MA, Rixen JJ, Wagoner MD, Schmidt GA, Stoeger CG, Straiko MD, et al. Diabetes mellitus increases risk of unsuccessful graft preparation in Descemet's membrane endothelial keratoplasty: A multicenter study. Cornea. 2014;33:1129-33.
120. Williams RS, Mayko ZM, Friend DJ, Straiko MD, Clay RD, Stoeger CG. Descemet's membrane endothelial keratoplasty (DMEK) tissue preparation: A donor diabetes mellitus categorical risk stratification scale for assessing tissue suitability and reducing tissue loss. Cornea. 2016;35:927-31.

5 Medicolegal Aspects of Eye Banking

M Vanathi, Rakhi Nathawat, Gurnarinder Singh, Rakesh Ahuja

INTRODUCTION

Laws have been enacted to allow eye banks to effectively perform the collection and distribution of eyes/corneas from donors to recipients. Eye donation and eye banking are associated with legal issues as well. This section reproduces key legal acts and documents that affect eye donation, eye banking, and operations.

In countries where organ and cornea transplantation were established long back, the legislation requires hospitals to play a vital role in the "required request law." In addition, the "Uniform Anatomical Gift Act" (UAGA) and "presumed consent" are in vogue, which covers human organ transplantation.

Eye banks in India were formerly regulated by the Bombay Corneal Grafting Act, 1957 and the Eyes Act 1982 until 1994. The enforcement of Transplantation of Human Organs Act (THOA) took place in 1994. In enacting the THOA, the "Eyes Act of 1982" got repealed, and the provisions of the Eyes Act were not even retained, thus demoting the eye banks in India to collection centers attached to keratoplasty units. THOA was amended in 2011, and the Transplantation of Human Organs (Amendment) Act, 2011 came into force on 10th January, 2014. The amended act is now named the Transplantation of Human Organs and Tissue Act (THOTA).

INTERNATIONAL LAWS ON EYE BANKING

Eye Banking Laws in USA

The Health Resources and Services Administration (HRSA) is the federal agency with responsibility for oversight of the transplant system in the United States.

To address the nation's critical organ donation shortage and improve the organ matching and placement process, the US Congress passed the National Organ Transplant Act in 1984. The act established the Organ Procurement and Transplantation Network (OPTN) to maintain a national registry for organ matching. The act also called for the network to be operated by a private, nonprofit organization under a federal contract. The United Network for Organ Sharing (UNOS), based in Richmond, VA, administers the OPTN.

Uniform Anatomical Gift Act

The UAGA was promulgated in 1968 by the Federal Government of the United States of America. It covers anatomical gifts including corneas for the purpose of transplantation. There were three versions of the UAGA that were enacted; the first was the UAGA of 1968, which was followed up with revisions in 1987. The most recent version was created in 2006. The UAGA has been established in some form, in every State and the District of Columbia (D.C.), as of 2017.

The Uniform Gift Act, USA states that:[1]

- Each acute care general hospital shall develop a method for identifying potential organ donors with the hospital staff.
- The acute care general hospitals shall initiate a request (to relatives of the deceased) and follow the designated procedure of the option to donate organs, tissues, or eyes. The person creating the request shall be an organ procurement organization representative or a designated requestor.
- The Department of Health, in association with organ procurement organizations, shall:
  - Formulate guidelines concerning efficient procedures facilitating the delivery of anatomical gift donations.
  - Formulate guidelines to assist hospitals in the selection and designation of tissue procurement providers (eye bank).

The quality of medical treatment is not affected if one is a known donor. Strict laws are in existence which protects the potential donor. Legal guidelines must be followed before death can be certified. The physician certifying a patient's death is not involved with the eye procurement or with the transplant. Also, it does not prohibit reimbursement for reasonable costs associated with the removal, storage, or transportation of a human body or part thereof according to an anatomical gift executed under this Act.

The UAGA was made because the following key problems that hinder organ donation were identified:

- Failure of persons to sign written directives
- Failure of police and emergency personnel to locate written directives at accident sites
- Uncertainty on the part of the public about circumstances and timing of organ recovery
- Failure on the part of medical personnel to recover organs on the basis of written directives
- Failure to systematically approach family members concerning donation
- Inefficiency on the part of some organ procurement agencies in obtaining referrals of donors
- High wastage rates on the part of some organ procurement agencies in failing to place donated organs
- Failure to communicate the pronouncement of death to next of kin
- Failure to obtain adequate informed consent from family members

Persons Who may Execute an Anatomical Gift

- Any individual of sound mind after the age of 18 years may decide to donate all or any part of the body for any purpose. Such a gift shall be effective upon the individual's death, and there is no requirement to obtain the consent of any survivor.
- An anatomical gift made by an agent of an individual, as authorized by the individual under the powers of attorney for healthcare law, as now or hereafter amended, is deemed to be a gift by that individual and takes effect without the need to obtain the consent of any other person.
- If no gift has been executed under subsection (a), any of the following persons may give all or any part of the deceased body after or immediately before death:
  - The decedent's agent under a power of attorney for health care which provides specific direction regarding organ donation.
  - The decedent's spouse, adult sons or daughters, either of the decedent's parents, any of the decedent's adult brothers or sisters, any adult grandchild of the decedent, the guardian of the decedent's estate, the decedent's surrogate decision-maker under the Health Care Surrogate Act, any person authorized or under obligation to dispose of the body.

In case the donor has actual notice of opposition to the gift by the deceased or any person in the highest priority class in which an available person can be found. In that case, no gift of all or any part of the decedent's body shall be accepted.

Revised Uniform Anatomical Gift Act, 2006

This revision retains the basic policy of the 1968 and 1987 anatomical gift acts by strengthening the "opt-in" system that honors the free choice of an individual to donate the individual's organ. This revision also preserves the right of other persons to make an anatomical gift of a decedent's organs if the decedent had not made a gift during life. And, it strengthens the right of an individual not to donate the individual's organs by signing a refusal that also bars others from making a gift of the individual's organs after the individual's death. The UAGA of 2006 clarifies words written in the law that formerly were not clear and confusing such as anatomical gift, record, refusal, guardian, prospective donor, reasonably available, and disinterested witness. This revision:

- Honors the choice of a person to be or not to be a donor and strengthens the language barring others from overriding a donor's decision to make an anatomical gift.
- Expands the list of those who may make an anatomical gift for another individual during that individual's lifetime to include healthcare agents and, under certain circumstances, parents or guardians.
- Empowers a minor eligible under other laws to apply for a driver's license to be a donor.
- Facilitates donations from an individual who made no lifetime choice by adding to the list of persons who can make a gift of the dead individual's organs and tissues. An adult who showed special care and concern for the decedent, the decedent's adult grandchildren, and/or the person acting as the decedent's agent under a power of attorney for health care at the time of the decedent's death.
- Permits a donation by any member of a class where, there is more than one person in the class so long as no objections by other class members are known. If an objection is known, it permits a majority of the members of the class to make the donation without having to take account of a known objection by any class member who is not reasonably available.
- Encourages and establishes standards for donor registries.
- Enables procurement organizations to get access to documents of gifts in medical records, records of a state motor vehicle department, or donor registries.
- Resolves the tension between a healthcare directive requesting the withholding or withdrawal of life support systems and anatomical gifts by permitting measures necessary to ensure the medical suitability of organs for intended transplantation.
- Expands and clarifies the rules relating to cooperation and coordination between coroners or medical examiners and procurement organizations.
- Recognizes anatomical gifts recognization made under the laws of other jurisdictions.
- Act updation to allow for electronic signatures and records.

Presumed Consent Law

Presumed consent law[2] allows for the harvesting of human organs for transplantation. This law allows, upon brain death, a person's organs to be made available automatically to be harvested for donation unless he or she has declared an opposite wish in writing or otherwise. Organs and tissue may be removed for transplantation or scientific purposes from cadavers of persons who did not, while living, indicate their refusal of donation.

Organ removal may be performed after death has been determined by two licensed physicians. The physicians in question must not be associated in any way with each other, with the transplant recipient, or with the transplant procedure. For the death of a minor or mentally incompetent person, organ donation must be approved by the patient's family or legal representative. The removal and transplantation of organs and tissues may be carried out only by a physician in a hospital. Organs, parts of organs, or any bodily tissue, may not be used for financial gain.

The 2006 revised UAGA has eliminated the presumed consent provisions of the 1987 UAGA and now recommends retrieval of corneas, other tissues, and organs only when there is actual consent by the dead person or by a family member of the decedent.

Eye Banking Laws in Australia[3]

In Victoria, (Australia) the relevant Act relating to the donation of organs and tissues is the Human Tissue Act, 1982, Human Tissue (Amendment) Act, 1987, and Coroners and Human Tissue Acts (Amendment) Act 2006.

The important features of the act are described here.

Consent of Next of Kin

Consent can be obtained from the deceased donor's spouse, adult son or daughter, either parent, adult brother or sister, or legal guardian—in that order of priority.

Verbal consent by the senior available next of kin is sufficient for donation to proceed. There is no requirement for written consent as long documentation of the consent is done accurately in the medical notes of the donor.

Any person can take consent as long as they accurately document their status (the person taking consent) and from whom consent was obtained and the time of consent.

There is no legal requirement to seek the consent of the next of kin if the wishes of the deceased are known. However, it is usual to approach the next of kin to determine if they are aware of the deceased's intention to be a donor. This may have been indicated by sticker on a driver's license, family discussion, signed donor card or registration on the Victorian Organ Donor Registry. It is advised to seek consent from the senior available next of kin, regardless of whether the wishes of the deceased are known or not. It is very unusual for the next of kin to go against the known wishes of a deceased. Conversely, a donation cannot proceed if the deceased had objected to donation prior to death.

Consent for the eyes is preferable, but only corneas can be donated. It should be documented if the consent was for eyes or only corneas.

Certification of Death

For donation after circulatory arrest, any medical practitioner can certify cardiac arrest death (but not brain death).

A formal death certificate does not have to be completed to proceed with eye/corneal donation. However, death should be adequately documented in the deceased's notes by the medical practitioner. If time and circumstances allow, a death certificate should be completed.

Coroner's Consent

In cases where a coronal inquiry is essential, tissue removal cannot proceed unless the coroners give consent. The eye bank will obtain this consent, but next of kin consent is first required.

A consent or direction must be given orally by a coroner and, if so issued, shall be confirmed in writing.

Designated Officer Authorization

A designated officer for a hospital may authorize the removal of tissue from the dead body of a person —(a) for the purpose of the transplantation of the tissue to a living person; or (b) for utilization of the tissue for other therapeutic usages or for scientific or medical purposes.

A designated officer could be a medical practitioner (e.g., admitting officer, medical administration), hospital administrator or a nurse appointed to this position. The role of the designated officer is to ensure:

- Documentation of the death by the medical officer
- That the donor had not objected to donation prior to death
- That consent given by the senior available next of kin
- When the next of kin cannot be located following all reasonable attempts to contact them have been made, the designated officer may also authorize the removal of tissue.
- That consent from the coroner has been obtained in cases where a referral is necessary.

Retrieval of Eyes/Corneas

It is no longer a requirement that the removal of eyes/corneas be carried out by a medical practitioner. The Act now states: "medical practitioner or prescribed person or class of persons to remove skin or ocular tissue or both."

Advertisements Relating to Buying Human Tissue Prohibited

As per the law, (a) a person shall not publish or disseminate by newspaper, book, broadcasting, television, cinematograph or other means whatever; (b) exhibit to public view in a house, shop or place; or (c) deposit in the area, yard, garden or enclosure of a house, shop or place, an advertisement relating to the buying in Australia of human tissue or of the right to take tissue from the bodies of persons. The penalty for the same is $1,000.

Eye Banking Laws in UK[4]

The retrieval and use of tissues for transplantation in the UK were governed by Human Tissues Act, 1961. Now it has been replaced with Human Tissues Act, 2004. Consent is required before the removal of tissues can proceed for the purposes of transplantation, research, or medical education. Either the donor must have made his/her wishes clear prior to death, or the donor's relatives must confirm to the best of their knowledge that the donor had not during his/her life objected to donation (In practice, a donor's relatives are always consulted). The Human Tissue Act, 2004 and the Human Tissue (Scotland) Act, 2006 (HT Acts) require specific consent/authorization for the donation and storage of tissue for transplantation and other specified usages including research and or training, clinical audit, and quality assurance. If a person has expressed a willingness to be a donor through the will or the National Organ Donor Register, that consent is supreme and cannot be overruled by the family. In case the prior consent is not available by a potential donor, consent may be given by a nominated representative of the potential donor or by a qualifying relationship/nearest relative. It is of utmost importance that consent/authorization is obtained according to the relevant legislation.

While the main purpose of eye donation will always be transplantation, there is also a need for tissue both for research into human eye disease and for teaching purposes. Relatives should therefore be asked to confirm the lack of objection to these uses as well as to transplantation.

Relatives should be apprised that not every cornea will be suitable for transplantation but that suitability cannot be determined before the eyes retrieval. Corneas and any other parts of the eye that are unsuitable for transplantation may be suitable for education, training, or research. If the eyes are not going to be utilized, family members should be made aware that the same will be disposed of in a lawful manner according to the HT Acts.

Approval should also be obtained for a sample of the donor's blood to be taken for serological testing of transmissible disease. Relatives should be told that they will be informed of any positive results that may have implications for their own health.

When an inquest is to be held in connection with the deceased or when the Coroner, or Procurator Fiscal in Scotland, requires a postmortem examination of the body, permission must be obtained from the Coroner/Procurator Fiscal before proceeding with eye collection, even though consent may have already been obtained from the relatives.

Opt-out System[5]

Organ donation in England has changed to an opt-out system. This means that all adults agree to become organ donors when they die, unless they have made it known that they do not wish to donate.

If a person have not recorded an organ donation decision and is not in one of the excluded groups, it will be considered that he/she agree to donate the organs after the death. This system is referred to as the opt-out system, deemed consent, presumed consent or Max and Keira's Law.

The individual can choose whether or not he/she want to be an organ donor when he/she dies by registering the decision and telling the family. The faith, beliefs, and culture of the individual will continue to be respected. Family consent will still be required for organs or tissues to be retrieved, both out of consideration for the family, and to make sure additional relevant information is gathered.

Corneal Tissue Act, 1986

It permits suitably trained National Health Service staff, who are not medically qualified, to remove eyes from donors. Training courses are run by corneal transplant service (CTS) eye banks.

Human Organ Transplant Act, 1989

It prohibits commercial dealings in human organs. The general standards governing eye donation and retrieval are set out in this act. Guidance on the removal of human eyes used in transplantation and research is issued by The Royal College of Ophthalmologists. It has been now replaced by Human Tissues Act, 2004.

EYE BANKING LAWS IN INDIA

The principal Act governing the donation of human organs in India is the THOA, 1994 and the Transplantation of Human Organs Rules, 1995. This Act legislated by the Government of India provides a legal framework for transplanting all human organs. Eye donation comes within its scope. THOA was amended in 2011, and the Transplantation of Human Organs (Amendment) Act, 2011 came into force on 10th January, 2014. The amended act is now named the THOTA.

The National Program for Control of Blindness and Visual Impairment (NPCBVI) has established Eye Banks in medical colleges to increase donor cornea collection. It now also extends support to various eye banks run by voluntary agencies. Eye Bank Association of India (EBAI) is the national level body focused on relieving corneal blindness. Among other goals, it aims to encourage the government to create and enforce a uniform legal framework for eye banking in the country. It has initiated action to persuade the government to amend the Human Organs Transplantation Act, 1994 to include eye donation and eye banks in the Act's framework.

Adoption of the Law

Since Health is a state subject, the State's act regarding organ and tissue donation needs to be adopted.

In the first instance, it applies to the whole of the States of Goa, Himachal Pradesh, and Maharashtra and to all the Union territories. State which adopts this Act by resolution passed in that behalf under clause (1) of Article 252 of the Constitution.

The Indian Human Organs Transplantation Act, 1994[6]

It is an Act to provide for the regulation of removal, storage, and transplantation of human organs for therapeutic purposes. It regulates the following actions:

- The government must register all hospitals or eye banks that collect eyes or other human organs after meeting specific service and medical standards.
- A procedure for obtaining the written consent of relatives of deceased persons has been laid down and has to be followed before eyes, or other organs are removed.
- *In India, even if a person when alive "wills" that his organs can be donated after death, such a will is not valid. Even in such cases Indian law states that no removal of organs is done without the consent of relatives. Hard punishment is specified for anyone removing organs without consent or using them for any purpose other than therapeutic purposes or buying and selling organs.*

Authority for the Removal of Human Organs

In such manner and subject to such conditions as may be prescribed, any donor may authorize the removal, before his death, of any human organ of his body for therapeutic purposes.

If any donor had, unequivocally authorized at any time before his death in writing and in the presence of two or more witnesses the retrieval of any human organ of body, after the death, for therapeutic usage, the lawful possessor of the donor shall, unless she/he has reasons to believe that the deceased had subsequently revoked the authority aforesaid, grant to a registered medical practitioner all reasonable facilities for the removal for therapeutic usage, of the human organ from the deceased body.

Where no authority, was made by any person before his death but such person also expressed no objection to any of his human organs being used after his death for therapeutic purposes, the person lawfully in possession of the dead body of such person may, unless he has reason to believe that any near relative of the deceased person has objection to any of the deceased person's human organs being used for therapeutic purposes, authorize the removal of any human organ of the deceased person for its therapeutic usage.

Where any human organ is to be removed from the body of a deceased person, the registered medical practitioner shall satisfy himself, before such removal, by a personal examination of the body from which any human organ is to be removed, that the person is dead, where, it appears to be a case of brainstem death.

Authority for Removal of Human Organs in Case of Unclaimed Bodies in Hospital or Prison

In the case of a dead body lying in a hospital or prison and not claimed by any of the near relatives of the deceased person within 48 hours from the time of the death of the concerned person, the authority for the removal of any human organ from the dead body which so remains unclaimed may be given, in the prescribed form, by the person in charge, for the time being, of the management or control of the hospital or prison, or by an employee of such hospital or prison authorized in this behalf by the person in charge of the management or control thereof.

No authority shall be given if the person empowered to give such authority has reason to believe that any near relative of the deceased person is likely to claim the dead body even though such near relative has not come forward to claim the body of the deceased person within the time.

Where the body of a person has been sent for postmortem examination:

- For medicolegal purposes by reason of the death of such person having been caused by accident or any other unnatural cause; or
- For pathological purposes

The person competent under this Act to give authority for the removal of any human organ from such dead body may, if he has reason to believe that such human organ will not be required for the purpose for which such body has been sent for postmortem examination, authorize the removal, for therapeutic purposes, of that human organ of the deceased person provided that he is satisfied that the deceased person, had not expressed, before his death, any objection to any of his human organs being used, for therapeutic purposes after his death or, where, he had granted an authority for the use of any of his human organs for therapeutic purposes after his death, such authority had not been revoked by him before his death. The doctor who removes the eyes for therapeutic purposes is protected against the charges of mutilating the dead body or offending religious or emotional sentiments which are considered offences under Section 297 of Indian Penal Code.

Offences and Penalties[7]

Any personnel working at the hospital, if found involved for the purpose of transplantation, associating with or helping in the removal of human organs and tissues without proper approvals shall be punishable with imprisonment for a term extending to 5 years and with a fine which may extend to ₹ 10,000.

Punishment for commercial dealings in human organs. Whoever:

- Making or receiving any payment for the supply of or an offer to supply any human organ
- Seeks to find a person willing to supply for payment any human organ
- Offers to supply any human organ for payment
- Initiates or negotiates any arrangement involving making any payment for the supply of, or for an offer to supply, any human organ
- Takes part in the management or control of a body of persons, firm or company, whose activities consist of or include the initiation or negotiation of any arrangement referred to in clause (d); or
- Publishes or distributes or causes to be published or distributed any advertisement:
  - Inviting persons to supply for payment of any human organ
  - Offering to supply any human organ for payment
  - Indicating that the advertiser is willing to initiate or negotiate any arrangement

These shall be punishable with imprisonment for a term which shall not be <2 years but which may extend to 7 years and shall be liable to fine which shall not be less than ₹ 10,000 but may extend to ₹ 20,000.

Required Request Law in India

After certification of brainstem death of the person, it is now compulsory by law for the medical practitioner to ask the near relative or person in lawful possession of the body of a person admitted in intensive care unit (ICU) that whether the donor had, in the presence of two or more witnesses (at least one of whom is a near relative of such person), authorized before his or her death as specified in Form 7 of THOTA, 2014, the removal of his or her organs or tissues after his or her death, for therapeutic purposes. If not, the relative should be made aware of the option of organ donation. Even if the donor has pledged his organs before death, the consent of a near relative or person in lawful possession of the body is also required.

Consent

The person with the power to give consent to the eye donation has been modified from time to time in the Indian law:

- *1994*: Daughter, father, mother, brother or sister
- *2011 Section 2(i)*: "Near relative" means spouse, son, daughter, father, mother, brother, sister, grandfather, grandmother, grandson or granddaughter
- *2014 Section 4(b)*: A near relative of the deceased or the person lawfully in possession of the body of the donor

Qualification of Transplant Coordinator

The transplant coordinator shall be employed by a registered hospital having qualifications such as:

- Graduate from any recognized system of medicine
- Nursing
- Bachelor's degree and preferably Master's degree in Social work or Psychiatry or Sociology or Social Science or Public Health Qualification.

Recovery of the Corneas

As per the law of India, "the technician who can enucleate cornea" means the technician with any of the below-mentioned qualifications and experience who can harvest corneas (enucleate eyeballs or excise corneas), namely:

- Ophthalmologists possessing a Doctor of Medicine (MD) or
- Master of Surgery (MS) in Ophthalmology or Diploma in Ophthalmology (DO); and
- Registered doctors from all recognized systems of medicine, Nurses, Paramedical Ophthalmic, Assistant, Ophthalmic Assistant, Optometrists, Refractionists, Paramedical Worker or Medical Technician with a recognized qualification from all recognized systems of medicine.

The person must be duly trained to enucleate a donated cornea or eye from a registered, authorized, and functional Eye Bank or Government Medical College. The certificate after training should mention that the person has acquired the required skills to independently conduct enucleation of the eye or retrieval of the cornea from a cadaver.

Recipient Information

All recipients shall be followed up and immediate and appropriate corrective and preventive actions taken in adverse events.

Processing Fee

As per THOTA, the expenses for recovery of organs or tissues, their preservation and transportation, shall be taken care of by the recipient or institution or Government or NGOs or society as per the decision of the state government or union territory administration. The donor family is not responsible for any of these expenses.

Distribution of Corneas

As per THOTA, 2014, the organs to be allotted as per the below sequencer:

1. State
2. Regional

3. National
4. Person of Indian Origin
5. Foreigner

REFERENCES

1. The National Conference of Commissioners on Uniform State Laws (2017). "Anatomical Gift Act (2006)". United States: Uniform Law Commission; 2017.
2. Orentlicher D. Presumed Consent to Organ Donation: Its Rise and Fall in the United States. (August 6, 2008). Rutgers Law Review. 2009;61:295.
3. Western Australia (1982). Human Tissue and Transplant Act 1982. [online] Available from: https://www.slp.wa.gov.au/statutes/swans.nsf/(DownloadFiles)/Human+Tissue+and+Transplant+Act+1982.pdf/$file/Human+Tissue+and+Transplant+Act+1982.pdf [Last accessed September, 2021].
4. Organ donation. (2020). Organ donation law in England. [online]. Available from: https://www.organdonation.nhs.uk/uk-laws/organ-donation-law-in-england/ [Last accessed September, 2021].
5. The guardian. (2020). All adults in England to be deemed organ donors in 'opt-out' system. [online]. Available from: https://www.theguardian.com/society/2020/may/19/deceased-uk-adults-to-be-deemed-organ-donors-in-opt-out-system [Last accessed September, 2021].
6. Sahay M. Transplantation of human organs and tissues Act-"Simplified". Indian J Transplant. 2018;12:84-9.
7. Notto. (2014). [online] Available from: https://notto.gov.in/WriteReadData/Portal/images/THOA-Rules-2014.pdf [Last accessed September, 2021].

6

Setting Up Corneal Transplant Center

Rakhi Nathawat, Namrata Sharma, Rasik B Vajpayee

INTRODUCTION

Corneal transplantation requires particular skill sets, specialized equipment, and extensive coordination. For these reasons, transplantation is only provided by top quality facilities.

A corneal transplant facility must offer top quality transplantation services, in all different types of corneal transplantation. It must employ specialized staff, right through from reception staff to corneal surgeons (**Fig. 1A**).

Many factors must be considered when setting up a corneal transplant facility. These include:

- Eye bank of choice, access to cornea
- Patient coordination and education
- Ward availability/staffing/education
- Anesthetic availability
- Specialty theater nurses
- Special equipment required
- Reception staff/emergency department staff training/education/availability
- Research
- Wet laboratory facilities

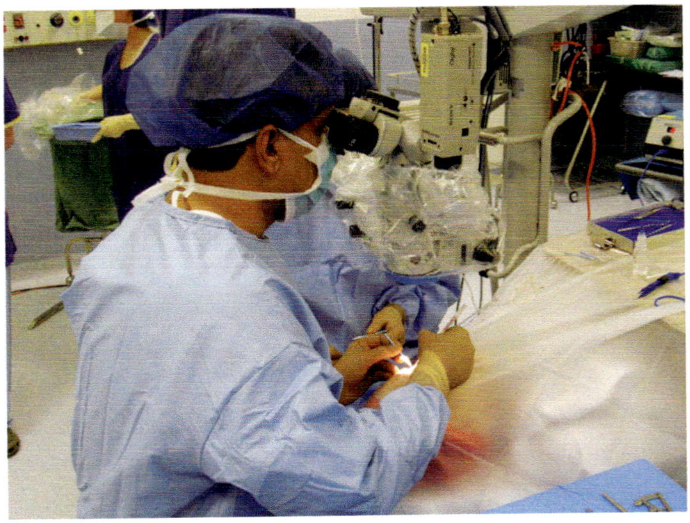

Fig. 1A: Operation theater in a corneal transplant center.

EYE BANK

The role of an eye bank is to provide safe and viable corneal tissue for transplantation. Tissue needs to be available, reliably and safely transported, of transplantable quality, and free of transmissible disease.

An onsite eye bank is most convenient, especially in developing countries, where same day transplantation may be arranged once serology has cleared, without the need for transport medium and storage. In the absence of an onsite eye bank, one should collaborate with as many eye banks as possible, and consider factors such as availability of tissue, culture medium used, transport issues, and waiting time.

It is imperative to maintain up-to-date waiting lists, including all patients awaiting corneal transplantation. Priority should depend upon the need for the surgery and visual acuity in that and the other eye. The lists could be divided into the following categories:

- General list/nonurgent cases
- Priority list/semiurgent cases
- Top priority list/urgent cases
- Emergency list

SCORING SYSTEM FOR PRIORITIZATION IN ALLOCATION OF OPTICAL GRADE TRANSPLANTABLE CORNEA

Scoring system for prioritization in allocation of optical grade has been described in **Table 1**.

Ideally, dates for elective, nonurgent cases would be specified at the time of booking tissue, however, emergency cases, of course, would be organized more quickly.

If a lamellar surgical procedure, such as Descemet stripping automated endothelial keratoplasty (DSAEK) or automated lamellar therapeutic keratoplasty (ALTK) has been planned, it is useful to cut the tissue one day prior to the case, in order to save time in the corneal theater on the day of surgery (**Fig. 1B**). This practice also allows for alternative arrangements to be made should there be any technical problems with the cutting of the tissue, and helps to avoid short notice cancellations.

Table 1: Scoring system for prioritization in allocation of optical grade.

S. No.	*Criteria for scoring*	*Points allocated*
1.	*Visual disability*: • Bilateral blindness, i.e., BCVA in better eye < 3/60 • Economic blindness, i.e., BCVA in better eye < 6/60 • Visual disability, i.e., BCVA in better eye < 6/18	 +3 +2 +1
2.	Bullous keratopathy or endothelial failure such as Fuchs' dystrophy eligible for endothelial keratoplasty with good visual prognosis	+3
3.	Primary donor failure	+4
4.	Age of recipient	+3, <6 years +2, 6–12 years +1, 12–18 years
5.	• Associated diseases affecting inferior outcome • Healed keratitis with deep vascularization in >2 quadrants or adherent leukoma • Associated with uncontrolled glaucoma • Expected poor visual potential due to posterior segment pathology/squint	 –2 –2 –2
6.	• Emergency graft with potential for good prognosis Impending perforation • Perforation progressive infective keratitis • If poor prognosis then nonoptical grade cornea can be directly utilized without waiting	+4

(BCVA: best-corrected visual acuity)

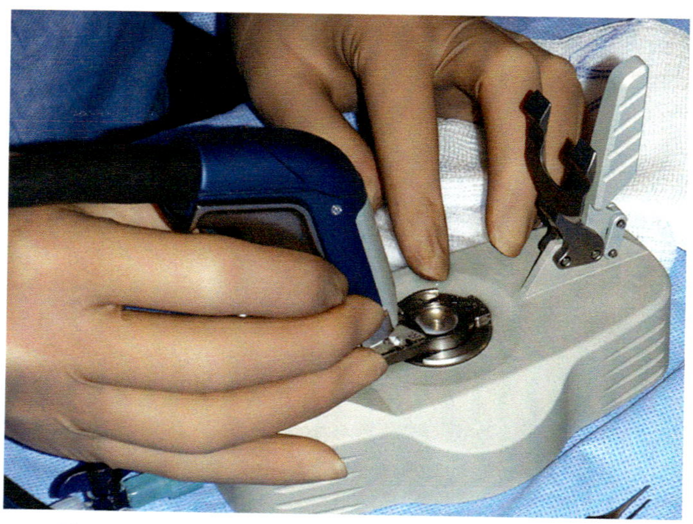

Fig. 1B: Precutting tissue for Descemet stripping automated endothelial keratoplasty.

PATIENT COORDINATION AND EDUCATION

Most corneal transplantation cases should be booked electively, with confirmation of tissue availability 3–4 days prior to the specified date. In more urgent cases, once a tissue is available, the patient will need to be notified of a time. They must fast for at least 6 hours preoperatively, and be aware of instructions requiring particular medications, particularly diabetic medications.

Patients should receive written information, in the form of a brochure, at the time of booking the case. This information should include:

- Place of arrival
- What to wear/bring
- Fasting instructions
- Instructions relating to any special medications, e.g., diabetic/anticoagulant
- Risks and benefits of corneal transplantation
- Theoretical risk associated with transplant material
- Possible day/time change at late notice due to unavailability of tissue
- Need for lifelong follow-up following the transplant
- Postoperative instructions, including importance of drops
- Symptoms of rejection/infection to look out for

WARD/STAFF EDUCATION

A corneal transplant facility should have the capacity to accommodate patients overnight, both pre- and postoperatively, when required. Occasionally, particularly in developing countries, patients may need to remain as inpatients while awaiting transplantation, and this may amount to many days on the ward.

Ward staff should be aware of different types of corneal transplantation, including the possibility of posturing post-operatively. They should be aware that severe pain, discomfort, nausea, or vomiting must be reported to the surgeon, or on-call ophthalmologist or resident. On-call staff should understand that there is a low threshold for contacting the corneal surgeon in case a problem arise. A corneal transplant facility must have an on-call ophthalmologist and also, if possible, a fellow or resident at all times, so that problems may be easily reported and patients assessed. Once assessed, a corneal fellow or corneal specialist should be notified of each presentation, to ensure management of the patient has proceeded effectively.

Anesthetic Staff

Anesthetic staff involved with a corneal transplant facility should be aware of the different types of corneal transplantation, and their anesthetic requirements. Ideally, written guidelines would be set by the anesthetic staff, outlining appropriate investigations to be performed prior to each case, as this may help to avoid delays at the time of surgery.

On booking a case, anesthetic preference should be considered. If the patient is considered to be of high anesthetic risk, preoperative assessment will be required by the anesthetist prior to surgery. Relevant bloods and echocardiograph should be considered. General or local anesthesia are appropriate for most patients undergoing corneal transplantation.

It is most important to liaise with the anesthetist when necessary, particularly for urgent cases.

OPERATING THEATER ISSUES

Specialty Theater Nurses

It is important to train ophthalmic nurses in the different types of corneal transplantation, as they will be able to assist the surgeon with each case, and ensure appropriate instruments are available. A corneal transplant facility should include relevant equipment, and a good selection of trephines and punches, as it may be difficult to adequately predict use prior to the case. At the time of booking a case, make sure the type of transplant to be performed, as well as any special equipment is clearly specified.

Provide the nursing staff with equipment lists for all types of corneal transplantation. Examples of such lists are shown in **Tables 1 to 5**. In this way, you will always have what you need within reach, and each surgery may run more quickly and efficiently.

LASERS IN CORNEAL SURGERY

Femtosecond laser-assisted anterior lamellar keratoplasty is an efficient and safe procedure for improving the quality of vision in patients with anterior corneal pathology. Femtosecond laser is now being used to perform many types of specialized corneal transplant surgeries. It is ideal to have the laser facility and the surgical facility in the same center, in order to avoid transport of patient's midprocedure. Due to financial and space constraints, however, this may not be possible for many transplant facilities. Even if separate locations are necessary, it may well still be possible to perform these femtosecond-assisted procedures.

SPECIAL EQUIPMENT

A corneal transplant facility must be set-up with all of the commonly required instruments. Less frequently used instruments or materials may be ordered on a case-by-case basis.

Equipment in the clinic would approach that usually required for an ophthalmology clinic. Medical photographic equipment such as slit-lamp mounted photographic equipment, corneal topography, specular microscopy, and anterior segment ocular coherence tomography is all required. A scan measurements, such as by IOLMaster, will be required for cataract or triple procedures.

Ideally, a transplant facility would be set-up for all types of corneal transplantation, including penetrating keratoplasty (PKP), ALTK, big bubble deep anterior lamellar keratoplasty (DALK), manual deep lamellar keratoplasty (DLK), DSAEK, tuck in lamellar keratoplasty (TILK), and femtosecond-assisted keratoplasty.

Provide the nursing staff with equipment lists for all types of corneal transplantation (**Tables 2 to 5 and Box 1**), and specify the exact type of transplant planned on the booking

Table 2: Equipment required for penetrating keratoplasty.

Drapes	*Consumables*
Sterile eye drape	• *Gloves*: Size X
Prep tray	• Disposable gown
Trays and instruments:	• Microscope drape
• Corneal graft tray:	• 15 degree blade
– Fine tooth forceps, e.g., Lim/ Hoskins	• Teflon block • Marking pen
– Right and left hand corneal scissors	• Spears
– Universal corneal scissors	
– Westcott scissors	• Disposable pot
– Vanas scissors:	
» Straight	
» Curved	• 10 Ml syringe × 1
– Needle holder	• 2 Ml syringe × 3
– Caliper	• All types of
• *Trephines*:	• Viscoelastics
– *Example*, Hessburg–Barron vacuum trephine and punch, size specified at start of case	• Nylon 10-0 suture with sharp point needle • Subconjunctival
– Phaco tray and equipment if triple procedure	• *Injections*: *Example*, Keflin, dexamethasone, lignocaine
Graft material: Check present	
Equipment:	• BSS 18 Ml
• Microscope with attached photographic and recording devices	• Fluorescein 2% minimum
• DVD recording device	• Rycroft cannula × 1

Table 3: Equipment required for ALTK or TILK in addition to that already listed for PKP.

Instruments	*Consumables*
• Artificial anterior chamber	• Tegaderm × 2
• Microkeratome console and tubing	• Microkeratome blade × 2
• ALTK lens applantor set	• Artificial AC tubing
• ALTK suction and cutting rings	• IV giving set
• ALTK anterior chamber bell	• BSS 500 mL
• ALTK lens applantor	
• Cutting heads 200/250/300 μm	• Donor tissue

(ALTK: automated lamellar therapeutic keratoplasty; PKP: penetrating keratoplasty; TILK: tuck in lamellar therapeutic keratoplasty)

Table 4: Equipment required for cutting tissue prior to automated lamellar transplantation procedures.

Drapes	**Consumables**
Sterile sheet *Instruments:* • Fine tooth forcep × 2 • Microkeratome console and tubing • Microkeratome motor and cutting head • *Artificial anterior chamber and tubing cutting heads*: 300 or 350 µm • Microkeratome blade • Operating microscope • Pachymeter	• Sterile gown • Sterile gauze • Spears • IV giving set • BSS 500 mL • Free standing • IV pole • 2 mL syringe • Marking pen • Sterile pot • Tegaderm • Microscope drape • Healon 0.4 mL

Table 5: Equipment required for DSAEK, in addition to that already listed for PKP.

Drapes	**Consumables**
None *Instruments:* • Busin glide • Busin forceps or end-gripping forceps • Descemet stripper • Descemet scorer • Bipolar cautery *Donor tissue:* Precut, preferably 1 day prior	• Bipolar leads • 3.2 mm keratome • Crescent blade • MVR blade • IV giving set, IV pole • BSS 500 mL • Anterior chamber • Maintainer • Vision blue • Miochol • 8-0 Vicryl suture • Steristrips × 1 packet

(DSAEK: Descemet stripping automated endothelial keratoplasty; MVR: microvitreoretinal; PKP: penetrating keratoplasty)

Box 1: Equipment required for DALK or DLK in addition to that on PKP list.

- Air filter
- 2 Ml Luer-lock syringe
- 26-g needle × 2
- Crescent blade
- Lamellar dissectors
- Vision blue

(DALK: deep anterior lamellar keratoplasty; DLK: deep lamellar keratoplasty; PKP: penetrating keratoplasty)

form. Exact equipment required will differ for different surgeons. For this reason, these lists are a guide only, and should be regularly updated and stored for each surgeon. In this way, an up-to-date list of equipment required for all different transplant procedures may be kept by the transplant facility for each surgeon, thus helping each surgery to run smoothly and efficiently (**Fig. 2**).

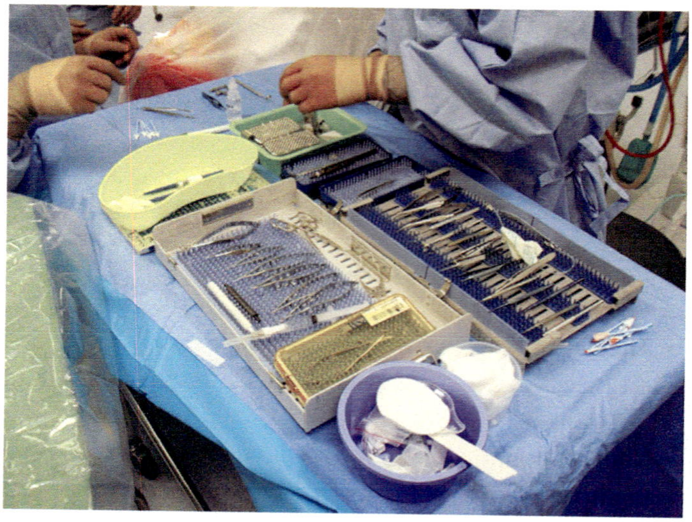

Fig. 2: Example of set-up for corneal transplantation.

FOLLOW-UP

A corneal transplant facility must have a clinic, and an emergency facility, in order to assess both pre- and postoperative patients. Referring practitioners would need to be aware of the presence of a transplant facility in their area. Services offered may be advertised to these referrers, by means of letter or pamphlet. An example of a list of services offered by a corneal transplant facility may include:

- Inpatient or outpatient management of acute corneal disease including:
  - Infectious keratitis
  - Neurotrophic keratitis
  - Corneal melt
  - Corneal perforation
- Inpatient or outpatient management of chronic corneal disease including:
  - Corneal dystrophy
  - Corneal ectasia
  - Low vision due to previous corneal disease
- Follow-up and management of all corneal conditions
- Emergency assessment, management, and treatment of corneal disease.

Patients must be aware of the procedure to be followed should an emergency develop, and the corneal fellow or specialist should be contacted following on-call ophthalmologist or resident assessment.

The major complications requiring immediate attention after a corneal transplant are infectious keratitis and graft rejection. A corneal transplant facility should develop management protocols and make them available to corneal fellows for the management of these cases.

A corneal transplant facility should aim to have photographs of all patients preoperatively, and at each follow-up visit, to aid in documentation of progression or improvement of disease.

CHECKLIST FOR BOOKING A CASE

- Tissue
  - Book with eye bank
  - Time of arrival
  - Courier if necessary
  - Place of delivery
  - Storage once delivered
  - Need to precut tissue for lamellar procedures
- Theater
  - Book case
  - Specify particular equipment required
- Notify specialty nursing staff
- Book ward bed
- Book anesthetist, and consider need for preoperative assessment
- Fast and notify patient
- Preoperative photograph
- Book follow-up

RESEARCH

It is essential that a corneal transplant facility will contribute to the progression of this rapidly expanding field. A good research facility can bring innovation to cornea transplant research programs. Research may be laboratory based or clinically based. A corneal transplant facility should aim to publish new techniques, as well as results or modifications to preexisting techniques. Make sure every surgical case is recorded and cataloged for future video production or education (**Fig. 3**). Our surgeons and researchers are actively engaged in various research topics from artificial corneas to treating keratoconus.

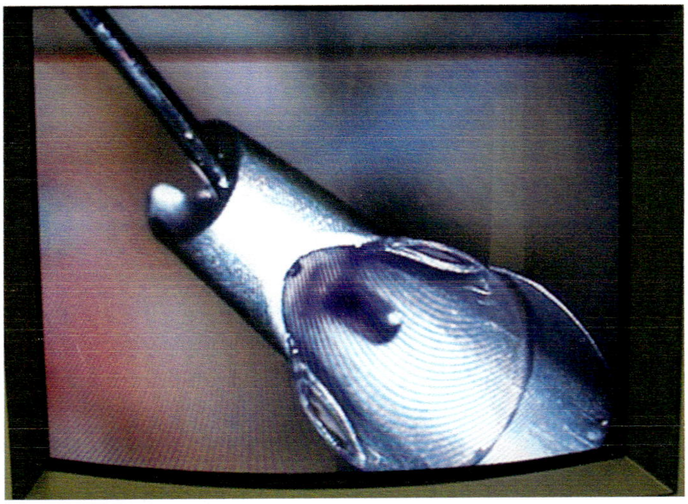

Fig. 3: Recording device.

BIOHAZARDOUS WASTE DISPOSAL

Human tissue and waste items shall be disposed of in such a manner as to minimize any hazard to medical personnel and the environment and comply with applicable regulations. Dignified and proper disposal procedures shall be used to obviate recognizable human remains.

WET LABORATORY

If possible, a corneal transplant facility should have a wet laboratory or skill development laboratory. Such a laboratory should have well-functioning operating microscopes, and appropriate instruments in order to practice the skills required for corneal transplant surgeries. Residents and fellows should aim to frequently practice their skills on animal eyes prior to performing live surgeries. Suturing, in particular, must be practiced in the wet laboratory. Practice of the various types of suturing is the best way to develop the skills of intricate wrist movements and optimal hand-eye coordination that are required for a corneal transplant surgeon.

Periodically, device companies may be invited to bring their corneal transplant instruments and machines to the wet laboratory to encourage residents and corneal fellows to practice newer transplantation techniques, and to learn how to prepare donor tissues for such surgeries.

PRECUT TISSUES

While many surgeons prefer to cut on their own the tissues for lamellar surgeries from whole corneas, eye banks have become very proficient at preparing the precut tissues. Thin, reproducible endothelial grafts can routinely be produced by trained technicians at their respective eye banks without significant concerns for an extended learning curve. This service can reduce perioperative surgical complexity, required surgical paraphernalia and theater times. The consistent preparation of single-pass, ultrathin precut corneas may have additional advantages for surgeons seeking to introduce lamellar techniques.

AUDIT AND OUTCOME MONITORING

An annual audit meeting should be arranged, involving all of the corneal transplant facility staff, in order to monitor the success of transplants performed at the facility, as well as to identify any problems occurring. A computerized database should be arranged, such that data may be easily entered at the time of surgery or follow-up, and so additional time is not required to gather large quantities of data at the end of each year. It is important to specify the indication for each surgery, surgeons involved, type of transplantation, date and time of transplantation, intra- or postoperative complications, and best corrected visual acuities for each clinic visit. In this way, success or problems may be easily highlighted, and changes made to address any issues arising.

It is also essential to send the recipient details, follow-up information and adverse reaction reports to the source eye bank.

Regular staff meetings should be held, involving all of the transplant facility staff, so that the facility may run effectively as a single unit. In this way, any problems arising will be dealt with quickly and efficiently, in order to achieve the best possible outcomes for as many patients as possible.

RECIPIENT FOLLOW-UP INFORMATION

The transplanting surgeon must send postoperative outcomes and recipient follow-up information concerning possible adverse reactions on all eye tissue used for transplantation. Eye banks may request that provision of this, and any additional follow-up information required, is mandatory for the supply of tissue. This information shall include the following (as a minimum):[1]

- Recipient's name
- Date of birth (or year of birth if a precise date of birth is unknown) or age
- Diagnosis, i.e., indication for transplant
- Name of surgeon receiving/transplanting tissue
- Date of surgery
- Location of surgery.

REFERENCE

1. Standards of Eye Banking in India 2020 by National Programme for Control of Blindness and Visual Impairment.

7 Setting Up an Eye Bank

Mukesh Taneja, Rakhi Nathawat, Prashant Garg, Usha Gopinathan

INTRODUCTION

It is estimated that about 100,000 corneal transplants yearly are needed to have a positive effect on the issue of corneal blindness in India. If the average utilization rate is considered an average of 50% based on the global experience, double the collection, i.e., 200,000 corneas, is required. To reach this figure, 50 eye banks are required for the entire nation with each eye bank processing 4,000 corneas annually. With the availability of the trained human resources and required equipment, this is possible ostensibly.

Each of these eye banks should be an autonomous organization, ideally with its own board and governance structure representing all the stakeholders in the community. All the major functions of an eye bank should be carried out, including public awareness, tissue harvesting, tissue evaluation (including serology and microbiology), tissue preservation and tissue distribution. Equitable distribution is key to long-term success, since this builds credibility in the community with all its subsequent benefits. The goal is to make safe and high-quality corneal tissue accessible to everyone who needs corneal transplantation in the community in an equitable manner. Essentially, this means that all those who require a corneal transplant for visual rehabilitation, irrespective of socioeconomic status, gender, religion, or choice of surgeon and institution, should have equal access to the eyes donated to eye banks on a first-come-first-served basis.

There should be one eye bank for every 20 million people, each of which should be linked to 40 eye donation centers (EDC)—eye banking units that are involved only in harvesting corneas.[1] In addition, each eye bank should develop a Hospital Cornea Retrieval Program (HCRP) in 10 major hospitals in the immediate community. Half (2000) of the harvesting should be achieved by the eye bank directly through the HCRP, and the other half (2000) should be through the contribution of EDCs, with 50 eyes (25 donors) from each EDC.

CORNEAL BLINDNESS: CURRENT SCENARIO

As per the National Blindness and Visual Impairment Survey India 2015–2019, the cataract continues to be the primary cause of blindness and responsible for 66.2% of blindness. Corneal blindness emerged as the second important cause of blindness.

The findings of the National Blindness and Visual Impairment Survey India 2015–2019 mention that:

- *Major causes of blindness in population aged ≥50 years*: Corneal opacity (including trachomatous) contributes 8.2%.
- *Major causes of blindness in population aged 0–49 years*: Corneal opacity contributes 37.5%.

EYE BANKING: PRESENT SCENARIO

There are >750 institutional members registered with the Eye Bank Association of India (EBAI). In the year 2019–2020, the total collection was 50,171. On average, each eye bank/EDC collected about 70 eyes in a year, up from 56 in 2013. Only about 250 of these organizations are active, and only about 15 eye banks, i.e., 2% of the 760 organizations, account for >80% of the total collection. About 30 eye banks, i.e., 4% of the 760 organizations, can be classified as full-fledged eye banks. Seven states of India contribute 74% of the total collection.

EYE BANK

An eye bank is a not-for-profit organization that obtains, medically evaluates, and distributes ocular tissue for transplant, research, and education. An eye bank is usually a society or trust registered under the Registrar of Societies Act. The functions of the eye bank are:

- Spread public awareness about eye donation
- Retrieval, preservation, processing, and evaluation of the donor corneas
- Serology testing of the cornea donor's blood sample

- Distribution of the donor corneas as per the waiting list
- Setting up of HCRP at the multispecialty hospitals
- Fundraising for covering the capital and recurring expenses.

EYE RETRIEVAL CENTER/EYE DONATION CENTER

Eye retrieval center/eye donation center (ERC/EDC) is affiliated with an eye bank and its role is to collect corneal tissue and blood sample for serological testing. The main responsibility is to transport the collected corneas safely to the eye bank and have a 24/7 availability of the man power for responding to the cornea collection calls.

The ERC/EDC's responsibility is to ensure the safe transportation of tissue to the parent eye bank and provide a round the clock public response system for eye donation. ERC/EDC work with the families of the cornea donors and hospitals for eye donation and organize the public and professional awareness on cornea donation.

FEASIBILITY STUDY[2]

Before taking the decision to establish an eye bank, a feasibility study must be completed covering the following aspects.

Existing Eye Banks and Eye Donation Centers in the City/Town/Suburban Area

In case the eye bank and EDCs in the area of operations are working satisfactorily, it is not desirable to start a new eye bank. This may lead to unnecessary proliferation and fragmentation of eye banks, which can be counterproductive.

Population of the City/Town/Suburban Area

The other important aspect is the population, as this will give you an estimate of the total potential for eye donation. 1% of the local death rate in the area, as an initial target for eye donation, gives a rough figure for potential in that area.

Multispecialty Hospitals in the City/Town/Suburban Area

Information of the multispecialty hospitals located in the area is essential as the establishment of HCRPs in these hospitals will ensure regular sourcing of corneas. Based on the mortality numbers of the hospitals, they can be classified as high mortality (>300 deaths per month), medium mortality (>100 and <300 deaths per month), and low mortality (<100 death per month). High mortality and medium mortality hospitals will require full-time eye donation counselors, while the low mortality hospitals can be covered through telephonic counseling.

Financial Viability

After determining the feasibility of establishing the eye bank, the next important step is to determine the requirements of setting up the eye bank (**Tables 1 to 3**). Substantial funds for equipment and operations and human resources are required to set up and sustain the facilities.

Table 1: Human resource requirement for eye bank and eye donation center.

	Human resources	
	Eye bank	***Eye donation center***
Panel of ophthalmic surgeons	1 statutory	
Medical director	1 statutory	1 desired
Back up medical director	1 desired	–
Eye bank manager/ administrator	1 desired	–
Recovery technician	1 statutory	1 statutory
Evaluation technician	1 statutory	1 desired
Eye donation counselor	1 statutory	1 desired

DECIDE YOUR LEVEL OF OPERATION

A full-fledged functional eye bank needs staff and facilities to collect donated corneas reliably on a 24-hour basis, space, equipment to evaluate the cornea quality, serology testing facility, and cornea distribution facility. In case the eye bank is situated within hospital premises, the resources may be shared.

However, in districts where some eye banks already exist within a range of transportation facilities, there is another simpler option—eye donation centers.

Eye donation center can be affiliated to the nearby eye banks and perform the supporting role of extending the community's reach of eye banking facilities. The EDC can efficiently focus on spreading awareness, responding to the telephone calls from donor families, and motivating the deceased's family for eye donation in nearby hospitals.

After the cornea recovery, the collected tissue shall be transported to the parent eye bank for testing and distribution. The local doctors and social workers can work together with fewer costs and overhead and fulfil the cornea collection's objective.

EYE BANK PERSONNEL AND GOVERNANCE

Eye Bank Director/Manager

The main aim of the eye bank director is to supervise all the eye bank's policies and procedures. The director/manager is appointed by the eye bank's board of directors. S/he shall be responsible for all administrative operations, including compliance with standards along with day-to-day operation of the eye bank. The director/manager shall work in consultation with the medical directors and shall provide all eye bank personnel with appropriate information to perform their duties in a safe and competent manner. Working with the board of directors eye bank manager also develop strategies for the growth including initiating new programs.

Table 2: Physical space requirement for the eye bank and eye donation center.

S. No.	Requirement	Eye bank	Eye donation center	Area (approximately)
1.	Serology laboratory (limited access laboratory for authorized personnel where blood serum samples are tested)	✓	×	12′× 10′
2.	Tissue processing laboratory (where tissues are evaluated, processed and prepared for packing and distribution, should have space for ultraviolet and laminar flow hood)	✓	×	15′× 10′
3.	Instrument cleaning area (limited access laboratory for authorized personnel where instruments are washed and sterilized)	✓	✓	8′× 10′
4.	Storage area	✓	✓	
5.	Record room (for long-term storage of all the documents)	✓	×	
6.	Administration area (should have a work desk, phone, computer, fax and cabinets)	✓	✓	10′× 10′
7.	Medical director's office	✓	×	10′× 10′

Table 3: Equipment/instrument requirement for the eye bank and eye donation center.

S. No.	Equipment/instrument	Eye bank (all values in INR)	Eye donation center (all values in INR)
1.	Slit lamp (**Fig. 1**)	2 lakhs	×
2.	Specular microscope (**Fig. 2**)	30 lakhs	×
3.	Laminar flow hood (**Fig. 3**)		×
4.	Medical refrigerator (**Fig. 4**)	90,000/-	×
5.	Refrigerator	25,000/-	25,000/-
6.	Autoclave for sterilization	1 lakh	Should have access
7.	Excision/enucleation instrument set	6 sets @10,000 per set	2 sets @10,000 per set
8.	Continuous temperature monitoring device	25,000/-	25,000/-
9.	UPS for electricity back up	50,000/-	×
10.	Computer with printer and scanner	60,000/-	×
11.	Geyser	15,000/-	15,000/-
12.	UV light	15,000/-	15,000/-
13.	Air conditioning	35,000/-	×
14.	Telephone	6,000 (2)	3,000 (1)
15.	Four-wheeler	4 lakhs	Should have access
16.	Two-wheeler	×	50,000/-

Costs are approximate and indicative.

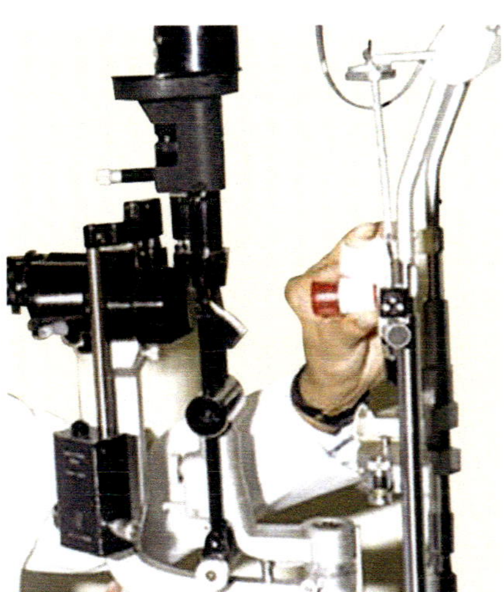

Fig. 1: Slit-lamp biomicroscopy.

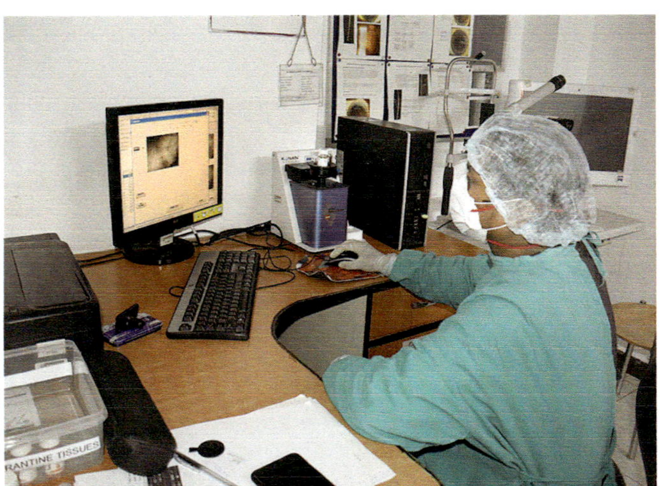

Fig. 2: Specular microscope to analyze the size, shape, and population of endothelial cells in cornea.

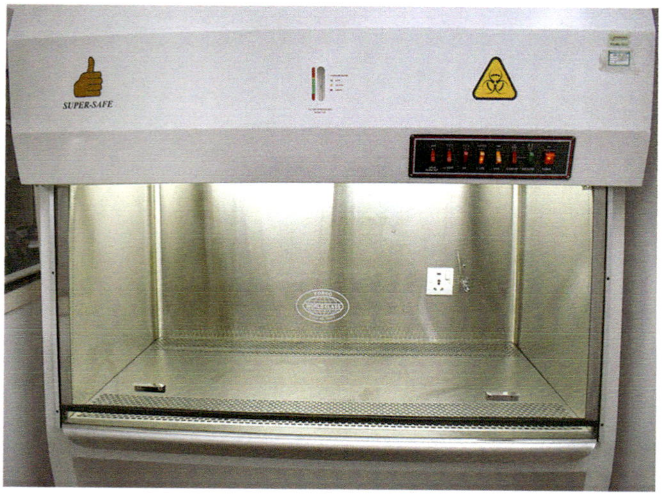

Fig. 3: Laminar flow hood.

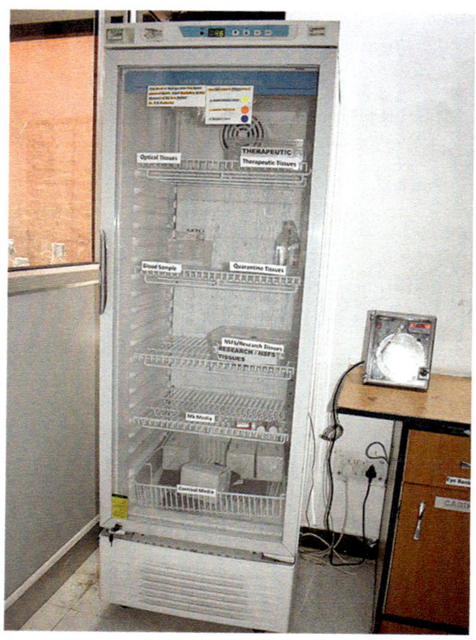

Fig. 4: Medical refrigerator for storage of tissues.

Eye Bank Medical Director

The eye bank must have a full-time medical director. If the medical director is on leave, a back-up medical director shall be designated by the eye bank on an interim basis.

The medical director must be a qualified ophthalmologist with a corneal fellowship or expertise in anterior eye disease, corneal transplantation, research, and teaching in cornea and/or external disease.

The medical director is responsible for overseeing and providing advice on all the eye bank operations' medical aspects. The responsibilities of the medical director are as follows:

- Formulation, approval, and implementation of eye bank policies and procedures
- Participate in training of the eye bank personnel
- Formulation of quality assurance program and periodic monitoring
- Participate in assessing and certification of the competency for tissue procurement and preservation by eye bank personnel.

Technical Staff

It is the responsibility of the director to appoint the technical staff with required skills and education. The director shall ensure that enough staff is available at the eye bank round the clock to perform all eye bank duties. The eye donation counselors shall be hired to timely counsel the next of kin of the deceased in a professional manner.

FINANCIAL ASSISTANCE FOR SETTING UP AN EYE BANK OR EYE DONATION CENTER3

The National Program for Control of Blindness and Visual Impairment (NPCBVI) provides a nonrecurring grant-in-aid for eye banks, which is up to a maximum of ₹4,000,000. The objective of the scheme is to promote eye banking all across the country through government facilities, non-governmental organizations (NGOs), and other stakeholders to procure adequate corneas for corneal transplantation.

Financial assistance: As per the scheme, financial assistance will be provided up to a maximum of ₹4,000,000 for the purchase of equipment and infrastructure.

1. *Eligibility criteria*: Only the eye banks functioning under the public sector are eligible for the scheme.
2. *Infrastructure requirement*:
   Manpower requirement:

Ophthalmologists	1
Eye recovery technician	1
Eye donation counselor	2

3. *Expected output for eye banks receiving nonrecurring grants shall*:
   - Utilize the entire grant within period of 12 months from receipt of the grant after following all necessary steps.
   - Provide and maintain detailed records of corneas collected and utilized in the prescribed format and submit a monthly report to the appropriate authorities.
   - The eye bank shall collect at least 200 corneas in the next 24 months. In case of difficult terrain (e.g., Northeastern states), relaxed standard of 100 cataract operations, together with other eye disease operations, shall be applicable.
4. *Procedure for approval of grants*:
   - The application would be submitted by the applicant eye bank along with necessary documents in support of qualifying criteria to the state program officer (SPO), NPCBVI.
   - The SPO will examine the proposal in terms of eligibility criteria and depute a team of expert(s) (2–3)

from the state to visit the eye bank to assess present facilities and requirements.

The complete process should be finished within a maximum of 3 months from the date of receipt of applications completion. The SPO need to forward his recommendation in the state program implementation plan (PIP) to the competent authority for final disposal.

Nonrecurring Grant-in-aid for Eye Retrieval Centers in Government

As per the scheme, the financial assistance will be provided up to a maximum of ₹100,000 (rupees one lakh only). The support is for the purchase of equipment.

Eligibility criteria for the grant:

- Should satisfy general eligibility conditions mentioned (except the 2-year clause, i.e., new organization can also apply)
- *Minimum requirement of the staff*:

S. No.	Staff role	No.
1.	Ophthalmic technician	1
2.	Eye donation counselor	1

- Required output for EDCs receiving nonrecurring grants shall:
  - Utilize the entire grant within a year from the receipt of grant money.
  - Detailed records of corneas collected and deposited in linked eye bank should be maintained in the prescribed format.
  - Monthly report submission to the District Health Society.
  - The center should be dedicated to collect at least 20 eyeballs/corneas in the next 24 months.

LEGAL REQUIREMENT[4]

As health is a state subject, the legal formalities may differ from state-to-state. As per Section 24(1) of the Transplantation of Human Organs and Tissues Act/Rules (THOTA), 2014, an application for registration shall be made to the appropriate authority as specified in the Form XV of THOTA 2014 for registration of eye banks and corneal transplant center. The application shall be accompanied by the fee applicable to the eye bank registration, payable to the appropriate authority through a bank draft.

For the renewal of registration, Form 17 of the THOTA Act needs to be submitted to the appropriate authorities.[5]

Eye donation centers need not apply for a THOTA registration, however, they must seek a consent from the state health authorities before functioning. They should have the required manpower, infrastructure and documentation and should be affiliated/have a MoU with an accredited eye bank.

REFERENCES

1. Rao GN. What is eye banking? Indian J Ophthalmol. 1996;44:1-2.
2. Guidelines and Project Report for setting up an Eye Bank or Eye Donation Centre, EBAI: 2003.
3. Standards of Eye Banking in India 2020 by National Programme for Control of Blindness & Visual Impairment (NPCBVI).
4. Transplantation of Human Organ Act (THOA), 1994.
5. The Transplantation of Human Organs (Amendment) Act 2011.

8 Accessing Human Corneal Tissue

Heather Machin, Collin Ross

INTRODUCTION

In the Chapter 4 (Eye Banking for Corneal Transplantation), Pollock provides an overview of the day-to-day eye banking practices. In this chapter, we will broaden the discussion by placing eye banking within the global contemporary healthcare context, and provide suggestions to facilitate increased and sustained access to corneal tissue (CT).

Global developments in eye banking and corneal transplantation are a relatively new and emerging area of investigation. As such, the recovery, allocation and distribution of donated CT for transplantation, research, and training, to-date, has been under reported within the human biological, eye bank (EB), and eye care fields. Very little is reported on how an EB allocates, how need is defined and met, how they function within the wider health system, or the economic mechanisms used to support their development, e.g., cost-recovery or for-profit or how CT is moved within complex supply lines from point of donation to point of use. Finally, there has been little reporting pertaining to how an EB interacts with other stakeholders; if and how they engage in the transnational movement (cross-border/jurisdictional import and export); or how EB humanitarian and capacity development processes are implemented. We suspect that this will be a growing field of investigation going forward.

COLLECTING DATA

Data is essential for understanding need, supply, and demand. Eye bankers, distributor-brokers, surgeons, hospitals, and governing agencies must co-manage the collection of data.

There is a dearth of data specifically pertaining to corneal transplantation at the local, national, and global level. A global report, based on 2012 voluntary data, indicated that there was an estimated 12.7 million persons potentially awaiting a corneal transplant,[1] mostly residing in low-middle income locations where there remains limited routine access to an adequate supply of donations. In addition, there is also a lack of consistency and clarity on reporting within the eye care and public health literature that defines need. Without clarity, and further reporting, it is unclear if this figure reported by Gain et al. (2016)[1] has increased, decreased, or remained consistent. We also note that there are no publicly available comprehensive assessment tools to effectively determine global need beyond this estimate.

DETERMINING NEED (DEMAND)

Need, which presents as demand, is determined by collecting and maintaining a transparent comprehensive data set at the local or nation level. Without adequate data, it is very difficult to effectively build corneal and EB services locally and nationally. Data required to determine need include information on recipients already scheduled for surgery, those yet to be scheduled, those requiring a regraft, and those yet to be referred by the primary eye care provider.

Need may be defined based on the provision of a basic minimum set of services, within the confines of available resources (e.g., health system caps). For example, a penetrating keratoplasty may be considered as the basic minimum service need. Additional services may be provided (e.g., endothelial keratoplasty, or precut or preloaded CT options) and may be considered as an extension to basic need. It is important to ascertain logistically, and practically where the base minimum standard rests within the confines of each jurisdiction and the expectations of the health system.

Depending on the location, need may encompass the provision of CT and other donations, for research or training. This can either be provided from donations that are not transplant-eligible or from CT that are recovered with intent for distribution to research and training. In some nations, donation consent requires the confirmation of consent for research and training prior to recovery and distribution. In other nations, recovery intended for research and training may actually be restricted or prohibited by law. Jurisdictions must assess the trade-offs involved in providing transplant-eligible CT for transplantation today or research to help those in the future. To date, there have been few efforts to integrate research and training tissue into the needs concept, and as such, there is no local, national, or global indication of the quantities of eye tissue allocated to these areas of need. In recent times, organizations, such as the Eye Bank Association of America and the American Research and Vision Organization are redefining this space, with the implementation of a research tissue national network program, *EyeFind*[2-4] which connects researchers and clinician-scientists with the participating EB who allocate the donation to the researcher.

Meeting the Need for Donation: Supply

There are two key misconceptions about supply and demand. Firstly, there is a belief that there is a lack of supply of CT. This is not correct. There is an abundance of supply, through the global potential donation of 55.3 million deaths per year.[5] The conversation around supply issues pertains to the lack of dedicated resources, and established services, to educate, consent, recover, allocate, and use the donation. The second misconception pertains to the concept that building an EB, will automatically provide a supply, and need will be met. This is not necessarily the case. Meeting need is dependent on several key factors: (1) The donation, (2) The surgeon, (3) The health system, and (4) The funding avenues. All elements need to be in alignment in order to meet need.

1. *The donation*: Without donors, there are no donation services. Therefore, donation management planning is an essential first step. As donation is also dependent on social, cultural, religious, and general awareness. In some locations, it may take several years to develop routine donation services and a common understanding within populations, regarding the options pertaining to donation. Donation is also dependent on the jurisdictional Tissue Act and Human Right Acts, which inform on the recovery and use of human donations, and on the systems engagement in presumed consent or opt-in donation programs.

   Educating the public, prior to the point of death and donation decision making is also necessary. Information can include: how to become a donor, what one can donate, how the donation is recovered, why it is recovered (describe the need), how it moves within the recovery and supply line, options for donating certain parts of the body, options for donating for transplant, research, and training, and consent for placement within for-profit-lines and/or for exportation. Transparency around how the EB and eye care sector transfers, moves, and uses human donations is necessary to ensure public trust in the EB, and health systems are maintained.

   Pollock in Chapter 4 has already outlined that donor eligibility is an essential feature to determining suitability for donation, however, where someone dies also impacts their donation ability. For instance, if someone dies in a location without an EB coordinator who is trained to recover their donation, then they will not be a donor. Predominantly in industrialized nations, people tend to die or have their body transferred to a health institution, such as a hospital, e.g., in the USA an estimated 80% of people die in institutionalized facilities, (60% acute hospitals, 20% nursing homes)[6] as opposed to dying in the home, which may be preferable to the individual, or as is traditionally favored elsewhere in the world. The institutional setting automatically increases the possibility (by proximity) of someone becoming a donor. Within institutions such as major comprehensive hospitals, where statistically more people are likely to die (e.g., they may house an intensive care unit), there is most likely a specialized donation coordinator (often a trained critical care nurse or counselor) who discusses the option of donation with the deceased's next of kin (NOK).[7] Some donation coordinators will consent the donor and then contact the EB (organ and tissue recovery team if applicable) to commence coordination of the recovery.

   Systems for identifying, screening, and consenting potential donors will vary from jurisdiction to jurisdiction, however, common types of systems include:

   i. Pledge card systems, in which potential donors are self-identified in advance through the submission of a signed pledge card to the governing agency or EB, indicating their desire to donate organs and tissues upon their death. When the donor does pass away, it is hoped that the NOK (or hospital designee) will contact the governing agency/EB, using the information printed on the pledge card, and initiate the donation process. These systems have the advantage of being simple and inexpensive to establish. However, donation rates produced by pledge card systems are generally low, as the system depends upon the donor NOK actually making the call to initiate the donation process at the time of death. If the pledge card is lost, forgotten, or the NOK simply decides not to honor the wishes, then the donation will not occur, and the EB will never have been made aware of the death. In some countries, the pledge is managed electronically on a registry, for example, the Australian government manages a national donation registry, for all organs and tissues.[8] The website is used to indicate intent to donate, rather than as a consent.
   ii. Donor registries are administered by national or state/provincial governments, are a sophisticated system for identifying and consenting potential donors. These registries are generally computerized, allowing ready access to the necessary information

before and during the donation process. In a registry-based donation system, a potential donor can sign up to the registry while still alive, indicating their wish to donate upon their death. In some jurisdictions, the donor actually provides legal consent for the donation when signing up on the registry (this is known as first-person consent). At the time of the donor's death, hospital and EB staffs are able to look up the donor on the registry, verify the intent to donate, and then the EB can proceed to screen the case. The EB can use the information on the registry to contact the NOK to confirm and obtain consent, unless the donor's jurisdiction allows the registry to provide for first-person consent. Having obtained consent, EB staff coordinate the recovery process with the hospital. Registry systems can be highly successful at increasing donation rates, but this success depends upon the development of sophisticated information systems and protocols on the part of the government, hospitals, and the transplant agencies.

iii. Hospital cornea recovery programs (HCRP), in this type of system, an EB donation coordinator works closely with a donor hospital (such as a large general hospital) to obtain information on recent or pending deaths, screen those cases as potential cornea donors, approach the NOK to obtain consent, and coordinates the recovery itself with the hospital. HCRP-based systems have the advantage of increasing donation rates versus pledge card systems, as trained EB staffs are able to have a direct and immediate role in identifying and pursuing likely donor cases. HCRP systems do entail a higher cost, however, mainly due to the need to hire and train a sufficient number of EB donation coordinators. In addition, cooperation between the hospital staff and the EB is absolutely essential to the success of an HCRP.

2. *The surgeon*: Corneal subspecialist training is essential for the effective use of donated CT, and to ensure recipients have the best possible postoperative outcome. As such, corneal training programs are an essential element of meeting need. Training programs, in principle, need to include competency-based training that encompasses: preoperative assessment and diagnosis, surgical performance, tissue handling and cutting techniques, and perhaps most importantly, the long-term postoperative management of transplant recipients. EB need to adapt their supply quotas to accommodate fluctuations in the number of corneal trained ophthalmologists, to ensure their EB services are keeping up with demand.
3. *The health system*: Access to associated health services and professionals is essential.

Firstly, primary eye care services need to effectively identify, triage, and refer forward potential corneal patients. Where cornea patients are not promptly identified and referred by the primary eye care system, this places greater pressures upon the supply of corneas for transplantation due to the effects of late presentation. In many cases, early identification and treatment of corneal conditions may reduce or redirect the need for a cornea tissue, (e.g., they may increase the transplant options for those currently unable to benefit from transplant services, such as making endothelial keratoplasty a more viable option), and may provide better clinical outcomes for the patient.

Secondly, access to operating theaters, pre- and post-operative clinics and finally, a supply of consumables (e.g., instruments, drapes, and antibiotics) for the procedural and postoperative aspects are essential. In addition, EB need access to appropriately trained and equipped pathology services, and materials necessary to confirm the eligibility of a donor and evaluate the integrity of the donation.

Workforce support is also a critical component to effectively developed services, to help meet need. Skill transfer to other professionals, such as nurses, who will free-the-hand of consultants, to perform higher-level intervention, assist in reducing operational backlog[9-11] are one area of effective workforce support. Another is how facilities schedule and how, staff and surgeon time is maximized within limited operating theaters and clinics time, e.g., by turning up on time, developing patient care flows with various healthcare providers, to transition patients through the various pre- and postoperative management phases, and how operating theater or instruments sets are turned-around and ready for the incoming patients.

The EB needs to adapt their supply quotas to meet changing availability of operating theaters and so on. While distribution to eye only facilities may be manageable, the EB needs to be mindful of fluctuating healthcare facility access and staff awareness, when distributing to general hospitals and ambulatory surgery centers. The EB must cultivate working relationships with the transplant facilities to ensure staff and surgeons are educated on CT storage, handing and use.[12]
4. *The funding avenues*: Economic management of donations is necessary.[13] In some nations, governing agencies (e.g., Medicare in Australia) or health insurance agencies, reimburse EB for the cost incurred to recover and provide the donation. Other nations may request the recipient to pay all or part of the fee. These funding avenues fundamentally impact the ability of a nation to work toward meeting their need. In some low-middle income locations or those without routine access to an adequate domestic supply of CT, civil societies (humanitarian agencies) may assist in providing short-term relief for

some immediate recipients, however, this may not necessarily provide long-term relief.

Most Tissue Acts stipulate that profit cannot be derived from the voluntary donation of human tissue and they cannot be sold. As such, those who recover donations must be registered as a not-for-profit organization. These organizations may be affiliated with government, benevolent, or stand-alone facilities. A nonprofit EB organization may be able to charge a fee for its services, or it may charge no fees, and be funded entirely through either government or charitable funding. Preferably, donations should remain in nonprofit supply lines. Some organizations may select to transfer (in exchange for funding) to a for-profit organization who facilitates one or more aspects of the processing, allocation, and distribution. For-profit organizations may be a nonrelated partner, owned by the not-for-profit, or the for-profit may own the not-for-profit. The validity of for-profit and patchwork supply-line models, we describe, remains unclear within the human biologicals field. As such, the general public, donors, healthcare providers, and recipients are relatively unaware of their involvement and impact.

Managing supply and demand is a balancing act[14] and they must move in unison. For example, the lack of supply suppresses demand, with surgeons and hospitals modifying need to match perceived supply. In turn, this impacts the ability of the surgeon, and their assisting staff, e.g., to retain their skills. Therefore, the expansion of EB must go hand-in-hand with surgeon, research and development, and health facility training, and resource expansion.

GUIDING DOCUMENTS AND GOVERNANCE

There are several guidance documents necessary when selecting to engage in the recovery and use of gifted human donations. They inform on sectorial and societal expectations with emphasis on the necessity for transparency and safeguards that simultaneously protect donors, recipients, the donation system, and the healthcare sector.

Firstly, jurisdictions need to be familiar with their Tissue Act and Human Rights Act, and any regulatory requirements. Secondly, global guidance documents including the *World Health Organization's Guiding Principles on human cells, tissue, and organ transplantation* (WHA63.22 2010),[15] the International Council of Ophthalmology's *Position Statement: Donation, Processing, Allocation, Advocacy, and Legislation Supporting Human Corneal Tissue for Ocular Transplant* (ICO 2017),[16] and Global Alliance of Eye Bank Associations', *The Barcelona Principles: An agreement on the use of human donated tissue for ocular transplantation, research and future technologies,* (GAEBA 2018)[17] provide an outline of what is expected of those engaged in accessing, processing, allocating, and using human donations. EB models, design and policy, benefit from adoption of these guidelines.

DOMESTIC ENGAGEMENT

The WHA63.22 (WHA63.22 2010)[15] advocates for need to be met in two stages. Firstly, to meet local need, and secondly, to meet national need. The intent is for domestic supply to service domestic need. These steps are proposed to assist in developing self-sufficient services.

TRANSNATIONAL ACTIVITY

Assuming a nation has met domestic need, then that nation may be in a position to assist others through transnational activity, otherwise termed as exportation and importation practice. To enact such an arrangement, an export nation must establish a relationship with an import nation which has self-identified that they are not meeting need and require assistance. In order for this type of arrangement to be possible, both nations must legally permit the movement of CT across national borders. It is advised that health authorities, regulators, and other peer professional bodies are consulted prior to engagement, to ensure such activity does not undermine or exploit either the export or import nation's ability to develop and maintain self-sufficiency.[18]

Transnational activity requires consideration of the ethical, legal, and economic implications, as well as the appropriateness of the transfer, particularly if CT is requested by expatriate civil societies to conduct voluntary short-visit surgical programs, via engagement of voluntary nonresident healthcare providers who exit the country after performing the surgery. This may place the postoperative recipient in a compromised position, in terms of limited access to postoperative trained physicians and further CT to facilitate further treats such as regrafts.

While transferring CT across-borders may be considered as a logistical, operational procedure, in reality, it is part of the wider health system planning process. Exporters and importers must confirm that permits and approvals have been met, the storage and logistical arrangements guarantee a safe arrival, that the transplant facility has the necessary instruments, consumables, and trained staff, the surgeon is qualified to perform the surgery, and most importantly, that there are qualified physicians to perform the long-term postoperative monitoring of the recipient. Nations must also ensure CT are not sold-onward and are appropriately distributed within clear agreed allocation guidelines. Therefore, tracking and monitoring are essential. In many instances, the export nation is required to track their international donations, as such importers must adhere to those requirements.

Transnational activity commenced in 1961 (King 1964),[19] however, to-date, it is not widely understood. There has been no examination pertaining to donor consent to export, recipient-consent to use imported material, the vetting system of exporters by importers and vice versa, how either nation economically justifies the transfer, and finally, the long-term implications of retaining such as system. Therefore, we propose that transnational activity be approached as a short-term mechanism to assist services, with the intent to review and scale-back periodically, to ensure import nations have the space necessary to develop their own self-sufficient service. Additionally, with the global reported need as 12.7 million,[1] transnational activity, which currently supports 22% of surgical need,[1] is unlikely to be an effective first-line option for most nations. This is especially so when cost, time, and the impact of movement while in transit (which contributes to endothelial cell loss)[20-22] making it difficult to access for many nations.

EVOLUTION OF EYE BANKS

The Eye bank will remain an important component of the healthcare services for some time, and will continually evolve to meet changes in demand. Preventative steps (e.g., corneal cross-linking and public safe-eye-care campaigns) and the emergence of biobanks will also play a dominant role in reshaping how EB function in the future. Biobank repositories in particular, will play a dominant role in research and development of stem cell, tissue engineering, and personalized medicine, however, today, they are reliant on the EB to allocate CT for research.

The emergence of new therapies and technologies within ophthalmology will continue to be a dominant force in the evolution of EB. In the coming years, emerging cellular and tissue-engineered therapies may have the potential to reduce the need for traditional cornea transplantation in the treatment of certain conditions. However, access to these therapies may present issues in both industrialized-economy nations (due to lengthy regulatory approval processes), and emerging-economy nations (due to costs and technological dependencies). At the same time, the EB has been, and will continue, to be a driving force in the development of these same innovations. Many have strong clinical and laboratory expertise (as well as being licensed processing facilities in some nations), with strong relationships with academic medical centers and other innovative practitioners. These qualities often make make the EB ideal partners in the development of new technologies and therapies in the cornea field.

BARRIERS TO ACCESS

While all countries will experience localized barriers, for the purposes of this chapter, we draw attention to several key barriers of global relevance.

Firstly, EB and corneal services do not operate in isolation. They must therefore keep abreast of developments in affiliated sectors and workforces. For example, it is estimated by 2030 that there will be a global shortage of 18 million healthcare workers.[10] This will have devastating consequence on all health services. Strategies to safeguard corneal services from a devastating dearth of these direct health carers require urgent address. Similarly, EB services are reliant on effective pathology and laboratory services, however, such affiliated services are not universally included in infrastructure and capacity development improvement programs.

Training for EB staff is also difficult to maintain due to the subspecialized nature of the niche profession. As such, pathways to employment are not well defined. EB training could be provided in conjunction with other tissues, or through its inclusion within other ophthalmic and healthcare profession training programs (e.g., optometry, nursing, or medical science). This could increase localized recovery groups in locations unable to manage an EB facility. In such an instance, these professionals could recover and transfer the donation to the EB for processing, however such a process requires skillful implementation to ensure the safe and timely passage to the EB processing facility. They also have an interconnected relationship with other donation services, e.g., tissues, artificial reproduction, milk, and organs. EB must foster effective interdonation service relations with these other donation groups as the general public and other healthcare providers may not differentiate between the peer groups. As such, a scandal or change in one area impacts another. For example, in 2014, a kidney allocation scandal in two hospitals in Germany, impacted national donation of CT, resulting in a decrease in domestic donation.[23] Impacted by similar regulations and regulatory constraints and resource limitations, these peer groups could, collectively, contribute to improving governance and policy in their jurisdictions, and develop pathways to improve donation by sharing resources, facility space and experience. While supporting and sharing resources and space is one consideration, such collaborations needs to ensure each human biological is managed separately. This will prevent one donation type (e.g., musculoskeletal) limiting the advancement of another donation type (e.g., CT) and vice versa. Each donation must be managed and resourced, based on the needs of that donation type.

As outlined in the Gain et al. (2016) report,[1] there is a global maldistribution of CT allocation. This indicates that EB and corneal services, globally, are not meeting equitable access to healthcare recommendations. This requires urgent address. Key stakeholders, inclusive of government, civil society, human biological (EB) and eye care providers must merge as one collective advocacy body, to develop and propose reform strategies to effectively influence policy and practice, and assist in transitioning toward a self-sufficient, ethical, safe and transparent EB, and corneal service.

Finally, transparency is a fundamental key element to safeguarding the access to donations for those in need. Barriers to transparency include organizational in-confidence contracts (which protect investor returns within commoditized models), cultural discomfort in sharing experiences and shortfalls which are necessary for transparent practice, and the lack of information available to the public. Without transparency and access to information, the sector cannot effectively evolve, develop appropriate development plans, or meet need or retain donor confidence and trust. All custodians (being the donation hospital/ agency, EB staff, surgeon, transplant hospital) must be transparent in order to effectively inform and safeguard access.

REFERENCES

1. Gain P, Jullienne R, He Z, Aldossary M, Acquart S, Cognasse F, et al. Global survey of corneal transplantation and eye banking. JAMA Ophthalmol. 2016;134(2):167-73.
2. Eye Bank Association of America (EBAA). (2019). EyeFind. [online] Available from: https://www.arvo.org/journals-and-publications/EyeFind/ [Last accessed September, 2021].
3. Association for Research in Vision and Ophthalmology. EyeFind. [online] Available from: https://www.arvo.org/journals-and-publications/EyeFind/ [Last accessed September, 2021].
4. Curcio CA. A New online portal will match eye banks with researchers seeking human ocular tissues. Invest Ophthalmol Vis Sci. 2018;59(12):4796-7.
5. Ecology Global Network. (2019). World Birth and Death Rates. [online] Available from: https://www.ecology.com/birth-death-rates/ [Last accessed September, 2021].
6. Stanford School of Medicine. (2019). Palliative Care. Where do Americans die? [online] Available from: https://palliative.stanford.edu/home-hospice-home-care-of-the-dying-patient/where-do-americans-die/ [Last accessed September, 2021].
7. Machin H, Pollock GA. Eye banking. In: Marsden J (Ed). Ophthalmic Care, 2nd edition. London: M&K Publishing; 2017.
8. Services Australia, Australian Government. (2019). Australian Organ Donor Register. [online] Available from: https://www.humanservices.gov.au/individuals/services/medicare/australian-organ-donor-register [Last accessed September, 2021].
9. Machin H, Vazquez Barrero A, Cosme E, Lansingh V, Marsden J, Raynel S, et al. Keeping trained ophthalmic nurses in eye care, improves services: Lifting the lid on the importance of effective subspecialty nurse rostering. Insight. 2019;44(3):15-20.
10. Britnell M. Human: Solving the Global Workforce Crisis in Healthcare. New York: Oxford University Press; 2019.
11. International Council of Ophthalmology. (2018). ICO Position on Training Teams to Meet Public Needs. [online] Available from: http://www.icoph.org/dynamic/attachments/resources/ico-position-training-teams_1.pdf [Last accessed September, 2021].
12. Eye Bank Association of Australia and New Zealand (EBAANZ). (2016). National guidelines: A resource for Australian hospitals, operating theatres and day surgery staff regarding the handling of human tissue for ocular transplantation. [online] Available from: https://ebaanz.org/wp-content/uploads/2021/05/EBAANZ-NATIONAL-GUIDELINES-2016-For-the-care-and-handling-of-HTO-FINAL.pdf [Last accessed September, 2021].
13. Hanna C. Eye bank finances in the 21st century: Tools to educate leaders for the eye bank of the future. Int J Eye Bank. 2016;4(1).
14. Sanchez Miller C, Abdullayev EE. Science of Comprehensive Eye Banking: Eye Bank Implementation and Operation Essentials. USA; Outskirts Press; 2014.
15. World Health Organization. (2010). WHO guiding principles on human cell, tissue and organ transplantation: Resolution WHA63.22. [online] Available from: https://www.who.int/transplantation/Guiding_PrinciplesTransplantation_WHA63.22en.pdf [Last accessed September, 2021].
16. International Council of Ophthalmology. (2017). Position statement: donation, processing, allocation, advocacy, and legislation supporting human corneal tissue for ocular transplant. [online] Available from: http://www.icoph.org/downloads/ICO%20Position%20Statement%20on%20Corneal%20Tissue%20for%20Ocular%20Transplant.pdf [Last accessed September, 2021].
17. The Barcelona Principles: An agreement on the use of human donated tissue for ocular transplantation, research, and future technologies©. Cornea. 2018;37(10):1213-7.
18. Martin DE, Kelly R, Jones GL, Machin H, Pollock GA. Ethical issues in transnational eye banking. Cornea. 2017;36(2):252-7.
19. King JH. American diplomacy eye to eye. Am J Ophthalmol. 1964;(85):5.
20. Ababneh OH, AlOmari AF. Outcomes of penetrating keratoplasty with imported corneas compared with local corneas. Cornea. 2016;35(9):1211-5.
21. Varssano D, Russ V, Linhart Y, Lazar M. Air transportation of corneal tissue: Experience with local compared to transatlantic donor corneas. Cornea. 2005;24(6):674-7.
22. Wang IJ, Hu FR. Effect of shaking on corneal endothelial preservation. Curr Eye Res. 1997;16(11):1111-8.
23. Röck D, Peterson P, Yoeruek E, Thaler S, Bartz-Schmidt KU, Röck T. Effect of organ scandal on corneal donation rate and organ donors at a German University Hospital. Ann Transplant. 2017;22:425-30.

SECTION

2

Penetrating Keratoplasty

9

Surgical Instruments for Penetrating Keratoplasty

Prakash Chand Agarwal, Rinky Agarwal, Namrata Sharma, Vishal Gupta

INTRODUCTION

The basic instruments for corneal grafting surgery include eye speculum, corneal trephines, needle holders, and a Pierse-Hoskin forceps. However in the recent past, the number of instruments available for corneal grafting has increased considerably. Many of the newer instruments are variations of the earlier designs.

Instruments specific for corneal transplantation surgery *can be divided into four categories:*

1. Instruments designed for optimal globe exposure.
2. Instruments specifically designed to cut the recipient and the donor cornea, such as trephines, punches, and blocks.
3. Instruments used to secure the donor cornea and to remove and replace lens implants such as forceps, scissors, and needle holders.
4. Instruments used to assist in the maintenance and reconstruction of the anterior segment such as cannulae, spatulas, and hooks.

Qualitative keratometers used intraoperatively to assess the corneal toricity.

The suitability and selection of instruments for corneal transplantation is based primarily on specific surgical technique, surgeon's preference, and the expertise.

INSTRUMENTS FOR GLOBE EXPOSURE

Eye Speculum

The transplant surgeons must have several speculums available in order to meet the needs of the various different anatomic configurations frequently encountered. The speculum should be light in weight, has minimum extraneous parts and avoid undue pressure over the globe which can increase intraocular pressure or distort the cornea (which can result in increased postoperative astigmatism). A wire lid speculum such as Barraquer eye speculum (**Fig. 1A**) or Kratz-Barraquer eye speculum is ideal for most cases. Barraquer eye speculum has open 14 mm blades and the blade spread is 20 mm. Eye specula used in children are of small size and tend to offer slightly less resistance to compression. The pediatric Barraquer eye speculum is open 11 mm of blade and the blade spread is 19 mm. Adjustable speculums contain a guard or a locking mechanism with a screw, by which the width of the open end of the speculum can be varied (**Fig. 1B**). The examples include Lieberman eye speculum (17 mm open blades and straight shaft, also available in pediatric sizes) Knapp eye speculum, Castroviejo eye speculum, etc. This is in contrast

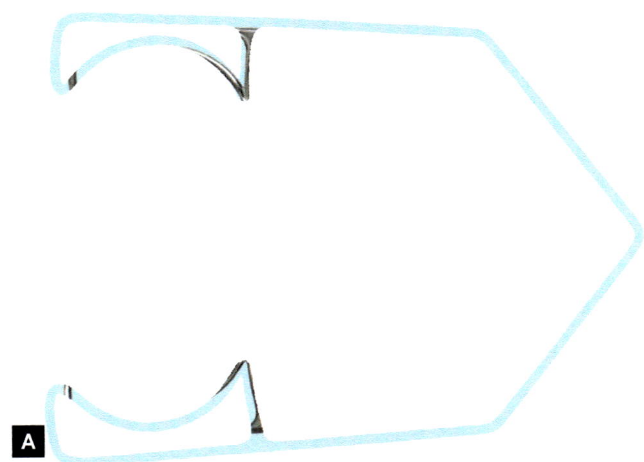

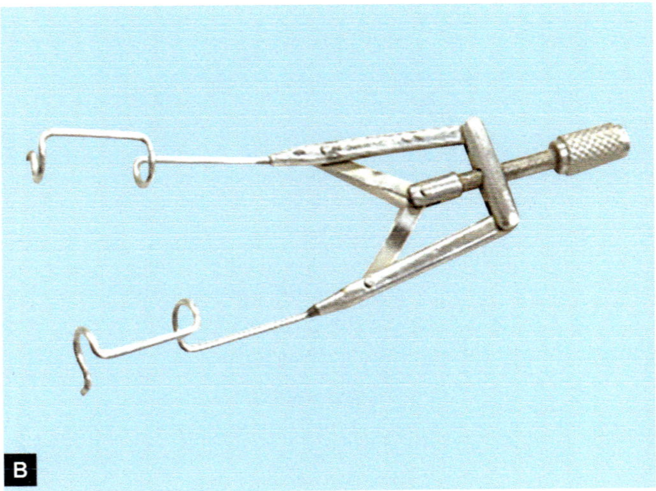

Figs. 1A and B: (A) Wire speculum; (B) Adjustable speculum.

to nonadjustable variety that usually function on a spring mechanism. Although adjustable speculums are self-retaining and provide a controlled lid retraction, these may raise the intraocular pressure by exerting extra pressure on the lids.

Globe Supporting Rings

The *Flieringa ring* (**Fig. 2**) is made of stainless steel and useful for maintaining the architecture of the globe once the host corneal button has been removed. Although, they are available in 11 sizes from 12 to 22 mm, the most commonly used sizes are the 17 and 18 mm. Use of globe supporting Flieringa rings has been advocated in aphakic eyes especially where vitrectomy has been performed, pseudophakic eyes and pediatric eyes as the eyeball has a tendency to collapse in these cases after the trephination. However, many surgeons do not choose to use these rings as they may transmit unequal traction forces to the host cornea.[1] This may distort the shape of the eyeball and cause an oval cut during trephination and subsequent high astigmatism. Occasionally subconjunctival hemorrhage may also occur while suturing these rings to the conjunctiva. *McNeill-Goldman ring* (**Fig. 3**) provides support with four strategically placed sutures. The ring features medial and temporal openings for greater access to the surgical field and two lid retractors to prevent eyelid closure by the patient. It is available in three sizes—(1) small, (2) medium, and (3) large.

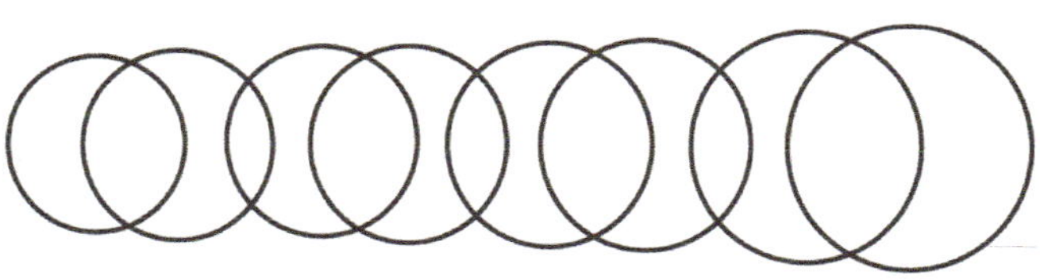

Fig. 2: Flieringa ring.
Courtesy: Katena products.

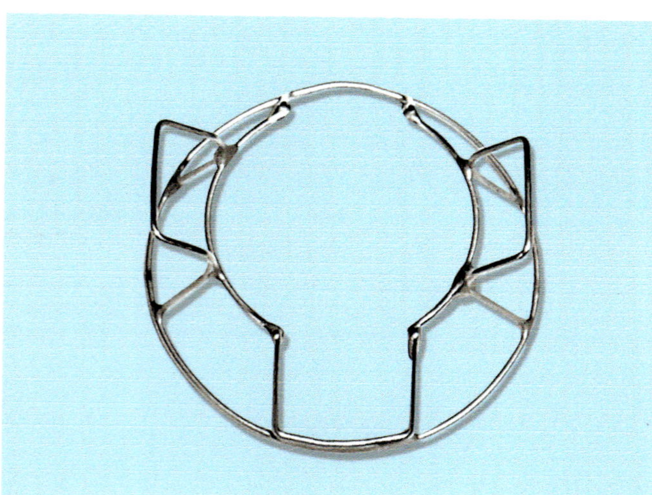

Fig. 3: McNeill–Goldman ring.
Courtesy: Katena products.

Corneal Marking Instruments

Castroviejo calipers (**Fig. 4**) are commonly used to measure corneal diameters immediately before surgery. These are portable dividers like instrument with one fixed arm that is attached to a graduated curved scale in millimeters and another movable arm. By accurately measuring the corneal diameter and the dimensions of corneal opacity/lesion, these guide selection of appropriate size of trephine during keratoplasty.

Various instruments like the radial keratotomy marker and the Vajpayee corneal marker (**Fig. 5A**) stained with gentian violet can be used to mark the donor cornea to aid in the optimal placement of the sutures in keratoplasty (*see* **Fig. 4**). Vajpayee corneal marker consists of 20 radial arms which guide the placement of the single continuous suture bites. Anis corneal marker (**Fig. 5B**) with 8 marks is also commonly used to guide the initial sutures.

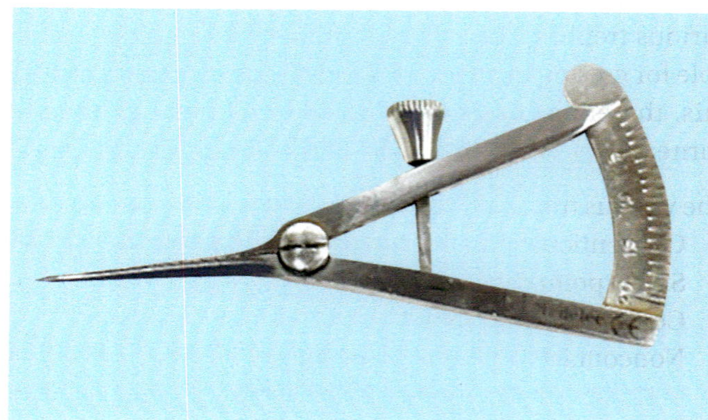

Fig. 4: Castroviejo calipers.

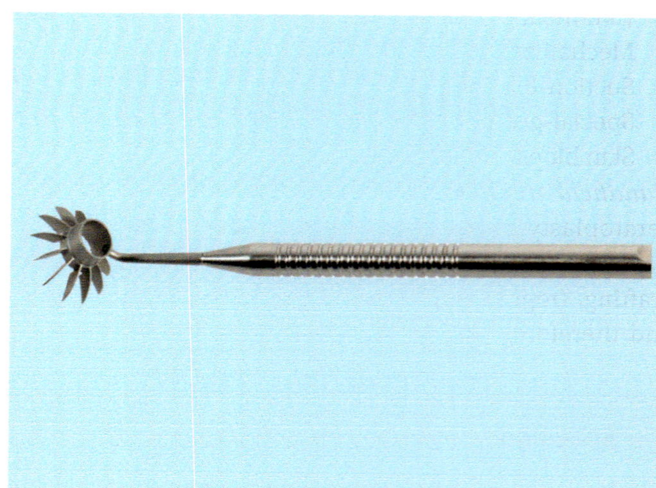

Fig. 5A: Vajpayee corneal marker.

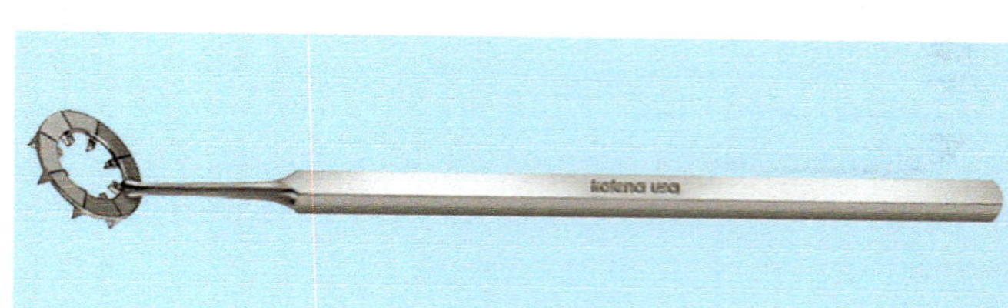

Fig. 5B: Anis corneal marker.
Courtesy: Katena products.

CORNEAL TREPHINES

A trephine is a stainless, sharp, cylindrical blade, which when used, creates a circular corneal incision (*see* **Fig. 4**). An ideal trephine is one that produces a sharp vertical cut without causing too much damage to the corneal tissues. The most common complication of corneal transplantation is postoperative astigmatism. A poor quality trephine may contribute substantially to the occurrence of this problem. It is important to have an ideal trephine that achieves the most accurate and reproducible cuts. Some trephines are available with handles to get a firm grip while cutting the corneal button (**Fig. 6**).

Types of Trephines

These may also be classified depending upon whether the host cornea or the donor button has to be cut. There are various trephines and trephination systems that are available for cutting the recipient and donor cornea. Apart from this, the endothelial punches are used to cut the donor cornea.

The various trephines are of following types:
- Conventional circular cutting trephines
- Single point cutting trephines
- Combination trephines
- Noncontact trephines (lasers)

Conventional Circular Trephines

There are five types of circular trephines:
1. Handheld
2. Mechanized
3. Suction-fixation type
4. Special-purpose type
5. Skin biopsy punches

Handheld trephines: Since the advent of microsurgical keratoplasty many modifications have occurred in the trephines over a period of time.[2-5] In the early era of corneal grafting, trephines did not have disposable cutting edges and therefore, required continual resharpening. This led to change in the original circular shape over a period of time, thus distorting the shape of the graft. Handheld circular disposable trephines remain the most commonly used trephines to cut *both the recipient and donor corneas*, particularly in the developing world. The handheld trephines are available in sizes ranging from 3 to 17 mm. The trephine is usually attached to a handle for greater stability, leverage, and control. The handle helps in securing the trephine and confers a mechanical advantage over simply holding the trephine blade by hand. The trephine handle may have a hollow core so as to allow observing the central cornea through the center of the trephines. In some trephines, there is a central obturator, which can be adjusted to select the depth of the corneal cut and hence an inadvertent entry into the anterior chamber can be avoided (**Fig. 7**). The handle of the obturator trephine offers a distinct advantage over the hollow core in allowing a fairly accurate depth measurement. However, the obturator does not allow the surgeons to view the central cornea through the trephine during its use. This may result in inaccurate centration during the trephination of the recipient's cornea.

The examples of handheld trephines with obturator are the *Castroviejo trephine* and the *Grieshaber-Franceschetti trephine*. The disadvantage of both the hollow core and the obturator type of handle is that each size trephine must be matched to the handle size and hence different handles are required to accommodate different trephine sizes. Hence, "Universal trephine" handle which accommodate various blade sizes was advocated. The advantage of this type of handle is that this single instrument will secure trephine sizes used in majority of cases. However, the disadvantage is that it is neither hollow for optimal visualization nor does it provide protection against inadvertent entry into the anterior chamber.

To overcome the problems of visualization associated with the obturator, certain trephine blades have been made long and can be easily grasped with the hand for a successful trephination both of the recipient cornea and the donor button. These *disposable trephines with long handle* do not

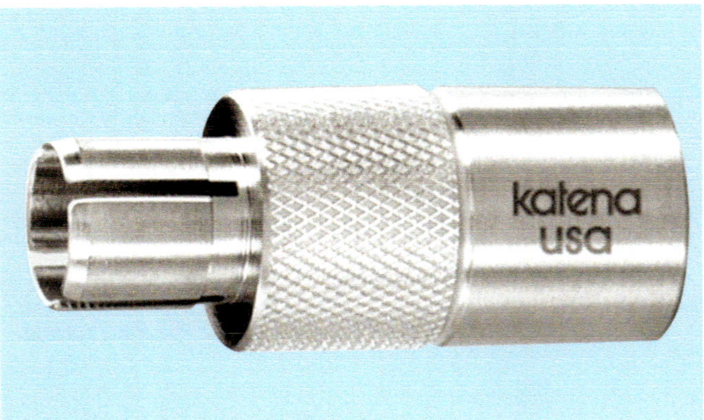

Fig. 6: Trephine handle.
Courtesy: Katena products.

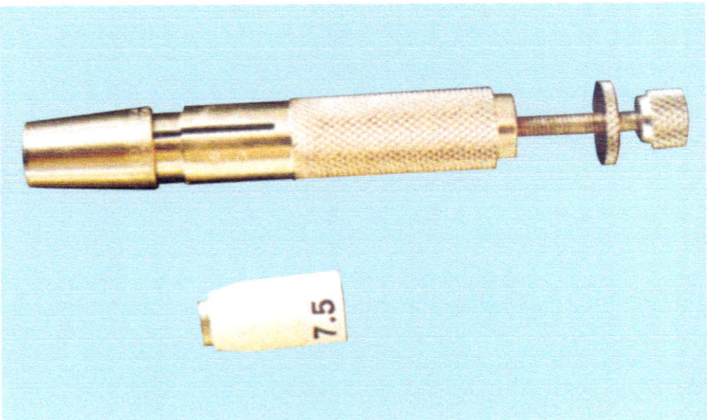

Fig. 7: Top—obturator-guided conventional circular trephine. Bottom—conventional circular, disposable trephine.

have provision for the obturator. These handheld trephines are disposable and made of razor blade and are see-through, easy to use and economical. However, the cut may be uncontrolled and there may be difficulty in centration. Additionally, the slippage of the trephine may lead to an uneven cut.

Mechanized corneal trephines: The cutting blade of this type of trephine is driven by a motor present in the main body. A circular trephine attached at the motor shaft end permits anterior chamber entry without damaging the intraocular structures. Some mechanized trephines make the use of limbal suction ring to assist in anterior chamber maintenance and protection during trephination. Microkeratron (Hans Geuder, Heidelberg), a commonly used mechanized trephine is used to *trephine recipient cornea* and it permits variation of rotation speed and has rapid braking within 0.1 second.

The disadvantages associated with motor driven trephines include corkscrew edge effect in the corneal stroma. However, less stromal disruption and a smoother interface has been reported with the use of a Microkeratron trephine (Hans Geuder, Heidelberg) which moves at the rate of 800 rpm in comparison to the manual trephines.[2]

Suction fixation corneal trephines: These trephines have been devised to obtain a perpendicular cut in the *recipient cornea*. These trephine systems essentially consist of an outer corneal suction ring for fixation and an inner circular cutting blade. Hessburg–Barron trephine is a prototype of this system (**Figs. 8A to C**). In Hessburg–Barron vacuum trephine, a spring-loaded disposable syringe creates the required negative pressure and the suction fixation provides the stability and an opportunity to cut perpendicularly to the limbal plane and hence diminishes the tilt of the trephine.[6] The newer model of this trephine includes the presence of a cross hair device for improved centration and an outer ring of corneal marks at equal intervals to assist in suture placement. The Barron radial vacuum trephine is available in diameters of 6.0–9.0 in 0.5 mm increments as well as diameter of 7.75 mm. For each spoke (90°) turned, the blade is lowered or raised approximately 0.06 mm. These trephine systems are used to trephine the host cornea. Its advantages are relatively low cost, consistency of the cut, control of depth, disposability and it is particularly useful for performing corneal grafting surgery in extremely soft and perforated eyes.[7] The Hessburg–Barron trephine appears to improve the accuracy of the cut. However, this trephine has a tendency to undercut and in the event of loss of suction during trephination, it can cause an asymmetrical cut. The vacuum fixation ring may also lead to endothelial damage.[8] The *Barron vacuum punch* features a solid stainless steel blade which is permanently mounted in a nylon housing. Four steel guide posts align with four corresponding holes in the cutting block base, automatically centering the blade over the donor cornea. The base of the punch features a circular groove for aspirating the epithelial side of the cornea, immobilizing it for cutting the button. The cutting block well has four small holes which can be inked with a sterile marking pen to identify the four quadrants of the cornea for cardinal suture alignment in the recipient bed.

The Olson calibrated cornea trephine system is a precise, reproducible trephine that can be used to trephinate *both the donor and recipient corneas*. The system consists of the anterior chamber maintainer, the reusable blade holder (with micrometer setting), and the suction ring. One revolution of the micrometer is equivalent to 500 μm. The trephine should be fully rotated at least three times to achieve a complete cut for penetrating keratoplasty. If planning a partial depth incision, select the desired depth by turning the micrometer, and tighten the set screw. To cut the donor tissue the anterior chamber maintainer is prepared. A small drop of viscoelastic is placed on the endothelium of the donor tissue and the donor cornea is centered onto the anterior chamber maintainer (epithelium-side up). The trephine is centered

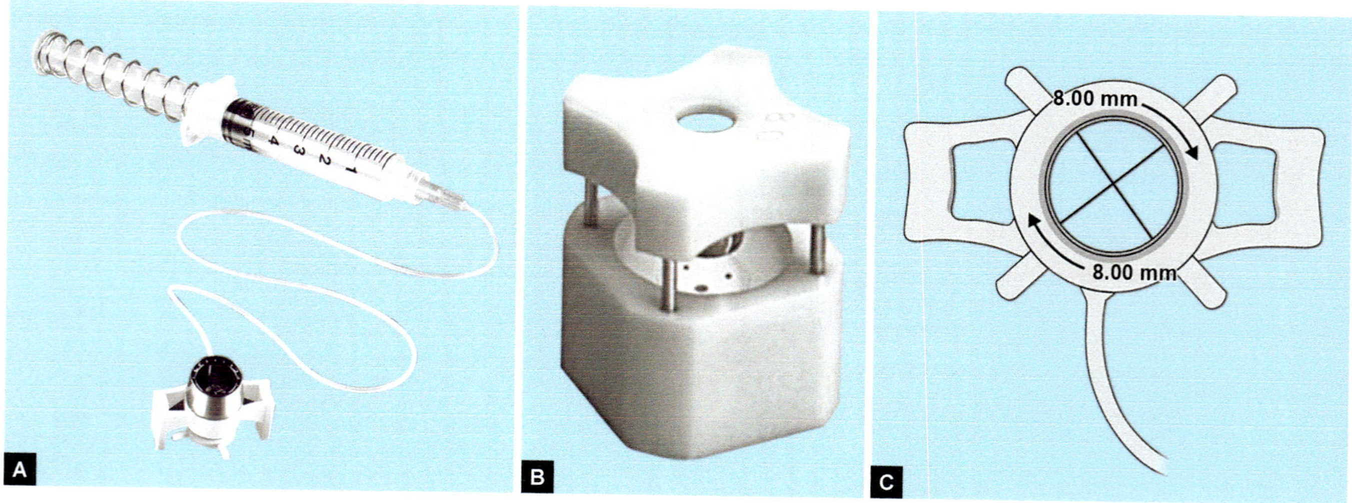

Figs. 8A to C: (A) Hessburg–Barron trephine; (B) Barron punch; (C) Trephine bottom view.
Courtesy: Katena products.

on the patient's cornea and releasing the syringe activates the suction. While holding the suction ring, the top of the trephine is turned to complete the cut. Using a different blade size, the recipient cornea can also be cut similarly.

After obtaining the donor button, it is placed in a graft holder (Paton spatula) (**Fig. 9**) over a viscoelastic and is kept covered till the recipient dissection is complete. Paton's spatula is a double-ended instrument with a 15 mm flat spatula at one end (that is angled 8 mm from tip) and a curved 6 mm teardrop-shaped spoon with three long openings at the other end. The spoon end is designed to snugly hold the donor button as openings in it drain excess viscoelastic substance and prevent slippage of the donor. The flat end aids in repositing iris and breaking iris adhesions. A trephine block can be used to cut the donor cornea from endothelial side (**Fig. 10**).

Special purpose trephines: These trephines are particularly useful to perform a transplant in cases of optical zone lacerations in the *recipient cornea*. This instrument helps in integrating two separate surgical procedures, that of initial repair and later transplantation into one. The lacerated cornea is supported from behind by protective plate, placed in anterior chamber and this avoids injury to the lens and iris during trephining. An upper plate is present above so that the cornea is securely placed between the two plates. The trephine then descends along the vertical shaft so that a circular cut is made without the underlying damage to the iris or the lens.

Skin biopsy punches: The skin biopsy punches, which have been used in dermatological practice, are especially useful in harvesting of small patch grafts used for tectonic purposes in cases of impending/frank perforation. These can be used for *both donor and recipient corneas.* The sizes of the most commonly used punches vary from 2.0 to 5.5 mm (**Fig. 11**). Additionally, a *Searcy chalazion trephine* 2.5 or 3.0 mm in size may be used to punch the patch grafts.

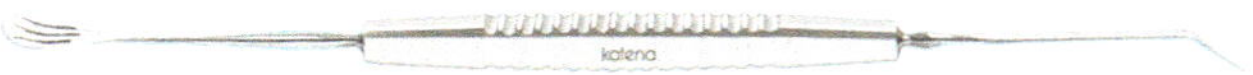

Fig. 9: Paton spatula.

Single Point Cutting Corneal Trephines

The single point cutter trephines were designed to decrease corneal torsion. In these trephines, fixation takes place at the limbus or on the sclera thereby reducing the corneal distortion. *Lieberman single point cutter* belongs to this class of trephines. It is composed of two cones. The outer cone is held by the fixation hand and contains the suction ring. The inner cone revolves and carries a disposable razor blade knife and is capable of making circular and oval perpendicular cuts with diameters of 2–8.5 mm. For 20° angle cuts, an interchangeable cutter may be used for lamellar cuts. This trephine can be used only on the eyeball for *trephining donor and recipient corneas.* As compared to other available trephines, single point corneal cutters do provide superior visibility under the microscope, the least distortion and potential for reproducible controlled cutting.

Combination Corneal Trephines

Over the period of time, new trephines have come up, that combine the best features of the previous trephines. *Hanna trephine system* has got a circular razor-cutting blade and incorporates many of the salient features of single point cutting trephines (**Fig. 12**).[6] This assembly can be used to trephine the *recipient as well as preserved donor cornea* since it has an artificial chamber maintainer system. It consists of two parts: (1) a limbal suction ring system and (2) a mechanical trephine fitted with a suction ring. The suction ring helps fixating the trephine perpendicular to the cornea. A preset depth of cut is selected and by rotation of the gear system, a cut of desired depth is obtained. Once the desired depth is reached, there is no further descent of the blade despite

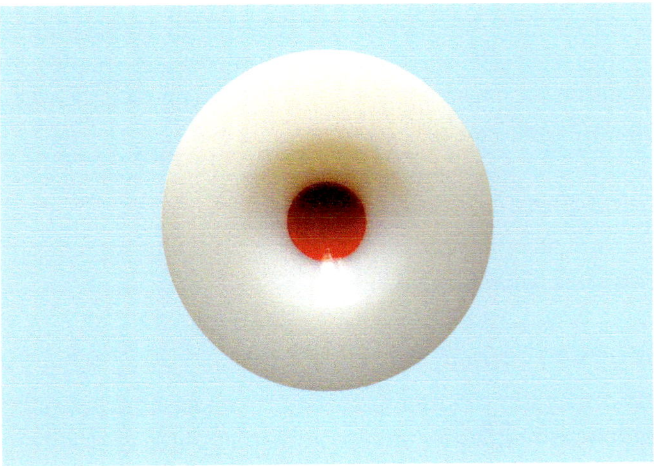

Fig. 10: Teflon block.
Courtesy: IOWA press.

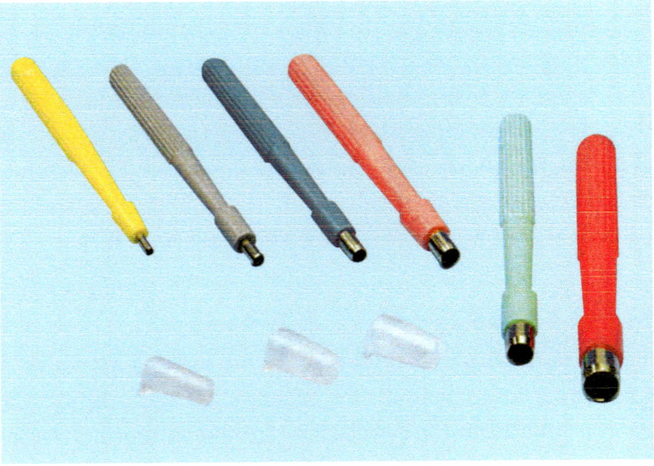

Fig. 11: Skin biopsy punches.

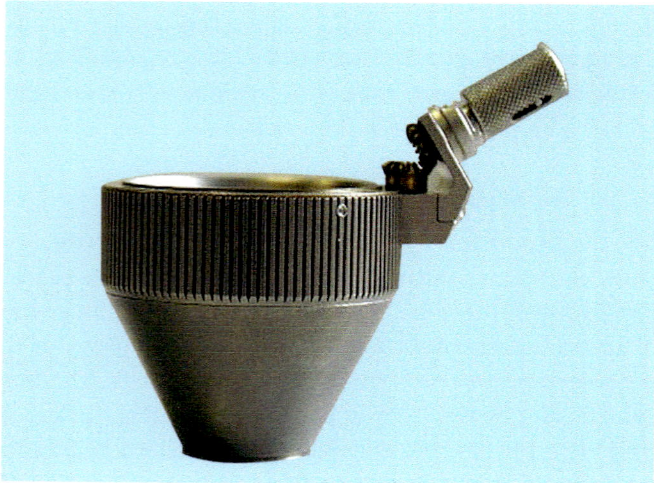

Fig. 12: Hanna's trephine.
Courtesy: IOWA press.

continued knob rotations. The Hanna vacuum trephine tends to produce less undercutting and smaller epithelial diameter than the Hessburg–Barron trephine.[6] Both the systems produce greater final graft curvature than the handheld trephines although there was no significant difference in the final keratometric results between the Hessburg–Barron trephine and the Hanna's trephine. Although better visual acuities were reported in patients who underwent keratoplasty with the Hanna trephine system compared with Hessburg-Barron trephine, the postoperative keratometric, and refractive astigmatism were not significantly different.[9] *Guided trephine system (GTS)* is another trephine system but with a different characteristic suction ring design. It uses a fixed glass obturator for corneal support and the cornea is trephined in an applanated state and thus enhances the perpendicularity of the corneal cuts.

Noncontact Trephines

They have got distinct advantages over other trephine systems in providing complete visualization, better centration, and eliminating the corneal topographic distortion. *Laser noncontact trephination eliminates* corneal topography distortion, provides the visualization of the entire cornea, and enhances centration. Comparative studies between mechanical and laser trephination with 193 nm reveal that there is no difference in the immunologic reactions following penetrating keratoplasty.[10] However, several concerns regarding endothelial injury, mutagenicity, and cost regarding use of these techniques remain.

GAUZE PIECE FIXATED EYEBALL

Gauze piece fixated eyeball can be used especially in developing countries where preservation techniques may not be available and the eyeball is stored in a moist chamber at 4°C.

EYE GLOBE FIXATION

Tudor Thomas Stand

The Tudor Thomas stand is used to fixate the whole eye globe prior to trephination. The whole eye globe is positioned in the Tudor Thomas stand and the trephination can be done both for full thickness as well as lamellar grafts.

CUTTING BLOCKS

The various cutting blocks available for corneal grafting are paraffin block, Teflon block, and polycarbonate and nylon blocks.[10,11]

An ideal cutting block attempts to approximate the corneal shape and reduces the tissue distortion. Previously, early models of blocks used to consist of different concavities of simple radius of curvature. But now, Teflon blocks with different radius of curvature are available. The available cutting blocks are as follows:

- *The Kaufmann corneal cutting block*: This is the simplest design which consists of a Teflon block with metal cover (*see* **Fig. 10**).
- *The Brightbill polytef cutting block*: This modern, compound curved block approximates the central, midperipheral, and peripheral curvature of donor. The Brightbill polytef cutting block uses three wells, each with a different radius of curvature and diameter. Two concentric inlays of colored polytef are present. The outer black polytef zone has a chord length of 12.5 mm and corresponds to the limbus and a second white polytef inlay with an 8 mm chord length corresponds to the central zone of the donor cornea.

Slippage of the moist donor cornea at the time of cutting can cause oval graft. This can be prevented by repeated drying of the well in which the donor is placed or by using a thin, slightly moistened layer of cotton in the well.

Corneal Endothelial Punches

To cut a donor button from endothelial side corneal punches are also available which use disposable trephine blades. The advantage of corneal punch is that they yield sharp vertical cuts without beveling.[8]

Cottingham Corneal Punch

It is a metal punch with a universal style handle. Additionally, it also has two replaceable base plugs.

Troutman Corneal Punch

It incorporates a centered block and a piston carrier with a central piston. The piston accommodates blades of 7–9 mm. This relies on the surgeon's thumb to incise the cornea.

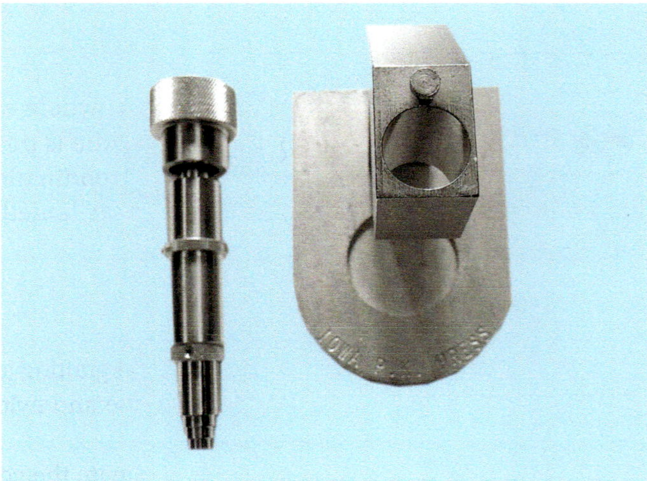

Fig. 13: IOWA PK press corneal punch.

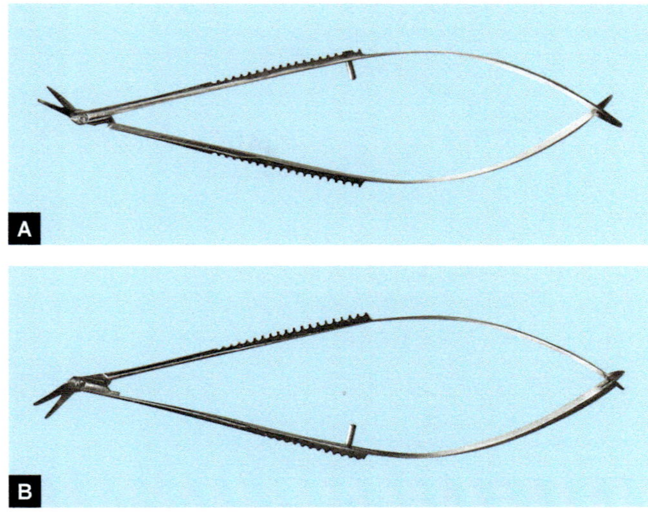

Figs. 14A and B: (A) Right Troutman scissors; (B) Left Troutman scissors.
Courtesy: Katena products.

IOWA PK Press Corneal Punch

It incorporates a spring-loaded piston with an expandable edge to accommodate 6–9.5 mm trephines to harvest various sizes the donor graft from the endothelial side. It has a unique two-color cutting block which aids in centration of the donor tissue. The recessed base assumes that the block is held centrally under the trephine block (**Fig. 13**).

Lieberman Gravity-action Punch

It is a guillotine-style punch with a heavy head, which uses the force of gravity rather than the surgeon's hand to punch the cornea.

Rothman–Gilbard Corneal Punch

It uses a piston which is not spring loaded. The suction block has eight evenly spaced suction holes which anchor the corneal button firmly so that there is minimal movement during trephination. The button has eight precisely placed marks and can be sutured into the host bed by suturing every mark on the button with the marks placed on the host bed.

There are four trephine assemblies, which use artificial anterior chamber. These include (1) Krumeich, (2) Hanna, (3) Olson and (4) Lieberman systems. This involves cutting the donor corneas from the epithelial side rather than the endothelial side. Pressure in the artificial anterior chamber is adjusted to the intraocular pressure with the help of attachments of the infusion tubings.

CUTTING INSTRUMENTS

Blade Breaker

A disposable razor blade is broken and mounted on the tip of a metallic pencil handle. This is one of the best instruments available for cutting tissues in straight or curved lines. Blade breaker is used to enter the anterior chamber in a controlled manner after a deep cut has been created in the recipient's cornea by a trephine. Blunt side of the blade can sometimes be used for blunt dissection of adherent iris. A microvitreoretinal blade can also be used for making a stab wound for initial intracameral entry.

Diamond Knife

This is the sharpest cutting instrument and available in various sizes and shapes. It is the most durable instrument and useful for stab incisions as well as to complete the trephine cuts.

Corneal Scissors

Ideally, all corneal scissors should have an immobile lower blade. Troutman microscissor (**Figs. 14A and B**) is the prototype, which has blades 5 mm in length and is curved on a radius of 5 mm. The lower handle, which controls the upper blade, has a flexible spring. This is a very light and fine scissors and mainly used to complete the cutting of the trephine incision. The blades should be kept vertical and must be curved to follow the curvature of the trephine, while cutting the host cornea. It is often used to remove the irregular tags from the wound margin. Corneal scissors are used to complete the trephination of the host cornea after creation of the circular cut following anterior chamber entry. Curved Vannas scissors can also be used for the same (**Fig. 15**).

Tenotomy/Conjunctival Scissors

These are used for delicate dissection, cutting and undermining of the conjunctiva, especially in eyes with shallow palpebral apertures due to conjunctival adhesions, symblepharon, and ocular surface disorders. Westcott tenotomy scissors have stout, yet lightweight handles with a spring mechanism and can have straight or curved blades

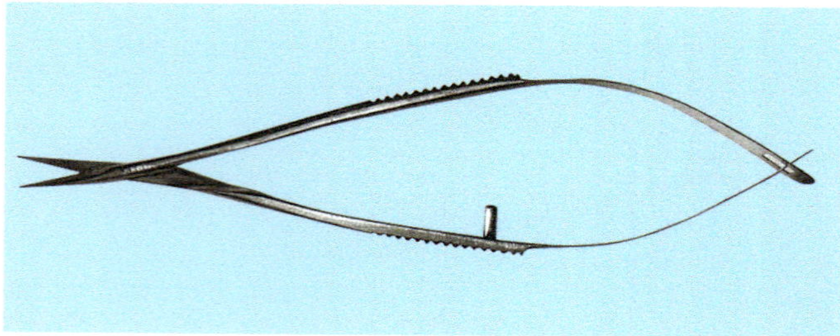

Fig. 15: Curved Vannas scissors.
Courtesy: Katena products.

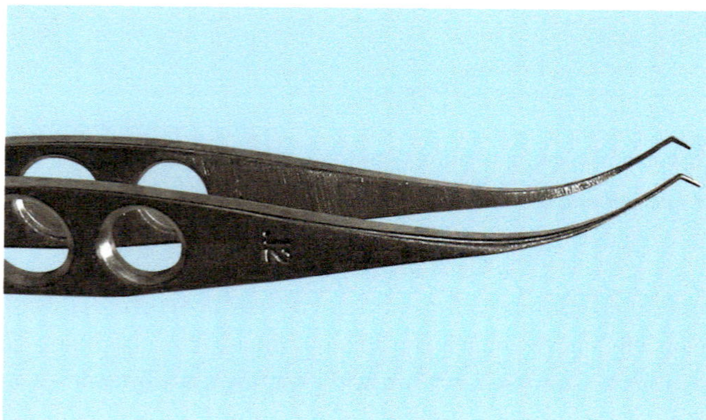

Fig. 16: Colibri forceps.
Courtesy: Katena products.

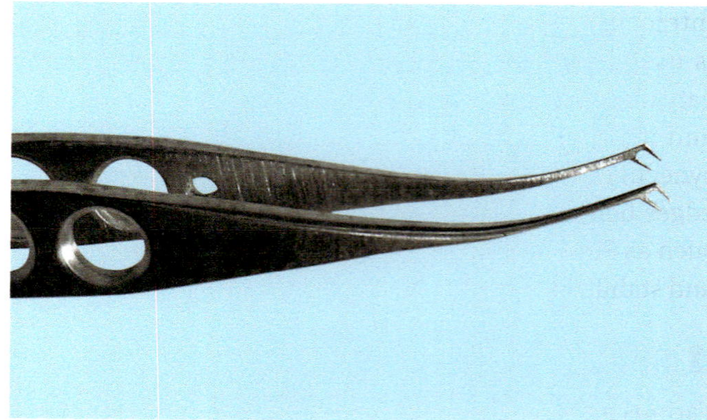

Fig. 17: Polack forceps.
Courtesy: Katena products.

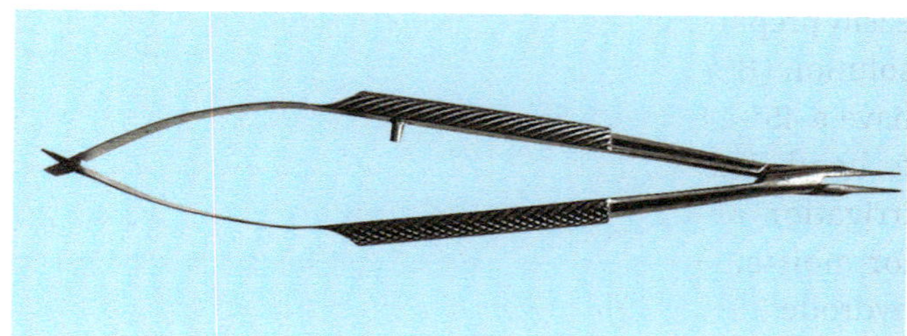

Fig. 18: Titanium needle holder.
Courtesy: Katena products.

with sharp or blunt tips. Stevens tenotomy scissors are ring type and have long handles with straight and curved blades with a blunt tip. The blunt tip helps in protecting the underlying and surrounding structures.

De Wecker's Iris Scissors

These are fine scissors with right-angled blades that are maintained in V-shape due to spring action. The right-angled configuration of the blades minimizes the trauma to surrounding tissue alongside providing a better field of vision. The scissors are slightly larger than the Vanna's scissors and are commonly used to perform iridectomy, and iridotomy, and to severe any prolapsed vitreous surgery.

GRASPING INSTRUMENTS

Varieties of forceps are used for penetrating keratoplasty. However, they can be broadly classified into toothed, nontoothed, or forceps used for special purposes.

Toothed Forceps

- *Pierse-Hoskin forceps*: It is a fine toothed tissue holding forceps and used to hold the corneal tissue firmly. Pierse-Hoskin forceps is the most frequently used tissue holding forceps in corneal grafting surgery. It is a 2 × 1 fine toothed lightweight instrument and extensively used for suture tying.
- *Colibri forceps*: This is another example of tissue holding forceps (**Fig. 16**).

Nontoothed Forceps

The nontoothed forceps have flat edges that help in holding or picking up structures like 10-0 nylon suture. McPherson forceps is the prototype of this variety. It can be used for suture tying and to bury the suture knots.

Forceps with Special Functions

- *Double corneal forceps, Colibri style*: It has two 2.75 mm long tips separated 1 mm with 0.4 mm Pierse tips. It is 72 mm long and has a serrated handle.
- *Colibri-style Polack double corneal forceps*: It is used for the first corneal suture. The cut edge of the graft is gently grasped at the junction of the epithelium and stroma with fine toothed forceps (**Fig. 17**).

HOLDING INSTRUMENTS

Needle holders used in ophthalmic microsurgery consists of two handles, which are supported between index finger and thumb. Needle holder (**Fig. 18**), which is lightweight, with nonslip curved handle and curved jaws is preferred for penetrating keratoplasty. The curvature of the jaw varies from a uniform smooth to a hockey stick shape. The jaws should be atraumatic to the steel needles but the grip should be firm. Barraquer's curved needle holder is an example.

SPATULAS AND HOOKS

These are mainly used in the reconstruction of the anterior chamber, the manipulation of the iris, and assistance in intraocular lens placement. A double-ended iris repositer is useful for lysis of synechiae between the iris and lens capsule, dissection of iris from retrocorneal membranes and iris supported implants, lysis of broad-based anterior synechiae, and sweeping the donor tissue to undermine its edges below the host tissue. Intraocular lens manipulators such as Sinskey and Lester hooks are very useful for placing and stabilizing an anterior chamber lens.

IRRIGATION AND ASPIRATION CANNULAS

Various instruments can be used for irrigation and aspiration of retained cortical matter or viscoelastic substance in the anterior chamber.[11,12]

Disposable 30G cannulas are cost-effective and can be easily prepared by mounting a 30-G needle on a balanced salt solution (BSS) syringe (**Fig. 19A**). These metallic cannulas have a 45°-angled tube, a blunt tip, and are 5 mm from tip to bend. These can be used for performing intracameral irrigation and aspiration and air/medications injection, for moistening the corneal surface, for hydrodissection/hydrodelineation during concomitant cataract extraction, and for wound hydration at the end of the procedure. Separate hydrodissection (23–30G, 32°-angled shaft, 8 mm from bend to tip, with flattened smooth oval-shaped tip) and viscoelastic cannulas (23–27G, blunt tip, 11 mm from bend to tip) are also available. Simcoe's irrigation-aspiration cannula (**Fig. 19B**) has a 15 mm long hollow metallic tube with a 0.3 mm diameter aspiration port, and a 21–23G front opening irrigation port. Aspiration of viscoelastic substance, cortical material or exudates/hypopyon is undertaken through a tubing hub attached to a 2–5 mL syringe, while intracameral irrigation is ensured through a lure-lock hub. An added advantage of this instrument is that it can be used for posterior capsule polishing also. Other variants such as reverse Simcoe and U-shaped Simcoe (right or left) cannulas are also available commercially. Even irrigation and aspiration probe (unimanual or bimanual) employed during phacoemulsification (**Fig. 19C**) can be used for this purpose.

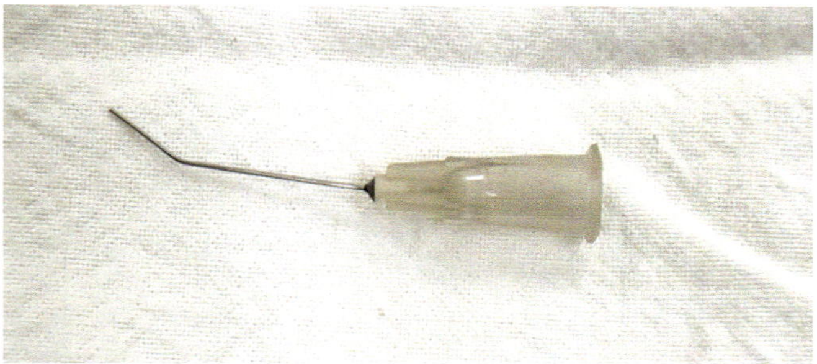

Fig. 19A: 30-G needle.

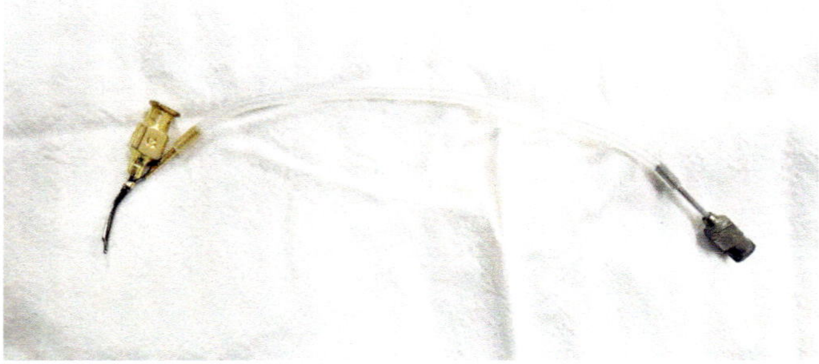

Fig. 19B: Simcoe's irrigation-aspiration cannula.

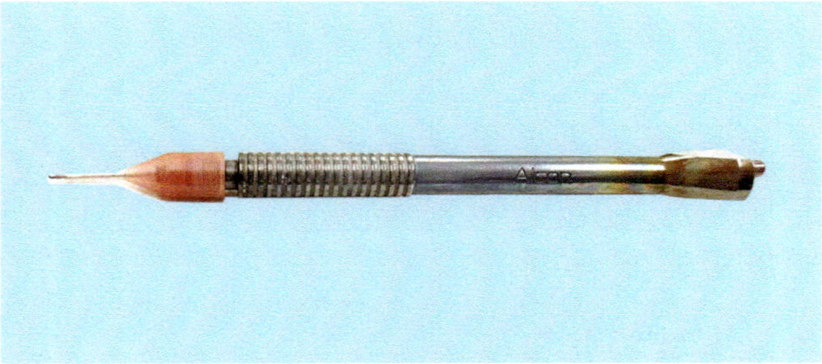

Fig. 19C: Irrigation and aspiration probe used during phacoemulsification.

QUALITATIVE KERATOMETERS

The keratometers are very helpful to assess the degree of corneal toricity at the end of the surgery. These can be of two types depending on whether they are attached to the microscope or they are handheld.

- *Keratometers with microscopic attachment*: There are a number of surgical keratometers like Smirmaul, Troutman, and Terry that are physically attached to the microscope and work by reflecting projected light off the surface of the cornea. However, these are not portable and require a regular smooth refracting surface to reflect the image and are quite expensive.
- *Handheld keratometer*: Simpler, cost-effective and portable methods as Mandel intraoperative keratometer and *Maloney* keratometer are available which work by reflecting a circle from the corneal surface. Maloney keratometer is a titanium cone-shaped instrument, which is designed to reflect the microscope light in rings on the cornea to detect astigmatism. In the absence of the expensive intraoperative surgical keratometers, a safety pin can also be used to monitor the intraoperative astigmatism. The circle of the safety pin is reflected off the corneal surface and any observed ovality implies excessive curvature in the axis of the shortest diameter of the oval. This is used for readjusting and replacement of the sutures and helps to reduce astigmatism intraoperatively and postoperatively.

EYE SHIELD

Eye shields provide impact resistance and are majorly used for protecting the eyeball from unexpected trauma and frequent rubbing in the immediate postoperative phase. These are saucer-shaped devices that are shaped specifically to cover either eye. These can be made of plastic or acrylic, can be translucent or opaque, ventilated or nonventilated, and

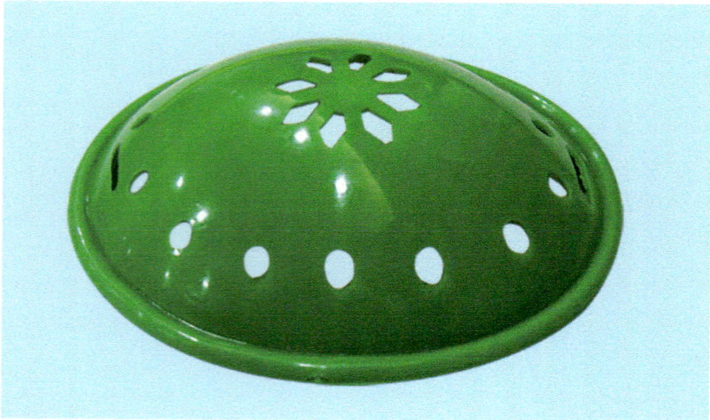

Fig. 20: Protective eye shield.

sterile or nonsterile. They are lightweight and cause minimal discomfort to the patient. They can also be temporarily dislodged form their place to instill medications (**Fig. 20**).

ACKNOWLEDGMENTS

- Dutch Ophthalmic Research Center, DORC Middle East, Dubai, UAE.
- Katena Products, Denville, NJ, USA.

REFERENCES

1. Vajpayee RB, Melki S. Three pearls to minimize penetrating keratoplasty astigmatism. In: Melki SA, Azar DT (Eds). 101 pearls in Refractive, Cataract and Corneal Surgery 2001. Thorofare, New Jersey: SLACK Inc.; 2001. pp. 161-2.
2. Schanzlin DJ, Robin JB, Spence DJ. Clinical and ultrastructure analysis of variable speed corneal trephination. Ophthalmic Surg. 1983;14(9):755-8.
3. Drews RC. Corneal trephine. Trans Am Acad Ophthalmol Otolaryngol. 1974;78:OP223-4.
4. Donaldson WB, Haining WM. A new corneal trephine. Trans Ophthalmol Soc U K. 1978;98(1):14-5.
5. Smirmaul H, Casey TA. A clear view trephine and lamellar dissector for corneal grafting. Am J Ophthalmol. 1980;90:92-4.
6. Wiffen SJ, Maguire LJ, Bourne WM. Keratometric results of penetrating keratoplasty with the Hessburg-Barron and Hanna trephine systems using a standard double-running suture technique. Cornea. 1997;16:306-13.
7. Ng JD, Nekola M, Parmley VC, Richardson M, Mader T. Comparison of three corneal trephines for use in therapeutic keratoplasties for large corneal perforations. Ophthalmic Surg. 1995;26:209-15.
8. Legeais JM, Parel JM, Simon G, Ren Q, Denham D. Endothelial damage by the corneal Hessburg-Barron vacuum trephine. Refract Corneal Surg. 1993;9:255-8.
9. Wilbanks GA, Cohen S, Chipman M, Rootman DS. Clinical outcomes following penetrating keratoplasty using the Barron-Hessburg and Hanna corneal trephination systems. Cornea. 1996;15:589-98.
10. Seitz B, Langenbucher A, Diamantis A, Cursiefen C, Küchle M, Naumann GO. Immunological graft reactions after penetrating keratoplasty—A prospective randomized trial comparing corneal excimer laser and motor trephination. Klin Monbl Augenheilkd. 2001;218:710-9.
11. Amsler M, Verry F. The removal of the graft for keratoplasty. Arch Ophthalmol (Paris). 1948;8:150.
12. Koplin RS. The Surgical Tray for Penetrating Keratoplasty. In: Koplin RS, Wu EI, Ritterband DC, Seedor JA (Eds). The Scrub's Bible. New York, NY: Springer; 2013. pp. 139-40.

10 Suture Materials and Needles

Mohamed Ibrahime Asif, Suman Lata, Namrata Sharma

SUTURE MATERIALS

The suture material is an important factor in the anatomical and functional outcomes of penetrating keratoplasty (PK). The choice of suture, suture placement techniques, and suture adjustment contribute to postoperative astigmatism postkeratoplasty. Braided silk sutures were used in PK before the advent of monofilament synthetic materials. The braided silk sutures had the advantage of greater tensile strength, extensibility, knot control, pliability, and more shear strength. At present, braided sutures have been completely replaced by nonabsorbable monofilament materials because of rapid degradation and excessive tissue reactivity of braided sutures.

The sutures can be divided into absorbable and nonabsorbable, braided or monofilament, high tensile strength and low tensile strength, and single-armed and double-armed (**Table 1**).

Nylon

Nylon is the suture of choice in keratoplasty surgeries. It has the advantage of low antigenicity, high elasticity, and prolonged tensile strength. Its monofilament nature permits a smooth passage through corneal tissue with a lesser tissue reaction. It is pliable and easy to handle. It maintains its tensile strength for >1 year allowing adequate time for wound healing. 10-0 is the most frequently used size because of its ease of placement and tensile strength, though 9-0 and 11-0 is also sometimes used.

Table 1: Classification of sutures based on the type of suture materials.

Absorbable		Nonabsorbable	
Braided	*Monofilament*	*Braided*	*Monofilament*
• Vicryl Rapide • Vicryl	• Fast absorbing gut • Plain gut • Monocryl • Chromic gut • PDS • Stratafix spiral (barbed)	• Silk • Nurolon	• Ethilon • Nylon • Prolene • Gore-Tex

(PDS: polydioxanone suture)

Nylon sutures can cause several complications if left in situ such as vascularization especially of become loose, induced astigmatism, accumulation of mucus, and breaking of sutures which can result in giant papillary conjunctivitis, limbitis, conjunctivitis, and even suppurative keratitis when the knot was not buried.

Thus, it is preferable to remove the sutures at an appropriate time interval.[1-4] 11-0 nylon suture is rarely used alone because of its lack of strength. It is most commonly used as a running suture in conjunction with 10-0 interrupted suture or as a double running suture.

Polypropylene (Prolene)

It is a nonabsorbable suture, which is used as haptic material for intraocular lenses. The tensile strength of this suture is excellent and maintained for many years. Hypothetically it has no tissue reaction and being the most inert material, it is well accepted by the tissues. It is highly elastic and can stretch up to 38% of its original length.[5,6] It does not adhere to the tissues, hence easy to remove. However, it is a stiff material and difficult to handle. Prolene resists microorganisms and tissue enzymes. Compared to nylon, it has a longer life since it does not undergo hydrolytic degradation. Therefore, unlike nylon, it does not produce long-term suture-related complications (loose or broken suture).[3,4] Prolene is rarely used as a single interrupted suture in keratoplasty. It can be used in a continuous interrupted pattern of suturing in keratoplasty. Good results have been reported with it because of its low tissue reactivity, high tensile strength and nonabsorbability.[6] Prolene is also used for iris repair or scleral fixation of posterior chamber lens.

Polyester (Mersilene)

It is a biodegradable material and thus allows long-term wound tension maintenance in keratoplasty surgeries.

Polyester is stronger as compared to nylon with lesser elasticity. It has a stretch factor of only 1%.[5] This helps in better control of intraoperative wound tension; thus, better control of postoperative astigmatism is possible by suture adjustment without the need for suture removal.

The polyester suture is stiff with difficulty in handling and requires precise tensioning. Moreover, its pale green color is difficult to differentiate from the background of the operative field. Early experience has shown that it has higher tissue reactivity. Case reports of necrotizing scleritis have been reported with the use of polyester suture.[7] It attracts particulate material and thus, requires a particle-free field. The rate of infiltration, infection, neovascularization, and handling complications such as exposed knots, loose and tight sutures, and wound leaks are higher with polyester suture.[8] It has been shown to have a fivefold increase in handling related complications and a twofold increase in tissue-related complications when compared to nylon.

Suture Removal

Nylon suture material gradually biodegrades over time hence to be removed on time. However, no standard guidelines described the ideal time for removal, to decrease suture-related complications and to get optimized results in terms of visual acuity and postkeratoplasty astigmatism. Studies have supported the removal of sutures from 6 months to 1-year postkeratoplasty.[9]

Suture-related Complications

Nylon suture material gradually biodegrades over time. Broken and exposed sutures lead to changes in astigmatism, vascularization, inflammation, subepithelial fibrosis, epithelial erosion, infectious keratitis, and endophthalmitis.[10,11]

NEEDLES

A good surgical needle should have the following characteristics:

- Strong enough to withstand mechanical deformation
- Sharp cutting edge
- Atraumatic
- Long enough to be passed through the wound and retrieved without the need to hold the point.
- The composition of the needle should provide enough strength to withstand mechanical force but should yield enough, not to get fractured.

Different Nomenclatures Used with Needles

- *Length*: It is the total distance of the needle from point to swage before bending.
- *Cord length*: It is a straight-line distance from a point to swage after bending.
- *Curvature*: It is that portion of circle to which the needle is bent.
- *Diameter*: It is the diameter of the original wire from which the needle is made. It is measured in thousands of an inch or mils (1 mil = 0.001 inches).
- *Regular cutting*: Regular cutting needle has a cross section of a triangle with the base down. It can easily traverse tougher tissues such as full-thickness scleral grafts and through corneal bites.
- *Reverse cutting*: It is a cross section of a triangle with apex down.
- *Spatulated*: Spatulated needle has a flattened reverse cutting point without a third cutting edge on the bottom. Spatulated needles work better for intralamellar work such as lamellar keratoplasty, cataract incision closure, etc.
- *Tapered circular cross section*: This needle has the advantage of causing a smaller tract in soft tissue and conjunctiva. It is difficult to penetrate cornea and sclera with this needle.

Keratoplasty needles are usually spatulated, reverse cutting with a smaller less traumatic point.

Types of Needles Used in Keratoplasty

There are various types of needles used in keratoplasty surgeries. These include:

- Full curve needles
- Mini curve needles
- Bi-curve needles
- Compound curve needles

Full Curve Needles

These are most frequently used needles in keratoplasty as well as in most of the anterior segment surgeries. Their curvature ranges from 140 to 180°. These needles achieve long and somewhat shallow bites, which require the surgeon to be vigilant in the presence of edematous tissues.

Mini Curve Needles

Mini curve needles have their cord length and radius of curvature significantly smaller than the full curve needles. These needles have the advantage of making shorter and deeper bites. However, they are difficult to handle because of the smaller size and tight radii.

Bi-curve Needles

Bi-curve needles achieve short and deep bites, easy to handle. The design has an average to flat radius of curvature from the swage to midportion and a much steeper or tighter radius from the midportion to the needlepoint. The architecture permits an easier handling and a rapid turn out after a deep bite.

Compound Curve Needles

It is a further modification of a bi-curve design. The needle has an initial flat curve changing to a steeper curve with a sharp straight point. The straight portion facilitates initial entrance and penetration to a depth and steep curve immediately behind the point and assures a rapid turnout.

NEWER HORIZONS

There have been several recent advances and development in the structure and functional aspect of the sutures. However, the clinical application of all these advances has not been established for suturing in the field of ophthalmology. Sutures with additional properties like modified with bioactive molecules (antibodies, DNA, proteins, drugs or growth factors) and antibacterial agents have been developed. There are few other modifications in the sutures such as stem cell-seeded sutures and smart sutures which are made from shape memory polymers.

- *Bioactive sutures:* With recent advances, it is possible to incorporate biologically active substances to enhance suture function and capability. It allows a controlled drug delivery to traumatic sites. These sutures are engineered to have controlled tissue interaction to optimize wound healing, in addition to their essential function in tissue approximation.[12,13]
- *Antibacterial-coated sutures*: Currently, only one product is commercially available in this category. Triclosan-coated polyglactin 910 (Vicryl Plus Antibacterial: Ethicon) has been found to reduce surgical site infection rate by 30%.[14] Handling and tension force of these sutures were found to be comparable to standard suture material. Although triclosan is relatively nontoxic, skin irritation, and the allergic reaction has been known to occur.

REFERENCES

1. Dana MR, Goren MB, Gomes JA, Laibson PR, Rapuano CJ, Cohen EJ. Suture erosion after penetrating keratoplasty. Cornea. 1995;14(3):243-8.
2. Sullivan LJ, Su C, Snibson G, Taylor HR. Sterile ocular inflammatory reactions to monofilament suture material. Aust N Z J Ophthalmol. 1994;22(3):175-81.
3. Landau D, Siganos CS, Mechoulam H, Solomon A, Frucht-Pery J. Astigmatism after mersilene and nylon suture use for penetrating keratoplasty. Cornea. 2006;25(6):691-4.
4. Bartels MC, van Rooij J, Geerards AJ, Mulder PG, Remeijer L. Comparison of complication rates and postoperative astigmatism between nylon and Mersilene sutures for corneal transplants in patients with Fuchs endothelial dystrophy. Cornea. 2006;25(5):533-9.
5. Alcon Laboratories. Manufacturers' specifications. Fort Worth, Tx: Alcon Laboratories; 1998.
6. Faggioni R, de Courten C. Short and long-term advantages and disadvantages of prolene monofilament sutures in penetrating keratoplasty. Klin Monbl Augenheilkd. 1992;200(5):395-7.
7. Stokes J, Wright M, Ramaesh K, Smith C, Dhillon B. Necrotizing scleritis after intraocular surgery associated with the use of polyester nonabsorbable sutures. J Cataract Refract Surg. 2003;29(9):1827-30.
8. Bertram BA, Drews-Botsch C, Gemmill M, Guell J, Murad M, Waring GO. Complications of Mersilene sutures in penetrating keratoplasty. J Refract Surg. 1992;8(4):296-305.
9. Yilmaz S, Ozdil MA, Maden A. Factors affecting changes in astigmatism before and after suture removal following penetrating keratoplasty. Eur J Ophthalmol. 2007;17(3):301-6.
10. Moorthy S, Graue E, Jhanji V, Constantinou M, Vajpayee RB. Microbial keratitis after penetrating keratoplasty: impact of sutures. Am J Ophthalmol. 2011;152(2):189-94.
11. Crawford AZ, Meyer JJ, Patel DV, Ormonde SE, McGhee CN. Complications related to sutures following penetrating and deep anterior lamellar keratoplasty. Clin Exp Ophthalmol. 2016;44(2):142-3.
12. Cummings SH, Grande DA, Hee CK, Kestler HK, Roden CM, Shah NV, et al. Effect of recombinant human platelet-derived growth factor-BB-coated sutures on Achilles tendon healing in a rat model: a histological and biomechanical study. J Tissue Eng. 2012;3(1):2041731412453577.
13. Fuchs TF, Surke C, Stange R, Quandte S, Wildemann B, Raschke MJ, et al. Local delivery of growth factors using coated suture material. ScientificWorldJournal. 2012;2012:109216.
14. Barbolt TA. Chemistry and safety of triclosan, and its use as an antimicrobial coating on Coated VICRYL* Plus Antibacterial Suture (coated polyglactin 910 suture with triclosan). Surg Infect (Larchmt). 2002;3(Suppl 1):S45-53.

11 Technique of Penetrating Keratoplasty

Nicholas York, Nagib Du Toit, Rasik B Vajpayee

INTRODUCTION

Penetrating keratoplasty (PK) is a corneal transplant procedure in which the full thickness, diseased, and host corneal tissue is excised and replaced with healthy donor corneal tissue. Over the past decade, there has been a significant trend away from PK toward partial thickness (lamellar) corneal procedures, aimed at replacing only the diseased layer of cornea.[1-6] However, PK still remains the technique of choice for pathology that involves the full thickness of the diseased cornea.

INDICATIONS

- Optical PK is performed to improve vision. The objective is to establish a clear corneal visual axis and reduction in refractive error in the setting of advanced corneal ectasia, full thickness corneal opacity, corneal dystrophy, bullous keratopathy, or corneal degeneration.
- Tectonic PK is aimed at restoring the structural integrity of the cornea in cases of severe thinning or perforation.
- Therapeutic PK removes infected corneal tissue in cases of microbial keratitis unresponsive to medical treatment.
- Other rare indications for PK include alleviating pain or improving cosmesis in the setting of a painful or unsightly blind eye where the cornea is significantly contributing to the patient's symptoms.

Penetrating keratoplasty is a major intraocular surgery and requires a meticulous surgical preparation of the patient, donor tissue, operating theater, instruments, and precise planning of surgical technique by the surgeon.

ESTABLISH REALISTIC PATIENT EXPECTATIONS

The definition of a successful PK is continuing to evolve, and the sole objective is no longer to simply maintain a clear cornea over time. Surgical techniques need to be continually refined in order to improve refractive outcomes, with the aim of achieving good best-corrected visual acuity and uncorrected visual acuity post-transplant.

It is critically important to have in-depth discussions with the patient (prior to any surgical planning) about the transplantation goals and to establish realistic expectations. Patients should be informed that healing takes at least 12–18 months after PK and in most cases, sutures would only be removed at that stage. Patients need to be informed that refractive errors such as myopia, hyperopia, and astigmatism commonly limit the uncorrected vision after the healing of a graft. This may require one or more modalities or procedures such as glasses, contact lenses, manual/femto-second arcuate keratotomies or topography-guided photorefractive keratectomy to achieve the best possible visual acuity.

PREOPERATIVE PREPARATION

Infection Control

Use of topical preoperative antibiotics may help to reduce the incidence of graft infection and endophthalmitis, although evidence for this in the literature is inconclusive.[7-9] Some surgeons would prescribe a fluoroquinolone such as ofloxacin 0.3% or ciprofloxacin 0.3% for 1–3 days prior to surgery. This has now been largely abandoned by many due to the lack of evidence, possibility of it promoting bacterial resistance, the increased cost, and risk of allergic reactions. The most common source of infection after a PK is usually from the patient's ocular and periocular flora.[10] Preexisting blepharitis and other factors that may lead to infection should be managed and eliminated prior to scheduling surgery.

Decrease in Corneal Neovascularization

Corneal neovascularization (NV) greatly increases the risk of graft rejection and ultimately graft failure in patients undergoing PK.[11] Multiple modalities have been tried with varying success to decrease the corneal NV, including preoperative steroids, electrocautery, and argon/YAG laser occlusion.[12,13] More recently, the topical and subconjunctival use of anti-VEGF agents, ranibizumab and bevacizumab have demonstrated good short-term efficacy in reducing corneal NV.[14,15] The inflammatory drive, which promotes recurrence of new vessels in the transplanted cornea, can be reduced by intensive postoperative topical steroid or cyclosporine usage.

Intraocular Pressure Control

Intraocular pressure (IOP) control in patients with preexisting glaucoma should be optimized prior to surgery. Limiting IOP and posterior vitreous pressure are vitally important in reducing the risk of complications during the open-sky phase of the PK procedure, such as lens or vitreous prolapse and expulsive choroidal hemorrhage.[16-18] The lack of positive pressure appears to also play a significant role in reducing endothelial cell loss after PK.[19] A good hypotony can be achieved preoperatively by means of digital massage, a Honan balloon or in high risk cases, and the use of preoperative intravenous Mannitol infusion. Honan balloon may be applied for 30 minutes at 30 mm Hg of pressure. Complete lid and extraocular muscle akinesia are also important to prevent intraoperative rises in IOP. This can be achieved by a good periocular anesthetic block or generalized muscle relaxant if the patient is under general anesthesia (GA). Positioning of a patient with increased body mass index in a reverse Trendelenburg position is also a useful consideration to reduce posterior pressure.

Pupillary Management

In cases of phakic keratoplasty without combined cataract surgery, two drops of 2.5% pilocarpine may be instilled 5 minutes apart before surgery to constrict the pupil and to protect the crystalline lens. If a combined cataract procedure is anticipated, the pupil is dilated as for cataract surgery—2.5% phenylephrine and 1% cyclopentolate drops every 5 minutes for three times. Intraocular acetylcholine chloride (Miochol) or carbachol can then be instilled after the cataract surgery portion of the procedure is completed, prior to performing the PK.

Donor Corneal Tissue Management

In the modern era of eye banking, extensive screening of corneal donors and donated corneal tissue is performed to exclude donors and corneas unsuitable for transplantation. Despite this, the surgeon still bears the ultimate responsibility for the safety and suitability of the tissue being transplanted. The surgeon should thus personally review the donor tissue, history, and results of screening investigations prior to surgery. The tissue should be examined to exclude defects such as infiltrates, retained glass, foreign debris, scars/lacerations, or other pathology. Some donor corneas may have undergone refractive surgical procedures like photorefractive keratotomy and laser in-situ keratomileusis (LASIK). This can be difficult to exclude without a history being supplied in the donor history. To be able to exclude use of such tissue, a videokeratography of the donor eyeball may have to be performed.

ANESTHESIA

Penetrating keratoplasty can be performed safely under local or GA with proper patient selection.[20,21]

General anesthesia is indicated in pediatric cases and in adults with mental impairment, deafness, aphasia, and language barriers, where intraoperative cooperation may prove difficult. It is also indicated in perforated corneas and in severely inflamed eyes where local anesthesia may be deemed unsafe. Finally, GA may be considered prudent in patients who are at increased risk of suprachoroidal hemorrhage. Risk factors include previous intraocular surgery, older age, glaucoma, systemic hypertension, arteriosclerosis, anticoagulant therapy, and history of previous suprachoroidal hemorrhage.[22-25] The incidence of suprachoroidal hemorrhage in PK is 0.56% with general anesthetic and 4.3% with local anesthetic.[22] It is, however, vitally important to check with the anesthetist immediately prior to the open-sky phase of the PK procedure, that the patient is deeply anesthetized and paralyzed. Bucking or coughing during the open-sky phase of the procedure could have devastating consequences.

Local anesthesia can be given by retrobulbar or peribulbar blocks.[20] Long-lasting anesthetic agent such as bupivacaine alone or combinations of bupivacaine with lidocaine should be used.[21] Complete lid and extraocular muscle akinesia are essential to eliminate intraoperative pressure elevations associated with muscle contraction. A good hypotony should be achieved preoperatively by means of digital massage or a Honan balloon, especially when local anesthesia is chosen.

SURGICAL PREPARATION

Cleaning and Draping

The surgical field should be cleaned and draped appropriately with the aim of providing a sterile field. The skin of the periorbital area may be painted with 5% povidone-iodine. The preoperative lid preparation should include removal of any residual lid margin debris, painting the lid margin, and lashes with 5% povidone-iodine solution. A single application of one drop of 1–5% iodine onto the ocular surface, for 3–5 minutes at the time of surgical preparation has been shown to significantly reduce the incidence of endophthalmitis.[26-29] An adhesive drape should be placed in such a manner that the lid margins as well as the eyelashes are kept out of the surgical field.

Exposure and Insertion of Lid-speculum

To be able to perform all the surgical maneuvers required for corneal transplantation surgery a good exposure of the eyeball is mandatory. Also, any inadvertent pressure exerted by the speculum should be avoided as it may raise the IOP and cause globe distortion that can lead to oval or irregular trephination, increased posterior pressure, poor suture alignment, and increased postoperative astigmatism.[30] We frequently use a Barraquer wire speculum as it is lightweight, easy to insert, and exposes the globe adequately. Additionally, in cases with small palpebral fissure, a lateral canthotomy may be performed to increase the area of exposure.

Placement of Scleral Fixation Ring

In pediatric patients and aphakic patients, low ocular rigidity can result in scleral collapse after the trephination of recipient cornea. The resultant displacement of iris, lens, and vitreous can cause extrusion of lens and vitreous loss. Even if there is no resultant complication, the collapse of the recipient corneal rim makes suturing very difficult. Most surgeons elect to use scleral-supporting devices in such patients. These scleral support rings include Flieringa ring, McNeill-Goldman scleral ring, and blepharostat ring. The size and the placement of any such ring must be such that it does not interfere with maneuvers required to perform the procedure of PK or distort the globe. The fixation ring diameter is sized to measure slightly less than the interpalpebral opening with the lid speculum in place. The ring should be sutured with only enough force to rest gently on, but not to depress the sclera. The scleral fixation ring is sutured with interrupted 7-0 vicryl sutures with bites of about 50% of the scleral thickness. These sutures should be passed from periphery to the limbus. Fixating the ring just peripheral to the limbus gives maximum scleral support. These rings can also be grasped during trephination to fixate the globe.

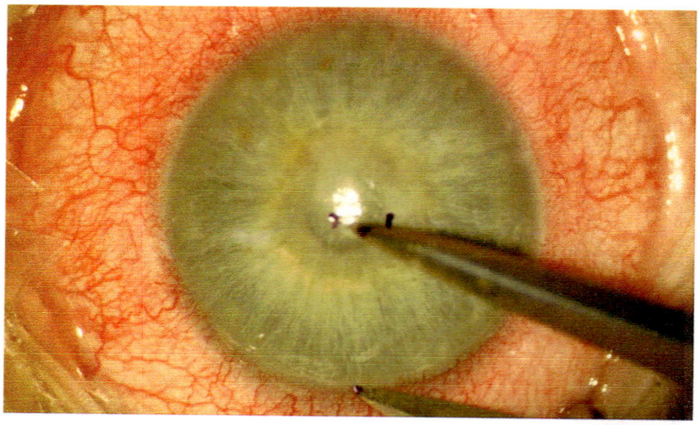

Fig. 1: Vernier calipers used for marking the geometric center.

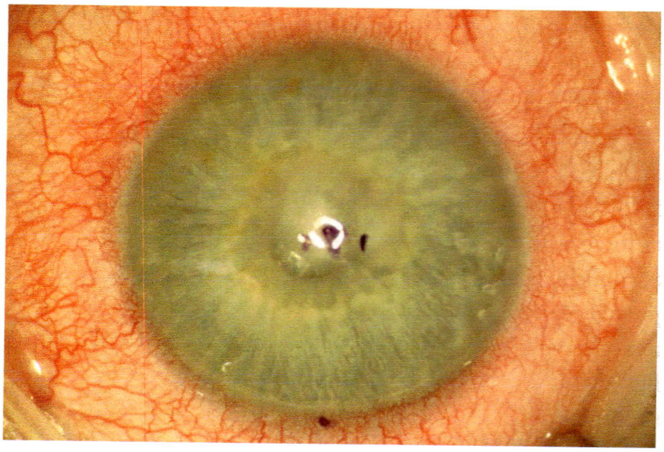

Fig. 2: Geometric center of cornea marked.

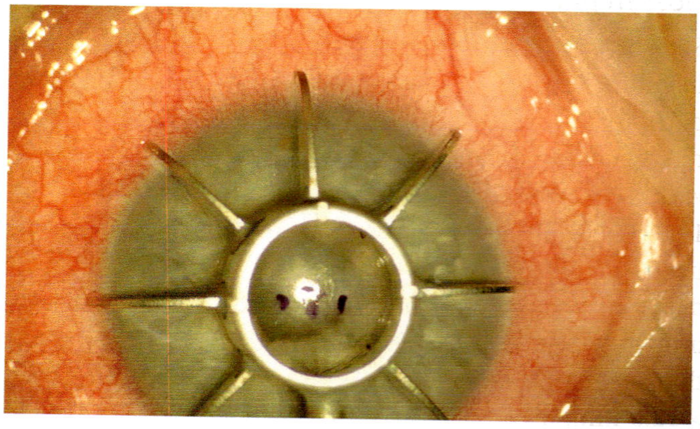

Fig. 3: Radial keratotomy marker used to apply symmetrical corneal markings.

MARKING THE HOST CORNEA

The centering of the graft is of utmost importance as any decentration may lead to high postoperative astigmatism, increased risk of graft-rejection and damage to the anterior chamber angle. The donor graft is usually centered on the geometric center of the host cornea or in some cases over the pupillary axis, which is often displaced slightly nasally.[31]

If there is significant disparity between the geometric center and the center of the pupil, then a point midway between the two may be chosen. The geometric center is located by measuring the horizontal and vertical diameter of the cornea with calipers (**Fig. 1**), halving each measurement and finding the point at which the horizontal diameter line bisects the vertical one. A centration mark is made on the anterior corneal surface with a surgical marking pen (**Fig. 2**).

After marking the geometric center of the cornea, radial keratotomy markers (8 arms and 16 arms) may be used for creating impression marks guiding exact suture placement in cases where interrupted sutures are planned (**Fig. 3**). In cases where the surgeon preference is to do a continuous suture, various corneal markers are available to aid suture placement, e.g., the Vajpayee's Corneal Marker, which has 20 radial marking arms and can be used to guide the placement of 20-bites single continuous sutures of various types such as torque, antitorque, and no torque.[32] The cornea should be thoroughly dried before placing the marker. The arms of the suture markers are stained with gentian violet and the marker is pressed on the corneal surface of the recipient (**Fig. 4**). While using such a marker, care should be taken

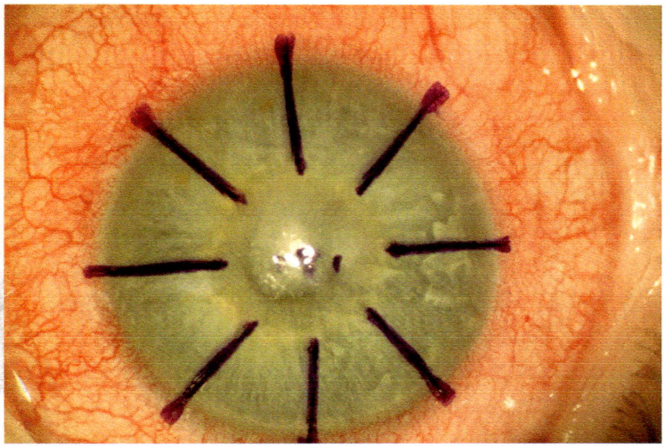

Fig. 4: Marks applied with suture marker using gentian violet.

to ensure that the center of the marker and the previously marked geometric center on the host cornea coincide.

A decentered graft may be preferred in certain situations such as a peripheral perforation or active microbial keratitis in order to ensure that the pathological area of the cornea is sufficiently excised.[33] In a cornea with peripheral pathology, a slightly decentered graft which encompasses the area of pathology and clears the pupil is preferred in comparison to a large and centered graft. If a previous decentered graft has failed, the previous keratoplasty wound is ignored and the second graft is centered on the geometric center of the cornea.

Selecting Sizes of Host and Donor Trephines

Host Trephine Sizing

Selecting the host trephine size depends on several factors including the host corneal diameter, the underlying corneal pathology, and the individualized rejection risk of the recipient. For patients with an average corneal diameter, with a horizontal white-to-white (WTW) measurement of 11.5–12.5 mm, an 8-mm host trephine is most commonly used. In patients with a smaller-than-average corneal diameter, with a horizontal WTW < 11.5 mm, a 7.5- or 7.75-mm host trephine is selected. In patients with a larger-than-average corneal diameter, with a horizontal WTW > 12.5 mm, an 8.25- or 8.5-mm host trephine is selected. The graft may also need to be oversized (and sometimes decentered) to encompass pathology, such as in cases of therapeutic excision of unresponsive microbial keratitis or tectonic PK in the setting of a more peripheral perforation. In patients with keratoconus, it is important to map the extent of the cone, which is often inferiorly displaced, and ensure that all of the thin ectatic cornea will be excised with the selected host trephine size. However, risk of rejection increases with host trephination of >8.5 mm in diameter and as the graft-host junction moves closer to the limbus.[34-38] Oversizing of grafts may be relatively contraindicated in patients with preexisting risk factors for rejection, such as young age, multiple previously failed grafts, and corneal NV.[39-41]

Donor Trephine Sizing

The selection of the donor trephine size depends on the planned diameter of the host cut. There are various factors which determine the graft-host disparity.

Barron has highlighted certain facts about the graft-host disparity, which are useful in guiding these decisions.[33]

- If the diameter of the recipient is between 7 and 9 mm and the eye is pseudophakic or phakic, the graft should be 0.25 mm larger than the host. However, if the eye is aphakic, the graft should be larger than the host by 0.5 mm.
- If the diameter of the recipient bed is larger than 9 mm or smaller than 7 mm, the graft should be larger than the host by 1 mm.
- With a 7.5-mm bed, a 0.25-mm oversized graft does not usually induce any refractive error.
- With the recipient bed of 7.5 mm, a 0.5-mm oversized graft induces myopia of 4 diopters; with an 8.0-mm recipient bed, a 0.5-mm oversized graft induces 2.5 diopters of myopia.
- A graft, which is the same sized or smaller than the recipient opening, decreases the myopia but can result in a flat cornea, which may not be amenable to contact lens fitting.

With the most commonly employed current trephine techniques, where donor corneal tissue is trephined from the endothelial side and the host cornea is trephined from the epithelial side, the donor tissue diameter achieved will be 0.25 mm less than the host corneal tissue cut with the same diameter trephine.[33,42-44] Most corneal surgeons will therefore use a 0.5-mm oversized graft for their routine cases (effectively oversizing by 0.25 mm). In certain situations like keratoconus, however, the graft-host disparity chosen is less, e.g., 0.25 mm (i.e., effectively same size), in order to compensate for the associated myopia. Some surgeons prefer to use a 0.5-mm oversized donor graft for all the cases including those with keratoconus. Additionally, patients with poor endothelial cell function such as Fuchs' dystrophy or pseudophakic or aphakic bullous keratopathy may benefit from increased number of endothelial cells in a larger graft. In cases with corneal scarring associated with severe corneo-iridic adhesions[42] and in pediatric eyes, we use 1 mm oversized grafts irrespective of the diameter of the host cut.[43]

TREPHINATION OF DONOR CORNEA

It is recommended that the donor corneal button be cut before the recipient cornea. This helps to ensure that a good quality and optimally prepared donor button is available prior to trephination of the recipient cornea. At times it has happened that the donor button has been cut in an irregular manner or has been damaged or lost during the trephining maneuvers. That is why it is important to first procure a good quality donor button before trephining the host cornea.

Harvesting the Donor Graft from a Preserved Corneoscleral Button

Depending on the availability and surgeon preference, one of the following techniques may be used to punch the preserved corneoscleral donor button.

Corneal Endothelial Punch Systems

Corneal endothelial punch systems incorporating the use of a disposable circular trephine are an ideal technique to harvest the graft from the donor button and most surgeons prefer to use these systems. Various corneal punches that can be used to harvest donor graft tissue include the Barron vacuum donor corneal punch, Cottingham punch, IOWA PK Press corneal punch, and Rothman-Gilbard corneal punch. These punches allow for accurate centration of the donor cornea and a sharp vertical cut. These punches can use trephine blades of various diameters. The basic method of punching is similar for all the trephine systems. The corneoscleral donor button is placed endothelial side up on a cutting block and a barrel mounted circular trephine is brought down through the central part of the system in a single motion cutting the donor button. Before lifting up the punch and releasing the downward pressure, a forceps is used to assess that the scleral rim is able to rotate freely, thus ensuring that the cornea has been punched through its full thickness. The functioning of the Barron vacuum donor cornea punch is slightly different. This punch consists of a nylon cutting block, a seating ring, and a blade. The cutting block has four holes into which the steel guidepost of the blade fits to ensure that the blade is perpendicular. The well of the cutting block has a diameter of 19 mm and a radius of curvature of 25.4 mm, except for the central 11 mm, which has a radius of curvature of 10 mm. The well has a central positioning hole, as well as four additional holes and a circular trough 12 mm in diameter that are connected by a silicone tube to a 5-mL syringe with a spring-loaded plunger. The syringe creates suction that holds the cornea in place as it is cut and ensures that the corneal button remains in the well, and not in the blade, after the cut has been made. When inked with gentian violet, the four holes in the well mark the cornea for accurate placement of the cardinal sutures.

Handheld Trephines

This technique is used in most developing countries, where the endothelial punches may not be available due to increased expense. The donor button is cut over a cutting block, which may be made of Teflon, Nylon, or Paraffin, and has a concave depression, or a well in which the donor cornea is placed with epithelial surface down.[45] Various trephines have been developed for cutting the donor cornea but a standard trephine consists of a disposable circular stainless steel blade on a handle. The blade should be properly secured on the handle and the obturator fully retracted to avoid its contact with the endothelium. Donor cornea should be cut by punching rather than rotating the blade.[45,46] Rotation of the blade results in more endothelial damage. The blade should always be held perpendicular to or centered on the cutting block. Slipping of the blade should be guarded against, as it can result in oblique cutting of the cornea with resultant irregular or oval button with a beveled or ragged edge. These irregularities can distort the wound and cause significant postoperative astigmatism. A uniform pressure should be applied over the blade with the thumb and an audible click signifies the complete through and through trephining of the donor button. The punched-cut corneal button either stays in the well of the Teflon block or may pass up into the barrel of the blade. If the donor button has been sucked inside the trephine, balanced salt solution (BSS) or a viscoelastic substance like 2% methyl cellulose is gently squirted into the barrel to dislodge the button. In order to confirm that the donor button has been cut circumferentially all around, the peripheral skirt of the corneoscleral rim may be retracted over the barrel of the trephine. The button is grasped with a forceps and placed epithelial surface down over the graft holder. The endothelium is covered by viscoelastic to prevent desiccation.

Trephining the Donor Cornea from the Epithelial Side Using an Artificial Anterior Chamber Maintainer and Suction Fixated Guided Trephine System

These systems consist of an anterior chamber maintainer, a reusable blade holder (with micrometer setting), and a suction ring attached to a syringe. A small drop of viscoelastic is placed on the top of the endothelium of the donor tissue and the tissue is centered on to the anterior chamber maintainer (epithelial side up). Once the scleral rim is securely fastened, air or BSS is used to create the anterior chamber. The suction ring is placed on the donor cornea and is activated by releasing the syringe. Following placement of the trephine (which consists of the blade holder with the blade) on the suction ring, the lever of the suction ring is pressed to lower the blade onto the donor tissue and the trephine is turned to complete the cut. The potential benefit of cutting the tissue from the epithelial side is that the donor corneal button is not undersized by 0.25 mm, as occurs with endothelial punch systems, and the angulation of the wound edge of the donor conforms better anatomically with the wound edge of the host's trephined cornea, as both are trephined from the same direction, resulting in better wound apposition and closure. Other potential benefits include less endothelial cell loss at the donor periphery.[47]

Harvesting the Donor Graft from a Whole Globe Stored in a Moist Chamber Using Handheld or Suction Fixation Trephines

In this technique, the donor graft is cut from the epithelial side and the grafts are the same size or 0.25 mm larger than the intended recipient opening. Many surgeons who do not have access to the McCarey-Kaufman preserved corneoscleral buttons, especially in developing countries, use the whole eye globe, which is fixated in a gauze piece or on a Tudor Thomas stand.

The globe in a moist sterile gauze piece is held in the nondominant hand, taking care that the cornea is perpendicular to the gauze piece. If the eye is tilted, the cut may be misdirected. Through a small stab incision in the limbus one may inject viscoelastic into the anterior chamber prior to trephination. Then using a sharp trephine in the dominant hand, the blade is placed centrally on the donor eye. Using counter pressure with one hand, the trephine is firmly placed into the cornea and rotated with the fingers while exerting pressure downward. A release of pressure will be noted when the anterior chamber is entered. Trephination must then stop immediately; otherwise the endothelium will come in contact with the iris. The initial cut is finished with the scissors, taking care not to shelve the edge. If minimal pressure is used, an air bubble will spontaneously fill the chamber and protect the endothelium from the iris and the lens. The cut is completed with the curved corneal scissors.

Once the donor button has been prepared by any of the above techniques, it should be kept submerged in storage medium or BSS, covered and placed at a safe and designated place while the surgeon moves on to preparation of the host corneal bed.

TREPHINATION OF THE RECIPIENT CORNEA

For cutting the recipient cornea, conventional handheld trephines as well as the suction and automated trephines have been used. Uniformity of the cuts varies with the trephine type and an ideal trephine, which provides straight cuts without any tissue distortion, is not yet available.

Trephining with Handheld Trephines

The "standard" handheld trephine, i.e. Castroviejo trephine consists of a circular blade on a handle. The circular blade can be used alone. The handle has an internal obturator, which limits the depth of the cut. The obturator, however, can distort the cornea and cause an irregular, noncircular cut if it comes in contact with the corneal apex before the blade touches the cornea. This can happen most frequently in patients with keratoconus. A disposable open-bladed trephine may be used as it trephines the recipient without distorting the cornea and simultaneously allows visualization of the optical centration mark.

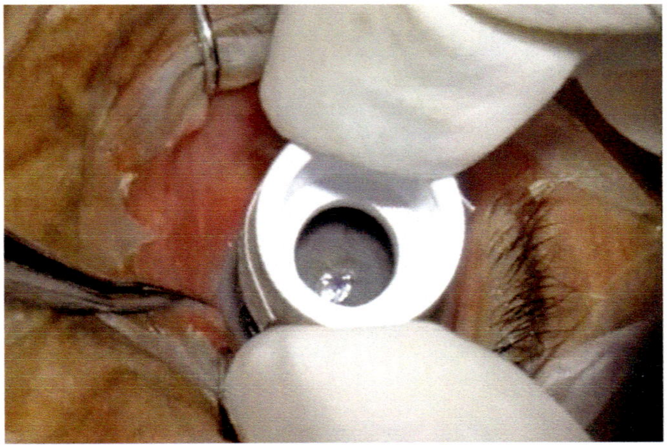

Fig. 5: Handheld trephine used for trephination.

The optical axis of the recipient's cornea is marked by the surgeon, using wherever possible the central point, as described earlier. The blade of the trephine should always be examined under the microscope to check for the regularity and sharpness of the edge before proceeding to trephination. The cornea should be thoroughly dried before trephining. The trephine is held perpendicular to the cornea and positioned by aligning the center of this blade with the centration mark on the cornea and checking the amount of cornea surrounding the blade (**Fig. 5**). The trephine is then rotated between the thumb and the forefinger maintaining a downward pressure. Care is taken to avoid applying undue external pressure on the eye with the trephine.

Some surgeons prefer to trephine almost to the full thickness whereas others recommend a guarded entry. In the former, the cut is perpendicular and allows easier removal of the host cornea. In the latter, a partial thickness cut up to the pre-Descemet's membrane is made first. A full thickness cut is generally avoided as it may cause an uneven entry into the anterior chamber, which may lead to its collapse; further pressure applied may lead to damage of iris or lens or extrusion of the lens. Once a partial thickness cut is made, anterior chamber entry is done with a blade, most conveniently at 11 o'clock position.

The escape of the aqueous should be carefully noted to ensure a full-thickness incision. If the aqueous humor is not seen, it is possible that the host's Descemet's membrane has been detached from the posterior stroma. This occurs most likely in patients with bullous keratopathy and congenital hereditary endothelial dystrophy (CHED) and if inadvertently left, may result in double anterior chamber postoperatively.

Trephining the Recipient Cornea with a Suction Trephine

Suction trephines (like the Barron radial vacuum trephine) can also be used for trephining the host corneas[48] (**Fig. 6**). These fixate the cornea by suction during trephination and

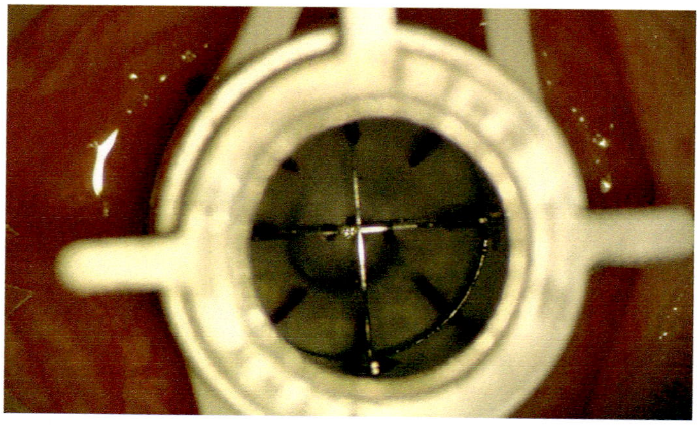

Fig. 6: Hessburg-Barron suction trephine used to trephinate the recipient bed.

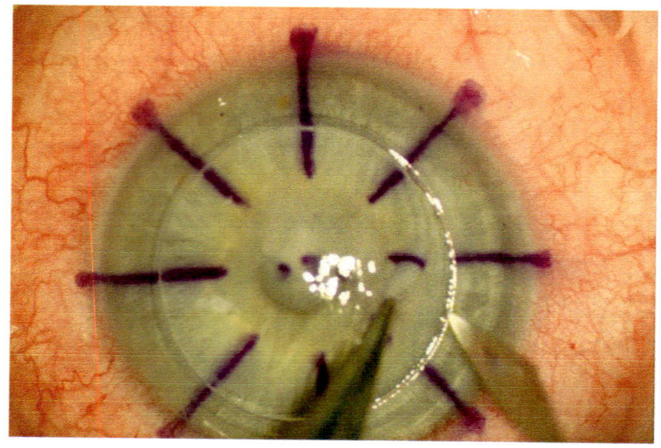

Fig. 7: 15° blade used to enter anterior chamber through partial thickness trephine.

are particularly useful in perforated corneas and result in less anterior chamber collapse and corneal distortion.[49-51] These create a sharper, deeper, and more perpendicular incision than free blades.

The Barron radial vacuum trephine is available in diameters of 6.0–9.0 mm, in 0.5 mm increments, as well as a diameter of 7.75 mm. This trephine consists of a body and a blade assembly. The body contains two plastic struts for holding and stabilizing the trephine, and a circular vacuum chamber is recessed slightly relative to the outer wall to account for the anterior corneal curvature. The vacuum chamber is connected by a silicone tube to a 5-mL syringe with a spring-loaded plunger. The blade assembly contains a blade, cross hairs for centering the trephine, and four plastic spokes for turning the blade. The inner wall of the body and the outer wall of the blade assembly are threaded so they fit together in a nut and bolt fashion. The blade is lowered or raised by turning the spokes clockwise or counterclockwise, respectively. For each one quarter turn, the blade is lowered or raised approximately 62.5 μm.

Before placement on the cornea, the trephine is examined under the microscope and the edge of the blade is aligned with the inner wall of the vacuum chamber. This position is called the zero position. The blade is then retracted approximately 187.5 μm by turning the spokes 270° (three quarter turns anticlockwise), which prevents the blade from hitting the cornea and interfering with suction as the trephine is placed on the eye.

The corneal surface should be wet with BSS prior to placement of the trephine. The plunger of the syringe is then pushed all the way in, the cross hairs of the trephine are aligned with the centration mark on the cornea, the trephine is pressed evenly, and the plunger is released abruptly. If suction has been obtained, the plunger stops at about the 3–4 mL mark on the syringe. If the plunger rebounds all the way out, suction has not been obtained and the above process is repeated. After suction has been obtained, the position of the trephine on the cornea is assessed by confirming that the cross hairs and centration mark are aligned and by checking the amount of cornea surrounding the outer wall of the vacuum chamber.

The trephine is stabilized by gently holding the struts, and the cornea is cut by turning the spokes in a clockwise direction. The suction orients the trephine perpendicular to the cornea. As the blade is lowered, the trephine is steadied but its angle to the cornea should not be forcibly changed. The initial three-quarter turns of the spokes lower the blade to the zero position. Because of the anterior corneal curvature, the cornea is cut slightly when the blade is lowered to this position. The number of spokes to turn further depends on the desired depth of cut and the corneal thickness—fewer for a shallow cut or a thin cornea and more for a deep cut or a thick cornea. An average of 6–8 quarter turns from the zero position (375–500 μm) is sufficient in most cases depending on the baseline corneal thickness. It is preferred that the cornea can be cut as close to the Descemet's membrane as possible, without entering the anterior chamber. The barrel of the trephine should be watched as the blade is lowered because if the anterior chamber is inadvertently entered, aqueous humor will appear in the barrel. If this occurs, the plunger of the syringe is pushed in all the way, which releases the suction and the trephine is removed from the eye. After the cut has been made up to 90% depth, the trephine is removed from the eye by pushing the plunger of the syringe in all the way, which releases the suction. Subsequently, the anterior chamber may be entered with a 15° blade (**Fig. 7**) and the cut is completed with corneoscleral scissors as described below.

Nonmechanical Laser Trephination of Donor and Host Corneal Tissue

Nonmechanical laser trephination can also be performed from the epithelial side on the donor and host using either an excimer or more recently a femtosecond laser. This avoids the mechanical distortion during trephination resulting in smooth almost perpendicular edges that are congruent in the donor and thus potentially improves the optical performance after transplantation.[52]

Excimer Laser Trephination

Trephination of the donor cornea is done using a 193-nm excimer laser. A circular round metal aperture mask consisting of 8 orientation teeth (diameter 7.6–8.1 mm; central opening 3 mm for centration) are positioned on a corneoscleral button (16 mm diameter) fixed in an artificial anterior chamber maintainer under microscopic control.[53] The pressure within the artificial chamber maintainer is adjusted to 20 mm Hg by attaching it to an infusion system. Using an automated rotation device for the artificial chamber (four rotations per minute), approximately 11,000 laser pulses are necessary to perforate the cornea focally. After perforation, the remaining stromal lamellae and the Descemet's membrane are cut with a curved corneal microscissors.

Trephination of the host cornea is performed using excimer laser along a metal mask (diameter 12.9 mm; central opening 7.5–8 mm; 8 orientation notches 0.15–0.3 mm), which is placed on the recipient cornea. Manually guided excimer laser is used. For focal corneal perforation on an average 7,000 laser pulses are required. To complete trephination, the remaining deep stromal lamellae and Descemet's membrane are cut with a curved corneal microscissors.[53]

Femtosecond Laser Trephination

Both recipient and donor trephination can now be performed with a femtosecond laser. The potential advantages of this technique include the ability to create more precise and accurate cuts, which may result in reduced astigmatism, and the possibility of creating various interlocking patterns in the host and donor corneal edges, e.g., zigzag, mushroom or top-hat patterns, which may improve wound stability and increase resistance to wound leakage. This may reduce the number of sutures required and the time required for sutures to remain in the eye prior to removal.[54-57] Disadvantages include both increased expense and the logistics of doing the femtosecond procedure immediately prior to the PK.

The uptake of excimer laser trephination was very limited due to the fact that most excimer lasers are performed in refractive suites away from operating theaters, making the logistics of excimer graft trephination very difficult. Femtosecond trephination has, however, been on the rise in recent years, especially as Femtosecond Laser Assisted Cataract Surgery has been performed with increased frequency resulting in more femtosecond lasers being setup in close proximity to operating theaters.

Completing the Excision of the Recipient Corneal Button with Corneal Scissors

Once the initial trephination is complete, a viscoelastic substance, such as hydroxypropyl methylcellulose (2%) or sodium hyaluronate (1%), is injected from the entry site to deepen the anterior chamber. This protects the iris and the lens against any possible trauma with the scissors' blade. Corneal scissors used to complete the cut should have a longer posterior blade and a blunt tip to protect iris and the lens (**Fig. 8A**). The blade of the corneal scissors should be held perpendicular to the cornea, so as to achieve a vertical cut. The cornea is cut full thickness along the trephine cut by closing the scissors as an upward pressure is applied. This is done to prevent the scissors from plunging posteriorly and damaging the iris and the lens. Some surgeons prefer to hold the scissors slightly obliquely to leave a small posterior ledge along the recipient cut. It helps in avoiding inadvertent cutting of the iris and the presence of a posterior ledge offers better apposition while suturing. The cornea must be stabilized with the forceps once half of it has been cut (**Fig. 8B**). Any iris or vitreous attachment to the posterior surface is severed with the scissors before lifting the corneal button.

In perforated corneas, the anterior chamber is frequently shallow and entering the anterior chamber through the cut

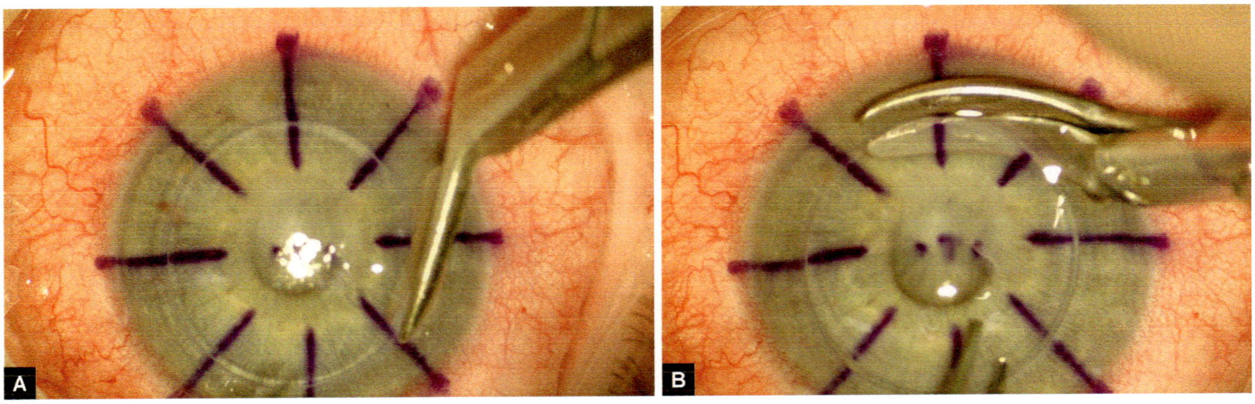

Figs. 8A and B: (A) Corneal scissors used to cut the corneal button; (B) Corneal scissors completes the excision of the recipient bed.

obtained by the trephine may cause damage to the underlying iris and the lens. In such cases, the posterior blade of the scissors may be inserted through the site of the perforation and cuts can be made radially toward the trephine cut like the spokes of the wheel, prior to completing the circular cuts along the trephine edge.

If some posterior tags of the corneal tissue are inadvertently left at the edges of the trephined area, these are trimmed with a curved corneal or Vannas scissors, but this must be done quickly and efficiently to limit open-sky time. Once the recipient bed has been completely prepared (**Fig. 9**), the focus of the surgeon shifts rapidly toward getting the new donor cornea onto the eye to limit the "open-sky" time and close the eye as soon as possible.

SUTURING OF DONOR CORNEA

Placement of the Donor Cornea on the Recipient

The anterior chamber of the host is then filled with a dispersive viscoelastic, which helps to maintain the dome of the donor button and its orientation for accurate suture placement, and further provides endothelial protection. BSS or air can be used for anterior chamber maintenance later in the suturing process, but they are not as effective as viscoelastic during the initial phases of the graft placement.

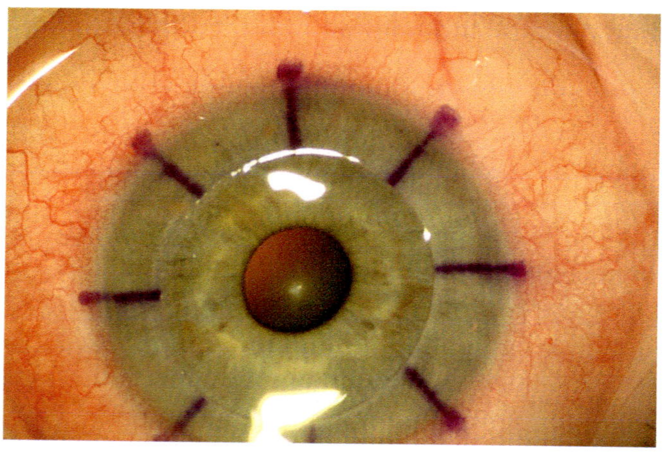

Fig. 9: Corneal recipient bed fully prepared and "open-sky".

The donor cornea is brought into the field of microscope on a Paton spatula (**Fig. 10A**). The edge of the button is placed on the inferior limbus and the spatula is slid down so that it too rests gently on the limbus (**Fig. 10B**). It is then rotated slightly further so that the anterior layers of the opposite end of the donor button can be grasped with a forceps at the junction of epithelium and stroma and transferred on to the recipient bed. Alternatively, the corneal button can be flipped completely over the corneal opening on to the bed of viscoelastic using the spatula. Inversion of the corneal button should be avoided by noting the orientation of the button in the well or by the curvature of the button. Care should be taken to avoid the endothelium of the donor button making contact with any instruments or surfaces.

Placement of the Four Cardinal Sutures

The button is grasped with a fine toothed, double-pronged forceps (e.g., the "Polack" forceps) at the epithelial-stromal junction and brought to the superior edge of the recipient corneal opening and sutured to the recipient cornea with 10-0 nylon suture on a spatulated side-cutting needle.

The first of the four cardinal sutures should be placed at the 12 o'clock position (**Fig. 11A**), followed by a 6 o'clock suture then 3- and 9 o'clock. The needle is passed between the two tips of Polack double-pronged corneal forceps exiting just anterior to Descemet's membrane. At the correct depth, Descemets, and the posterior stroma will tent forward from the posterior edge of the donor as the suture is being passed through. The needle is then passed through the recipient cornea at the radial marks and should exit at 1 mm from the edge. The suture is tied with a double- or triple-throw, followed by two single throws (2:1:1 or 3:1:1). A 2:1:1 technique provides a smaller knot, which is easier to turn, bury, and remove. An alternative option is to use a slipknot to allow precise modulation of suture tension prior to locking the knot.

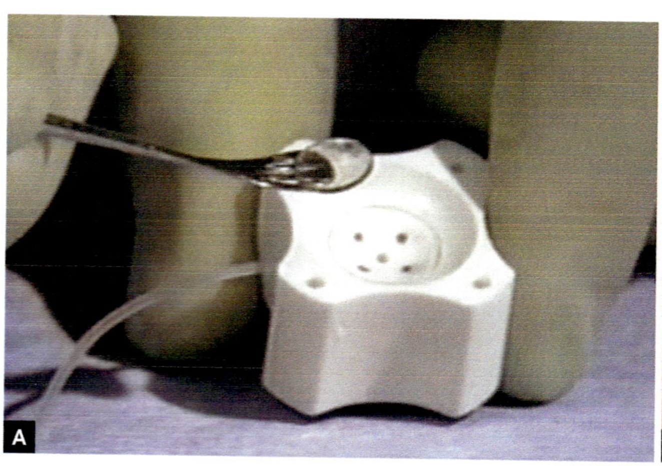

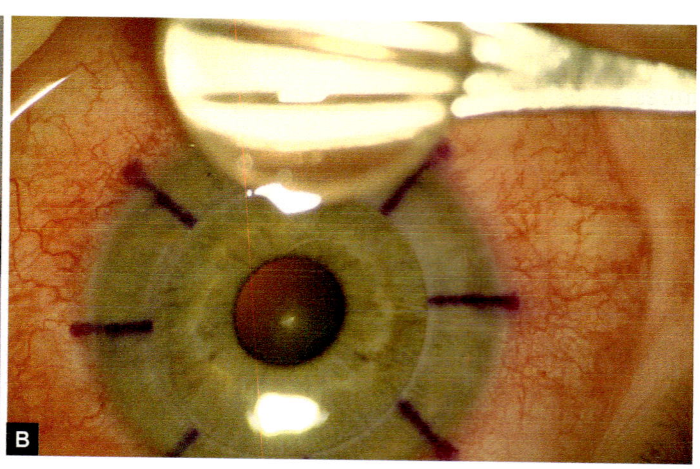

Figs. 10A and B: (A) Paton spatula used to lift donor corneal button; (B) Paton spatula used to position graft at the inferior limbus before placing it on to the recipient bed.

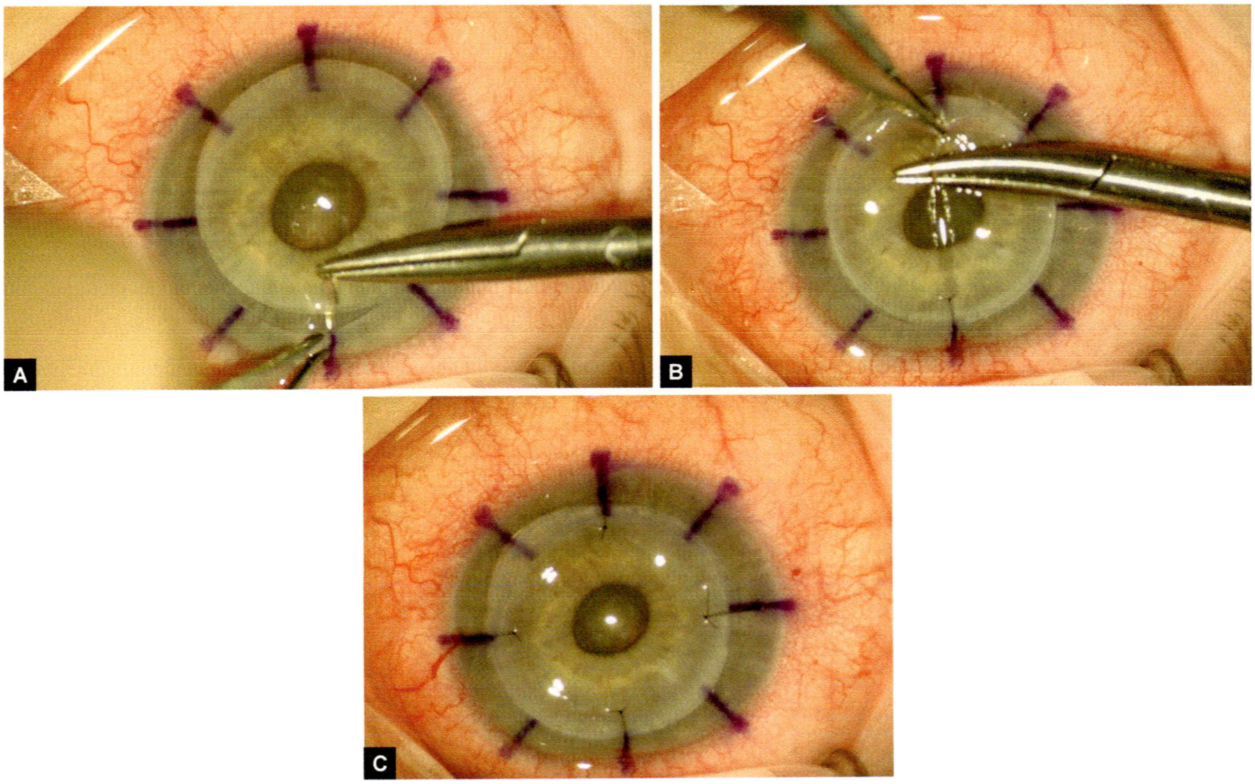

Figs. 11A to C: (A) Placing the first cardinal suture; (B) Second cardinal suture passed 180° from first; (C) Four cardinal sutures in place.

The second cardinal suture is placed 180° from the first suture at 6 o'clock and is the most important suture in PK. This suture plays a vital role in establishing an equal distribution of tissue on either side of the midline (**Fig. 11B**). It is improper placement can cause poor tissue alignment and significant postoperative astigmatism. The prior placement of radial marks helps to eliminate this problem. The third and fourth sutures are then placed at 3- and 9 o'clock, through the marks 90° from the first two sutures. These first four sutures are known as the cardinal sutures. The correct tension and equal spacing of the cardinal sutures should be such that a diamond-like shape appears in the donor cornea after their placement (**Fig. 11C**).

Completion of Corneal Sutures

The rest of the sutures may be placed as single interrupted sutures, a single running suture, or double running sutures. Long-term follow-up shows no significant difference in astigmatism between the suture techniques.[58]

- *Single interrupted sutures* are recommended in infants and children, highly vascularized corneas, cases of previous rejection, inflammatory conditions and in therapeutic keratoplasty for infectious keratitis. Many surgeons now consider this as the standard in keratoplasty. They have the advantage of selective individual suture removal if need arises, e.g., loose-suture, vascularized suture, suture-induced astigmatism or suture abscess. Interrupted sutures are placed in a manner similar to that used for cardinal sutures. The needle should pass anterior to the Descemet's membrane. The suture length should be about 2 mm, 1 mm on each side of the graft-host junction. Full-thickness passes should be avoided as these cause more endothelial trauma and increase risk of aqueous leaks through the suture tracts postoperatively. A total of 16 sutures are usually placed, with the second four sutures equidistant between the first four sutures and the second eight equidistant between the first eight sutures.[36] Besides being equidistant, these sutures should be placed one at a time in quadrants opposite each other so as to improve the chances of making the tension across the different meridians equal and thus potentially reduce astigmatism. Additional sutures may be required for larger grafts, pediatric cases or in patients with thin recipient corneas. The knot ends are trimmed short and buried just beneath the epithelium of the donor cornea using tying forceps and a quick flicking motion in an eye which has been firmed with BSS. We prefer to bury the knots in the donor cornea so that they are well away from the limbus. If buried on the recipient side, they may stimulate vascularization and increase rejection risk because of closer proximity to the limbus. Before the final suture is placed, a simcoe cannula should be inserted into the anterior chamber to ensure that all viscoelastic material is washed out of the eye in order to prevent postoperative pressure rise. This could alternatively be done through the preexisting limbal paracentesis wound after suturing is complete.

Continuous sutures: An alternative to interrupted sutures involves placing only 4–8 interrupted sutures, followed by a continuous running suture. The first bite of a running suture is usually placed radially into the recipient corneal rim, adjacent to and clockwise from the 12 o'clock cardinal suture, and then subsequent bites divide the spaces between the further interrupted sutures evenly. Suture tension can be evenly distributed by continually adjusting the tension of each bite with tying forceps. The final bite will be taken at the same site as the initial bite but will only involve a radial pass through the donor tissue. The two ends of the continuous suture are then tied in a 3-1-1 fashion and the knot will be buried inside the graft-host junction next to the 12 o'clock cardinal suture. If a single running suture technique is used a 10-0 nylon suture is placed after the cardinal sutures are in position and 20–24 bites are taken instead of 16. When a single running suture is used, torque, anti-torque or no-torque suturing techniques can be used (**Fig. 12**). In a double running suture technique, after an initial 16 bites running suture is placed, a second 11-0 nylon suture may be placed between each bite of the 16 bites of 10-0 nylon suture. Each of these continuous suturing techniques is amenable to suture adjustment in cases of astigmatism.

Check for Wound Leakage

After the completion of the suturing and burying of all knots, the wound is tested for water tightness. This is done after drying the surface with a cellulose sponge pressing at the limbus and observing the wound for leakage of aqueous humor. Topical fluorescein is a better method of evaluation for wound leakage. Here the fluorescein is instilled at the wound margins. In the presence of wound leak, a darker track of aqueous fluid leak can be observed due to dilution of the surrounding green fluorescein dye. If a wound leak is present, additional sutures should be applied appropriately. If there is a suture tract leak (**Fig. 13**) this is an indication that the suture was placed full thickness and this suture should be removed and replaced with a suture at 90% depth as described above.

Intraoperative Adjustment for Astigmatism

An intraoperative keratoscope may be helpful in reducing postoperative astigmatism by recognizing steep or flatter meridians. A suture adjustment may be done until regular mires are obtained. Intraoperative keratoscopes available include those with microscope attachment, e.g., Terry's keratometer or those which are based on the reflection of the mires from the corneal surface (**Fig. 14**), such as Maloney's and Mandel's keratometer. Alternatively, the round end of a safety pin may be used and the reflex of the circular image may be evaluated to adjust the suture placement and hence correct for astigmatism intraoperatively. If the reflected mires are circular, this indicates that minimal astigmatism is present. If, however, the reflected mires appear oval, this indicates uneven suture tension is inducing astigmatism. The sutures should thus be adjusted in such a manner so as to achieve circular shape of the mires. In cases with interrupted sutures, the tight sutures (which are present along the shorter diameter of the oval) may be replaced by the sutures that have optimal tension. Similarly, if a continuous suture is used, the loop along the largest diameter of the oval may be manipulated toward the smallest diameter of the oval so that a circular mire is obtained.

Newer technological advancements for intraoperative astigmatism assessment include the various intraoperative aberrometry platforms such as optiwave refractive analysis (ORA) (Alcon Laboratories, Inc., Fort Worth, Texas, USA) and innovative illumination devices such as the Illuminating Surgical Keratoscope known as the Ring Light (Mastel, Rapid City, South Dakota, USA).

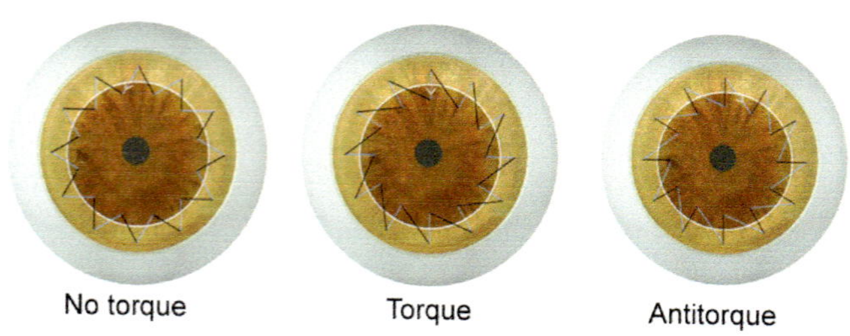

Fig. 12: Types of continuous suturing.

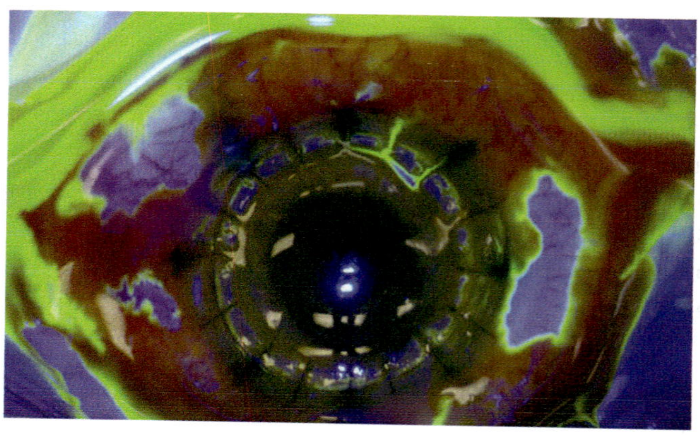

Fig. 13: Suture tract leak at 2 o'clock suture.

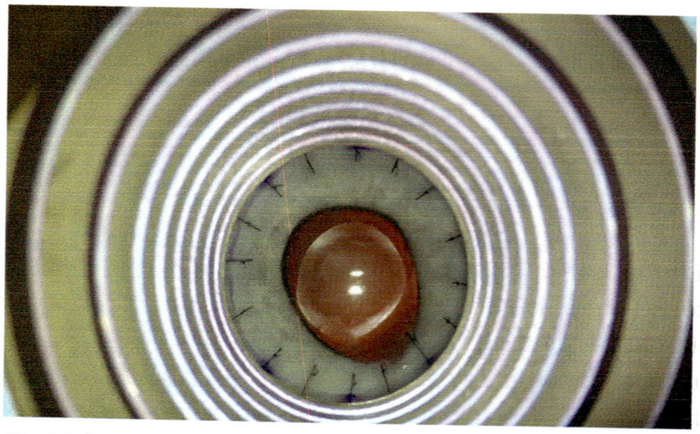

Fig. 14: Intraoperative keratometer to assess for corneal astigmatism.

INTRAOPERATIVE MEDICATIONS

A subconjunctival injection of an antibiotic (e.g., cefazolin 50 mg) and steroid (e.g., dexamethasone 4 mg) combination is given in the inferior fornix at the end of the surgery and the patient is given a pad and hard plastic protective eye shield for 24 hours.

POSTOPERATIVE REGIME

Antibiotics

Routine Cases

Topical antibiotic such as chloramphenicol or ofloxacin 0.3% is used four times a day for 1 week postoperatively or until the epithelium is healed.

Special Cases

Fortified antibiotics such as fortified tobramycin 1.3% or cefazolin 5% may be given in cases where therapeutic PK has been performed for uncontrolled infectious keratitis varying in frequency from 30 minutes to 4 hourly which can be tapered over a 2–3 weeks period once the infection is controlled. In therapeutic PK for fungal keratitis, 5% natamycin or voriconazole drops may be used postoperatively for several weeks. In cases of PK with a history of herpes simplex virus keratitis, oral acyclovir should be given (400 mg 5 times/day) for 1–3 weeks postoperatively and then decreased to maintenance dose (400 mg bd) for several months in order to reduce risk of recurrence in the new graft.

Systemic antibiotics such as ciprofloxacin 500–750 mg twice daily may be considered perioperatively for 3–5 days after the surgery in the following conditions:

- Preexisting external eye infection
- Prosthesis use in the fellow eye
- Penetrating trauma
- Combined procedures, especially with vitrectomy or intraocular lenses (IOLs).

Corticosteroids

Topical corticosteroids such as 1% prednisolone acetate or 0.1% dexamethasone sodium phosphate may be used 2–4 hourly for the first month post-transplant. These are then tapered slowly over several months.

In cases with significant ocular surface disease or limbal stem cell deficiency resulting in delayed epithelial healing, preservative-free dexamethasone or prednisolone should be considered.

In high-risk keratoplasties, topical steroids should be administered 1–2 hourly for the first month and systemic corticosteroids, i.e., prednisolone 1 mg/kg/day should be started 1–2 days before surgery and tapered over 2–3 weeks. In some high-risk cases, long-term systemic steroid-sparing immunosuppressive agents may be considered, such as T-cell inhibitors, e.g., cyclosporine A or antimetabolites, e.g., mycophenolate mofetil. This should be done in close consultation with a physician to ensure regular and adequate monitoring for potential systemic side effects.

Antiglaucoma Medications

Prophylactic antiglaucoma medication such as timolol maleate 0.5% twice a day may be considered in the following cases:

- Preexisting glaucoma
- Penetrating keratoplasty combined with:
  - Cataract surgery
  - Vitrectomies
  - Lysis of synechiae
  - Anterior segment reconstruction

Intraocular pressure should be measured at each subsequent postoperative visit, as patients who have undergone PK are at increased risk of synechial angle closure and steroid induced glaucoma and this should be screened for and managed appropriately.

Cycloplegics

Short-acting agents such as tropicamide 1% or cyclopentolate 1% may be given for early postoperative pain and inflammation control and to reduce the risk of postoperative aqueous misdirection. Strong agents such as atropine should be avoided in cases of keratoconus because of reports of increased risk of permanent pupillary dilation (Urrets-Zavalia syndrome). Wide dilation of the pupil in cases of posterior chamber IOL may increase the risk of formation of synechiae to the posterior capsule and capture of the edge of the lens with iris. Wide dilation should also be avoided in cases where large grafts have been used as this may cause crowding at the angle and adherence to the posterior edge of the wound.[33] Dilation should be used in cases where tectonic grafts are performed (patients with preoperative shallow anterior chambers) and in these cases, peripheral iridectomies should be cut intraoperatively as there is an increased risk of aqueous misdirection.

Lubricants

In routine keratoplasties, preservative-free lubricants may be given at 2 hourly to 4 times daily dosage. Epitheliotoxic drugs such as nonsteroidal anti-inflammatory drugs and topical aminoglycosides should be avoided. In cases with severe ocular surface issues or lagophthalmos, a temporary suture tarsorrhaphy or botulinum-toxin-induced ptosis may be of benefit in promoting epithelial healing over the graft.

POSTOPERATIVE SUTURE MANAGEMENT

Corneal sutures are routinely only removed between 12 and 18 months postoperatively to ensure adequate time for a strongly adherent wound to have developed joining the host and recipient corneas. This can be performed at the slit-lamp or with the patient supine under a microscope in a procedure room. After instillation of local anesthetic drops and diluted povidone iodine solution, the sutures may be cut using a 25-G needle and then removed using a corneal tying forceps. Try to prevent pieces of suture breaking off and being left behind in the cornea. If a suture does break, ensure that the broken suture ends are buried underneath the corneal surface and not left exposed. Experience has shown that the sutures may be removed over two sessions to reduce the risk of dehiscence and to allow improved patient comfort. A topical antibiotic such as chloramphenicol should be used for 1 week post-removal to prevent infection developing in the areas of disturbed epithelium. The final shape of the cornea and degree of astigmatism will only be established after removal of all the corneal sutures and visual acuity often improves after suture removal because of a reduction in irregular astigmatism.[59]

If corneal astigmatism is negligible and the patient has good uncorrected vision with the sutures in place, then many surgeons will opt to leave the sutures in permanently unless the patient develops an indication for removal, such as vascularization, suture breakage, infection, or patient discomfort.

During the initial 12–18 months prior to removal of sutures, any loose sutures should be removed. This is because a loose suture is providing no structural support to the wound and loose or broken sutures have been shown to be the leading cause of postkeratoplasty graft infections.[60]

Postoperative suture adjustment is also beneficial in terms of reduction of corneal astigmatism and visual rehabilitation. A tight interrupted suture will cause increased central steepness along the meridian of the suture. Removing tight sutures on the axis of steep curvature will flatten the central cornea along this axis. Removal of sutures along the steep axis can significantly reduce the amount of corneal astigmatism and improve the uncorrected and best-corrected visual acuity. If this is performed before wound healing is complete, then collagen remodeling can alter the final shape of the cornea even after final removal of the remaining sutures at 12–18 months.

POSTOPERATIVE PATIENT EDUCATION

Proper patient education on life, post a corneal graft, is vital in terms of the long-term survival and outcomes after PK. Patients should be informed of the importance of complying with postoperative drop instructions and the regular follow-up visits in the postoperative period. Clear instructions and handouts should be given detailing their postoperative regime. Protective eyewear should be recommended for any recreational or occupational situations that may carry increased risk of potential ocular trauma. Contact sports should be avoided. Patients should also be well educated on the symptoms and signs of rejection, infection, or loose sutures and be advised to follow up urgently if these symptoms occur. A well-educated patient can make all the difference between a graft that survives for decades and one that fails soon after surgery because of delayed presentation.

REFERENCES

1. Melles GR, Eggink FA, Lander F, Pels E, Rietveld FJ, Beekhuis WH, et al. A surgical technique for posterior lamellar keratoplasty. Cornea. 1998;17(6):618-26.
2. Terry MA, Ousley PJ. Deep lamellar endothelial keratoplasty visual acuity, astigmatism, and endothelial survival in a large prospective series. Ophthalmology. 2005;112(9):1541-8.
3. Gorovoy MS. Descemet-stripping automated endothelial keratoplasty. Cornea. 2006;25(8):886-9.
4. Price FW Jr, Price MO. Descemet's stripping with endothelial keratoplasty in 200 eyes. Early challenges and techniques to enhance donor adherence. J Cataract Refract Surg. 2006;32(3):411-8.
5. Melles GR, Ong TS, Ververs B, van der Wees J. Preliminary clinical results of Descemet membrane endothelial keratoplasty. Am J Ophthalmol. 2008;145(2):222-7.
6. Anwar M, Teichmann KD. Big-bubble technique to bare Descemet's membrane in anterior lamellar keratoplasty. J Cataract Refract Surg. 2002;28(3):398-403.
7. Starr MB. Prophylactic antibiotics for ophthalmic surgery. Surv Ophthalmol. 1983;27(6):353-73.
8. Hughes DS, Hill RJ. Infectious endophthalmitis after cataract surgery. Br J Ophthalmol. 1994;78(3):227-32.
9. Chitkara DK, Manners T, Chapman F, Stoddart MG, Hill D, Jenkins D. Lack of effect of preoperative norfloxacin on contamination of anterior chamber aspirates after cataract surgery. Br J Ophthalmol. 1994;78(10):772-4.
10. Speaker MG, Milch FA, Shah MK, Eisner W, Kreiswirth BN. Role of external bacterial flora in the pathogenesis of acute postoperative endophthalmitis. Ophthalmology. 1991;98(5):639-50.
11. The Collaborative Corneal Transplantation Studies (CCTS). Effectiveness of histocompatibility matching in high-risk corneal transplantation. The Collaborative Corneal Transplantation Studies Research Group. Arch Ophthalmol. 1992;110(10):1392-403.
12. Lim KJ, Wee WR, Lee JH. Treatment of corneal neovascularization with argon laser. Korean J Ophthalmol. 1993;7(1):25-7.
13. Nirankari VS, Baer JC. Corneal argon laser photocoagulation for neovascularization in penetrating keratoplasty. Ophthalmology. 1986;93(10):1304-9.
14. Stevenson W, Cheng SF, Dastjerdi MH, Ferrari G, Dana R. Corneal neovascularization and the utility of topical VEGF inhibition: ranibizumab (Lucentis) vs bevacizumab (Avastin). Ocul Surf. 2012;10(2):67-83.
15. Cheng SF, Dastjerdi MH, Ferrari G, Okanobo A, Bower KS, Ryan DS, et al. Short-term topical bevacizumab in the treatment of stable corneal neovascularization. Am J Ophthalmol. 2012; 154(6):940-8.e1.
16. Kirsch RE, Steinman W. Digital pressure, an important safeguard in cataract surgery. AMA Arch Ophthalmol. 1955;54(5):697-703.
17. Quist LH, Stapleton SS, McPherson SD Jr. Preoperative use of the Honan intraocular pressure reducer. Am J Ophthalmol. 1983;95(4):536-8.
18. Jay WM, Carter H, Williams B, Green K. Effect of applying the Honan intraocular pressure reducer before cataract surgery. Am J Ophthalmol. 1985;100(4):523-7.
19. Bourne WM. Reduction of endothelial cell loss during phakic penetrating keratoplasty. Am J Ophthalmol. 1980;89(6):787-90.
20. Feibel RM. Current concepts in retrobulbar anesthesia. Surv Ophthalmol. 1985;30(2):102-10.
21. Atkinson WS. Local anesthesia in ophthalmology. Am J Ophthalmol. 1948;31(12):1607-18.
22. Ingraham HJ, Donnenfeld ED, Perry HD. Massive suprachoroidal hemorrhage in penetrating keratoplasty. Am J Ophthalmol. 1989;108(6):670-5.

23. Speaker MG, Guerriero PN, Met JA, Coad CT, Berger A, Marmor M. A case-control study of risk factors for intraoperative suprachoroidal expulsive hemorrhage. Ophthalmology. 1991; 98(2):202-10.
24. Price FW Jr, Whitson WE, Ahad KA, Tavakkoli H. Suprachoroidal hemorrhage in penetrating keratoplasty. Ophthalmic Surg. 1994;25(8):521-5.
25. Purcell JJ Jr, Krachmer JH, Doughman DJ, Bourne WM. Expulsive hemorrhage in penetrating keratoplasty. Ophthalmology. 1982;89(1):41-3.
26. Apt L, Isenberg S, Yoshimori R, Paez JH. Chemical preparation of the eye in ophthalmic surgery. III. Effect of povidone-iodine on the conjunctiva. Arch Ophthalmol. 1984;102(5):728-9.
27. Isenberg SJ, Apt L, Yoshimori R, Khwarg S. Chemical preparation of the eye in ophthalmic surgery. IV. Comparison of povidone-iodine on the conjunctiva with a prophylactic antibiotic. Arch Ophthalmol. 1985;103(9):1340-2.
28. Speaker MG, Menikoff JA. Prophylaxis of endophthalmitis with topical povidine-iodine. Ophthalmology. 1991;98(12):1769-75.
29. Nentwich MM, Ta CN, Kreutzer TC, Li B, Schwarzbach F, Yactayo-Miranda YM, et al. Incidence of postoperative endophthalmitis from 1990 to 2009 using povidone-iodine but no intracameral antibiotics at a single academic institution. J Cataract Refract Surg. 2015;41(1):58-66.
30. Olson RJ. The effect of scleral fixation ring placement and trephine tilting on keratoplasty wound size and donor shape. Ophthalmic Surg. 1981;12(1):23-6.
31. Uozato H, Guyton DL. Centering corneal surgical procedures. Am J Ophthalmol. 1987;103(3 Pt 1):264-75.
32. Vajpayee RB, Sharma V, Sharma N, Panda A, Taylor HR. Evaluation of techniques of single continuous suturing in penetrating keratoplasty. Br J Ophthalmol. 2001;85(2):134-8.
33. Barron BA. Penetrating keratoplasty. In: Kaufman HE, Barron BA, McDonald MB (Eds). The Cornea. Boston: Butterworth-Heinemann; 1998. pp. 805-46.
34. Bourne WM, Davidson JA, O'Fallon WM. The effects of oversize donor buttons on postoperative intraocular pressure and corneal curvature in aphakic penetrating keratoplasty. Ophthalmology. 1982;89(3):242-6.
35. Wiffen SJ, Maguire LJ, Bourne WM. Keratometric results of penetrating keratoplasty with the Hessburg-Barron and Hanna trephine systems using a standard double-running suture technique. Cornea. 1997;16(3):306-13.
36. Waring GO 3rd. Management of pseudophakic corneal edema with reconstruction of anterior ocular segment. Arch Ophthalmol. 1987;105(5):709-15.
37. Sharif KW, Casey TA. Penetrating keratoplasty for keratoconus: complications and long-term success. Br J Ophthalmol. 1991;75(3):142-6.
38. Tuft SJ, Gregory WM, Davison CR. Bilateral penetrating keratoplasty for keratoconus. Ophthalmology. 1995;102(3):462-8.
39. Alldredge OC, Krachmer JH. Clinical types of corneal transplant rejection. Their manifestations, frequency, preoperative correlates, and treatment. Arch Ophthalmol. 1981;99(4):599-604.
40. Boisjoly HM, Bernard PM, Dubé I, Laughrea PA, Bazin R, Bernier J. Effect of factors unrelated to tissue matching on corneal transplant endothelial rejection. Am J Ophthalmol. 1989;107(6):647-54.
41. Maguire MG, Stark WJ, Gottsch JD, Stulting RD, Sugar A, Fink NE, et al. Risk factors for corneal graft failure and rejection in the collaborative corneal transplantation studies. Ophthalmology. 1994;101(9):1536-47.
42. Vajpayee RB, Dada T, Ray M, Tandon R, Sethi A, Turaka K. Oversized corneal grafts for corneal opacities with iridocorneal adhesions. Ophthalmology. 2001;108(11):2026-8.
43. Vajpayee RB, Ramu M, Panda A, Sharma N, Tabin GC, Anand JR. Oversized grafts in children. Ophthalmology. 1999;106(4):829-32.
44. Olson RJ. Variation in corneal graft size related to trephine technique. Arch Ophthalmol. 1979;97(7):1323-5.
45. Brightbill FS, Polack FM, Slappey T. A comparison of two methods of cutting donor corneal buttons. Am J Ophthalmol. 1973;75(3):500-6.
46. Tanne E. A new donor cutting block for penetrating keratoplasty. Ophthalmic Surg. 1981;12(5):371-2.
47. Radner W, Skorpik CH, Loewe R, Mudrich C, Radner G, Mallinger R. Effect of trephination technique on the ultrastructure of corneal transplants: guided trephine system v posterior punch technique. Br J Ophthalmol. 1999;83(10):1172-7.
48. Verdier DD. Penetrating keratoplasty. In: Krachmer JH, Mannis MJ, Holland EJ (Eds). Cornea Surgery of the Cornea and Conjunctiva. Vol. III. St. Louis: Mosby; 1997. pp. 1581-92.
49. Cohen SW, Benko W. Automated motorized penetrating keratoplasty. Ann Ophthalmol. 1977;9(11):1461-6.
50. Weiner M, Alvis Y. Transplantation of cornea by means of a mechanically obtained beveled- edge segment. Am J Ophthalmol. 1940;23(8):877-81.
51. Legeais JM, Parel JM, Simon G, Ren Q, Denham D. Endothelial damage by the corneal Hessburg- Barron vacuum trephine. Refract Corneal Surg. 1993;9(4):255-8.
52. Seitz B, Langenbucher A, Kus MM, Küchle M, Naumann GO. Nonmechanical corneal trephination with the excimer laser improves outcome after penetrating keratoplasty. Ophthalmology. 1999;106(6):1156-65.
53. Langenbucher A, Seitz B, Kus MM, Vilchis E, Naumann GO. Graft decentration in penetrating keratoplasty: nonmechanical trephination with the excimer laser (193 nm) versus the motor trephine. Ophthalmic Surg Lasers. 1998;29(2):106-13.
54. Farid M, Kim M, Steinert RF. Results of penetrating keratoplasty performed with a femtosecond laser zigzag incision initial report. Ophthalmology. 2007;114:2208-12.
55. Cheng YY, Tahzib NG, van Rij G, van Cleynenbreugel H, Pels E, Hendrikse F, et al. Femtosecond laser-assisted inverted mushroom keratoplasty. Cornea. 2008;27(6):679-85.
56. Bahar I, Kaiserman I, Lange AP, Levinger E, Sansanayudh W, Singal N, et al. Femtosecond laser versus manual dissection for top hat penetrating keratoplasty. Br J Ophthalmol. 2009;93(1):73-8.
57. Price FW Jr, Price MO. Femtosecond laser shaped penetrating keratoplasty: One-year results utilizing a top-hat configuration. Am J Ophthalmol. 2008;145(2):210-4.
58. Filatov V, Alexandrakis G, Talamo JH, Steinert RF. Comparison of suture-in and suture-out postkeratoplasty astigmatism with single running or combined and interrupted sutures. Am J Ophthalmol. 1996;122(5):696-700.
59. Kagaya F, Tomidokoro A, Tanaka S, Amano S, Oshika T. Fourier series harmonic analysis of corneal topography following suture removal after penetrating keratoplasty. Cornea. 2002;21(3):256-9.
60. Fong LP, Ormerod LD, Kenyon KR, Foster CS. Microbial keratitis complicating penetrating keratoplasty. Ophthalmology. 1988; 95(9):1269-75.

12 Suturing Techniques in Penetrating Keratoplasty

C Banu Cosar, Peter R Laibson

INTRODUCTION

Obtaining a clear graft in penetrating keratoplasty (PK) has become almost expected. For most eyes undergoing PK, the success rate for a clear graft exceeds 90%.[1,2] However, postoperative astigmatism still remains a problem that can prevent the functional success of clear graft.[3] There are many factors contributing to astigmatism after PK, including preexisting corneal thinning and vascularization, eccentric trephination of the donor or host, oversized grafts, preexisting keratoconus, quality of wound healing, and astigmatism of donor eye. Tension, length, depth, and configuration of corneal sutures have also been implicated as causative factors.[4]

There are mainly four types of suturing techniques in PK:
1. Interrupted sutures
2. Combined interrupted and continuous sutures
3. Single continuous sutures
4. Double continuous sutures

Many authors have compared the effectiveness of these suturing techniques in terms of astigmatism, visual outcome, and complications.[5-13] However, it is difficult to corroborate the results of these various studies because of the differences in techniques, indications, timing of suture adjustment and removal, and follow-up periods. However, all suturing techniques have been used successfully to secure the wound and create a relatively smooth corneal contour. Therefore, specific suturing technique is mainly dictated by the expertise and preference of the surgeon, and by the presence or absence of localized disease (**Table 1**).

Table 1: Advantages and disadvantages of various suturing techniques.

Suturing technique	*Advantage*	*Disadvantage*
Single interrupted sutures	• Easiest to place • Permit partial or complete suture removal such as in pediatric keratoplasty, vascularization in host cornea, multiple previous rejections, and inflammatory conditions	Only adjustment possible is removal, therefore, flattening
Combined continuous and interrupted sutures	• Continuous suture maintains wound apposition whenever the interrupted sutures are removed • Earlier visual rehabilitation	Interrupted sutures are difficult to remove after several years
Single continuous suture	• Adjustment is possible without removal • Adjustment can be repeated more than once • Earlier visual rehabilitation	• Requires more technical expertise • Removal of the suture is an all or none phenomenon
Double continuous suture	• Adjustment is possible without removal • Remaining continuous suture maintains wound apposition whenever the other continuous suture is removed • Adjustment can be repeated more than once	Requires more technical expertise

SUTURING TECHNIQUES

Single Interrupted Suturing Technique

Interrupted sutures are commonly used by many corneal surgeons[14] because they are easy to place and permit partial or complete suture removal in one region of the graft if necessary.

In very young pediatric keratoplasty, interrupted sutures are used almost exclusively. For older children some surgeons advocate a running closure providing there is no asymmetric vascularization.[15,16] Single interrupted sutures are also indicated in vascularization in the host cornea so that partial suture removal may be performed earlier in these vascularized areas in the postoperative course. Multiple previous rejections, inflammatory conditions that may predispose to localized vascularization, rejection, or ulceration are other indications for single interrupted sutures.[17]

Interrupted sutures are placed with 10-0 nylon. Sixteen is the average number of interrupted sutures placed for a typical 8 mm diameter graft. Twenty-four or 32 sutures may be necessary in larger grafts. An 8-blade RK marker can be used as a guide (**Fig. 1**). The first cardinal suture is placed at 12 o'clock position. The second cardinal suture, placed 180° away at 6 o'clock, is the most critical in terms of tissue alignment and subsequent astigmatism. It should be placed so that an equal amount of tissue is distributed on either side. Then, cardinal sutures at 3 o'clock and 9 o'clock are placed followed by other sutures. The sutures should be placed as radially and as evenly spaced as possible, with the ideal depth of each suture bite 90%. They should neither be too loose nor too tight (**Figs. 2 and 3**). The knots can be buried either in the host tissue or the donor tissue. We prefer to bury the knots in the donor tissue to induce less vascularization in the graft.[18] Some surgeons bury the knots in the host tissue so that after the knots are cut and the suture is pulled, there is less tension on the graft-host junction, reducing the chance of dehiscence if the sutures are removed during the early stages of postoperative wound healing.[19]

Combined Continuous and Interrupted Suturing Technique

This technique is most often performed using 12 interrupted 10-0 nylon sutures and a 12-bite continuous 10-0 or 11-0 nylon running suture with bites of the continuous suture placed between each of the interrupted sutures (**Fig. 4**). The needle pass of the continuous suture bites should be made close to the interrupted suture so that the epithelial portion of the continuous suture lies across the wound between the interrupted sutures. If suture bites are made halfway between the interrupted sutures, the superficial segment will lie across the interrupted sutures, providing little additional wound supports. The ideal depth of the suture bites is 95%. 11-0 Mersilene® suture has also been reported to be an effective suture material in this technique for either interrupted or the running suture.[20,21]

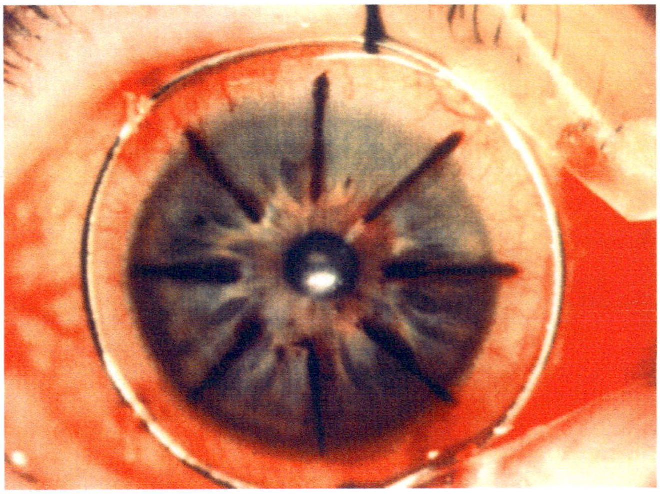

Fig. 1: Eight-blade RK marks on the cornea to assist in suture placement. The Flieringa ring is in place.

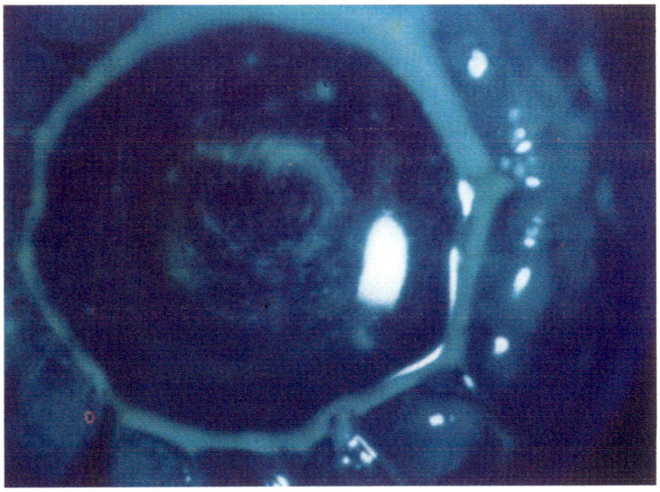

Fig. 3: Penetrating keratoplasty with 16 interrupted sutures which are too tight. Note guttering of fluorescein at the host-donor junction and whorl superficial punctate keratopathy of the donor cornea.

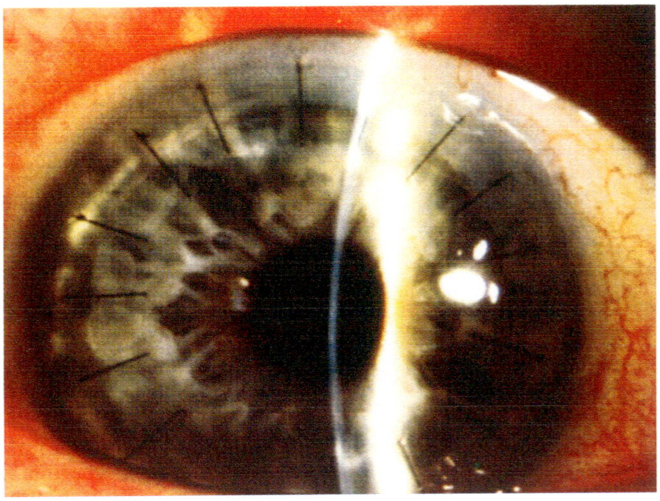

Fig. 2: Penetrating keratoplasty with 16 interrupted sutures. Note the smooth contour of the host-donor junction with the slit illumination.

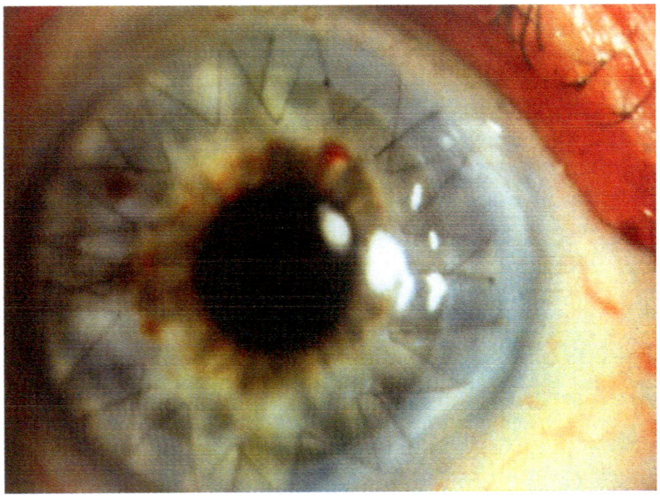

Fig. 4: Combined technique, using 8 interrupted and 16-bite running 10-0 nylon sutures.

Single Continuous Suturing Technique

There are three types of single continuous suturing techniques: (1) torque, (2) antitorque, and (3) no torque (**Fig. 5**). The torque pattern rotates the corneal graft counter-clockwise by 0.7 ± 0.1 mm at the wound or 11°; the antitorque pattern rotates the corneal graft clockwise by 0.7 ± 0.1 mm at the wound or 11°; and the no-torque pattern, the bites of which form an isosceles triangle, produces no rotational effect.[22] In the antitorque suturing technique, the distortion occurs more in the deeper layers of cornea and does not contribute much to postoperative corneal astigmatism. However, with the torque suturing technique, the oblique overlying suture segment causes distortion of anterior corneal surface contributing to corneal astigmatism postoperatively. In the no-torque technique, since the intrastromal bytes and the overlying sutures are at equal inclination, they act as a splint and cause less corneal distortion.[22,23] Vajpayee RB et al. evaluated these three single continuous suturing techniques in PK and found that the torque suturing technique showed the highest astigmatism although the difference among the three was not significant.[23]

A single continuous suture is technically more difficult than interrupted sutures because one irregular bite can impair the integrity of the closure and cannot be removed without removing the entire suture. The four cardinal sutures are placed in the regular manner followed by a 24-bite continuous suture with 10-0 nylon with a 95% depth. The continuous suture is knotted temporarily at 12 o'clock while the four interrupted cardinal sutures are carefully removed. The anterior chamber is inflated with balanced salt solution plus (BSS plus). The continuous suture is tightened and is then permanently knotted at 12 o'clock (**Fig. 6**). If the continuous suture is tightened when the eye is soft, "barrel topping" of the graft with a topographically flat donor cornea results.[17] 11-0 Mersilene® has also been reported to be an effective suture material for the single continuous suturing technique.[24]

Double Continuous Suturing Technique

After the four cardinal sutures are placed, a 12-bite 10-0 nylon suture is placed with bites at approximately 80% depth. The suture is then knotted superiorly and the knot is buried in the host cornea. A second continuous suture (either 10-0 or 11-0 nylon) is then placed. The bites should alternate between each 10-0 bite for 360°. The second 10-0 or 11-0 is placed approximately 50–60% the corneal depth (**Fig. 7**).

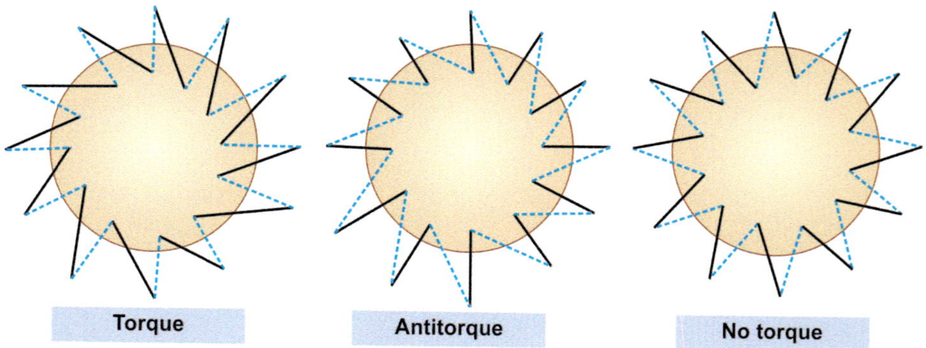

Fig. 5: Three types of single continuous suturing technique in penetrating keratoplasty.

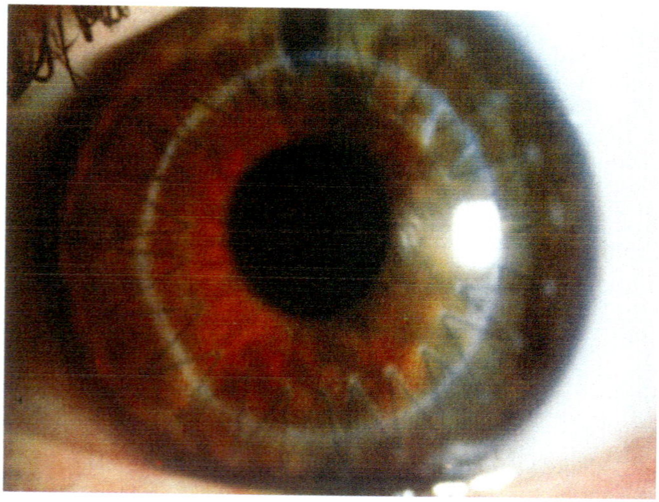

Fig. 6: Twenty-four-bite single continuous 10-0 nylon suture.

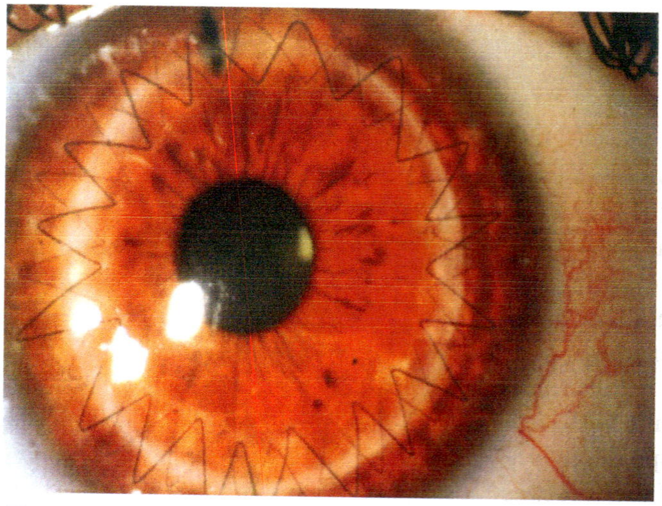

Fig. 7: Double continuous technique with 10-0 and 11-0 nylon sutures.

SUTURE ADJUSTMENT AND SUTURE REMOVAL

The purpose of suture adjustment is to minimize postoperative astigmatism. Postoperative suture adjustment is less effective in reducing spherical refractive errors. Final suture removal may induce either hyperopization or corneal steepening.[25,26]

Many studies have been performed previously to address the ideal timing for suture removal. A study comparing intraoperative suture adjustment, early postoperative suture adjustment (<2 weeks) and late postoperative suture adjustment (>1 month) concluded that early postoperative suture removal was more effective than late postoperative suture removal. The same study found that intraoperative suture adjustment may further reduce final astigmatism and the necessity for postoperative suture manipulation.[27] Whereas, another study compared early suture removal (<18 months after surgery), late suture removal (≥18 months after surgery) and leaving the sutures in place, and concluded that final refractive error and net change in refractive and keratometric astigmatism are not dependent on the timing of suture removal.[28]

Suture adjustment or removal should be performed as early as possible to provide early visual rehabilitation. A previous study tested the hypothesis that the cornea becomes fixed more than 1 year after PK so that desirable refractive results will remain when all sutures are eventually removed. However, when the remaining sutures were removed 1–6 years after PK, corneal astigmatism changed unpredictably and by large amount.[29]

Topographical analyses using keratometry, photokeratoscopy, or videokeratography, individually or in combination, are helpful in planning suture adjustment.[30] However, often there is a disagreement between the topographically determined steep axis and sutures to be removed, and that is determined by keratometry and refraction. Agreement between refraction, keratometry, and topography is associated with greater change in vector-corrected astigmatism. Disagreement between refraction, keratometry, and topography is associated with less vector-corrected astigmatism, but patients in the disagreement group have a greater chance of improvement than worsening following suture removal.[31]

Suture adjustment can take the form of removal of all sutures, partial suture removal, or adjustment in the tension of a running suture. If corneal astigmatism is satisfactory with sutures in place, sutures should remain until there is some indication for removal, such as scarring, vascularization, suture breakage, loose interrupted sutures, and pronounced inflammation, or infiltration around sutures.[17]

The suture removal or adjustment is performed at the slit lamp with topical anesthesia guided by the computerized topography, or keratometry or refraction, or by a combination of the three, as well as slit lamp evaluation. One drop of antibiotic is placed in the eye after removal or adjustment. The patient is given antibiotic drops and antibiotic ointment at bed time for 3 days or 4 days.

The topographic changes induced by suture removal occur immediately. However, continued shifting in corneal curvature takes place over the subsequent 4–6 weeks.[32] Astigmatic errors become stable, with less than 1 D of change between successive examinations within 6 months after suture removal.[33]

Single Interrupted Sutures

The only adjustment possible with single interrupted sutures is removal and therefore flattening. We start removing the sutures at 1 year after the surgery unless otherwise indicated. A very tight suture can be removed as early as 6 weeks. In the case of a suture that loosens or becomes undone in the first few weeks after keratoplasty, if there is a wound gape this suture can be replaced under topical anesthesia. The suture at the steepest meridian indicated by computerized topography analysis is cut either with a razor blade fragment or a disposal 27-gauge needle. It is removed with a tying forceps or a jeweler's forceps. A sudden jerk is more effective at removing the interrupted suture than slower and less forceful pressure.

In pediatric keratoplasty, every other interrupted 10-0 nylon suture is removed in the early postoperative period, followed by complete removal of sutures at a later date. All sutures in patients less than a year are usually removed within 8 weeks.

Combined Continuous and Interrupted Sutures

At approximately 2–3 months after PK, corneal topography is evaluated and a very tight interrupted suture can be removed. Usually this does not occur until 6 months from the time of surgery. A disadvantage of combined continuous and interrupted sutures (CCIS) adjustment is that only the tight suture can be removed; therefore, only the steep axis can be flattened. Another disadvantage is that interrupted sutures are very difficult to remove after several years.

Single Continuous Suture

Adjustment of the single continuous suture can change corneal topography and still support the wound. The suture is very carefully advanced from the flat to the steep meridian, simultaneously flattening the steep meridian and steepening the flat meridian. Adjustment can be repeated more than once if desired. Acceptable astigmatism with sutures allows the patient to achieve early visual rehabilitation.

The risk of breakage during the adjustment procedure should be considered seriously but is not common. Suture breakage can result in wound dehiscence and requires prompt repair in the operating room. Consequently, suture adjustment of the single continuous suture should not be attempted unless facilities are available to make the repair.

Double Continuous Sutures

Double continuous suture technique may involve a 10-0 and an 11-0 nylon suture or a double 10-0 running suture. The deeper and tighter 10-0 suture may be removed or adjusted. And the shallower 11-0 or 10-0 suture is left in place as a safety net.

CONCLUSION

All suturing techniques have been used successfully to secure the wound and create a relatively smooth corneal contour. Suture adjustment can be performed intraoperatively and postoperatively. Sutures should be left in place once the suture has been adjusted to achieve suitable topography.

REFERENCES

1. Price FW Jr, Whitson WE, Collins KS, Marks RG. Five-year corneal graft survival. Arch Ophthalmol. 1993;111(6):799-805.
2. Thompson RW Jr, Price MO, Bowers PJ, Price FW Jr. Long-term graft survival after penetrating keratoplasty. Ophthalmology. 2003;110(7):1396-402.
3. Hardten DR, Lindstrom RL. Surgical correction of refractive errors after penetrating keratoplasty. Int Ophthalmol Clin. 1997;37(1):1-35.
4. Riddle HK Jr, Parker DA, Price FW Jr. Management of postkeratoplasty astigmatism. Curr Opin Ophthalmol. 1998;9(4):15-28.
5. Karabatsas CH, Cook SD, Figueiredo FC, Diamond JP, Easty DL. Combined interrupted and continuous versus single continuous adjustable suturing in penetrating keratoplasty: a prospective, randomized study of induced astigmatism during the first postoperative year. Ophthalmology. 1998;105(11):1991-8.
6. Spadea L, Cifariello F, Bianco G, Balestrazzi E. Long-term results of penetrating keratoplasty using a single or double running suture technique. Graefes Arch Clin Exp Ophthalmol. 2002;240(5):415-9.
7. Javadi MA, Naderi M, Zare M, Jenaban A, Rabei HM, Anissian A. Comparison of the effect of three suturing techniques on postkeratoplasty astigmatism in keratoconus. Cornea. 2006;25(9):1029-33.
8. Busin M, Mönks T, al-Nawaiseh I. Different suturing techniques variously affect the regularity of postkeratoplasty astigmatism. Ophthalmology. 1998;105(7):1200-5.
9. Murta JN, Amaro L, Tavares C, Mira JB. Astigmatism after penetrating keratoplasty. Role of the suture technique. Doc Ophthalmol. 1994;87(4):331-6.
10. Filatov V, Steinert RF, Talamo JH. Postkeratoplasty astigmatism with single running suture or interrupted sutures. Am J Ophthalmol. 1993;115(6):715-21.
11. Assil KK, Zarnegar SR, Schanzlin DJ. Visual outcome after penetrating keratoplasty with double continuous or combined interrupted and continuous suture wound closure. Am J Ophthalmol. 1992;114(1):63-71.
12. Solano JM, Hodge DO, Bourne WM. Keratometric astigmatism after suture removal in penetrating keratoplasty: double running versus single running suture techniques. Cornea. 2003;22(8):716-20.
13. Ramirez M, Hodge DO, Bourne WM. Keratometric results during the first year after keratoplasty: adjustable single running suture technique versus double running suture technique. Ophthalmic Surg Lasers. 2001;32(5):370-4.
14. Rapuano CJ, Luchs JI, Kim T. Anterior segment surgery and complications. In: Krachmer JH (Ed). Anterior Segment: The Requisites in Ophthalmology. St. Louis: Mosby; 2000. pp. 232-85.
15. Stulting RD. Penetrating keratoplasty in children. In: Brightbill FS (Ed). Corneal Surgery: Theory, Technique, and Tissue. St. Louis: Mosby; 1993.
16. Dana MR, Moyes AL, Gomes JA, Rosheim KM, Schaumberg DA, Laibson PR, et al. The indications for and outcome in pediatric keratoplasty: a multicenter study. Ophthalmology. 1995;102(8):1129-38.
17. Van Meter W, Katz DG. Keratoplasty suturing techniques. In: Krachmer JH, Mannis MJ, Holland EJ (Eds). Cornea: Surgery of the Cornea and Conjunctiva, 2nd edition. St. Louis: Mosby; 2005. pp. 1481-92.
18. Dana MR, Schaumberg DA, Kowal VO, Goren MB, Rapuano CJ, Laibson PR, et al. Corneal neovascularization after penetrating keratoplasty. Cornea. 1995;14(6):604-9.
19. Melles GR, Binder PS. A comparison of wound healing in sutured and unsutured corneal wounds. Arch Ophthalmol. 1980;108(10):1460-9.
20. Bigar F, Uffer S. The unsolved problem of transplant astigmatism. Klin Monbl Augenheilkd. 1992;200(5):401-3.
21. Ramselaar JA, Beekhuis WH, Rijneveld WJ, van Andel MV, Dijk F, Jongebloed WL. Mersilene (polyester), a new suture for penetrating keratoplasty. Doc Ophthalmol. 1992;82(1-2):89-101.
22. Au YK, Mahjoub SB, Hart JC. Suture patterns and corneal graft rotation in the cadaver eye. Ophthalmic Surg. 1990;21(7):472-4.
23. Vajpayee RB, Sharma V, Sharma N, Panda A, Taylor HR. Evaluation of techniques of single continuous suturing in penetrating keratoplasty. Br J Ophthalmol. 2001;85(2):134-8.
24. Touzeau O, Borderie VM, Allouch C, Scheer S, Laroche L. Effects of penetrating keratoplasty suture removal on corneal topography and refraction. Cornea. 1999;18(6):638-44.
25. Mathers WD, Gold JB, Kattan H, Lemp MA. Corneal steepening with final suture removal after penetrating keratoplasty. Cornea. 1991;10(3):221-3.
26. Frueh BE, Brown SI, Feldman ST. 11-0 mersilene as running suture for penetrating keratoplasty. Am J Ophthalmol. 1992;114(6):675-9.
27. Shimazaki J, Shimmura S, Tsubota K. Intraoperative versus postoperative suture adjustment after penetrating keratoplasty. Cornea. 1998;17(6):590-4.
28. Serdarevic ON, Renard GJ, Pouliquen Y. Randomized clinical trial of penetrating keratoplasty. Before and after suture removal comparison of intraoperative and postoperative suture adjustment. Ophthalmology. 1995;102(10):1497-503.
29. Davis EA, Azar DT, Jakobs FM, Stark WJ. Refractive and keratometric results after the triple procedure: experience with early and late suture removal. Ophthalmology. 1998;105(4):624-30.
30. Mader TH, Yuan R, Lynn MJ, Stulting RD, Wilson LA, Waring GO 3rd. Changes in keratometric astigmatism after suture removal more than one year after penetrating keratoplasty. Ophthalmology. 1993;100(1):119-27.
31. Strelow S, Cohen EJ, Leavitt KG, Laibson PR. Corneal topography for selective suture removal after penetrating keratoplasty. Am J Ophthalmol. 1991;112(6):657-65.
32. Sarhan AR, Dua HS, Beach M. Effect of disagreement between refractive, keratometric, and topographic determination of astigmatic axis on suture removal after penetrating keratoplasty. Br J Ophthalmol. 2000;84(8):837-41.
33. Goren MB, Dana MR, Rapuano CJ, Gomes JA, Cohen EJ, Laibson PR. Corneal topography after selective suture removal for astigmatism following keratoplasty. Ophthalmic Surg Lasers. 1997;28(3):208-14.

13

Postoperative Care after Penetrating Keratoplasty

Raj Maini, Rinky Agarwal, Urmimala Ghatak, Hugh R Taylor

INTRODUCTION

The postoperative care of a corneal graft is probably more important in determining the long-term outcome of the graft than the surgery itself. A lack of careful attention to prevention of early detection and prompt treatment of rejection episodes may lead to graft failure in an otherwise technically perfect graft.

The postoperative care in penetrating keratoplasty (PK) is far more complex than after cataract surgery. With the advent and increasing popularity of endothelial keratoplasty and deep anterior lamellar keratoplasty techniques for lower risk indications, the postoperative care for the more complex patients requiring full-thickness grafts becomes even more crucial.

Routine postsurgical care involves the use of topical antibiotics until epithelial defects are healed. The use of topical steroids to minimize postoperative inflammation, reduce immune sensitivity, and chance of rejection must be carefully tailored. Frequent clinical assessments in the early postoperative period are directed at prevention and early recognition of the myriad of complications that can occur after PK. This can make the difference between surgical success and failure.

It is very important to instruct the patient regarding symptoms of rejection, but even having done this, a significant proportion of episodes of clinically evident rejection are picked up during routine postoperative visits.[1]

Increased pain, irritation, redness, decreased vision, and photophobia are important symptoms. Patients should seek referral immediately in the event that they experience any of these and should be examined within 24 hours of symptom onset.

It is also important that the patient avoids any situation that may produce trauma to the eye, such as heavy lifting, eyelid squeezing, contact sports, etc.

STANDARD POSTOPERATIVE CARE

This section covers postoperative care in uncomplicated corneal grafting in non-neovascularized eyes, typically with keratoconus or corneal dystrophy (**Fig. 1 and Table 1**).

Early Postoperative Management

At the completion of surgery, subconjunctival corticosteroid, and antibiotic of choice can be administered. Though intracameral antibiotic injection is gaining popularity as this has been shown to be safe and efficacious in cataract surgery,[2] there is a paucity of data in this regard for PK. The eye may be patched for 24 hours with antibiotic ointment. We prefer to use fluoroquinolone ointment. We also instill a single drop of short-acting mydriatic (tropicamide 1%) along with antibiotic ointment in eyes subjected to iris manipulation, combined lens extraction, or vitrectomy. A mild analgesic can also be administered in the immediate postoperative period to reduce periocular pain. However, need for stronger analgesics should raise the suspicion of possible complications.[3,4]

The oral carbonic anhydrase inhibitor acetazolamide may be used to prevent a rise in intraocular pressure (IOP), especially if viscoelastic has been used. Topical carbonic anhydrase inhibitors, e.g., dorzolamide may controversially interfere with endothelial function and should be avoided.

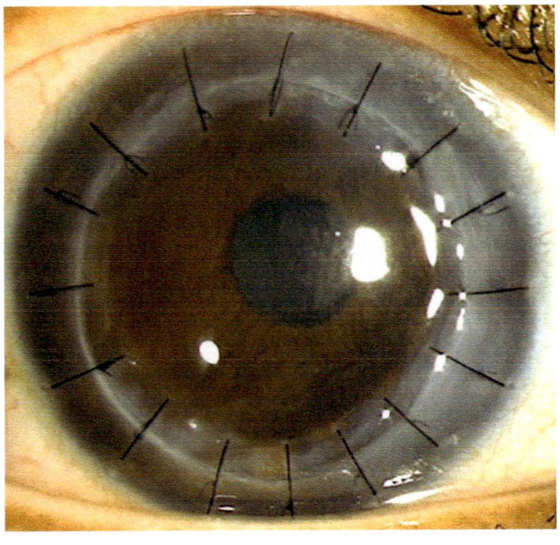

Fig. 1: 1 month postoperative appearance of an eye with a full thickness graft, with all sutures intact and buried.

Table 1: Follow-up schedule.

1 week	*1 month*	*3 months*	*6 months*	*1 year*
• Visual acuity • Graft clarity and thickness • Status of corneal epithelium • Graft infection • *Sutures*: Tight/loose/ broken, infiltrates • Wound leak • AC depth, inflammation • Lens status • Fundus • IOP	• Visual acuity and astigmatism • Graft clarity and thickness • Sutures • AC depth, inflammation • Lens status • PAS release • Fundus • IOP • Corneal topography ± suture adjustment	• Visual acuity and astigmatism • Graft clarity and thickness • Sutures • AC depth, inflammation • Lens status • PAS release • Fundus • IOP • Corneal topography ± suture adjustment • Selective suture removal	• Visual acuity and astigmatism • Graft clarity and thickness • Sutures • AC depth, inflammation • Lens status • Fundus • IOP • Corneal topography ± suture adjustment • Selective suture removal	• Visual acuity and astigmatism • Graft clarity and thickness • Sutures • AC depth, inflammation • Lens status • Fundus • IOP • Corneal topography ± suture adjustment • Suture removal • Refractive correction

(AC: anterior chamber; IOP: intraocular pressure; PAS: peripheral anterior synechiae)

Patients are commonly encouraged to have soft foods, plenty of oral fluids, and change over to comfortable body posture soon after the surgery depending on their recovery from the effects of anesthesia. The patients are also instructed to avoid direct trauma to the eye. In children and in individuals with mental disturbances, we use a rigid metallic or plastic eye shield to protect the eyeball from unnecessary trauma. We generally encourage the family members to actively involve themselves in the postoperative care of the patient.

Criteria for discharging the patient from hospital (in a daycare setting) include:

- Stable vital signs
- Return to the preoperative mental state
- Absence of nausea
- Absence of unusual pain
- Availability of an escort
- Review of postsurgical care with the patient and/or escort, including medication dosage
- Prearranged follow-up appointment
- Written postoperative instructions

First Postoperative Day

The eye pad is removed at first dressing, but the eye should be protected during sleep with a shield for the first 4–6 weeks and the patient's head should be slightly elevated ("higher than the patient's heart"). During the daytime, the patient can wear spectacles having appropriate optical correction for the fellow eye. Dark glasses are not mandatory. Activities of daily living can be resumed depending on the visual recovery of the patient and their physical status. However, any direct injury to the eye and unusual degrees of physical strain should be avoided during the first few weeks after surgery. Simultaneously, ocular hygiene should be maintained to prevent infection.[3,4]

At this stage, it is mandatory to assess:

- Visual acuity
- Degree of pain
- Slit-lamp examination

  At slit-lamp examination particular attention must be paid to:

  - The presence of a wound leak-relative hypotony, unusual stromal swelling, and a shallow anterior chamber should alert you to the possibility of this. Assess the leak with the Seidel test; treatment may require insertion of a therapeutic (bandage) contact lens or aqueous production inhibitors. If the leak persists for >3 days, wound resuture should be considered
  - Pupil shape
  - Corneal epithelial status
  - Extreme anterior chamber shallowing or iris incarceration in the wound—requires immediate surgical management
  - Elevated IOP—treat medically in the first instance
  - Early signs of infection or endophthalmitis—this requires aggressive medical and/or surgical management.

  Topical medication should be commenced:

  - *Topical antibiotic*: Fluoroquinolone eye drops four times daily until epithelium is healed—usually within 7–14 days
  - *Topical steroid*: The use of topical corticosteroids is universal, but the dose requirements may vary widely between individual cases. fluorometholone acetate 0.1% or prednisolone acetate 1% are generally used 4–6 times daily initially.

Fluorometholone acetate 0.1% may be considered as first-line treatment because it has less epithelial toxicity than prednisolone acetate 1% and is less likely to result in elevation of IOP. Recently, rimexolone 1% has been touted as a potent topical anti-inflammatory agent without the potential IOP problems encountered with topical dexamethasone. Other topical steroid preparations, such as prednisolone sodium phosphate are not potent enough to produce adequate therapeutic effect.

In uncomplicated corneal grafts, the topical steroid medication may be gradually reduced as the inflammation within the eye diminishes. A typical regimen is outlined in **Table 2**.

Intraocular pressure and the status of the lens must be monitored carefully, for as long as the steroids are used.

Postoperative Visits

There are many postoperative care regimens; the key to them all is a careful slit-lamp examination. In addition to the signs outlined above (day 1 assessment), the patient must be assessed for the signs of rejection: corneal stromal thickening, fine epithelial edema, aqueous flare and cell, keratic precipitates (KPs) and the presence of Khodadaust line (**Fig. 2**). The presence of a few, fine KPs when there were none at previous visits, is indicative of early rejection and must be treated vigorously with hourly topical corticosteroids. Keratic precipitates can only be assumed to be "old pigmented KP" if they do not resolve with intensive treatment. The use of pulsed high-dose systemic immunosuppression[5,6] is not universal.[7]

Deturgescence of the graft in the short- to medium-term can be monitored serial measurements of graft thickness using anterior segment optical coherence tomography.

Table 2: Use of topical steroids in penetrating keratoplasty.

Month 1	*Month 2*	*Month 3*	*Month 4*	*Month 5*	*Month 6*	*Month 7*
Fluorometholone acetate 0.1%				Fluorometholone alcohol 0.1%		
4–6 hourly	4x/day	3x/day	2x/day	4x/day	3x/day	2x/day

Eyes with non-reversal of corneal edema following intensive administration of corticosteroids lead on to develop established graft failure (**Fig. 3**) requiring future keratoplasty.

Fundoscopy should be undertaken within the first month after surgery to assess the optic nerve (glaucomatous damage, atrophy), macula (age-related degeneration, scarring), and peripheral retina (retinal tears or detachment).

The presence of a nonhealing corneal epithelial defect for >14 days increases the risk of stromal ulceration with subsequent corneal stromal thinning, perforation or scarring. These patients should be carefully assessed for ocular surface disease and lid malposition, in particular dry eye, exposure, rosacea, and blepharitis, which must be treated. Lubrication, patching, a bandage contact lens, botulinum toxin, surgical ptosis, or tarsorrhaphy may be required. It is good to check for both ocular surface drug toxicity and exposure of lagophthalmos with some lissamine green.

The status of sutures should be evaluated at every follow-up visit. Loose sutures associated with vascular ingrowth should be removed as early as possible to prevent the possible occurrence of immune-mediated graft failure (**Fig. 4**). Use of a little fluorescein helps to detect even slightly loose sutures as it tend to pool around them (**Fig. 5**). Loose sutures may be secondary to poor surgical technique, wound contraction, suture breakage, or cheese wiring. They trap mucous and can result in infection or stimulate graft rejection or giant papillary conjunctivitis. They do not contribute to wound integrity and should be removed. Vascularization along suture tracks indicates a healed wound and these sutures may also be removed safely. Any loose suture with surrounding vascularization should be removed without any delay.

Patients who are grafted for corneal dystrophy must be examined for recurrence of the dystrophy within the graft tissue; fungal, viral, and amebic infections may all recur

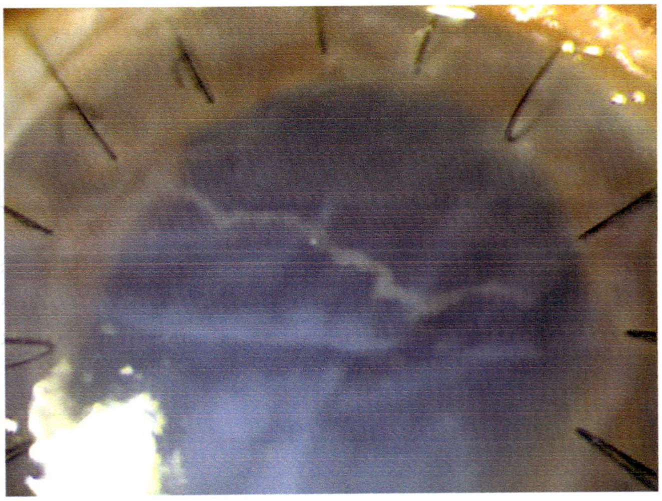

Fig. 2: Early graft rejection manifesting as an endothelial (Khodadoust) rejection line.

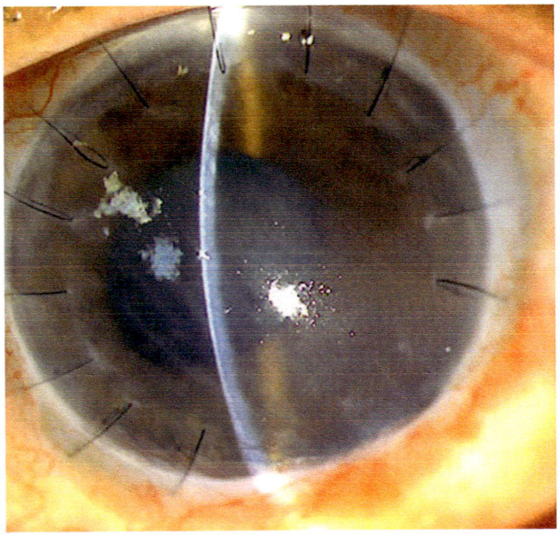

Fig. 3: Established graft failure.

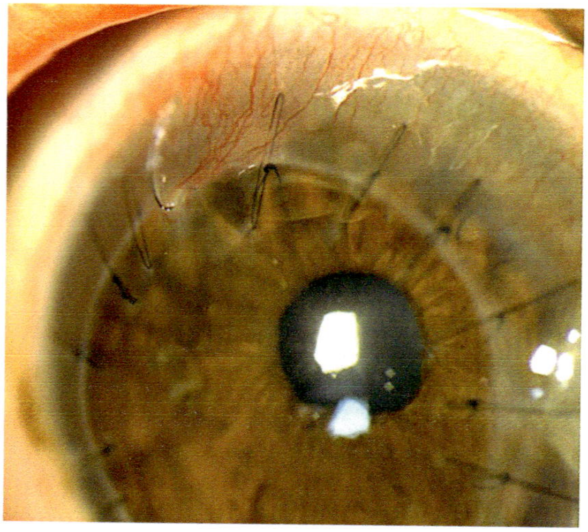

Fig. 4: Loose sutures over a graft, inciting vascularization.

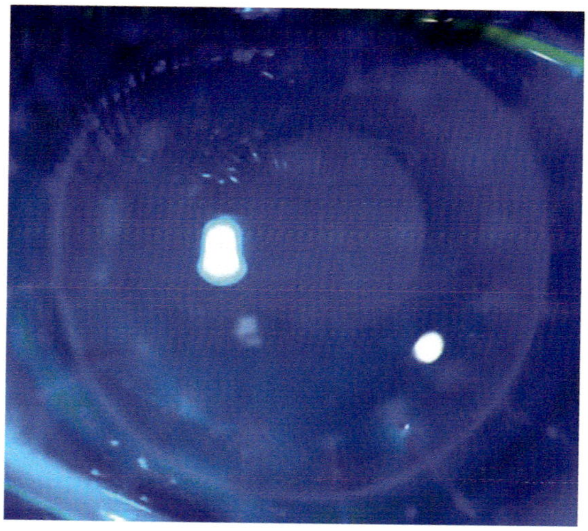

Fig. 5: Subtle fluorescein staining at 5 o'clock position, suggestive of suture loosening.

within corneal grafts and treatment should be directed toward the causative agent. Another important concern following a keratoplasty is to look for any evidence of graft infection (**Fig. 6**). Such signs should be carefully picked up and patient should be advised routine microbiological evaluation in order to start appropriate antimicrobial therapy.

A patient without signs or symptoms of complications should be examined on a regular basis for 18–24 months (**Table 3**). Progress of improvement and the course of complications should be documented by detailed clinical drawings or anterior segment photography at each visit.

Graft clarity and visual acuity should begin to improve in the early postoperative period. Persistent graft edema from the first dressing and continuing in the absence of inflammation may indicate primary graft failure—this may be confirmed with pachymetry and specular microscopy.

After suture removal, the patient will not require more planned appointments. Patients should however, still be instructed to consult an ophthalmologist promptly in the event of any rejection symptoms. If a patient has

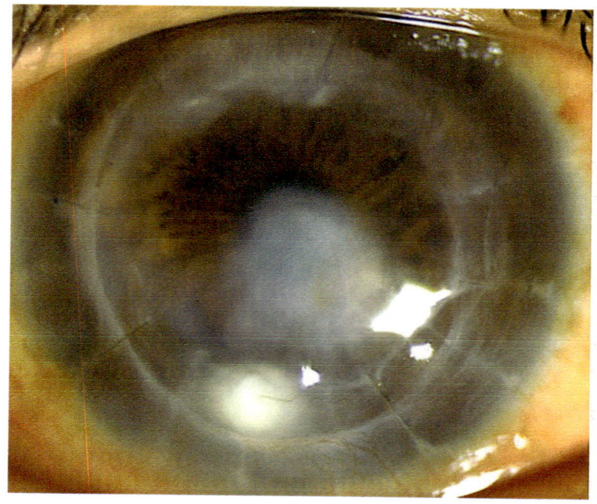

Fig. 6: Broken suture over a graft with adjacent stromal infiltration.

Table 3: Postoperative penetrating keratoplasty outpatient schedule.

Month 1	*Month 2*	*Months 3–12*	*Months 13–24*
Every 2 weeks	Every 4 weeks	Every 6 weeks	Every 6–12 weeks until all sutures are removed

had a rejection episode, an argument can be made to continue long-term, low-dose topical steroid such as fluorometholone 0.1% once or twice a day.

The prescription of spectacles or contact lenses depends on a number of factors. The patient's visual needs are paramount, but the healing process, the amount of astigmatism, the presence of sutures, and the stability of the refractive error may all be important factors. Refraction and computerized topographic mapping with suture adjustment will aid visual rehabilitation in the first year. Selective suture removal may be indicated where, interrupted sutures have been used. Temporary spectacles may be prescribed within a few months of surgery to aid with the rehabilitation process.

The final spectacles are prescribed when the sutures have been removed and the refraction and corneal curvature have stabilized. Occasionally, residual or irregular astigmatism may require rigid gas-permeable contact lens fitting.

CORNEAL GRAFTING IN OCULAR SURFACE DISEASES

This section includes management of keratoplasty in lagophthalmos, entropion, lid scarring, dry eye, chemical burns, and ocular cicatricial pemphigoid.

Overview

Penetrating keratoplasty in these conditions presents a considerable management challenge, primarily aimed at optimizing the health of the ocular surface.

The integrity of the corneal epithelium after keratoplasty is vital for graft survival. The normal intact corneal epithelium provides an optical interface with the tear film and a barrier to the external environment, noxious substances, and microorganisms. The presence of an epithelial defect interferes with vision and increases the risk of rejection, infection, thinning, and perforation. Epithelial defects occur frequently on the first postoperative day in donor corneas stored in both McCarey-Kaufman (MK) medium and organ culture medium.

Toxic topical medication and preservatives may have an adverse effect on epithelial wound healing because of the inhibition of epithelial migration, epithelial mitosis, or epithelial attachment to the underlying basement membrane; if these problems are encountered the patient should be switched to unpreserved medication or commenced on these immediately postoperatively.

Abnormalities of the tear film from decreased aqueous secretion, rapid evaporation, mucin deficiency, blepharitis, poor lid position or movement and lagophthalmos can influence epithelial healing and wound healing. Some systemic medications may exert an indirect effect on the corneal epithelium through effects on tear secretion and epithelial cell wound healing.

Local primary ocular surface disease, for example, ocular cicatricial pemphigoid, Stevens-Johnson syndrome or chemical burns may prevent normal epithelial wound healing secondary to lid scarring, resulting in entropion and trichiasis. Disturbed anatomy with symblepharon, ankyloblepharon, and goblet cell deficiency with resultant tear film abnormalities, or intrinsic epithelial abnormalities can also delay healing.

Patients may present with inadvertent self-inflicted epithelial damage through mechanical trauma with fingernails, mascara brushes, or curling irons and through the abuse of topical medication.

It is critical for the survival of the donor corneal epithelium that existing dry eye or local ocular surface disease, such as ocular pemphigoid, be recognized, treated, and controlled before surgery.

Aberrant lashes (trichiasis) should be eliminated either by electrolysis or cryotherapy. Lid margin entropion or ectropion, lagophthalmos, and lid scarring should be surgically corrected prior to PK.

Blepharitis, whether from local or systemic disease, such as rosacea, must be controlled with lid hygiene, topical lubrication, antibiotic, and steroid if needed. Topical cyclosporine 0.05% emulsion has been used in the management of posterior blepharitis and ocular rosacea.[8] The value of systemic tetracyclines in the treatment of rosacea should not be forgotten.

Postoperative Prevention of Epithelial Problems

Careful clinical examination for lash, lid abnormalities, and abnormalities of the ocular surface is mandatory.

Trichiasis

Epilation is temporary as lashes normally regrow within 2–3 weeks. Electrolysis works well only for removing a few lashes. Cryotherapy is the treatment of choice to remove ingrowing lashes.

Dry Eye

Punctal occlusion may be of benefit for patients with keratoconjunctivitis sicca to prevent epithelial ulceration postkeratoplasty. Punctal occlusion increases tear retention and resultant increase in the tear volume to surface area (TVSA) ratio. Options include temporary punctal occlusion using punctal plugs or permanent punctal closure with laser, cautery, or diathermy.

Topical cyclosporine 0.05% shows beneficial effects in all categories of dry eye disease.[9]

Lagophthalmos

Surgical options to correct this include *lateral tarsorrhaphy or lateral canthal sling procedures.*

The therapeutic effect of these procedures is attributable to the decrease in exposed ocular surface area, which increases the TVSA ratio, protecting the epithelial surface and promotes spreading of the tear film.

The ocular surface should be kept well lubricated with artificial tears, if required more frequently than 4–6 times daily. Unpreserved solutions should be used to minimize epithelial toxicity. Unpreserved drops can be used every hour or more frequently if needed. However, if required more than every 2 hours, punctal plugs should be considered. Carbomer gel-based medication (e.g., Viscotears) and ointments without preservative are retained in the conjunctival fornices for longer and may also be used four times a day and supplemented with unpreserved tears and/or punctal plugs.

Patients with sensitivity to lanolin or wood should avoid lanolin-containing ointment.

Topical antibiotics, antivirals, timolol, and steroids may all exert a toxic effect on the epithelium and should not be used indiscriminately.

Botulinum toxin ptosis is another treatment for persistent epithelial defect: 7.5 units are injected into the orbital roof, adjacent to levator palpebrae superioris. The ptosis develops in 2–3 days, resolves in 6–8 weeks and injections can be repeated.

Platelet rich plasma and autologous serum tears containing vitamin A, epidermal growth factor and transforming growth factor-β have been shown to be of benefit in persistent epithelial defects;[10] they can be administered 4–6 times daily.

CORNEAL GRAFTING IN GLAUCOMA

One of the major causes of corneal graft failure is inadequate control of elevated IOP. Significant endothelial cell loss occurs because of acute and greatly elevated IOP.

This is encountered secondary to severe anterior chamber reaction and may require treatment with topical β-blockers, such as timolol maleate 0.5% twice daily; α-blockers (e.g., brimonidine) in those with relative contraindications to β-blockers may be considered.

Topical prostaglandin analogs are controversial and may theoretically stimulate graft rejection, although this has not been borne out in practice and these useful drugs are in widespread use after PK. Dorzolamide may affect the donor endothelial function and result in prolonged graft edema and should be avoided postkeratoplasty.

Miotics are known to dilate the ocular blood vessels and break down the blood-aqueous barrier inducing chronic iridocyclitis. Miotic use in aphakic patients is associated with increased risk of retinal tear and subsequent retinal detachment. Systemic carbonic anhydrase inhibitors (e.g., acetazolamide) must be used with great caution in elderly keratoplasty patients as they may trigger a malaise symptom complex consisting of fatigue, depression, anorexia, and weight loss; the diuretic effect of this drug must also be considered in patients with cardiovascular disease.

If seclusio pupillae develops secondary to posterior synechiae, laser iridotomy may be needed to prevent or treat pupil block.

Anti-inflammatory therapy can result in steroid-induced glaucoma and topical medication should be carefully tailored to avoid this.

CORNEAL GRAFT IN INFLAMED EYES (HOT EYES)

Special precautions should be taken in cases of rheumatoid arthritis, collagen diseases, perforation, and trauma.

Postoperative care in these cases is often governed by how well the ocular inflammation has been controlled preoperatively; the chances of a successful outcome being inversely proportional to the inflammatory status of the eye at surgery.

The presence of active systemic vasculitis has a bearing on long-term outcome of grafting and should be monitored and treated aggressively in the perioperative period; this may necessitate the use of systemic as well as intensive topical immunosuppression (see below—high-risk keratoplasty).

Tight control of the systemic disease is necessary to maximize graft survival and should be undertaken in conjunction with a rheumatologist or immunologist.

Penetrating keratoplasty for noninflammatory perforation or trauma requires antibiotic cover postoperatively to minimize the risk of infection and endophthalmitis.

CORNEAL GRAFT IN INFECTED EYES

Corneal blindness secondary to infective keratitis is a major problem in most parts of the world. Early diagnosis, better understanding of pathogenesis, and the availability of potent antimicrobial drugs have improved the success rate for medical control of corneal infections, particularly those of bacterial origin. However, virulent and resistant forms of some bacteria, fungi and *Acanthamoeba* can progress inexorably, even with maximal medical therapy, and these may necessitate PK.

Bacterial Keratitis

Postkeratoplasty, in the presence of active keratitis, antimicrobial treatment is directed against the offending microbe. If an etiologic diagnosis has not been established, antibiotic coverage with combination therapy or with a broad-spectrum medication should be undertaken.

Where, the sensitivities are known, the topical antibiotic with the least toxicity, to which the organism is most sensitive, should be administered frequently until sterilization is achieved.

In cases where, the organism and/or sensitivity is unknown, combination therapy (e.g., fortified cefazolin/vancomycin and tobramycin) or a broad-spectrum antibiotic (such as a fluoroquinolone) should be given. Cycloplegics are used to alleviate discomfort and minimize posterior synechiae, and antiglaucoma medication used as required.

To minimize the risk of rejection, topical corticosteroids may be used judiciously. If sensitivities are known, hourly or 2 hourly fluorometholone acetate 0.1% or prednisolone acetate 1% can be used under sufficient antibiotic cover; in the absence of confirmed sensitivities more cautious use of topical medication is recommended, e.g., fluorometholone acetate 0.1% four times daily.

If perforation occurs, structural integrity can be maintained with tissue adhesive (cyanoacrylate or fibrin "glue") until the infection and inflammation has receded, when regrafting can be safely undertaken.

Fungal Keratitis

Filamentous (molds), e.g., *Aspergillus*, *Fusarium*, the following regimens are currently recommended:

- Topical natamycin 5% every hour initially
- Fluconazole 200–400 mg daily or topical preparation 1% Cyclosporine A (CsA) topically four times daily

Nonfilamentous (yeasts), e.g., *Candida*

- Topical amphotericin B 0.075–0.15% every hour initially
- Cyclosporine A four times daily

In patients not responding to conventional antifungal therapy, voriconazole (oral 200 mg BD, 2 hourly 1% topical eye drops, intrastromal injection 50 μg/0.1 mL) and topical caspofungin (0.5%, 1%) may be used.[11-13] Topical corticosteroids are mostly contraindicated in the postoperative phase and are used only under extremely special conditions in which removal of the entire infected area has been ensured.

Acanthamoeba Keratitis

- Topical amebicidal drugs
- Polyhexamethylene biguanide (PHMB) 0.02% every 2 hours
- Propamidine isethionate (Brolene) 0.1% every 2 hours
- Chlorhexidine every 2 hours
- Neosporin every 2 hours
- Topical corticosteroids may be given judiciously
- Systemic steroids and itraconazole may be required
- Oral nonsteroidal anti-inflammatory agent
- Cycloplegic
- Topical anti-acanthamoeba medication is often required for many months to eradicate the encysted form of amoeba.

Herpes Simplex

Recurrence of herpes simplex infection in the graft may lead to or mimic a rejection episode. It is often difficult to distinguish between the two and treating a recurrence as a rejection with intensive topical steroid will allow uncontrolled proliferation of the virus. Therefore, treatment should be aimed at both, balancing the epithelial toxicity of the antiviral medication with the deleterious effect of the steroid on the virus infection.

Acyclovir given orally 200 mg four times daily for 4/12, then twice daily for 4/12 may prevent recurrences of epithelial keratitis [the Herpetic Eye Disease study (HEDS) demonstrated this effect while treatment continued].[14] It has therefore been suggested (especially for monocular patients) that systemic acyclovir treatment may be required on an indefinite basis for patients at high-risk of recurrent epithelial HSK. Such patients require frequent renal function monitoring. The HEDS study did not examine the effect of topical acyclovir as this preparation is not available in the USA, it may have a role in prevention of recurrent disease in patients with a good fellow eye.

Valacyclovir 500 mg OD for 1 year has been found to have equal efficacy as oral acyclovir 400 mg BD in the prevention of recurrent lesions in immunocompetent individuals with ocular herpes simplex virus (HSV) disease.[15] Prophylactic oral valacyclovir treatment is also at least as effective as oral acyclovir in preventing recurrence in patients who underwent corneal transplantation for herpetic keratitis.[16]

Cyclosporine A—one drop four times daily may also be useful in controlling inflammation.

REPEAT CORNEAL GRAFT/HIGH-RISK CORNEAL GRAFT

Immunosuppression in High-risk Keratoplasty (Table 4)

Two approaches can be taken to prevent immune-mediated rejection and ultimately failure in high-risk corneal transplantation:

- Suppression of the host immune response.
- Making the donor tissue less antigenic: Animal studies have demonstrated reduced rejection rates for corneal allografts after pretreatment with ultraviolet B irradiation[17] and the use of anti-CD4 receptor antibodies.[18]

These are difficult cases and should be managed in conjunction with an immunologist. The role of human leukocyte antigen class I and II matching is at present unproven in most populations.

Options for immunosuppression (these may be used as single agents or in combination) include:

Corticosteroids

Topical: Topical steroids continue to be the primary immunosuppressive agents in the postoperative management of high-risk keratoplasty:

Topical fluorometholone acetate 0.1% or prednisolone acetate 1% every 2 hours is most commonly used.

Table 4: Side effects of immunosuppressive agents in high-risk penetrating keratoplasty.

Topical steroid	*Systemic steroids*	*Topical CsA*	*Systemic CsA*	*Azathioprine*
• Glaucoma, cataract • Delayed wound • Healing, infectious • Keratitis	• Weight gain • Hypertension • Hyperglycemia • Peptic ulcer • Growth retardation • Mental changes • Cataract • Osteoporosis • Susceptibility to infections • Avascular hip necrosis	• Ocular discomfort • Conjunctival injection • Punctate keratopathy	• Hypertension • Nephrotoxic • Neurotoxic • Hepatotoxic • Hirsutism • Gingival hyperplasia, reactivation of latent • Infections	• Anemia • Thrombocytopenia • Leukopenia, • Bone marrow suppression • Alopecia • Gastrointestinal • Toxicity

(CsA: cyclosporine A)

Systemic: Systemic steroids can be used as an adjunct to topical therapy in high-risk keratoplasty to minimize risk of rejection.

Methylprednisolone 125–250 mg intravenously at the time of surgery followed by oral prednisolone 1 mg/kg/day slowly tapered in 3–6 months may be useful in high-risk cases.

Alternatively, prednisolone 100 mg orally for 2–3 days, then tapered over 2 weeks may be used.

Severe or refractory rejection may also respond to systemic immunosuppression. The role of pulsed intravenous methylprednisolone for severe rejection is not proven and may only be of benefit if the patient presents early in the rejection episode;[5] some surgeons prefer to use short-term high-dose oral prednisolone in these cases: A single intravenous dose of methylprednisolone 500 mg[3] or oral prednisolone 80 mg daily[6] for 5–7 days may be considered.

Both are given in addition to hourly topical fluorometholone acetate 0.1% or prednisolone acetate 1%.

Cyclosporine A

Topical: Cyclosporine A 2% in castor oil or 1% in artificial tears four times daily.

At present, the penetration of this drug into the anterior chamber or deeper corneal layers is not proven. Combined treatment with cyclosporine 2% and topical corticosteroids offered better rejection-free graft survival rates over use of topical corticosteroids alone in a study evaluating results of pediatric keratoplasty.[19]

Systemic: Some success has been achieved with the use of systemic cyclosporine in high-risk keratoplasty:[20]

- 4–5 mg/kg once or two divided doses daily
- Blood cyclosporine A level should be between 100 and 300 ng/mL.

All patients using cyclosporine A need close monitoring of blood pressure, renal function including serum creatinine and liver enzymes.

Azathioprine

- 50 mg daily increasing to a maintenance dose of 75–100 mg daily.
- Used as a "steroid sparing" agent in rejection for high-risk keratoplasty.

Renal, hepatic, and bone marrow function must be monitored. Reversible leukopenia may occur in up to 20% of patients.

Mycophenolate Mofetil

- 2,000–3,000 mg daily
- Suppresses lymphocyte proliferation in a similar manner to azathioprine
- Used successfully to treat refractory rejection in renal transplantation, it has a low incidence of significant adverse effects and is better tolerated than azathioprine.

It may increasingly have a role in the management of rejection in high-risk keratoplasty.[21]

Tacrolimus

This is a macrolide immunosuppressant that is a fungal metabolite and suppresses both humoral and cellular immune responses.

Liver transplantation studies have shown that it may reduce the need for adjunctive immunotherapy for treatment of rejection episodes compared to cyclosporine-based regimens.

Renal function must be monitored and neurological adverse effects have been documented (more so with intravenous preparations).

It may surpass cyclosporine as the "steroid sparing" agent of choice in the future. Recent studies have confirmed its efficacy in the management of high-risk keratoplasty.[22,23]

Topical tacrolimus 0.03% ointment seems to be a promising second-line immunosuppressant in management of high-risk grafts.[24]

As corneal neovascularization is also considered an important risk factor for allograft rejection after PK, antiangiogenic therapies such as laser or fine-needle thermal cauterization of these vessels and subconjunctival injection of bevacizumab may also be tried in the postoperative period to improve graft survival.[25]

SUMMARY

Intense care and vigilance are required during routine postoperative care after PK. High-index of suspicion must be maintained and patients be warned against the symptoms and signs of serious complications such as graft rejection, graft infection, and endophthalmitis. Special care is required for patients subjected to high-risk and emergency PK. It is always wise to actively involve the family members in the routine postoperative care of the patient.

REFERENCES

1. Kamp MT, Finnk NE, Enger C, Maguire MG, Stark WJ, Stulting RD, et al. Patient-reported symptoms associated with graft reactions in high-risk patients in the collaborative corneal transplantation studies. Collaborative Corneal Transplantation Studies Research Group. Cornea. 1995;14:43-8.
2. Barry P, Seal DV, Gettinby G, Lees F, Peterson M, Revie CW, et al. ESCRS study of prophylaxis of postoperative endophthalmitis after cataract surgery: Preliminary report of principal results from a European multicenter study. J Cataract Refract Surg. 2006;32:407-10.
3. Saini JS. Postoperative management of corneal graft. Indian J Ophthalmol. 1994:42:215-7.

4. Shimmura-Tomita M, Shimmura S, Satake Y, Shimazaki-Den S, Omoto M, Tsubota K, et al. Keratoplasty postoperative treatment update. Cornea. 2013;32 Suppl 1:S60-4.
5. Hill JC, Maske R, Watson PG. The use of a single pulse of intravenous methylprednisolone in the treatment of corneal graft rejection. A preliminary report. Eye. 1991;5:420-24.
6. Hill JC, Maske R, Watson PG. Corticosteroids in corneal graft rejection. Oral versus single pulse therapy. Ophthalmology. 1991;98:329-33.
7. Hudde T, Minassian DC, Larkin DF. Randomized controlled trail of corticosteroid regimens in endothelial corneal allograft rejection. Br J Ophthalmol. 1999;83:1348-52.
8. Donnenfeld E, Pflugfelder SC. Topical ophthalmic cyclosporine: pharmacology and clinical uses. Surv Ophthalmol. 2009; 54(3):321-38.
9. Perry HD, Solomon R, Donnenfeld ED, Perry AR, Wittpenn JR, Greenman HE, et al. Evaluation of topical cyclosporine for the treatment of dry eye disease. Arch Ophthalmol. 2008;126(8):1046-50.
10. Tsubota K, Goto E, Shimmura S, Shimazaki J. Treatment of persistent corneal epithelial defect by autologous serum application. Ophthalmology. 1999;106:1984-9.
11. Lee SJ, Lee JJ, Kim SD. Topical and oral voriconazole in the treatment of fungal keratitis. Korean J Ophthalmol. 2009;23(1):46-8.
12. Prakash G, Sharma N, Goel M, Titiyal JS, Vajpayee RB. Evaluation of intrastromal injection of voriconazole as a therapeutic adjunctive for the management of deep recalcitrant fungal keratitis. Am J Ophthalmol. 2008;146(1):56-9.
13. Sahay P, Singhal D, Nagpal R, Maharana PK, Farid M, Gelman R, et al. Pharmacologic therapy of mycotic keratitis. Surv Ophthalmol. 2019;64(3):380-400.
14. Herpetic Eye Study Group. Oral acyclovir for herpes simplex virus eye disease: effect on prevention of epithelial keratitis and stromal keratitis. Arch Ophthalmol. 2000;118:1030-6.
15. Miserocchi E, Modorati G, Galli L, Rama P. Efficacy of valacyclovir vs. acyclovir for the prevention of recurrent herpes simplex virus eye disease: a pilot study. Am J Ophthalmol. 2007;144(4):547-51.
16. Goldblum D, Bachmann C, Tappeiner C, Garweg J, Frueh BE. Comparison of oral antiviral therapy with valacyclovir or acyclovir after penetrating keratoplasty for herpetic keratitis. Br J Ophthalmol. 2008;92(9):1201-5.
17. Niederkorn JY, Callanan D, Ross JR. Prevention of allospecific cytotoxic T lymphocyte and delayed-type hypersensitivity responses by ultraviolet irradiation of corneal allografts. Transplantation. 1990;50:281-86.
18. Pleyer U, Milani JK, Dukes A, Chou J, Lutz S, Rückert D, et al. Effect of topically applied anti-CD4 monoclonal antibodies on orthotopic corneal allografts in a rat model. Invest Ophthalmol Vis Sci. 1995;36:52-61.
19. Cosar CB, Laibson PR, Cohen EJ, Rapuano CJ. Topical cyclosporine in pediatric keratoplasty. Eye Contact Lens. 2003;29(2):103-37.
20. Hill JC. Systemic cyclosporine in high-risk keratoplasty: long-term results. Eye (Lond). 1995;9:422-8.
21. Reis A, Reinhard T, Voiculescu A, Kutkuhn B, Godehardt E, Spelsberg H, et al. Mycophenolate mofetil versus cyclosporine A in high-risk keratoplasty patients: a prospectively randomized clinical trial. Br J Ophthalmol. 1999;83:1268-71.
22. Sloper CM, Powell RJ, Dua HS. Tacrolimus (FK506) in the management of high-risk corneal and limbal grafts. Ophthalmology. 2001;108:1838-44.
23. Joseph A, Raj D, Shanmuganathan V, Powell RJ, Dua HS. Tacrolimus immunosuppression in high-risk corneal grafts. Br J Ophthalmol. 2007;91(1):51-5.
24. Dhaliwal JS, Mason BF, Kaufman SC. Long-term use of topical tacrolimus (FK506) in high-risk penetrating keratoplasty. Cornea. 2008;27(4):488-93.
25. Hos D, Le VNH, Hellmich M, Siebelmann S, Roters S, Bachmann BO, et al. Risk of corneal graft rejection after high-risk keratoplasty following fine-needle vessel coagulation of corneal neovascularization combined with Bevacizumab: A Pilot Study. Transplant Direct. 2019;5(5):e452.

14 Postkeratoplasty Contact Lens Fitting

Rajesh Sinha, Suman Lata, Jeewan S Titiyal

INTRODUCTION

Contact lens can be used for either visual or therapeutic purposes after a successful penetrating keratoplasty.[1-3] For optimal visual rehabilitation, contact lenses may be required when there is marked postoperative astigmatism, anisometropia, or aphakia. On the other hand, bandage soft contact lenses are used to promote surface healing in the presence of persistent epithelial defect.

Advances in microsurgical techniques and postoperative care have made it possible to achieve a high rate of clear graft in a number of clinical conditions. Despite all these advances, many corneal surfaces remain irregular and have high degrees of astigmatism following penetrating keratoplasty.[4] In most of the studies, postoperative astigmatism ranges between 4 and 5 D.[5-7] Excessive astigmatism decreases potential uncorrected visual acuity, reduces best-corrected spectacle acuity, and is associated with asthenopic symptoms when patients are given spectacles. The astigmatism can be caused by factors such as the configuration of trephine incisions, donor-recipient graft disparity, irregular and tight suturing, and differences in thickness of donor and recipient wound edges creating a step.

Various approaches have been tried to reduce postoperative irregular astigmatism, which includes suture adjustment, selective suture removal, and occasionally refractive surgery. The nonsurgical approaches to the management of postkeratoplasty astigmatism can be spectacles, rigid gas permeable (RGP) contact lens, soft toric contact lens, contact lens and spectacle combination, piggyback, and hybrid contact lenses. RGP contact lenses are usually the correction of choice for such patients because of the need to correct regular and irregular astigmatism with due consideration to improved oxygen transmission.[8]

INDICATIONS

Contact lenses of various types remain an important tool in the visual rehabilitation of patients after penetrating keratoplasty. Around 10–25% of the postkeratoplasty patients require contact lens for visual rehabilitation.[1,6,9] Therapeutic contact lenses are used for short-term to enhance graft resurfacing.[10] Long-term use of contact lenses is mainly for optical purposes.

Short-term Indications

Therapeutic contact lenses may be useful in the presence of epitheliopathy following keratoplasty. Most graft epithelial defects heal within 48–72 hours. Certain conditions where the epithelial defect persists beyond 72 hours, use of a bandage contact lens may help to promote epithelial healing. It is also indicated in the presence of a persistent punctate epitheliopathy in the graft. Soft (hydrogel) contact lenses are the ones that are used in such conditions.

There are certain clinical conditions wherein epithelial healing is impaired. Patients being transplanted for Stevens-Johnson syndrome, alkali burns and herpetic neurotrophic ulcers require cover for the epithelium as early as possible after surgery to promote and maintain epithelialization.[10] Again, therapeutic lenses may play a role in patients who have lagophthalmos. It is also indicated in certain lid or conjunctival deformities such as keratinized conjunctiva, irregular lid margins, and cobblestone papillae from vernal catarrh, that do not need plastic surgery before grafting but that may traumatize the epithelium of the fresh graft.

Although trichiatic lashes should be removed before corneal surgery, lash deviation, often in association with spastic entropion, may create problems in the postoperative period. A bandage contact lens may be useful temporarily in such cases. At times, therapeutic contact lens can be used to prevent trauma to the graft by the lids, e.g., if there is slight graft override (misalignment) or if the edge of the graft is elevated by edema in the suture compression zone. Such lenses will allow defects on the elevated portions of the graft to heal and may also prevent dellen formation in the adjacent concave areas where wetting by lid may not be proper.[10] Finally, it has been seen on rare occasion that small wound leaks can be sealed by temporary placement of a therapeutic lens.

Long-term Indications

Optical correction is the primary aim of long-term use of contact lenses following penetrating keratoplasty. The primary indication for visual rehabilitation using contact lenses is high corneal toricity, irregular astigmatism, anisometropia, and uniocular aphakia.

The increasing use of triple procedure (penetrating keratoplasty, extracapsular cataract extraction, and intraocular lens implantation) in dealing with combined corneal and lens pathology is based on providing visual correction without the need of contact lens use. However, contact lenses do have a role when the graft has high or an irregular astigmatism. In some such cases, rigid contact lens may be a better alternative to corrective refractive surgery.

Either rigid or soft contact lens may be employed for visual purposes, depending on a variety of factors. The options from which a physician has to decide are a rigid contact lens, a daily wear or an extended wear soft contact lens, piggyback, or hybrid lenses. The indications for a specific lens type depend mainly on the refractive status of the eye, the degree of corneal toricity, and the specific needs of the patient.

In an aphakic patient, with a graft of low toricity (<2.5 D), the physician may consider either a rigid contact lens or a soft lens. In the presence of high corneal toricity or irregular astigmatism, either a rigid lens or a piggyback system can be employed.

In most of the phakic graft patients, contact lens correction can be achieved with rigid lenses or with daily wear soft lenses if corneal toricity is not excessive. If there is high toricity in the graft, rigid lens is the sole alternative. Most of the cases of keratoconus have high postoperative graft toricity and require rigid contact lens for visual rehabilitation.[9]

TYPE OF CONTACT LENS

Soft Contact Lenses

In the phakic or aphakic graft with low toricity, daily wear soft contact lenses can be used. The use of extended wear soft contact lenses is more problematic as most studies have shown that the corneal graft tolerates the extended wear contact lens poorly and that its use in such patients is associated with corneal vascularization. This increases the risk of graft rejection and hence graft failure. On the contrary, some studies have shown that extended wear contact lenses can be fitted in such patients with long-term success.[5,11] Regardless of the findings of various studies, the indication for an extended wear lens in the graft patients must be based not only on visual need but also on those factors that may play a significant role in the success of the lens, including lid function, tear quality and production, hygiene, and patient reliability. There has to be a serious commitment on part of both patient and physician to monitor lens wear closely. Soft contact lens especially extended wear has very limited use in postkeratoplasty contact lens rehabilitation.

Rigid Contact Lenses

As mentioned earlier, rigid lenses play a significant role in visual rehabilitation of phakic, aphakic, and pseudophakic graft patients with high corneal toricity.[11,12-14] One such group comprises the patients of keratoconus. These patients are often excellent rigid contact lens candidates, since they have often worn rigid lenses for many years previously under less optimal fitting conditions, and they are usually rigid contact lens corrected in the nongrafted eye.[15] Studies indicate that such postkeratoplasty patients can be fitted in the early postoperative period even in the presence of sutures, that acuity and lens tolerance are good and that prekeratoplasty experience is an important factor in the rapid rehabilitation of these patients.

CONTACT LENSES FITTING METHOD

Although lenses can be fitted when sutures are in place, rigid lenses are usually fitted after suture removal, 12–18 months postoperatively (**Fig. 1**). Prior to lens fitting, K readings and manifest refraction should be stable over a period of a couple of months.

Prefitting Physiologic and Topographic Considerations

The penetrating keratoplasty patient presents with an unusual physiologic status. The patient's donor button is entirely repopulated with host epithelium and keratocyte replacement has begun by the time contact lens fitting is initiated. Unfortunately, corneal innervation is permanently altered by penetrating keratoplasty,[16] and endothelial function may differ significantly from the preoperative status.[17] Again, the impact of contact lens wear on both corneal innervation,[12]

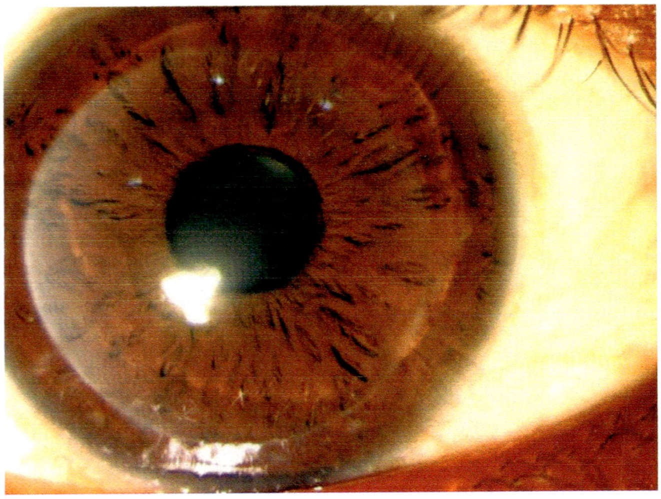

Fig. 1: Clear graft after suture removal.

and endothelial function[13] has been well documented. For this reason, the physician has to select a lens design that has a minimal impact on corneal physiology. In meeting this objective, ensuring adequate oxygen transmissibility is a major priority. The RGP lenses, owing to their high oxygen transmissibility, are an obvious choice (**Fig. 2**). To date, fluorosilicone acrylates are recommended because of their good oxygen transmission characteristics.[14]

When a silicone hydrogel lens is indicated, the physician should consider an extended wear variety worn on a daily basis. The limited oxygen profiles of hybrids and piggyback designs make each a less logical first choice. If these lens designs are indicated for other reasons, then a limited wearing time may be recommended.

Another factor of serious consideration in keratoplasty patients is that of corneal neovascularization.

If the patient's preexisting corneal disease is marked by severe inflammation, neovascularization may actually precede surgery. Often neovascularization develops as part of the postoperative healing phase. Aggressive corneal neovascularization can predispose an individual toward graft rejection.[18] In contact lens patients, neovascularization has been associated with intracorneal hemorrhage and lipid leakage, both of which can impair vision. Again, long-term use of contact lens itself can cause corneal vascularization. Although the exact mechanism of contact lens-induced corneal neovascularization is not known, the importance of adequate oxygenation and minimal inflammation is evident.[19] In an effort to satisfy these needs, a gas permeable lens design is often utilized.

Silicone hydrogel, hybrid, and piggyback designs are less desirable for the vascularized corneal graft, as they cover a large portion of the peripheral cornea. This additional coverage can result in a tight fit, hypoxia, and tear stagnation, inducing further encroachment of the vessels.

Another important consideration regarding the physiologic status of the graft patient involves the corneal surface disease. In view of the significantly altered corneal topography, a keratoplasty patient often manifests an irregular tear film. This is most often observed at the graft host junction and at the site of suture tracks. The compromised tear film may predispose these individuals toward ocular surface disease, including keratitis sicca, contact lens-induced erosions, and infectious keratitis.

No single material or design is most beneficial in managing the dry eye. While selecting an RGP lens it is wise to avoid high silicone-content lenses.[14] With hydrogel lenses, high water lens options and ultrathin designs are usually contraindicated.[20] The use of prophylactic lid hygiene, ocular surface lubricants, and punctal occlusion should be considered if the patient remains symptomatic. The potential for ocular surface erosion is increased if an RGP lens is fitted on a highly irregular graft surface. Erosion is often the result of focal lens bearing and can be sometimes managed by altering lens design. If epithelial erosion persists despite lens design alterations, the most prudent solution involves refitting into a silicone hydrogel or piggyback design.

In addition to these physiologic concerns of fitting the penetrating keratoplasty patient, there are obvious topographic considerations. Patients after penetrating keratoplasty often manifest a topographic profile that differs considerably from the normal cornea. This is often the result of many factors that includes preoperative corneal pathology, donor-recipient topographic discrepancies, surgical technique, and wound healing. With the corneal graft patient a significant discrepancy can exist between the donor and recipient topographies. The resultant cornea may manifest unusual asphericities, irregular optic zones, and a dramatically displaced apex. These topographic alterations result in postoperative visual disturbances which present as a specific challenge to the contact lens fitter. Historically, corneal topography measurements were limited to keratometry. In recent years, these measurements have been expanded to include automated keratometry and photokeratoscopy.[21] These days computer-assisted topographic analysis is advantageous to assess the topography of regular and irregular corneas,[22-29] monitor contact lens-induced corneal warpage,[30] and as baseline measurements for fitting cosmetic, keratoconic, and postsurgical contact lenses.[31-33] Recent software enhancements now allow the use of corneal topography to design rigid lenses.

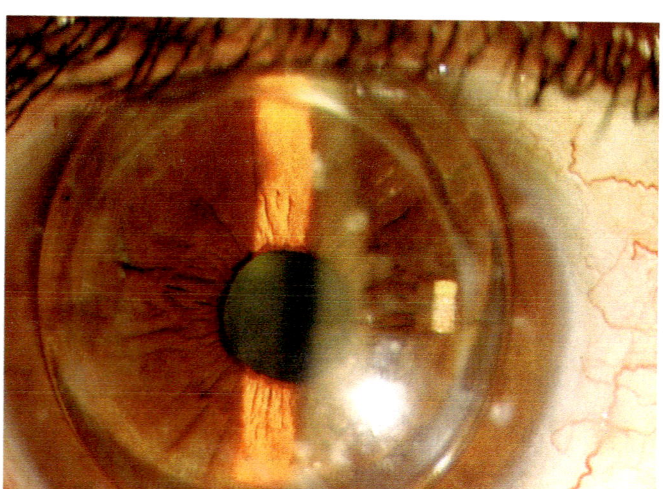

Fig. 2: Rigid gas permeable contact lens after penetrating keratoplasty.

Contact Lens Options

The aims of contact lens fitting after penetrating keratoplasty involve correction of residual refractive error, comfort commensurate with a reasonable wearing time, and maintenance of ocular health. It has long been accepted that such goals are to be achieved by utilizing a variety of contact lens options and by employing fitting techniques, that are as much an art as a science.

Gas Permeable Lenses

Although lenses can be fitted when sutures are in place, rigid lenses are usually fitted after suture removal (*see* **Figs. 1 and 2**), 12–18 months postoperatively. Enhanced oxygen transmissibility is desirable in the presence of a graft. Because of astigmatism and ocular surface irregularity, it is often impossible to achieve a perfect lens fit. Use of gas permeable materials appears to improve the patient's tolerance of lenses having areas of corneal touch where the fit is fairly flat. Lens flexure and poor wetting can be minor problems with gas permeable lenses, but these can be alleviated through modifications in the lens design and use of appropriate wetting agents and topical lubrication.

Goals

The goals in rigid contact lens fitting after keratoplasty are to achieve adequate lens centration and movement, optimal visual acuity, and good lens tolerance. Proper lens centration is difficult to obtain, owing to asymmetry of the graft wound. Often there is a tendency for the lens to gravitate toward one aspect of the wound, and lens also tends to ride high. Perfect centration is not necessary, but it is important to avoid decentration to the extent that the lens passes over the limbus during blink-induced movement. Lens contact with the limbus is usually associated with discomfort (**Fig. 3**).

Lenses should be fit loosely enough to ensure 1–2 mm of movement with each blink. Initially, there is often reflex tearing, so the lens movement must be evaluated after at least 30 minutes of lens wear. Lens movement is necessary for tear exchange under the lens, which in turn, is important not only for the delivery of oxygen that can pass through the lens but also for the removal of exfoliated material from under the lens.

Lens flexure or rocking can reduce acuity by several lines. Sometimes lens flexure is diminished with a larger or thicker lens. Lens rocking is often associated with edge lift, which can be reduced through the use of either a steeper or a smaller lens. Lens fit as well as lens power affect visual acuity in the presence of a graft.

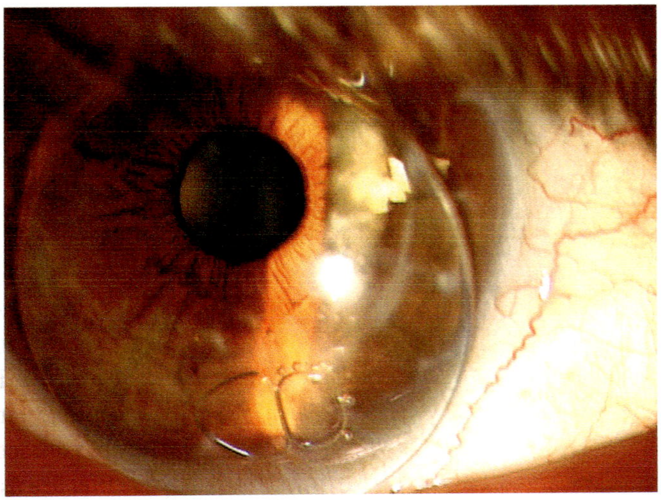

Fig. 3: Poorly fit contact lens.

The most important goal in contact lens fitting is to achieve good lens tolerance. The patient should be able to wear the lens with reasonable comfort for 10–14 hours per day. Gas permeable lenses with adequate centration and movement are usually well-tolerated despite an imperfect fit over an irregular graft surface.

Fitting Method

There are certain guidelines for selecting an initial trial lens, but experience and trial and error are factors in the selection of subsequent trial lenses. Unfortunately, the graft topography is often a challenge for the clinician who fits an RGP lens. To gain a better perspective on lens material and design considerations we will look at each variable.

Lens Materials

Among the RGP materials, fluorosilicone acrylate offers the greatest margin of safety. This material provides excellent oxygen transmission, improved surface characteristics, and acceptable flexure resistance in comparison to other materials.

Lens Overall Diameter

Most clinicians agree that lenses with an overall diameter of at least 9.0 mm are indicated in graft patients.[34] The earlier concept of a small (7.0–8.0 mm) lens fitted inside the graft-host junction has been abandoned. Difficulties with lens position, poor comfort, and easy displacement have accounted for this designs disfavor. Longer overall diameters of 9.5–11.0 mm are necessary if the corneal apex is grossly decentered and the lens centration is a problem. These larger designs may also facilitate lid attachment. In general, flatter corneas are fit with larger lenses and steeper corneas with smaller ones.

Optic Zone

The optic zone diameter should be modified according to overall lens diameter. Ideally, optic zone diameter should be as large as possible to facilitate lens centration and minimize glare, but not so large as to create harsh bearing or result in lens binding. The optic zone diameter should equal the base curve when both are expressed in millimeters. For example, a contact lens with a base curve of 42.50 D would have an optic zone of 7.95 mm.

Base Curve and Peripheral Curve Systems

Keratometry (K) provides a useful starting point for rigid lens fitting but is of limited value in the final lens selection. After keratoplasty, a wide range in curvature is present. The mires often are distorted making accurate measurement difficult. Routine keratometry measures only a small area of the central cornea. Because the shape of cornea near the graft-host junction is equally important in lens fitting, corneal topography, which provides more information about surface topography than does keratometry, is useful. Computerized videokeratoscopy software programs have the capability to design initial RGP lens parameters and simulate contact lens fluorescein patterns. Such programs allow the physician to choose posterior lens curvature, an overall and optic zone diameter, edge lift and power in some instances.

Usually, the first trial lens used is on or near flat K. Using videokeratography, the average of the two flattest readings at a point 1.5 mm superior to the visual axis can be used to select the base curve of the initial trial lens. When astigmatism is >5 D, the selected initial trial lens is steeper than flat K. The physician should modify base curve selection to facilitate a divided support fit. In this strategy, the clinician strives for a lens-cornea fitting relationship in which there is approximately one-third surface area-bearing and two-thirds surface area clearance.[35] Toric base curve options should be reserved for patients whose grafts are highly astigmatic. Although many are of the opinion that approximately 7 D of postoperative astigmatism is average,[2] the irregular nature of this astigmatism precludes routine use of back toric designs. As aspheric lens designs have long been recognized for their ability to accommodate atypical topographies, this option seems to be another logical choice. Recent work with a biaspheric back surface design has proven beneficial for penetrating keratoplasty patients.[36]

There is no clear consensus regarding the appropriate peripheral curve system for fitting the penetrating keratoplasty patient. As the central-peripheral corneal topography relationship is so dramatically altered in these patients, a traditional base curve-peripheral curve relationship may no longer be indicated. There is one definite situation in which the peripheral curve system is of paramount importance. This involves the patient with a plateau graft and difficulty with lens centration. In such cases, an unusually steep peripheral curve system is indicated. Such situation may require RGP design in which the secondary curve is steeper than the base curve.

One recent study has reported the use of tetra-curve contact lens with an overall diameter of 12.0 mm in postkeratoplasty patients.[37] The lens was well tolerated in all patients for >13 hours daily.

Lens Thickness

Whenever possible the thinnest design should be used to enhance lens comfort, centration, and optimum oxygen transmission. Thicker lenses should be reserved for problem with flexure, warpage, or frequent lens damage.

Lens Power

Refraction with spheres over a trial lens of appropriate base curve and diameter is necessary to determine which lens power to order. It is helpful, if a trial lens that approaches the correct power can be used. Ideally, the lens power should be compatible with the manifest refraction expressed in minus cylinders. Sometimes, it is not possible to obtain excellent visual acuity with an over refraction.

Immediately after fitting a trial lens, slit-lamp examination should be performed. A superior lens position with good lens movement (1–2 mm) is the goal of fitting. A fluorescein pattern indicating a relatively flat fit is preferred. A tight lens fit should be avoided in keratoplasty patient.

Rose-K Contact Lens

Rose-K design of RGP contact lens has been successfully fitted in eyes with keratoconus[38,39] and is now becoming increasingly popular for postkeratoplasty fitting as well (**Figs. 4A and B**). The Rose-K system has set optical zones to maximize vision while maintaining good corneal health. A separate set of postgraft trial lenses (Rose-K2 postgraft) is available for fitting Rose-K contact lens after keratoplasty.

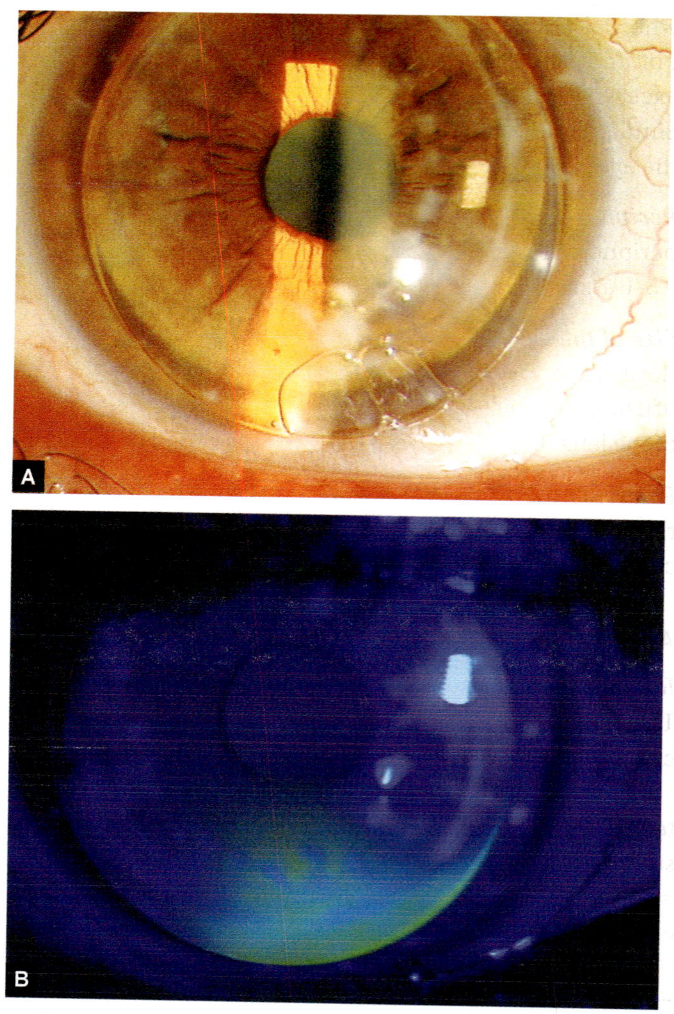

Figs. 4A and B: Rose-K contact lens fitting over a corneal graft.

Unlike normal corneas, the postgraft cornea has irregularity on its surface and to achieve optimal alignment with the cornea, many curves are required on the back surface of the lens.

Rose-K Postgraft Fitting Procedure

There are certain guidelines for fitting Rose-K lens in postkeratoplasty patients.

Prefitting examination: A thorough history of the patients should be taken that should include the motivation of the patient toward using the contact lens. A detailed examination of the eye should be done in view of the suitability for fitting contact lens.

Initial base curve selection: The initial base curve is 0.3 mm steeper than the average K reading. If the patient is already wearing an RGP contact lens, a base curve similar to the present lens may initially be tried.

Central fit: Adequate time should be given for the lens to equilibrate on the eye and also to minimize watering in the eye. The central fit is evaluated by fluorescein pattern immediately after blink when the lens is centered. A central pooling of 0.2–0.3 mm is acceptable in early flatter graft where the donor tissue is still flatter than the host tissue but an alignment of 0.1 mm in older grafts is aimed. An excessive amount of fluorescein may give a false picture. Similar situation can arise if there is excessive watering in the eye.

Peripheral fit: Once a good central fit is achieved, the peripheral edge lift is assessed. An even fluorescein band of 0.5–0.7 mm is aimed.

Size of the lens: The standard overall diameter in postgraft Rose-K2 contact lens for initial trial is 10.4 mm. The purpose of using large diameter lenses is to achieve a better centration of the lens.

Power: Once the base curve has been determined, over refraction is done to determine the correct power of the contact lens.

Advanced Models of Rose-K Lenses

Rose-K2 lens: These lenses curves on back surface of lens. These lenses minimize aberrations by applying very small changes to the curve on both front and back of the lens.

Rose-K2 postgraft lens: Based on asymmetric corneal technology (ACT), that is, inferior quadrant of the lens is steeper than the superior quadrant, hence leads to more accurate fit at 6 o'clock position. These lenses are based on reverse curve geometry and available in large diameter (10.40 mm). These lenses come with a better edge design and better optics and have a perfect repeatability of design as in trial lens. Five different edge lift values (+0.6, +1.2, –0.5, –1.0, and standard lift) are available to fit all types of corneas. Fitting is determined by keratometry, base curve, central fitting, peripheral fitting, centration or mobility, and power of lens.

Rose-K2 irregular cornea (IC) lens: These lenses have a reverse design with base curve >7.20. These lenses have a larger optical zone. Edge lift is steeper than conventional Rose-K lenses. Five different edge lift values (+0.6, +1.2, –0.5, –1.0, and standard lift) are available to fit all types of corneas. These lenses are used for larger areas of corneal distortion. It fits accurately to irregular corneas that do not respond to small diameter fits. In majority of postkeratoplasty eyes, the irregular cornea design of Rose-K lens fits well and is well acceptable to the patient in terms of visual improvement as well as comfort (**Fig. 5**).

Rose-K2 XL miniscleral lens: These lenses are recommended in patients who are not able to tolerate gas permeable corneal lenses, e.g., in patients with significant corneal distortion after undergoing penetrating keratoplasty.

Miniscleral design: These are large RGP lenses with diameter ranging from 14 to 18 mm. These lenses are particularly indicated in grafts, where there is very high irregular astigmatism and in conditions where in the graft-host junction is very steep in one meridian. The lens vaults the cornea and rests on sclera and creates a fluid-filled environment hence provides a better visual acuity and improved comfort to the patient (*see* **Fig. 5**).

Soft Contact Lens Fitting

Silicone Hydrogel Lenses

Soft contact lenses are fitted following keratoplasty more frequently for therapeutic purposes to promote surface healing than for visual purposes.

Aphakia is one indication for corrective daily-wear and extended-wear soft contact lens fitting. Extended wear soft contact lenses are used in elderly aphakic patients who are

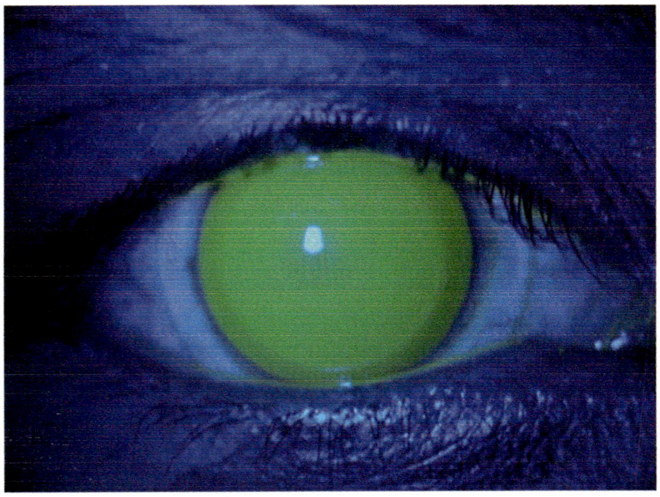

Fig. 5: Miniscleral contact lens.

unable to manipulate daily-wear lenses and who have only a low or moderate amount of astigmatism. Another indication for silicone hydrogel lens is an atypical graft-recipient geometry with attending RGP lens instability. Unfortunately, these cases may concomitantly manifest significant amount of astigmatism and require adjunctive spectacle correction.

In prescribing for a corneal graft patient, a balance between oxygen permeability and good surface characteristics is important. For myopic correction, this generally involves a thin design with low water content.

The clinician may wish to consider a toric hydrogel lens to cover for the astigmatism in keratoplasty patients. However, these patients manifest significant amount of irregular astigmatism on corneal topographic analysis and may cause a problem in fitting a back toric design.

The primary reason why silicone hydrogel lenses are not fitted in a corneal graft patient involves poor visual outcome. Another factor why it is relatively unacceptable is the potential for neovascularization.[24] Soft lenses are worn in an extended wear mode; the incidence of infectious keratitis can be expected to increase significantly.

Therapeutic Soft Contact Lens Fitting

Bandage soft contact lenses are useful in management of postkeratoplasty epithelial defects and persistent superficial punctate keratitis. Patients with ocular surface diseases and neurotrophic keratitis prior to keratoplasty are predisposed to nonhealing epithelial defects postoperatively. However, many graft patients without these conditions also have significant superficial punctate keratitis. This is caused by poor wetting due to abnormal corneal topography near the wound and, in some cases, due to drug toxicity. When topical lubrication or patching do not result in surface healing, bandage lenses are often beneficial. A variety of plano lenses with variable water content depending on the indication, can be used. Patients wearing therapeutic lenses can be maintained on topical medications as needed for the underlying condition. Lens fit must be checked after 1 hour, 1 day, and 1 week of lens wear, and then monthly to ensure that the lens moves 1–2 mm with the blink, the eye is white and quite, and the graft is tolerating the lens.

Piggyback Lenses

When an RGP or hydrogel lens alone does not suffice, a combination of the two may be indicated. The "piggyback" involves using a silicone hydrogel lens for surface smoothing and then employing a rigid lens for visual restoration.

Materials

The potential for oxygen debt is significant when one considers the simultaneous use of a silicone hydrogel and rigid contact lens. Therefore, high-oxygen transmission materials should routinely be prescribed. During lens adaptation, the clinician should carefully monitor biomicroscopy and adjust wearing time accordingly.

Design

The two major determinations in selection of silicone hydrogel lens are corneal topography and prescription. If the patient has a flat graft, then a mid-plus range lens design is selected. This particular carrier lens will accommodate the anticipated need for plus power correction while providing for a steeper topography on which to place the rigid lens. If the patient has a steep graft, then an ultrathin mid-minus range lens design is indicated. This carrier lens will lessen the amount of minus power required in the rigid lens while providing a flatter topography on which to fit the rigid lens. In either of these situations, the value of incorporating some of the refractive power into the silicone hydrogel lens allows the use of a thinner and lighter rigid lens.

The actual fitting of a "piggyback" lens design begins with evaluation of the underlying silicone hydrogel lens. The lens should be allowed to equilibrate and then evaluated for centration and lens movement. Optimal to slightly excessive lens movement is encouraged, as once the rigid lens is placed over the silicone hydrogel, its movement is almost certainly diminished. Once, a satisfactory silicone hydrogel lens fit is obtained, over-keratometry is performed. The result of over-keratometry serves as a starting point for rigid lens selection. The average of flat and steep over-keratometric value is often a reasonable starting point for rigid lens selection. Final base curve, overall diameter, optic zone, peripheral curve, power, and thickness determinations are best accomplished by diagnostic fitting. High molecular weight fluorescein can be utilized to assess optical clearance of the rigid lens relative to its hydrogel carrier. Care must be taken to avoid a tightly fitted rigid lens, as this often traps interfacial debris.

Hybrid Lenses

Hybrid lenses were designed to combine the comfort and centering capabilities associated with hydrogel lenses with the visual acuity offered by a rigid lens. The SoftPerm (SBH Corp. Sunnyvale, CA) lens is a hybrid lens made from a single button containing a copolymerized hydrophilic skirt with an RGP center molecularly bonded at the transition zone.

The overall diameter of the lens is 14.3 mm and the rigid optical zone diameter is 8 mm. A single base curve is selected from a diagnostic set of trial lenses based upon the mean central keratometry reading. The greater the increased corneal toricity, the steeper the base curve selected. Because the RGP center diameter is 8.0 mm, one typically fits steeper than the flattest K to achieve a parallel sagittal depth in relationship to the cornea. The final base curve must be selected by diagnostic fitting, with each trial lens allowed to equilibrate for a minimum of 15 minutes. Regardless of a good visual response and positive patients acceptance, adequate lens movement is essential. Once an optimal fit is achieved, an over refraction is performed to determine exact lens power. Certain clinicians believe that this lens permits a more over refraction free from the unstable and inconsistent vision that can be associated with RGP lenses that have been fit over corneas with irregular astigmatism.[40]

COMPLICATIONS

Any keratoplasty patient fitted with contact lens has to be monitored carefully for possible complications. A corneal graft fitted with contact lens is prone to develop certain specific complications owing to altered corneal surface physiology and topography. There is high-risk of ocular surface erosion particularly if an RGP lens has been fitted on a highly irregular graft surface. Erosion is often the result of focal lens bearing and can sometimes be managed by altering lens design. Bad ocular surface and compromised tear film may further aggravate the existing situation. The use of ocular surface lubricants and lid hygiene should be considered. Infectious keratitis is the most dreaded consequence of ocular surface disease. The propensity of certain bacteria to colonize epithelial defects in contact lens users is well documented.[41] This consideration is especially important among patients of penetrating keratoplasty, as the graft-host junction and suture tracks are highly prone to infection and the eye may be immunocompromised as a result of long-term steroid usage. The significance of epithelial erosion, loose sutures, improper contact lens hygiene, bacterial invasion, compromised host immunity, and delayed treatment is obvious in establishing condition for potential infectious keratitis.

A keratoplasty patient fitted with silicone hydrogel lenses is prone to develop corneal neovascularization resulting in a high chance of graft rejection. Again, optical quality of silicone hydrogel lenses is not as good as RGP. Moreover, as these lenses are used for extended wear, there is always the risk of infection.

The complications that can be associated with piggyback and hybrid designs are corneal edema, neovascularization, contact lens adherence, acute red eye episodes, infectious keratitis, and graft rejection. Another problem with hybrid designs is difficulty in inserting and removing the lens and a high percentage of lens separation. Because of the difficulty in removing the lens and the presence of a junction between the optical center and hydrogel skirt, the lens can tear relatively easily.

Many contact lens designs may be employed for the refractive management of a graft patient. These include RGP, silicone hydrogel, hybrid, and piggyback lenses. The specific design selected is dependent on a number of factors, which includes corneal graft physiologic status, corneal topography, refractive error, desired wearing schedule and patient handling capabilities. Each of these factors must be weighed independently to ensure the greatest likelihood of contact lens success.

REFERENCES

1. Cohen EJ, Adams CP. Postkeratoplasty fitting for visual rehabilitation. In: Dabezies OH Jr (Ed). Contact Lenses: The CLAO Guide to Basic Science and Clinical Practice. New York: Grune and Stratton; 1984.
2. Genvert GI, Cohen EJ, Arentsen JJ, Laibson PR. Fitting gas permeable lenses following penetrating keratoplasty. Am J Ophthalmol. 1985;99:511-4.
3. McDonald M, Baldone JA. Postkeratoplasty fitting to enhance re-epithelialisation. In: Dabezies OH Jr (Ed). Contact Lenses: The CLAO Guide to Basic Science and Clinical Practice. New York: Grune and Stratton; 1984.
4. Binder PS. The effect of total suture removal on postkeratoplasty astigmatism. Am J Ophthalmol. 1988;105:637-45.
5. Cayanaugh HD, Leveille AS. Extended wear contact lenses in patients with corneal grafts and aphakia. Ophthalmology. 1980;89:643-50.
6. Jensen AD, Maumenee AE. Refractive error following keratoplasty. Trans Am Ophthalmol Soc. 1970;72:123-31.
7. Troutman RC, Gaster RN. Surgical advantages and results of keratoconus. Am J Ophthalmol. 1980;90:131-6.
8. Bennett ES, Weissman BA. Clinical Contact Lens Practice. Philadelphia: JB Lippincott Company; 1991. pp. 9-10.
9. Buxton JN. Contact lenses in keratoconus. Contact Intraocular Lens Med J. 1978;4:74-85.
10. Casey TA, Mayer DJ. Contact lenses and keratoplasty. Corneal Grafting. Philadelphia: WB Saunders; 1984. pp. 281-8.
11. Dangel ME, Kracher GP, Stark WJ, Maumenee AE, Martin NF. Aphakic extended-wear contact lenses after penetrating keratoplasty. Am J Ophthalmol. 1983;95:156-60.
12. Millodot M. Effect of the length of wear of contact lenses on corneal sensitivity. Acta Ophthalmol (Copenh). 1976;54:721-30.
13. Holden BA, Sweeny DF, Vannas A, Kotow M, Hood KM, Grant T, et al. Contact lens induced endothelial polymegathism. Invest Ophthalmol Vis Sci. 1987;26(suppl.):275.
14. Tomlinson A. Choice of materials—a material issue. Contact Lens Spectrum. 1990;5:27.
15. Mannis MJ, Zadnik K, Deutch D. Rigid contact lens wear in the corneal transplant patient. CLAO J. 1986;12:39-42.
16. Ruben M, Colebrook E. Keratoconus keratoplasty curvatures and contact lens wear. Br J Ophthalmol. 1979;63:268-73.
17. Bron AJ, Brown NA. Endothelium of the corneal graft. Trans Ophthalmol Soc U K. 1974;94:863-73.
18. Lemp MA. The effect of extended-wear aphakic hydrophilic contact lenses after penetrating keratoplasty. Am J Ophthalmol. 1980;90:331-5.
19. McMonnies CW. Risk factors in the etiology of contact lens induced corneal vascularisation. Int Contact Lens Clin. 1984;11:286-93.
20. Helton DO, Walton LS. Hydrogel contact lens dehydration rates determined by thermogravimetric analysis. CLAO J. 1991;17:59-61.
21. Gormley D, Gerston M, Koplin RS, Lubkin V. Corneal modeling. Cornea. 1988;7:30-5.
22. Dingledein SA, Klyce SD. The topography of normal corneas. Arch Ophthalmol. 1989;107:512-8.
23. Dingledein SA, Klyce SD. Imaging of the cornea. Cornea. 1988;7:170-82.
24. Wilson SE, Klyce SD. Advances in the analysis of corneal topography. Surv Ophthalmol. 1991;36:269-77.

25. Bogan SJ, Waring GO 3rd, Ibrahim O, Drews C, Curtis L. Classification of normal corneal topography based on computer-assisted videokeratography. Arch Ophthalmol. 1990;108:945-9.
26. Wilson SE, Lin D, Klyce SD. Corneal topography of keratoconus. Cornea. 1991;10:2-8.
27. McMohan TT, Robin JB, Scarpulla KM, Putz JL. The spectrum of topography found in keratoconus. CLAO J. 1991;17:198-204.
28. Wilson SE, Friedman RS, Klyce SD. Contact lens manipulation of corneal topography after penetrating keratoplasty: a preliminary study. CLAO J. 1992;18:177-82.
29. Strelow S, Cohen EJ, Leavitt KG, Laibson PR. Corneal topography for selective suture removal after penetrating keratoplasty. Am J Ophthalmol. 1991;112:657-65.
30. Wilson SE, Lin DT, Klyce SD, Reidy JJ, Insler MS. Rigid lens decentration: a risk factor for corneal warpage. CLAO J. 1990;16:177-82.
31. Wasserman D, Itzkowitz J, Kamenar T, Asbell PA. Corneal topographic data: Its use in fitting aspheric contact lenses. CLAO J 1992;18:83-5.
32. Rabinowitz YS, Garbus JJ, Garbus C, McDonnell PJ. Contact lens selection for keratoconus using a computer-assisted videokeratoscope. CLAO J. 1991;17:88-93.
33. Lopatynsky M, Cohen EJ, Leavitt KG, Laibson PR. Corneal topography for rigid gas permeable lens fitting after penetrating keratoplasty. CLAO J. 1993;19:41-4.
34. Zadnik K. Post-surgical contact lens alternatives. Int Contact Lens Clin. 1988;15:211-20.
35. Shovlin J, Kame R, Weissman B, DePaolis M. How to fit an irregular cornea? Rev Optom. 1987;124:88.
36. Weiner B. Contact lens correction of the post-penetrating keratoplasty patient. Contact Lens Update. 1989;8:61.
37. Eggink FA, Nuijts RM. A new technique for rigid gas permeable contact lens fitting following penetrating keratoplasty. Acta Ophthalmol Scand. 2001;79:245-50.
38. Betts AM, Mitchell GL, Zadnik K. Visual performance and comfort with the Rose K lens for keratoconus. Optom Vis Sci. 2002;79(8):493-501.
39. Jain AK, Sukhija J. Rose K contact lens for keratoconus. Indian J Ophthalmol. 2007;55(2):121-5.
40. Binder PS, Kopecky L. Fitting the short-term contact lens after keratoplasty. CLAO J. 1992;18:170-2.
41. Reichert R, Stern G. Quantitative adherence of bacteria to human corneal epithelial cells. Arch Ophthalmol. 1984;102:1394-5.

SECTION

3

Penetrating Keratoplasty: Management of Complications

15 Complications of Penetrating Keratoplasty

Mohamed Ibrahime Asif, Ritu Nagpal, Sarath S, Namrata Sharma

INTRODUCTION

Several clinical and technological advances in corneal transplantation during the last few decades resulted in improved visual outcomes, better graft survival rates and lesser number of complications. But we should remember the fact that complications are bound to occur in any surgical procedure and having a knowledge of all possible complications and appropriate management of the same can ultimately result in improved graft survival. The complications of penetrating keratoplasty may be broadly categorized as intraoperative or postoperative. Postoperative complications can be early or late. Early postoperative complications developing within the first 4 weeks of surgery while the term late is applied to changes occurring after the 4 week period.

INTRAOPERATIVE COMPLICATIONS

Poor Anesthesia and Positive Vitreous Pressure

Both analgesia and akinesia which lasts throughout the surgical time is a prerequisite for shifting the patient to the operating table. Retrobulbar and peribulbar anesthesia are known to cause a rise in the intraocular pressure (IOP) and vitreous upthrust by increasing the intraorbital volume. Intraoperatively, this upthrust could result in a difficult dissection of the host corneal button, capsulorhexis, cortical matter removal and IOL implantation; however, the most dreaded complication, expulsive choroidal hemorrhage could also occur due to sudden decompression.

Prevention: General anesthesia, in general, reduces the IOP and is hence, preferred over retrobulbar or peribulbar blocks.[1] Positive vitreous pressure can be reduced by preoperative intravenous mannitol 1–2 g/kg administered, 20–30 minutes before the peribulbar block. Oral acetazolamide 15 mg/kg can also be used 1–2 hours before surgery. A super pinky applied for 5–10 minutes or an adequate digital massage after peribulbar block could reduce the vitreous pressure. A self-retaining speculum is preferred over a wire speculum to avoid undue pressure on the globe.

Management: In cases anticipated to have high vitreous pressure, a pars plana 25-G single port anterior vitrectomy can be done before trephination.[2] Vitreous upthrust after the host corneal button removal can be managed by automated anterior vitrectomy via anterior route, especially if the anterior vitreous phase is disrupted.

Scleral Perforation while Scleral Fixation Rings

Flieringa rings and McNeill-Goldman Blepharostat are used by some surgeons to prevent scleral collapse, especially in cases with low scleral rigidity such as in children, aphakic or vitrectomized eyes. These rings are secured using sutures. Inadvertent scleral perforation can happen while securing the rings, resulting in bleeding from the underlying vascular choroid. This is, however, self-limiting and usually requires no treatment.

Improper Trephination

Reversed Host and Donor Trephines

In most cases of corneal transplants, a graft host disparity of 0.5 mm is kept for better graft host apposition and maintenance of angle anatomy. However, inadvertent trephination of both the host and donor cornea using the same size trephine or reversal of host and donor trephines could sometimes happen, leading to tight suturing, shallow anterior chamber, and a flatter cornea. Collapse of the angles and trabecular meshwork could result in a rise in postoperative IOP.[3] Tight sutures also causes hyperopic shift due to corneal flattening.[4]

Management: Ideally in these scenarios, another tissue should be trephined with an appropriately sized trephine if a backup is available. In case of non-availability of back up tissue, management depends upon the stage at which the mishap is detected. If the host has not been trephined or only partially trephined, without entering the anterior chamber and the donor button has been cut inadvertently with a smaller trephine, a trephine 0.25 mm smaller than used on the donor cornea may be used on the host, provided it completely encompasses the lesion.[5] If the donor has been prepared and the host anterior chamber entry is complete, the smaller button may be used. If an intraocular lens is planned, the power of the lens may be adjusted to account for 2–3 D of induced hyperopia.

Eccentric, Oval, and Irregular Host Trephination

Improper centration of the graft during trephination could result in oval or eccentric trephination resulting in high postoperative astigmatism.[6] This happens due to improper stabilization during trephination resulting in sliding of the trephine during the process. The use of blunt trephines results in irregular trephined margins. Scleral fixation rings can also cause oval trephination due to irregular pull caused by scleral sutures.

Prevention and management: Marking the lesion with a calipers and gentian violet dye and visualization of all marks through the center of trephine can avoid irregular trephination. Adequate fixation with Hessburg-Barron vacuum trephine and use of sharp disposable single-use trephines can avoid most trephining problems. If the eccentric cut is less than one-third of the stromal depth, the trephine can be replaced, and the initial incision may be ignored. If the cut is deeper, it may be necessary to use a slightly larger trephine, so that the resultant opening encompasses the previous eccentric cut and remains central (**Fig. 1**). Some surgeons do not prefer to use scleral fixation rings to avoid oval trephination.[7] Recently excimer laser has been used to create circular, well-centered cuts.[8]

Damaged Donor Button

In a penetrating keratoplasty donor tissue has to be prepared before host trephination. Donor tissue can get damaged right from transportation till the end of surgery. There are incidences where donor tissue has been slipped and lost while transferring from media, during trephination and while transferring from operating table to the eye. The use of distilled water could also potentially damage the endothelium resulting in primary graft failure. Endothelial cell loss occurs more in phakics than in aphakics due to endothelial iris contact.[9]

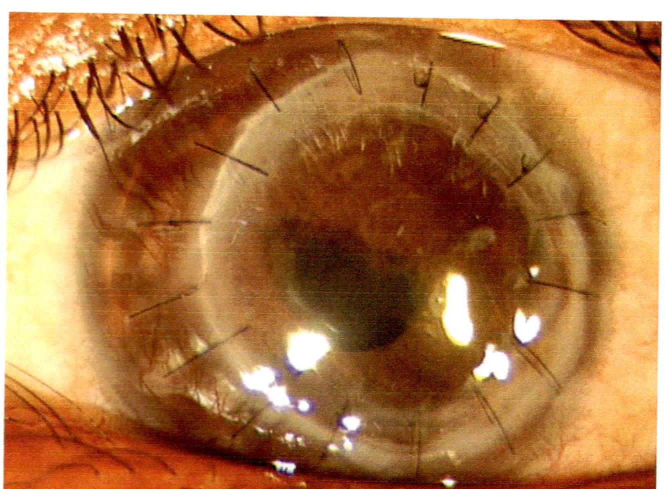

Fig. 1: Eccentric graft.

Prevention: Every possible effort should be made to prevent damage to the endothelium. Careful handling of the tissue during the transfer and process should be ensured. Sharp new trephines or disposable trephines should be used to prevent damage during the trephination.

A graft holder should always be used to transfer the donor cornea to the recipient bed to avoid graft loss. Never use any tissue which gets contaminated by accidental fall on the floor as it can lead to multidrug-resistant graft infections, endophthalmitis, etc. The ideal way is to suture the patient's host cornea and the case may be rescheduled.[10] Very rarely in an aphakic eye, it is possible to lose the graft in the vitreous.[11] An oversized graft reduces the risk of this disastrous hazard. Viscodispersive agents such as Viscoat should be used to protect the endothelium while placing donor over the recipient bed.

Inversion of the Graft

Inversion of corneal button can rarely occur. In one instance, the graft was sutured with the endothelial side facing upward.[12] This can occur in cases of small sized grafts and patch grafts where the corneal curvature can not be made out.

Prevention and management: The epithelial and endothelial surfaces can be easily identified by the orientation of button in the well, the curvature of the button and marks on the epithelial surface if the button has been previously marked.

Excessive Bleeding

Minimal bleeding which settles intraoperatively is something not to be worried, however, inflamed ocular surfaces such as in therapeutic keratoplasty or vascularized corneas could result in excessive bleeding. Vigorous synechiolysis or inadvertent iatrogenic iris damage could also result in excessive bleeding. Iridodialysis can occur due to iris manipulation during surgery or while explanting closed-loop anterior chamber lenses, adhered posterior chamber lenses resulting in excessive bleeding from the angle vessels.[13] Excessive bleeding during the surgery can cause increased postoperative inflammation, inflammatory membranes in the anterior chamber and a rise in IOP. Postoperative long-standing hyphema can cause corneal staining.

Prevention and management: Hemorrhage may be controlled with cautery, compression with viscoelastic or tamponade with sponges/swab sticks soaked with epinephrine 1:1,000 dilution.[13] Intracameral epinephrine should be avoided in aphakic eyes as it leads to increased risk for cystoid macular edema. Care should be taken to prevent seepage of blood into the vitreous, especially in aphakic patients, as this absorbs very slowly. Iris tissue should be minimally manipulated to release any adhesions/synechiae to avoid excessive bleeding. Any visible hyphema at the end of the surgery should be carefully washed to avoid corneal staining.

Retained Descemet's Membrane

This happens when the surgeon inadvertently enters the Descemet plane while making an incision in the host cornea or while injecting ocular viscoelastic devices. It is more common in cases with adherent leucoma, thick and edematous corneas as seen in congenital hereditary endothelial dystrophy and interstitial keratitis. Since the Descemet's membrane is transparent, visually it may not be possible to recognize this complication intraoperatively. The iris architecture should be carefully inspected after trephination of such corneas and this tissue should be gently picked up with a forceps.[11] Failure to grasp the iris is a conclusive sign of the presence of retained Descemet's membrane. Postoperatively, anterior segment optical coherence tomography (OCT) may be used to demonstrate the presence of a retained Descemet's membrane as well as document successful management of the same (**Fig. 2**).[14,15]

Management: If detected intraoperatively, the retained Descemet's can be removed with capsulorhexis forceps after injecting viscoelastic behind it.

Complete removal should be ensured until the graft-host junction. In the postoperative period, the membrane appears as a sheet posterior to the graft and opacifies with time so that it can be confused with a retrocorneal membrane. However, an attempt should be made to salvage the graft by making an opening with neodymium-doped yttrium aluminium garnet (Nd: YAG) laser, i.e., Nd: YAG descemetotomy. We can use 0.1% trypan blue dye to stain this membrane to improve its visualization so that tearing of the membrane, i.e., "descemetorhexis" can be undertaken easily.[16] Repeat grafting should be done if this fails and graft rejection occurs.

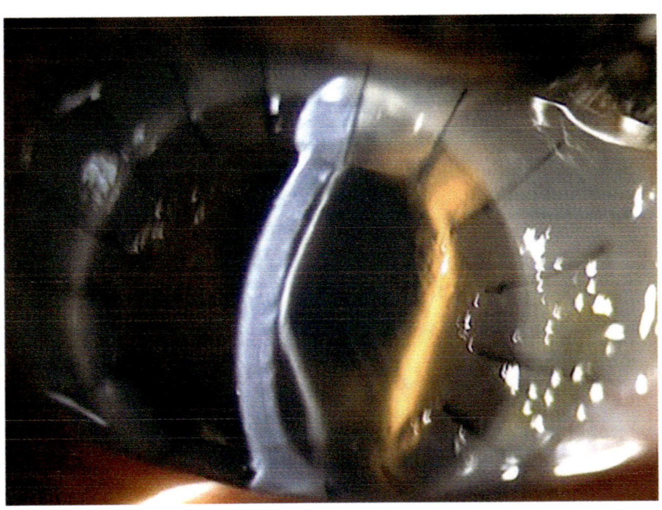

Fig. 2: Day 1 postoperative image of patient with retained Descemet's membrane.

Injury to Iris-lens Diaphragm

Injury to the lens-iris diaphragm can occur during trephination as well as while dissecting out the host button. This usually occurs in *thinned or perforated corneas*. Intracameral miosis with pilocarpine 1% and the use of viscocohesive OVD can prevent inadvertent lens damage.

This can also be prevented by attempting a partial depth trephination, filling the anterior chamber with an OVD through a paracentesis followed by making a controlled entry through the partial groove using a microvitreoretinal blade. The host bed can then be cut with curved corneal scissors. The use of lamellar dissection technique can also effectively save the iris from undergoing severe damage during trephination especially in cases of adherent leucoma.[17] Any inadvertent iris damage and iridodialysis should be repaired with a 10-0 polypropylene suture as far as possible. Damage to the anterior lens capsule that occurs *during trephination* should be recognized immediately and extracapsular cataract extraction should be undertaken combined with placement of a posterior chamber intraocular lens.[5]

Hirst et al.[18] described the combined use of viscoelastic for anterior chamber reformation and cyanoacrylate glue assisted closure of the perforation before attempting trephination in eyes with perforated corneas.[5]

Posterior Capsular Tear and Vitreous Prolapse

During the combined procedure of penetrating keratoplasty with extracapsular cataract extraction, the posterior capsule may be torn inadvertently during aspiration of the lens matter. The incidence of posterior capsular tear with vitreous loss has been reported to vary from 0 to 16%.[18,19]

Management: A regular small posterior capsular tear, can be converted into a posterior continuous curvilinear capsulorhexis and a foldable posterior chamber IOL can be implanted in the bag. In a case where the tear is large, an anterior vitrectomy should be performed with and a three piece IOL is placed in the ciliary sulcus. In cases with no sulcus support and low risk for glaucoma and endothelial decompensation, an open-loop Kelman multiflex anterior chamber intraocular lens may be implanted with a peripheral iridectomy.

Suture-related Complications

Problems with Suturing Graft to the Host

Improper suturing can cause unequal graft tissue distribution and can lead to severe postkeratoplasty astigmatism. *The second suture (6'o clock) is considered the most important one in a case of keratoplasty.* The donor tissue should be firmly grasped, and the first suture should be passed directly beneath the forceps, which grasps the graft to prevent any undue torque. The depth of the suture should be almost up to the Descemet's membrane (90%) to ensure optimal wound closure and prevent posterior wound gaping. The donor button may be rotated/spun in any direction before the application of the first suture. The second suture should be placed exactly opposite to the first one, as even a slight deviation will result in torsion of the graft and consequently astigmatism. The formation of a diamond after placing four cardinal sutures is an indication of equal distribution of tension. One must ensure that the anterior chamber is well-formed while passing each suture.

Broken/Loose/Tight Sutures

Sutures that are loose, tight, or improperly oriented can break while burying as well result in postoperative astigmatism. Tight sutures especially can cause radiating folds and can result in persistent epithelial defects. Loose sutures can lead to the accumulation of debris, mucus resulting in increased chances of graft infections. Suture knots could get bulky and fail to get buried especially if the technique is not proper. All sutures should be assessed properly after forming the anterior chamber under balanced salt solution (BSS).

Management: All broken, tight, and loose interrupted sutures should be replaced. Any suture which does not bury should be immediately replaced. Caution is required, especially when using a continuous suture. The continuous suture may be accidentally cut while attempting to remove the cardinal sutures. The use of double-armed suture allows suturing in a direction opposite the first when needed.

Iris Incarceration

While suturing donor cornea with host tissue iris can get incarcerated leading to pupillary peaking or an irregular pupil. This can lead to bleeding into the anterior chamber, poor wound healing, uveitis due to low-grade inflammation and peripheral anterior synechiae which can ultimately lead to graft failure.

Prevention and management: This can be avoided by lifting the wound edge slightly before passing the suture through the host, always visualizing the graft-host junction while passing each suture and keeping a well-formed AC under viscoelastic or air tamponade. If iris incarceration occurs, then that suture had to be released and the anterior chamber must be formed and then suturing should be carried out. Pilocarpine could also assist in constriction of pupil and stretching of iris, thereby preventing this complication.

Shallow Anterior Chamber

A shallow anterior chamber during penetrating keratoplasty may occur due to the presence of floppy iris, such as in cases of corneoiridic scars, positive vitreous pressure, cataractous lens, and use of a small graft.

In cases such as corneoiridic scar[20] and pediatric cases[21] where a shallow anterior chamber is anticipated, oversized grafts should be used to prevent the occurrence of a shallow anterior chamber. At the end of keratoplasty, the anterior chamber should be formed with BSS to prevent the occurrence of posterior synechiae and endothelial damage. Peripheral anterior synechiae should be released completely as much as possible to restore angle anatomy and floppy iris should be managed by pupilloplasty.

Failure to reform the anterior chamber usually signifies a wound leak from poorly apposed corneal edges or irregular suturing and hence should be appropriately managed. A cataractous lens should be removed and chamber IOL should be implanted. Air has higher surface tension than water and may actually seal and thereby hide a wound leak. Therefore, while checking for such a leak, *BSS should replace the air* in the anterior chamber. A shallow anterior chamber may also occur due to positive vitreous pressure in the absence of wound leak. Anterior vitrectomy via pars plana route with 25-G cutter can be done to reduce vitreous pressure.

Wound Leak

Following completion of suturing the donor to the host, one must always check for the presence of wound leaks with an anterior chamber formed with BSS. *Fluorescein dye* (Seidel's test) can be applied to the surface of the cornea and tight manual pressure should be applied to the globe. Alternatively, the wound may be dried with one cellulose sponge and the limbus may be gently pressed with another dry sponge so that the presence of wound leak is easily detected. If a wound leak is noted, *additional sutures* may be applied, or sutures can be replaced, if there is poor graft host apposition. If suture tract leak is present, a 10-0 prolene suture can be placed perpendicular to the suture tract. This is especially important in pediatric keratoplasty, where there are more chances of wound leak due to a less rigid cornea or if a suture has been placed multiple times at a particular area.

Suprachoroidal Hemorrhage

This is a rare and the *most dreaded* complication of penetrating keratoplasty.[22] The incidence of suprachoroidal hemorrhage varies from 0.47 to 3.3%.[5] Uncontrolled bleeding into the suprachoroidal space may result in the expulsion of intraocular contents through the trephined area. The condition can be promptly diagnosed by progressive anterior bulging of vitreous along with direct observation of choroidal detachment. The mechanism of suprachoroidal hemorrhage is sudden and prolonged decompression of the globe resulting in rupture of fragile choroidal vessels due to either traction on the vitreous or elevated transmural pressure gradient. Various risk factors include preexisting glaucoma, hypertension, high myopia, inflammation, sudden cough, previous surgery, previous traction, and Valsalva maneuver.[23,24] Injection of an excessive amount of retrobulbar local anesthetic may also predispose to it by increasing the episcleral venous pressure.[23]

Prevention and management: Suprachoroidal hemorrhage can be prevented by preoperative lowering of IOP, controlling hypertension, and preventing any Valsalva maneuver during surgery. Patient's head can be slightly elevated. Trephination should be performed gently so that the IOP is not markedly elevated by downward pressure with the trephine and then rapidly reduced when the anterior chamber is opened. However, if intraoperative hemorrhage occurs, the emergency management includes occlusion of the host corneal opening and sealing of the eye to provide a good tamponade. Management of expulsive hemorrhage depends on immediate recognition and prompt action.

If the hemorrhage occurs immediately or *shortly after entering the globe, a posterior sclerotomy* via a stab incision through the conjunctiva and sclera is performed. The inferotemporal quadrant is the most readily accessible. Multiple sclerotomies may be required. However, if the hemorrhage occurs during the open-sky phase of keratoplasty, management becomes difficult. A temporary keratoprosthesis, if available, or even a finger can be used for occlusion. Intravenous mannitol should be started immediately and one or more sclerotomies made to facilitate drainage. Donor button is then sutured in place with 8-0 nylon suture as rapidly as possible. Visual prognosis is usually poor and depends on the extent of hemorrhage, concurrent involvement of retina and efficiency of intraoperative management.

POSTOPERATIVE COMPLICATIONS

Early Postoperative Complications

Complications in the early postoperative period vary from minor to true ophthalmic emergencies resulting in the loss of eye. Hence, a meticulous follow-up, early diagnosis, and timely interventions are mandatory.

Shallow Anterior Chamber and Wound Leak

A shallow anterior chamber along with low IOP on the first postoperative day usually signifies a wound leak or a serous choroidal detachment. IOP may be normal or even high especially in eyes with malignant glaucoma or hemorrhagic choroidal detachment. Site of the leak can be identified by Seidel's test. The test is performed by placing concentrated fluorescein dye 2% on the eye and observing under cobalt blue filter on a slit lamp. A change in color from green to black, occurs due to the dilution of dye by th leaking aqueous and confirms the presence of a wound leak. A prolonged shallow anterior chamber may result in the formation of peripheral anterior synechiae, anterior bulging of the lens with endothelial touch, and secondary glaucoma. Graft survival is dependent on early diagnosis and quick reformation of the anterior chamber. The likely *causes of wound leak* are mentioned in **Box 1**.

Box 1: Common causes of wound leak.

- Broken, loose or misplaced sutures
- *Suture track leak*
- Sutures passed through thin or necrotic tissue
- Excessive gap between sutures
- Unequal thickness of graft and host
- Increased vitreous pressure

Prevention and management: If the anterior chamber is flat and a suture tract leak is present, immediate surgical repair is required. If the anterior chamber remains formed in the presence of a wound leak a pressure bandage or bandage contact lens may be given which aids in reapposition of the wound, tamponades the leak, and decreases the trauma caused by the lids to the wound. Additionally, acetazolamide may be prescribed to decrease aqueous production.

If the wound does not seal in 24 hours, it must be resutured. In case of interrupted sutures, any loose or broken sutures should be replaced. An additional suture can be placed in the area of the leak. In case of a continuous suture, loosening the tight area and tightening the area of the leak may redistribute the tension over the wound. In case of a broken continuous suture in the early postoperative period, a new segment of 10-0 nylon suture must be added, making several bites across the wound.

Suture track leak caused by full-thickness sutures usually closes spontaneously. An additional mattress suture may be applied perpendicular to the suture which is causing the suture track leak. The leak caused by suturing through necrotic tissue is very difficult to manage, as resuturing is nearly impossible. Corneal glueing and bandage contact lens placement may be tried in such cases. Choroidal detachments usually resolve once the chamber is formed.

Iris Incarceration

Iris incarceration may occur due to collapse of the anterior chamber or from wound leak. This may occur in cases where penetrating keratoplasty has been undertaken in inflamed eyes and the iris is swollen and flaccid. It can also occur due to poorly placed sutures causing incarceration of iris, especially if the lens-iris diaphragm herniates forward. The presence of incarcerated iris may incite postoperative inflammation. It closes the angles at the site of incarceration and can cause glaucoma and graft failure. Large adhesions at the graft-host junction may lead to localized edema of the graft and attract vascularization.

Management: Argon laser iridoplasty may be undertaken to release the iris if the incarceration is minimal. However, if conservative management fails, surgical intervention is necessary. Iris tissue is separated from all attachments and swept out of the wound with an iris repositor. A viscoelastic can be injected into the anterior chamber by making a separate stab wound entry and the iris tissue may be rotated away from the wound gently using the viscoelastic cannula. In case, the iris cannot be separated from the wound, the suture may be the culprit, in which case suture must be replaced.

Wound Dehiscence

Wound dehiscence in the postoperative period may occur immediately or several years after penetrating keratoplasty. Young patients, especially males, should be made aware that their eye, after keratoplasty, will always be vulnerable to injury. High-risk situations should be avoided if possible. Older patients at particular risk should have adequate risk reduction strategies, social support, and supervision, in particular, to minimize the risk of falls.[25] A wound dehiscence in the immediate postoperative period usually occurs secondary to technical problems such as a thin, necrotic recipient bed. It may also occur due to a postoperative rise in the IOP or after suture removal. The incidence of wound dehiscence after suture removal requiring repair has been reported to be 2.4–2.9%.[26,27]

Causes of wound dehiscence are mentioned in **Box 2.**[28-31] Spontaneous wound dehiscence may occur in the elderly or patients of keratoconus. Generally, traumatic wound dehiscence following penetrating keratoplasty occurs at the donor-recipient interface. Eyes with traumatic wound dehiscence have worse visual outcome than those with dehiscence after suture removal. Patients should be cautioned about the risks and consequences of wound dehiscence. The suture may be left in place longer in older patients or when corneal edema is the indication for grafting.[32]

Full-thickness wound dehiscence must be repaired immediately. Wound dehiscence is the leading indication for resuturing following penetrating keratoplasty.[33] If iris prolapse is present which is <24 hours duration and the iris tissue appears healthy, it should be replaced into the anterior chamber. If the prolapsed tissue appears necrotic or if the duration of iris prolapse is >24 hours, iris tissue abscission should be done with scissors held flush to the wound.

Box 2: Causes of wound dehiscence.[28-31]

- Trauma
- Infectious keratitis
- Suture breakage
- Spontaneous wound separation

Additional procedures such as lensectomy, vitrectomy, and IOL explantation may be required, and in some cases, regrafting may be necessary.

Low Intraocular Pressure

Low IOP after penetrating keratoplasty is not uncommon. Following are the possible causative factors:

- Wound leak
- *Iridocyclitis*: Ciliary shock
- Cyclodialysis
- Choroidal detachment
- Retinal detachment.

Postoperative wound leak is suspected when a shallow anterior chamber coexists with low IOP. A positive Siedel's test confirms the diagnosis. Management of the wound leak has been discussed previously. Postoperative iridocyclitis is also an important etiologic factor for low IOP due to ciliary shutdown. Iridocyclitis decreases the aqueous humor produced by the ciliary body. Topical steroids usually control the inflammation in 1–2 weeks and IOP returns to normal as the aqueous production resumes. A cyclodialysis is a separation of the ciliary body from the scleral spur. Iatrogenic cyclodialysis cleft created could result in low IOP due to excessive drainage of the aqueous into the supraciliary space. The condition is difficult to diagnose, as graft oedema or hazy graft-host junction prevents the visualization of the angle by gonioscopy. Fortunately, in most cases, the resolution occurs spontaneously. Choroidal detachment as a cause of low IOP is suspected when a postoperative flat anterior chamber is associated with the absence of wound leak. Ultrasonography B-scan confirms the diagnosis. Most choroidal detachments resolve spontaneously without any sequelae. Commonly used treatment regimens for choroidal detachment include topical and systemic corticosteroids. If the anterior chamber angle is compromised for more than 48–72 hours and the choroidal detachment is persistent, surgical drainage of the suprachoroidal space with a reformation of the anterior chamber is recommended.

Suture-related Problems

Various suture-related complications observed include *exposed suture knots, broken, tight or loose sutures, unraveled suture knots, suture-related infiltrates* and suture-induced vascularization (**Figs. 3–5**).

Exposed suture knots are important causal factors for foreign body sensation, photophobia, excessive mucous production, giant papillary conjunctivitis, and corneal vascularization thereby increasing the risk of rejection. An exposed suture also acts as a nidus for microbial infection. In a study by Christo et al., the incidence of broken or loose sutures requiring surgical repair was found to be 8.3%.[26] Sutures should be placed with appropriate tension since both tight as well as loose sutures are a cause for concern.

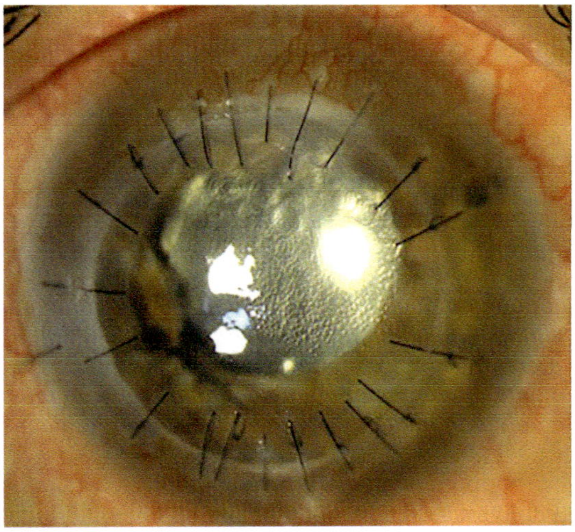

Fig. 3: Loose sutures with adjacent area of epithelial edema in honey comb pattern.

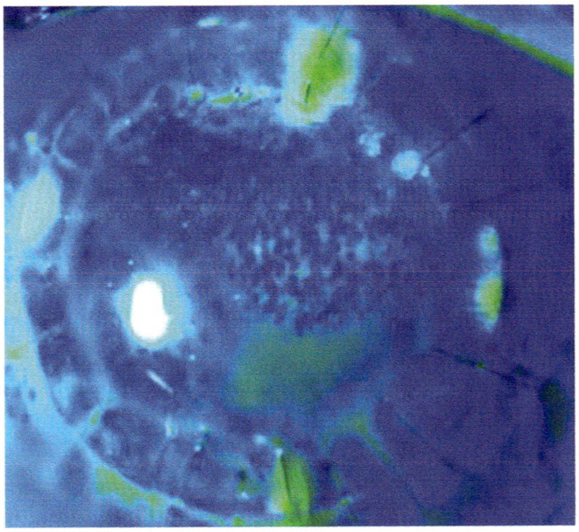

Fig. 4: Loose sutures with adjacent pooling of the fluorescein dye and punctate staining of the graft surface.

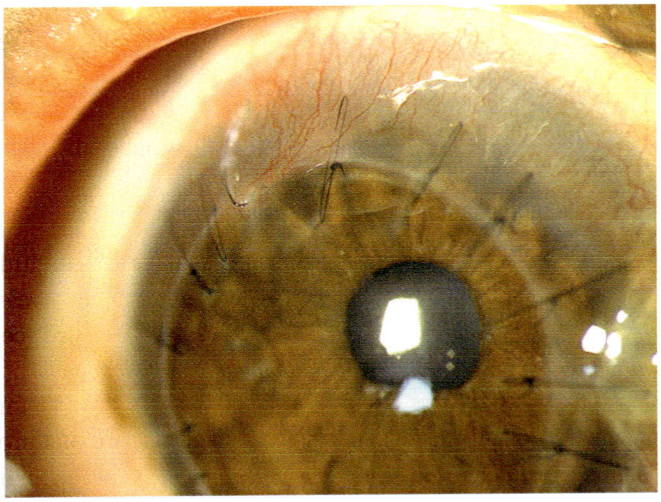

Fig. 5: Suture induced vascularization.

A tight suture can cause persistent epithelial defect and induce a high amount of astigmatism. In contrast, loose sutures, fail to undergo epithelialization and tend to remain exposed. It acts as a nidus for collection of mucous and tear debris and may become a focus for infection. Occasionally, a *suture knot may unravel*, which is more common when the suture is not squarely tied, the ends of the suture are trimmed too close to the knot or the knot is not buried in the cornea. Corneal deturgescence, wound remodeling, scar contraction, and biodegradation caused by enzymatic factors and ultraviolet light exposure occur during wound healing and as these proceed, the sutures get loosen, become exposed and may serve as a nidus for infection.[25]

Table 1: Comparison between features of immune and infectious suture infiltrates.

Immune suture infiltrates:	*Infectious suture infiltrates*:
• Usually multiple and small • Are limited to the on host side only • Not associated with epithelial defects	• Solitary • May occur on either host or on the graft side • Epithelial defect is commonly seen overlying the infiltrate

Suture-related infections are related to suture exposure, use of soft bandage contact lenses, and topical steroids. Suture abscesses are considered a poor prognostic factor for the survival of graft since even when treated aggressively, they can result in wound dehiscence, graft failure secondary to infection, corneal scarring, and endophthalmitis.

Suture-related immune infiltrates occur as a result of an immunological reaction to either suture material or to talc from the surgical gloves, which get adhered to the sutures. These must be differentiated from infectious infiltrates (**Table 1**). These are usually seen in relation to the sutures, which come in contact with the margins of the upper as well as the lower eyelid. In such situations, it is seen as a hypersensitivity reaction to *Staphylococcus albus*, which colonizes the lid margins, particularly in the patients with ocular surface disorders such as blepharitis.

Management: Any tight or loose suture in the immediate postoperative period should be replaced. In case of an exposed suture knot, suture rotation should be done. If suture rotation is not possible, the suture with the exposed knot should be replaced and the knot buried. Suture abscess should be treated energetically because of their deleterious consequences. Suture abscess roof should be opened up with the help of a 26-gauge needle and the material should be sent for microbiological examination. The removed sutures should also be subjected to microbiological evaluation including smear examination and culture sensitivity. If the affected suture is a running suture, removal is based upon whether additional sutures are present for support. The patient should be started on broad-spectrum fortified antibiotics until the organism is identified and antibiotic sensitivity is known. The frequency of topical corticosteroids may be temporarily reduced in the early stages of treatment. During this period, many surgeons have used systemic corticosteroids to protect against possible graft rejection, although the role of systemic steroids in the prevention of graft rejection is not clear. Once the infection is controlled, topical corticosteroids may be increased cautiously. The treatment of choice for immune related suture infiltrates is corticosteroids. The frequency of topical corticosteroids is increased with careful monitoring of epithelial healing. The associated blepharitis should be addressed.

Descemet's Membrane Detachment

This may be a consequence of improper graft handling at the time of trephination or suturing or develop later as a result of trauma during repeated introduction and removal of instruments.

Prevention: Gentle handling of donor tissue and careful instrument manipulation helps minimize the risk of this complication.

Management: Options include intracameral injection of air or viscoelastic, transcorneal suturing, and graft exchange for persistent cases. Intracameral injection with either sulfur hexafluoride (20% SF6) or perfluoropropane (14% C3F8) gas is being increasingly used.

Epithelial Defects

During the early postoperative course of penetrating keratoplasty, re-epithelialization and maintenance of intact epithelium is essential for postoperative wound healing. Epithelial defect heals by a sliding movement of the cells from periphery towards the center. Survival of a corneal graft is critically dependent on an intact epithelial barrier. A persistent corneal epithelial defect is a full-thickness loss of cells that fails to show the expected rate of healing. An epithelial defect failing to close by the 14th postoperative day, is considered as persistent epithelial defect. Average time for complete epithelialization of a corneal graft is 4–6 days.[34,35]

The risk factors for a persistent epithelial defect are outlined in **Box 3**.

Box 3: Risk factors for persistent epithelial defect.

- Ocular surface disorders
- *Lid abnormalities:* Ectropion, entropion, lagophthalmos
- Infection and inflammation (e.g., herpes simplex virus infection)
- Neurogenic
- *Iatrogenic:* Tight sutures, drying of the ocular surface, poorly apposed graft-host junction
- *Epitheliotoxic drugs:* Gentamicin, timolol maleate, ciprofloxacin, neomycin, diclofenac sodium, prednisolone acetate, dorzolamide
- Damaged donor epithelium
- Basement membrane disorders
- *Intrinsic epithelial disorder:* Stem cell deficiency secondary to chemical and thermal burns, Stevens–Johnson syndrome, ocular cicatricial pemphigoid
- Trauma
- *Poor nutrition:* Vitamin A deficiency, protein-calorie malnutrition
- Metabolic eye disease such as diabetes in the donor as well as the host

A persistent epithelial defect (**Figs. 6 and 7**) can give rise to graft ulceration, stromal melting, perforation, and even graft failure.[36]

Prevention and treatment

Preoperative: Significant ectropion, entropion, lagophthalmos or other potential causes of corneal exposure should be corrected before undertaking a keratoplasty. Patients with significant loss of stem cells secondary to chemical burns, thermal burns, Stevens-Johnson syndrome, or other ocular surface diseases should be considered for limbal stem cell transplantation, along with keratoplasty either as a staged procedure or in one setting. Dry eye disease should be addressed by medical treatment or punctal occlusion.

The incidence of persistent epithelial defects in herpetic keratitis varies from 0 to 44%. Surgical incision of the trigeminal nerve reactivates latent herpes virus.[37,38] In cases of penetrating keratoplasty performed for herpes keratitis, use of perioperative oral acyclovir (400 mg twice daily) may decrease the risk of persistent epithelial defects associated with active herpes disease. In cases of persistent

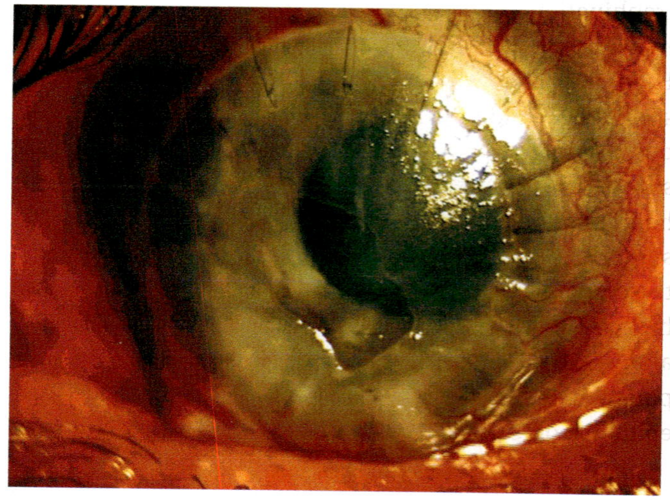

Fig. 6: Epithelial defect following penetrating keratoplasty.

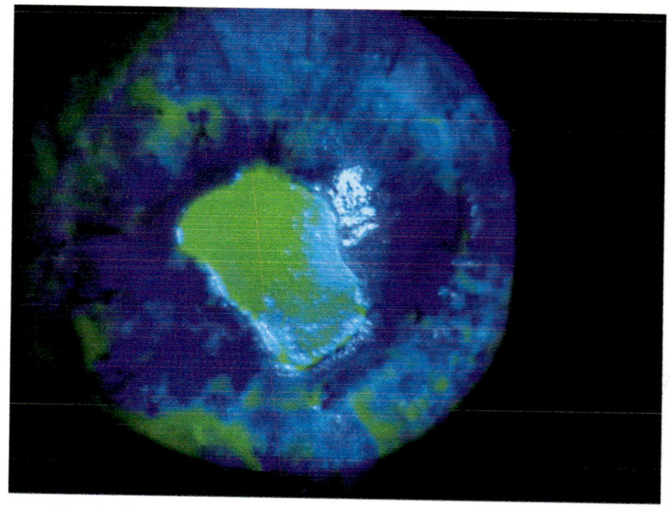

Fig. 7: Fluorescein staining of the epithelial defect following penetrating keratoplasty.

epithelial defects not amenable to treatment, the possibility of recrudescence of herpetic keratitis should always be considered in cases of previous herpetic scars.

Herpes simplex keratitis may also develop after penetrating keratoplasty without a prior history of herpetic keratitis in the host.[39] The incidence of newly acquired herpetic keratitis after penetrating keratoplasty has been reported to be 1.2 per 1,000 person-years in one study.[40] The defect usually begins at the graft-host junction and may not resemble a typical herpetic epithelial keratitis.

Intraoperative: In patients in whom problems with epithelialization are anticipated, the use of donor tissue with a epithelium is warranted. Prolonged donor preservation time and increased death preservation time are associated with a higher incidence of epithelial defects.[41] Fresh corneal tissue preferably a shorter death preservation time may be used in high-risk patients. Intraoperatively, damage to the donor epithelium should be avoided.

Any rough areas on the Teflon block should be inspected for and slippage of the donor cornea during trephination should be avoided. The cornea must be kept moist to preserve the epithelial cells as much as possible. Excessive irrigation may be detrimental to the graft and should be avoided. Use of viscoelastic substances over the donor cornea intraoperatively is a useful option. Any tight sutures must be replaced, and any misalignment of graft-host junctions should be carefully avoided by meticulous surgery. A bandage soft contact lens or even a temporary tarsorrhaphy at the end of surgery may be considered in high-risk cases. Addition of amniotic membrane transplants along with penetrating keratoplasty can be done in cases of poor ocular surface and severe dry eye to prevent persistent epithelial defects.

Postoperative management: Most topical medications are epitheliotoxic and therefore, their benefits must be weighed against their possible adverse effects. Preservative-free can also be performed as an office procedure topical antibiotics, lubricants, and steroids may be used to prevent the occurrence of epithelial toxicity in high-risk cases. Use of ointment form of chloramphenicol is also recommended as it provides lubrication. Frequent use of lubricants is necessary to promote epithelial healing.

A bandage soft contact lens can be used if epithelial healing is not complete by the first week of surgery. Placing a contact lens protects the migrating epithelial cells from eyelid trauma enhances the healing process. Recently extended wear fluid ventilated gas-permeable scleral contact lenses have been tried.[42] However, prolonged use of a bandage contact lens is discouraged because of the potential risk of infection and vascularization. The frequency of topical antibiotic drops should be increased to 3 or 4 hourly when a bandage contact lens is used.

Amniotic membrane transplantation can also be done for a persistent epithelial defect after penetrating keratoplasty.[43] It contains a thick basement membrane and an avascular stromal matrix. The basement membrane facilitates migration of the epithelial cells, reinforces adhesion of basal epithelial cells, and promotes epithelial differentiation. The basement membrane is also important in preventing epithelial apoptosis.

Autologous serum can be used to enhance the healing of epithelial defects. The various concentrations which have been used range from 20 to 100%.[44-46] Epidermal growth factor is present in both tears and serum and has found to be helpful in the healing of epithelial defects, possibly due to its antiapoptotic properties. Further, fibronectin and vitamin A are also present in the serum which aid in epithelialization. Umbilical cord serum has demonstrated faster healing of the persistent corneal epithelial defects refractory to all medical management compared to autologous serum.[47]

The use of topical agents such as *recombinant epidermal growth factor* and *fibronectin* for enhancement of epithelial healing has not been conclusively proven.[48,49] Additional clinical trials are required to determine the use of these agents in future. Multifocal phototherapeutic keratectomy (PTK) has also been tried for persistent epithelial defects. A focal excimer laser PTK with a 1.0-mm diameter and 150–200 pulse ablations at the edge of the epithelial defect is performed.[50] The excimer laser is used to smoothen the elevated margins of the epithelial defect so that the epithelial cells can easily slide in and cover the defect.

If healing is not complete by the second postoperative week, a *temporary tarsorrhaphy* is considered.[51] The tarsorrhaphy should be performed in a manner that results in maximum coverage of epithelial defect. If the defect is located on the temporal cornea, a lateral tarsorrhaphy should be performed and if it is nasal, a medial tarsorrhaphy should be done. Temporary cyanoacrylate glue tarsorrhaphy can also be performed as an office procedure. Anterior chemodenervation of the levator palpebrae superioris may be performed using 10–15 units of botulinum toxin type A (Botox) injected transcutaneously, thereby creating iatrogenic ptosis and obviating the need for a surgical tarsorrhaphy.[52]

Filamentary Keratitis

Filaments consist of an abnormal collection of mucus and corneal epithelial cells. The reported incidence of filamentary keratitis after penetrating keratoplasty is 27% as reported in one of the series.[53] Patients complain of redness and foreign body sensation. Filaments are usually seen in the early post-operative period and develop at the graft-host junction along the suture tracts. They stain brilliantly with rose-bengal stain. Management consists of treating the underlying dry eye disease and addressing the filaments. Proposed treatments include nonpreserved lubricants, topical steroidal and nonsteroidal anti-inflammatory agents, punctal plugs for aqueous-deficient dry eye, mechanical removal of filaments, hypertonic saline, mucolytic agents, and application of a bandage contact lens.[54]

Primary Graft Failure

Graft failure that develops immediately after keratoplasty and without being preceeded a period of clearing is labeled as primary graft failure. It is the faulty donor tissue that results in irreversible graft edema in the immediate postoperative period. The possible factors responsible for primary graft failure are listed below:

- Prolonged death preservation time
- Poor donor endothelial count
- Aphakic and pseudophakic donor
- Elderly donor
- Inadequate preservation
- Surgical trauma
- Herpes simplex virus infection.

Unhealthy donor endothelium, inadequate tissue preservation, and surgical trauma are the major causes of primary graft failure.[55] Primary graft failure has also been attributed to donor tissue contamination with herpes simplex virus.[56,57] Edema usually develops on the first postoperative day after surgery and is unresponsive to hypertonic saline or steroids. However, to make the diagnosis of primary graft failure, other causes of corneal edema, e.g., severe hypotony and intense inflammation must be excluded. Hyposecretion of aqueous humor, which is common after penetrating keratoplasty, may result in graft edema due to decreased supply of metabolites to the endothelium. The endothelial function improves once the aqueous production is restored and cornea begins to clear. The incidence of primary graft failure is <5%.[55]

Prevention: Primary graft failure can be minimized by proper donor selection, good preservation and by avoiding endothelial injury during donor processing and during surgery. A major goal of corneal preservation and transplantation is to maintain high postoperative endothelial count. Long-term graft survival depends on postoperative endothelial cell count and quality. Good technique is essential when removing the corneoscleral rim from the donor globe. All corneas should be examined preoperatively with a slit lamp for any possible endothelial damage. McCarey-Kaufman medium is used in most of the eye banks in India, which can preserve the donor tissue up to 72 hours. During storage, endothelial cells are lost at variable degrees. Optimum results are obtained if the surgery is performed at the earliest, with lesser donor preservation time.

During suturing of corneal graft, most of the endothelial damage occurs at the beginning when the graft encounters the host corneal rim tissue and the iris. Endothelial loss can be avoided by using sufficient OVD preferably Viscoat (Alcon Labs, Fort Worth, TX) which consists of 4% chondroitin sulfate and 3% sodium hyaluronate). During surgical manipulation, distortion of the donor corneal tissue should be minimized, and no surgical instruments should come in contact with the endothelium. Endothelial cell damage may also occur from excessive irrigation of the anterior chamber.

Management: Once the diagnosis of primary graft failure is made, regrafting should be performed as early as possible. A case of primary graft failure should be preferably observed for 3–4 weeks for any signs of graft clearing before proceeding with the second surgery.[58] All cases should be investigated thoroughly to determine possible factors responsible for primary graft failure.

Graft Rejection

It is a specific process in which a graft, which has been clear for at least 2 weeks, suddenly succumbs to graft edema in conjunction with inflammatory signs due to some immunologic process[59,60] (**Fig. 8**). This will be discussed in detail under the sub-section corneal graft rejection (Section 3).

Hyphema

The postoperative occurrence of hyphema is rare after penetrating keratoplasty. Incidence of hyphema increases with intraoperative manipulations such as extensive synechiolysis, iridoplasty, or iridotomy. Most of the postoperative hyphema clears spontaneously without treatment. It may, however, be associated with an elevated IOP that should be treated aggressively.

Management: If topical β-blockers alone not adequate to control IOP, systemic carbonic anhydrase inhibitor should be used. Weak mydriatics to prevent posterior synechiae

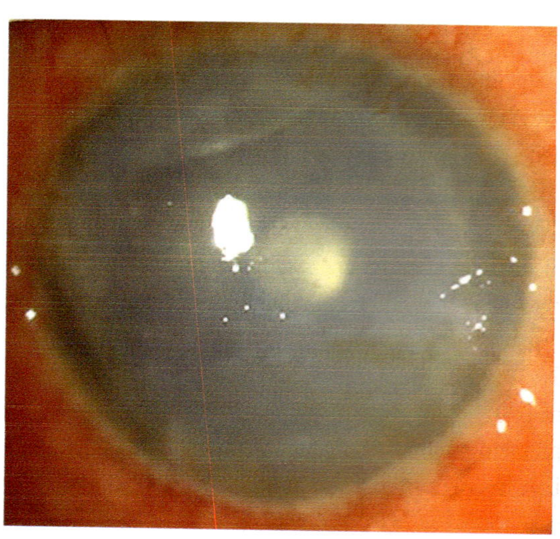

Fig. 8: Corneal edema due to graft rejection.

and topical steroids to control intraocular inflammations are recommended.

The presence of elevated IOP, refractory to medical management or prolonged persistence of hemorrhage may necessitate surgical intervention in the form of clot irrigation and aspiration through the limbal incision. The use of thrombolytic agents, e.g., streptokinase, tissue plasminogen activator to dissolve blood clots or ε-aminocaproic acid to prevent rebleeds have not been adequately studied in penetrating keratoplasty.[61]

High Intraocular Pressure and Pupillary-block Glaucoma

Several factors can contribute to early elevation of IOP after penetrating keratoplasty.[62,63] The major factors involved are:

- Residual viscoelastic anterior chamber
- Uveitis
- Hyphema
- Crowding of the anterior chamber angle
- Pupillary block
- Forward movement of the iris lens diaphragm

Prevention and management: Viscoelastic material, which is left inside the anterior chamber, is one of the most common causes of early postoperative rise of IOP. Irrigation at the end of surgery removes most of the viscoelastic and prevents postoperative pressure rise. However, excessive irrigation can cause endothelial damage and must be avoided. Postoperative uveitis is controlled by intensive treatment with topical steroids such as 1% prednisolone acetate or 0.1% dexamethasone sodium phosphate given 2 hourly. Systemic steroids, such as oral prednisolone 1–2 mg/kg body weight may be started. Further, short-acting cycloplegics, such as 1% tropicamide may be given. Crowding of the anterior chamber angle gives rise to both immediate and long-term elevation of IOP. It is more common in aphakic keratoplasty when trabecular meshwork collapses due to lack of lenticular support. The relatively small size of the donor button and tight sutures are other important factors. Use of a slightly oversized graft in aphakic patients and avoiding tight sutures may prevent the postoperative rise of IOP in these cases. Presence of a flat or shallow anterior chamber and a securely closed wound, confirmed by Siedel's test, suggest the presence of pupillary block, ciliary block, or a choroidal detachment. The pupillary block or ciliary block is usually associated with high IOP whereas, low IOP is recorded in cases of serous choroidal detachment. The presence of posterior synechiae or vitreous protruding through the pupil with a peripheral shallowing of the chamber confirms the diagnosis of a pupillary block, whereas in ciliary block both the central as well as the peripheral anterior chamber are shallow due to anterior shifting of the entire lens iris diaphragm. Air should not be used to form the chamber, especially in aphakes, as this may lead to pupillary-block glaucoma. Sometimes a diffuse wound leak results in anterior displacement of the lens-iris diaphragm, which plugs both leak as well as the anterior chamber angle. This again raises the IOP. Treatment of pupillary block includes vigorous attempt to dilate the pupil pharmacologically and concurrent use of antiglaucoma medications. In situations where the pupillary block is unresponsive to the pharmacological dilatation, a peripheral iridectomy should be considered. This may be undertaken with the help of laser if the peripheral cornea is clear or a surgical iridectomy may be done if the peripheral cornea is hazy.

Urrets–Zavalia Syndrome

This is an unexplained syndrome which was described by Alberto Urrets-Zavalia,[64] characterized by wide and rigid pupils, multiple posterior synechiae and iris atrophy following penetrating keratoplasty in patients with keratoconus.[65] Typically, the mydriasis is unresponsive to miotics. This syndrome has also been reported following deep lamellar keratoplasty for keratoconus.[66,67] Although the aetiology is unknown, possible risk factors are increased IOP during or after surgery, use of mydriatics such as atropine, retained OVD, and postoperative anterior chamber inflammation. Severe iris ischemia has been demonstrated by anterior segment fluorescein angiography.

Spontaneous partial recovery might be possible. Peripherally painted contact lens with clear optic zone may be helpful in these patients to prevent photophobia and glare associated with the syndrome. This syndrome can be avoided by monitoring the patient postoperatively by adequately treating the raised IOP and by avoiding the use of atropine postoperatively.

Herpes Simplex Keratitis

Recurrence of herpes simplex keratitis in the graft is not uncommon. The infection can recur any time between 1 and 15 years postoperatively.[39] There is a unique relationship between herpes simplex keratitis and graft rejection. The keratitis can incite graft rejection and vice versa. Sometimes it is very difficult to distinguish the graft rejection and herpes simplex keratitis. It is relatively easier to diagnose herpes simplex keratitis when it presents with classical dendritic or geographic form. However, stromal involvement which presents with graft edema and keratic precipitates is almost impossible to distinguish from graft rejection. The features which help to distinguish recrudescence of epithelial herpetic keratitis from graft rejection include the classical epithelial dendrite, focal involvement, and propensity of herpes to occur at the host-graft junction. Besides the epithelium shows a granular appearance. The characteristic feature of graft rejection—Khodadoust line is not seen in herpes keratitis.

Management: Herpes simplex keratitis is treated with topical antiviral agents, e.g., acyclovir (3%) five times daily along with supportive therapy. Stromal keratitis is treated with topical corticosteroids along with topical antiviral agents, i.e., prednisolone acetate 1% 2–4 hourly in combination with 3% acyclovir five times daily. Topical antivirals are epitheliotoxic and therefore, patients should be monitored frequently.

The recurrence of herpes simplex keratitis can be reduced by prophylactic use of antivirals.[67,68] Topical acyclovir (five times daily) is given postoperatively for 2 weeks. Maintenance dose of acyclovir 400 mg BD has been shown to reduce allograft rejection and graft failure after penetrating keratoplasty in patients with herpes. Vajpayee et al.[69] compared systemic versus topical acyclovir therapy for preventing recurrence of herpetic keratitis following penetrating keratoplasty and found that systemic acyclovir is more effective in the prevention of recurrence of herpetic keratitis.

Valacyclovir 500 mg OD for 1 year has also been found to be effective in preventing recurrent lesions in immunocompetent individuals with ocular herpes simplex virus disease.[70] Prophylactic oral valacyclovir treatment has also been found to be as effective as oral acyclovir in preventing recurrence in patients who undergo corneal transplantation for herpetic keratitis.[71]

Microbial Keratitis

Post-penetrating keratoplasty microbial keratitis is characterized by either infection within the graft or infection along the suture tracts at the graft-host junction. Infections within the graft or at the graft-host junction can produce an inflammatory reaction in the eye with the initiation of graft rejection and can cause graft failure, melting of the graft and even endophthalmitis with subsequent loss of vision. The incidence of microbial keratitis in corneal grafts ranges from 1.76 to 4.9% in western countries. In developing countries, it has been reported to be as high as 11.9%.[72] Increased risk of graft infection is associated with preoperative herpes simplex keratitis and grafts performed for complications of previous infectious keratitis.[72] Postoperative infectious keratitis may also be caused by intraoperative contamination, recurrent host disease or poorly preserved donor material (**Fig. 9**). Suture-related problems and persistent epithelial defect are the most common risk factors predisposing to graft infection.[73] It is important to ensure that all sutures are secure, knots are buried, and sutures are nicely covered by epithelium postoperatively. If the sutures are not properly tied and secured or knots are not buried, it can lead to loosening, broken sutures and exposed knots in the early postoperative period with increased risk of suture abscesses.[72,74] Corneal graft sutures may erode through the overlying epithelium. Wound remodeling, scar contracture, and cheese-wiring of sutures may loosen and expose the previously secured sutures. The superficial loop of an intrastromal embedded nylon suture tends to undergo biodegradation earlier than does the deeper aspect of the sutures. Loose sutures breach the normal epithelial barrier and thus initiates the infectious cascade providing a direct route for the entry of infection into the stroma. Broken and exposed ends of a suture can accumulate mucus and foreign debris and act as an "infectious wick". The surgeon and the assistants should wash their gloves to avoid postoperative talc-related suture infiltrates. Suture fragments, cotton fibers or any debris trapped by the sutures must be removed meticulously as they serve as a potential source of infection. Patients should be kept in close follow-up and any loose suture must be removed as soon as possible and replaced if necessary.

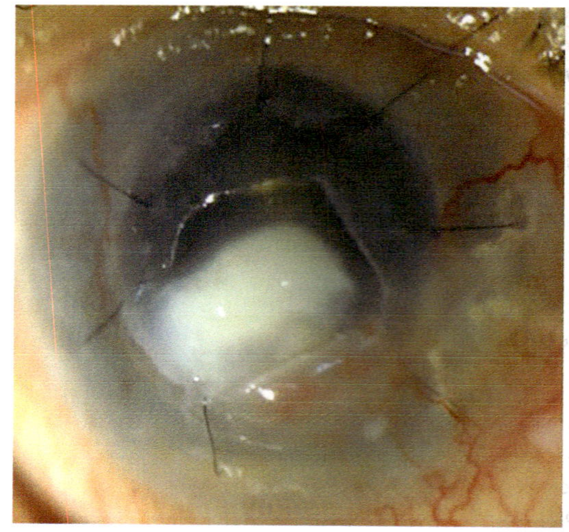

Fig. 9: Infectious keratitis over a full-thickness graft.

Various possible risk factors for postoperative graft infection have been enlisted in (**Box 4**).

About half of the infections occur within the first 6 months of surgery, with the majority occurring within the first year. Gram-positive bacterial infections, especially *Staphylococcus* species are more common than gram-negative ones. *Pneumococcus* species and *Staphylococcus aureus* are the most common microorganisms in the developed world, whereas *Staphylococcus epidermidis* is the most frequently detected microorganism in the developing world.[74]

Fungal infections, although less common, are prevalent in countries with warm and humid weather. Common causative organisms include *Aspergillus, Fusarium* and *Candida*.[75] In the majority of studies, the incidence of fungal keratitis varied from 0 to 14%. The high incidence of fungal keratitis in the series reported by Harris et al. was attributed to possible

Box 4: Possible risk factors for postoperative graft infection.

- *Faulty preservation*:
  - Contamination of preservative media
  - Lack of asepsis during tissue processing
- *Faulty grafts*:
  - Suture-related problems
  - Persistent epithelial defect
  - Use of contact lens
  - Graft failure
  - Wound dehiscence
- *Preexisting ocular disease*:
  - Dry eye syndrome
  - Herpes simplex keratitis
  - Chemical burns
  - *Lid abnormalities*: Ectropion, entropion
- *Cicatricial diseases:* Stevens–Johnson syndrome
- Topical steroids
- *Systemic diseases*:
  - Diabetes mellitus
  - Immunosuppression

geographic variation and high risk patients with significant ocular surface disorders or altered immune function. Fungal infections tend to recur more frequently than bacterial infections. *Acanthamoeba* infection, on the other hand, is a rare but devastating infection with a 30% chance of recurrence. The recurrence is manifested either by a peripheral stromal infiltration or by a coarse elevated epithelial line. The latter should not be confused with an epithelial rejection line.

Management: Meticulous tissue processing in a sterile environment and optimum use of antibiotics in proper concentration reduce the risk factors related to faulty preservation. Any change in the color of preservative media is an indication of contamination and the donor tissue must be discarded. The use of contact lens can incite severe infection in the graft. Patients should be educated about contact lens care and instructed to report early if there is pain, irritation, or foreign body sensation. Preexisting ocular diseases should be treated preoperatively. Every attempt should be made to improve the ocular surface with tear substitutes, punctal occlusions or lid surgery. Though topical corticosteroids suppress ocular inflammation, they impair the host defense mechanism and promote bacterial super-infection.

Diagnosis and treatment of microbial keratitis in a graft is analogs to the management of corneal ulcers in general. Corneal scrapings are obtained for smear and culture-sensitivity and vigorous antimicrobial therapy should be started. Therapy can be modified based on smear and culture reports and therapeutic response. The initial therapy consists of either a fluoroquinolone, 0.5% gatifloxacin eye drops or combination therapy of concentrated cefazolin 5% and concentrated tobramycin 1.3% eye drops, in 1 hourly dosage round the clock. Additional supportive therapy includes cycloplegics as well as antiglaucoma medications. In cases unresponsive to medical management, therapeutic regraft should be undertaken at the earliest.[75] If the infection is caused by *Acanthamoeba* topical amebicidal drugs including polyhexamethylene biguanide (PHMB) 0.02%, propamidine isethionate (Brolene) 0.1%, chlorhexidine and Neosporin must be used. The medical treatment must be continued several months after keratoplasty to reduce the risk of recurrence.

Endophthalmitis

Endophthalmitis following keratoplasty, though rare, is a sight-threatening complication with an incidence ranging from 0.1 to 0.7%.[76-81] Endophthalmitis may occur in the immediate (usually within 72 hours) or in the late postoperative period after PK. Reported risk factors for immediate postoperative endophthalmitis include contamination of donor material or storage media, prolonged storage, donor with sepsis, any break in the sterility of surgical technique or use of contaminated irrigating solutions.[21] Additional risk factors include vitrectomy during the time of surgery, placement of an intraocular lens especially with polypropylene haptics or a history of drug allergy. A study by Kloess et al.[82] revealed that contaminated donor tissue is the major cause of post-keratoplasty endophthalmitis. In this study, donor rim cultures were positive for the same organism causing endophthalmitis in 75% of cases. Though endophthalmitis is more likely with a culture-positive donor rim, positive culture do not predict endophthalmitis correctly and have a limited value as a screening test. In a study by Kloess et al. 55% of endophthalmitis were gram-positive, 19% were gram-negative and 21% were fungal. In a study by Kunimoto et al., most common isolates included gram-positive cocci (*Streptococcus* sp. and *Staphylococcus* sp.) followed by gram-negative organisms (*Proteus mirabilis, Serratia marcescens*). Approximately 75% of the post-PK endophthalmitis cases reported in the literature are bacterial and another 20% are fungal in origin. Though gentamicin is present in preservative storage media like M-K medium, but the offending organisms have been found to be resistant in some studies.[82–84]

To minimize this serious complication, the donor tissue should be routinely screened and evaluated for microbial contamination. All recipients should be treated with prophylactic intraoperative subconjunctival and postoperative broad-spectrum antibiotics. Suture removal requires strict asepsis and continuation of topical antibiotics for several days after the procedure. Any wound dehiscence must be repaired as early as possible.

Management: A full-fledged case of endophthalmitis is diagnosed by clinical signs and confirmed by ultrasound B-scan. Management includes vitreous tap for smear and culture-sensitivity and intensive topical, intravitreal and systemic antibiotics are prescribed as given in any other endophthalmitis patient. Pars plana vitrectomy should be done at the earliest with regrafting for fulminant cases.

Late Postoperative (Months, Years)

Infectious Crystalline Keratopathy

Infectious crystalline keratopathy (ICK) is a chronic, progressive corneal infection occurring mostly in the anterior lamella of the grafts without any clinically evident stromal inflammation. The clinical appearance of ICK includes crystalline branching opacities in the anterior and midstroma due to intralamellar aggregates of gram-positive cocci occurring several months following penetrating keratoplasty.[84,85] The characteristic lesions are associated with a persistent epithelial defect, use of topical corticosteroids, herpes simplex keratitis, and contact lens use. The pathogenesis of ICK is not well understood. Bacteria are thought to gain access to the corneal stroma via epithelial ingrowth into a suture track or by direct access through an epithelial defect. Administration of topical corticosteroid serves to protect the organism from the marked inflammatory response. The most common organism causing ICK is *Streptococcus viridans*. Rarely other organisms such as *Staphylococcus*, *Enterococcus*, *Haemophilus*, fungal species such as *Candida* have been implicated. Fastidious bacteria which do not get a full nutrient supply and form a biofilm around them have been particularly implicated.

Management: Management of ICK requires laboratory evaluation including corneal scraping for smears and cultures. Appropriate antibiotics can be formulated based on investigations. Often the lesion is too deep for material to be obtained by scrapings. A corneal biopsy may be necessary and can be performed by lamellar dissection over the lesion or with a biopsy punch. Treatment of ICK begins with fortified antibiotic regimen given in an intensive dosage schedule. Concentrated vancomycin and cefazolin (both 50 mg/mL) are the most commonly used regimen. Therapy can be modified based on the culture report. Superficial lamellar keratectomy to remove or debride infected tissue can be curative. Therapeutic ablation by the excimer laser is successful in very superficial ICK.[86] Some cases have shown poor response to antibiotics and eventually required regrafting.[87,88] Disruption of the intrastromal crystals using Nd: YAG laser has hastened resolution of keratopathy unresponsive to topical antibiotics.[89]

Corneal Membranes

Epithelial ingrowth: Corneal and conjunctival epithelium may enter the anterior chamber through a gap at the host-graft junction. Predisposing factors for epithelial ingrowth are:[90]

- Poorly healed wound
- Fistulous tract
- Wound dehiscence with iris incarceration
- Trauma
- Previous intraocular surgery
- *Epithelial seeding in the anterior chamber by*:
  - Full-thickness suture
  - Surgical instrument
  - Foreign body

Epithelial ingrowth progresses over the posterior surface of the cornea, anterior chamber angle and the iris in a sheet-like fashion. Ingrowth over the posterior surface of cornea results in endothelial dysfunction, corneal edema, and hazy graft.[90] Epithelial invasion into the anterior chamber angle, especially trabecular meshwork hinders the aqueous drainage and ultimately results in intractable glaucoma and severe vision loss. Epithelial ingrowth over the iris causes pupillary distortion, heterochromia, iritis and rarely iris inclusion cyst. The epithelial ingrowth can be distinguished from other retrocorneal membranes by applying laser burns over the iris. In this case, the tissue "takes" the laser, identified by white, blanched lesions whereas the iris produces dark burns. Other lesions do not take up the laser.

Confocal microscopy imaging technique seems to be a useful tool in the early diagnosis of epithelial ingrowth after penetrating keratoplasty.[91]

Management: Meticulous surgery and a secure wound are necessary to prevent epithelial ingrowth. Treatment is extremely difficult. Cryotherapy gives a better result but can lead to phthisis bulbi. In general, in extensive cases, the treatment includes large en-bloc removal of the involved ocular structures along with corneoscleral grafts. In case of intractable rise of IOP, glaucoma implant surgery may be tried. Use of 5-fluorouracil is a potentially effective treatment of epithelial ingrowth, particularly in eyes with extensive involvement, in which the risks of traditional ablative therapeutic modalities are considerable.[92]

Fibrous Ingrowth

This represents a fibrous proliferation of subepithelial connective tissue or corneal stromal fibroblasts and invasion of these tissues around the surgical site. Clinical risk factors are similar to epithelial downgrowth; however, a fistulous tract is not a pre-requisite for fibrous ingrowth. They are much lesser aggressive than the epithelial downgrowth in its proliferation. Clinically, a translucent membrane with irregular edges on the posterior surface of the cornea near the wound could be seen. This membrane is usually vascular, unlike epithelial downgrowth. There may be associated Descemet's membrane breaks with fibro cellular proliferation through the break, suggesting corneal stroma as the source of the ingrowth.

Confocal reveals a hyper-reflective fibrous-appearing layer. Glaucoma may be frequent; however, less aggressive than epithelial downgrowth. The clinical course of fibrous ingrowth is variable and depends on the extent of the factors promoting ingrowth. Frequently it runs an insidious course with little discomfort and the membrane is often noted as

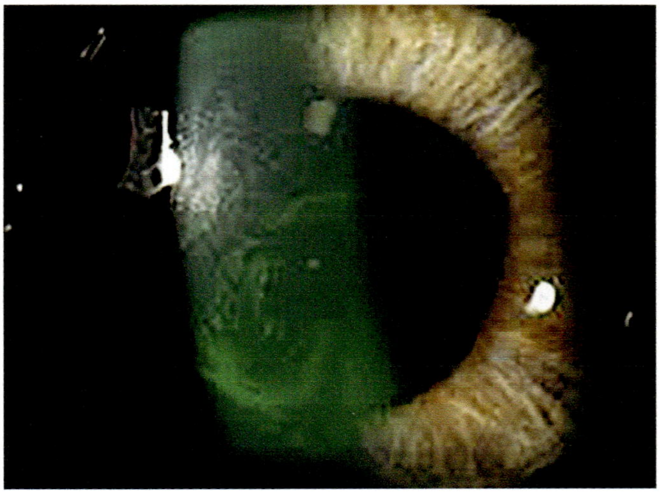

Fig. 10: Hurricane keratopathy.

an incidental finding. Less commonly, patients present with decreased visual acuity caused by a fibrous membrane or symptoms related to uveitis, glaucoma or rarely retinal detachment. The diagnosis of fibrous ingrowth should be made based on preceding clinical features and distinguished from epithelial ingrowth by argon laser burns. Graft becomes hazy and edematous in penetrating keratoplasty when affected by fibrous ingrowth.

Management: Medical management of inflammation, glaucoma and corneal edema is sufficient in most cases. Unlike epithelial downgrowth, complete removal of proliferating tissue is not required. Clearing the visual axis is usually a successful option. Steroids and radiation therapy are not effective. Cyclodestructive procedures for glaucoma and a repeat PK could sometimes benefit.

Hurricane (whorl) keratopathy: "Hurricane keratopathy" is the name given to the whorl pattern, highlighted with fluorescein, seen in situations where corneal epithelial cell turnover is exaggerated (**Fig. 10**). The terms "vortex keratopathy" and "hurricane keratopathy" describe two similar conditions affecting the corneal surface. In the former, a vortex or whorl pattern is seen on the corneal surface and is due to the deposition of substances such as pigment, iron or drugs in the epithelial cells. In the latter, a similar pattern is presented by migrating epithelial cells but, unlike the former, the pattern is rendered more visible by fluorescein staining. Both represent the migratory pattern of normal epithelial cells which is otherwise not visible due to the slow rate of epithelial turnover and migration. The whorl pattern has a clockwise predisposition in majority of cases and is hypothesized to be due to the influence of ocular electromagnetic fields on the migrating epithelial cells.[93,94]

Cataract

Cataract is a common cause of decreased visual acuity in a patient with successful corneal grafting. A preexisting senile cataract may progress rapidly after penetrating keratoplasty[95] (**Fig. 11**). The incidence of cataract in various studies after penetrating keratoplasty varies from 25 to 80%.[95,96]

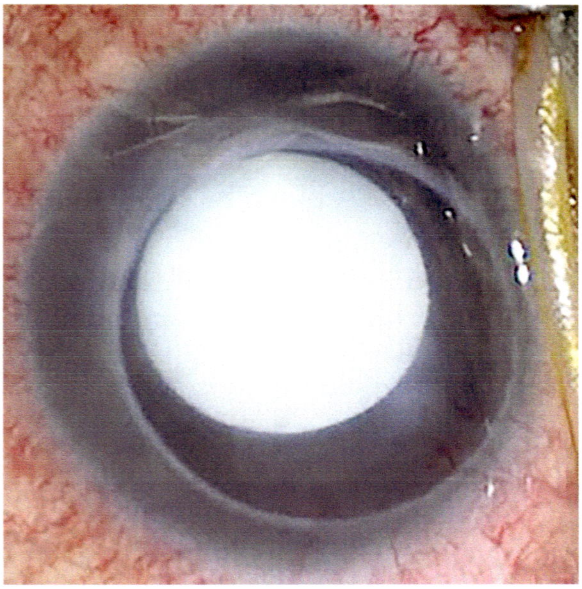

Fig. 11: Postkeratoplasty total cataract.

Following three major mechanisms are involved the causation of postkeratoplasty cataract.

1. *Poor surgical technique*:
   i. Anterior capsular injury
   ii. Excessive iris manipulation
   iii. Excessive irrigation
2. *Altered lens metabolism*:
   i. Persistent inflammation
   ii. Hyphema
3. *Toxic*:
   i. Corticosteroids (topical and systemic)
   ii. Anticholinesterase

Prevention: To reduce lenticular injury a good viscoelastic can be used which prevents anterior capsular contact by maintaining a deep anterior chamber. Preoperative or intraoperative pilocarpine can provide a good mechanical barrier by constricting the pupil. One should strongly consider combined cataract surgery and penetrating keratoplasty in patients with early senile cataractous changes. Postoperative inflammation must be controlled, and corticosteroids dose should be tapered to a minimum maintenance dose.

Management: Cataract can be extracted through a separate incision after the wound is healed. Endothelium must be protected by a good viscoelastic.

Astigmatism

Improvements in microsurgical techniques and instrumentation, surgical training, eye-banking procedures, and management of postoperative complications have enabled corneal surgeons to expect a very high rate of clear grafts after PK. An anatomically successful graft may fail optically if postoperative astigmatism is too high. Average post-keratoplasty astigmatism measured by keratometry ranges from 4 to 5 diopters. High postoperative astigmatism is expected in eyes with scarring/thinning due to healed keratitis. Other cases are solely related to surgical techniques of keratoplasty.[97,98] Possible factors that give rise to high postoperative astigmatism are as follows:

- Donor-related factors—age of donor tissues (infant donors induce high astigmatism), scarring, thinning in donor tissue, undetected ectatic disorders in the host.
- Recipient-related factors—ectatic disorders, aphakic eyes, recipient bed vascularization, scleral rigidity.
- Intraoperative surgical factors—tilted/eccentric trephination, eccentric graft, malalignment of graft, faulty suturing techniques (improper placement of the second suture, unequal depth, non-radial sutures, tight sutures, unequal distribution of tension in a continuous suture).

Prevention: While cutting the recipient cornea the surgeon must ensure that the trephine is centerd properly and perpendicular to the iris plane. The cutting edge of the trephine can be checked under a microscope and a sharp trephine must be used. Blunt trephines causes slippage and irregular cuts. While suturing the graft, the second suture is most important because it determines the proper distribution of corneal tissue.[98,99] The second suture should be exactly at the opposite meridian of the first suture. Even slight misplacement of the second suture can cause torsion of the graft and subsequent severe astigmatism. A tight suture causes peripheral flattening and central steepening of the cornea. Non-radial sutures can distort the graft and cause postoperative astigmatism. Intraoperative use of a keratometer/placido disc facilitate in the evaluation of astigmatism and which can be adjusted intraoperatively by modifying the sutures.

There are controversies regarding different suturing techniques and their long-term refractive outcome. Several suturing techniques such as interrupted, single running, double running, or a combination of interrupted and running are used to secure a keratoplasty wound. A comparison of torque, anti-torque and no-torque techniques of single continuous suturing revealed a higher proportion of prolate corneal topography maps with the anti-torque suturing technique.[100] Some studies report the highest astigmatism with interrupted sutures technique; however, selective suture removal and adjustment are easier with interrupted sutures. Final astigmatism is almost same with single running and double running suturing technique. Suture adjustment is an effective method of reducing post-PK astigmatism.[101] In general, the outcome mostly depends on the expertise and efficiency of the operating surgeon. The running sutures can also be adjusted postoperatively to reduce astigmatism. Some surgeons advocate a combination of interrupted and single running suture. As the running suture supports the wound, the astigmatic error can be reduced by selectively removing the interrupted sutures starting 3–4 weeks post-surgery. Corneal topography performed 30–40 minutes after suture removal can identify the next set of sutures requiring removal. This can be used as a guide to remove more sutures at the same visit, thereby expediting post-keratoplasty visual rehabilitation and reducing the number of follow-up visits.[102] In the double running suture technique, ideally one 10-0 and the other 11-0 monofilament nylon are used. Early visual rehabilitation is achieved by removing the 10-0 suture about 3 months after surgery. Stable refraction is usually possible with 11-0 sutures in place.

Management: The management of post-PK astigmatism can be done in two stages: (1) suture-in (when the sutures are still in place) and (2) suture-out (after removal of all sutures). Suture adjustment could be useful in the early postoperative period from as early as 1 day up to 6 weeks. Visual rehabilitation either by spectacles or contact lenses can be done irrespective of the suture status. Spectacle have a limited role in the presence of astigmatism more than 3D, irregular astigmatism or significant ametropia, hence, contact lenses, especially rigid lenses or scleral lenses are very useful. Before fitting contact lenses, one must be sure that all suture knots are buried. Patients using contact lenses must be monitored closely for possible complications. A variety of surgical options are available for patients with high astigmatism following complete suture removal and for those who can not tolerate glasses or contact lenses. These include astigmatic keratotomy (AK), relaxing incisions with or without compression sutures, wedge resection, excimer laser and toric intraocular lenses/toric phakic intraocular lenses. Among various AK techniques, transverse and arcuate incisions are most commonly practised. They are placed in the donor graft, graft-host junction or on the host cornea. It is usually preferred to place these incisions central to the graft-host junction at a 7 mm optical zone. This causes flattening along the axis and steepening in the axis perpendicular to it, known as the "coupling effect". Compression sutures are placed across the flatter axis and are usually combined along with arcuate incisions. Wedge resection involves the excision of a wedge of corneal tissue along the flatter axis and the shortened tissue is apposed with tight sutures resulting in steepening of that axis. Although the astigmatic part could be corrected, the associated myopia and hyperopia can not be corrected by the above methods. Laser *in situ* keratomileuses (LASIK) and photorefractive keratectomy (PRK) have been used more commonly for the correction of myopia, myopic astigmatism and less commonly for hypermetropia and hyperopic astigmatism. Mitomycin-C (MMC) should be combined with surface ablation to prevent haze. LASIK has the advantage of correcting a wider range of refractive errors. All sutures should be removed before LASIK and the minimum interval between PK and LASIK should be 1 year. Preoperative evaluation includes refraction, slit-lamp biomicroscopy, corneal topography, and specular microscopy. LASIK for post-PK eyes is usually carried out as a 2-step approach by many surgeons. They claim that significant astigmatic changes occur following flap formation,[103] therefore, in the first step, the flap is created, reposited back and allowed to heal. In the second session, the flap is lifted, and laser correction is done. However, there are increased chances of epithelial ingrowth compared to the one-step LASIK. Augmentation with arcuate cuts on the stromal bed and topographically guided LASIK are also some modifications for refractive correction. Improvement in both uncorrected visual acuity and spectacle-corrected visual acuity, as well as a decrease in spherical equivalent, cylinder, and anisometropia, has been reported in various studies.[104] Arcuate keratotomies performed with the femtosecond laser are effective in reducing post-keratoplasty astigmatism.[105] Toric IOLs are good options in patients who have contraindications for keratorefractive surgeries, and have cataract along with corneal thinning or ectasias.[106]

Glaucoma

Penetrating keratoplasty, using modern techniques of tight wound closure, can be complicated by IOP elevation in both early and late postoperative periods. Sustained elevation of IOP not only damages the optic nerve head but also has a deleterious effect on the corneal endothelium.[106] High IOP is also responsible for occasional wound dehiscence and ectasia. Factors related to early postoperative glaucoma have already been discussed. Following are the major risk factors for late postoperative glaucoma.

- Preexisting glaucoma
- Aphakic and pseudophakic eyes
- Pigment dispersion syndrome
- Prolonged severe inflammation
- Tight and deep sutures
- Peripheral anterior synechiae
- Epithelial and fibrous ingrowth
- Long-term use of steroids

Gradual flattening of the anterior chamber, several months after aphakic keratoplasty has been described. Compression of the anterior chamber angle may be caused by the conventional technique of penetrating keratoplasty.[106,107] This may lead to early postoperative IOP rise as well as subsequent chronic glaucoma resulting from peripheral anterior synechiae. A tightly sutured wound can contribute to crowding of the anterior chamber angle and thus increases the IOP. Pigment dispersion is more common with pseudophakic keratoplasty or keratoplasty combined with cataract extraction and intraocular lens implantation. Postoperative use of corticosteroids may elevate IOP in some patients.[108] The incidence is further increased in patients with preexisting glaucoma, diabetes mellitus, and high myopia.[109]

Prevention: Prevention of post-penetrating keratoplasty glaucoma begins with adequate preoperative control of IOP. IOP in most cases can be controlled by antiglaucoma medication. However, if filtering surgery is necessary, it is better to combine it with keratoplasty. An oversize graft can minimize postoperative glaucoma in aphakic and pseudophakic eyes. Smaller trephine size should be used when possible.[106] Intraoperative considerations include release of all synechiae, iridoplasty to make iris-diaphragm taut and sutures should not be too tight, too long or too deep. Inadvertent overtightening of the suture can be avoided by maintaining a consistently deep anterior chamber throughout the procedure. Postoperatively steroids with less IOP rising effects can be used especially in high-risk cases.[109]

Management: Medical therapy should be tried first in all cases of established postkeratoplasty glaucoma. Medical therapy involves the use of systemic and topical antiglaucoma medications, topical β-adrenergic antagonists, like timolol, drops twice daily, being the first choice. However, corneal epithelial toxicity sometimes prevents the use of topical β-blockers. Topical parasympathetic agents should be used very cautiously in eyes with severe peripheral anterior synechiae, as they tend to reduce uveoscleral outflow, which is a major pathway of drainage in these eyes. Latanoprost is a better choice in such eyes.

Surgical therapy is indicated when either the optic nerve or the graft is threatened by persistent elevation of IOP. Traditional filtering procedures have a high failure rate in postkeratoplasty eyes. Use of antimetabolites such as mitomycin-C or 5-fluorouracil to maintain the filtering bleb may be effective but there is a high risk of graft failure from epithelial toxicity. Selective laser trabeculoplasty may be considered as a valuable therapeutic method that limits invasive surgery for the treatment of secondary glaucoma after penetrating keratoplasty.[110] Different glaucoma implants such as Molteno, Ahmed and Baerveldt[111] can be used to treat refractory glaucoma. Cyclodestructive procedures may be used to control IOP in eyes, with poor visual potential. Diode laser trans-scleral cyclophotocoagulation appears to be a safe and effective procedure in these eyes.[112] Cyclocryotherapy destroys the ciliary body by external application of cryoprobe. Although the success rate is quite high, the procedure is not without complications. Apart from pain, redness and chronic inflammation, there are chances of graft failure and phthisis bulbi. Alternately Nd:YAG laser can be used for cyclodestruction with relatively fewer complications. Further details of these complications are discussed in Chapter 16.

Recurrence of the Original Corneal Pathology

Several corneal dystrophies are known to recur in grafts even decades after keratoplasty. The probable mechanism is the migration of recipient keratocytes into the graft stroma. Initial recurrence occurs at the graft periphery and small size grafts are most frequently involved. The following lesions are known to recur frequently in grafts.

- Stromal dystrophies:
  - Granular: 100% at 4 years[113]
  - Macular: 5.2%[114]
  - Lattice: 48%[115]
- Reis-Bückler's dystrophy
- Central crystalline dystrophy
- Posterior polymorphous dystrophy

Management: The answer is a repeat graft. Superficial keratectomy or excimer laser PTK can be considered if the lesion is superficial.

Disease Transmission from Donor Cornea

Transmission of original donor diseases has been discussed in detail in Chapter 4.

Vitreoretinal Problems

Retinal detachment: Retinal detachment after penetrating keratoplasty is a rare but well-known complication. The incidence increases with the complexity of the surgical procedure, especially after vitreous manipulation. Eyes that had undergone concomitant anterior vitrectomy are four times more likely to develop retinal detachment than eyes that had not. Using a proper vitrectomy instrument rather than sponge vitrectomy can lessen the risk of development of postoperative retinal detachment. A high cutting rate and a moderate suction are helpful in meticulous removal of vitreous.

Early diagnosis gives a better prognosis, although surgical reattachment rate after keratoplasty is poor. The main reason for failure is poor visualization of peripheral retina. High-risk cases must be monitored closely with frequent indirect ophthalmoscopy or ultrasound B-scan if indicated. Preexisting retinal detachment may be managed by placing a temporary keratoprosthesis to allow visualization of retina and completing the keratoplasty after the retinal procedure is over. Retinal reattachment surgery requires tremendous manipulation of the globe often results in graft failure.

Maculopathy: Macular edema is a common cause of nonimprovement of vision despite a clear graft after penetrating keratoplasty. Incidence of macular edema from keratoplasty itself is unknown because it may be preexisting. Aphakic and pseudophakic bullous keratopathy, trauma, and virtually any previous intraocular surgery may predispose to macular edema. Anterior vitrectomy at the time of surgery greatly increases the incidence. Similarly, the incidence is expectedly more in eyes undergoing combined cataract surgery and penetrating keratoplasty.

Prevention and management: Prophylactic use of nonsteroidal anti-inflammatory drugs such as indomethacin (both topical and systemic) can reduce the incidence of macular edema. The treatment should be continued for at least 2 weeks postoperatively. Chronic macular edema is more difficult to treat than the acute one. Every attempt should be made to control the intraocular inflammation. Intravitreal injection of triamcinolone acetonide may be used as an additional tool in the management of refractory cystoid macular edema after penetrating keratoplasty.[116] Some cases of macular edema may resolve spontaneously. Macular edema and visual acuity continue to improve for 1–2 years. However, overall prognosis remains sub-optimal.

REFERENCES

1. Jasien JV, Girkin CA, Downs JC. Effect of anesthesia on intraocular pressure measured with continuous wireless telemetry in Nonhuman primates. Invest Ophthalmol Vis Sci. 2019;60(12):3830-4.
2. Illif CE. A surgical soft eye by posterior sclerotomy. Am J Ophthal. 1966;61:276-7.
3. Zimmerman T, Olson R, Waltman S, Kaufman H. Transplant size and elevated intraocular pressure. Postkeratoplasty. Arch Ophthalmol. 1978;96:2231-33.
4. Wilson SE, Bourne WM. Effect of recipient-donor trephine size disparity on refractive error in keratoconus. Ophthalmology. 1989;96:299-305.
5. Purcell JJ. Intraoperative complications of penetrating keratoplasty. In: Krachmer JH, Mannis MJ, Holland EJ (Eds). Cornea: Surgery of the Cornea and Conjunctiva. St. Louis, MO: Mosby; 1997. pp. 1639-44.
6. Wilson SE, Kaufman HE. Graft failure after penetrating keratoplasty. Surv Ophthalmol. 1990;34:325-56.
7. Vajpayee RB, Melki S. Three pearls to minimize penetrating keratoplasty astigmatism. In: Melki SA, Azar DT (Eds). 101 Pearls in Refractive, Cataract and Corneal Surgery. Thorofare, New Jersey: SLACK Inc.; 2001. pp. 161-2.
8. Cruz GK, Ferreira Júnior MA, Azevedo IC, Santos VE, Flores VG, Gonçalves ED. Clinical and surgical factors and intraoperative complications in patients who underwent penetrating keratoplasty. Rev Lat Am Enfermagem. 2019;27.e3141.
9. Bourne WM, O'Fallon WM. Endothelial cell loss during penetrating keratoplasty. Am J Ophthalmol. 1978;85:760-6.
10. Abad JC. Kornmehl intraoperative complications of penetrating keratoplasty. In: Brightbill FS (Ed). Corneal Surgery: Theory, Technique, and Tissue. St. Louis: Mosby; 1999. pp. 358-64.
11. Casey TA, Mayer DJ. Corneal grafting—principles and practice. London: WB Saunders; 1984. p. 291.
12. Ohlrich S, Hirst LW, Harrison M, Green WR, Bancroft BJ. Inadvertent corneal button inversion during penetrating keratoplasty. Cornea. 1992;11:586-8.
13. Koenig SB, McDermott ML, Hyndiuk RA. Penetrating keratoplasty and intraocular lens exchange for pseudophakic bullous keratopathy associated with a closed-loop anterior chamber intraocular lens. Am J Ophthalmol. 1989;108:43-8.
14. Vengayil S, Vanathi M, Panda A, Khokhar S. Anterior segment OCT-based diagnosis and management of retained Descemet's

membrane following penetrating keratoplasty. Cont Lens Anterior Eye. 2008;31:161-3.
15. Ide T, Yoo SH, Kymionis GD, Shah PA, O'Brien TR. Diagnosis of residual Descemet's membrane after Descemet's stripping endothelial keratoplasty with anterior segment optical coherence tomography. Ophthalmic Surg Lasers Imaging. 2008;39:422-5.
16. Sinha R, Vajpayee RB, Sharma N, Titiyal JS, Tandon R. Trypan blue assisted descemetorhexis for inadvertently retained Descemet's membranes after penetrating keratoplasty. Br J Ophthalmol. 2003;87:654-5.
17. Hirst LW, De Juan E Jr. Sodium hyaluronate and tissue adhesive in treating corneal perforations. Ophthalmology. 1982;89:1250-3.
18. Taylor DM, Stern AL, McDonald P. The triple procedure: 2 to 10 year follow-up. Trans Am Ophthalmol Soc. 1986;84:221-49.
19. Crawford GJ, Stulting RD, Waring GO 3rd, Van Meter WS, Wilson LA. The triple procedure. Analysis of outcome, refraction, and intraocular lens power calculation. Ophthalmology. 1986;93:817-24.
20. Vajpayee RB, Dada T, Ray M, Tandon R, Sethi A, Turaka K. Oversized corneal grafts for corneal opacities with iridocorneal adhesions. Ophthalmology. 2001;108:2026-8.
21. Vajpayee RB, Ramu M, Panda A, Sharma N, Tabin GC, Anand JR. Oversized grafts in children. Ophthalmology. 1999;106:829-32.
22. Taylor DM. Expulsive hemorrhage. Am J Ophthalmol. 1974;78:961-6.
23. Ingraham HJ, Donnenfeld ED, Perry HD. Massive suprachoroidal hemorrhage after penetrating keratoplasty. Am J Ophthalmol. 1989;108:670-5.
24. Price FW Jr, Whitson WE, Ahad KA, Tavakkoli H. Suprachoroidal hemorrhage in penetrating keratoplasty. Ophthalmic Surg. 1994;25:521-5.
25. Williams MA, Gawley SD, Jackson AJ, Frazer DG. Traumatic graft dehiscence after penetrating keratoplasty. Ophthalmology. 2008;115(2):276-8.e1.
26. Christo CG, van Rooij J, Geerards AJ, Remeijer L, Beekhuis WH. Suture-related complications following keratoplasty: a 5-year retrospective study. Cornea. 2001;20:816-9.
27. Binder PS, Abel R Jr, Polack FM, Kaufman HE. Keratoplasty wound separations. Am J Ophthalmol. 1975;80:109-15.
28. Tseng SH, Lin SC, Chen FK. Traumatic wound dehiscence after penetrating keratoplasty: clinical features and outcome in 21 cases. Cornea. 1999;18:553-8.
29. Oshry T, Lifihitz T. Traumatic wound dehiscence after corneal graft. Ophthalmic Surg Lasers. 2001;32:470-3.
30. Raber IM, Arentsen JJ, Laibson PR. Traumatic wound dehiscence after penetrating keratoplasty. Arch Ophthalmol. 1980;98:1407-9.
31. Renucci AM, Marangon FB, Culbertson WW. Wound dehiscence after penetrating keratoplasty: clinical characteristics of 51 cases treated at Bascom Palmer Eye Institute. Cornea. 2006;25:524-9.
32. Das S, Whiting M, Taylor HR. Corneal wound dehiscence after penetrating keratoplasty. Cornea. 2007;26:526-9.
33. Jeganathan SV, Ghosh S, Jhanji V, Lamoureux E, Taylor HR, Vajpayee RB. Resuturing following penetrating keratoplasty: a retrospective analysis. Br J Ophthalmol. 2008;92:893-5.
34. Friedenwald JS, Buschke W. Mitotic and wound healing activities of the corneal epithelium. 1944;32:410-3.
35. Kuwabara T, Perkins DG, Cogan DG. Sliding of the epithelium in experimental corneal wounds. Invest Ophthalmol Vis Sci. 1976;15:4-14.
36. Kim T, Palay DA, Lynn M. Donor factors associated with epithelial defects after penetrating keratoplasty. Cornea. 1996;15:451-6.
37. Pazin GJ, Ho M, Janetta PJ. Reactivation of herpes simplex virus after by decompression of the trigeminal nerve root. J Infect Dis. 1978;138:405-9.
38. Carton CA, Kilbourne ED. Activation of latent herpes simplex by trigeminal by sensory-root section. N Engl J Med. 1952;246:172-6.
39. Mannis MJ, Plotnik RD, Schwab IR, Newton RD. Herpes simplex dendritic keratitis after keratoplasty. Am J Ophthalmol. 1991;111:480-4.
40. Remeijer L, Doornenbal P, Geerards AJ, Rijneveld WA, Beekhuis WH. Newly acquired herpes simplex virus keratitis after penetrating keratoplasty. Ophthalmology. 1997;104:648-52.
41. Chou L, Cohen EJ, Laibson PR, Rapuano CJ. Factors associated with epithelial defects after penetrating keratoplasty. Ophthalmic Surg. 1994;25:700-3.
42. Rosenthal P, Cotter JM, Baum J. Treatment of persistent corneal epithelial defect with extended wear of a fluid-ventilated gas-permeable scleral contact lens. Am J Ophthalmol. 2000;130:33-41.
43. Prabhasawat P, Tesavibul N, Komolsuradej W. Single and multilayer amniotic membrane transplantation for persistent corneal epithelial defect with and without stromal thinning and perforation. Br J Ophthalmol. 2001;85:1455-63.
44. Tsubota K, Goto E, Shimmura S, Shimazaki J. Treatment of persistent corneal epithelial defect by autologous serum application. Ophthalmology. 1999;106:1984-9.
45. Ferreira de Souza R, Kruse FE, Seitz B. [Autologous serum for otherwise therapy resistant corneal epithelial defects—Prospective report on the first 70 eyes]. Klin Monbl Augenheilkd. 2001;218:720-6.
46. Poon AC, Geerling G, Dart JK, Fraenkel GE, Daniels JT. Autologous serum eye drops for dry eyes and epithelial defects: clinical and in vitro toxicity studies. Br J Ophthalmol. 2001;85:1188-97.
47. Vajpayee RB, Mukerji N, Tandon R, Sharma N, Pandey RM, Biswas NR, et al. Evaluation of umbilical cord serum therapy for persistent corneal epithelial defects. Br J Ophthalmol. 2003;87:1312-6.
48. Ho PC, Elliott JH. Kinetics of corneal epithelial regeneration. II. Epidermal growth factor and topical corticosteroids. Invest Ophthalmol. 1975;14:630-3.
49. Nishida T, Nakagawa S, Nishibayashi C, Tanaka H, Manabe R. Fibronectin enhancement of corneal epithelial wound healing of rabbits in vivo. Arch Ophthalmol. 1984;102:455-6.
50. Kim MS, Song SW, Kim JH, Woo HM. Multifocal photo-therapeutic keratectomy for the treatment of persistent epithelial defect. J Cataract Refract Surg. 2000;26:1753-7.
51. Donnenfeld ED, Perry HD, Nelson DB. Cyanoacrylate temporary tarsorrhaphy in the management of corneal epithelial defects. Ophthalmic Surg. 1991;22:591-3.
52. Naik MN, Gangopadhyay N, Fernandes M, Murthy R, Honavar SG. Anterior chemodenervation of levator palpebrae superioris with botulinum toxintype-A (Botox) to induce temporary ptosis for corneal protection. Eye (Lond). 2008;22:1132-36.
53. Rotkis WM, Chandler JW, Forstot SL. Filamentary keratitis following penetrating keratoplasty. Ophthalmology. 1982;89:946-9.
54. Albietz J, Sanfilippo P, Troutbeck R, Lenton LM. Management of filamentary keratitis associated with aqueous-deficient dry eye. Optom Vis Sci. 2003;80:420-30.
55. Wilhelmus KR, Stulting RD, Sugar J, Khan MM. Primary corneal graft failure. A national reporting system. Medical advisory board of Eye Bank Association of America. Arch Ophthalmol. 1995;113:1497-502.
56. Biswas S, Suresh P, Bonshek RE, Corbitt G, Tullo AB, Ridgway AE. Graft failure in human donor corneas due to transmission of herpes simplex virus. Br J Ophthalmol. 2000;84:701-5.
57. De Kesel RJ, Koppen C, Ieven M, Zeyen T. Primary graft failure caused by herpes simplex virus type 1. Cornea. 2001;20:187-90.
58. Van Rensburg PD, Raber IM, Laibson PR, Eagle RC Jr. Management of primary corneal graft failure. Cornea. 1998;17:208-11.

59. Mader TH, Stulting RD. The high risk penetrating keratoplasty. Ophthalmol Clin North Am. 1991;4:411-26.
60. Alldredge OC, Krachmer JH. Clinical types of corneal transplant rejection: their manifestations, frequency, preoperative correlates and treatment. Arch Ophthalmol. 1981;99:599-604.
61. Parker A, Folk JC, Weingeist TA, Goldsmith JC. Procoagulant effects of intraocular sodium hyalunorate. Am J Ophthalmol. 1985;100:479.
62. Levenson JE, Imperia PS. Viscoelastic materials. In: Brightbill FS (Ed). Corneal Surgery: Theory, Technique, and Tissue. St Louis: Mosby; 1993.
63. Simmons RB, Stern RA, Teekhasaenee C, Kenyon KR. Elevated intraocular pressure following penetrating keratoplasty. Trans Am Ophthalmol Soc. 1989;87:79-91; discussion 91-3.
64. Urrets-Zavalia A Jr. Fixed, dilated pupils, iris atrophy and secondary glaucoma. Am J Ophthalmol. 1963;56:257-65.
65. Maurino V, Allan BD, Stevens JD, Tuft SJ. Fixed dilated pupil (Urrets-Zavalia syndrome) after air/gas injection after deep lamellar keratoplasty for keratoconus. Am J Ophthalmol. 2002;133:266-8.
66. Minasian M, Ayliffe W. Fixed dilated pupil following deep lamellar keratoplasty (Urrets-Zavalia syndrome). Br J Ophthalmol. 2002;86:115-6.
67. Foster CS, Pavan-Langstorn D. Corneal wound healing and antiviral medication. Arch Ophthalmol. 1977;95:2062-7.
68. Barney NP, Foster CS. A prospective randomized trial of oral acyclovir after penetrating keratoplasty for herpes simplex keratitis. Cornea. 1994;13:232-6.
69. Ghosh S, Jhanji V, Lamoureux E, Taylor HR, Vajpayee RB. Acyclovir therapy in prevention of recurrent herpetic keratitis following penetrating keratoplasty. Am J Ophthalmol. 2008;145:198-202.
70. Miserocchi E, Modorati G, Galli L, Rama P. Efficacy of valacyclovir vs acyclovir for the prevention of recurrent herpes simplex virus eye disease: a pilot study. Am J Ophthalmol. 2007;144:547-51.
71. Goldblum D, Bachmann C, Tappeiner C, Garweg J, Frueh BE. Comparison of oral antiviral therapy with valacyclovir or acyclovir after penetrating keratoplasty for herpetic keratitis. Br J Ophthalmol. 2008;92:1201-5.
72. Fong LP, Omerod LD, Kenyon KR, Foster CS. Microbial keratitis complicating penetrating keratoplasty. Ophthalmology. 1988;95:1269-75.
73. Vajpayee RB, Sharma N, Sinha R, Agarwal T, Singhvi A. Infectious keratitis following keratoplasty. Surv Ophthalmol. 2007;52:1-12.
74. Harris DJ, Stulting RD, Waring GO, Wilson LA. Late bacterial and fungal keratitis after penetrating keratoplasty. Ophthalmology. 1988;95:1450-7.
75. Shi W, Li S, Liu M, Jin H, Xie L. Antifungal chemotherapy for fungal keratitis guided by in vivo confocal microscopy. Graefes Arch Clin Exp Ophthalmol. 2008;246:581-6.
76. Vajpayee RB, Boral SK, Dada T, Murthy GV, Pandey RM, Satpathy G. Risk factors for graft infection in India: a case-control study. Br J Ophthalmol. 2002;86:261-5.
77. Pardos GJ, Gallagher MA. Microbial contamination of donor eyes. A retrospective study. Arch Ophthalmol. 1982;100:1611-3.
78. Leveille AS, McMullan FD, Cavanagh HD. Endophthalmitis following penetrating keratoplasty. Ophthalmology. 1983;90:38-9.
79. Guss RB, Koenig S, De La Pena W, Marx M, Kaufman HE. Endophthalmitis after penetrating keratoplasty. Am J Ophthalmol. 1983;95:651-8.
80. Taban M, Behrens A, Newcomb RL, Nobe MY, McDonnell PJ. Incidence of acute endophthalmitis following penetrating keratoplasty: a systematic review. Arch Ophthalmol. 2005;123:605-9.
81. Kloess PM, Stulting RD, Waring GO 3rd, Wilson LA. Bacterial and fungal endophthalmitis after penetrating keratoplasty. Am J Ophthalmol. 1993;115:309-16.
82. Kunimoto DY, Tasman W, Rapuano C, Recchia F, Busbee B, Pearlman R, et al. Endophthalmitis after penetrating keratoplasty: microbiologic spectrum and susceptibility of isolates. Am J Ophthalmol. 2004;137:343-5.
83. Lam DS, Kwok AK, Chew S. Post-keratoplasty endophthalmitis caused by Proteus mirabilis. Eye. 1998;12:139-40.
84. Stern GA. Infectious crystalline keratopathy. Int Ophthalmol Clin. 1993;33:1-7.
85. Sharma N, Vajpayee RB, Pushker N, Vajpayee M. Infectious crystalline keratopathy. CLAO J. 2000;26:40-3.
86. Eiferman RA, Forgey DR, Cook YD. Excimer laser ablation of infectious crystalline keratopathy. Arch Ophthalmol. 1992;110:18.
87. Salabert D, Robinet A, Colin J. [Infectious crystalline keratopathy occurring after penetrating keratoplasty]. J Fr Ophthalmol. 1994;17:355-7.
88. Lam S, Meisler DM, Krachmer JH. Enterococcal infectious crystalline keratopathy. Cornea. 1993;12:273-6.
89. Daneshvar H, MacInnis B, Hodge WG. Nd:YAG laser corneal disruption as adjuvant treatment for infectious crystalline keratopathy. Am J Ophthalmol. 2000;129:800-1.
90. Sugar A, Meyer RF, Hood I. Epithelial downgrowth following penetrating keratoplasty in aphakia. Arch Ophthalmol. 1977;95:464-7.
91. Forseto Ados S, dos Santos MS, Sampaio A, Mascaro V, Nosé W. Diagnosis of epithelial ingrowth after penetrating keratoplasty with confocal microscopy. Cornea. 2006;25:1124-7.
92. Lai MM, Haller JA. Resolution of epithelial ingrowth in a patient treated with 5-fluorouracil. Am J Ophthalmol. 2002;133:562-4.
93. Dua HS, Gomes JA. Clinical course of hurricane keratopathy. Br J Ophthalmol. 2000;84:285-8.
94. Dua HS, Singh A, Gomes JA, Laibson PR, Donoso LA, Tyagi S. Vortex or whorl formation of cultured human corneal epithelial cells induced by magnetic fields. Eye (Lond). 1996;10:447-50.
95. Martin TP, Reed JW, Legault C, Oberfeld SM, Jacoby BG, Yu DD, et al. Cataract formation and cataract extraction after penetrating keratoplasty. Ophthalmology. 1994;101:113-9.
96. Rathi VM, Krishnamachary M, Gupta S. Cataract formation after penetrating keratoplasty. J Cataract Refract Surg. 1997;23:562-4.
97. Musch DC, Mayer RF, Sugar A, Soong HK. Corneal astigmatism after penetrating keratoplasty. The role of suture technique. Ophthalmology. 1989;96:698-703.
98. Heidemann DG, Sugar A, Meyer RF, Musch DC. Oversized donor grafts in penetrating keratoplasty; A randomized trial. Arch Ophthalmol. 1985;103:1807-11.
99. Sharma V, Sharma N, Vajpayee RB, Titiyal JS, Sinha R. Study of corneal topographic patterns with single continuous suturing techniques in penetrating keratoplasty. Cornea. 2003;22:5-9.
100. Vajpayee RB, Sharma V, Sharma N, Panda A, Taylor HR. Evaluation of techniques of single continuous suturing in penetrating keratoplasty. Br J Ophthalmol. 2001;85:134-8.
101. Sarhan AR, Fares U, Al-Aqaba MA, Miri A, Otri AM, Said DG, et al. Rapid suture management of post-keratoplasty astigmatism. Eye (Lond). 2010;24:540-6.
102. Dada T, Vajpayee RB, Gupta V, Sharma N, Dada VK. Microkeratome-induced reduction of astigmatism after penetrating keratoplasty. Am J Ophthalmol. 2001;131:507-8.
103. Vajpayee RB, Sharma N, Sinha R, Bhartiya P, Titiyal JS, Tandon R. Laser in-situ keratomileusis after penetrating keratoplasty. Surv Ophthalmol. 2003;48:503-14.
104. Nubile M, Carpineto P, Lanzini M, Calienno R, Agnifili L, Ciancaglini M, et al. Femtosecond laser arcuate keratotomy for the correction of high astigmatism after keratoplasty. Ophthalmology. 2009;116:1083-92.
105. Borkenstein AF, Reuland A, Limberger IJ, Rabsilber TM, Auffarth GU. Transscleral fixation of a toric intraocular lens to correct aphakic keratoplasty with high astigmatism. J Cataract Refract Surg. 2009;35:934-8.

106. Charlin R, Polack FM. The effect of elevated intraocular pressure on the endothelium of corneal grafts. Cornea. 1982;1:241-9.
107. Sekhar JC, Vyas P, Nagrajan R. Post-penetrating keratoplasty glaucoma. Indian J Ophthalmol. 1993;41:181-4.
108. Olson RJ, Kaufman HE. A mathematical description of causative factors and prevention of elevated intraocular pressure after keratoplasty. Invest Ophthalmol Vis Sci. 1977;16:1085-92.
109. Foulks GN. Glaucoma associated with penetrating keratoplasty. Ophthalmology. 1987;94:871-4.
110. Nakakura S, Imamura H, Nakamura T. Selective laser trabeculoplasty for glaucoma after penetrating keratoplasty. Optom Vis Sci. 2009;86:e404-6.
111. Witmer MT, Tiedeman JS, Olsakovsky LA, Conaway MR, Prum BE. Long-term Intraocular Pressure Control and Corneal Graft Survival in Eyes With a Pars Plana Baerveldt Implant and Corneal Transplant. J Glaucoma. 2010;19:124-31.
112. Ocakoglu O, Arslan OS, Kayiran A. Diode laser transscleral cyclophotocoagulation for the treatment of refractory glaucoma after penetrating keratoplasty. Curr Eye Res. 2005;30:569-74.
113. Lyons CJ, McCartney AC, Kirkness CM, Ficker LA, Steele AD, Rice NS. Granular corneal dystrophy. Visual results and pattern of recurrence after lamellar or penetrating keratoplasty. Ophthalmology. 1994;101:1812-7.
114. Al-Swailem A, Al-Rajhi M. Wagoner MD. Penetrating keratoplasty for macular corneal dystrophy. Ophthalmology. 2005;112(2):220-4.
115. Meisler DM, Fine M. Recurrence of the clinical signs of lattice corneal dystrophy (type I) in corneal transplants. Am J Ophthalmol. 1984;97:210-4.
116. Jonas JB, Kamppeter B. Intravitreal triamcinolone acetonide for persisting cystoid macular edema after penetrating keratoplasty. Cornea. 2006;25:240-1.

16

Post-penetrating Keratoplasty Glaucoma

Viney Gupta, Shikha Gupta, Jonathan G Crowston

INTRODUCTION

There are no standard definitions for postkeratoplasty glaucoma, with different publications using different criteria to define the condition. Some of the commonly used criteria include: (1) ocular hypertension (>21 mm Hg) after penetrating keratoplasty; (2) ocular hypertension (>21 mm Hg) after penetrating keratoplasty, requiring a glaucoma surgery or medications to lower intraocular pressure (IOP); (3) persistently elevated IOP > 21 mm Hg or >10 mm Hg above baseline, requiring antiglaucoma medications or surgical intervention at any time. In patients with preexisting glaucoma, it has been defined as uncontrolled IOP with the original treatment regime requiring treatment escalation after penetrating keratoplasty. These criteria do not include fundus evaluation or visual field assessment owing to the difficulty in their assessment in such eyes.

Secondary ocular hypertension after penetrating keratoplasty is not uncommon. However, with the introduction of less invasive surgical techniques for keratoplasty, the incidence of postkeratoplasty rise of IOP has reduced significantly. IOP elevation can have serious consequences after keratoplasty, such as endothelial cell loss, early graft rejection, graft failure, and optic nerve damage over time.[1,2] Experimental evidence indicates that corneal endothelium from grafted tissues is more susceptible to IOP-induced damage than healthy nongrafted corneal endothelium.[3] Hence, early detection of IOP elevation and its control is important to promote graft survival. Elevation of IOP has been associated with graft rejection episodes, though a causal association is not known.[4] One large series found elevated IOP to be the third most common cause of graft failure, other risk factors being rejection and infection.[5] In addition to the corneal decompensation, raised IOP may, of course, also result in progressive visual impairment due to optic nerve damage which may go unrecognized especially in a failing graft with hazy cornea.

INCIDENCE

The 10-year cumulative incidence of postkeratoplasty glaucoma is reported to be approximately 20%.[6,7]

The incidence of post-penetrating keratoplasty glaucoma (PPKG) ranges from 11 to 38% in phakic eyes and 42 to 89% in aphakic eyes.[8-10]

Post-penetrating keratoplasty glaucoma occurs at different time periods depending upon the pathogenic factor; however, almost half of such cases arise in the early postoperative period after keratoplasty. In most cases, the IOP elevation occurs within the first year of surgery during which it must be monitored closely. The incidence of IOP elevation and glaucoma is lesser with lamellar keratoplasty procedures than with penetrating keratoplasty probably due to less angle distortion from partial retention of the corneal layers and lesser duration of steroid use in the former.[11]

FACTORS ASSOCIATED WITH IOP ELEVATION IN EYES WITH KERATOPLASTY

Preoperative

The presence of glaucoma prior to the keratoplasty is an important risk factor despite adequate control.[2,8,12,13] Glaucoma following keratoplasty is more common in aphakic eyes as compared to phakic eyes.[9] In pseudophakic eyes the rise in IOP is more frequent than in phakic eyes, but less as compared to aphakic eyes (**Fig. 1**).[14] While keratoplasty in patients with a keratoconus is less likely to be associated with a raised IOP, the highest risk of glaucoma postkeratoplasty was reported for eyes with aphakic/pseudophakic bullous keratopathy.[15] This may be because of intraocular lens (IOL) material, inflammatory response after penetrating keratoplasty, the effects of aphakia and pseudophakia on the angle structures, and the synechiae formation postkeratoplasty.

Keratoplasty performed for tectonic reasons, especially grafts performed for perforated corneal ulcers have also been found to lead to high rates of IOP elevation,

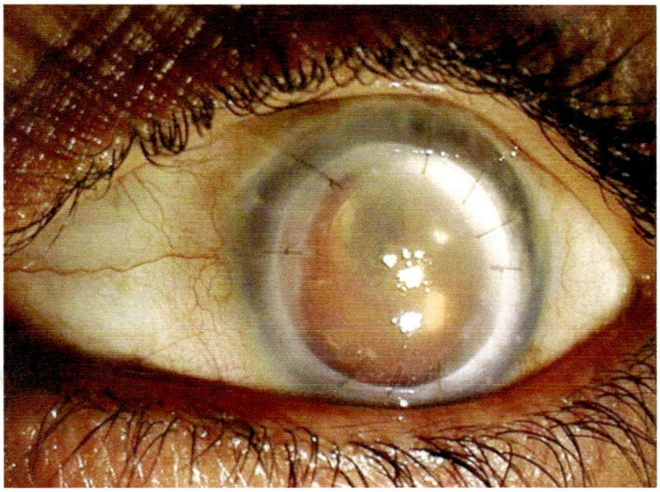

Fig. 1: Post-penetrating keratoplasty glaucoma.

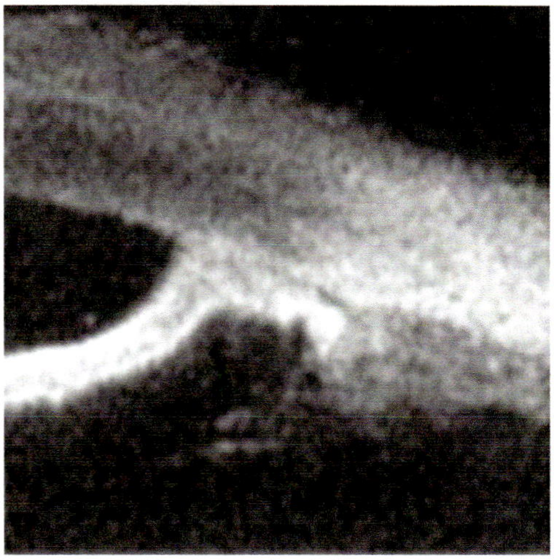

Fig. 2: Ultrabiomicroscopy shows peripheral anterior synechiae.

with glaucoma being the most common complication postoperatively.[8,14,16] The longer the period between the perforation and therapeutic keratoplasty, the greater the likelihood of developing glaucoma. Eyes with corneo-iridic scars (adherent leukomas) preoperatively have also been found to be at high risk of development of glaucoma postkeratoplasty.[17] Other indications of keratoplasty associated with high risk of glaucoma development include preoperative diagnosis of inflammatory diseases such as graft thinning [relative risk (RR) = 4.96], traumatic scar formation (RR = 2.66), graft abscess (RR = 2.62), graft rejection (RR = 2.61), bullous keratopathy (RR = 2.59), and corneal abscess (RR = 1.52).[18]

According to the largest published systematic review, strong risk factors for PPKG include preexisting glaucoma and aphakia, modest predictors include pseudophakia, regrafting, and preoperative diagnosis of bullous keratopathy and trauma.[19]

Intraoperative

Using a donor transplant that is 0.5 mm larger than the recipient's bed has been found to be less likely to cause IOP elevation than if same size donor graft is used especially in aphakic keratoplasties.[20] Using same-sized donor tissue as the recipient results in compression of the corneolimbal angle thus compromising the trabecular meshwork. Tighter sutures, longer bites, larger trephine size, small total recipient corneal diameter during surgery and increased peripheral corneal thickness, increase distortion of the angle leading to a raised IOP.[10,21]

Other intraoperative factors that can cause raised IOP postkeratoplasty include the use of viscoelastics and additional surgical procedures performed with the corneal grafting. Mac Rae et al. demonstrated in primate studies, IOP elevation as high as 67 mm Hg, 90 minutes after intracameral injection of 1% sodium hyaluronate.[22] Hence, it is recommended that the viscoelastic agents should be replaced with balanced saline solution at the end of the surgery though an IOP elevation >50 mm Hg even after satisfactory removal of the viscoelastic at the end of the procedure has been reported in the early postoperative period.[23] The risk of IOP elevation and glaucoma increases with additional procedures like lens extraction and IOL insertion or even a secondary IOL implantation.[24]

Postoperative

Shallow anterior chamber or the presence of an air bubble can trigger pupillary block glaucoma postoperatively. Pupil block glaucoma has also been reported to occur as a complication of Descemet's stripping automated endothelial keratoplasty (DSAEK).[25,26] Immediate postoperative wound leaks with shallow anterior chamber can also lead to malignant glaucoma.[27] Both early and delayed suprachoroidal hemorrhage is known to complicate a penetrating keratoplasty.[28,29]

An IOP elevation postkeratoplasty may also accompany herpes simplex virus (HSV) uveitis in eyes that have undergone keratoplasty for herpetic keratitis. This IOP elevation is related to the trabeculitis and is short lived.[4]

Progressive angle closure due to development of fine peripheral anterior synechiae (PAS) can lead to postkeratoplasty glaucoma and is one of the important causes of late IOP rise after corneal transplants (**Fig. 2**).[30]

Epithelial and fibrous downgrowth, though uncommon, can lead to a refractory postkeratoplasty glaucoma. Finally, secondary ocular hypertension should be suspected to be steroid induced in eyes on intensive steroid therapy especially for graft rejection. Use of steroids might contribute to a 21–22% proportion of intraocular hypertension or glaucoma after penetrating keratoplasty.[19]

DIAGNOSIS

Clinical signs: One of an indirect indicator of raised IOP following keratoplasty is a thinning of corneal stroma. This is followed by epithelial edema and if not treated leads to progressive thickening of the stroma due to endothelial cell damage.[21,31]

Tonometry: IOP measurement is critical, though difficult in postkeratoplasty eyes. Unrecognized IOP elevation can lead to progressive optic nerve damage. Biomechanical changes in the cornea that may affect its flexural rigidity, can influence IOP measurement. Technical difficulties exist in measuring IOP with Goldmann applanation tonometry (GAT) due to irregular astigmatism and hence formation of distorted mires. Also the measurements with GAT vary significantly with corneal properties such as corneal curvature, thickness, hysteresis, edema, scarring, etc. Hence, the pneumotonometer, Tonopen, and the dynamic contour tonometer (DCT) are alternatives to GAT for IOP measurement in eyes with scarred corneas, post keratoplasty. All the three instruments have been found to give higher IOP reading than the GAT in postkeratoplasty eyes.[32-34] While Rao et al.[35] in their study found the pneumotonometer not to be affected by central corneal thickness (CCT) and a useful alternative to GAT, Browning et al. found it to be most affected by CCT in eyes with other corneal pathologies.[32] The DCT may give more realistic IOP readings in grafted eyes compared to GAT as the measurements take into account the corneal thickness variability, though there are no large studies using the DCT in grafted eyes.[34] In general, Tonopen and pneumotonometer appear to be the most reliable for measuring IOP in eyes with scarred or irregular cornea and DCT and ocular response analyzer seem to be the best in cases with deviant corneal thickness.

Fundus evaluation: IOP measurement should be performed at all visits after keratoplasty and optic disk assessed whenever possible, if IOP is elevated.[36]

MANAGEMENT

Medical

Medical therapy remains the initial management of postkeratoplasty glaucoma unless surgically treatable cause like pupillary block is found.

Beta-adrenergic blocking agents (timolol, levobunolol, and betaxolol) and alpha-2 adrenergic agonist (brimonidine) by decreasing adequate aqueous humor production are useful in the treatment of postkeratoplasty glaucoma although there are conflicting reports in the literature.[37,38] Adverse effects of beta-adrenergic blockers such as superficial punctate keratitis, corneal anesthesia, dry eye, and subconjunctival fibrosis may, however, compromise graft function. Brimonidine is also to be used with caution as it may cause allergic reactions, dry eyes, and superficial punctate keratitis.

Prostaglandin analogs (latanoprost, travoprost, and bimatoprost) which decrease IOP by increasing uveal outflow may be used alone or in combination with beta-adrenergic blocking agents or alpha-2 adrenergic agonists. Precautions should be taken as they have been reported to cause cystoid macular edema in patients with a past history of uveitis and patients with aphakia and pseudophakia.[39] Wand et al. reported recurrence of herpetic infections in patients with herpes simplex keratitis.[40] Hence, care needs to be taken in instituting prostaglandins in eyes grafted for HSV keratitis.

Carbonic anhydrase inhibitors (dorzolamide, brinzolamide, and acetazolamide): Topical therapy may be tried as a second- or third-line agent, however, they are not recommended as they also suppress the carbonic anhydrase enzyme in the corneal endothelium and may lead to graft decompensation.[41]

Systemic carbonic anhydrase inhibitors (acetazolamide) are useful in the treatment of immediate postoperative pressure spikes but their long-term therapy is limited by their side effects of nausea, gastrointestinal disturbances, paresthesia, fatigue, depression, anorexia, and weight loss. There have been reports however of its limited efficacy.[42]

Miotics (pilocarpine) are of little value in the presence of PAS and are best avoided as they breakdown the blood-aqueous barrier and can cause graft rejection.[43] In the immediate postoperative period, they can cause shallowing of the anterior chamber and can promote synechiae formation.

Most topical medications have preservatives, which can lead to punctate epithelialopathy.[44] Preservative-free medications are therefore preferable in eyes postkeratoplasty as these patients already have a compromised cornea. Certain alternatives such as nonpreserved formulation of timolol, brimonidine preserved with Purites, and travoprost formulation preserved with SofZias instead of benzalkonium chloride can be used.

Hyperosmotic agents (mannitol) may be indicated for the temporary relief of the high rise in IOP in the early postoperative period.[42]

Topical steroids are part and parcel of the treatment following penetrating keratoplasty. One should always consider the possibility of steroid-induced glaucoma, either decreasing the dose/frequency of steroids or using less potent topical steroids, like fluorometholone, are potential ways to decrease the IOP elevation associated with steroid use. Topical immunomodulators like cyclosporine A in conjunction with topical glaucoma medications can help lowering IOP in steroid responders.

Lasers

Laser Iridotomy

Laser iridotomy may be performed if a component of pupillary block is suspected in postkeratoplasty glaucoma.

It presents as iris bombe with a very shallow peripheral anterior chamber.

Laser Trabeculoplasty

The role of laser trabeculoplasty is limited in eyes with PPKG due to the presence of PAS and poor visibility of the trabecular meshwork, through the corneal transplant. Furthermore, there is limited data on the efficacy of trabeculoplasty in glaucoma following keratoplasty.

Surgical

Managing PPKG can be difficult. However, a planned and stepwise approach should be adopted to attain the best outcomes.

Gonioscopy-assisted transluminal trabeculotomy (GATT): It has been described for one patient with steroid-induced glaucoma PPKG.[45] Because of the presence of widespread PAS, the feasibility of this procedure in general for nonsteroid-induced PPKG remains poor.

Trabeculectomy

Trabeculectomy is indicated when medical management has failed and the optic nerve head or the graft is threatened by persistent elevation of IOP. Trabeculectomy with mitomycin C has better success for eyes with postkeratoplasty glaucoma who have minimal conjunctival scarring, absence of PAS, and open angles. The success rate for IOP control in patients with postkeratoplasty glaucoma undergoing trabeculectomy with mitomycin C has been reported to be between 67 and 91% and that of graft failure between 12 and 18%.[39,46] An overall 70% success over a 3-year follow-up for IOP < 21 mm Hg is described for trabeculectomy with mitomycin C in eyes with postkeratoplasty glaucoma.[47] Hence, trabeculectomy with mitomycin C as a filtering surgery should be preferred as first-line surgical treatment. However, caution should be taken in administering subconjunctival 5-fluorouracil injections postoperatively to prevent bleb scarring in these eyes in view of its corneal epithelial toxicity.

Glaucoma Drainage Devices

Glaucoma drainage devices (GDDs) may be considered in patients where trabeculectomy with mitomycin C is not an option or has a high likelihood of failure, is contraindicated or in patients with a previously failed trabeculectomy with mitomycin C. The average success of GDDs to control glaucoma in patients following keratoplasty in a series was 84%, however, a 10–51% incidence of graft failure is reported to occur in different series with varying follow-up times.[43,48,49] In a retrospective interventional comparative study, Ahmed glaucoma valve (AGV) implant controlled IOP more effectively than trabeculectomy with mitomycin C. However, GDDs result in higher rates of corneal graft failure in a shorter duration of time.[50,51] Early AGV implantation, within a month of diagnosis of PPKG resulted in a statistically significant better success rates when compared with implantation occurring >1 month of diagnosis. Factors associated with a high risk of failure include preexisting angle-closure glaucoma, a history of previous PKP, and a preoperative IOP > 21 mm Hg. The most common surgical complications, aside from graft failure, was hyphema.[52]

The optimal location for the drainage tube remains controversial; but graft clarity is more for tubes placed in pars plana region (83%) compared with anterior chamber tube placement (48%) with no difference in IOP control between the two tube locations.[53] Vitreal placement of the tube necessitates a complete vitrectomy with careful removal of the vitreous skirt, thereby preventing vitreous from occluding the tube. However, pars plana tube placement may have greater risk of retinal detachment and suprachoroidal hemorrhage.[54] Besides tube placement in the ciliary sulcus is also associated with significantly lesser risk of corneal endothelial cell loss versus anterior chamber placement.

Cyclodestructive Procedures

Trans-scleral diode laser cyclophotocoagulation is the treatment of choice among the available cyclodestructive procedures. Graft failure following GDDs and cyclodestructive procedures is about the same, however, there may be a higher incidence of permanent visual loss and hypotony with cyclodestructive procedures.[36] Shah et al. in a series of 28 patients followed up from 18 to 38 months found an incidence of 16% for graft failure after cyclodiode.[55] The procedure needs to be repeated for the desired IOP control. It is generally reserved if other interventions have failed in eyes with poor visual potential.

Managing Preexisting Glaucoma

Preexisting glaucoma is a high-risk factor for the development of postkeratoplasty glaucoma and also leads to higher incidence of graft failure in patients undergoing glaucoma surgery following keratoplasty.[2,15,56] Hence, patients with uncontrolled glaucoma or those on maximal medical management should ideally be treated with either trabeculectomy aided with antifibrotic agents or GDDs prior to keratoplasty or may be combined with planned corneal transplant.[2,15,56] Staging the trabeculectomy before the transplant however, has the risk of bleb failure due to inflammation and progressive synechiae formation after keratoplasty.[57]

Reducing Postkeratoplasty Glaucoma in Future

The survival of the graft depends on minimum complications, hence, it is important to take measures to prevent the development or reduce the incidence of glaucoma rather than to treat it. One important measure is to perform lamellar keratoplasties wherever possible which less frequently distort the angle and therefore predispose less to the development of glaucoma. Another technique is to use femtosecond-aided host and donor button to improve wound architecture (zigzag, top-hat, or mushroom patterns), and limit astigmatism as the wounds require less number of sutures for closure thus limiting angle distortion.[58]

REFERENCES

1. Aldave AJ, Rudd JC, Cohen EJ, Rapuano CJ, Laibson PR. The role of glaucoma therapy in the need for repeat penetrating keratoplasty. Cornea. 2000;19(6):772-6.
2. Chien AM, Schmidt CM, Cohen EJ, Rajpal RK, Sperber LT, Rapuano CJ, et al. Glaucoma in the immediate postoperative period after penetrating keratoplasty. Am J Ophthalmol. 1993;115(6):711-4.
3. Charlin R, Polack FM. The effect of elevated intraocular pressure on the endothelium of corneal grafts. Cornea. 1982;1(3):241-9.
4. Adams GG, Stevenson KE, Kirkness CM, Steele AD, Rice NS. Is raised intraocular pressure a bad prognostic sign in acute corneal graft rejection? Eye (Lond). 1991;5(Pt 4):412-9.
5. Williams KA, Muehlberg SM, Lewis RF, Coster DJ. How successful is corneal transplantation? A report from the Australian Corneal Graft Register. Eye (Lond). 1995;9(Pt 2):219-27.
6. Ing JJ, Ing HH, Nelson LR, Hodge DO, Bourne WM. Ten-year postoperative results of penetrating keratoplasty. Ophthalmology. 1998;105(10):1855-65.
7. Patel SV, Hodge DO, Bourne WM. Corneal endothelium and postoperative outcomes 15 years after penetrating keratoplasty. Am J Ophthalmol. 2005;139(2):311-9.
8. Foulks GN. Glaucoma associated with penetrating keratoplasty. Ophthalmology. 1987;94(7):871-4.
9. Irvine AR, Kaufman HE. Intraolar pressure following penetrating keratoplasty. Am J Ophthalmol. 1969;68(5):835-44.
10. Karesh JW, Nirankari VS. Factors associated with glaucoma after penetrating keratoplasty. Am J Ophthalmol. 1983;96(2):160-4.
11. Borderie VM, Loriaut P, Bouheraoua N, Nordmann JP. Incidence of intraocular pressure elevation and glaucoma after lamellar versus full-thickness penetrating keratoplasty. Ophthalmology. 2016;123(7):1428-34.
12. Goldberg DB, Schanzlin DJ, Brown SI. Incidence of increased intraocular pressure after keratoplasty. Am J Ophthalmol. 1981;92(3):372-7.
13. Simmons RB, Stern RA, Teekhasaenee C, Kenyon KR. Elevated intraocular pressure following penetrating keratoplasty. Trans Am Ophthalmol Soc. 1989;87:79-91; discussion-3.
14. Zaidman GW, Goldman S. A prospective study on the implantation of anterior chamber intraocular lenses during keratoplasty for pseudophakic and aphakic bullous keratopathy. Ophthalmology. 1990;97(6):757-62.
15. Kirkness CM, Ficker LA. Risk factors for the development of postkeratoplasty glaucoma. Cornea. 1992;11(5):427-32.
16. Sukhija J, Jain AK. Outcome of therapeutic penetrating keratoplasty in infectious keratitis. Ophthalmic Surg Lasers Imaging. 2005;36(4):303-9.
17. Sihota R, Sharma N, Panda A, Aggarwal HC, Singh R. Post-penetrating keratoplasty glaucoma: risk factors, management and visual outcome. Aust N Z J Ophthalmol. 1998;26(4):305-9.
18. Karadag O, Kugu S, Erdogan G, Kandemir B, Eraslan Ozdil S, et al. Incidence of and risk factors for increased intraocular pressure after penetrating keratoplasty. Cornea. 2010;29(3):278-82.
19. Wu S, Xu J. Incidence and risk factors for post-penetrating keratoplasty glaucoma: A systematic review and meta-analysis. PLoS One. 2017;12(4):e0176261.
20. Zimmerman T, Olson R, Waltman S, Kaufman H. Transplant size and elevated intraocular pressure. Postkeratoplasty. Arch Ophthalmol. 1978;96(12):2231-3.
21. Olson RJ, Kaufman HE. Intraocular pressure and corneal thickness after penetrating keratoplasty. Am J Ophthalmol. 1978;86(1):97-100.
22. Mac Rae SM, Edelhauser HF, Hyndiuk RA, Burd EM, Schultz RO. The effects of sodium hyaluronate, chondroitin sulfate, and methylcellulose on the corneal endothelium and intraocular pressure. Am J Ophthalmol. 1983;95(3):332-41.
23. Barron BA, Busin M, Page C, Bergsma DR, Kaufman HE. Comparison of the effects of Viscoat and Healon on postoperative intraocular pressure. Am J Ophthalmol. 1985;100(3):377-84.
24. Sekhar GC, Vyas P, Nagarajan R, Mandal AK, Gupta S. Post-penetrating keratoplasty glaucoma. Indian J Ophthalmol. 1993;41(4):181-4.
25. Cheng YY, Hendrikse F, Pels E, Wijdh RJ, van Cleynenbreugel H, Eggink CA, et al. Preliminary results of femtosecond laser-assisted descemet stripping endothelial keratoplasty. Arch Ophthalmol. 2008;126(10):1351-6.
26. Koenig SB, Covert DJ. Early results of small-incision Descemet's stripping and automated endothelial keratoplasty. Ophthalmology. 2007;114(2):221-6.
27. Greenlee EC, Kwon YH. Graft failure: III. Glaucoma escalation after penetrating keratoplasty. Int Ophthalmol. 2008;28(3):191-207.
28. Duncker GI, Rochels R. Delayed suprachoroidal hemorrhage after penetrating keratoplasty. Int Ophthalmol. 1995;19(3):173-6.
29. Price FW Jr, Whitson WE, Ahad KA, Tavakkoli H. Suprachoroidal hemorrhage in penetrating keratoplasty. Ophthalmic Surg. 1994;25(8):521-5.
30. Lass JH, Pavan-Langston D. Timolol therapy in secondary angle-closure glaucoma post penetrating keratoplasty. Ophthalmology. 1979;86(1):51-9.
31. Ytteborg J, Dohlman CH. Corneal edema and intraocular pressure. II. Clinical results. Arch Ophthalmol. 1965;74(4):477-84.
32. Browning AC, Bhan A, Rotchford AP, Shah S, Dua HS. The effect of corneal thickness on intraocular pressure measurement in patients with corneal pathology. Br J Ophthalmol. 2004;88(11):1395-9.
33. Geyer O, Mayron Y, Loewenstein A, Neudorfer M, Rothkoff L, Lazar M. Tono-Pen tonometry in normal and in post-keratoplasty eyes. Br J Ophthalmol. 1992;76(9):538-40.
34. Ismail AR, Lamont M, Perera S, Khan-Lim D, Mehta R, Macleod JD, et al. Comparison of IOP measurement using GAT and DCT in patients with penetrating keratoplasties. Br J Ophthalmol. 2007;91(7):980-1.
35. Rao VJ, Gnanaraj L, Mitchell KW, Figueiredo FC. Clinical comparison of ocular blood flow tonometer, Tonopen, and Goldmann applanation tonometer for measuring intraocular pressure in postkeratoplasty eyes. Cornea. 2001;20(8):834-8.
36. Ayyala RS. Penetrating keratoplasty and glaucoma. Surv Ophthalmol. 2000;45(2):91-105.
37. Nissenkorn I, Wood TO. Intraocular pressure following aphakic transplants. Ann Ophthalmol. 1983;15(12):1168-71.
38. Olson RJ, Kaufman HE, Zimmerman TJ. Effects of timolol and Daranide on elevated intraocular pressure after aphakic keratoplasty. Ann Ophthalmol. 1979;11(12):1833-6.
39. Ayyala RS, Cruz DA, Margo CE, Harman LE, Pautler SE, Misch DM, et al. Cystoid macular edema associated with latanoprost in aphakic and pseudophakic eyes. Am J Ophthalmol. 1998;126(4):602-4.
40. Wand M, Gilbert CM, Liesegang TJ. Latanoprost and herpes simplex keratitis. Am J Ophthalmol. 1999;127(5):602-4.
41. Konowal A, Morrison JC, Brown SV, Cooke DL, Maguire LJ, Verdier DV, et al. Irreversible corneal decompensation in patients treated with topical dorzolamide. Am J Ophthalmol. 1999;127(4):403-6.

42. Wood TO, West C, Kaufman HE. Control of intraocular pressure in penetrating keratoplasty. Am J Ophthalmol. 1972;74(4):724-8.
43. Beebe WE, Starita RJ, Fellman RL, Lynn JR, Gelender H. The use of Molteno implant and anterior chamber tube shunt to encircling band for the treatment of glaucoma in keratoplasty patients. Ophthalmology. 1990;97(11):1414-22.
44. Fraunfelder F. Drugs used primarily in Ophthalmology. In: Meyer SM (Ed). Drug-induced Ocular Side Effects and Drug Interactions, 3rd edition. Philadelphia: Lea & Febiger; 1989.
45. Nazarali S, Cote SL, Gooi P. Gonioscopy-Assisted Transluminal Trabeculotomy (GATT) in Postpenetrating Keratoplasty Steroid-induced Glaucoma: A Case Report. J Glaucoma. 2018; 27(10):e162-e4.
46. Figueiredo RS, Araujo SV, Cohen EJ, Rapuano CJ, Katz LJ, Wilson RP. Management of coexisting corneal disease and glaucoma by combined penetrating keratoplasty and trabeculectomy with mitomycin-C. Ophthalmic Surg Lasers. 1996;27(11):903-9.
47. Ishioka M, Shimazaki J, Yamagami J, Fujishima H, Shimmura S, Tsubota K. Trabeculectomy with mitomycin C for post-keratoplasty glaucoma. Br J Ophthalmol. 2000;84(7):714-7.
48. Binder PS, Abel R Jr, Kaufman HE. Cyclocryotherapy for glaucoma after penetrating keratoplasty. Am J Ophthalmol. 1975;79(3):489-92.
49. Rapuano CJ, Schmidt CM, Cohen EJ, Rajpal RK, Raber IM, Katz LJ, et al. Results of alloplastic tube shunt procedures before, during, or after penetrating keratoplasty. Cornea. 1995;14(1):26-32.
50. Elhofi A, Helaly HA. Graft survival after penetrating keratoplasty in cases of trabeculectomy versus Ahmed valve implant. J Ophthalmol. 2018;2018:9034964.
51. Kwon YH, Taylor JM, Hong S, Honkanen RA, Zimmerman MB, Alward WL, et al. Long-term results of eyes with penetrating keratoplasty and glaucoma drainage tube implant. Ophthalmology. 2001;108(2):272-8.
52. Tai MC, Chen YH, Cheng JH, Liang CM, Chen JT, Chen CL, et al. Early Ahmed glaucoma valve implantation after penetrating keratoplasty leads to better outcomes in an Asian population with preexisting glaucoma. PLoS One. 2012;7(5):e37867.
53. Arroyave CP, Scott IU, Fantes FE, Feuer WJ, Murray TG. Corneal graft survival and intraocular pressure control after penetrating keratoplasty and glaucoma drainage device implantation. Ophthalmology. 2001;108(11):1978-85.
54. Sidoti PA, Mosny AY, Ritterband DC, Seedor JA. Pars plana tube insertion of glaucoma drainage implants and penetrating keratoplasty in patients with coexisting glaucoma and corneal disease. Ophthalmology. 2001;108(6):1050-8.
55. Shah P, Lee GA, Kirwan JK, Bunce C, Bloom PA, Ficker LA, et al. Cyclodiode photocoagulation for refractory glaucoma after penetrating keratoplasty. Ophthalmology. 2001;108(11):1986-91.
56. Reinhard T, Kallmann C, Cepin A, Godehardt E, Sundmacher R. The influence of glaucoma history on graft survival after penetrating keratoplasty. Graefes Arch Clin Exp Ophthalmol. 1997;235(9):553-7.
57. Lee RK, Fantes F. Surgical management of patients with combined glaucoma and corneal transplant surgery. Curr Opin Ophthalmol. 2003;14(2):95-9.
58. Jonas JB, Vossmerbaeumer U. Femtosecond laser penetrating keratoplasty with conical incisions and positional spikes. J Refract Surg. 2004;20(4):397.

17 Corneal Graft Rejection

Robin G Abell, Ben Connell, Michael S Loughnan

DEFINITION OF GRAFT FAILURE VERSUS REJECTION

The most common cause of corneal graft failure is allogeneic rejection, despite the unique immune privilege of the cornea. Corneal graft rejection refers to specific immunologic response mechanisms of the recipient to the corneal donor tissue. It is importaWnt to distinguish corneal graft rejection from other forms of nonimmune-mediated graft failures. A rare cause of nonimmune-mediated graft failure is primary graft failure, which is distinguished from early rejection by the presence of a clear graft in the early postoperative weeks. This type of graft failure is rarely due to an immunogenic mechanism and is usually due to poor eye banking or surgical trauma with damage to the endothelial surface. Secondary graft failure occurs in a graft that has functioned in the immediate postoperative period. Unless specifically stated graft failure refers to secondary graft failure.

CAUSES OF SECONDARY GRAFT FAILURE

Graft failure is due to any cause of endothelial cell loss such as aphakia, older style anterior chamber intraocular lenses, uncontrolled intraocular pressure, or ongoing inflammation. The most common cause of secondary graft failure is an immune-mediated process termed allogeneic graft rejection.[1] One large study found that one-third of corneal graft failures in high-risk grafts were due to graft rejection.[2] Not all episodes of allogeneic graft rejection, however, progress to secondary graft failure. The reversal of a rejection episode in many cases is possible with endothelial function returning and stromal edema improving. Less is known regarding effective prophylaxis in corneal graft patients who are at high risk of rejection.

Allogeneic graft rejection will subsequently be referred to as graft rejection in this chapter. Primary graft failure is not considered further.

TYPES OF GRAFT REJECTION

The three transplanted tissue components in penetrating keratoplasty are: (1) epithelium, (2) stroma, and (3) endothelium. Rejection can be directed at any of these three layers in isolation or combination.[3] Donor epithelium can persist for up to 15 months post graft, hence rejection can occur at any time during this period.

Stromal keratocytes persist indefinitely and are the antigenic stimulus for stromal rejection. They are replaced gradually over a period of years, (which explains why stromal dystrophies eventually recur in the graft) but some keratocytes persist. Hence, stromal rejection can potentially occur for the life of the graft. Endothelial cells are nonreplicatory and persist indefinitely.

Hence, rejection can occur at any time against this layer. Allogeneic graft rejection refers to a cell-mediated immune reaction directed against the corneal allograft. It is directed against major histocompatibility complex (MHC) alloantigens present on donor cells. Endothelial graft rejection is the most common type of rejection. Graft rejection generally refers to this unless specifically stated.

PREVENTION OF GRAFT REJECTION

Careful Case Selection

It has been demonstrated that there is little benefit with performing visual grafts for unilateral disease,[1] unless patient is motivated to wear a contact lens unilaterally to achieve the full visual benefit. This is especially the case in high-risk situations such as chemical burns and following herpes simplex keratitis. Even grafting for low-risk unilateral keratoconus has marginal benefit.

As such, it is always important to address the question of whether a patient really does require a corneal graft. Alternatively no surgery or some other surgery such as lens extraction in Down syndrome patients with a high degree of induced myopia may be more appropriate.

Identifying High-risk Corneal Grafts

The latest report from the Australian Corneal Graft Registry[1] has again demonstrated clearly that the occurrence of at least one corneal rejection episode significantly reduces the probability of corneal graft survival. The same report detected other major risk factors for graft failure:

- Inflammation before or at the time of grafting
- Recipient corneal neovascularization at the time of grafting, with the magnitude of risk proportional to the number of quadrants vascularized.
- History of raised intraocular pressure in the grafted eye
- Number of previously failed grafts

Postgraft events associated with graft failure were:

- Donor vascularization (inversely proportional to the vascularity[4])
- Number of rejection episodes
- Postoperative rise in intraocular pressure

The registry also demonstrated the indication for the graft influenced survival. The presence of glaucoma, trauma, past or current herpes simplex virus (HSV) infection, other infections such as acanthamoeba, bacteria, fungi, and corneal thinning all had negative effects on graft survival. Comparatively, grafts performed for keratoconus and corneal dystrophies had a better prognosis. Graft diameter also influenced survival with larger diameter grafts having higher rates of failure.[1] This is likely due to proximity of limbal blood vessels and higher numbers of antigenic Langerhans cells in the peripheral cornea.[2]

Topical Corticosteroids

Topical corticosteroids provide some prophylaxis against rejection, however, carry a risk of side effects such as raised intraocular pressure, cataract, and inhibition of wound healing. Many do not advocate lifelong corticosteroids for noninflammatory indications such as keratoconus, non-HSV corneal scars, or corneal dystrophies. Long-term infrequent (once or twice daily) corticosteroid drops should be considered in patients where there is a high risk of graft failure (past HSV, other infections, corneal ulcer, thinning, or previous graft failure) or where there has been more than one rejection episode.

Suture removal can often precipitate graft rejection. Frequent topical corticosteroid should therefore be given for 1 week post removal. Our institution uses prednisolone acetate or dexamethasone acetate four times per day for a period of 1 week.

Systemic Corticosteroid Sparing Immunosuppression

There is only limited evidence of increased graft survival with systemic cyclosporine A for high-risk grafts.[5] This finding has not been supported by other studies.[6] Despite this systemic immunosuppression, most commonly cyclosporine,[7] could be considered in high-risk grafts, particularly where the consequences of rejection and failure are high such as poor vision in the other eye.

Newer agents, such as tacrolimus and rapamycin have some evidence of a benefit,[4] with a low rate of systemic side-effects. Given the lipophilic nature of the compounds, these drugs achieve higher corneal penetration than cyclosporine A, with a similar mechanism of action.[4]

Tissue Matching

The matching of MHC and blood group antigens has also been examined in several major studies including the Collaborative Corneal Transplantation Studies (CCTS).[8] This failed to establish any benefit from matching for class 1 or class 2 antigens for high-risk grafts. Consequently, while matching of host and donor MHC antigens is widely practiced in other solid organ transplants, it is infrequently in ophthalmology. Most eye banks are not set up for this facility.

Interestingly, the CCTS did demonstrate a significant reduction in the frequency of allograft rejection in high-risk cases where the ABO blood group was matched. Despite this, matching for these antigens is not routinely performed in current clinical practice.

Antiviral Prophylaxis where there is a History of Herpes Simplex Virus Disease

Patients who have had a corneal graft with prior HSV corneal infection represent a group at particular risk of developing inflammation and subsequent rejection. This is not due to the high risk of recurrence of HSV, but rather the stromal vascularization that results from the disease process.[2]

Much of rationale for prophylactic antiviral therapy postcorneal grafts has been derived from studies of HSV stromal prophylaxis in populations with no history of corneal surgery. The Herpetic Eye Disease Study (HEDS)[9] demonstrated that acyclovir 400 mg twice daily provided a 45% reduction in the recurrence of HSV stromal disease. This benefit ceased when the acyclovir was stopped.

The morbidity from systemic antivirals therapy is low. Most patients with past HSV should therefore receive ongoing prophylactic dose systemic antivirals.

CLINICAL PRESENTATION

Symptoms

Graft rejection can present with any combination of the following symptoms: blurred vision, a red eye, pain, discomfort, irritation, and/or photophobia. Many episodes, however, are asymptomatic.[10] Rejection typically occurs in the first postoperative year.[11]

Rejection has typically been classified into three types: (1) epithelial, (2) stromal, and (3) endothelial.[3] A clinical rejection episode however, rarely fits discretely into one of these three entities. In many there is overlap with the presentation taking components from more than one type.

Signs

Epithelial rejection typically presents in the first year, on average 3 months post-surgery,[11] as a raised line of epithelium, staining with fluorescein or rose bengal. The line advances across the graft replacing donor with recipient epithelial cells leaving damaged cells in its wake (**Fig. 1**). This must not be confused with normal epithelial degenerative changes seen near the suture line in new corneal transplants due to alteration in tissue contour, known as Kaye's dots.[12]

Krachmer[13] described graft rejection manifesting as anterior stromal nummular inflammatory lesions in the donor, similar to those seen in epidemic keratoconjunctivitis (**Fig. 2**). Stromal rejection has been described in the New Zealand rabbit and is seen infrequently in humans as an isolated clinic entity. Most commonly, it is associated with endothelial rejection. Stromal rejection manifests as full-thickness corneal haze and circumcorneal hyperemia.

Endothelial rejection manifests as new keratic precipitates, either in a line (**Fig. 3**) or in diffusely arranged (**Fig. 4**). The first entity described by Khodadoust[3] is a line of keratic precipitates across the endothelium representing the advancing front of rejection. The line advances across the relatively healthy donor endothelium, leaving a wake of damaged donor endothelial cells and stromal swelling.

Alternatively, endothelial rejection can present as increased number of diffusely arranged keratic precipitates. A more diffuse stromal swelling ensues as endothelial cell density and function is diminished.

Numbers of keratic precipitates should therefore be followed closely, since increased numbers are likely to represent recent inflammation and probable graft rejection. Keratic precipitates with time become pigmented and develop sharper borders compared with the acute and fluffy edged precipitates associated with recent rejection.

Stromal swelling due to endothelial damage usually occurs with endothelial rejection although not in all cases.[14]

Modern portable, often handheld, pachymetry units allow corneal thickness to be measured accurately and quickly. Corneal thickness can be used as a marker for endothelial function. Serial pachymetry can be combined

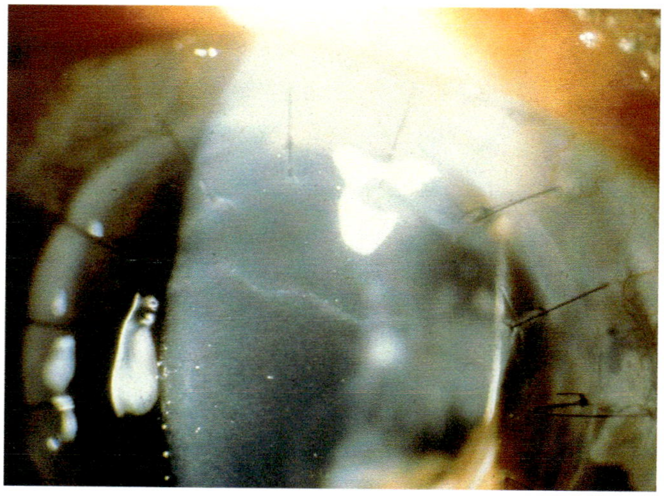

Fig. 1: Epithelial rejection.

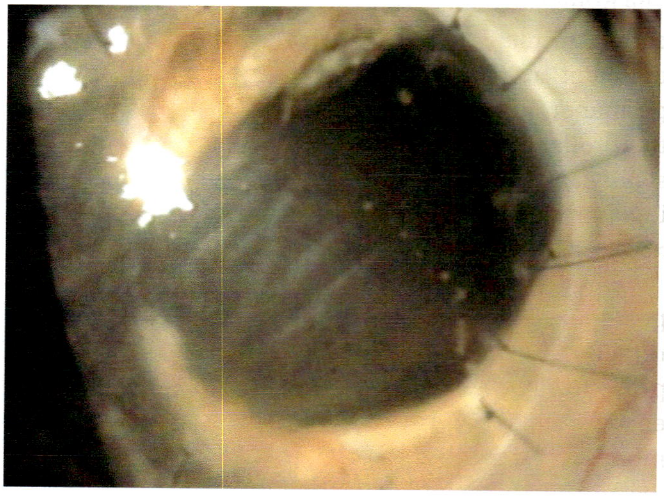

Fig. 3: Khodadoust endothelial rejection line.

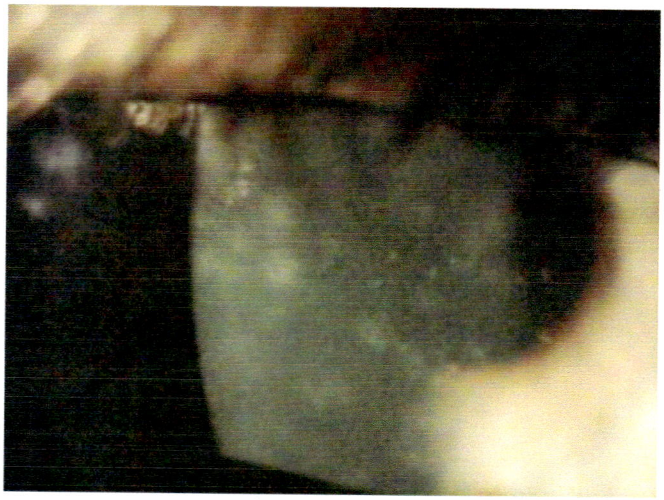

Fig. 2: Subepithelial infiltrates.

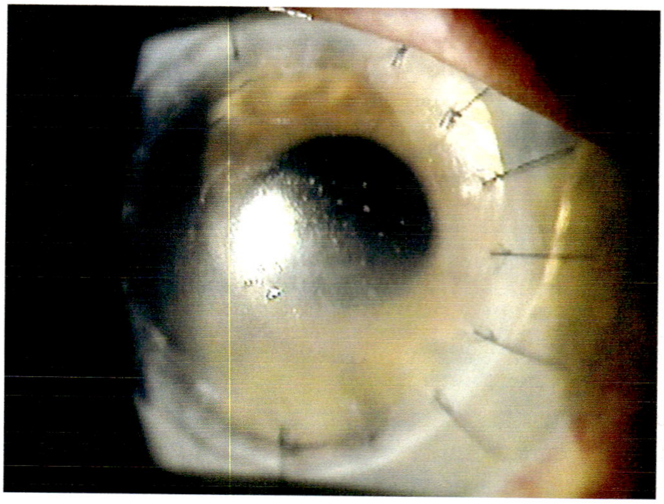

Fig. 4: Diffuse keratic precipitates in endothelial rejection.

with slit-lamp findings to improve the diagnostic accuracy of early graft rejection. Minor increases in thickness with increased keratic precipitates suggest low-grade rejection. Corneal pachymetry can also be used to provide an objective measure of resolution after an episode of graft rejection.

Endothelial rejection is usually accompanied by anterior chamber inflammation, ranging from a minimal to marked reaction and rarely, hypopyon.

Rejection in Subsequent Grafts after Graft Failure

It is important to note, rejection in recipients with a history of graft failure may appear differently to first-time grafts. The rejection may occur within the first 2 weeks of grafting due to a presensitized host and a second set of immune phenomena.[2] The rejection may involve the margin of the host bed, and a higher chance of graft failure exists despite adequate therapeutic measures.[2]

TREATMENT OF REJECTION

Early Recognition

The principle of successful management of graft rejection is early presentation, diagnosis, and prompt commencement of potent corticosteroid drops. Early treatment minimizes permanent endothelial cell loss and therefore improves the probability of graft clarity returning. Risk factors for significant endothelial cell loss include a delay in initiating antirejection treatment >24 hours, and recipient age >60 years.

Early diagnosis occurs through clear pre- and postoperative counseling regarding symptoms of graft rejection, emphasizing the importance of prompt presentation should they arise. Patients should be encouraged to have a low threshold for presenting. Acting promptly and presenting immediately to an ophthalmologist the same day as symptoms arise is extremely important. Any potential graft recipient needs to understand that the risk of rejection is lifelong. The ophthalmologist also needs to understand the implications for this in terms of accessibility to their patient.

Minimum Treatment for Allogeneic Graft Rejection

The minimum treatment for a rejection episode is topical corticosteroids drops. The corticosteroid should be combined with a lipophilic base vehicle such as an acetate allowing high corneal epithelial penetration. Examples are prednisolone acetate 1%, dexamethasone, or fluorometholone acetate.

The following is our institution's protocol for treatment of allogeneic corneal graft rejection: Prednisolone acetate 1% or dexamethasone hourly day and night for 2 days.

Where there is a clinical response, the drops can be tapered according to the following regime:

- Continue hourly during the day (8 am to 10 pm) and less frequently overnight for 2–5 days.
- Where frequent overnight drop administration is logistically difficult and the rejection episode is resolving, overnight drops can substituted with a corticosteroid ointment such as hydrocortisone acetate.
- The drops should be tapered to four times daily over a period of 1 month as the resolution process continues.

As discussed earlier, those at particular risk of further rejection, episodes should be considered for long-term infrequent (once or twice daily) corticosteroid drops.

Where there is no immediate clinical improvement, they should be continued frequently for at least 2–3 weeks.

Both epithelial and stromal rejection, while less common, are significant in that they can progress to endothelial rejection. In isolation, they are less significant clinically, and are unlikely to result in endothelial cell loss. Given the risk of concurrent or subsequent endothelial rejection, both conditions should still be treated aggressively.

Role of Oral Corticosteroids and Steroid Sparing Agents

Systemic corticosteroids such as oral prednisolone 1 mg/kg daily can be considered where the consequence of rejection progressing to failure is particularly significant, inflammation is severe or there is lack of response to initial therapy. For example, a patient experiencing a rejection episode in an "only eye" with previous grafts. The morbidity associated with systemic corticosteroids needs to be considered and balanced against limited evidence for their efficacy.

Intravenous pulsed administration of corticosteroids can be used as an alternative, with one dose on presentation, with another repeated after 48 hours.[2] The anti-inflammatory effect usually lasts 4–7 days, although this may confer no additional benefit over topical corticosteroids alone in patients without other risk factors for graft failure.[2]

Cyclosporine has relatively good T cell specificity. Topical preparations are limited in their ability to penetrate the cornea, and blood levels are negligible, however monitoring of renal and liver function is required. Our institution demonstrated no benefit in a randomized control trial of cyclosporine for treatment of acute allogeneic graft rejection. Other studies have found that topical cyclosporine treatment is effective in reduces the numbers of infiltrating T lymphocytes, thereby reducing the risk of allograft rejection in high-risk patients.[2]

Keratoconus and Allergic Eye Disease

Patients undergoing keratoplasty for keratoconus with a history of atopy rarely develop an aggressive sclerokeratitis up to 10 days postoperatively.[15] Sutures cheese wire through the graft, attract mucous and the donor moves anteriorly rarely dehiscing completely. These patients generally require high-dose oral prednisolone (1 mg/kg/day) and rarely oral cyclosporine.[16] The long-term prognosis for this condition is generally good once the acute episode has resolved.

REJECTION POST LAMELLAR KERATOPLASTY

Anterior lamellar keratoplasty involves transplantation of a donor anterior lenticule to a recipient posterior lamellar bed. The most common indications are keratoconus and anterior stromal opacities or dystrophies, where there is a healthy recipient endothelium. By maintaining the host's own endothelium, the risk of immune-mediated endothelial rejection is avoided, the most common and most significant type of rejection. Very good visual results have been demonstrated with this technique, almost comparable to penetrating keratoplasty.[17] Typical epithelial and stromal rejection have both been demonstrated in anterior lamellar transplantation, often the former progressing to the latter.[18] Treatment of these episodes is the same as for rejection post-penetrating keratoplasty.

In posterior lamellar keratoplasty, a posterior donor lenticule is transplanted onto the recipient after Descemet's membrane and endothelium stripping or lamellar dissection. Relatively low postoperative astigmatism, faster visual rehabilitation, and tectonic benefits are making this a more popular procedure for patients with endothelial dysfunction. Both stromal and endothelial rejection has been reported with this procedure.[19] The highest concentration of corneal stromal keratocytes is in the anterior stroma, decreasing posteriorly. Hence, less stromal tissue in the posterior lamellar keratoplasty is likely to lead to less rejection. Rejection rates have proven to be much lower than that after penetrating keratoplasty.[20]

DIFFERENTIAL DIAGNOSIS OF GRAFT REJECTION

The following diagnoses need to be considered:

Graft Failure

The absence of inflammation is the main sign distinguishing graft failure from rejection. Signs of inflammation can be subtle and easily missed. In some patients provisionally diagnosed with graft failure, stromal swelling resolves with treatment for rejection. As a general principle, patients diagnosed with graft failure should be given an empirical trial of rejection treatment. There should be a low threshold for initiating graft rejection treatment, particularly in the group with risk factors for rejection.

Loose Sutures and Secondary Microbial Keratitis

All loose sutures need to be removed immediately as they provide no tectonic function and if left, can precipitate graft rejection. Frequent topical corticosteroid should be used for at least 1 week after removal of any suture as prophylaxis against graft rejection. Where a loose suture is associated with inflammation, the clinician should have a low threshold for diagnosing early graft rejection and initiating frequent topical corticosteroids.

A loose suture associated with a stromal infiltrate or new stromal tissue loss (even in the absence of a "typical" infiltrate) should be assumed due to microbial keratitis. The suture should be sent for microbiological culture, a corneal scrape performed and hourly broad-spectrum antibiotic drops initiated for at least 48 hours. In principle, frequent topical corticosteroids should be used since treating the inflammation takes precedence over any small risk of promoting spread of the infection. Suture-related infections are usually due to gram-positive cocci. These generally do not respond adversely to topical corticosteroids.

Microbial Keratitis

Chronic low-grade infection such as infectious crystalline keratopathy or those caused by organisms such as *Candida*[21] can also present in a similar manner or even cause graft rejection. The organism could be either acquired, or where the graft indication was therapeutic, due to persistence. Inflammation in the graft in these scenarios could be due to infection. Such occult, chronic infections often respond badly to frequent corticosteroid drops.

Treatment involves the competing needs of adequate corticosteroid administration to treat the rejection episode, and resisting the use of high-dose corticosteroids, which may potentiate the infection.

The primary clinical goal is to adequately treat the infection, while protecting the graft long enough to minimize endothelial cell loss.

Herpes Simplex Virus Keratitis

This condition can be difficult to distinguish from allograft rejection. Keratic precipitates in HSV stromal disease are not confined to the graft unlike endothelial rejection. Additionally, virus reactivation can precipitate rejection and vice versa. Activation of HSV epithelial disease should be confirmed with laboratory testing. Polymerase chain reaction, where available, has a high sensitivity for HSV since small quantities of HSV antigen are amplified. Where a diagnosis of HSV has been made, the viral replication process can be treated with a therapeutic dose of antiviral medication, such as acyclovir 400 mg orally five times per day.

Graft inflammation where there is suspected or coexistent HSV should still be treated aggressively with frequent topical corticosteroids. The concern regarding activation of epithelial disease is less significant compared with ongoing graft inflammation. Oral acyclovir penetrates the tear film well and is as efficacious as topical acyclovir.

Herpes Zoster Virus Inflammation

Zoster-related graft inflammation causes stromal swelling and increase anterior chamber inflammation. Similar to HSV reaction, keratic precipitates should not confined to the donor. There is no evidence for use of prophylactic oral antivirals in patients with previous herpes zoster ophthalmicus.

Epithelial Downgrowth

An advancing wave of epithelial downgrowth can spread across the endothelial surface similar to the spread of an endothelial rejection line. When downgrowth spreads over the anterior surface of the iris, the condition is distinguished from endothelial rejection. Iris tissue blanching as a reaction to argon laser distinguishes this condition from fibrous downgrowth. Epithelial downgrowth has a poor prognosis, not responding to topical corticosteroids. Some newer modalities such as low-dose intracameral 5-fluorouracil may prove some benefit over aggressive surgical debridement, but are yet to be studied in vivo apart from case reports.

Postsurgical Inflammation

Postgraft patients having further surgery will usually develop inflammation, often quite intense, depending on the type of surgery. For example, cyclodiode laser for glaucoma often results in a strong postoperative inflammatory response. When used postkeratoplasty, the inflammation can be difficult to distinguish from graft rejection. Similarly, other types of postkeratoplasty surgery can precipitate graft rejection. The differential diagnosis of postoperative inflammation is therefore graft rejection. Inflammation of either cause needs to be treated with frequent topical corticosteroids.

PROGNOSIS

The most frequent complication of allograft rejection is failure. Inflammation from endothelial rejection results in endothelial cell loss. Where endothelial reserve is sufficient and treatment commenced promptly, rejection is reversed. Stromal swelling resolves, graft clarity returns, and a subjective improvement ensues. Where premorbid endothelial function was borderline at maintaining graft clarity, a relatively minor rejection episode can result in graft failure. Where treatment for a rejection episode is ineffective and the graft fails, there is no role for ongoing corticosteroids and they should be ceased.

REFERENCES

1. Williams KA, Keane MC, Coffey NE, Jones VJ, Mills RA, Coster DJ. The Australian Corneal Graft Registry 2018 Report. Adelaide, Australia: Department of Ophthalmology, Flinders University, South Australian Health and Medical Research Institute; 2018.
2. Bartels MC, Doxiadis II, Colen TP, Beekhuis WH. Long-term outcome in high-risk corneal transplantation and the influence of HLA-A and HLA-B matching. Cornea. 2003;22:552-6.
3. Khodadoust AA, Silverstein AM. Transplantation and rejection of individual cell layers of the cornea. Invest Ophthalmol. 1969;8:180-95.
4. Panda A, Vanathi M, Jumar A, Dash Y, Priya S. Corneal graft rejection. Surv Ophthalmol. 2007;52(4):375-96.
5. Hill JC. Systemic cyclosporine in high-risk keratoplasty. Short- versus long-term therapy. Ophthalmology. 1994;101(1):128-33.
6. Poon AC, Forbes JE, Dart JK, Subramaniam S, Bunce C, Madison P, et al. Systemic cyclosporin A in high risk penetrating keratoplasties: a case-control study. Br J Ophthalmol. 2001;85:1464-9.
7. Barker NH, Henderson TR, Ross CA, Coster DJ, Williams KA. Current Australian practice in the prevention and management of corneal allograft rejection. Clin Exp Ophthalmol. 2000;28:357-60.
8. The collaborative corneal transplantation studies (CCTS). Effectiveness of histocompatibility matching in high-risk corneal transplantation. The Collaborative Corneal Transplantation Studies Research Group. Arch Ophthalmol. 1992;110:1392-403.
9. Acyclovir for the prevention of recurrent herpes simplex virus eye disease. Herpetic Eye Disease Study Group. N Engl J Med. 1998;339:300-6.
10. Kamp MT, Fink NE, Enger C, Maguire MG, Stark WJ, Stulting RD. Patient-reported symptoms associated with graft reactions in high-risk patients in the collaborative corneal transplantation studies. Collaborative Corneal Transplantation Studies Research Group. Cornea. 1995;14:43-8.
11. Alldredge OC, Krachmer JH. Clinical types of corneal transplant rejection. Their manifestations, frequency, preoperative correlates, and treatment. Arch Ophthalmol. 1981;99:599-604.
12. Kaye DB. Epithelial response in penetrating keratoplasty. Am J Ophthalmol. 1980;89:381-7.
13. Krachmer JH, Alldredge OC. Subepithelial infiltrates: a probable sign of corneal transplant rejection. Arch Ophthalmol. 1978;96:2234-7.
14. McDonnell PJ, Enger C, Stark WJ, Stulting RD. Corneal thickness changes after high-risk penetrating keratoplasty. Collaborative Corneal Transplantation Study Group. Arch Ophthalmol. 1993;111:1374-81.
15. Lyons CJ, Dart JK, Aclimandos WA, Lightman S, Buckley RJ. Sclerokeratitis after keratoplasty in atopy. Ophthalmology. 1990;97:729-33.
16. Daniell MD, Dart JK, Lightman S. Use of cyclosporin in the treatment of steroid resistant post-keratoplasty atopic sclerokeratitis. Br J Ophthalmol. 2001;85:91-2.
17. Watson SL, Ramsay A, Dart JK, Bunce C, Craig E. Comparison of deep lamellar keratoplasty and penetrating keratoplasty in patients with keratoconus. Ophthalmology. 2004;111:1676-82.
18. Watson SL, Tuft SJ, Dart JK. Patterns of rejection after deep lamellar keratoplasty. Ophthalmology. 2006;113:556-60.
19. Terry MA, Wall JM, Hoar KL, Ousley PJ. A prospective study of endothelial cell loss during the 2 years after deep lamellar endothelial keratoplasty. Ophthalmology. 2007;114:631-9.
20. Allan BD, Terry MA, Price FW Jr, Price MO, Griffin NB, Claesson M. Corneal transplant rejection rate and severity after endothelial keratoplasty. Cornea. 2007;26(9):1039-42.
21. Morrison DA, Fahy GT, Brown LJ. Unsuspected infections crystalline keratopathy masquerading as corneal graft rejection. Br J Ophthalmol. 1997;81:608.

18 Surgical Management of Refractive Errors Following Corneal Transplantation

Haitham Al-Mahrouqi, Shokufeh Tavassoli, Mohammed Ziaei

INTRODUCTION

Since the first successful corneal graft in 1905 by Eduard Zirm,[1] corneal transplantation has evolved dramatically over the last century to include anterior and posterior lamellar keratoplasties to averse the problems associated with penetrating keratoplasty (PKP), including graft rejection or failure, ametropia, and suture-related complications.[2]

While a clear graft is achieved in most patients following keratoplasty, ametropia continues to be one of the most critical factors affecting the visual acuity of patients despite the significant advancement in instrumentation and surgical technique.[3] Ametropia is resultant from a mixture of lower and higher-order aberrations which occur after corneal transplantation. Lower-order aberrations (myopia, hypermetropia, and regular astigmatism) are important for the Snellen visual acuity; while higher-order aberrations (spherical aberration, coma, and secondary astigmatism) are important for subjective visual quality. Most patients needing corneal transplants usually have a significant preoperative reduction in Snellen visual acuity and are therefore happy to achieve good corrected distance visual acuity (CDVA). An exception to this is posterior lamellar keratoplasty for early Fuchs endothelial dystrophy.[4]

Following suture removal, the mean reported refractive astigmatism post-PKP is 3–5 diopters (D) with a mean myopic spherical equivalent (SE) of around 1–3 D.[5-8] Similar results have also been reported following deep anterior lamellar keratoplasty (DALK).[9,10]

The causes for ametropia following corneal transplantation are numerous and can be divided as preoperative, intraoperative, and postoperative (**Table 1**).[11]

PENETRATING VERSUS LAMELLAR KERATOPLASTY

A recent meta-analysis of 16 clinical studies involving 6,625 eyes with keratoconus (1,185 eyes in DALK group, and 5,440 eyes in PKP group) found that DALK and PKP had similar outcomes in terms of SE and astigmatism after 6 months.[9]

In contrast to anterior lamellar keratoplasty, endothelial keratoplasty results in very little refractive change. Early studies evaluating Descemet stripping automated endothelial keratoplasty (DSAEK) reported a slight hypermetropic shift of about 0.5–1 D.[12,13] However, with the recent advent of ultrathin DSAEK and Descemet membrane endothelial keratoplasty (DMEK), and the utilization of small and potentially self-sealing corneal/scleral incisions, virtually no change in refraction is induced.[14,15]

GENERAL APPROACH TO THE MANAGEMENT OF REFRACTIVE ERROR FOLLOWING KERATOPLASTY

A holistic approach is essential in correcting refractive error following corneal transplantation. First and foremost, it is vital to ascertain the needs of the patient. Older patients may not be medically fit or potentially less willing to undergo surgical intervention. In such cases, spectacles or contact lenses offer a safe and practical method of visual rehabilitation. If a surgical option is pursued, the potential CDVA in the operated and nonoperated eye, subjective refraction, corneal topography as well as ocular aberrometry need to be evaluated. Prior to suture removal, continuous suture adjustment and selective removal of sutures may be

Table 1: Factors associated with ametropia following corneal transplantation.

Preoperative factors	*Intraoperative factors*	*Postoperative factors*
• Shape of the donor and recipient corneas • Preexisting axial ametropia in recipient • Preexisting thinning, ectasia and scarring	• Decentered or abnormal trephination of donor/recipient • Graft diameter • Suturing technique	• Rejection • Scarring • Vascularization • Ectasia • Wound healing and dehiscence

tried. However, the effect may only be temporary as the overall refraction can change significantly when all the sutures are removed. After suture removal, orthogonal astigmatism, which is fully corrected with spectacles, is amenable to interventions such as compression sutures, arcuate keratotomy, or toric intraocular lenses (IOLs). Ametropia, which is not correctable with spectacles, normally infers the presence of irregular astigmatism and higher-order aberrations. Such patients typically would benefit from rigid gas permeable (RGP) contact lenses as well as topography or wavefront-guided excimer laser ablation in an attempt to regularize the cornea. Revision of the wound can be considered where there is wound misalignment or thinning. In the presence of very high levels of ametropia, significant irregular astigmatism, poor endothelial cell counts, or where there are clinical signs of graft failure, a repeat graft may be contemplated.

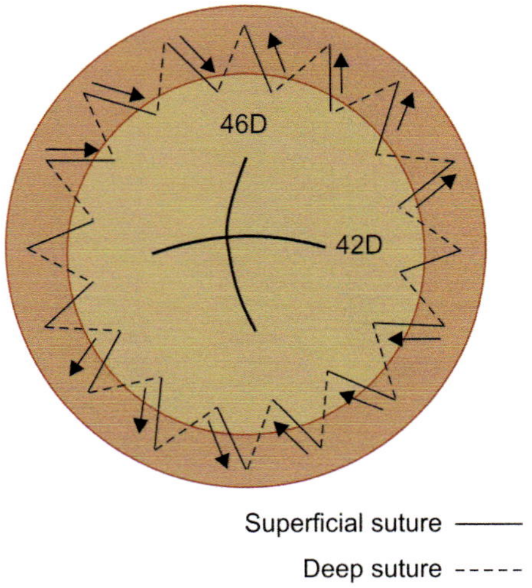

Fig. 1: Adjustment of running suture. The sutures are grasped from the exposed superficial arms in the flat meridian and pulled toward the steep meridian (vertical in this figure) to create a slack. This is done from all four quadrants as depicted by the arrows.

SURGICAL OPTIONS

Suture Adjustment and Selective Removal of Sutures

While the sutures are in place, running suture adjustment, and selective removal of sutures can be used to correct ametropia. Adjustment of running sutures was first described by Roper-Hall in 1982.[16] This method aims to control astigmatism in the early postoperative period up to 6 weeks in individuals with more than 3D of astigmatism.[17] After obtaining reliable corneal topography, keratometry, and manifest refraction, the running suture is loosened in the steep meridian and tightened in the flat meridian (**Fig. 1**).

Running suture adjustment has been reported to result in less postoperative astigmatism in the early postoperative period, fewer suture manipulations per patient, and faster visual rehabilitation.[18] The technique also has the advantage of being adjustable. The single running suture has also been reported to be superior to combined running and simple interrupted sutures for correcting postoperative astigmatism.[17] Adjusting astigmatism when there are only two running sutures is slightly more complex. The deeper and tighter suture should be removed.[19] If different calibers of sutures were used (i.e., 11-0 nylon and 10-0 nylon), then the larger caliber suture is typically removed.[20] Nevertheless, adjusting running sutures carries a small risk of suture breakage and possible post suture manipulation complications such as infectious keratitis, endothelial rejection, and possible endophthalmitis.

In the technique of simple interrupted suture removal, the sutures corresponding to the steep meridian are removed, resulting in flattening in that meridian and a coupled effect of steepening in the opposite meridian. Simple interrupted sutures can be removed as early as 2 months as long as only one suture is removed at a time.[21] Nonadjacent sutures can be removed after a follow-up period of 4–6 weeks.

Sequential selective same-day topography-guided suture removal has also been described and reported to be effective.[22] In this technique, sutures are removed after a period of at least 6 months following surgery, with sutures removed along the steep axis based on corneal topography. Topographic evaluation is repeated after 45 minutes, and the next set of sutures are removed. In a study involving 20 eyes, a net reduction in astigmatism of 50% was reported using vector analysis. Where there is agreement between refraction, keratometry, and topography, results of suture removal are more favorable.[23]

It should be noted that there is still no good evidence to date on the effect of selective suture removal in the early postoperative period on the final refractive outcome of patients following complete suture removal.

Astigmatic Keratotomy

Astigmatic keratotomies are either arcuate (**Figs. 2A and B**) or transverse. These are also sometimes called relaxing incisions. Arcuate incisions are superior to transverse incisions as they exert forces which are distributed equally on the optical zone. The incisions are typically carried out for large degrees of astigmatism, typically >6 D and are done at least 3 months after complete suture removal.[24] The incisions can be placed on the graft, graft-host junction, or the host with multiple nomograms such as the Hanna,[25] Nordan,[26] and more recently, the Saint-Clair nomogram[26] described.

Incisions placed in the host cornea are less effective as the scarring at the graft-host junction forms a "new limbus", making the optical effects of such incisions less pronounced. Incisions can be made up to 90% depth, based on preoperative pachymetric, tomographic, or optical coherence tomograph (OCT)-based thickness calculations; however, many surgeons aim for a depth of

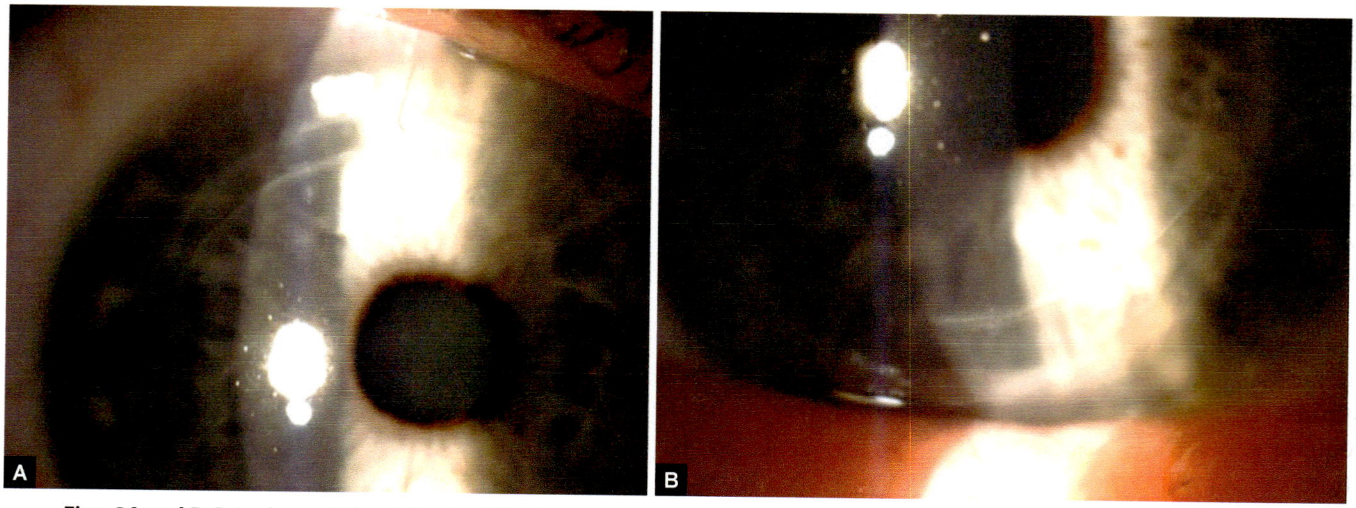

Figs. 2A and B: Paired arcuate keratotomies following penetrating keratoplasty (PKP) resulting in a 3.5 D reduction of astigmatism.

75–80% to avoid perforations. The effect is more prominent with central, paired, long, and deep incisions. Interestingly, increasing age and male sex are also associated with a more pronounced effect.[27] The incisions can be made manually using a diamond knife, the Hanna arcitome or using a femtosecond laser. The femtosecond laser provides the added advantage of more accurate incision depth planning with the use of intraoperative OCT, thus making decentration or perforations less likely.[28] The femtosecond laser has also been utilized to make intrastromal astigmatic keratotomies.[29] This technique has been reported to have reasonable outcomes and avoids an anterior wound, thus reducing the chance of infection, dehiscence, and epithelial ingrowth.[29]

The results of astigmatic keratotomy are best achieved when the astigmatism is orthogonal. This is because of the coupling effect where the relaxing incision flattens the steep meridian while also steepening the opposite flat meridian, thus preserving the overall SE.

A systematic review[24] of astigmatic keratotomy found that visual and refractive results were somewhat unpredictable due to the presence of a significant nonorthogonal astigmatism component in many postkeratoplasty patients as well as the diversity of nomograms used. Nevertheless, astigmatic keratotomies resulted in a 30–72% reduction in residual astigmatism, with most patients with ≥6 D of astigmatism corrected to ≤3 D, making them amenable to laser vision correction or IOL implantation.

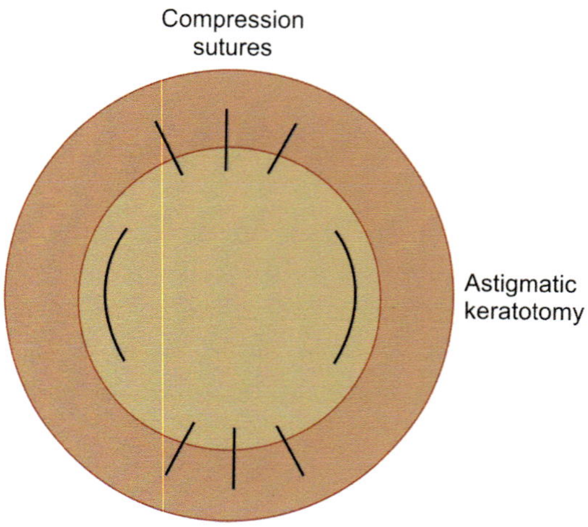

Fig. 3: The opposite placement of compression sutures from the astigmatic arcuate keratotomies.

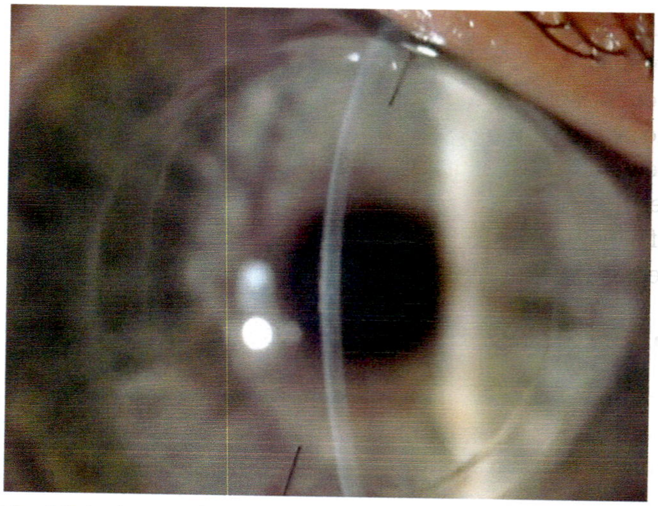

Fig. 4: Paired arcuate keratotomies with compression sutures following penetrating keratoplasty (PKP) resulting in a 8 D reduction in astigmatism.

Compression Sutures

Compression sutures are employed alone or with adjuvant astigmatic keratotomies in cases of high astigmatism, typically >6 D (**Figs. 3 and 4**).[30] Compression sutures alone usually correct low degrees of astigmatism and therefore are used when the astigmatism is in the region of 3–4 D.[31]

The effect is typically temporary and lasts until the suture loosens or is removed, although sutures can be left long term, especially in older patients. The result is accentuated when compression sutures are placed 90° away from astigmatic keratotomies, with the compression sutures placed on the flat meridian and astigmatic keratotomies on the steep meridian. Jacobi et al.[30] reported results on 25 eyes treated with astigmatic keratotomies and compression sutures. Mean astigmatism decreased from 11.7 ± 4.9 D preoperatively to 6.2 ± 2.7 D postoperatively, a net reduction of 47%. Others have reported up to two-thirds reduction in net astigmatism.[32] It must be noted that during surgery, a 50% overcorrection of the intended astigmatic correction is planned to counter the regression effect which takes place in the early postoperative period. To further refine results, surgery should be performed with the aid of intraoperative keratoscopy or topography. Postoperatively, the effect can be modified by the selective removal of the compression sutures. The suture material used in compression sutures requires attention. Nylon sutures have a higher tendency to stretch, loosen or break compared to Prolene or Mersilene sutures.[33,34] Nevertheless, Mersilene can be difficult to handle, leading to higher complications in the early postoperative period.[35] Overall, the results of compression sutures are difficult to predict and require significant expertise to tailor the effect accordingly.

Wedge Resection

Wedge resection is a subtractive surgical option used to correct extreme levels of astigmatism, typically over 10 D.[11] In this procedure, the flat meridian is identified, and the graft-host junction is opened down to Descemet membrane. A corneal wedge of 3 clock hours is excised from the graft or host tissue, and the two edges are then opposed with tight sutures initially aiming for an overcorrection of up to 50%.[11] It is believed that for every 0.1 mm excised, there is a reduction of 1–2 D.[36] Since this procedure is typically carried out for astigmatism of >10 D, a 0.5–1.0-mm wedge is typically excised. Not only width, but length, location, and depth of the excised wedge play a role in determining outcomes. Unfortunately, this procedure is highly surgeon-dependent and subsequently unpredictable, and there are no available nomograms to produce reproducible outcomes. Few studies in the literature, however, have shown promising results with a two-thirds or more reduction in the amount of astigmatism.[37,38] With high astigmatism, wedge resection seems to be a good alternative to regrafting.[39]

Revision of the Graft-host Junction

Revision of graft-host junction should always be considered where there is a significant misalignment of the donor and host tissue resulting in irregular and high astigmatism. In this procedure, the graft-host junction is opened down to Descemet membrane and resutured to achieve good alignment (**Fig. 5**). The use of preoperative and intraoperative OCT can help the surgeon determine the depth of dissection and avoid perforations. The predictability of this procedure is also poor, with potential complications such as intraoperative perforation, microbial keratitis, and rejection.

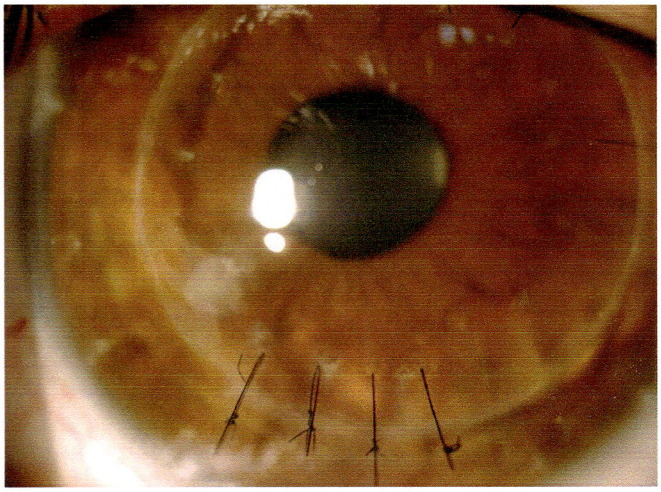

Fig. 5: Revision of graft-host junction. Astigmatism reduced from 14 to 5 D.

Refractive Surgery

Excimer Laser

The excimer laser has the potential to treat a range of keratoplasty-induced refractive error, including myopia, hyperopia, and astigmatism. The technology offers the corneal surgeon a unique opportunity to simultaneously correct refractive error and remove subepithelial fibrosis or scarring.[11,40]

Surface Ablation

Photorefractive keratectomy (PRK) and laser-assisted subepithelial keratectomy (LASEK) have been widely reported to treat refractive error following keratoplasty. Initial studies evaluating PRK, reported variable outcomes with a high incidence of regression, irregular astigmatism induction, corneal haze, and scarring.[41,42] Bilgihan et al. treated 16 patients with PRK and reported a 24% reduction in SE and a 42% reduction in manifest astigmatism but encountered late haze in 25% of patients with a resulting loss of final visual acuity.[43]

In an effort to reduce the incidence of haze, LASEK as an advanced surface ablation technique was attempted to improve outcomes, but Huan et al.[44] reported no difference in visual and refractive outcomes as well as haze formation between the two techniques. The use of mitomycin C (MMC) has been advocated as a means of modifying the corneal wound-healing response with good outcomes reported. Ward et al. reported an uncorrected distance visual acuity (UDVA) of 20/40 or better in 65% of patients after 0.02% MMC application for 12 seconds. The group also reported an 82% reduction in SE and a 41% reduction in astigmatism with no significant haze formation.[45]

More modern techniques such as transepithelial,[46] as well as topography[47] or wavefront-guided PRK[48] have also been reported in treating postkeratoplasty ametropia with good outcomes. Bizrah et al.[47] reported the outcome of 54 eyes undergoing topography-guided PRK with a mean follow-up of 31 months and demonstrated a mean astigmatism reduction of 55% with no cases of clinically significant haze but no improvement in CDVA was achieved.

Laser in situ Keratomileusis

Laser in situ keratomileusis (LASIK) seems to offer a lower risk for haze development in patients following keratoplasty as well as the ability to treat a larger degree of refractive error. LASIK in this clinical setting however, has a steep learning curve and can result in complications related to the lamellar flap creation and retention, particularly in corneas with poor endothelial function. Some authors recommend a two-staged procedure with the creation of a flap in the first instance followed by flap lift and excimer ablation 8–12 weeks later as it has been hypothesized that flap creation can induce a refractive error, requiring a change of treatment.[49]

Buzard et al.[9] reported the outcome of 26 eyes undergoing LASIK after corneal grafting and found a significant improvement in UDVA, a 93% reduction in SE and a 61% reduction in astigmatism. Hardten et al. also reported good outcomes but reported a higher rate of complications compared to virgin eyes, such as epithelial ingrowth (16%), loss of two or more lines of CDVA (7%), with 9% of treated patients requiring repeat keratoplasty.

Small incision lenticule extraction: In an effort to avoid flap-related complications associated with LASIK and perform a single-step surgical procedure, small incision lenticule extraction (SMILE), has been attempted in postkeratoplasty patients. Masoud et al. reported a vector analysis of 10 patients undergoing SMILE, demonstrating a mean astigmatism reduction at the intended axis of 67%, a correction index of 0.81 and a stable postoperative SE. The authors reported a high safety and efficacy index for the procedure and noted no intraoperative or postoperative complications.[50]

There are, however, reports of rejection as well as infectious keratitis following all forms of refractive surgery in postkeratoplasty patients.[43,51] Therefore, a course of prophylactic steroid and antibiotic therapy, as well as close monitoring of patients in the early postoperative period, is recommended following any graft manipulation to minimize the risk of such complications. Larger studies comparing PRK, LASIK, and SMILE are also required to further refine the case selection for each of the above refractive procedures in postkeratoplasty patients.

Intracorneal Ring Segments

Intracorneal ring segments (ICRSs) have been reported as a method to treat moderate to high degrees of postkeratoplasty astigmatism of up to 11 D.[52] Implantation of the ICRS can be performed using a manual mechanical technique or with a femtosecond laser.[52-54] ICRS implantation has several advantages over laser refractive surgery in the correction of postkeratoplasty astigmatism. There is relative sparing of the central visual axis of the cornea, thereby minimizing the potential risk of opacification caused by scarring of the visual axis. Furthermore, it is a reversible procedure; the ICRS can be explanted if the desired outcome is not achieved.[55]

In a study evaluating the clinical outcomes of ICRS (Ferrara ring; Ferrara ophthalmics Inc.) implantation in 59 post-PKP eyes of 54 patients, with corneal astigmatism ranging from 3 to 5 D, an improvement in CDVA and a decrease in refractive error was reported at 1 year review.[56] CDVA (logMAR) improved from 0.45 ± 0.17 to 0.30 ± 0.17 with 47.4% of the patients gaining two or more lines of CDVA. No patient lost visual acuity. SE improved from –6.34 ± 3.40 D preoperatively to –2.66 ± 2.52 D postoperatively. The mean corneal topographic astigmatism decreased from 3.37 ± 1.51 D preoperatively to 1.69 ± 1.04 D postoperatively. However, 47.5% of eyes remained with >3 D of refractive astigmatism.[56] ICRS implantation is also reported to be a useful option for the correction of astigmatism after DALK, with significant improvement in visual, topographic, and refractive results.[57]

To avoid the risk of graft-host dehiscence during manual stromal tunnel dissection, it is recommended to wait at least 2 years after PKP and at least a year after suture removal.[58,59] The use of the femtosecond laser is preferable to the mechanical technique in postkeratoplasty eyes, and may help minimize the risk of graft-host interface disruption.[55] No complications were reported in a study of 14 eyes with high astigmatism after PKP, implanted with ICRS (Keraring; Mediphacos, Inc.) by a femtosecond laser.[55]

In order to avoid close proximity of the ICRS to the graft-host junction, where the graft has a diameter of 7.5 mm or smaller, it is recommended to avoid using ICRS with a large optical zone (6.0 or 7.0 mm).[56] An ICRS with an optical zone of 5.0 mm is generally preferred in such cases to allow the ICRS to be further away from the graft-host junction, thereby minimizing the risk of interface dehiscence or vascularization.[56] One disadvantage of the smaller optical zone ICRS, however, is that they may induce greater optical phenomena such as glare and halos.[56] A nomogram for ICRS implantation with the femtosecond laser, proposed using two segments with a small apical diameter of 5 mm, for astigmatism up to 6 D and a larger apical diameter of 6 mm, for astigmatism >6 D.[52] A 90° arc was used for small errors and a 120° arc for the higher ones.[52] In a study of 32 eyes with previous PKP, ICRS (Keraring; Mediphacos, Inc.) implantation with femtosecond laser tunnel creation resulted in a CDVA of better than 20/40 in 96.9% of eyes and 20/25 or better in 56.2% of eyes, at 6 months postoperatively.[52] Furthermore,

SE and astigmatism components were significantly reduced after ICRS implantation.

Intraocular Procedures: Implantable Collamer Lens

Phakic IOLs (PIOLs) have been successfully used for the correction of both spherical and cylindrical refractive errors following corneal transplantation.[60-63] PIOLs, including the iris-fixated Artisan (Ophtec; Groningen, Netherlands) and Verisyse (Abbott Medical Optics; Santa Ana, CA, USA), and the posterior chamber sulcus-supported Visian implantable collamer lens (ICL; STAAR Surgical Company; Monrovia, CA, USA), can be used. These phakic lenses can treat higher degrees of refractive error; -3 to -20 D in the United States, and +3 to +12 D outside the United States, with up to 4 D of cylindrical error for the toric form of the ICL. In comparison to laser refractive surgery, PIOLs have a reduced potential for corneal haze, dry eye, and have the added benefit of being reversible (**Fig. 6**).[64]

The ICL (STAAR Surgical Company; Monrovia, CA, USA), in either the myopic or toric form, depending on the refractive error, was found to be effective in the correction of high ametropia (-2 to -17 D myopia, or -1.5 to -7 D astigmatism), in 15 eyes of 15 patients, 3.35 ± 2.34 years (mean ± SD) after PKP.[61] The Artisan or Artiflex toric PIOL (Ophtec; Groningen, Netherlands) was found to be effective for correcting high ametropia in 11 eyes of 11 patients after DALK, with good stability over a minimum 3-year follow-up period.[63] There are, however, concerns of increased endothelial cell loss with PIOL use in postkeratoplasty eyes.[63] For the ICL, the rate of endothelial cell loss was reported as 8.1% at 24 months in post-PKP eyes.[63] For the Artisan lens, the endothelial cell loss reported was 8.7% at 1 year in post-DALK eyes.[63] In eyes with corneal transplantation, the endothelial cell loss rate is reported to be 7.8% per year at 3–5 years[65] and approximately 4.2% at 5–10 years,[66] in comparison to the reported rate of approximately 0.5% per year loss in normal corneas without any prior surgery.[65] A further concern may be cataract formation, although this was not identified at 24-month follow-up with the ICL in post-PKP eyes.[61] Thus, PIOLs may be considered for younger patients with a clear lens. However, the potential need for cataract surgery in the future and the risk of graft failure should be discussed with the patient.

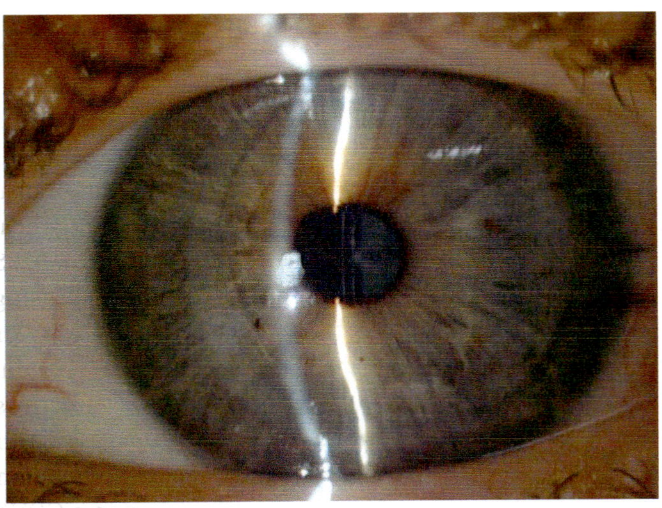

Fig. 6: Implantable collamer lens (ICL) implantation to correct 4 D of myopia and 6 D of astigmatism in a patient following penetrating keratoplasty (PKP).

Intraocular Procedures: Clear Lens Extraction/Cataract Surgery

Cataract extraction, in the presence of a cataract, or clear lens extraction, in the absence of a cataract, may be considered in the management of post-transplant astigmatism in cases where the cornea graft is otherwise clear.[67,68] When the cataract extraction is combined with corneal transplantation as a "triple" procedure, a spherical IOL should be used. However, when performing lens based surgery at a later stage, correction of any residual astigmatism can be achieved through the use of a toric IOL alone[69] or in combination with AK.[70] If performing AK, a staged approach is recommended; first performing the AK followed by cataract surgery at a later date, to ensure accurate IOL power calculation.[70] Cataract surgery should be performed once all sutures are removed and the refraction is stable for at least 4–6 months. Direct keratometry (K) readings can be obtained from tomography, and compared to that from the biometer, to optimize IOL power calculations. It is recommended to use low-energy phacoemulsification settings, along with generous amounts of dispersive viscoelastic to protect the endothelium during surgery.[71] In a study of 26 eyes with prior PKP, the post-operative mean endothelial cell density reported at 6-months following cataract surgery was found to be significantly lower with phacoemulsification compared to extracapsular cataract extraction.[71] Thus, extracapsular cataract extraction may be preferable if the cataract is dense to help protect the endothelial cells, particularly if preoperative endothelial cell counts are already compromised.[71] Preoperative specular microscopy is considered helpful in the surgical planning of such cases.

In a study of 21 eyes of PKP patients with residual astigmatic error, phacoemulsification with implantation of a toric IOL resulted in a UDVA of 20/30 or better in 67% of eyes (CDVA of 20/30 or better in 90% of eyes) and a predicted postoperative manifest astigmatism within 1 D or better in 76.2% of eyes.[67] No IOL repositioning or explantation was required. One patient underwent LASIK after toric IOL implantation to correct a large increase in corneal astigmatism following cataract surgery. The use of a toric IOL to treat residual astigmatism in post-DALK eyes undergoing phacoemulsification has also been reported.[68] In 10 eyes, 1 month after phacoemulsification, all had a UDVA and CDVA of ≥20/40 and ≥20/25 respectively, with a residual SE of

0.00 ± 0.84 D.[68] There was good rotational stability 1 month after implantation, reported as 1.8 ± 1.5° rotation from the intended position. Endothelial cell loss was reported as 5.8 ± 1.8% at 1-year follow-up. Thus, toric IOL implantation may be considered in the management of postgraft astigmatism.[72] Prior to undertaking cataract extraction, patients should be consented for the risk of graft failure, as well as the potential need for further refractive correction postoperatively. The potential risk of postoperative toric IOL rotation should also be discussed with the patient.[73,74]

Regraft

A regraft may be the optimal approach if there is high residual astigmatism.[53] In particular, for cases where the graft is edematous or has failed, or in older grafts that may have historically been of smaller diameter. In such cases, the regraft would require trephination of the cornea with a larger size than the original graft, and the transplantation of a larger diameter graft.

CONCLUSION

Despite significant advancements in the field of corneal transplantation, ametropia remains a significant barrier toward visual rehabilitation of patients. Optimizing visual outcomes requires a customized approach which begins at the preoperative assessment stage and continues through surgical techniques and postoperative management of the graft. Multiple techniques are available to minimize astigmatism levels following surgery and a typical approach involves optical correction followed by a stepladder approach of increasing levels of invasive surgery. Modern techniques such as topography or wavefront-guided excimer ablations, femtosecond-assisted astigmatic keratotomies as well as astigmatic correcting IOLs provide the surgeon with an excellent breadth of choice in the visual rehabilitation process.

REFERENCES

1. Zirm E. Eine erfolgreiche totale Keratoplastik. Graefes Arch Ophthalmol. 1906;64:580-93.
2. Arenas E, Esquenazi S, Anwar M, Terry M. Lamellar corneal transplantation. Surv Ophthalmol. 2012;57(6):510-29.
3. Williams KA, Keane MC, Coffey NE, Jones VJ, Mills RA, Coster DJ. The Australian Corneal Graft Registry 2018 Report. Australia; South Australian Health and Medical Research Institute; 2018. [online]. Available from https://dspace.flinders.edu.au/xmlui/handle/2328/37917 [Last accessed December, 2021].
4. van der Meulen IJ, Patel SV, Lapid-Gortzak R, Nieuwendaal CP, McLaren JW, van den Berg TJ. Quality of vision in patients with fuchs endothelial dystrophy and after descemet stripping endothelial keratoplasty. Arch Ophthalmol. 2011;129(12):1537-42.
5. Troutman RC, Lawless MA. Penetrating keratoplasty for keratoconus. Cornea. 1987;6(4):298-305.
6. Olson RJ, Pingree M, Ridges R, Lundergan ML, Alldredge C Jr., Clinch TE. Penetrating keratoplasty for keratoconus: a long-term review of results and complications. J Cataract Refract Surg. 2000;26(7):987-91.
7. Sutton G, Hodge C, McGhee CN. Rapid visual recovery after penetrating keratoplasty for keratoconus. Clin Exp Ophthalmol. 2008;36(8):725-30.
8. Kirkness CM, Ficker LA, Steele AD, Rice NS. The success of penetrating keratoplasty for keratoconus. Eye (Lond). 1990;4(Pt 5):673-88.
9. Liu H, Chen Y, Wang P, Li B, Wang W, Su Y, et al. Efficacy and safety of deep anterior lamellar keratoplasty vs. penetrating keratoplasty for keratoconus: a meta-analysis. PLoS One. 2015;10(1):e0113332.
10. Keane M, Coster D, Ziaei M, Williams K. Deep anterior lamellar keratoplasty versus penetrating keratoplasty for treating keratoconus. Cochrane Database Syst Rev. 2014;(7):CD009700.
11. Fares U, Sarhan AR, Dua HS. Management of post-keratoplasty astigmatism. J Cataract Refract Surg. 2012;38(11):2029-39.
12. Price MO, Price FW Jr. Descemet's stripping with endothelial keratoplasty: comparative outcomes with microkeratome-dissected and manually dissected donor tissue. Ophthalmology. 2006;113(11):1936-42.
13. Koenig SB, Covert DJ. Early results of small-incision Descemet's stripping and automated endothelial keratoplasty. Ophthalmology. 2007;114(2):221-6.
14. Agha B, Ahmad N, Dawson DG, Kohnen T, Schmack I. Refractive outcome and tomographic changes after Descemet membrane endothelial keratoplasty in pseudophakic eyes with Fuchs' endothelial dystrophy. Int Ophthalmol. 2021;41(8):2897-904.
15. Mencucci R, Favuzza E, Marziali E, Cennamo M, Mazzotta C, Lucenteforte E, et al. Ultrathin Descemet stripping automated endothelial keratoplasty versus Descemet membrane endothelial keratoplasty: a fellow-eye comparison. Eye Vis (Lond). 2020;7:25.
16. Roper-Hall MJ. Control of astigmatism after surgery and trauma. Br J Ophthalmol. 1982;66(9):556-9.
17. Filatov V, Steinert RF, Talamo JH. Postkeratoplasty astigmatism with single running suture or interrupted sutures. Am J Ophthalmol. 1993;115(6):715-21.
18. Van Meter WS, Gussler JR, Soloman KD, Wood TO. Postkeratoplasty astigmatism control. Single continuous suture adjustment versus selective interrupted suture removal. Ophthalmology. 1991;98(2):177-83.
19. McNeill JI, Kaufman HE. A double running suture technique for keratoplasty: earlier visual rehabilitation. Ophthalmic Surg. 1977;8(4):58-61.
20. Young SR, Olson RJ. Results of a double running suture in penetrating keratoplasty performed on keratoconus patients. Ophthalmic Surg. 1985;16(12):779-86.
21. Feizi S, Zare M. Current Approaches for management of postpenetrating keratoplasty astigmatism. J Ophthalmol. 2011;2011:708736.
22. Fares U, Mokashi AA, Elalfy MS, Dua HS. Sequential selective same-day suture removal in the management of post-keratoplasty astigmatism. Eye (Lond). 2013;27(9):1032-7.
23. Sarhan AR, Dua HS, Beach M. Effect of disagreement between refractive, keratometric, and topographic determination of astigmatic axis on suture removal after penetrating keratoplasty. Br J Ophthalmol. 2000;84(8):837-41.
24. Ho Wang Yin G, Hoffart L. Post-keratoplasty astigmatism management by relaxing incisions: a systematic review. Eye Vis (Lond). 2017;4:29.
25. Hanna KD, Hayward JM, Hagen KB, Simon G, Parel JM, Waring GO 3rd. Keratotomy for astigmatism using an arcuate keratome. Arch Ophthalmol. 1993;111(7):998-1004.
26. Nordan LT. Quantifiable astigmatism correction: concepts and suggestions, 1986. J Cataract Refract Surg. 1986;12(5):507-18.
27. Price FW, Grene RB, Marks RG, Gonzales JS. Astigmatism reduction clinical trial: a multicenter prospective evaluation of the predictability of arcuate keratotomy. Evaluation of surgical

nomogram predictability. ARC-T Study Group. Arch Ophthalmol. 1995;113(3):277-82.

28. Hoffart L, Proust H, Matonti F, Conrath J, Ridings B. Correction of postkeratoplasty astigmatism by femtosecond laser compared with mechanized astigmatic keratotomy. Am J Ophthalmol. 2009;147(5):779-87, 787.e1.
29. Wetterstrand O, Holopainen JM, Krootila K. Treatment of postoperative keratoplasty astigmatism using femtosecond laser-assisted intrastromal relaxing incisions. J Refract Surg. 2013;29(6):378-82.
30. Jacobi PC, Hartmann C, Severin M, Bartz-Schmidt KU. Relaxing incisions with compression sutures for control of astigmatism after penetrating keratoplasty. Graefes Arch Clin Exp Ophthalmol. 1994;232(9):527-32.
31. Limberg MB, Dingeldein SA, Green MT, Klyce SD, Insler MS, Kaufman HE. Corneal Compression Sutures for the Reduction of Astigmatism After Penetrating Keratoplasty. Am J Ophthalmol. 1989;108(1):36-42.
32. Mandel MR, Shapiro MB, Krachmer JH. Relaxing incisions with augmentation sutures for the correction of postkeratoplasty astigmatism. Am J Ophthalmol. 1987;103(3 Pt 2):441-7.
33. Bartels MC, van Rooij J, Geerards AJ, Mulder PG, Remeijer L. Comparison of complication rates and postoperative astigmatism between nylon and mersilene sutures for corneal transplants in patients with Fuchs endothelial dystrophy. Cornea. 2006;25(5):533-9.
34. Gimbel HV, Raanan MG, DeLuca M. Effect of suture material on postoperative astigmatism. J Cataract Refract Surg. 1992;18(1):42-50.
35. Bertram BA, Drews-Botsch C, Gemmill M, Guell J, Murad M, Waring GO 3rd. Complications of Mersilene sutures in penetrating keratoplasty. Refract Corneal Surg. 1992;8(4):296-305.
36. Hardten DR, Lindstrom RL. Surgical correction of refractive errors after penetrating keratoplasty. Int Ophthalmol Clin. 1997;37(1):1-35.
37. Mejía LF, Gil JC, Naranjo S. Long-term results of corneal wedge resection for high postkeratoplasty astigmatism. Cornea. 2020;39(5):535-9.
38. Ezra DG, Hay-Smith G, Mearza A, Falcon MG. Corneal wedge excision in the treatment of high astigmatism after penetrating keratoplasty. Cornea. 2007;26(7):819-25.
39. Ilari L, Daya SM. Corneal wedge resection to treat progressive keratoconus in the host cornea after penetrating keratoplasty. J Cataract Refract Surg. 2003;29(2):395-401.
40. Alio JL, Abdou AA, Abdelghany AA, Zein G. Refractive surgery following corneal graft. Curr Opin Ophthalmol. 2015;26(4):278-87.
41. Amm M, Duncker GI, Schroder E. Excimer laser correction of high astigmatism after keratoplasty. J Cataract Refract Surg. 1996;22(3):313-7.
42. Deschenes J, Jovkar S, Balazsi G, Thompson P. Photorefractive keratectomy for correction of astigmatism after penetrating keratoplasty. Int Ophthalmol Clin. 1996;36(4):113-8.
43. Bilgihan K, Ozdek SC, Akata F, Hasanreisoglu B. Photorefractive keratectomy for post-penetrating keratoplasty myopia and astigmatism. J Cataract Refract Surg. 2000;26(11):1590-5.
44. Huang PY, Huang PT, Astle WF, Ingram AD, Hèbert A, Huang J, et al. Laser-assisted subepithelial keratectomy and photorefractive keratectomy for post-penetrating keratoplasty myopia and astigmatism in adults. J Cataract Refract Surg. 2011;37(2):335-40.
45. Ward MS, Wandling GR, Goins KM, Sutphin JE, Kitzmann AS, Wagoner MD. Photorefractive keratectomy modification of postkeratoplasty anisometropic refractive errors. Cornea. 2013;32(3):273-9.
46. Spadea L, Visioli G, Mastromarino D, Alexander S, Pistella S. Topography-guided trans-epithelial no-touch photorefractive keratectomy for high irregular astigmatism after penetrating keratoplasty: A prospective 12-months follow-up. Ther Clin Risk Manag. 2021;17:1027-35.
47. Bizrah M, Lin DTC, Babili A, Wirth MA, Arba-Mosquera S, Holland SP. Topography-guided photorefractive keratectomy for postkeratoplasty astigmatism: long-term outcomes. Cornea. 2021;40(1):78-87.
48. Sorkin N, Kreimei M, Einan-Lifshitz A, Mednick Z, Belkin A, Chan CC, et al. Wavefront-guided photorefractive keratectomy in the treatment of high astigmatism following keratoplasty. Cornea. 2019;38(3):285-9.
49. Alio JL, Javaloy J, Osman AA, Galvis V, Tello A, Haroun HE. Laser in situ keratomileusis to correct post-keratoplasty astigmatism; 1-step versus 2-step procedure. J Cataract Refract Surg. 2004;30(11):2303-10.
50. Massoud TH, Ibrahim O, Shehata K, Abdalla MF. Small Incision Lenticule Extraction for Postkeratoplasty Myopia and Astigmatism. J Ophthalmol. 2016;2016:3686380.
51. Hashemi H, Aghamirsalim M, Asgari S. Stromal Rejection After SMILE for the Correction of Astigmatism After Graft. J Refract Surg. 2019;35(11):737-9.
52. Lisa C, Garcia-Fernandez M, Madrid-Costa D, Torquetti L, Merayo-Lloves J, Alfonso JF. Femtosecond laser-assisted intrastromal corneal ring segment implantation for high astigmatism correction after penetrating keratoplasty. J Cataract Refract Surg. 2013;39(11):1660-7.
53. Ahmadi M, Javadi MA. Corneal regrafts for correction of post-keratoplasty anisometropia and high astigmatism in two patients with keratoconus. Bina J Ophthalmol. 2005;10(2): 236-41.
54. Ziaei M, Barsam A, Shamie N, Vroman D, Kim T, Donnenfeld ED, et al. Reshaping procedures for the surgical management of corneal ectasia. J Cataract Refract Surg. 2015;41(4):842-72.
55. Prazeres TM, Souza AC, Pereira NC, Ursulino F, Grupenmacher L, de Souza LB. Intrastromal corneal ring segment implantation by femtosecond laser for the correction of residual astigmatism after penetrating keratoplasty. Cornea. 2011;30(12):1293-7.
56. Coscarelli S, Ferrara G, Alfonso JF, Ferrara P, Merayo-Lloves J, Araújo LP, et al. Intrastromal corneal ring segment implantation to correct astigmatism after penetrating keratoplasty. J Cataract Refract Surg. 2012;38(6):1006-13.
57. Arantes JCD, Coscarelli S, Ferrara P, Araújo LPN, Avila M, Torquetti L. Intrastromal Corneal Ring Segments for Astigmatism Correction after Deep Anterior Lamellar Keratoplasty. J Ophthalmol. 2017;2017:8689017.
58. Arriola-Villalobos P, Diaz-Valle D, Güell JL, Iradier-Urrutia MT, Jiménez-Alfaro I, Cuiña-Sardiña R, et al. Intrastromal corneal ring segment implantation for high astigmatism after penetrating keratoplasty. J Cataract Refract Surg. 2009;35(11):1878-84.
59. Ziaei M, Vellara HR, Gokul A, Ali NQ, McGhee CNJ, Patel DV. Comparison of corneal biomechanical properties following penetrating keratoplasty and deep anterior lamellar keratoplasty for keratoconus. Clin Exp Ophthalmol. 2020;48(2):174-82.
60. Park JC, Mundasad MV, Tole DM. Piggyback intraocular lens implant to correct severe refractive error after penetrating keratoplasty in pseudophakes. Br J Ophthalmol. 2009;93(2):272.
61. Alfonso JF, Lisa C, Abdelhamid A, Montes-Mico R, Poo-Lopez A, Ferrer-Blasco T. Posterior chamber phakic intraocular lenses after penetrating keratoplasty. J Cataract Refract Surg. 2009;35(7):1166-73.
62. Tiveron MC Jr, Alió Del Barrio JL, Kara-Junior N, Plaza-Puche AB, Abu-Mustafa SK, Zein G, et al. Outcomes of toric Iris-claw phakic intraocular lens implantation after deep anterior lamellar keratoplasty for keratoconus. J Refract Surg. 2017;33(8): 538-44.
63. Malheiro L, Coelho J, Neves MM, Gomes M, Oliveira L. Phakic intraocular lens implantation after deep anterior lamellar keratoplasty: Retrospective case series analysis with long-term follow-up. Clin Ophthalmol. 2019;13:2043-52.

64. Kohnen T, Kook D, Morral M, Guell JL. Phakic intraocular lenses: part 2: results and complications. J Cataract Refract Surg. 2010;36(12):2168-94.
65. Bourne WM, Hodge DO, Nelson LR. Corneal endothelium five years after transplantation. Am J Ophthalmol. 1994;118(2):185-96.
66. Ing JJ, Ing HH, Nelson LR, Hodge DO, Bourne WM. Ten-year postoperative results of penetrating keratoplasty. Ophthalmology. 1998;105(10):1855-65.
67. Wade M, Steinert RF, Garg S, Farid M, Gaster R. Results of toric intraocular lenses for post-penetrating keratoplasty astigmatism. Ophthalmology. 2014;121(3):771-7.
68. Scorcia V, Lucisano A, Savoca Corona V, De Luca V, Carnevali A, Busin M. Deep anterior lamellar keratoplasty followed by toric lens implantation for the treatment of concomitant anterior stromal diseases and cataract. Ophthalmology @ Point of Care. 2017;1(1):oapoc.0000008.
69. Srinivasan S, Ting DS, Lyall DA. Implantation of a customized toric intraocular lens for correction of post-keratoplasty astigmatism. Eye (Lond). 2013;27(4):531-7.
70. Feizi S, Javadi MA. Corneal graft curvature change after relaxing incisions for post-penetrating keratoplasty astigmatism. Cornea. 2012;31(9):1023-7.
71. Acar BT, Buttanri IB, Sevim MS, Acar S. Corneal endothelial cell loss in post-penetrating keratoplasty patients after cataract surgery: phacoemulsification versus planned extracapsular cataract extraction. J Cataract Refract Surg. 2011;37(8):1512-6.
72. Lockington D, Wang EF, Patel DV, Moore SP, McGhee CN. Effectiveness of cataract phacoemulsification with toric intraocular lenses in addressing astigmatism after keratoplasty. J Cataract Refract Surg. 2014;40(12):2044-9.
73. Meyer JJ, Kim BZ, Ziaei M, McGhee CN. Postoperative rotation of supplementary sulcus-supported toric intraocular lenses. J Cataract Refract Surg. 2017;43(2):285-8.
74. Ziaei M, Meyer JJ, Patel DV, McGhee CN. Scleral suture fixation of supplementary sulcus-based toric intraocular lenses to prevent rotational instability. Clin Exp Ophthalmol. 2018;46(5):570-3.

SECTION 4

Lamellar Keratoplasty

A: Anterior Lamellar Keratoplasty Techniques

- **Surgical Instruments for Lamellar Keratoplasty**
  Namrata Sharma, Sohini Mandal, Prakash Chand Agarwal, Rasik B Vajpayee
- **"Dry" Manual Technique for Deep Anterior Lamellar Keratoplasty**
  Paolo Rama, Karl Anders Knutsson
- **Automated Lamellar Therapeutic Keratoplasty**
  Namrata Sharma, Sohini Mandal, Ritu Nagpal, Sameer Kaushal
- **Superficial Anterior Lamellar Keratoplasty**
  Giuseppe Giannaccare, Angeli Christy Yu, Massimo Busin
- **Deep Anterior Lamellar Keratoplasty: The Melles Technique**
  Keamela Vasanthananthan, C Maya Tong, Gerrit RJ Melles
- **Deep Anterior Lamellar Keratoplasty: Big Bubble Technique**
  Luigi Fontana, Antonio Moramarco
- **Deep Anterior Lamellar Keratoplasty: Double Bubble Technique**
  Vishal Jhanji, Ritu Nagpal, Sarath S, Namrata Sharma, Rasik B Vajpayee
- **Large-diameter Deep Anterior Lamellar Keratoplasty**
  Angeli Christy Yu, Asaf Friehmann, Massimo Busin
- **Cannula-assisted Big Bubble Deep Anterior Lamellar Keratoplasty**
  Rajesh Fogla
- **"Groove and Peel" Deep Anterior Lamellar Keratoplasty**
  Rishi Swarup
- **Diamond Knife-assisted Deep Anterior Lamellar Keratoplasty**
  Sri Vatsa Sehra, Prafulla K Maharana, Elsie Chan, Namrata Sharma, Rasik B Vajpayee
- **"Tuck in" Lamellar Keratoplasty**
  Namrata Sharma, Vishal Jhanji, Sohini Mandal, Rahul Kumar Bafna, Rasik B Vajpayee

B: Endothelial Keratoplasty Techniques

- **Surgical Instruments for Endothelial Keratoplasty**
  Priyadarshini K, Ritu Nagpal, Namrata Sharma, Rasik B Vajpayee
- **Descemet's Stripping Automated Endothelial Keratoplasty**
  Marianne O Price, Sohini Mandal, Francis W Price Jr
- **Thin Lenticule Descemet's Stripping Automated Endothelial Keratoplasty**
  Prabhakar Singh, Sohini Mandal, Namrata Sharma
- **Ultrathin Descemet Stripping Automated Endothelial Keratoplasty**
  Angeli Christy Yu, Asaf Friehmann, Massimo Busin
- **Manual DSEK: "Manual Dissection" Technique of Descemet Stripping Endothelial Keratoplasty**
  Samar K Basak, Soham Basak
- **Pre-Descemet's Endothelial Keratoplasty**
  Amar Agarwal
- **Tectonic Descemet Stripping Automated Endothelial Keratoplasty**
  Vincenzo Scorcia, Angeli Christy Yu, Massimo Busin
- **Descemet's Stripping Automated Endothelial Keratoplasty: Triple Procedure**
  Vishal Jhanji, Sarath S, Ritu Nagpal, Rasik B Vajpayee
- **Descemet's Membrane Endothelial Keratoplasty**
  Denisse Pinkus, Marianne O Price, Francis W Price Jr

19

Surgical Instruments for Lamellar Keratoplasty

Namrata Sharma, Sohini Mandal, Prakash Chand Agarwal, Rasik B Vajpayee

INTRODUCTION

The instruments required for lamellar keratoplasty are used to dissect the donor cornea as well as the recipient bed.

INSTRUMENTS FOR GLOBE EXPOSURE

Eye Speculum

It should be lightweight with minimum extraneous parts to avoid undue pressure on the globe. A wire lid speculum such as Barraquer eye speculum is ideal for most cases (**Fig. 1**). The ones that are used in children are of small size that tend to offer less resistance to compression.

Globe Supporting Rings

The Flieringa ring (**Fig. 2**) is made of stainless steel and is useful in maintaining the architecture of the globe after removal of the host button. The most commonly used sizes are 17 and 18 mm. They are advocated in aphakic, vitrectomized eyes, pseudophakic, and pediatric eyes as the eyeball has a tendency to collapse in these cases after trephination.

McNeill-Goldman ring provides support with four strategically placed sutures. It has two inbuilt lid retractors to prevent lid closure during surgery and medial and temporal openings for greater access to surgical field (**Fig. 3**).

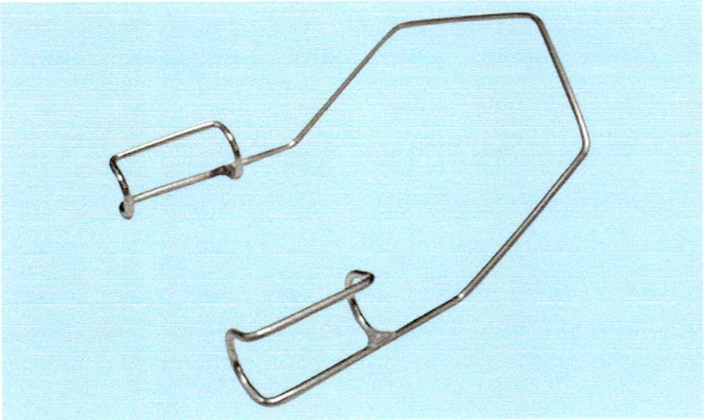

Fig. 1: Universal metallic wire speculum.

INSTRUMENTS FOR RECIPIENT CORNEA DISSECTION

Corneal Trephines

A trephine is a stainless sharp cylindrical blade which is used to create a circular corneal incision. An ideal trephine is one that produces a sharp vertical cut without causing too much damage to the corneal tissues.

- *Handheld disposable trephine*: These are the most commonly used trephine to cut both the donor and

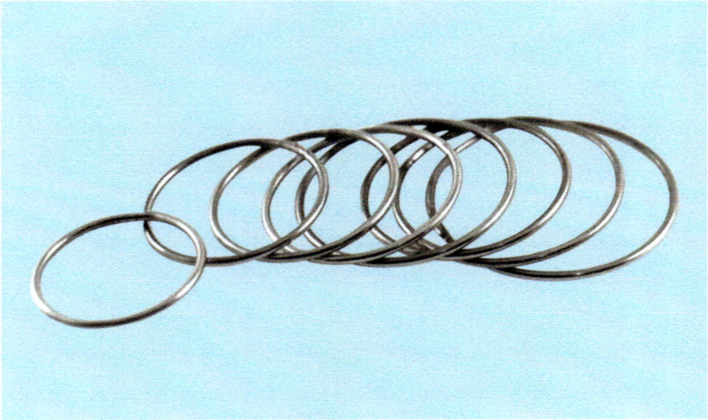

Fig. 2: Flieringa ring.
Courtesy: Katena products.

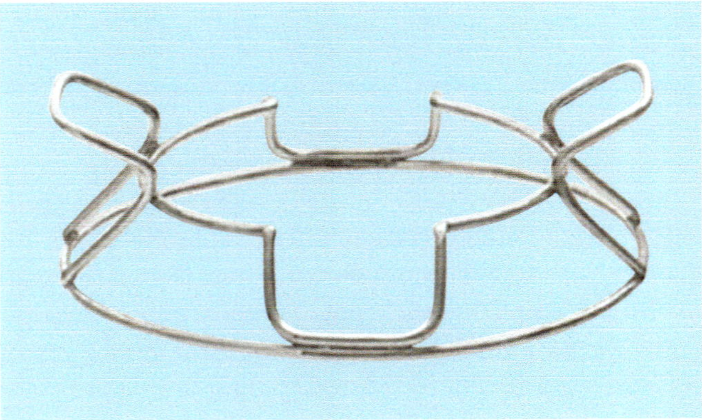

Fig. 3: McNeill–Goldman ring.
Courtesy: Katena products.

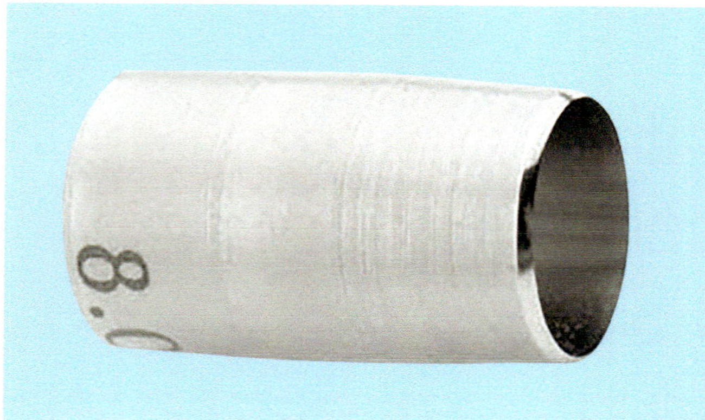

Fig. 4: Disposable handheld trephine.

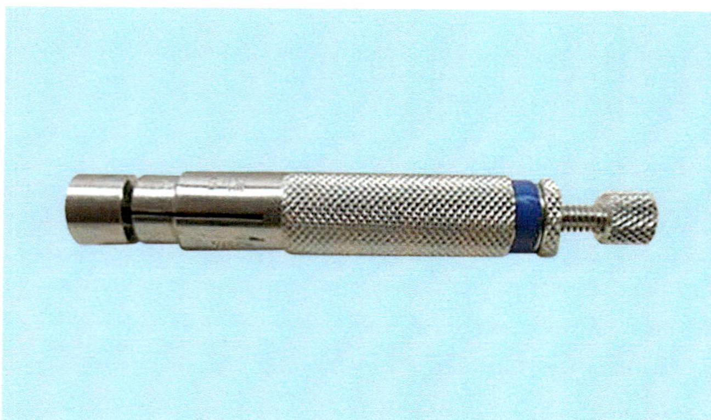

Fig. 5: Handheld trephine with obturator.

recipient corneas. They are usually attached to a handle for greater stability and control. They might have a central hollow core for visualization of the central cornea (**Fig. 4**). In some, there is a central obturator which can be adjusted to select the depth of the corneal cut (**Fig. 5**). **Castroviejo trephine** is a prototype of handheld trephine with obturator.

- *Mechanized corneal trephine*: The cutting blade is driven by a motor present in the main body. A circular trephine is attached at the motor shaft end that allows anterior chamber entry without damaging the intraocular structures. *Microkeratron* (Hans Geuder, Heidelberg) is a prototype to trephine the recipient cornea.
- *Suction fixation corneal trephine*: These are used to make the initial trephination so as to reach a depth of 60–70%. Hessburg-Barron trephine is a prototype of the suction system (**Figs. 6A and B**). It consists of an outer corneal suction ring for fixation and an inner circular cutting blade. A spring loaded disposable syringe creates negative pressure and the suction fixation provides the stability to cut perpendicularly to the limbal plane. The newer model incorporates cross hair device to enable centration and an outer ring of corneal marks to help in suture placement. For each spoke turned, i.e., 90°, the blade is lowered or raised by 0.06 mm.
- *Skin biopsy punches*: They are useful in harvesting small grafts such as in patch grafts (**Fig. 7**). They can be used for both donor and recipient corneas with sizes varying from 2 to 5.5 mm.

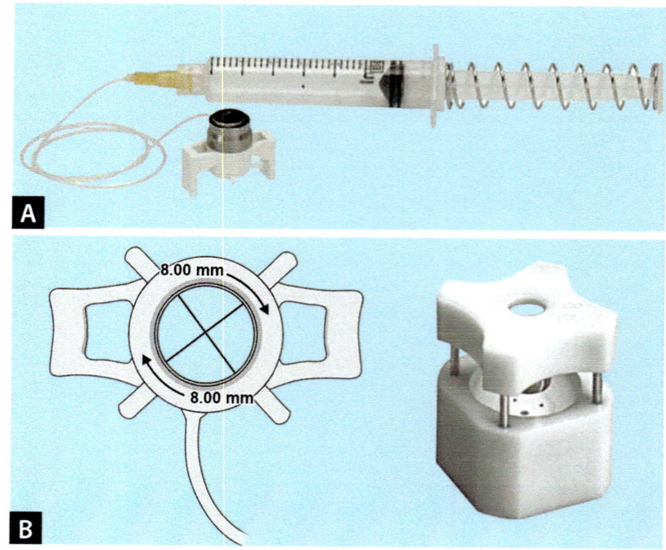

Figs. 6A and B: Hessburg–Barron trephine.

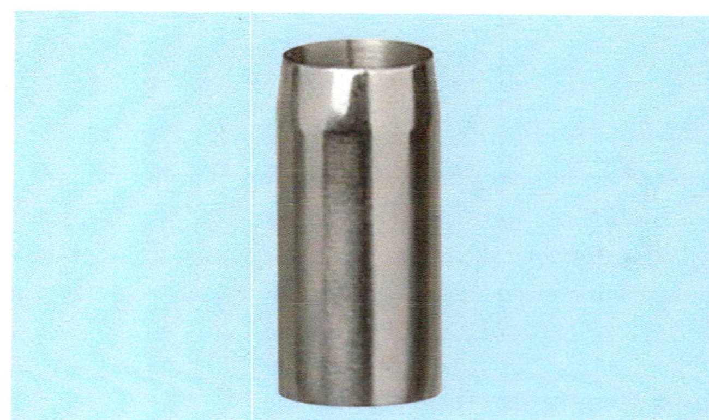

Fig. 7: Skin biopsy punch.

- *Combination corneal trephine*: Hanna trephine system has got a circular razor cutting blade and can be used for both recipient and donor cornea since it has an artificial chamber maintainer system. It consists of two parts: (1) limbal suction ring system and (2) mechanical trephine fitted with a suction ring. By rotation of the gear system, a cut of the desired depth is achieved.
- *Noncontact trephines*: They have distinct advantages in providing complete visualization, better centration, and eliminate topographic distortion. However, there are several concerns regarding endothelial injury, mutagenicity, and cost.

INSTRUMENTS FOR DONOR CORNEA DISSECTION

The instruments used to dissect donor cornea include various artificial anterior chambers and clamps. Herein, the donor corneoscleral rim is fixed in the artificial anterior chamber (**Fig. 8**) or in the King's clamp (**Fig. 9**).

Trephines and lamellar dissectors can then be used to dissect the lamellar disk.

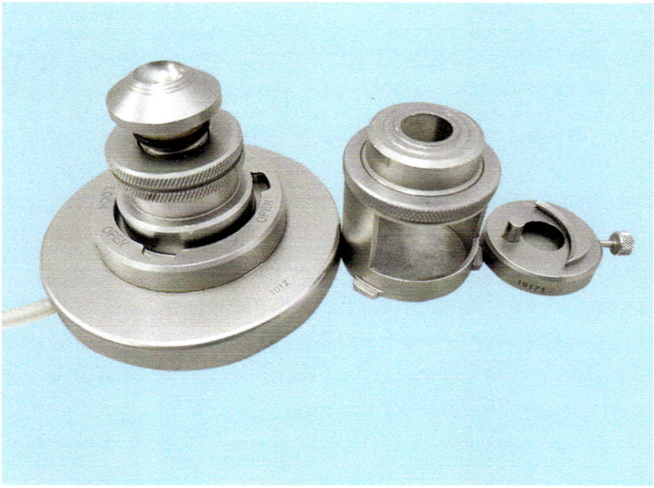

Fig. 8: Moria artificial anterior chamber.
Courtesy: Katena products.

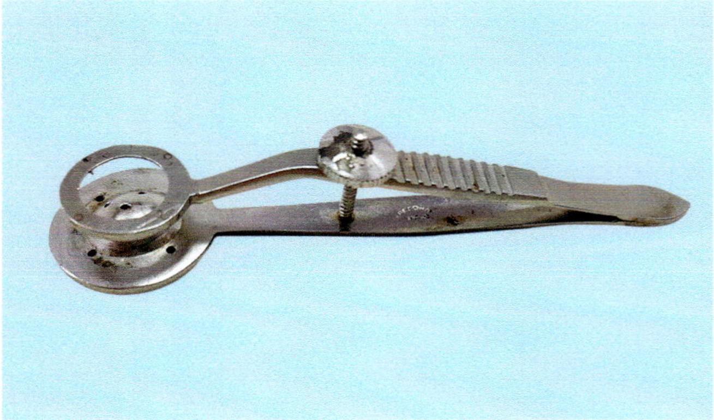

Fig. 9: King's clamp.

There are other methods also described to harvest the partial thickness donor lenticule. A simple technique harvesting the donor lamellar lenticule from the corneoscleral rim using a 3-point fixation has been used.[1] Wong et al.[2] described another method of obtaining the donor lamellar tissue. Two layers of sterile fine-weave fabric were wrapped tightly around a glass orbital implant. The corneoscleral button was sutured firmly at its scleral rim onto the fabric. The lamellar graft was then dissected in the regular fashion. During the dissection, the donor cornea and its supporting fabric-covered glass ball were easily handled, and there was minimal risk of perforation of the posterior lamella of the donor cornea.

Lamellar Dissectors

In lamellar keratoplasty, a fine thin blade is necessary to split the stroma in the correct plane. The instrument must be lightweight, have a fine edge and have a curve that conforms to the curvature of the cornea with a handle to allow for firm grip for rotation. Various types of lamellar dissectors have been designed according to different functions.

- *Tooke's knife*: The pocket for the initiation of the lamellar dissection may be performed with a Tooke's knife. Its overall length is 119 mm and it has a flat serrated handle. It has a 3 mm × 18 mm smooth blade at one end, which can be inserted intralamellarly to create the pocket (**Fig. 10**).
- *Paufique's knife*: It has a double-edged 1.5 × 3 mm sharp-angled blade simultaneously helps in outlining the graft, making the pocket, and in dissecting the lamellar planes (**Fig. 11**).
- *Desmarre's lamellar dissector*: It is used in the open type of dissection, which has a curve in its vertical meridian and it is used to sweep across the fibers in a cutting and teasing motion (**Fig. 12**). A duckbill shape lamellar dissector is used for closed type of dissection, which is curved in the horizontal dimension.
- *Gill's lamellar dissector*: It has a 3 mm wide blade which can be either straight or curved (**Fig. 13**).

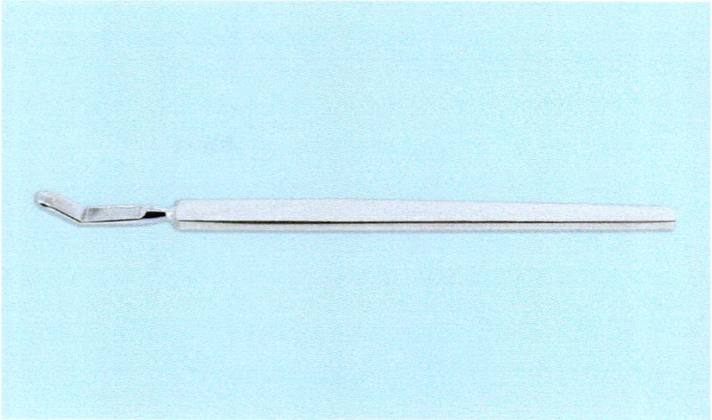

Fig. 10: Tooke's knife.

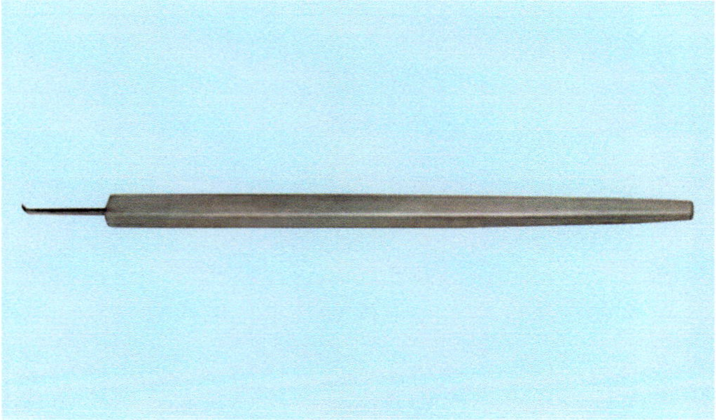

Fig. 11: Paufique's lamellar dissector.

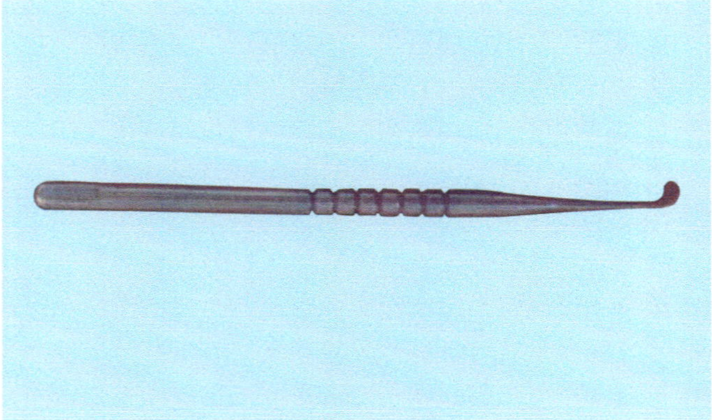

Fig. 12: Desmarre's lamellar dissector.

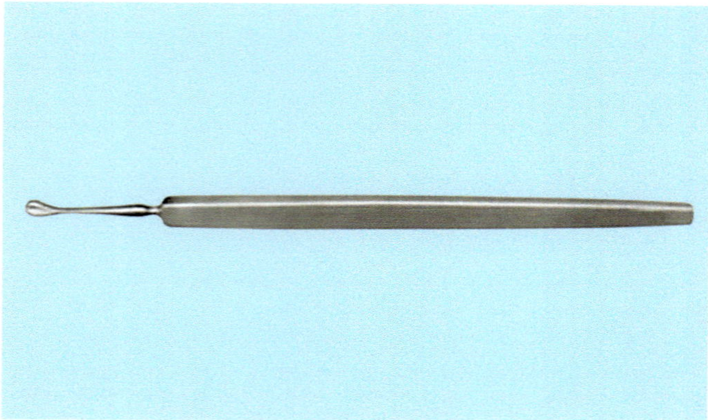

Fig. 13: Gill's straight lamellar dissector.

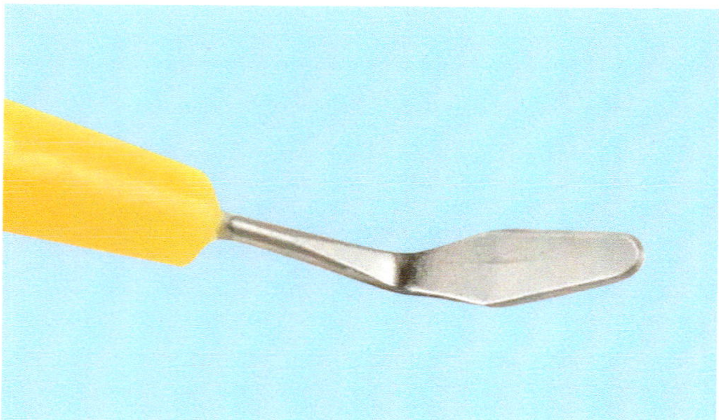

Fig. 14: Crescent knife.

- *Guarded diamond knife*: The micrometer adjusted, guarded diamond knife has made free hand, irregularly shaped lamellar grafts easier and safer to accomplish.
- *Crescent knife*: This is another useful instrument for the lamellar dissection. It has a 2.0 mm blade (**Fig. 14**).

The Melles deep anterior lamellar keratoplasty (DALK) spatula dissection set consists of a red, white and blue spatula. The *red spatula* is a short, triangled spatula used to dissect downward into the cornea till desired stromal depth is obtained. The *white spatula* is half length, curved spatula with a rounded tip to make dissection up to two-thirds of cornea. The *blue spatula* is a full length, curved spatula used to complete the dissection over 360° of cornea.[3] (**Figs. 15A to C**). With the continued development of lamellar keratoplasty newer instruments are being designed to make the surgical procedure easy and safe. The pioneers of Descemet stripping automated endothelial keratoplasty (DSAEK) have developed various instruments which have been rightly named after them. With various available instruments lamellar surgeries for different corneal pathology can be performed.

CUTTING INSTRUMENTS

Blade Breaker

A disposable razor blade is broken and mounted on the tip of pencil handle. It is used to enter the anterior chamber in a controlled manner after partial thickness trephination (**Fig. 16**).

Diamond Knife

It is available in various shapes and sizes. It is useful for stab incisions as well as to complete the trephine cuts.

Corneal Scissors

Troutman microscissors is the prototype which has blades 5 mm in length and is curved on a radius of 5 mm (**Figs. 17A and B**). This light and fine scissors is used to complete the cutting of the trephine incision. The blades should be kept vertical and should be curved to follow the curvature of the trephine while dissection of the host cornea. It is usually used to remove the irregular tags from the margin.

GRASPING INSTRUMENTS

Pierse–Hoskin's Forceps

It is a fine toothed tissue holding forceps used to hold the corneal tissue and extensively used for suture tying (**Fig. 18**). Colibri forceps is another example of tissue holding forceps (**Fig. 19**).

McPherson Forceps

It is a non-toothed forceps with flat edges that is used for suture tying and burying of suture knots (**Fig. 20**).

Graft Holder (Paton Spatula)

After obtaining the donor button, it is placed in a graft holder (Paton spatula) (**Fig. 21**) over a viscoelastic and is kept covered till the recipient dissection is complete.

AUTOMATED LAMELLAR THERAPEUTIC KERATOPLASTY MACHINE

We use the Moria automated lamellar therapeutic keratectomy microkeratome system (**Figs. 22A and B**, ALTK; Moria, Antony, France). It utilizes the CBm microkeratome and an artificial chamber which is manually driven by the surgeon. Multiple microkeratome heads may be used to achieve dissection of various thicknesses ranging from 130 to 350 (130, 150, 250, 300, 350 μm). The Moria ALTK artificial anterior chamber does require a donor scleral rim that is symmetrically >16 mm (maximum 19 mm) in diameter to provide proper vacuum during the microkeratome pass. The surgical time is greatly reduced as compared to manual dissection technique. Rotational microkeratome can be used to dissect the diseased host tissue to a predetermined depth in cases of epithelial stromal dystrophies and Salzmann nodular degenerations where sutureless anterior lamellar keratoplasty is the preferred technique (**Figs. 23A and B**).

Other machines available are the Amadeus II microkeratome (**Fig. 24**) with an artificial anterior chamber (AAC; Ziemer Group) and **Gebauer microkeratome** (**Figs. 25 and 26**). The assembly unit of Amadeus II comes

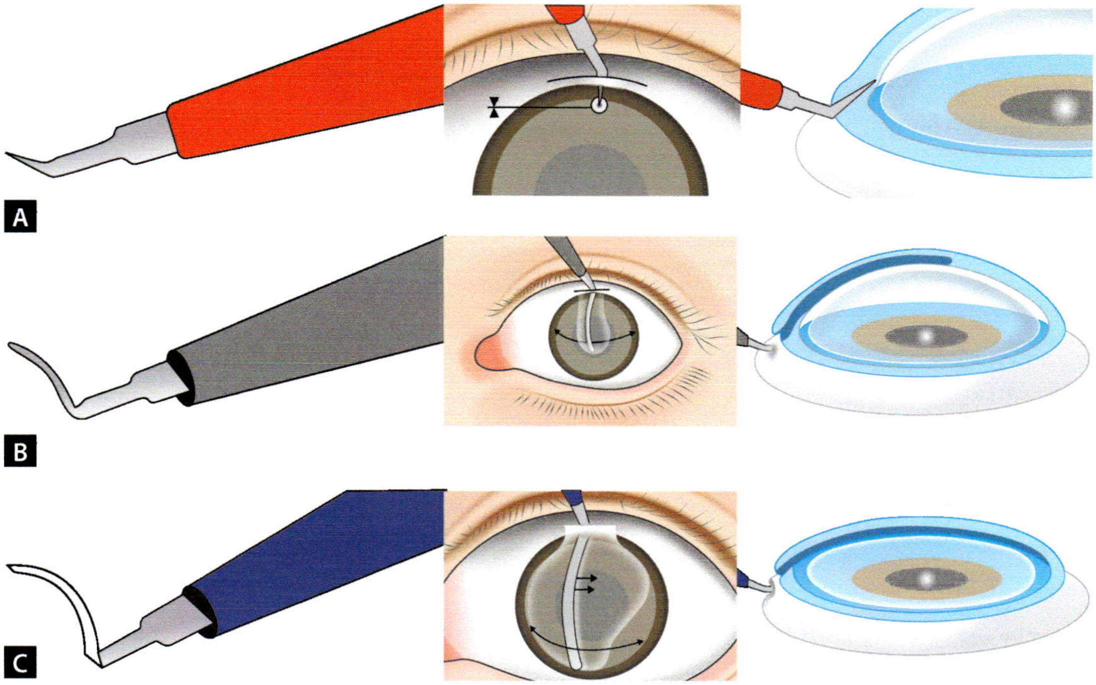

Figs. 15A to C: (A) Red spatula; (B) White spatula; (C) Blue spatula.
Courtesy: DORC products.

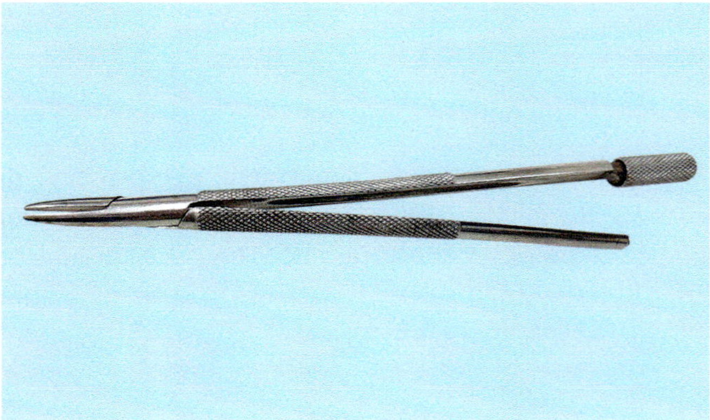

Fig. 16: Blade beaker.

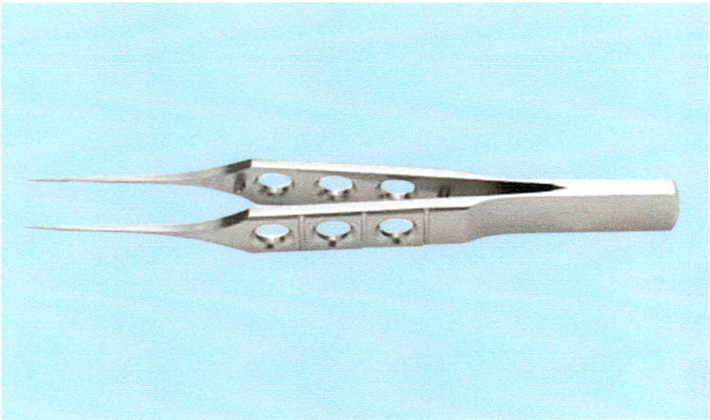

Fig. 18: Pierse–Hoskin's forceps.
Courtesy: Katena products.

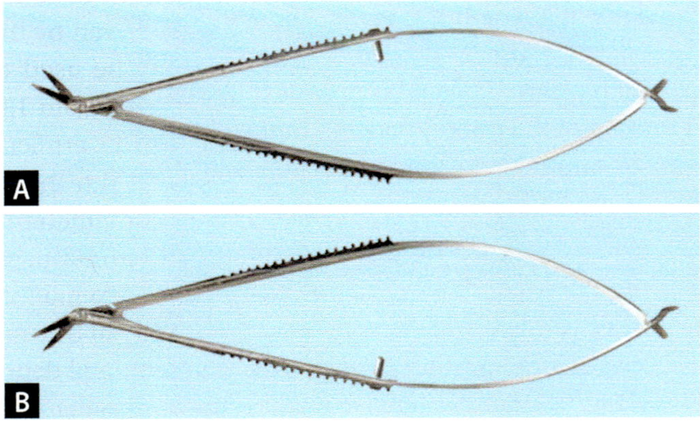

Figs. 17A and B: Right and left Troutman scissors.
Courtesy: Katena products.

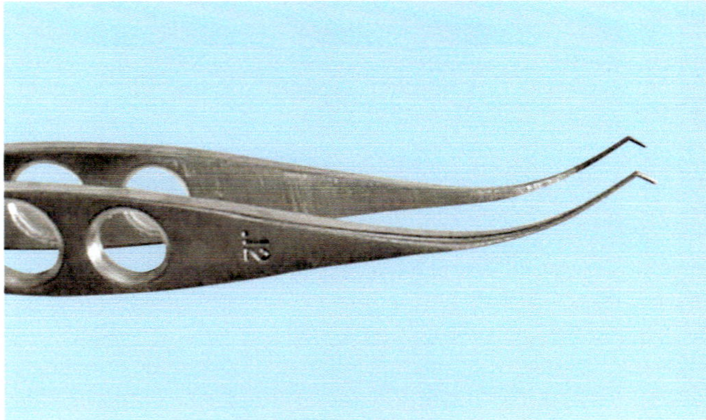

Fig. 19: Colibri forceps.
Courtesy: Katena products.

equipped with four interchangeable suction units (with diameters of 8.5, 9.0, 9.5, and 10.0 mm) and a choice of five blade holders (for a flap thickness of 200, 250, 350, 400, or 450 μm). The AAC body has an inset type in which to place the donor cornea. To obtain the ideal pressure inside the AAC, we create a direct link between the inset type and a phacoemulsification machine. Once assembled, the motor unit should cover the 16 mm diameter of the scleral rim. This

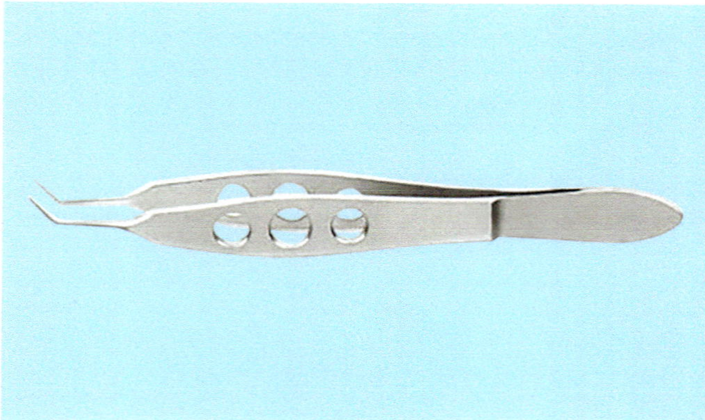

Fig. 20: McPherson forceps.
Courtesy: Katena products.

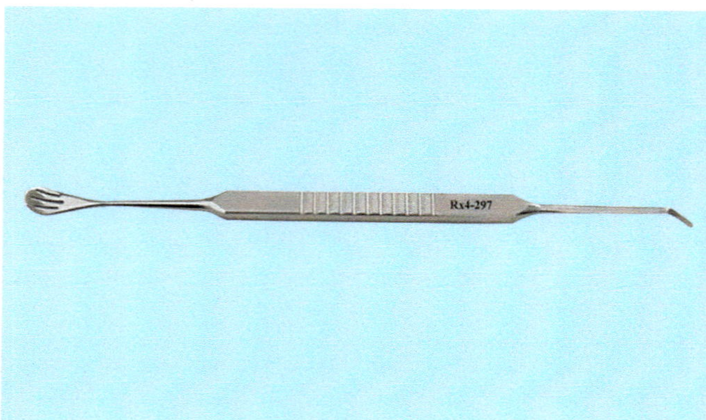

Fig. 21: Paton spatula.

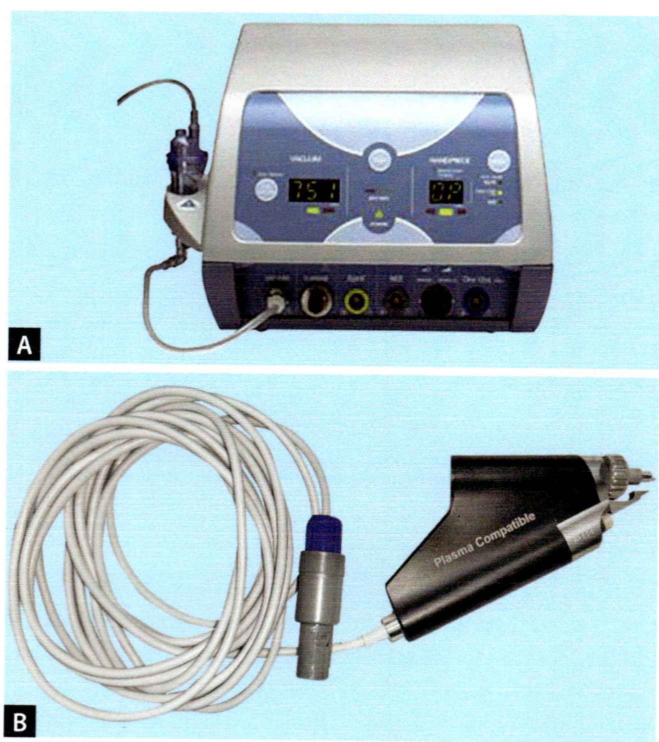

Figs. 22A and B: Automated lamellar therapeutic keratoplasty machine for dissection of donor lenticule.
Courtesy: Moria, Paris, France.

closing mechanism assures a watertight anterior chamber—comparable to a human eye—for a stretched donor cornea; the pressure inside the chamber is checked with a 65 mm Hg tonometer (Barraquer). The microkeratome cuts the button into two parts. The posterior button can be used for DSAEK.

MORIA PUNCH BLOCK

The corneoscleral rim is placed on a 7.5 mm Moria punch block which has been specially designed for partial thickness trephination of Descemet's membrane endothelial keratoplasty (DMEK) tissue. The tissue is then positioned on the block to comfortably incorporate the S-stamp into the punch.

S-STAMP

The mark is typically stamped with gentian violet ink, minimizing loss of the endothelial cells under the mark. Stromal marking can be associated with very minimal cell loss and greatly facilitates proper graft orientation in endothelial keratoplasty surgeries and prevents graft failure (**Fig. 27**).

DESCEMET STRIPPING AUTOMATED ENDOTHELIAL KERATOPLASTY SPATULA (STRIPPER)

The DSAEK spatula, made of surgical steel is designed to strip the recipient's Descemet's membrane during the DSAEK or DMEK procedure. The DSAEK strippers (**Fig. 28**) are available in 45 and 90° angled models, in both irrigating and nonirrigating versions. The angled tips facilitate effective dissection and removal of Descemet's membrane without inadvertent damage to the stroma.

BUSIN GLIDE

The donor lenticule can be inserted into the anterior chamber by pull through technique by a specially designed glide known as the Busin glide (**Fig. 29**). It allows insertion of the donor lenticule (folded in the form of a taco) through 3.2 mm incision. It facilitates graft unfolding and ensures centration of the donor lenticule in the anterior chamber. It helps to minimize intraoperative manipulation of the graft and the possibility of endothelial cell loss.

DESCEMET STRIPPING AUTOMATED ENDOTHELIAL KERATOPLASTY BUSIN FORCEPS

It is a microincision forceps with 20-G diameter and distal action (**Fig. 30**). It is designed to position the graft in the glide and to pull it from the glide into the anterior chamber. Its tips have been designed specifically to contact the periphery of the graft such that the endothelial and the stromal surfaces remain untouched in the optical zone. The size of the tips is perfectly adapted to the glide to prevent endothelial cell damage during the pull-through maneuver (**Fig. 31**).

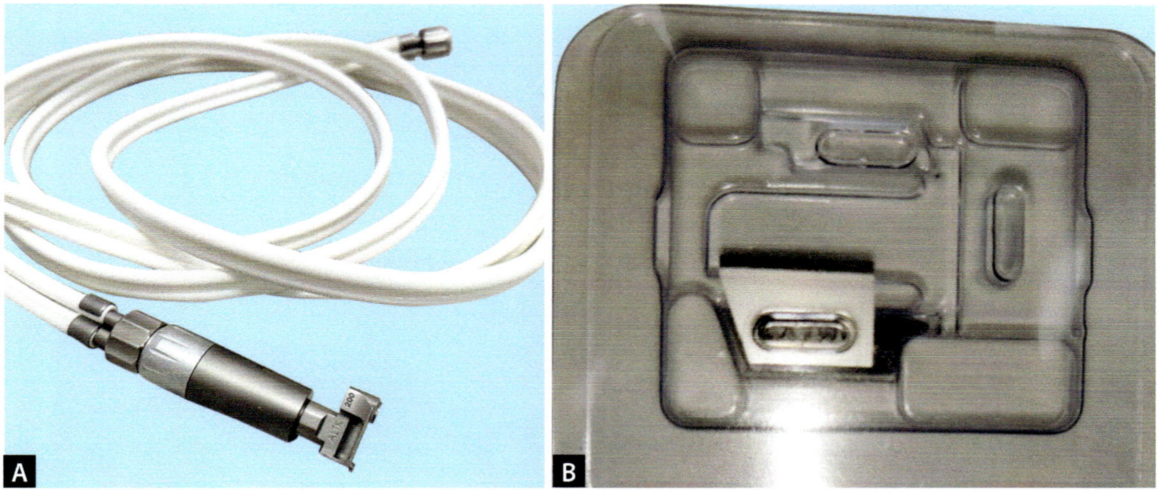

Figs. 23A and B: Automated lamellar therapeutic keratoplasty machine used a rotational microkeratome in sutureless anterior lamellar keratoplasty.
Courtesy: Moria, Paris, France.

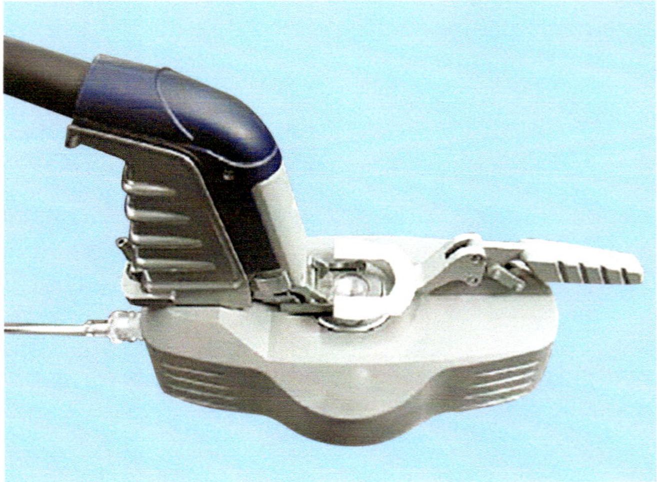

Fig. 24: Amadeus II microkeratome.

ONE CORNEAL PUNCH

A new corneal punch (**Fig. 32**) is available which is disposable and has ultra-sharp razor trephine for straight walled cuts. The punch is a two-piece device with a preload, recessed blade. It is packaged sterile for single use.

FORCEPS

The tips of the forceps remain separated when the handles are closed, to minimize injury to the folded donor tissue. The folded graft is then easily released into the anterior chamber (**Fig. 33**).

CORNEAL MARKER

An 8.0–9.0 mm marker is available to mark the area of the recipient's cornea to be stripped. The anterior surface of the recipient cornea is marked with gentian violet blue or surgical marker pen (**Fig. 34**).

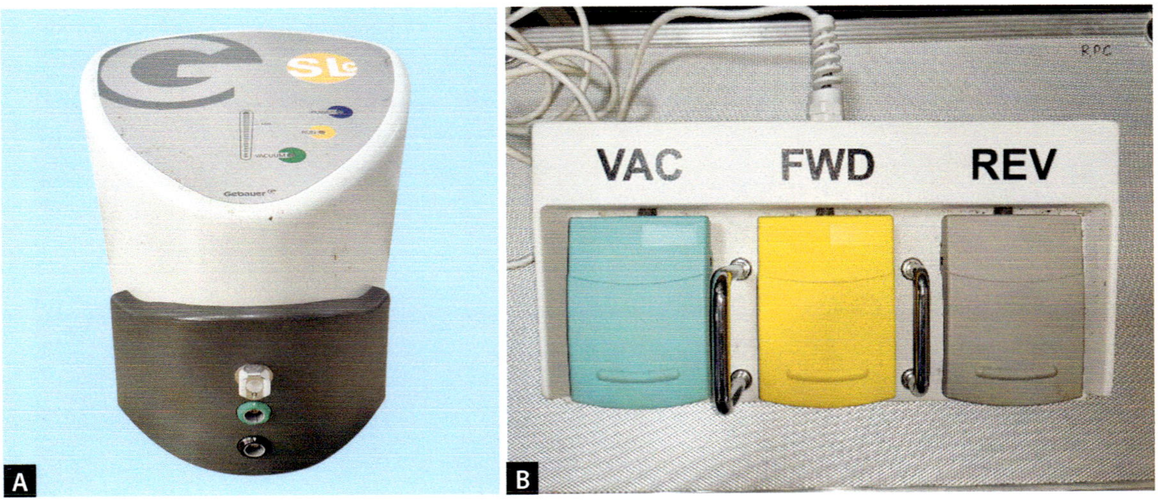

Figs. 25A and B: Automated lamellar therapeutic keratoplasty machine.
Courtesy: Gebauer/Medizintechnik GmbH, Neuhausen, Germany.

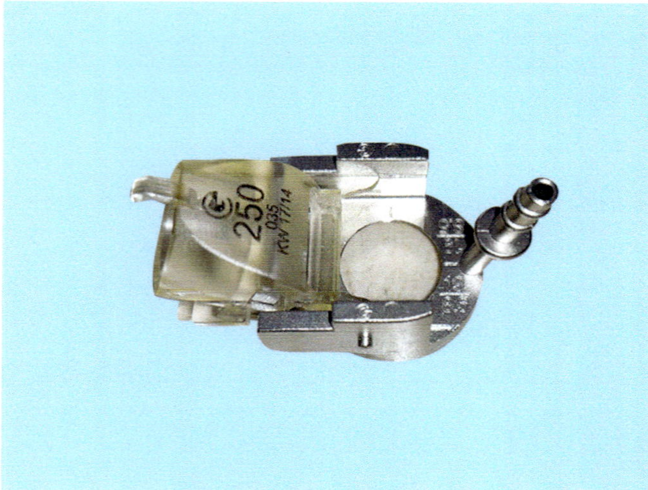

Fig. 26: Gebauer microkeratome head.

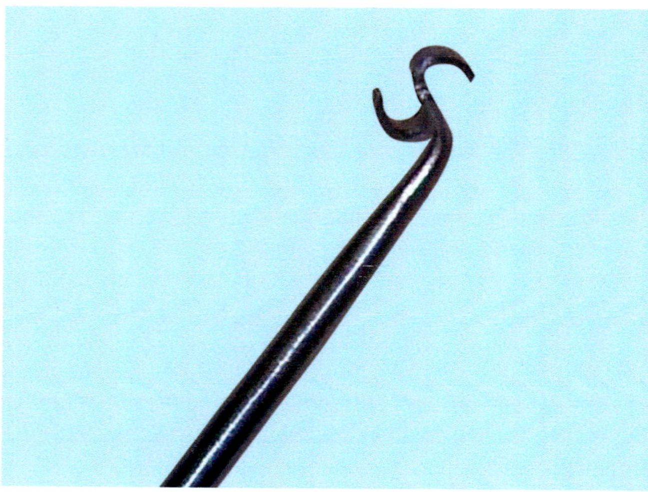

Fig. 27: S-stamp.

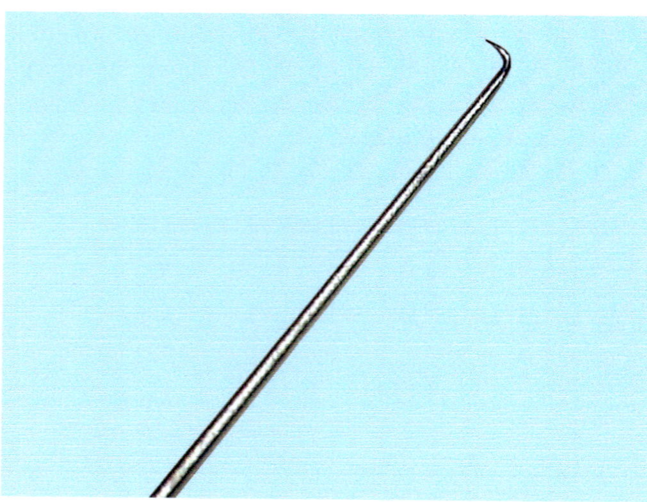

Fig. 28: Descemet stripping automated endothelial keratoplasty spatula (stripper).

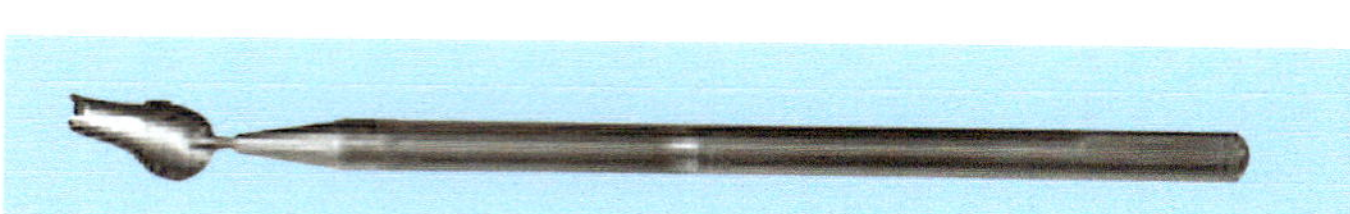

Fig. 29: Busin glide.
Courtesy: Moria SA, France.

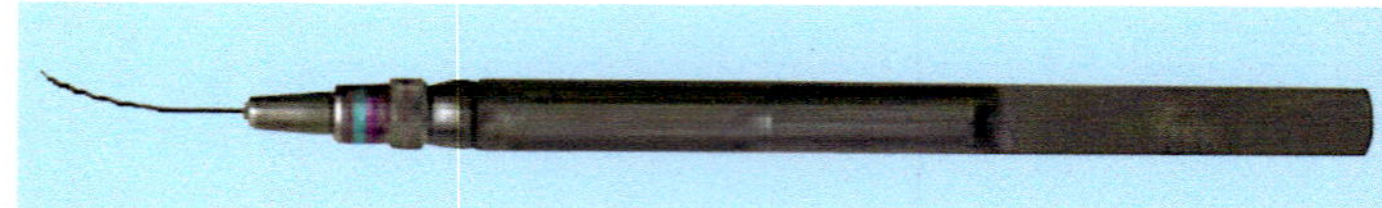

Fig. 30: Descemet stripping automated endothelial keratoplasty Busin forceps.
Courtesy: Moria SA, France.

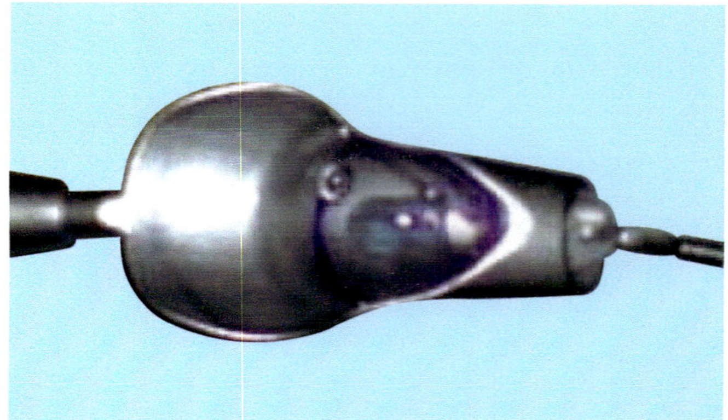

Fig. 31: Pulling the graft with Descemet stripping automated endothelial keratoplasty Busin forceps.
Courtesy: Moria SA, France.

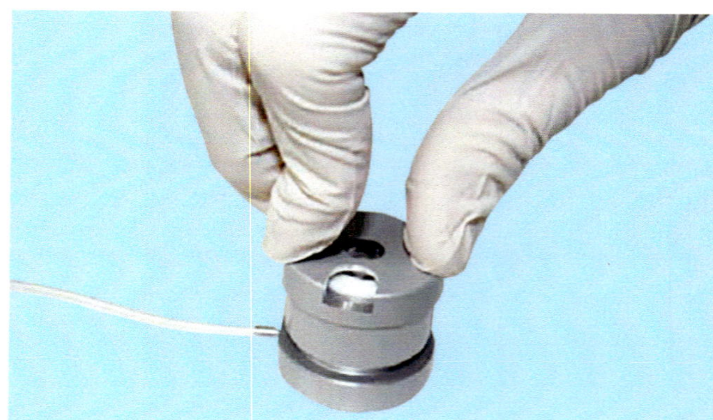

Fig. 32: One corneal punch.
Courtesy: Moria SA, France.

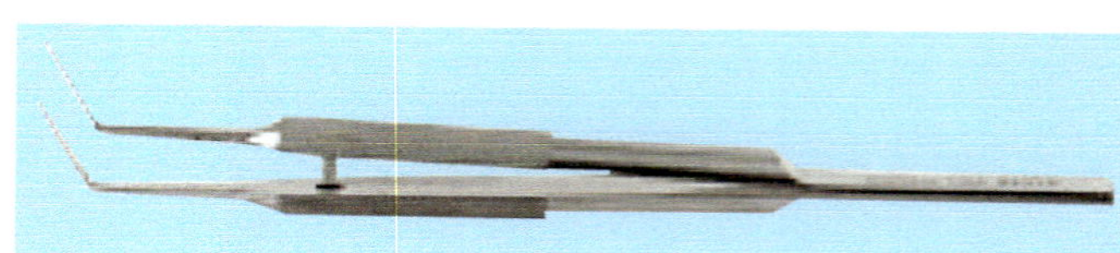

Fig. 33: Forceps for donor insertion.
Courtesy: Moria SA, France.

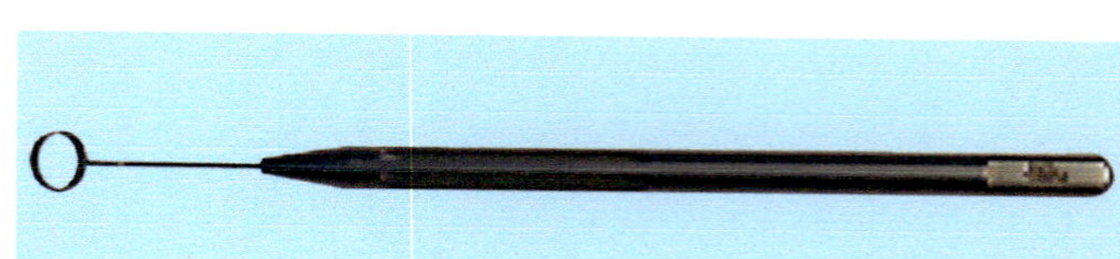

Fig. 34: Corneal marker.
Courtesy: Moria SA, France.

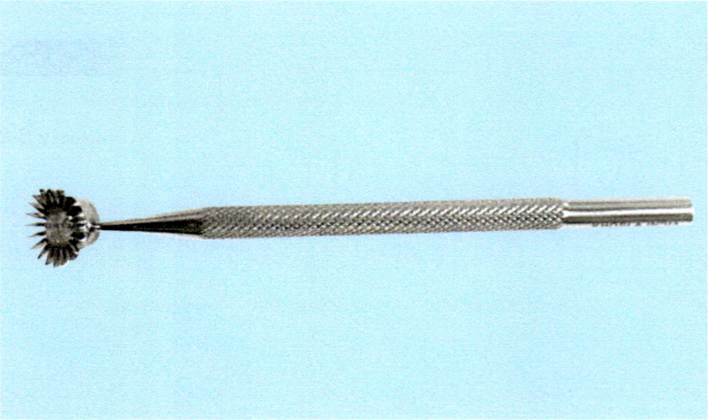

Fig. 35: Vajpayee's modified keratoplasty suture marker.

CORNEAL MARKING INSTRUMENT

Various instruments such as the radial keratotomy marker (16 radial arms), Anis corneal marker (8 radial arms), and the Vajpayee corneal marker stained with gentian violet can be used to mark the recipient cornea to aid in the ideal suture placement in keratoplasty. The "Vajpayee corneal marker" which consists of 20 radial arms, guide the placement of the single continuous suture bites (**Fig. 35**).

DESCEMET STRIPPING AUTOMATED ENDOTHELIAL KERATOPLASTY ANTERIOR CHAMBER MAINTAINER

Descemet stripping automated endothelial keratoplasty anterior chamber maintainer has a 20-G threaded tip, supplied with silicone tubing and adaptor (**Fig. 36**).

Fig. 36: Descemet stripping automated endothelial keratoplasty anterior chamber maintainer.
Courtesy: Moria SA, France.

STRAIKO INJECTOR

This transparent injector is loaded with the DMEK roll directly from the corneoscleral rim so as to minimize touching and damaging the donor tissue. The tip of the injector is placed bevel up into the corneoscleral rim and positioned so that the tip of the bevel is beneath one end of the DMEK scroll. The graft is then gently aspirated into the modified Jones tube until it is in the tube's distal flared midsection. The tip of the modified Jones tube is briskly inserted into the main incision with bevel down until it is snugly seated against the walls of the main wound and injected into the anterior chamber. The intraocular lens injector attached with a 5 cc syringe can alternatively be used for this purpose as well.

REFERENCES

1. Vrabec M, Jordan J, Lawlor P. Lamellar keratoplasty performed with a corneal scleral button. Ophthalmic Surg. 1994;25:389-91.
2. Wong D, Chan W, Tan D. Harvesting a lamellar graft from a corneoscleral button: A new technique. Am J Ophthalmol. 1997;123:688-9.
3. Jhanji V, Sharma N, Vajpayee RB (Eds). Deep Anterior Lamellar Keratoplasty Different Strokes. New Delhi: Jaypee Brothers Medical Publishers; 2011.

20 "Dry" Manual Technique for Deep Anterior Lamellar Keratoplasty

Paolo Rama, Karl Anders Knutsson

INTRODUCTION

Lamellar keratoplasty (LKP) is the surgical procedure currently indicated when the endothelium is not affected/involved. It presents several advantages compared to penetrating keratoplasty (PKP): (1) it is an extraocular procedure; (2) there is no risk of endothelial rejection, the major cause of graft failure in PKP, requiring shorter treatment with topical steroids; (3) superior wound strength; (4) sutures can be removed earlier; (5) selection criteria for donor tissue are less strict and donor tissue used for Descemet membrane (DM) endothelial keratoplasty can be shared for LKP. The main concern regarding LKP is aberrations due to the interface between the graft and the recipient stromal bed.

Deep anterior lamellar keratoplasty (DALK) has been proposed to reduce interface scarring. It consists of removal of the stroma down to the pre-Descemetic or Descemetic plane and transplantation of the donor button without endothelium. DALK proves to result in similar visual acuity compared to PKP and better visual acuity when confronted with conventional LKP, while maintaining the same advantages. The main concern regarding DALK is that it is technically difficult, resulting in a steep learning curve. The most feared intraoperative complication is perforation of the DM which occurs more often when the overlying stroma is completely removed.

Recent developments in surgical techniques have favored approaches such as the "big bubble" technique[1] with the objective of removing all of the corneal stroma to obtain better visual results. However, the big bubble technique can be technically challenging when the air bubble is not formed, requiring completion of the procedure using manual dissection of stromal layers that have been altered by the injection of air. It is also not clear whether full stromal removal provides better results than cases in which a small portion of posterior stroma is left in place.[2,3] Sugita and Kondo (1997)[4] and other authors later, have shown that manual DALK, leaving a small amount of stroma, may give same visual recovery while reducing the risk of perforation.[5-8]

In this chapter, we describe a modified manual technique in which a Descemetic or pre-Descemetic plane is reached through a "dry" blunt dissection, without the aid of air or fluid. The most relevant step is the calibrated diamond blade incision (set at 20 μm less than the full corneal thickness) utilized as a guide to target a deep dissection plane, reaching the pre-Descemetic layer. More recently, we have used the same principals to develop a modified big bubble technique.[9] The same diamond incision has been used in a modified version of the big-bubble technique allowing the insertion of a cannula for air injection so that a correct deep plane can be promptly identified. The deep plane allows a facilitated conversion to manual dissection in the presence of unsuccessful bubble formation. Interestingly a study group from Brazil independently developed a similar technique termed "pachy-bubble".[10]

INDICATIONS TO DRY MANUAL DEEP ANTERIOR LAMELLAR KERATOPLASTY

The following scheme illustrates the rationale behind the indications:

- *Optical*:
  - When we aim to reduce the risk of perforation as much as possible, such as in ocular surface disorders, for example.
  - In pediatric patients, where it is known that Descemet's membrane is firmly attached to the stroma and thus difficult to be detached with air or fluid.
  - In case of unsuccessful bubble formation
- *Tectonic*:
  - Decreased corneal thickness
    - Chemical burns
    - Leukomas
    - Advanced ectasias
  - Small perforations
- *Therapeutic*:
  - Infections
  - Tumors
- *Esthetic*:
  - Corneal tattoos in blind eyes

SURGICAL TECHNIQUE

The surgical technique can be summarized in the following steps:

- Pilocarpine (2%) may be used to constrict the pupil and avoid direct damage of the lens in case of perforation.
- Local or general anesthesia should be chosen according to the patient and surgeon preference.
- Eyelids and conjunctiva are disinfected with povidone iodine (5%).
- The cornea is marked with the diameter of trephination and intraoperative pachymetry is taken 1–2 mm inside the marked diameter, where the keratotomy will be performed (**Fig. 1**).
- A 2 mm keratotomy is performed with a calibrated diamond knife 1–2 mm inside the marked circumference. The depth of the incision is 20 μm less than the corneal thickness in the particular point of incision (measured with ultrasonic pachymetry) (**Fig. 2**).
- The calibrated corneal trephine is used to cut at approximately 70% of the central corneal thickness and a crescent knife is used to remove the superficial lamella (**Figs. 3 and 4**).
- A peripheral pocket is created using a 360° disk-knife starting from the location of the previously created deep incision (**Figs. 5 and 6**).

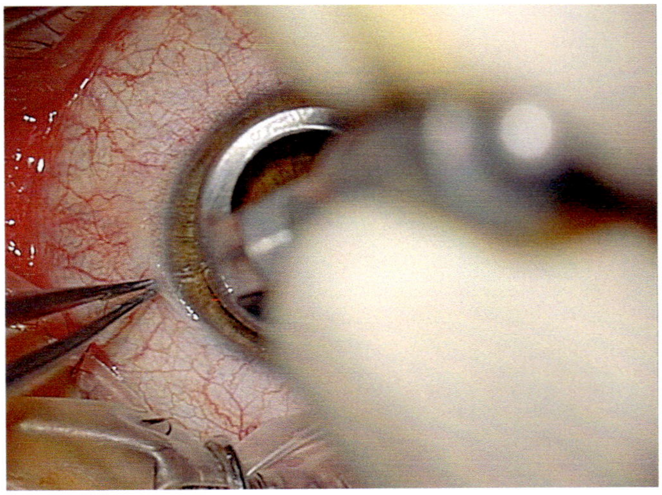

Fig. 1: Corneal diameter (in this case 8.5 mm) and central cornea are marked.

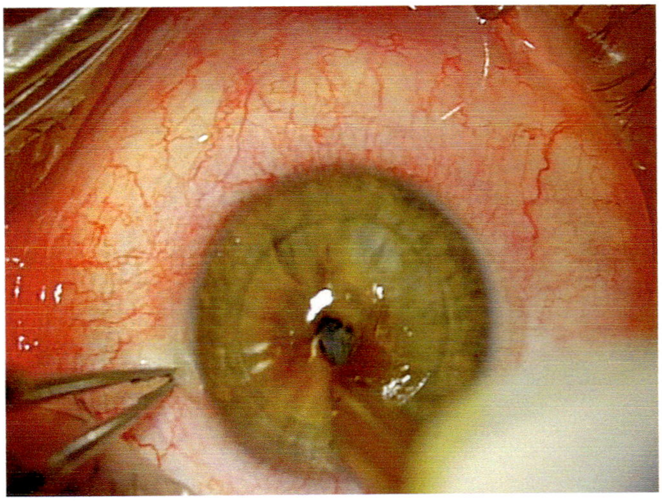

Fig. 2: Deep incision is performed at 12 o'clock using a diamond calibrated knife.

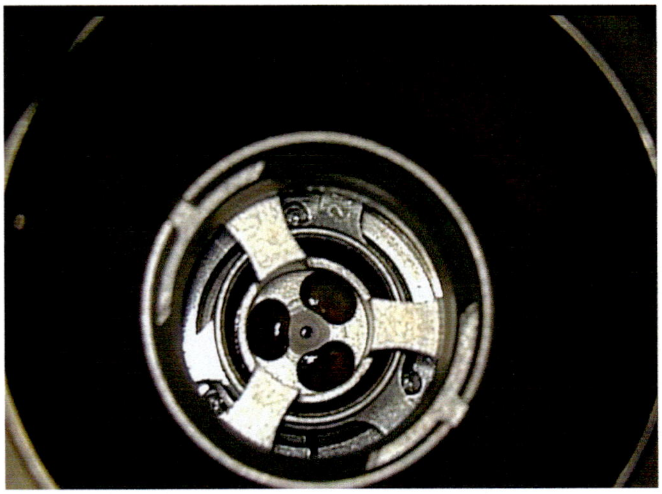

Fig. 3: Calibrated corneal trephine is set to cut at 70% of the corneal thickness and used to prepare a superficial lamella of tissue.

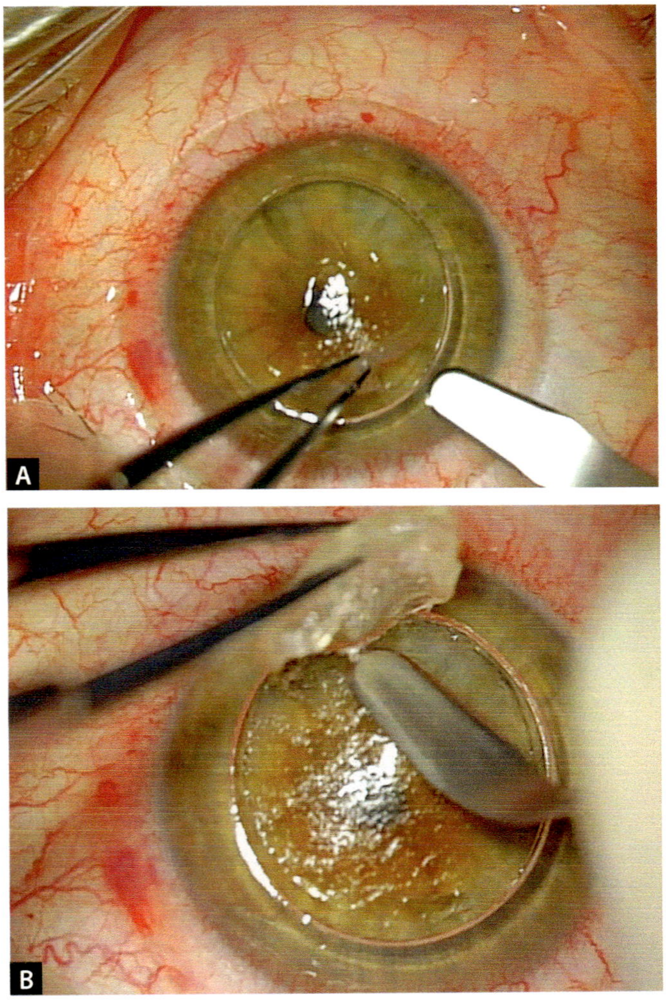

Figs. 4A and B: The superficial lamella is removed using a crescent knife (BD Medical, Franklin Lakes, NJ, USA).

- Vannas scissors are used to cut at the aimed depth for 360° (**Fig. 7**).
- Removal of deeper layers, starting from the initial incision is obtained utilizing a blunt spatula until a pre-Descemetic plane is reached in the optical zone of the cornea (approximately the central 7 mm) (**Fig. 8**).
- The donor graft is prepared using a punch from the endothelial side. The donor size is 0.25 mm greater than the recipient bed.
- The Descemet membrane and endothelium are removed from the donor graft.
- Four cardinal sutures (nylon 10.0) are applied to fix the donor graft firmly to the recipient bed.
- A continued suture (nylon 10.0) is applied.
- Before tying the suture, a paracentesis of the anterior chamber is performed in order to achieve a better fit of the graft on the recipient bed and to decrease suture tension.
- Cardinal sutures are removed.
- Suture tension and astigmatism are regulated using a manual keratoscope (**Fig. 9**).
- Subconjunctival injection of betamethasone 4 mg/2 mL.
- Topical instillation of antibiotic eye drops (ciprofloxacin 0.3%) and application of eye patch.

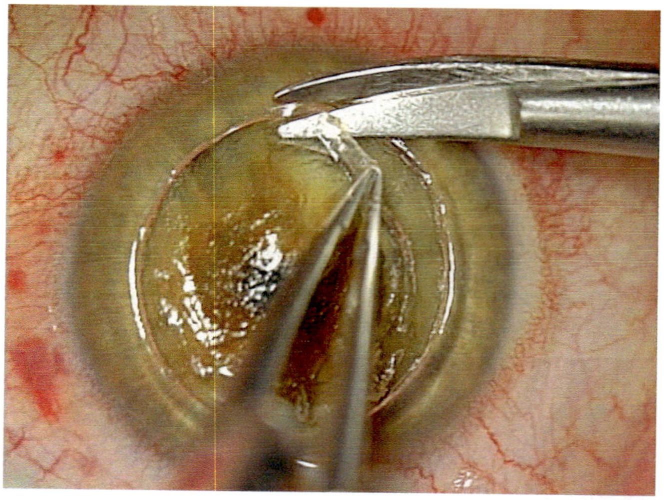

Fig. 7: Vannas scissors (Janach J4201) are used to cut at the aimed depth for 360°.

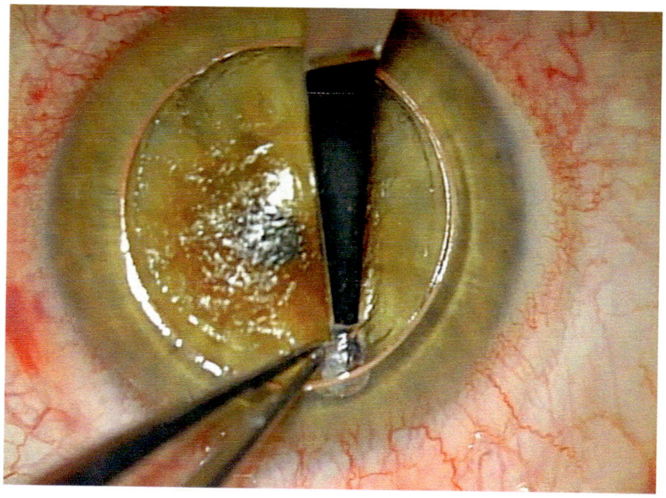

Fig. 5: A disk knife (Alcon, Fort Worth, TX, USA) is used to create a peripheral pocket starting from the deep incision.

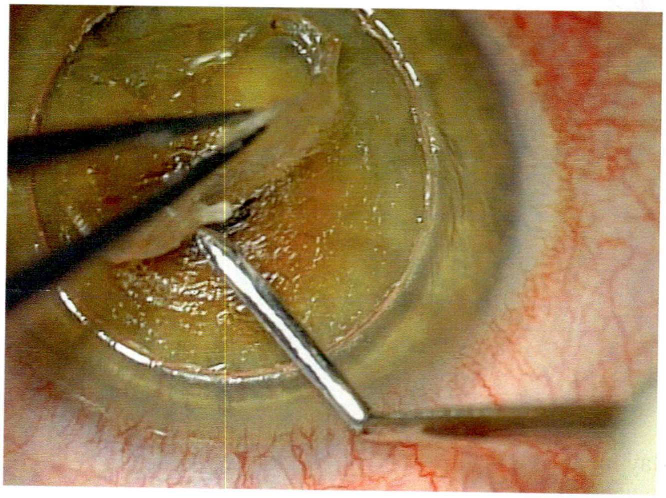

Fig. 8: Removal of deeper layers, starting from the initial incision is obtained utilizing a blunt spatula (Janach model J2401.1a, Como, Italy) until a pre-Descemetic plane is reached.

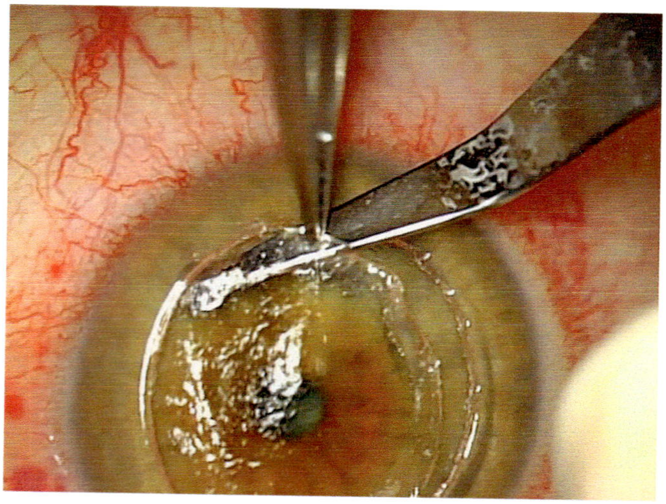

Fig. 6: Peripheral pocket formation is continued for 360°.

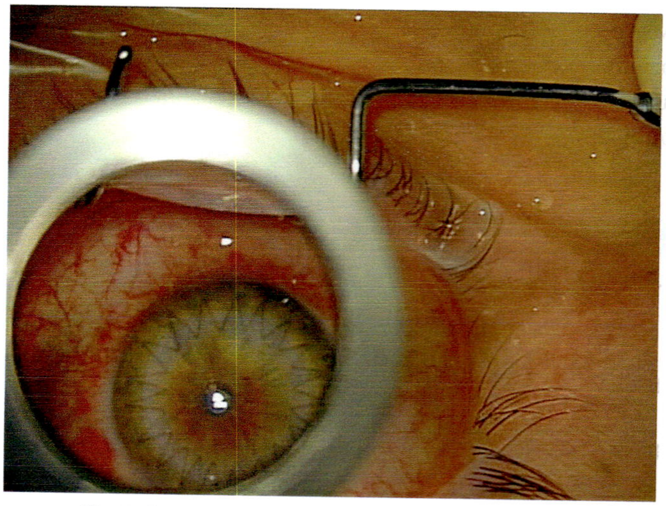

Fig. 9: Corneal astigmatism is checked after suturing.

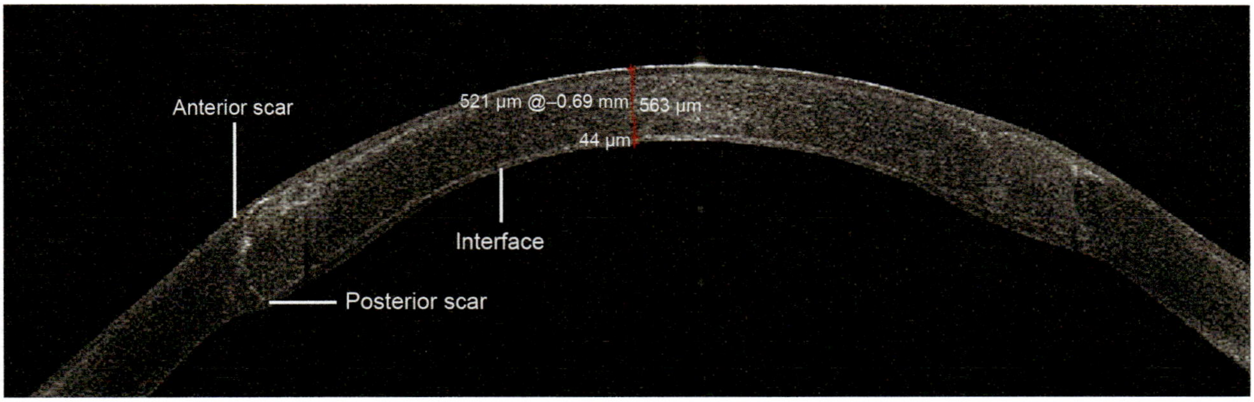

Fig. 10: Anterior segment optical coherence tomography (OCT) image of the lamellar graft. Arrows indicate the anterior and posterior scars and the interface area between the stromal recipient bed and the donor graft.

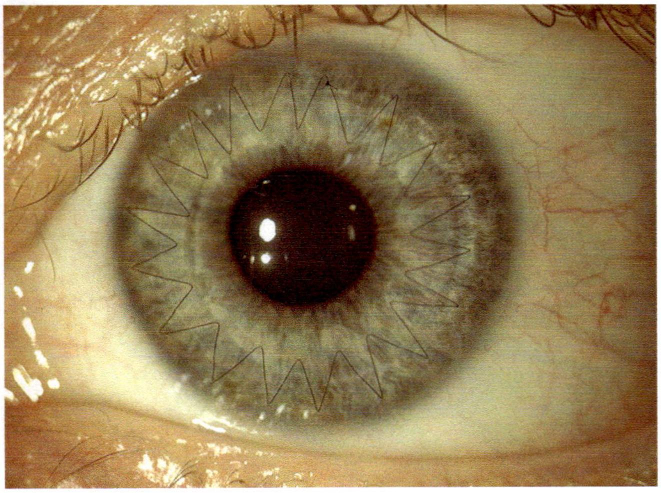

Fig. 11: Dry manual deep anterior lamellar keratoplasty (DALK) 6 months postoperative.

Postoperative therapy was topical levofloxacin 3 times a day for 15 days, and topical dexamethasone (0.15%) 3 times a day for 15 days, tapering the quantity to 2 times a day for 15 days and once a day for 30 days.

RESULTS

More than 400 patients have been operated with our original lamellar technique (**Figs. 10 and 11**). Data analysis and postoperative follow-up of a group of cases have been published.[6,9]

Indications were keratoconus in most of the cases (keratoconus 90.2%, postinfective leukomas 3.8%, leukomas from other causes 3.1%, postrefractive surgery ectasia 1.3%, corneal dystrophies 1.6%).

The diameter of the donor graft, punched from the endothelium side, was always 0.25 mm larger, and graft trephination were 8.25 mm or 8.5 mm in most of the cases. The minimum trephination diameter was 7.50 mm and the maximum was 8.75 mm. The suture was removed at an average of 8.69 ± 5.54 months.

A postoperative best spectacle-corrected visual acuity (BSCVA) similar to a "big bubble" DALK or a PKP may be achieved when the residual stroma is regular and <40–60 µm thick. Refractive error measured by spherical equivalent, refractive astigmatism, and topographic astigmatism was also similar (**Tables 1 and 2**).

Perforation occurred in 3.0% of the cases.[1,3,5,6,8,11-13]

CONCLUSION

In conclusion, "dry" manual DALK can be a valid alternative to other DALK techniques. It gives comparable visual results of "big bubble" DALK when the residual stroma is <40–60 µm. Leaving some residual stroma might be safer compared to Descemetic-DALKs in risky cases, such as in children or in ocular surface disease. It can be used when the bubble is not reached, and the good reproducibility of this technique has allowed surgeons to use the same deep plane, created

Table 1: Postoperative LogMAR visual acuity. Mean values ± standard deviation (fifth; 95th percentiles).

Acuity	*2 months*	*6 months*	*1 year*	*2 years*
UCVA	0.741 ± 0.311 (1.301; 0.222)	0.637 ± 0.326 (1.30; 0.100)	0.573 ± 0.305 (1;0.097)	0.545 ± 0.334 (1; 0.069)
BSCVA	0.312 ± 0.192 (0.699; 0.046)	0.216 ± 0.180 (0.523; 0)	0.160 ± 0.143 (0.398; 0)	0.131 ± 0.087 (0.301; 0)
BCVA	0.174 ± 0.133 (0.398; 0.046)	0.130 ± 0.120 (0.325; 0)	0.102 ± 0.099 (0.222; 0)	0.097 ± 0.078 (0.222; 0)

(BCVA: best-corrected visual acuity; BSCVA: best spectacle-corrected visual acuity; UCVA: uncorrected visual acuity)

Table 2: Postoperative refraction (diopters). Mean values ± standard deviation.

	2 months	*6 months*	*1 year*	*2 years*
Spherical equivalent	−2.99 ± 3.48 (−9; 2)	−3.03 ± 3.32 (−9.29; 1.90)	−2.86 ± 3.03 (−8.18; 1.50)	−2.70 ± 3.30 (−8.5; 2)
Refractive astigmatism	−3.57 ± 2.47 (−8; 0)	−3.33 ± 2.51 (−8; 0.025)	−2.94 ± 1.77 (−6; −0.75)	−2.22 ± 2.52 (−6; 3.5)
Topographic astigmatism	3.99 ± 2.49 (0.72; 8.22)	3.66 ± 2.34 (0.72; 8.87)	2.96 ± 1.69 (0.79; 6.37)	2.87 ± 1.57 (0.81; 6.10)

with the calibrated-diamond incision, for air injection in a modified version of the big-bubble technique. The deep plane might increase the chances of a bubble formation, and allows a facilitated conversion to manual dissection in the presence of unsuccessful bubble formation.

REFERENCES

1. Anwar M, Teichmann K. Big-bubble technique to bare Descemet's membrane in anterior lamellar keratoplasty. J Cataract Refract Surg. 2002;28:398-403.
2. Feizi S, Javadi MA, Rastegarpour A. Visual acuity and refraction after deep anterior lamellar keratoplasty with and without successful big-bubble formation. Cornea. 2010;29:1252-5.
3. Fontana L, Parente G, Tassinari G. Clinical outcomes after deep anterior lamellar keratoplasy using the big-bubble technique in patients with keratoconus. Am J Ophthalmol. 2007;143:117-24.
4. Sugita J, Kondo J. Deep lamellar keratoplasty with complete removal of pathological stroma for vision improvement. Br J Ophthalmol. 1997;81:184-8.
5. Marchini G, Mastropasqua L, Pedrotti E, Nubile M, Ciancaglini M, Sbabo A. Deep lamellar keratoplasty by intracorneal dissection: a prospective clinical and confocal microscopic study. Ophthalmology. 2006;113:1289-300.
6. Rama P, Knutsson KA, Razzoli G, Matuska S, Viganò M, Paganoni G. Deep anterior lamellar keratoplasty using an original manual technique. Br J Ophthalmol. 2013;97:23-7.
7. Vajpayee RB, Maharana PK, Sharma N, Agarwal T, Jhanji V. Diamond knife-assisted deep anterior lamellar keratoplasty to manage keratoconus. J Cataract Refract Surg. 2014;40:276-82.
8. Ardjomand N, Hau S, McAlister J, Tuft S. Quality of vision and graft thickness in deep anterior lamellar and penetrating corneal allografts. Am J Ophthalmol. 2007;143:228-35.
9. Knutsson KA, Rama P, Paganoni G. Modified big-bubble technique compared to manual dissection deep anterior lamellar keratoplasty in the treatment of keratoconus. Acta Ophthalmol. 2015;93:431-8.
10. Ghanem RC, Ghanem MA. Pachymetry-guided intrastromal air injection ("pachy-bubble") for deep anterior lamellar keratoplasty. Cornea. 2012;31:1087-91.
11. Feizi S, Javadi MA, Jamali H, Mirbabaee F. Deep anterior lamellar keratoplasty in patients with keratoconus: big-bubble technique. Cornea. 2010;29:177-82.
12. Han DC, Mehta JS, Por YM, Htoon HM, Tan DT. Comparison of outcomes of lamellar keratoplasty and penetrating keratoplasty in keratoconus. Am J Ophthalmol. 2009;148:744-751.e1.
13. Fogla R, Padmanabhan P. Results of deep lamellar keratoplasty using the big-bubble technique in patients with keratoconus. Am J Ophthalmol. 2006;141:254-9.

21

Automated Lamellar Therapeutic Keratoplasty

Namrata Sharma, Sohini Mandal, Ritu Nagpal, Sameer Kaushal

INTRODUCTION

Automated lamellar therapeutic keratoplasty (ALTK) is a modification of the manual technique of lamellar keratoplasty (LK) wherein a microkeratome is used to perform donor as well as host corneal stromal dissection. Use of an automated microkeratome allows removal of the pathological part of the host cornea at a predetermined depth.[1]

The ALTK system (Moria, Paris, France) consists of a microkeratome with interchangeable heads and an artificial anterior chamber for mounting the donor corneoscleral rim. This was specifically developed and marketed for the purpose of therapeutic LK.[2] The entire assembly can be autoclaved, ensuring absolute sterility of the surgical procedure.

Microkeratomes allow corneal surgeons to safely and reproducibly dissect corneal stroma at a desired thickness and with a smooth interface. The other advantage of this surgical technique is the ease of dissection, compared to manual keratoplasty.

INDICATIONS OF AUTOMATED LAMELLAR THERAPEUTIC KERATOPLASTY

Automated lamellar therapeutic keratoplasty has been performed with promising outcomes both in children as well as in adults.

The indications include pathologies involving anterior to midstromal layers of corneal stroma with retained endothelial function.[3,4] These include patients with anterior stomal dystrophies, postherpetic scarring, keratoconus, superficial chemical burns, post-traumatic and postinfections leukomas, trachomatous keratopathy, Salzmann nodular degeneration, and postexcimer laser corneal haze.[5-7] It has also been used for tectonic purposes in patients with significant corneal thinning and impending perforation.[8] A modified microkeratome with a redesigned head has also been evaluated for limbal stem cell harvesting and transplantation.[9]

CONTRAINDICATIONS OF AUTOMATED LAMELLAR THERAPEUTIC KERATOPLASTY

The contraindications of ALTK include patients with endothelial dysfunction, eyelid abnormalities such as ectropion, entropion, trichiasis, lagophthalmos, severe blepharitis, and keratoconjunctivitis sicca. Patients with deep set eyes or small palpebral apertures pose challenge in terms of difficult microkeratome placement over the host bed. Another limitation of performing microkeratome-assisted dissection is in eyes with eccentrically steep or thin corneas, since they are at increased risk of corneal perforation during host bed preparation.[3]

Patients with underlying collagen vascular diseases and history of keloid formation are also contraindications for surgery due to abnormal wound healing response.

PREOPERATIVE EVALUATION

Preoperative evaluation includes assessment of the exact depth of lesion in order to select a suitable microkeratome head. Anterior segment optical coherence tomography is a reliable tool to estimate the depth of corneal involvement.

Intraoperatively, ultrasound pachymetry and microscope-integrated optical coherence tomography (MIOCT) help to precisely determine the central as well as the peripheral corneal thickness. This is specifically helpful to confirm the depth and location of thinnest point, in eyes with irregular cornea. This helps in selecting a suitable microkeratome head, thereby avoiding inadvertent intraoperative host bed perforation.

SURGICAL TECHNIQUE

Preparation of Recipient Bed

The recipient lamellar bed is prepared using a suction ring and an automated microkeratome in a manner similar to laser-in-situ keratomileusis (**Figs. 1 and 2**). The suction ring determines the size of lenticule obtained. It is available in sizes from +2, +1, 0 to –1, producing small to large size lenticules respectively

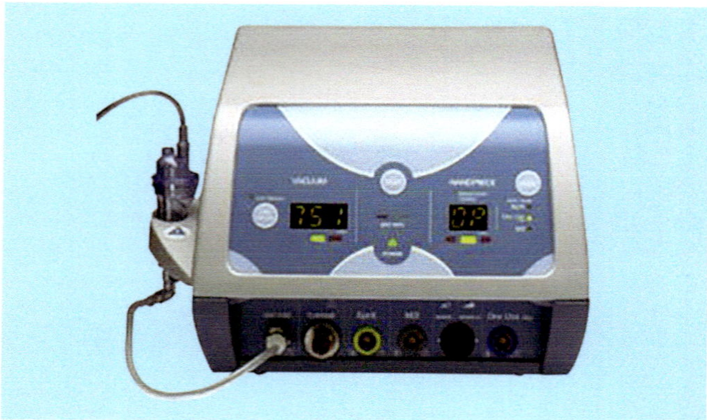

Fig. 1: Automated lamellar therapeutic keratoplasty machine. *Courtesy*: Moria SA France.

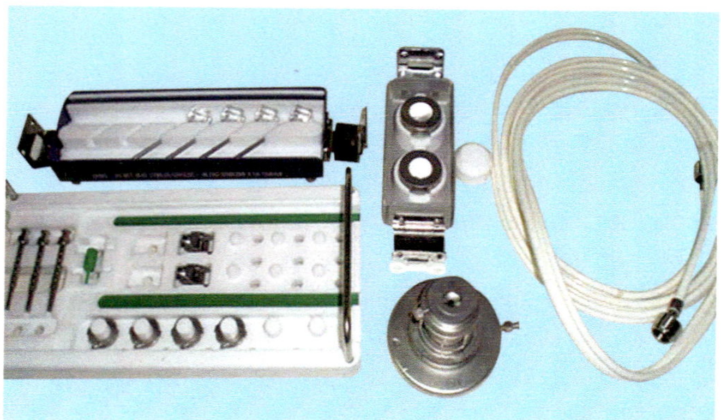

Fig. 2: Automated lamellar therapeutic keratoplasty (ALTK) surgical trolley.

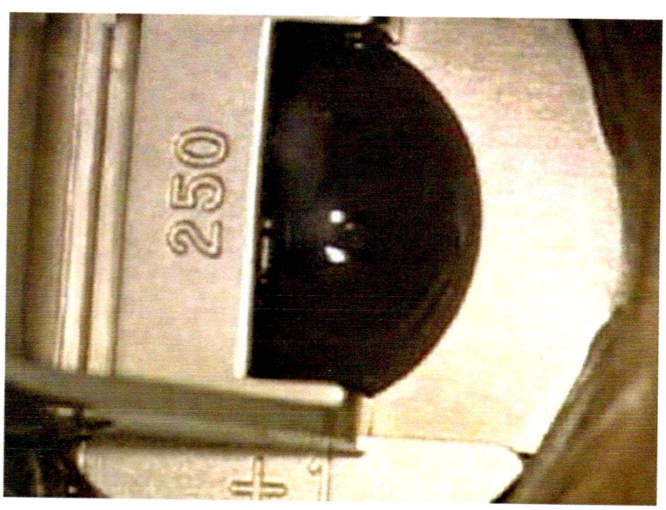

Fig. 3: Host cut made with a 250 µm microkeratome head.

for the same keratometry. The automated microkeratome is used as a cutting instrument. The advancement of the microkeratome over the suction ring can be either motor driven or manual. The microkeratome is available in various head sizes such as 120, 180, 250, and 350 µm, which can be used depending on the depth of the lamellar cut desired (**Fig. 3**). Once the disk is removed, the recipient bed is washed with balanced salt solution and dried using a sponge (**Fig. 4**).

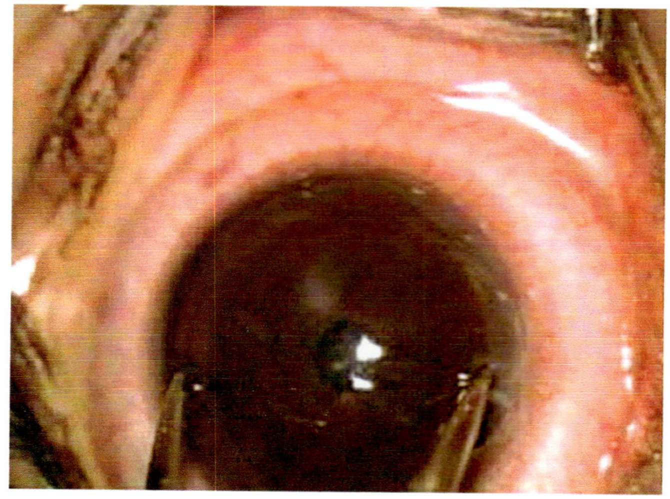

Fig. 4: Measurement of the diameter of host cut after the microkeratome cut.

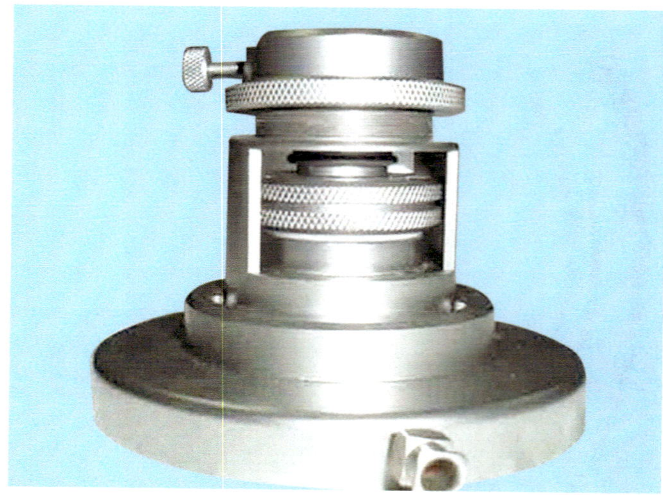

Fig. 5: Artificial anterior chamber.

Preparation of Donor Lenticule

The donor lenticule is dissected from a corneoscleral rim, mounted on an artificial anterior chamber system. The scleral frill should be at least 4 mm wide to allow proper positioning over the anterior chamber maintainer. The artificial anterior chamber is made of stainless steel and has three screw type safety rings. The lower ring sustains a metal device that covers the superficial sclera and maintains a tight fit on the metal base of the chamber to avoid leakage. A second ring in an intermediate position approximates the chamber on the former structure to tighten the sclera from above. The third ring, located superiorly is adjusted to modify the height of the microkeratome plate. This plate is a gearless track to guide the microkeratome head translation at a constant height along the corneal pass (**Fig. 5**). Depending on the height at which this plate is positioned, more (lower position) or less (higher position) of the cornea is exposed, resulting in a larger or smaller lenticule diameter, respectively. The chamber is connected to an infusion system with a reservoir of saline solution, placed 1.2 m above the chamber level. An expansion air chamber is located within the infusion line at a distance

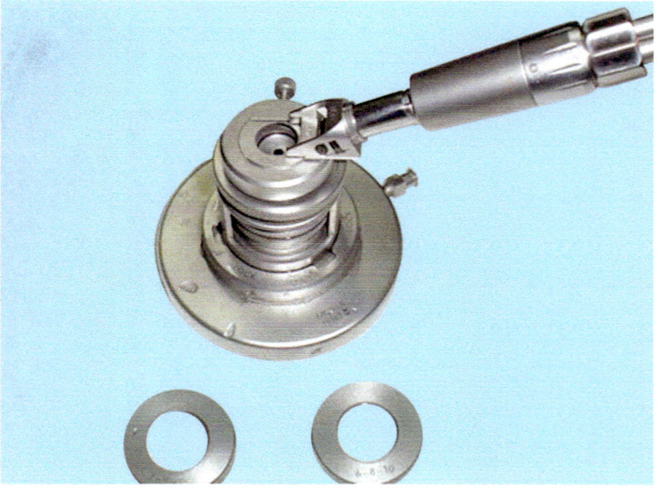

Fig. 6: Microkeratome head applanation lenses.

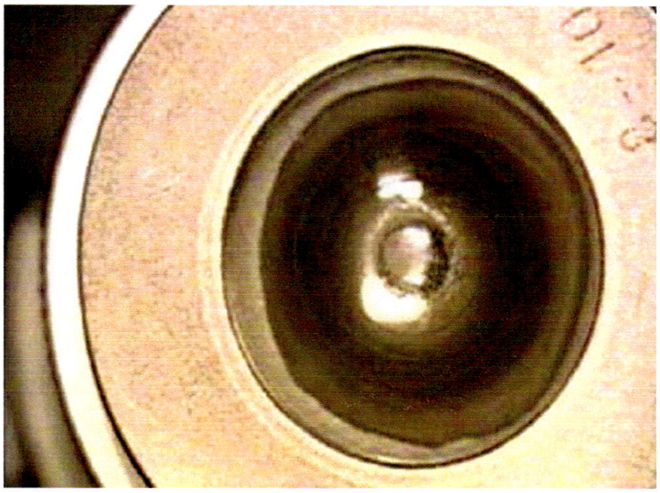

Fig. 8: Desired diameter is adjusted by using an applanation lens.

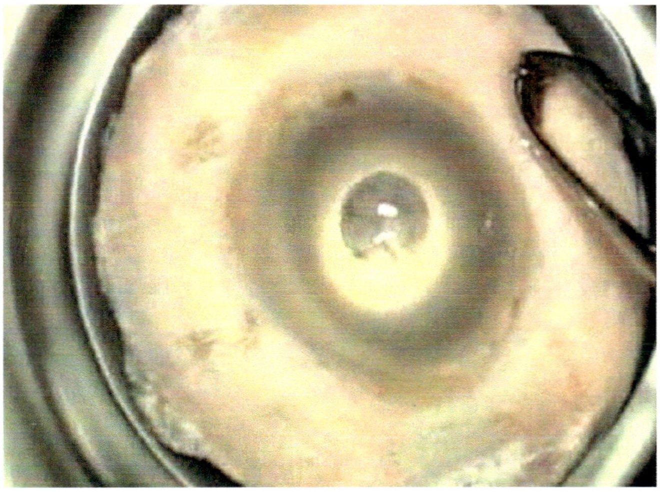

Fig. 7: Donor placement over the anterior chamber.

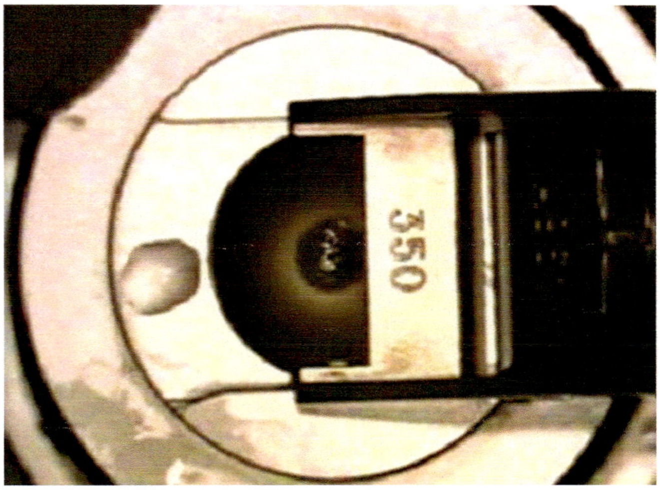

Fig. 9: 350 μm microkeratome head used for donor dissection.

of 10.0 cm from the connecting point with the chamber. The pressure should be kept at >60 mm Hg and should be checked with a Barraquer tonometer. Pressure as high as 95 mm Hg has been suggested to ensure a donor lenticule with more consistent thickness.

We use LSK microkeratome (Moria) to perform automated LK. It consists of a single piece metal head connected to a nitrogen-gas-driven hand piece. The blade oscillates at a rate of 15,000 oscillations/min with an orientation of 25° to the cut plane. The grooves on the base plate of the artificial anterior chamber are designed to fit onto the microkeratome head, to allow uniform passage through the cornea (**Fig. 6**).

To reduce the number of air bubbles beneath the cornea, rims are placed on the chamber base once, the infusion is released (**Fig. 7**). Once the cornea is stabilized and centered and the absence of air bubbles is confirmed, the infusion is closed, the superior metal support is placed and locked by turning the first ring clockwise, and the second ring is turned anticlockwise to elevate the chamber height and tighten the scleral skirt between the support and chamber.

The applanation lens is then placed on the cornea to determine the plate height for the desired diameter, turning the second ring counter clockwise, or clockwise depending on the guiding circle marks on the lenses (**Fig. 8**). Drops of saline solution are placed on the cornea and keratectomy is performed by passing the microkeratome head with its oscillating blade at a relatively constant speed along the plate (**Fig. 9**). The diameter of the flap which has been cut, is then measured (**Fig. 10**). Behrens et al. report that the precision and accuracy of this system varies according to the attempted thickness and diameter. Greater precision is obtained if the diameter of the cut is <8 mm or if the flaps are thinner.[10]

DONOR RECIPIENT APPOSITION

The donor lenticule is transferred over the recipient bed. Although some surgeons leave the donor lenticule adhered to the recipient bed without any sutures, we prefer to put at least 8 interrupted sutures with 10-0 monofilament nylon sutures. The eye is than patched for 24 hours. Use of fibrin

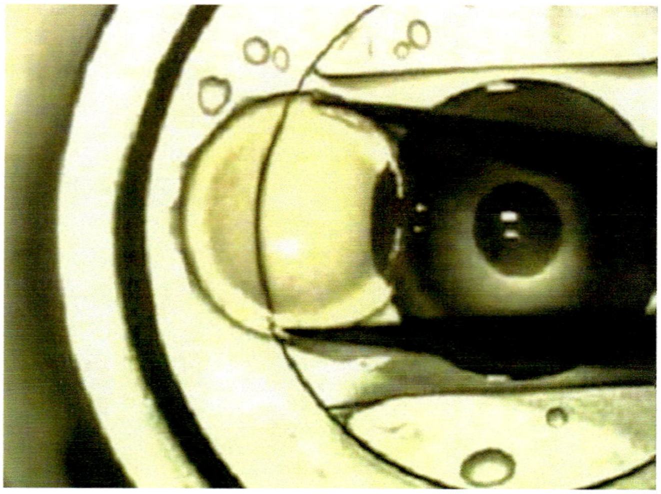

Fig. 10: Assessing the diameter of donor button using a callipers.

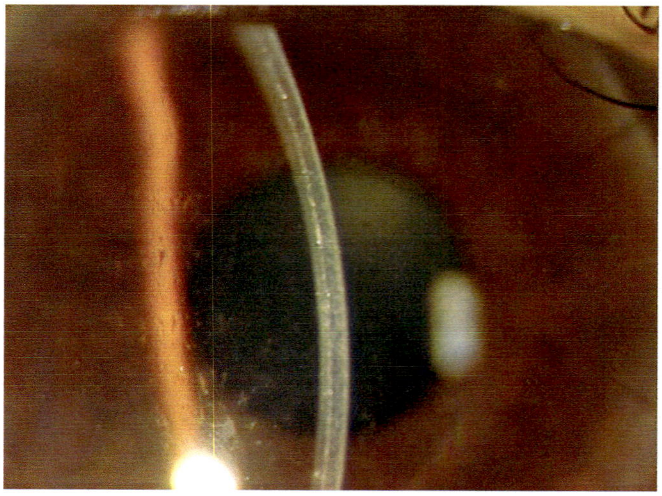

Fig. 11: Cross-sectional slit lamp view showing a smooth graft-host interface, after microkeratome-assisted automated lamellar keratoplasty.

glue instead of sutures has also been suggested for securing the donor lenticule over the host bed.[11]

Postoperatively, the patient is prescribed topical antibiotics, corticosteroids in tapering doses and preservative-free lubricants.

FEMTOSECOND-ASSISTED AUTOMATED LAMELLAR KERATOPLASTY

Femtosecond is the latest addition in the armamentarium available for lamellar corneal procedures. The main advantages over an automated microkeratome are better safety, reproducibility, predictability, and flexibility of femtosecond laser. Use of femtosecond laser for automated lamellar keratoplasty has been reported although larger studies are required to better understand the full scope of utility provided by the femtosecond laser.[12]

ADVANTAGES

An automated microkeratome allows the surgeon to obtain corneal lenticules with parallel faces that are almost identical in the donor and the recipient corneas. These factors result in optical and refractive results that are better than those obtained with the manual technique. The cut made by an automated microkeratome is regular and homogeneous producing a smooth surface (**Fig. 11**) without significant chatter lines as seen with scanning electron microscope.[13] This prevents irregular astigmatism that occurs following manual procedure because of the horizontal adherence of the disk to the donor tissue. Further, the surgical time is shortened and fewer sutures are required for shorter periods of time, which reduces suture-related complications.[14] The procedure may be combined with phacoemulsification if a significant cataract is present. Removal of anterior diseased corneal tissue allows better visualization for phacoemulsification.

COMPLICATIONS

Complications associated with ALTK are usually microkeratome related. The most dreaded but uncommon complication is corneal perforation during recipient bed preparation.[3] It usually occurs in eyes with steep and irregular cornea. Precise assessment of lesion depth and appropriate selection of microkeratome head and suction ring can help to avoid this complication.

Incomplete pass of the microkeratome may result in partial flap formation. This may result from resistance to the movement of the microkeratome or loss of suction. Patients with deep set eyes and small palpebral apertures are especially predisposed. Another complication is significant discrepancy in the size and thickness of the host bed and donor lenticule. It has been shown that almost 85% of recipient beds have diameter within 0.5 mm of the desired lenticule diameter but a few cases may have too high or too low diameter due to improper choice of suction ring or abnormal keratometry. The donor cornea used may have significant edema during preparation of the lenticule.

The donor lenticule thus prepared will further reduce in thickness during the postoperative period.[10]

There are several things a surgeon should consider when using this technique. It is important to obtain lenticules with same diameter and thickness so that the fit is perfect and future epithelial ingrowth is avoided. Epithelial ingrowth can occur after significant trauma even after many years of surgery.[15] Epithelium of the donor should be kept intact as far as possible. It gets replaced by the recipient epithelium during the first week, postoperatively.

Other complications are similar to manual LK. Incidence and severity of interface haze is likely to be less in ALTK due to a smoother interface. Although endothelial rejection does not occur, possibility of stromal rejection or epithelial rejection should always be kept in mind.[16]

OUTCOMES OF AUTOMATED LAMELLAR THERAPEUTIC KERATOPLASTY

Automated lamellar therapeutic keratoplasty was undertaken in 48 eyes at our center for various indications which included cases such as keratoconus (**Figs. 12A and B**), corneal stromal (**Figs. 13A and B**), Salzmann nodular degeneration (**Figs. 14A and B**), impacted corneal foreign bodies (**Figs. 15A and B**), and healed bacterial (**Figs. 16A and B**) and fungal keratitis (**Figs. 17A and B**). The donor corneal size ranged from 8.5 to 10 mm (thickness 350 μm) and the host cut size ranged

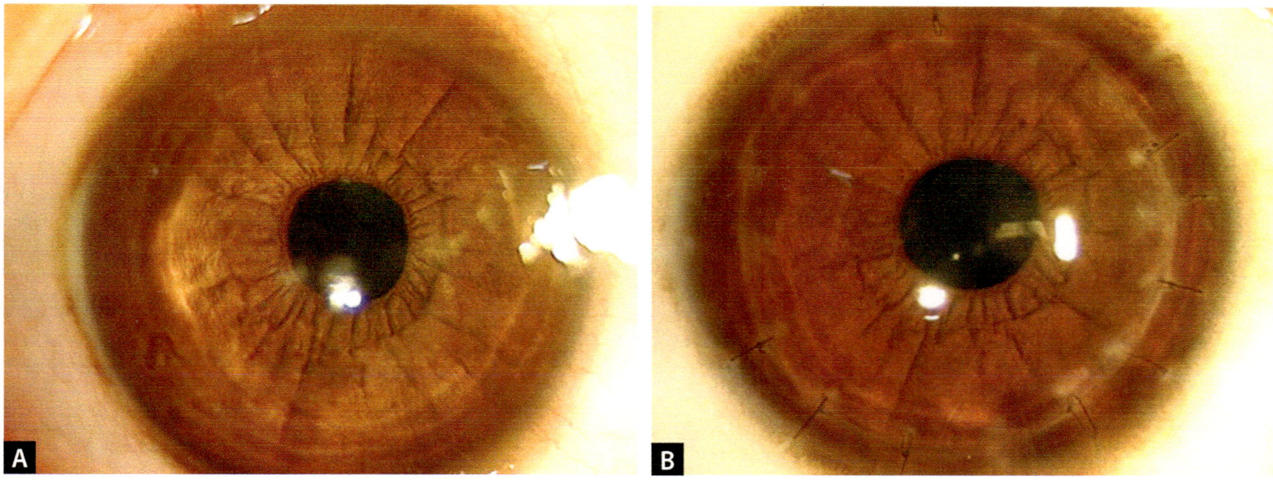

Figs. 12A and B: (A) Slit-lamp photograph of the left eye of a patient with keratoconus; (B) Postoperative slit-lamp photograph of the same eye, 6 months following automated lamellar therapeutic keratoplasty showing a smooth and regular corneal surface.

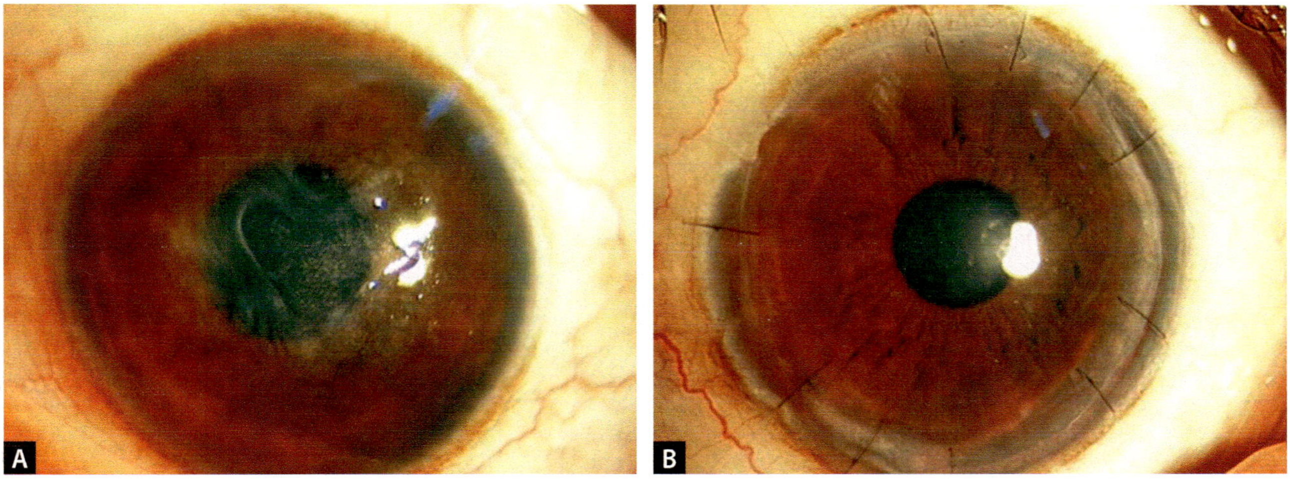

Figs. 13A and B: (A) Slit-lamp photograph of the right eye of a patient with lattice corneal dystrophy; (B) Postoperative slit-lamp photograph of the same eye, 3 months following automated lamellar therapeutic keratoplasty.

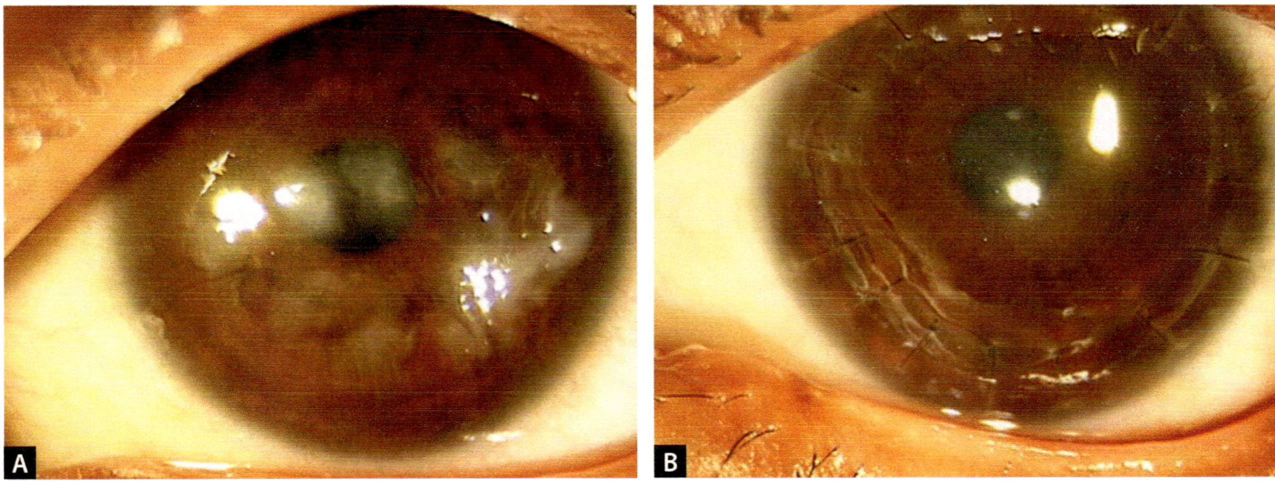

Figs. 14A and B: (A) Slit-lamp photograph of the left eye of a patient with Salzmann nodular degeneration; (B) Postoperative slit-lamp photograph of the same patient, 6 months following automated lamellar therapeutic keratoplasty.

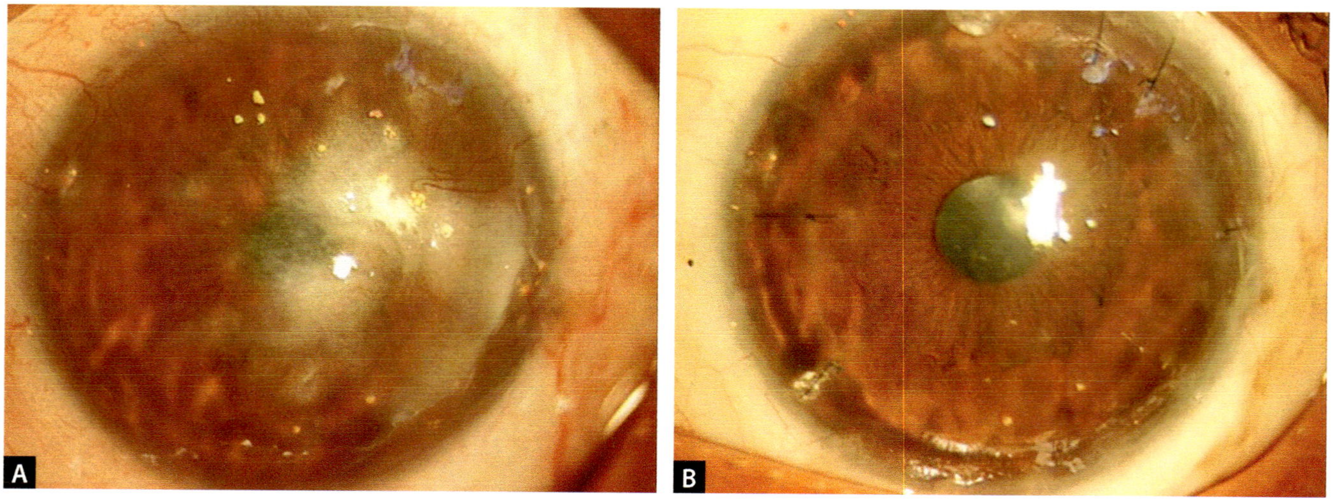

Figs. 15A and B: (A) Slit-lamp photograph of the right eye of a patient with multiple corneal foreign bodies; (B) Postoperative slit-lamp photograph of the same patient, 9 months following automated lamellar therapeutic keratoplasty.

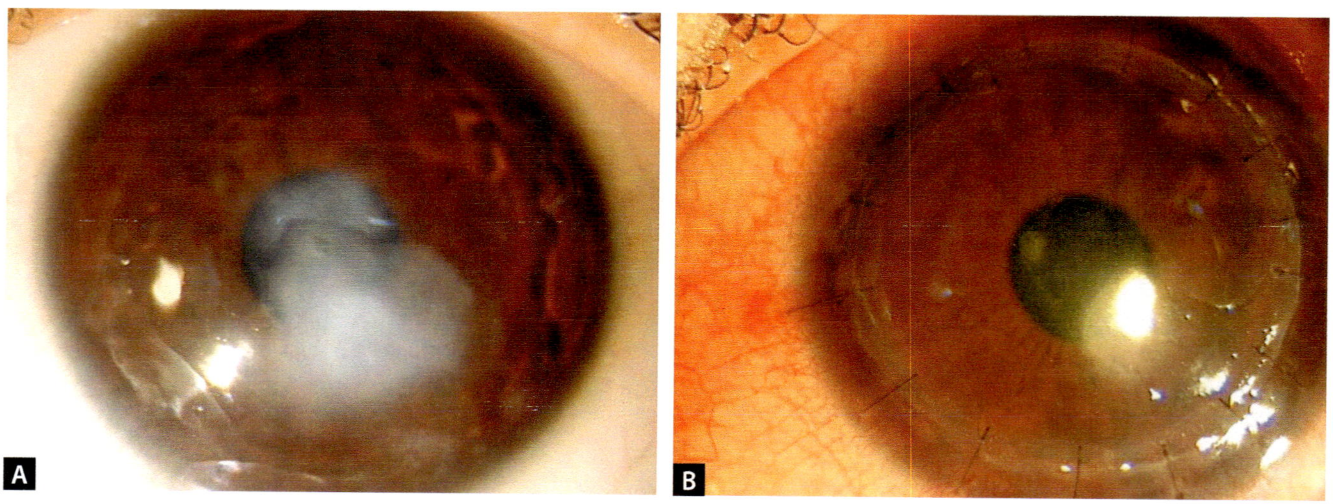

Figs. 16A and B: (A) Slit-lamp photograph of the left eye of a patient with resolved bacterial keratitis; (B) Postoperative slit-lamp photograph of the same eye, 1 month following automated lamellar therapeutic keratoplasty.

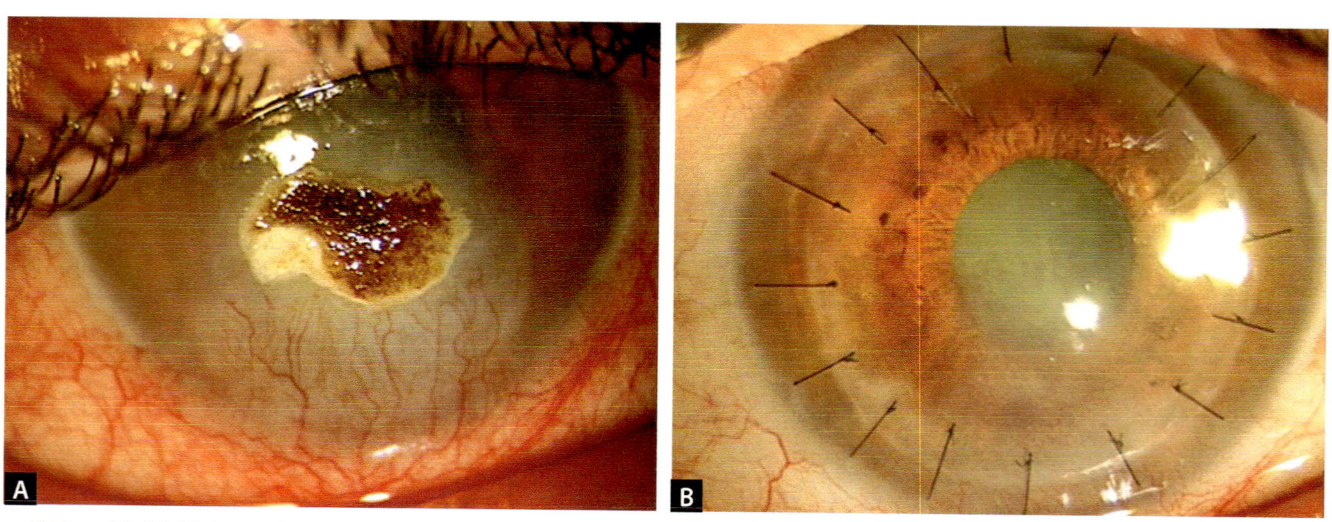

Figs. 17A and B: (A) Slit-lamp photograph of the right eye of a patient with demateaceous fungal keratitis; (B) Postoperative slit-lamp photograph of the same eye, 1 month following automated lamellar therapeutic keratoplasty.

from 8 to 9.5 mm (thickness 250 μm). Sixteen to twenty four interrupted sutures using 10-0 monofilament nylon sutures applied (*see* **Fig. 4**). The mean central corneal thickness was 503 mm. From a preoperative visual acuity of ≤2/60 in all eyes, a postoperative visual acuity of ≥6/18 was achieved in 32 out of 48 patients. The mean epithelialization time was 3 days (range 1–10 days). No cases of interface scarring were seen after a follow-up of 6 months. However, the long-term problems of interface scarring need to be ascertained.

In the largest and longest follow-up study reported by Guber I et al., ALTK was performed in 37 adult and 16 juvenile eyes.[17] The outcomes were evaluated as a function of age. Visual impairment due to corneal scarring was the predominant indication for surgery. Mean age of enrolled patients was 34.8 years, ranging from 3 months to 88 years. Mean follow-up period was 35 months. A 250 μm microkeratome head was used to cut both the donor as well as host cornea. The grafts were secured either with a standard suturing technique or using overlay sutures. Mean LogMAR visual acuity was 0.55 in adult eyes and 0.45 in juvenile eyes, which was comparable. Overall, juvenile eyes had greater number of complications and required significantly more number of surgical revisions.

Although we did not encounter any major complications, there are risks associated, including delayed epithelialization, epithelial ingrowth, corneal vascularization, and dry eye.[15,17] Edema or melting of the lenticule can also occur. Although an endothelial rejection will not occur, an epithelial and stromal rejection may occur.[16] Finally, the original disease may recur. Optical LK, performed with an automated microkeratome, is an easy, simple, and accurate technique. It produces good visual results and is a good alternative to penetrating keratoplasty especially for the treatment of anterior corneal stromal pathology.

REFERENCES

1. Jimenez-Alfaro I, Perez-Santonja JJ, Telleria GG, Palcin B, Puy P. Therapeutic lamellar keratoplasty with an automated microkeratome. J Cataract Surg. 2001;27:1161-5.
2. Springs CL, Joseph MA, Odom JV, Wiley LA. Predictability of donor lamellar graft diameter and thickness in an artificial anterior chamber system. Cornea. 2002;21:696-9.
3. Vajpayee RB, Vasudendra N, Titiyal JS, Tandon R, Sharma N, Sinha R. Automated lamellar therapeutic keratoplasty (ALTK) in the treatment of anterior to mid-stromal corneal pathologies. Acta Ophthalmol Scand. 2006;84:771-3.
4. Jiménez-Alfaro I, Pérez-Santonja JJ, Gómez Tellería G, Bueno Palacín JL, Puy P. Therapeutic lamellar keratoplasty with an automated microkeratome. J Cataract Refract Surg. 2001;27:1161-5.
5. Tan DT, Ang LP. Modified automated lamellar therapeutic keratoplasty for keratoconus: a new technique. Cornea. 2006;25:1217-9.
6. Chen W, Qu J, Wang Q, Lu F, Barabino S. Automated lamellar keratoplasty for recurrent granular corneal dystrophy after phototherapeutic keratectomy. J Refract Surg. 2005;21:288-93.
7. Tan DT, Ang LP. Automated lamellar therapeutic keratoplasty for post-PRK corneal scarring and thinning. Am J Ophthalmol. 2004;138:1067-9.
8. Wiley LA, Joseph MA, Springs CL. Tectonic lamellar keratoplasty utilizing a microkeratome and an artificial anterior chamber system. Cornea. 2002;21:661-3.
9. Chuck RS, Behrens A, McDonnell PJ. Microkeratome-based limbal harvester for limbal stem cell transplantation: preliminary studies. Am J Ophthalmol. 2001;131:377-8.
10. Behrens A, Dolorico AM, Kara DT, Novick LH, McDonnell PJ, Chao LC, et al. Precision and accuracy of an artificial anterior chamber system in obtaining corneal lenticules for lamellar keratoplasty. J Cataract Refract Surg. 2001;27:1679-87.
11. Chen W, Qu J, Lu F, Zhu RY. Sutureless lamellar keratoplasty by microkeratome combined with fibrin tissue adhesive in rabbits. Zhonghua Yan Ke Za Zhi. 2004;40:331-6.
12. Hoffart L, Proust H, Matonti F, Catanèse M, Conrath J, Ridings B. Femtosecond-assisted anterior lamellar keratoplasty. J Fr Ophtalmol. 2007;30:689-94.
13. Victor G, Sousa SJ, Alves MR, Nosé W. Evaluation of a new system for obtaining donor lamellar grafts. Cornea. 2007;26(2):151-3.
14. Maia NC, Chamon W, Castelo Branco B. Evaluation of performance, efficacy and safety of semi-automated lamellar keratoplasty. Arq Bras Oftalmol. 2006;69:795-804.
15. Wang TJ, Wang IJ, Hou YC, Hu FR. Giant epithelial ingrowth induced by blunt injury after automated lamellar keratoplasty. J Formos Med Assoc. 2005;104:279-81.
16. Kawashima M, Mochizuki H, Kawakita T, Hatoh S, Shimazaki J, Yamada M. Presumed stromal graft rejection after automated lamellar therapeutic keratoplasty: case report. J Med Case Rep. 2007;1:10.
17. Guber I, Bergin C, Othenin-Girard P, Munier F, Majo F. 12-year outcomes of microkeratome-assisted anterior lamellar therapeutic keratoplasty (ALTK) for disorders of the anterior part of the corneal stroma—A comparative review of adult and children. Klin Monbl Augenheilkd. 2018;235(4): 404-8.

22

Superficial Anterior Lamellar Keratoplasty

Giuseppe Giannaccare, Angeli Christy Yu, Massimo Busin

INTRODUCTION

In the past, penetrating keratoplasty (PK) was considered the main surgical option for corneal diseases not amenable to conservative management. With improved instrumentation, recent years have seen a dramatic shift in surgical trends, now favoring selective lamellar keratoplasty.

Moreover, the introduction of the mechanical microkeratome system has not only revolutionized the field of refractive surgery but has also led to significant innovations in corneal transplantation. Its successful use in laser in situ keratomileusis (LASIK) has allowed the development of improved techniques for lamellar keratoplasty such as microkeratome-assisted superficial anterior lamellar keratoplasty (SALK).[1-4]

SALK is indicated for the treatment of superficial corneal opacities resulting from previous refractive surgical procedures, infections, trauma, degenerations, and dystrophies (**Fig. 1A**). The use of SALK for the various indications have been well-described in literature.[1-9] Modifications of SALK including combined excimer laser ablation,[5,6] and femtosecond laser-assisted techniques have also been proposed.[8,9] However, aside from the additional costs for the use of the laser, laser-assisted dissection is technically possible only in cases with good corneal transparency since the laser may not penetrate well through opacified tissue and fails to work immediately when bleeding occurs. Thus, we prefer the use of microkeratome-assisted dissection technique for SALK in these cases.

OPERATIVE TECHNIQUE

Anesthesia and akinesia can be obtained by means of peribulbar injection. A 130 μm or 200 μm head is chosen depending on the depth of involvement of the corneal stromal lesion. Using a pivoting microkeratome with a size "0" suction ring, a 9 mm diameter superficial free cap is cut from a recipient cornea with intact epithelium. To ensure a planar cut with the intended diameter, dissection must be performed through a continuous, slow advancement of the microkeratome with counter-rotation of the fixation ring.

The donor cornea is mounted on the artificial anterior chamber of an automated lamellar therapeutic keratoplasty system. The anterior donor lamella is dissected by means of a 90 or 130 μm microkeratome head. The thickness of the donor lamella does not need to exactly match the one of the excised donor stroma. Using a microkeratome cutting head that is 40 μm less for the donor compared with the host cornea results in uniform apposition in all cases without the need for sutures. More importantly, the thickness of the residual recipient bed must be at least 250 μm, in order to avoid postoperative ectasia.

As the donor graft is particularly thin, it may be difficult to distinguish between anterior and posterior surfaces. Therefore, it is advisable to mark the anterior surface of the donor cornea. The donor tissue is placed on the cutting block and punched to the same size as the recipient bed using a Hessburg-Barron punch. In SALK, a slightly undersized graft may be preferable over larger grafts. If a graft with a diameter smaller than that of the recipient bed is used, the recipient epithelium usually covers the annular area of bare stroma. However, when a graft that is larger than the recipient bed is used, an epithelial ingrowth within the graft-host interface may develop, albeit rarely, and compromise the results of surgery.

Once prepared, the graft is then simply laid onto the recipient bed. The interface should be copiously irrigated to remove any blood or any debris that can cause interface haze. As with any lamellar technique, interface haze or scarring may compromise the functional recovery. Cauterization of the bleeding vessels may be performed or topical epinephrine may be applied to achieve hemostasis.

Similar to a LASIK flap, the graft adheres to the recipient cornea even without fixation sutures. As no hinge is present to keep the graft in place, bandage contact lens can be used to secure the graft. Alternatively, overlay sutures can be used to keep the graft in place by passing the needle through the periphery of the recipient cornea at three equidistant points and then suturing over the graft. The edges of the graft must be examined to ensure that there is no over-riding or under-riding. Attention to suture tension is particularly

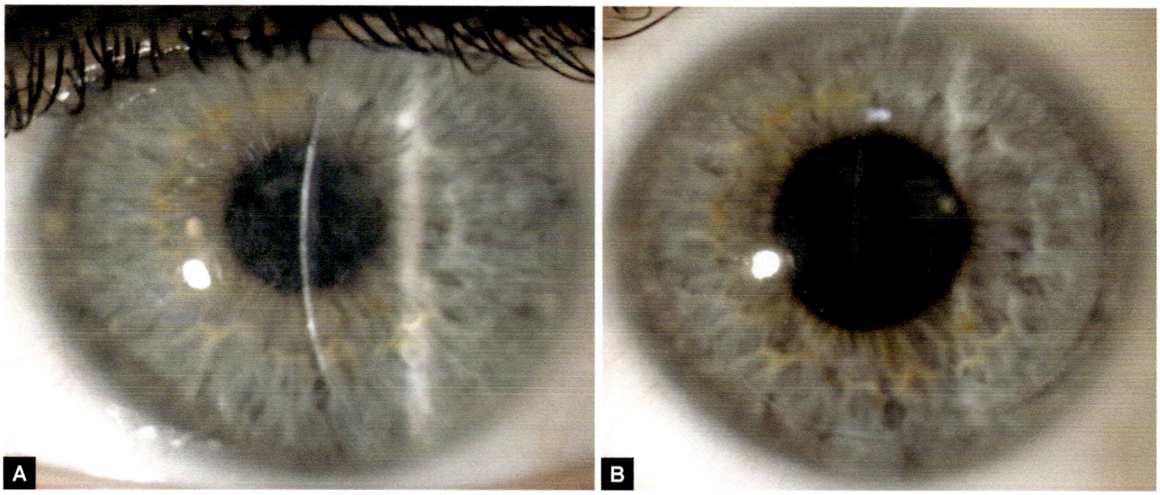

Figs. 1A and B: (A) Preoperative clinical photo of an eye that developed corneal haze after photorefractive keratectomy; (B) Postoperative clinical photo of the same eye following superficial anterior lamellar keratoplasty.

important for achieving good outcomes. Excessively tight sutures and/or delayed suture removal tend to create permanent folds in the graft and act as a physical barrier against normal re-epithelialization of the graft surface. It is also important to make sure that all portions of the sutures lie on the surface rather than in the interface. Radial sutures are contraindicated in this procedure, as they would distort the thin graft and induce high and irregular astigmatism. The overlay sutures must be removed within 7 days of surgery. **Figure 1B** illustrates the appearance after suture removal.

DISCUSSION

Superficial anterior lamellar keratoplasty shares several advantages with other forms of lamellar keratoplasty. As an extraocular procedure, devastating complications of open-sky surgery including suprachoroidal hemorrhage and iatrogenic injury to various intraocular structures are avoided. With preservation of the host endothelium, this procedure carries no risk of immunologic endothelial rejection regardless of graft diameter. Should an episode of epithelial or stromal rejection occur, complete reversal is possible though topical steroidal therapy alone without adverse effects on both graft survival and visual outcomes.

Considering the relative ease of use of the microkeratome in the absence of particular surgical skills, SALK is a rapid and fairly reproducible procedure with a more easily surmountable learning curve over that of deep anterior lamellar keratoplasty (DALK). In addition, microkeratome dissection facilitates the removal of diseased corneal stroma and produces a smooth, regular graft-host interface independent of tissue clarity, consistency or vascularization. Thus, SALK results in significant visual recovery in a shorter period of time postoperatively.[1-3]

Since the largest contributing component of the overall corneal optical power is the anterior corneal curvature, the use of large-diameter 9 mm grafts maximizes the refractive benefits of SALK.[1-3] Moreover, by limiting the dissection to the superficial stroma, the biomechanics of the host cornea is maintained. In cases of surface ablation-related corneal haze after phototherapeutic keratectomy (PTK), sutureless SALK provides excellent visual outcomes with refractive astigmatism that is correctable with spectacles alone.[3]

It is important to recognize the limitations of SALK. Eyes with significant pathology extending into the posterior half of the stroma would require DALK or even a PK. If the patient's cornea is irregular with areas of elevation or thinning, these would be reproduced by the microkeratome when creating the recipient flap. Nonetheless, SALK is a safe and effective procedure for superficial corneal opacities.

REFERENCES

1. Busin M. Microkeratome-assisted superficial anterior lamellar keratoplasty. Tech Ophthalmol. 2006;4(2):64-8.
2. Patel AK, Scorcia V, Kadyan A, Lapenna L, Ponzin D, Busin M. Microkeratome-assisted superficial anterior lamellar keratoplasty for anterior stromal corneal opacities after penetrating keratoplasty. Cornea. 2011;31(1):101-5.
3. Myerscough J, Bovone C, Thomas PBM, Mimouni M, Aljassar F, Padroni S, et al. Sutureless superficial anterior lamellar keratoplasty for recurrent corneal haze after repeat excimer laser surface ablation. Br J Ophthalmol. 2020;104(3):341-4.
4. Jimenez-Alfaro I, Perez-Santonja JJ, Gomez Telleria G, Bueno Palacin JL, Puy P. Therapeutic lamellar keratoplasty with an automated microkeratome. J Cataract Refract Surg. 2001;27(8):1161-5.
5. Alio JL, Javaloy J, Merayo J, Galal A. Automated superficial lamellar keratectomy augmented by excimer laser masked PTK in the management of severe superficial corneal opacities. Br J Ophthalmol. 2004;88:1289-94.
6. Wiley LA, Joseph MA, Pemberton JD. Microkeratome-assisted anterior lamellar keratoplasty. Arch Ophthalmol. 2008;126:404-8.
7. Fogla R, Knyazer B. Microkeratome-assisted two-stage technique of superficial anterior lamellar keratoplasty for Reis-Bücklers corneal dystrophy. Cornea. 2014;33:1118-22.
8. Alió JL, Agdeppa MCC, Uceda-Montanes A. Femtosecond laser-assisted superficial lamellar keratectomy for the treatment of superficial corneal leukomas. Cornea. 2011;30:301-7.
9. Shousha MA, Yoo SH, Kymionis GD, Ide T, Feuer W, Karp CL, et al. Long-term results of femtosecond laser-assisted sutureless anterior lamellar keratoplasty. Ophthalmology. 2011;118:315-23.

23

Deep Anterior Lamellar Keratoplasty: The Melles Technique

Keamela Vasanthananthan, C Maya Tong, Gerrit RJ Melles

INTRODUCTION

Deep anterior lamellar keratoplasty (DALK) is a surgical procedure in which pathologic corneal stroma is replaced by donor tissue leaving the recipient's Descemet membrane (DM) and endothelium intact. DALK can be successfully performed with two surgical techniques, one relying on injection and one relying on manual dissection. The Melles manual DALK (mmDALK) technique belongs to the latter group and facilitates precise dissection down to the level of the DM by using the phenomenon of the *air-endothelial reflex*.[1,2]

BACKGROUND

Although the concept of anterior lamellar keratoplasty (ALK) was first introduced over 150 years ago and early attempts of lamellar dissection near the DM were made by Hallermann in the 1950s, surgeons have long preferred to perform a penetrating keratoplasty (PK).[3,4] Initially, a PK was easier to perform and had better visual outcomes.[5] Lamellar transplants often had decreased best corrected visual acuity due to irregular astigmatism and/or scarring at the donor-to-recipient interface because the total removal of the recipient's stroma, down to the DM, was difficult to achieve with manual dissection. The stroma left behind would interact with the donor tissue, producing haze at the graft's interface and restrict the visual outcome.[6] Despite these initial challenges, lamellar procedures have become increasingly popular as they carry the advantages of avoiding most complications associated with "open-sky" surgery. These include easier postoperative management, less risk of allograft rejection, and other long-term complications.

In the early 1990s, Anwar et al. showed that injecting saline into the deep corneal stroma often resulted in a cleavage plane just above the DM.[7-10] This technique was further refined by using air instead of saline, and constituted the basis for the big-bubble DALK technique.[11] Around the same time, it was demonstrated that injection of viscoelastics could yield similar results.[12,13]

However, formation of a big bubble can be challenging. A major problem with these techniques was that up to 10–50% of the attempts resulted in an overt perforation of the DM.[14-20] If perforation occurs, completion of the stromal dissection can be difficult. The donor button may have to be sutured into an imperfectly prepared recipient bed, or the DALK may be aborted and the procedure converted into a PK requiring donor tissue with good endothelium, which may not always be available. With this in mind, a technique with visually controlled dissection of the recipient stroma from its DM was developed, and ultimately resulted in the mmDALK technique.[1,2]

THE MELLES MANUAL DEEP ANTERIOR LAMELLAR KERATOPLASTY SURGICAL TECHNIQUE

Visualization and Dissection Depth during Surgery

Although an intraoperative anterior optical coherence tomography (OCT) can be used to analyze the depth of the corneal incision and the lamellar stromal dissection plane, this technology is not readily available to all surgeons. The mmDALK technique is more applicable and depends on a single intraoperative observation with the operating microscope and a special set of instruments.

Insertion of air in the anterior chamber (AC) will create an optical interface at the posterior corneal surface due to a difference in refractive index. When instruments are inserted from the peripheral cornea, a reflection can be observed at the tip of these instruments. The deeper the indentation of the instrument is during incision of the cornea, the closer the reflection appears at the tip of the instrument. When the two are nearly touching each other, a stromal dissection at the plane anterior to the posterior corneal surface can be made. This air-endothelial reflex is always present. It provides immediate visual feedback to the surgeon, and allows for a controlled and precise manual dissection of host stroma from the underlying DM (**Figs. 1 and 2**).

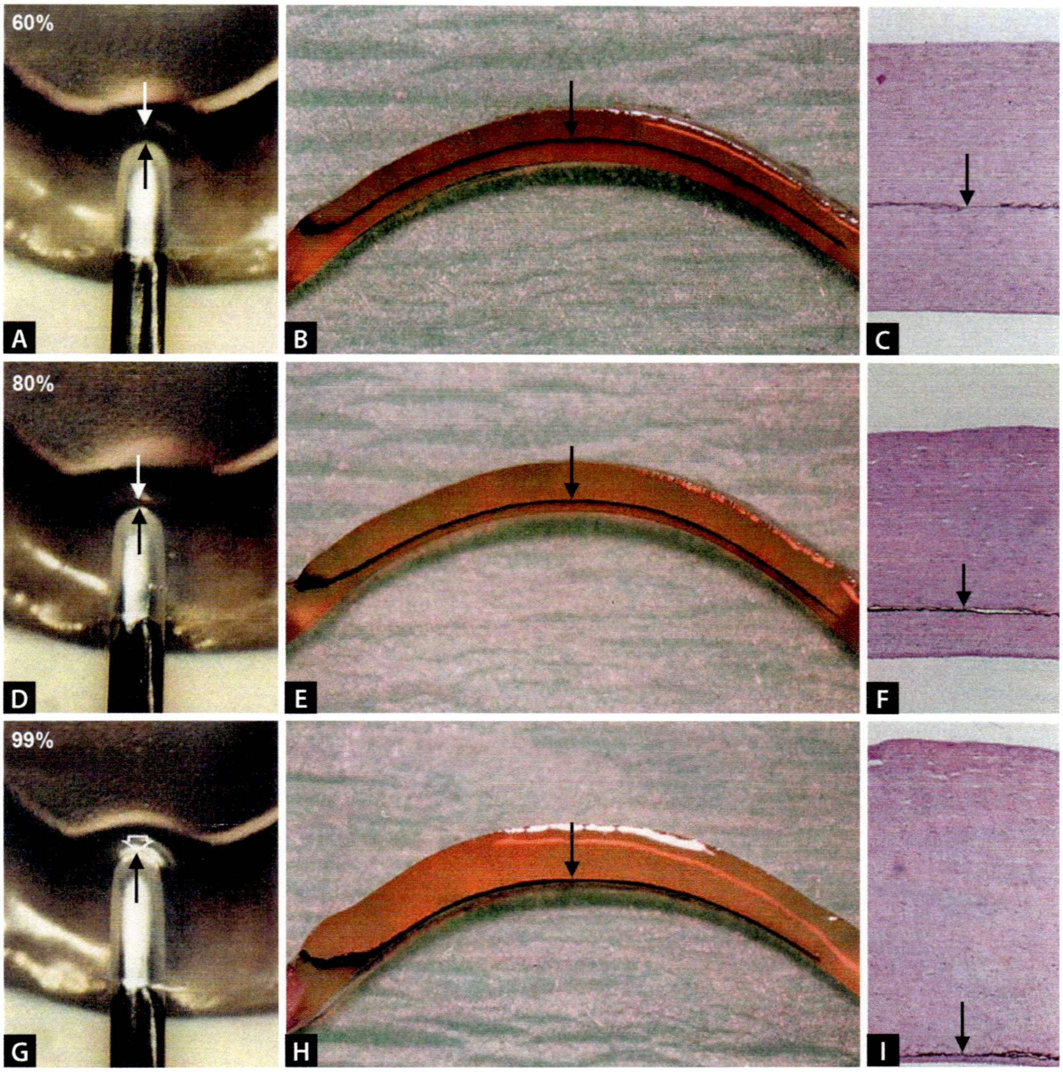

Figs. 1A to I: Clinical, macroscopic, and light microscopic pictures of lamellar dissections made at an intended depth of (A to C) 60%, (D to F) 80%, and (G to I) 99%. A "dark band" is visible between the blade tip (arrow) and the semicircular light reflex at the air-to-endothelium interface (open arrow). Note how the amount of nonincised tissue underneath the blade tip in A, D and G compares to the dissection depth in B/C, E/F and H/I. Thus, the achieved dissection depth (thick arrows) can be estimated by the thickness of the dark band adjacent to the blade tip.
Courtesy: Modified with permission from Melles GR, Rietveld FJ, Beekhuis WH, Binder PS. A technique to visualize corneal incision and lamellar dissection depth during surgery. Cornea. 1999;18:80-6.

Surgical Steps

A superior peritomy is performed and a corneoscleral tunnel is made using a 5-mm crescent knife. The AC is filled with air to support the air-endothelial reflex. Using the air-endothelial reflex as a guide, the recipient cornea should be dissected from limbus to limbus, 360° around, using a specialized set of spatulas: the Melles spatula set (DORC International BV, Zuidland, the Netherlands). This set consists of three spatulas with (1) red, (2) white, and (3) blue handles corresponding to their increasing lengths and curvatures (**Figs. 3A to C**). After the stromal dissection is completed, the air is removed from the AC and viscoelastic is injected into the dissected stromal pocket. The anterior cornea is be trephined away, and the donor lamellar graft sutured in place (**Figs. 4A to I**).[1,2]

Preparation of Donor Tissue

Ordering a full-thickness donor cornea from the providing eye bank has two advantages. The first is that a full-thickness graft can be available in the event that the case requires conversion to PK. Second, premature removal of DM can result in stromal edema and thickening, making the graft difficult to suture securely at the time of surgery.

The posterior surface of the donor cornea is stained with vision blue (VisionBlue, DORC International BV). The DM and endothelium are completely removed by gentle swabbing with a cellulose sponge. The donor corneoscleral rim is mounted epithelial side down onto a punch block, and a 0.25-mm-oversized donor button is cut with a punch trephine (Ophtec, Groningen, the Netherlands).

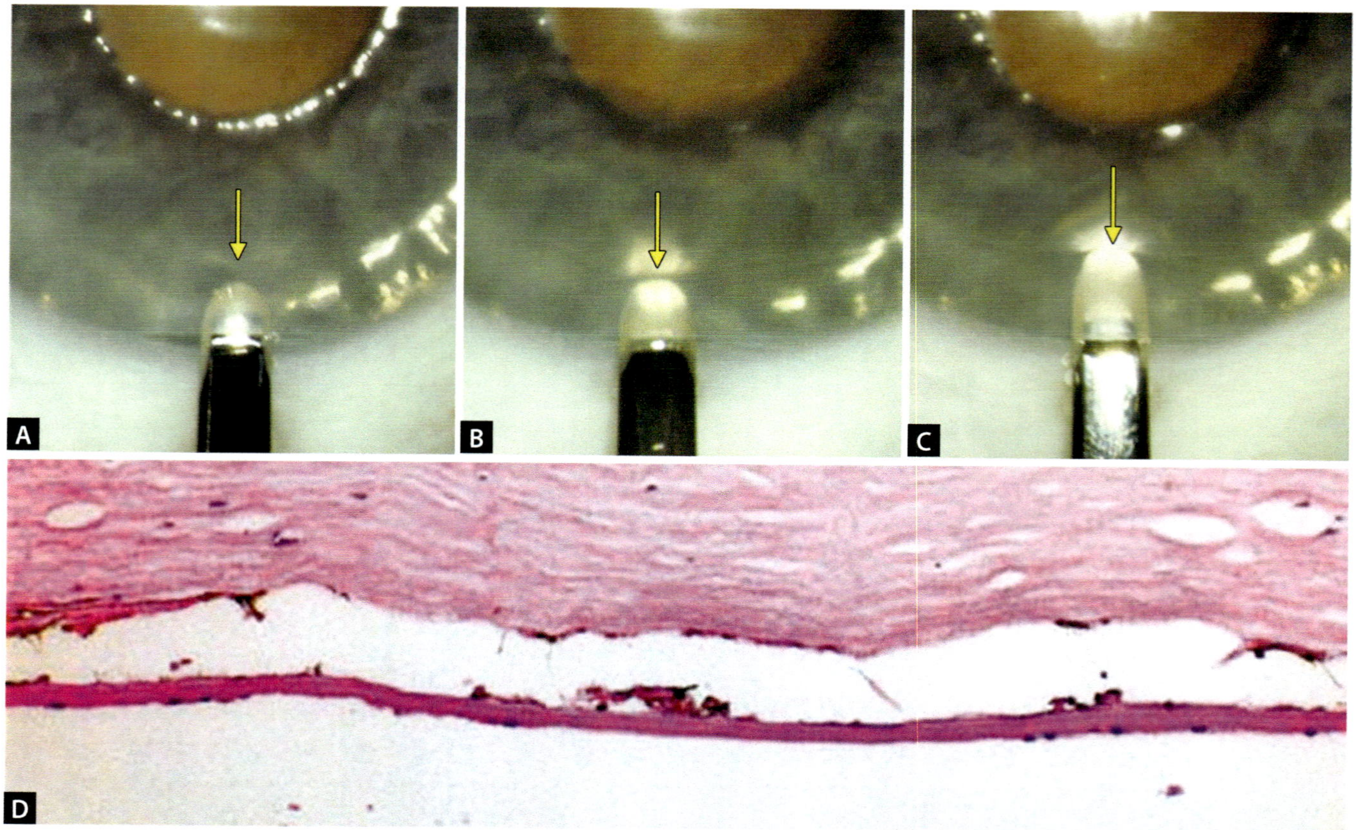

Figs. 2A to D: Demonstration of the surgical technique in a human eye bank eye. (A) The anterior chamber has been filled with air. In-between the blade tip and the air-to-endothelial interface light reflex, a dark band is visible. (B) Because the dark band reflects nonincised posterior corneal tissue, the dark band decreases in width when the blade is advanced into the deeper stromal layers. (C) When the blade appears to touch the air-to-endothelium interface, a stromal dissection level just anterior to the posterior corneal surface is reached. (D) Light microscopy of a deep lamellar dissection through a scleral incision in a human eye bank eye. A deep stromal dissection level is seen (98% corneal depth). Few stromal lamellae are visible between the stromal dissection and Descemet's membrane (hematoxylin-eosin, original magnification × 35 and × 450).

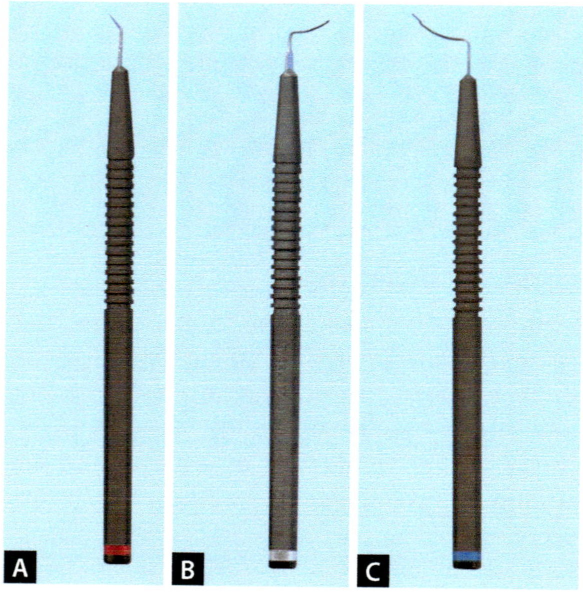

Figs. 3A to C: Lamellar dissectors for deep lamellar keratoplasty; the Melles spatula set (DORC International BV, Zuidland, the Netherlands).

Suturing Technique

Multiple suturing techniques have been described for PK, most often with 10-0 nylon sutures, with an interrupted, running or a combined method. Interrupted sutures have the advantages that closely monitored astigmatism which can be easily controlled by selective suture removal. In case of loose sutures requiring removal, the remaining sutures left in place are usually sufficient for fixation of the transplant. Single or double running sutures have the advantages that suture placement is easier and can be performed faster, and that the astigmatism may be controlled by suture adjustment. However, loose sutures may require additional surgical intervention.

In contrast to PK, that requires the sutures to be in situ for at least 1 year, the sutures may be removed at 4–6 months after lamellar keratoplasty. Therefore, a suturing technique with the least surgical time, the least amount of astigmatism, and sufficient fixation of the graft in the event of inadvertent suture loosening would a double running 8-bite 10-0 nylon anti-torc suture (**Fig. 5**).

This can be performed quickly and easily, without the need for cardinal fixation sutures. After marking four corneal meridians with an eight-radial marker, the needle is placed obliquely in the donor button at an ink mark, then inserted into the dissection plane present in the peripheral recipient cornea and moved upward. Care should be taken to bury

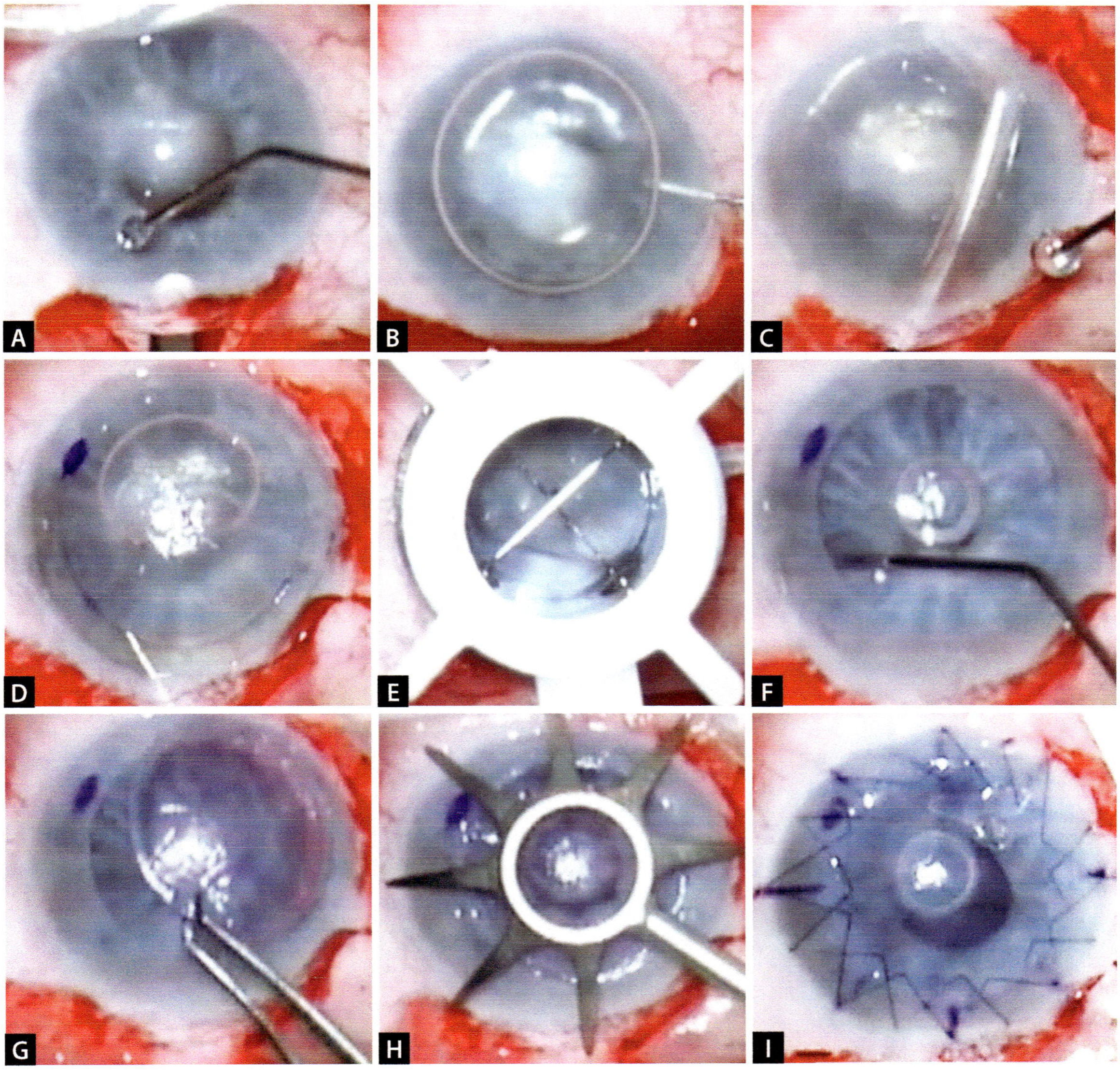

Figs. 4A to I: Surgical stills demonstrating the Melles manual deep anterior lamellar keratoplasty (DALK)-technique. (A) After a superior peritomy is performed and a 5-mm corneoscleral tunnel is fashioned using a crescent blade, (B) the anterior chamber is filled with air through a side port. (C) Then a deep stromal dissection up to the limbus over 360° is completed with spatulas. The thin black line alongside the spatula serves as an indication for dissection depth. (D) Most of the air has been removed from the anterior chamber and the dissected pocket is filled with viscoelastic to separate the Descemet membrane from the posterior stroma. (E) Next, with a Hessburg–Barron trephine, the anterior corneal lamella is trephined until the viscoelastic escapes, and (F) excised while leaving the Descemet membrane in situ, note the smooth recipient bed, which is rinsed with balanced salt solution, (G) before an anterior lamellar donor button is placed onto the recipient bed. (H) Finally, the donor and recipient corneal surfaces are marked with an eight incision radial keratotomy marker and (I) the donor button is sutured in place with two running sutures.

the knots at the 12 o'clock position, as unburied knots may cause continuing discomfort for the patient and may serve as a nidus for infection. Theoretically, a double running 8-bite 10-0 nylon anti-torc suture may induce little astigmatism, because the forces exerted by each bite are counteracted by an opposing bite. If suture loosening occurs after surgery, the graft is usually fixated well by the remaining suture. In our series, secondary suture placement has not been necessary.[1,2] Finally, removal of this 8-bite running 10-0 suture can easily be performed behind the slit lamp.

Topical and Systemic Therapy

A standard therapy regimen for PK patients is preoperative gentamicin ointment in the evening before surgery, and postoperative chloramphenicol 0.5% three times daily for 1 month and dexamethasone 0.1% six times daily for 1 month, tapering to one time daily at 1 year. In our series of DALK patients, the same perioperative therapy regimen was followed. Steroid therapy may be tapered sooner because the risk of endothelial allograft rejection is minimized for DALK recipients.

PREOPERATIVE CONSIDERATIONS

The main indications for mmDALK are patients with conventionally treated hydrops, advanced keratoconus, and less commonly postherpetic or traumatic corneal scars and a variety of stromal corneal dystrophies.[21-23]

The corneal endothelium of patients should be in good health to be suitable for a DALK procedure. Psychological

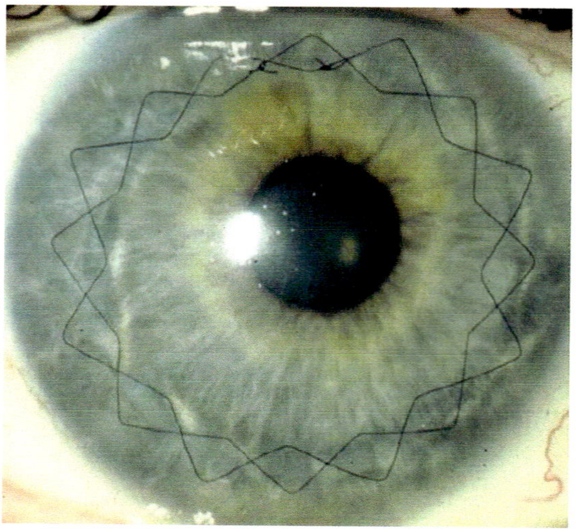

Fig. 5: Slit-lamp photograph 6 months after deep anterior lamellar keratoplasty (DALK). A clear lamellar corneal transplant is visible, with a deep stromal donor-to-recipient interface.

surveys have shown that patient satisfaction after corneal replacement for keratoconus depends on the operated eye becoming the better seeing eye, rather than the absolute level of visual improvement.[24-26] Therefore, the best candidates would be patients with two severely visually impaired eyes. Few studies on pediatric cases of DALK (of any technique) have shown that the operative success depends on patients' ability and willingness to cooperate.[27,28]

The mmDALK is an extraocular procedure and can be considered minimally invasive, therefore, it can be performed with retrobulbar anesthesia. The most important preoperative step is to obtain a soft eye after retrobulbar anesthesia as significant posterior pressure will make manual stromal dissection substantially more difficult and increases the risk of inadvertent DM perforation.[2,23] Therefore, it is advised to perform digital ocular massage and a Honan balloon after an effective retrobulbar block. Intraoperatively, care should be taken to place the patient in proper anti-Trendelenburg position, and to ensure that the eyelid speculum is not too tight.

POSTOPERATIVE RESULTS

The visual outcome of mmDALK depends on whether deep stromal dissection is successfully achieved. In these cases, with an average best-spectacle corrected vision of 20/40 (0.5), this may equal the results achieved with PK and big-bubble DALK.[29-36] The endothelial cell density after mmDALK is higher compared to that seen after big-bubble DALK, suggesting that rapid expansion due to the air bubble might be traumatic to the recipient corneal endothelium.[37,38]

After DALK, corneas are steeper compared to PK, resulting in higher postoperative myopia, on average 2D. This may be due to the fact that during DALK no intraoperative collapse of the AC and angle occurs as during PK.[39-41] Myopia might be reduced by using the same size graft instead of an oversized graft. For PK, 10% of the patients require rigid contact lenses postoperatively to achieve satisfactory visual results. No comparable research study has been published for DALK to date.[42-47]

Compared to PK, DALK results in earlier suture removal and visual stability.

POSTOPERATIVE CONSIDERATIONS AND COMPLICATIONS

The most common intraoperative complication is DM perforation which occurs in approximately 10% of the cases with both Melles manual and big-bubble DALK techniques.[11,13,15,16,34,48] When DM perforation occurs with the big-bubble technique, the DALK usually needs to be converted to PK, as large corneal incisions have already been made by the time air is injected after partial thickness surface trephination.[49,50] Some recent studies show that with early identification and adequate management of the DM rupture, conversion is not always needed.[16,51,52] When DM perforation occurs with mmDALK the operation can be aborted, permitting the DM perforation to heal and enabling another attempt of DALK in future.

Graft failure remains a controversial topic, mostly because of indistinct definition. Originally, it referred to corneal decompensation due to donor endothelial cell death or depletion.[53] This type of graft failure is very rare with DALK. The average life expectancy of ALK after uncomplicated surgery is 50 years, compared to 18 years with PK.[54] Recently, some studies have used the term *failed graft* to describe an optically undesirable result, for example dense interface haze that limits visual performance.[55] Therefore, caution is needed when comparing rates or incidences of graft failure, and to clearly distinguish between cellular and optical graft failure.[56] No comparative studies yet exist between mmDALK and the big-bubble DALK for allograft reaction or cellular graft failure. Considering that cell densities tend to be higher after mmDALK compared to the big-bubble technique, and the occurrence of DM perforation are lower, graft survival may be longer in the manual method.[35,36,50]

Another consideration for both PK and DALK is that both techniques do not prevent recurrence of ectasia in the transplanted tissue or the graft-host tissue junction.[57-65] The mechanism behind this recurrence is proposed as infiltration of the donor tissue with pathologic recipient keratocytes.[66] If this is the case, then DALK might have a slightly elevated risk of recurrence compared to PK as more recipient cornea is left in-situ.

FUTURE OF LAMELLAR KERATOPLASTY

Since its introduction in 2007, UV-cross-linking (UV-CXL) has revolutionized treatment of keratoconus. Several studies have demonstrated that UV-CXL may slow or halt the progression of keratoconus. UV-CXL has contributed to

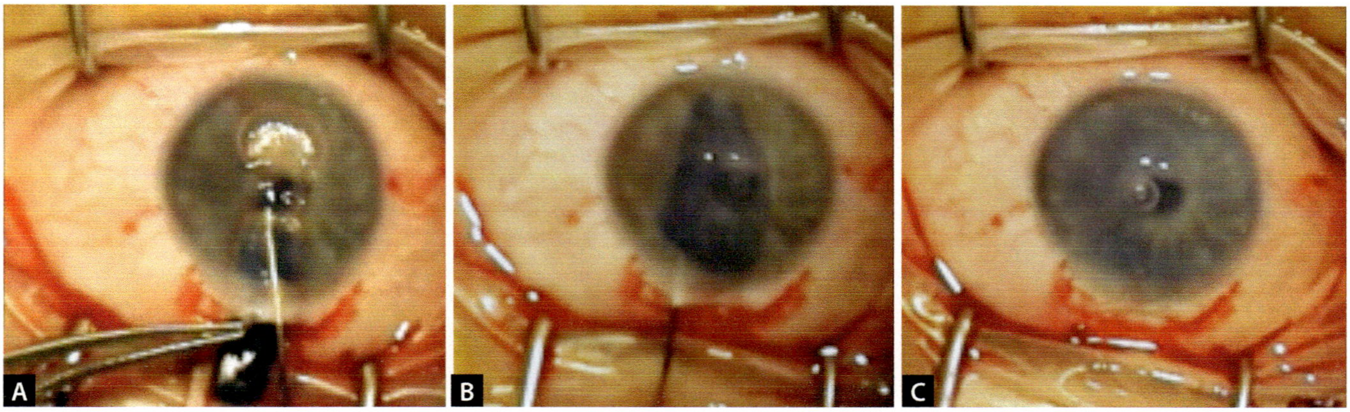

Figs. 6A to C: Surgical views of an eye during Bowman layer (BL) transplantation. After the creation of a midstromal pocket using the Melles manual deep anterior lamellar keratoplasty (mmDALK) dissection technique, (A) a stained BL graft is inserted into the pocket through a glide and (B) carefully unfolded and centered with a 30-gauge air cannula. (C) At the end of the surgery, the BL graft is sandwiched between the anterior and posterior stromal layers. No sutures are required to fixate the graft or to close the tunnel incision.

a 25% decrease of DALK surgery in the Netherlands in the years following the nationwide introduction.[67,68]

Even though DALK has advantages over conventional PK, it still requires a large surface incision in the recipient cornea, long-standing corneal sutures, and cellular donor material, leading to an ongoing risk of allograft reaction and graft rejection which demands extended follow-up examinations.[69-72] A new alternative for eyes with progressive advanced keratoconus may be Bowman layer (BL) transplantation which was design to arrest the progression of disease and flatten the cornea in patients who are not candidates for UV-CXL or corneal ring segments.[73,74]

The BL surgery is performed by making a manual, midstromal dissection within the recipient cornea using the standard mmDALK dissection spatulas. An isolated BL graft is inserted and unfolded within this created corneal pocket at a depth of approximately 50% (**Figs. 6A to C**).[73,74]

Bowman layer transplantation was shown to halt the progression of corneal ectasia in approximately 90% of the transplanted eyes, and flattening the cornea by about 8 D after surgery, and decreasing the risk of allograft and graft rejection while suture-related complication cannot occur. In case the outcome is not desirable, the operation can still be reversed and a DALK or PK can always be performed on a later date. Therefore, BL transplantation might be amenable for patients whose corneas are too thin for UV-CXL or corneal ring segments.[73-75]

CONCLUSION AND RECOMMENDATIONS

The biggest advantage of mmDALK over the big-bubble DALK and other manual techniques is the unequaled level of direct visual feedback and control that this technique offers. Once it has been successfully learned, this method is reproducible and safe; however, it is skill-dependent and relies on meticulous attention to detail as the depth of dissection must be continuously monitored. Also, a special set of dissection instruments is required. Compared to big-bubble DALK, the mmDALK technique might be more time consuming.

The biggest drawback of DALK surgery is related to (postoperative) problems of surface incision, sutures, haze formation, and the use of cellular donor material. These complications are inherent to the DALK technique and would require a fundamentally new approach in order to be avoided. This was the motivation that inspired for a less interventionist, more specific treatment for patients with advanced keratoconus, namely the BL transplantation. The first cases are now 8 years removed from surgery and the results are promising. This operation might replace the nearly full-thickness keratoplasty for patients with advanced keratoconus like the endothelial keratoplasty has displaced PK for patients with Fuchs' endothelial dystrophy.

REFERENCES

1. Melles GR, Rietveld FJ, Beekhuis WH, Binder PS. A technique to visualize corneal incision and lamellar dissection depth during surgery. Cornea. 1999;18:80-6.
2. Melles GR, Lander F, Rietveld FJ, Remeijer L, Beekhuis WH, Binder PS. A new surgical technique for deep stromal, anterior lamellar keratoplasty. Br J Ophthalmol. 1999;83:327-33.
3. Mühlbauer FX. Ueber transplantation der cornea; Gekrönte Preisschrift. München, Jos. Lindauer, 1840. (Abstract) In: Schmidt CC (Ed). Jahrbücher der in und Ausländischen Gesamten Medizin. Germany: Leipzig, Otto Wigand; 1842. pp. 267-8.
4. Hallermann W. Verschiedenes über Keratoplastik. Klin Monbl Augenheilkd. 1959;135:252-9.
5. Morrison JC, Swan KC. Full-thickness lamellar keratoplasty: A histologic study in human eyes. Ophthalmology. 1982;89:715-9.
6. Krachmer JH, Mannis MJ, Holland EJ. Cornea: Fundamentals, Diagnosis, and Management. St. Louis, MO: Mosby Elsevier; 2011.
7. Amayem AF, Anwar M. Fluid lamellar keratoplasty in keratoconus. Ophthalmology. 2000;107:76-9.
8. Chau GK, Dilly SA, Sheard CE, Rostron CK. Deep lamellar keratoplasty on air with lyophilised tissue. Br J Ophthalmol. 1992;76:646-50.

9. Archila EA. Deep lamellar keratoplasty dissection of host tissue with intrastromal air injection. Cornea. 1984-1985;3:217-8.
10. Price FW Jr. Air lamellar keratoplasty. Refract Corneal Surg. 1989;5:240-3.
11. Anwar M, Teichmann KD. Big-bubble technique to bare Descemet's membrane in anterior lamellar keratoplasty. J Cataract Refract Surg. 2002;28:398-403.
12. Manche EE, Holland GN, Maloney RK. Deep lamellar keratoplasty using viscoelastic dissection. Arch Ophthalmol. 1999;117:1561-5.
13. Melles GR, Remeijer L, Geerards AJ, Beekhuis WH. A quick surgical technique for deep anterior lamellar keratoplasty using visco-dissection. Cornea. 2000;19:427-32.
14. Den S, Shimmura S, Tsubota K, Shimazaki J. Impact of the Descemet membrane perforation on surgical outcomes after deep lamellar keratoplasty. Am J Ophthalmol. 2007;143:750-4.
15. Feizi S, Javadi MA, Jamali H, Mirbabaee F. Deep anterior lamellar keratoplasty in patients with keratoconus: big-bubble technique. Cornea. 2010;29:177-82.
16. Leccisotti A. Descemet's membrane perforation during deep anterior lamellar keratoplasty: prognosis. J Cataract Refract Surg. 2007;33:825-9.
17. Goweida MB. Intraoperative review of different bubble types formed during pneumodissection (big-bubble) deep anterior lamellar keratoplasty. Cornea. 2015;34:621-4.
18. Michieletto P, Balestrazzi A, Balestrazzi A, Mazzotta C, Occhipinti I, Rossi T. Factors predicting unsuccessful big bubble deep lamellar anterior keratoplasty. Ophthalmologica. 2006;220:379-82.
19. Feizi S, Faramarzi A, Javadi MA, Jafarinasab MR. Modified big-bubble deep anterior lamellar keratoplasty using peripheral air injection. Br J Ophthalmol. 2014;98:1597-600.
20. Feizi S, Daryabari SH, Najdi D, Javadi MA, Farimian F. Big-bubble deep anterior lamellar keratoplasty using central vs peripheral air injection: a clinical trial. Eur J Ophthalmol. 2016;26:297-302.
21. Millar MJ, Maloof A. Deep lamellar keratoplasty for pellucid marginal degeneration review of management options for corneal perforation. Cornea. 2008;27:953-6.
22. Kawashima M, Kawakita T, Den S, Shimmura S, Tsubota K, Shimazaki J. Comparison of deep lamellar keratoplasty and penetrating keratoplasty for lattice and macular corneal dystrophies. Am J Ophthalmol. 2006;142:304-9.
23. Karimian F, Feizi S. Deep anterior lamellar keratoplasty: Indications, surgical techniques, and complications. Middle East Afr J Ophthalmol. 2010;17:28-37.
24. Mendes F, Schaumberg DA, Navon S, Steinert R, Sugar J, Holland EJ, et al. Assessment of visual function after corneal transplantation: The quality of life and psychometric assessment after corneal transplantation (Q-PACT) study. Am J Ophthalmol. 2003;135:785-93.
25. Uiters E, van den Borne B, van der Horst FG, Völker-Dieben HJ. Patient satisfaction after corneal transplantation. Cornea. 2001;20:687-94.
26. Williams KA, Ash JK, Pararajasegaram P, Dipl H, Coster DJ. Long-term outcome after corneal transplantation: visual result and patient perception of success. Ophthalmology. 1991;98:651-7.
27. Singh D, Vanathi M, Gupta C, Gupta N, Tandon R. Outcomes of deep anterior lamellar keratoplasty following autologous simple limbal epithelial transplant in pediatric unilateral severe chemical injury. Indian J Ophthalmol. 2017;65:217-22.
28. Harding SA, Nischal KK, Upponi-Patil A, Fowler DJ. Indications and outcomes of deep anterior lamellar keratoplasty in children. Ophthalmology. 2010;117:2191-5.
29. Fontana L, Parente G, Sincich A, Tassinari G. Influence of graft-host interface on the quality of vision after deep anterior lamellar keratoplasty in patients with keratoconus. Cornea. 2011;30:497-502.
30. Funnell CL, Ball J, Noble BA. Comparative cohort study of the outcomes of deep lamellar keratoplasty and penetrating keratoplasty for keratoconus. Eye (Lond). 2006;20:527-32.
31. Han DC, Mehta JS, Por YM, Htoon HM, Tan DT. Comparison of outcomes of lamellar keratoplasty and penetrating keratoplasty in keratoconus. Am J Ophthalmol. 2009;148:744-51.
32. Javadi MA, Motlagh BF, Jafarinasab MR, Rabbanikhah Z. Outcomes of penetrating keratoplasty in keratoconus. Cornea. 2005; 24:941-6.
33. Jones MN, Armitage WJ, Ayliffe W, Larkin DF, Kaye SB; NHSBT Ocular Tissue Advisory Group and Contributing Ophthalmologists (OTAG Audit Study 5). Penetrating and deep anterior lamellar keratoplasty for keratoconus: A comparison of graft outcomes in the United Kingdom. Invest Ophthalmol Vis Sci. 2009;50:5625-9.
34. Kim MH, Chung TY, Chung ES. A retrospective contralateral study comparing deep anterior lamellar keratoplasty with penetrating keratoplasty. Cornea. 2013;32:385-9.
35. Smadja D, Colin J, Kreuger RR. Outcomes of deep anterior lamellar keratoplasty for keratoconus: Learning curve and advantages of the big bubble technique. Cornea. 2012;31:859-63.
36. Keane M, Coster D, Ziaei M, Williams K. Deep anterior lamellar keratoplasty versus penetrating keratoplasty for treating keratoconus. Cochrane Database Syst Rev. 2014;22:CD009700.
37. Borderie VM, Werthel AL, Touzeau O, Allouch C, Boutboul S, Laroche L. Comparison of techniques used for removing the recipient stroma in anterior lamellar keratoplasty. Arch Ophthalmol. 2008;126:31-7.
38. Cheng YY, Visser N, Schouten JS, Wijdh RJ, Pels E, van Cleynenbreugel H, et al. Endothelial cell loss and visual outcome of deep anterior lamellar keratoplasty versus penetrating keratoplasty: A randomized multicenter clinical trial. Ophthalmology. 2011;118:302-9.
39. Amayem AF, Hamdi IM, Hamdi MM. Refractive and visual outcomes of penetrating keratoplasty versus keep anterior lamellar keratoplasty with hydrodissection for treatment of keratoconus. Cornea. 2013;32:e2-e5.
40. Borderie VM, Georgeon C, Borderie M, Bouheraoua N, Touzeau O, Laroche L. Corneal radius of curvature after anterior lamellar versus penetrating keratoplasty. Graefes Arch Clin Exp Ophthalmol. 2014;252:449-56.
41. Kim KH, Choi SH, Ahn K, Chung ES, Chung TY. Comparison of refractive changes after deep anterior lamellar keratoplasty and penetrating keratoplasty for keratoconus. Jpn J Ophthalmol. 2011;55:93-7.
42. Geerards AJ, Vreugdenhil W, Khazen A. Incidence of rigid gas-permeable contact lens wear after keratoplasty for keratoconus. Eye Contact Lens. 2006;32:207-10.
43. Lim L, Pesudovs K, Coster DJ. Penetrating keratoplasty for keratoconus: Visual outcome and success. Ophthalmology. 2000;107:1125-31.
44. Price FW Jr, Whitson WE, Marks RG. Progression of visual acuity after penetrating keratoplasty. Ophthalmology. 1991;98:1177-85.
45. Severinsky B, Behrman S, Frucht-Pery J, Solomon A. Scleral contact lenses for visual rehabilitation after penetrating keratoplasty: Long-term outcomes. Cont Lens Anterior Eye. 2014;37:196-202.
46. Silbiger JS, Cohen EJ, Laibson PR. The rate of visual recovery after penetrating keratoplasty for keratoconus. Cont Lens Anterior Eye. 1996;22:266-9.
47. Sutton G, Hodge C, McGhee CN. Rapid visual recovery after penetrating keratoplasty for keratoconus. Clin Experiment Ophthalmol. 2008;36:725-30.
48. Villarrubia A, Fuentes-Páez G, Dapena I, Palacín E. Deep anterior lamellar keratoplasty with Melles' technique: Mid-term clinical outcome. J Emmetropia. 2010;1:182-6.

49. Anwar HM, El-Danasoury A, Hashem AN. The use of fibrin glue to seal Descemet membrane microperforations occurring during deep anterior lamellar keratoplasty. Cornea. 2012;31:1193-6.
50. Sutiga J, Kondo J. Deep lamellar keratoplasty with complete removal of pathological stroma for vision improvement. Br J Ophthalmol. 1997;81:184-8.
51. Kodavoor SK, Deb B, Ramamurthy D. Outcome of deep anterior lamellar keratoplasty patients with intraoperative Descemet's membrane perforation: A retrospective cross-sectional study. Indian J Ophthalmol. 2018;66:1574-9.
52. Sarnicola E, Sarnicola C, Cheung AY, Panico E, Panico C, Sarnicola V. Total or subtotal full thickness recipient bed cut to repair donor-recipient curvature disparity in cases of DM rupture with manual DALK. Eur J Ophthalmol. 2020;30:1172-8.
53. Sharma N, Kandar AK, Singh Titiyal J. Stromal rejection after big bubble deep anterior lamellar keratoplasty: Case series and review of literature. Eye Contact Lens. 2013;39:194-8.
54. Borderie VM, Sandali O, Bullet J. Long-term results of deep anterior lamellar versus penetrating keratoplasty. Ophthalmology. 2012;119:249-55.
55. Coster DJ, Lowe MT, Keane MC, Williams KA; Australian Corneal Graft Registry Contributors. A comparison of lamellar and penetrating keratoplasty outcomes: A registry study. Ophthalmology. 2014;121:979-87.
56. Baydoun L, Melles GR. Refining the terminology of graft failure in reports on endothelial keratoplasty outcomes. JAMA Ophthalmol. 2016;134:125-6.
57. Bechrakis N, Blom ML, Stark WJ, Green WR. Recurrent keratoconus. Cornea. 1994;13:73-7.
58. Dang TQ, Molchan RP, Taylor KR, Reilly CD, Panday VA, Caldwell MC. Novel approach for the treatment of corneal ectasia in a graft. Cornea. 2014;33:310-2.
59. Fukuoka S, Honda N, Ono K, Mimura T, Usui T, Amano S. Extended long-term results of penetrating keratoplasty for keratoconus. Cornea. 2010;29:528-30.
60. Hayes S, Young R, Boote C, Hawksworth N, Huang Y, Meek KM. A structural investigation of corneal graft failure in suspected recurrent keratoconus. Eye (Lond). 2010;24:728-34.
61. Lim L, Pesudovs K, Goggin M, Coster DJ. Late onset post-keratoplasty astigmatism in patients with keratoconus: indications and outcomes. Br J Ophthalmol. 2004;88:371-6.
62. Nirankari VS, Karesh J, Bastion F, Lakhanpal V, Billings E. Recurrence of keratoconus in donor cornea 22 years after successful keratoplasty. Br J Ophthalmol. 1983;67:23-8.
63. Niziol LM, Musch DC, Gillespie BW, Marcotte LM, Sugar A. Long-term outcomes in patients who received a corneal graft for keratoconus between 1980 and 1986. Am J Ophthalmol. 2013;155:213-9.
64. Patel SV, Malta JB, Banitt MR, Mian SI, Sugar A, Elner VM, et al. Recurrent ectasia in corneal grafts and outcomes of repeat keratoplasty for keratoconus. Br J Ophthalmol. 2009;93:191-7.
65. Yeniad B, Alparslan N, Akarcay K. Eye rubbing as an apparent cause of recurrent keratoconus. Cornea. 2009;28:477-9.
66. Bourges JL, Savoldelli M, Dighiero P, Assouline M, Pouliquen Y, BenEzra D, et al. Recurrence of keratoconus characteristics: a clinical and histological follow-up analysis of donor grafts. Ophthalmology. 2003;110:1920-5.
67. Godefrooij DA, Gans R, Imhof SM, Wisse RP. Nationwide reduction in the number of corneal transplantations for keratoconus following the implementation of cross-linking. Acta Ophthalmol. 2016;94:675-8.
68. Sandvik GF, Thorsrud A, Raen M, Ostern AE, Saethre M, Drolsum L. Does corneal collagen cross-linking reduce the need for keratoplasties in patients with keratoconus? Cornea. 2015;34:991-5.
69. Williams KA, Muehlberg SM, Lewis RF, Coster DJ. How successful is corneal transplantation? A report from the Australian Corneal Graft Register. Eye (Lond). 1995;9:219-7.
70. de Toledo JA, de la Paz MF, Barraquer RI, Barraquer J. Long-term progression of astigmatism after penetrating keratoplasty for keratoconus: evidence of late recurrence. Cornea. 2003;22:317-23.
71. Elder MJ, Stack RR. Globe rupture following penetrating keratoplasty: how often, why, and what can we do to prevent it? Cornea. 2004;23:776-80.
72. Nagra PK, Hammersmith KM, Rapuano CJ, Laibson PR, Cohen EJ. Wound dehiscence after penetrating keratoplasty. Cornea. 2006;25:132-5.
73. van Dijk K, Parker J, Tong CM, Ham L, Lie JT, Groeneveld-van Beek EA, et al. Midstromal isolated Bowman layer graft for reduction of advanced keratoconus: A technique to postpone penetrating or deep anterior lamellar keratoplasty. JAMA Ophthalmol. 2014;132:495-501.
74. van Dijk K, Liarakos V, Parker J, Ham L, Lie JT, Groeneveld-van Beek EA, et al. Bowman layer transplantation to reduce and stabilize progressive, advanced keratoconus. Ophthalmology. 2015;122:909-17.
75. Tong CM, van Dijk K, Melles GR. Update on Bowman layer transplantation. Curr Opin Ophthalmol. 2019;30:249-55.

24 Deep Anterior Lamellar Keratoplasty: Big Bubble Technique

Luigi Fontana, Antonio Moramarco

INTRODUCTION

Anterior lamellar keratoplasty involves the heterotopic lamellar replacement of the anterior layers of the cornea while retaining the posterior layers of the recipient cornea, including Descemet's membrane (DM) and endothelial layer. Main disadvantage of anterior lamellar keratoplasty compared to penetrating keratoplasty (PK) for optical purpose is the potential irregularity of the recipient stromal bed that may ensue after manual lamellar dissection, potentially limiting the final visual acuity. Different approaches have been devised to overcome this problem, including the use of a microkeratome[1,2] to obtain a regular lamellar dissection or excising the diseased stroma until baring the DM.[3] To obviate to this problem, a variety of surgical techniques have been described for performing "maximum depth" deep anterior lamellar keratoplasty (DALK), in which complete stromal removal with exposure of the DM, in the central visual axis, is attempted.[3-8]

These techniques include the use of viscoelastic,[9,10] fluids, or air injected into the deep stroma to cleave the stroma from the DM[3] (**Fig. 1**).

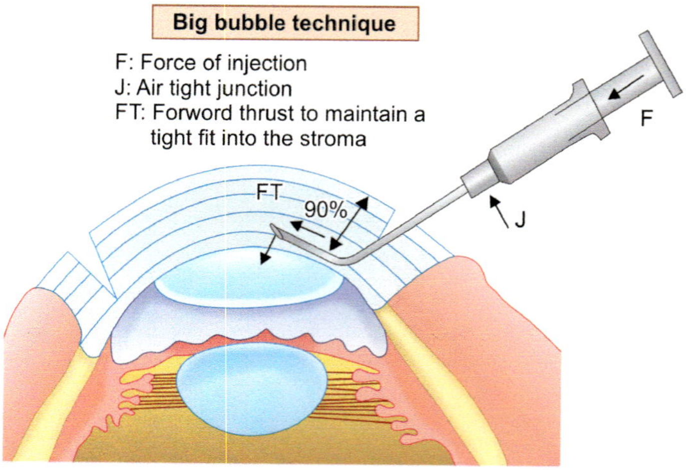

Fig. 1: A 27-gauge needle bent with the bevel facing down is inserted into the deep stroma through the trephination groove. The needle is directed halfway between tangential and radial direction, avoiding the center of the cornea. A syringe filled with air is tightly connected to the needle.

The Anwar's "big bubble" technique for DALK consists in the cleavage of DM or recently defined pre-Descemetic (pre-DM) layer from the overlying stroma by mean of a forceful injection of air into the deep stroma with a needle or a cannula[4] (**Fig. 2**).

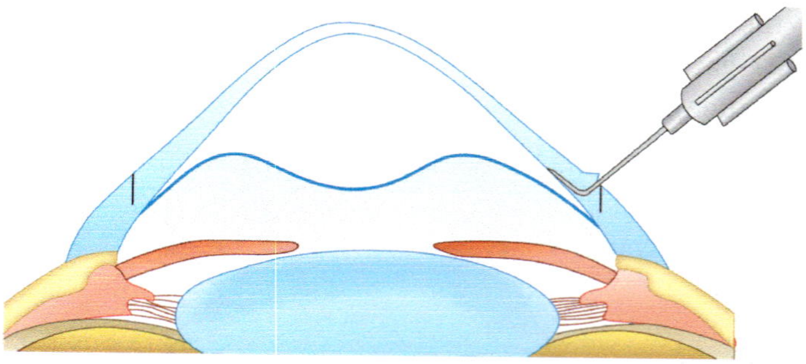

Fig. 2: Big bubble formation characterized by a semiopaque disk with a near-circular outline. Air detaches the central Descemet's membrane that protrudes into the anterior chamber.

To successfully obtain separation of the DM from stroma, the needle or cannula should be positioned close to the DM so that air may reach the correct cleavage plane.[11,12] This technique has a steep learning curve and is contraindicated in some diseases where the DM may be interrupted or involved in deep stromal scarring.[3] Successful DM cleavage separation using the big bubble technique has been reported in 60–70% of cases using a needle and 80–90% of cases when a dedicated blunt tip cannula for air injection is eployed.[13,14]

Big bubble technique for DALK carries good visual outcomes in keratoconus patients. This may be due to the presence of a regular donor-to-recipient interface between the DM or pre-DM layer and the donor stroma, minimizing graft-host interface irregularities.

The most critical step in achieving successful big-bubble formation remains the insertion of the needle or cannula into the stroma: a too superficial position usually results in diffuse corneal emphysema without big bubble formation, whereas too deep insertion can lead to accidental DM perforation, requiring conversion to PK.[15] Several techniques have been suggested to judge the depth of dissection, including air or triamcinolone injected into the anterior chamber, slit lamp coupled to a surgical microscope, and recently, intraoperative anterior segment optical coherence tomography (AS-OCT) combined with femtosecond laser technology to guide the insertion of the cannula near to the pre-DM plane.[11,16,17]

In cases when big bubble cleavage does not succeed, DALK can still be carried out by manual dissection. Manual dissection DALK may also be considered the procedure of choice in full thickness corneal scars or in cases where DM has been torn, such as in corneal perforations, previous hydrops, and after radial keratotomy.[3]

SURGICAL TECHNIQUE

Shortly before surgery, few drops of tropicamide 1% (Visumidriatic 1%; Visufarma Spa, Italy) are instilled into the lower fornix to obtain mydriasis. Pupil dilation results in a bright red reflex, useful for the trephine centration and localization of a deep stromal plane for air injection.

After marking the geometric center of the cornea, a circular partial thickness trephination of desired diameter (8–9 mm diameter) up to 80% of the total corneal thickness is conducted using an adjustable depth suction trephine (one step; Moria, Antony, France). A pointed dissector (Moria, Antony, France) is used to penetrate the stroma right at the base of the trephination and advanced 1–2 mm centripetally. A red line (fold) is noted ahead of the dissector tip; the width of this line corresponds to the thickness of the residual underlying stromal bed[18] (**Video 1**). At this point, the dissector is further advanced and deepened, reducing the width of the red line until it disappears. Then, a blunt 27-gauge cannula (Fontana cannula, Moria, Antony, France), connected with a 5 mL Luer-lock syringe filled with air, is inserted into the stromal channel and advanced toward the center of the cornea for further 2–3 mm. As the cannula advances into the stroma, the surgeon may initially perceive some resistance, then suddenly, a giveaway sensation, with effortless progression of the cannula, indicates reaching of the desired point for injection. Air is gently injected until the big bubble is initially formed, always starting at the center of the cornea and expanding centrifugally (**Video 2**). At this point, air injection is suspended. A vertical paracentesis is performed at the limbus using a slit knife to release some aqueous and lower the intraocular pressure. Air injection is resumed allowing enlargement of the big bubble until it reaches or slightly exceeds the margin of the trephination. Further aqueous may be evacuated from the anterior chamber to lower the intraocular pressure if necessary.

The big bubble expands, occupying space inside the anterior chamber. As a result of air stromal infiltration (stromal emphysema), the central cornea becomes partially white and opaque and visualization of the anterior chamber is dimmed centrally but it is possible at the periphery that usually remains clear. To confirm the presence of the big bubble, a small quantity of air may be injected into the anterior chamber through a paracentesis. When the big bubble is present, air bubbles in the anterior chamber are displaced in the periphery by the space-occupying big bubble. When a big bubble is not formed, small air bubbles are passing from the peripheral cornea through the trabecular meshwork inside the anterior chamber gather centrally under the emphysematous cornea. These bubbles are free to move across the anterior chamber with the eye movements[19] (**Video 3**). In this case, the surgeon knows that DM is attached to the posterior stroma and can decide whether to make further attempts to induce cleavage separation of the DM with more injections of air, or viscoelastics or try to expose the DM using a layer-by-layer stromal dissection technique.

In cases of successful bubble formation, an anterior lamellar keratectomy is performed to remove 30–40% of the anterior using a crescent knife. The anterior wall of the big bubble is cut with a slit knife collapsing of the big bubble (**Fig. 3**). Through the same stromal slash, blunt-tipped corneal scissors are used to cut and divide the residual stroma into four quadrants that are then excised baring the pre-DM layer across the trephination diameter (**Fig. 4**).

When the big bubble is not achieved, surgery may completed by manual dissection of the residual stromal bed (**Video 4**). In this case, after removal of an anterior stromal lamella, a radial stromal cut of about 2 mm is performed within the trephination using any sharp instrument of

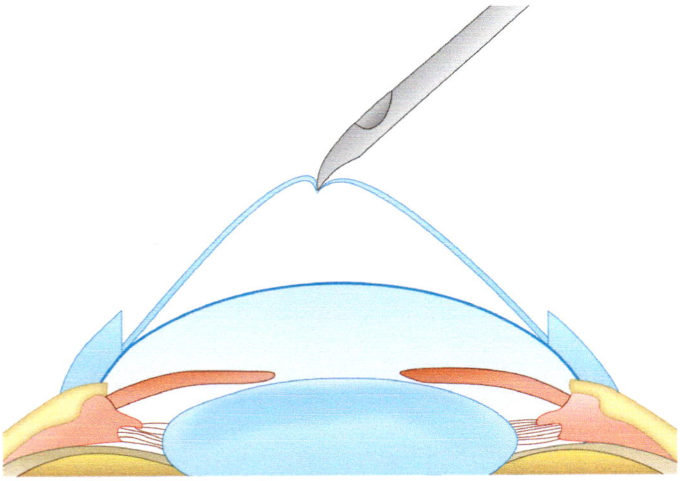

Fig. 3: The big bubble is pierced with a point knife creating an opening of 1 mm or larger.

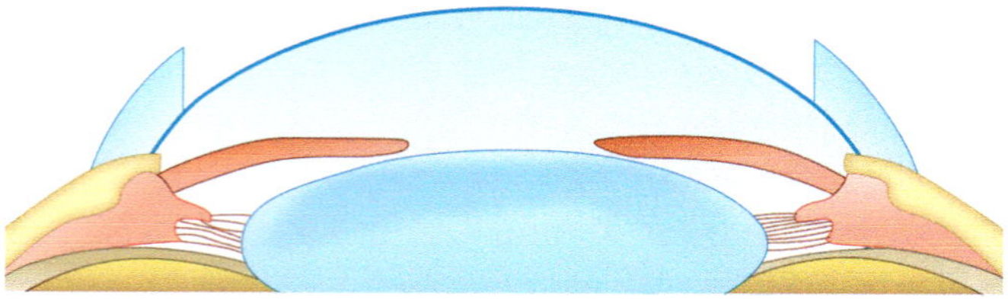

Fig. 4: The stroma is excised using blunt tip corneal scissors and the Descemet's membrane is exposed.

preference. The cut should be progressively deepened in order to approach the DM. Progressive fading of the white emphysematous stroma and the appearance of a dark reflex from iris through the translucent DM layer indicate the proximity to a deep stromal plane. Once a satisfactory deep plane has been reached, any instrument of choice for blunt stromal dissection is introduced in the bottom of the radial cut and advanced along the plane to dissect the stroma clockwise or anticlockwise. The dissection should proceed starting from the midperiphery and extending beyond the trephination margin, and then to the center of the cornea. Once a quadrant or more has been dissected, blunt corneal scissors are introduced in the depth of the pocket to cut and excise the stroma along the trephination margin in circular fashion for 360°. Often times, upon completion of dissection, should the transparency of the residual stromal plane result unsatisfactory, a second circular dissection can be performed to achieve a deeper stromal excision closest possible to the DM.

A donor cornea, of the same diameter as the trephination, is punched from the endothelial side with a suction donor punch (Moria, Antony, France). The endothelium and DM are gently stripped with a dry Weck-Cel sponge after staining the endothelial surface with 0.06% trypan blue dye (VisionBlue; D.O.R.C., Zuidland, Netherlands) to better visualize the DM (**Video 5**). Four interrupted 10-0 nylon cardinal sutures are used to secure the donor on the recipient bed and the graft is sutured with 2 running 10-0 nylon sutures.

Descemet's membrane folds frequently occur after DALK particularly in keratoconus patients due to the redundant DM compressed by the sutured in place donor graft (**Fig. 5**). In these cases the so called DM-tucking technique may be used as soon as central DM folds are noted after graft placement and suture tensioning. In the area of approach, the donor epithelium is removed using a dry Weck-Cel sponge to avoid epithelium seeding into the graft-host junction. Under physiological intraocular pressure, a blunt tip spatula (J2192.32A, E. Janach, Como, Italy) is introduced vertically into the trephination cut, 90° away from the main direction of the DM folds, and advanced until it touches the host layer. Gentle pressure is applied sufficiently enough to stretch the DM layer and tucking the redundant host layer in the periphery. The tucking maneuver may be repeated at different clock hours, with the aim of obtaining a uniform stretching of the redundant DM tissue with gathering toward the graft margin. The maneuver is stopped when a regular graft-host interface is obtained and there are no visible central DM folds[20] (**Video 6**).

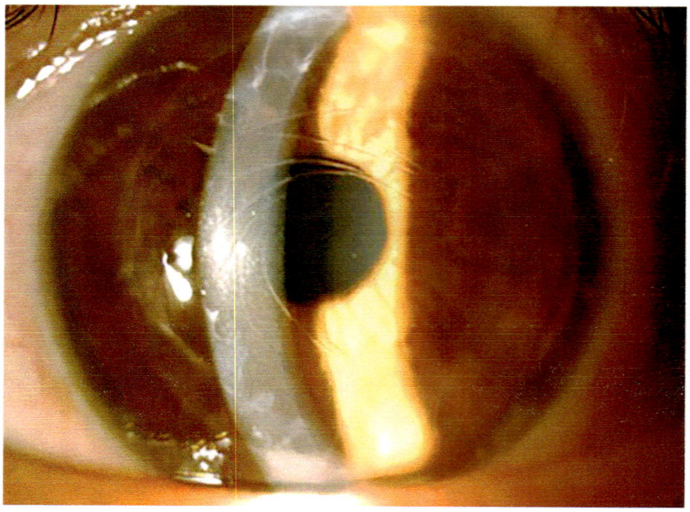

Fig. 5: An example of central Descemet's membrane folds after deep anterior lamellar keratoplasty for keratoconus.

REFERENCES

1. Tan DT, Ang LP. Modified automated lamellar therapeutic keratoplasty for keratoconus: a new technique. Cornea. 2006;25:1217-9.
2. Tan DT, Ang LP. Automated lamellar therapeutic keratoplasty for post-PRK corneal scarring and thinning. Am J Ophthalmol. 2004;138:1067-9.
3. Anwar M, Teichmann KD. Deep lamellar keratoplasty: surgical techniques for anterior lamellar keratoplasty with and without baring of Descemet's membrane. Cornea. 2002;21:374-83.
4. Anwar M, Teichmann KD. Big-bubble technique to bare Descemet's membrane in anterior lamellar keratoplasty. J Cataract Refract Surg. 2002;28:398-403.
5. Archila EA. Deep lamellar keratoplasty dissection of host tissue with intrastromal air injection. Cornea. 1984-85;3:217-8.
6. Sujita J, Kondo J. Deep lamellar keratoplasty with complete removal of pathologic stroma for vision improvement. Br J Ophthalmol. 1997;91:184-9.
7. Melles GR, Lander F, Rietveld FJ, Remeijer L, Beekhuis WH, Binder PS. A new surgical technique for deep stromal, anterior lamellar keratoplasty. Br J Ophthalmol. 1999;83:327-33.
8. Tsubota K, Kaido M, Monden Y, Satake Y, Bissen-Miyajima H, Shimazaki J. A new surgical technique for deep lamellar keratoplasty with single running suture adjustment. Am J Ophthalmol. 1998;126:1-8.
9. Melles GR, Remeijer L, Geerards AJ, Beekhuis WH. A quick surgical technique for deep, anterior lamellar keratoplasty using visco-dissection. Cornea. 2000;19:427-32.
10. Shimmura S, Shimazaki J, Omoto M, Teruya A, Ishioka M, Tsubota K. Deep lamellar keratoplasty (DLKP) in keratoconus patients using viscoadaptive viscoelastics. Cornea. 2005;24:178-81.
11. Scorcia V, Busin M, Lucisano A, Beltz J, Carta A, Scorcia G. Anterior segment optical coherence tomography-guided big-bubble technique. Ophthalmology. 2013;120(3):471-6.

12. Dua HS, Faraj LA, Said DG, Gray T, Lowe J. Human corneal anatomy redefined: a novel pre-Descemetd layer (Duaye layer). Ophthalmology. 2013;120(9):1778-85.
13. Fogla R. Deep anterior lamellar keratoplasty in the management of keratoconus. Indian J Ophthalmol. 2013;61(8):465-8.
14. Romano V, Iovieno A, Parente G, Soldani AM, Fontana L. Long-term clinical outcomes of deep anterior lamellar keratoplasty in patients with keratoconus. Am J Ophthalmol. 2015; 159(3):505-11.
15. Jhanji V, Sharma N, Vajpayee RB. Intraoperative perforation of Descemet's membrane during "big bubble" deep anterior lamellar keratoplasty. Int Ophthalmol. 2010;30:291-5.
16. McKee HD, Carley FM, Jhanji V, Brahma AK. Use of triamcinolone to judge needle depth in big-bubble deep anterior lamellar keratoplasty. Cornea. 2011;30:1499-501.
17. Buzzonetti L, Laborante A, Petrocelli G. Standardized big-bubble technique in deep anterior lamellar keratoplasty assisted by the femtosecond laser. J Cataract Refract Surg. 2010;36:1631-6.
18. Scorcia V, Lucisano A, Pietropaolo R, Savoca Corona V, Scorcia G, Busin M. Red Reflex-guided big-bubble deep anterior lamellar keratoplasty: A simple technique to judge dissection depth. Cornea. 2015;34(9):1035-8.
19. Fontana L, Parente G, Tassinari G. Simple test to confirm cleavage with air between Descemet's membrane and stroma during big-bubble deep anterior lamellar keratoplasty. J Cataract Refract Surg. 2007;33(4):570-2.
20. Neri A, Moramarco A, Iovieno A, Fontana L. Management of Descemet membrane's folds after deep anterior lamellar keratoplasty: Descemet membrane-tucking technique. Cornea. 2019;38(6):772-4.

25 Deep Anterior Lamellar Keratoplasty: Double Bubble Technique

Vishal Jhanji, Ritu Nagpal, Sarath S, Namrata Sharma, Rasik B Vajpayee

INTRODUCTION

Deep anterior lamellar keratoplasty (DALK) is a technique of corneal transplantation that entails the replacement of only the diseased stroma without replacing the healthy endothelial layer. The procedure completely eliminates the risk of immunological graft rejection and other inherent complications related to full-thickness corneal transplantation. Although DALK has been described for various corneal stromal disorders,[1] keratoconus is by far its most common indication.[2,3] The classical technique of DALK involves layer by layer removal of the host tissue, until the Descemet's membrane (DM) is exposed. Techniques such as intrastromal air injection or segmental removal of host stroma help to improve the visibility of DM. Melles et al. were the first to inject air into the anterior chamber (AC) to create a mirror reflex which helps to guide the entry of surgical instruments into the space between DM and the posterior stroma.[4] Archila et al. demonstrated the use of intrastromal air injection to facilitate the removal of affected stroma.[5] Anwar et al. modified the technique of air injection by performing about 60–70% of initial trephination before injecting the "big bubble" into the corneal stroma.[6] The "big bubble" technique of DALK is a novel method for achieving complete baring of DM from the posterior stroma.

In order to make this technique more reproducible, corneal surgeons have proposed modifications of the standard surgical technique. Parthasarathy et al. reported injecting a small air bubble into the AC to help determine if a successful big bubble has been formed.[7] Foroutan et al. described the "shifting bubble sign"[8] wherein, a small bubble of air is injected into the AC after injection of air into the corneal stroma. Following decompression of the big bubble, the small air bubble in the AC moves to its central part. In spite of all these modifications, it may be difficult to ascertain the formation of a big bubble in the supra-Descemet's plane. In our technique of "double bubble" DALK, a small amount of air is injected into the AC before injecting air into the cornea stroma. As soon as a big bubble is formed, there is a sudden peripheral movement of the air from the central part of the AC due to inward bulging of the DM. Being a dynamic sign, this sudden movement of the air bubble is easily appreciated by the surgeon. Also, the decompression of AC prior to the injection of small bubble reduces resistance and provides space for the DM to bulge inward upon formation of a big bubble.

INDICATIONS

Similar to "big bubble" DALK, "double bubble" DALK can be successfully performed to treat corneal pathologies that do not involve the DM or endothelium. The indications for "double bubble" DALK are as follows:

- Keratoconus
- Corneal stromal dystrophies
- Corneal stromal scars sparing the DM

SURGICAL TECHNIQUE

Preparation of the Patient

The surgery should preferably be performed under general anesthesia. It is best to avoid a Lieberman speculum as it can cause too much pressure over the globe and can lead to bulging of the DM, increasing the chances of intraoperative perforation. A wire speculum should preferably be used in these cases.

Corneal Trephination

After marking the center of the cornea, a Hessburg–Barron suction trephine is used to perform partial-thickness trephination of the host cornea up to an approximate depth of 60–70% of the minimum corneal thickness. Subsequently a self-sealing paracentesis wound is created using a 15-degree surgical blade, just posterior to the limbus at 11 o'clock, and some aqueous humor is expressed out. A small amount of air measuring about 0.08–0.1 cm^3 in volume, is injected into the AC through the same paracentesis wound using a Rycroft

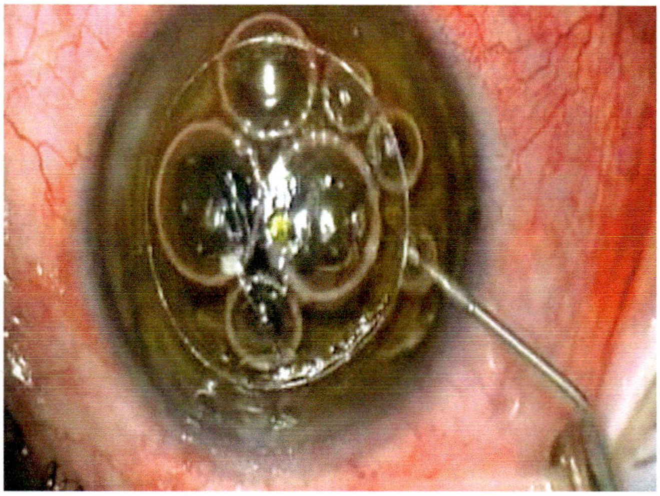

Fig. 1A: A small amount of air (3–4 mm in diameter) is injected into the anterior chamber through the paracentesis wound using a Rycroft cannula.

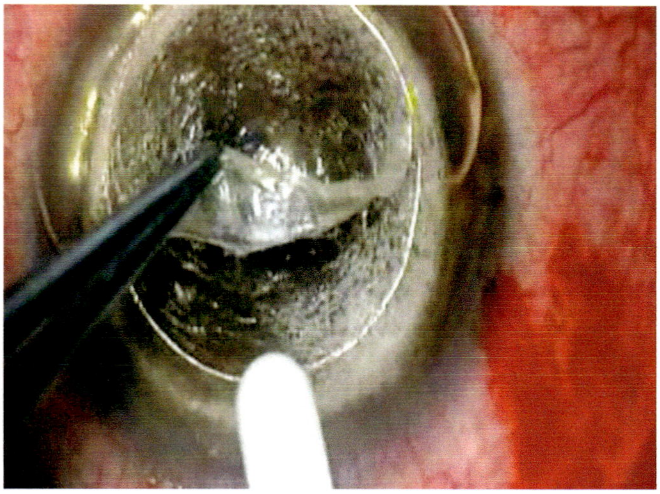

Fig. 1C: Anterior two-thirds of the corneal stroma is debulked leaving a thin layer of posterior corneal stroma.

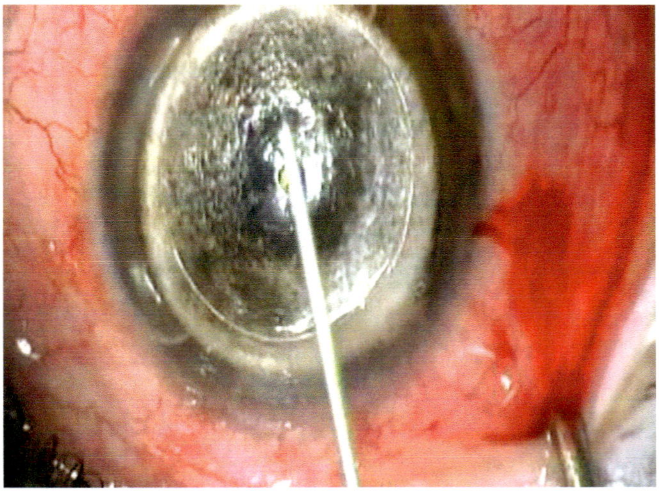

Fig. 1B: Air is injected into the corneal stroma, until peripheral movement of the first air bubble injected in the anterior chamber, is observed.

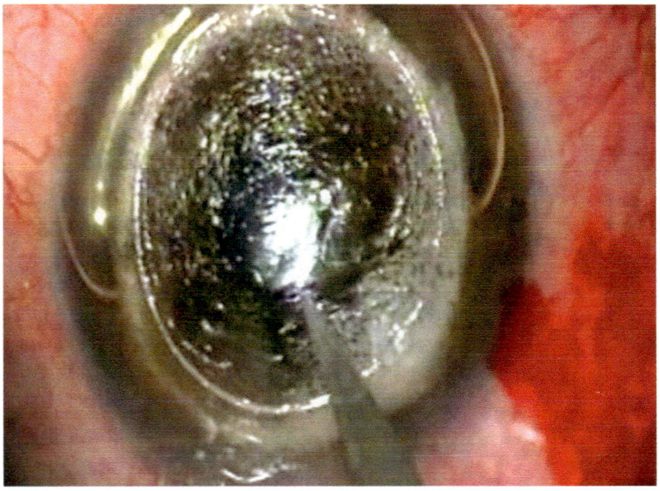

Fig. 1D: A 15-degree blade stained with gentian violet is used to create a shelved opening, into the potential space between the Descemet's membrane and the posterior stroma.

cannula, to achieve an air bubble of 3–4 mm in diameter (**Fig. 1A**). This is referred to as the "first air bubble" of our "double bubble" technique.

Injection of Air into the Corneal Stroma

Following this, a 27-gauge disposable needle, attached to a 2 cm^3 syringe is used to inject air into the corneal stroma to form a big bubble. The needle is bent at an angle of 70° away from the direction of the bevel. The needle tip, with the bevel facing down, is inserted tangentially into the paracentral corneal stromal tissue at a depth of 60–70%, through the previously created partial trephination wound (**Fig. 1B**). Under direct visual control, the needle is advanced in the corneal stroma for about 2 mm and air is injected slowly until the bubble present in the AC moves to the periphery (**Figs. 2A and B**). This sudden peripheral movement of the air bubble in the AC is an indication of successful formation of a "big bubble" in the supra-Descemetic space (**Figs. 1B and 2C**). This is the 'second air bubble' of our "double bubble" technique.

CONFIRMATION OF BIG BUBBLE FORMATION

At this stage, the formation of big bubble can be confirmed by rotating the eye in all quadrants. The big bubble formation can be confirmed by the confinement of all air bubbles present in the AC to its peripheral part. Since, the central part of the DM bulges into the AC, it prevents the migration of air bubbles towards the central part of AC. The next step involves debulking of the anterior two-thirds of the corneal stroma central to the trephination mark using a crescent blade (**Fig. 1C**). This leaves a thin layer of posterior corneal stroma above the big bubble. The debulking of corneal stroma helps in preventing inadvertent perforation of DM while excising the overlying stromal tissue. The AC is

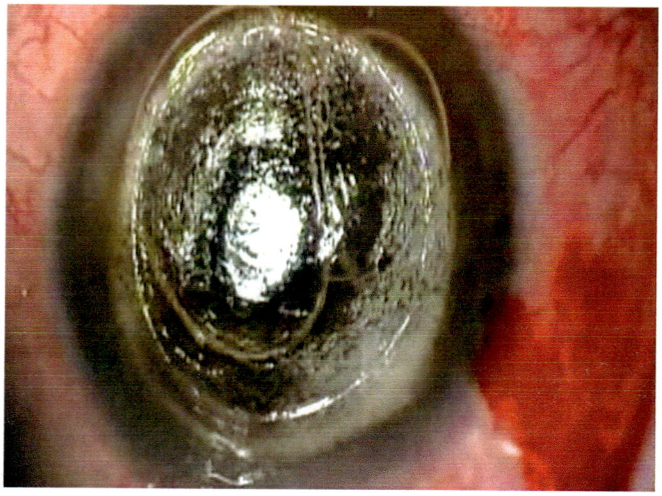

Fig. 1E: Entry into the supra-Descemetic space is identified by the dynamic movement of small air bubbles from the periphery of the anterior chamber back to its central part.

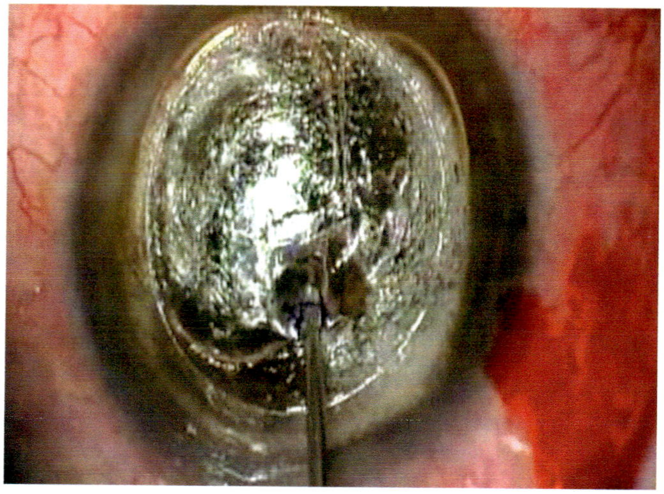

Fig. 1F: Subsequent to the central migration of air bubbles in the anterior chamber, 2% hydroxypropyl methylcellulose is injected through the opening into the potential space above the Descemet's membrane.

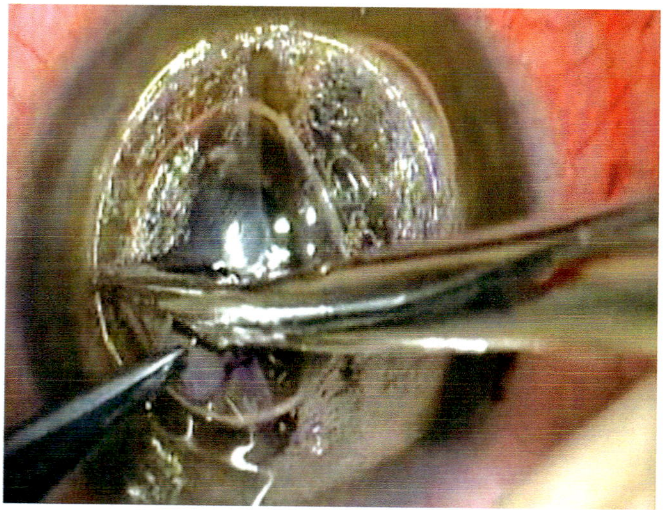

Fig. 1G: A pair of blunt-tipped curved Vannas scissors is then used to divide the thin layer of posterior corneal stromal tissue into four quadrants.

decompressed again to reduce tension over the DM and a 15 degree blade stained with gentian violet is used to create a shelved opening into the potential space between the DM

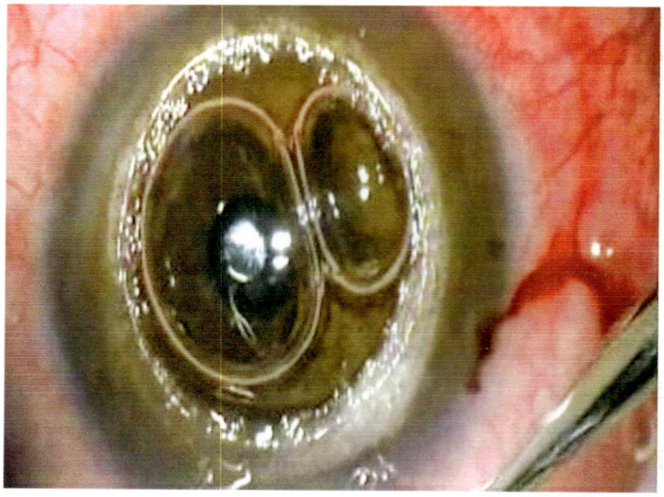

Fig. 1H: Each quadrant of posterior corneal stromal tissue is excised and the Descemet's membrane is completely bared.

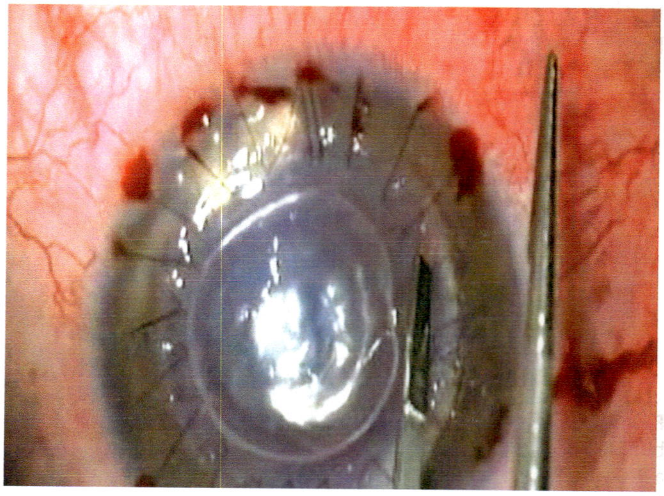

Fig. 1I: Donor lenticule is secured on to the host cornea with sixteen 10-0 monofilament nylon interrupted sutures.

and the posterior stroma (**Fig. 1D**). Entry into this space is identified by the sudden movement of the air bubble from the periphery of the AC back into the central part (**Fig. 1E**). At this point, the incision is immediately discontinued and 2% hydroxypropyl methylcellulose is injected through the opening into the potential space to keep the DM away from the rest of the stroma (**Fig. 1F**). A pair of blunt-tipped curved Vannas scissors is used to divide the thin layer of posterior corneal stromal tissue into four quadrants (**Fig. 1G**), and each quadrant is subsequently excised, baring the DM (**Fig. 1H**).

PREPARATION OF THE DONOR LENTICULE AND SUTURING

A 0.25 mm oversized donor lenticule is punched from the endothelial side and its DM is removed after staining with 0.06% trypan blue dye. The hydroxypropyl methylcellulose overlying the bare DM of the host cornea is washed with balanced salt solution, and the donor lenticule is secured using 16 10-0 monofilament nylon sutures (**Fig. 1I**). As in a penetrating keratoplasty (PKP), standard suturing techniques can be using either interrupted, running, or a combination of interrupted and running sutures.

POSTOPERATIVE FOLLOW-UP

Postoperatively, all patients are prescribed topical antibiotics (3 times a day) for a period of 3 weeks and topical corticosteroids in tapering doses for a duration of approximately 1 year.

Suture Removal

Selective suture removal is performed for any suture-related complication and for managing astigmatism. All sutures are however removed only after a period of 1 year.

COMPLICATIONS

The complications of "double bubble" DALK are similar to that of the standard technique of big bubble DALK. Briefly, they can be divided into the following categories:

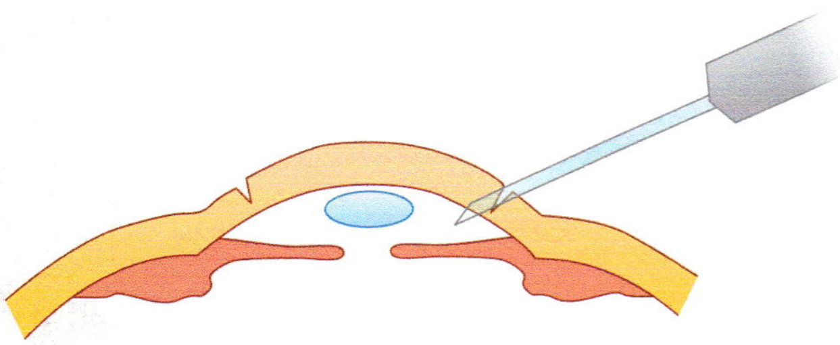

Fig. 2A: Schematic diagram depicting the injection of small first air bubble into the anterior chamber through the paracentesis wound using a Rycroft cannula.

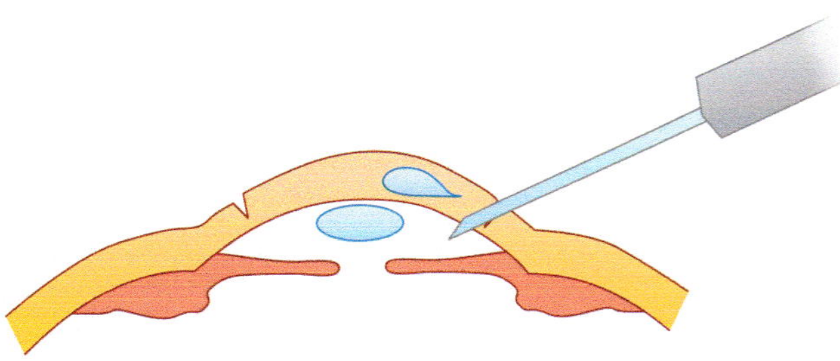

Fig. 2B: Schematic diagram depicting the injection of second air bubble into the corneal stroma using a 27-gauge needle.

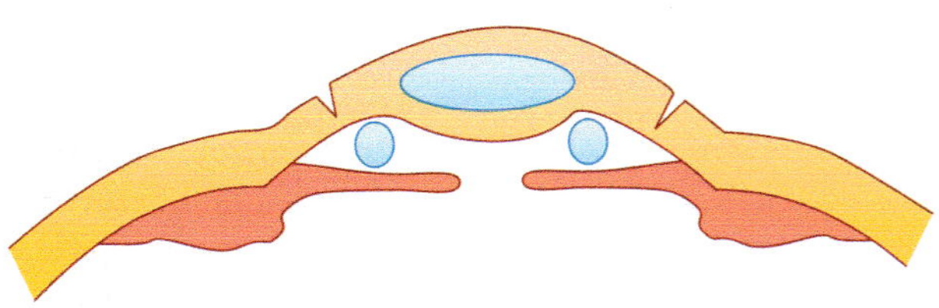

Fig. 2C: Schematic diagram depicting the movement of small air bubbles toward the peripheral part of the anterior chamber subsequent to air injection in the corneal stroma, due to inward bulging of the Descemet's membrane.

Intraoperative Complications

Failure of big bubble formation: Sometimes during the injection of air into the corneal stroma, the air can keep infiltrating the central corneal disk without an evident bubble formation. This usually happens if the needle is placed in the superficial part of the corneal stroma. In such cases, the surgeon should stop further air injection, in order to preserve some clear areas of stromal tissue. The needle should be withdrawn and re-introduced at another point, at a relatively deeper level, staying within the perimeter of the trephination. If the big bubble fails to form even after 2–3 such attempts, an anterior lamellar keratectomy can be carried out and repeat stromal air injection should be attempted through the debulked corneal stroma.

Perforation of DM: Intraoperative perforation of DM is the most feared complication during a DALK procedure. The management depends upon the stage of the surgery at which the perforation has occurred, and also on the size of perforation. If the cornea is perforated during initial trephination, the wound can be sutured and the surgery can either be postponed, or a layer-by-layer dissection be attempted. If the perforation occurs while the corneal stroma still covers the DM, a careful layer-by-layer dissection can be carried out leaving some stroma intact, above the area of perforation. Injection of air, a mixture of SF6 with air, or a mixture of C3F8 with air into the AC can be used for temporary closure of microperforations.[9] In case of a macroperforation, conversion to a full-thickness keratoplasty is inevitable. In such a situation, trypan blue dye may be used to highlight the remnants of the ruptured DM in order to ensure complete removal of the DM.[10]

Postoperative Complications

Formation of a double anterior chamber: The occurrence of a microperforation intraoperatively may lead to the formation of double AC in the postoperative period. Although some cases may resolve spontaneously, nonresolution may necessitate the use of tamponading agents such as air, SF6, or C3F8. Injection of any of these into the AC causes sealing of the microperforation and allows the fluid to get absorbed eventually from the double AC. Injection of longer acting agents such as SF6 and C3F8 may require a peripheral iridotomy in order to prevent pupillary block glaucoma.

Corneal stromal graft rejection: Although the risk of endothelial rejection is eliminated after DALK, the risk of immune-mediated stromal rejection remains. Presumed stromal graft rejection after lamellar keratoplasty presents with diminished visual acuity and corneal stromal edema. The clinical features of stromal rejection after DALK are similar to those seen in rejections occurring after a PKP. It is imperative to rule out recurrence or a new episode of herpetic graft infection in such cases. Management of rejection involves use of intensive topical corticosteroids in tapering doses and prophylactic antibiotics with serial monitoring of graft thickness.

SUMMARY

Our technique of "double bubble" DALK is a simple and effective surgery that helps in easy recognition of big bubble formation in the supra-Descemetic space. This helps in successful performance of a Descemet's baring DALK with preservation of the host's endothelial layer.

REFERENCES

1. Vajpayee RB, Tyagi J, Sharma N, Kumar N, Jhanji V, Titiyal JS. Deep anterior lamellar keratoplasty by big bubble technique for treatment corneal stromal opacities. Am J Ophthalmol. 2007;143:954-7.
2. Noble BA, Agrawal A, Collins C, Saldana M, Brogden PR, Zuberbuhler B. Deep Anterior Lamellar Keratoplasty (DALK): visual outcome and complications for a heterogeneous group of corneal pathologies. Cornea. 2007;26:59-64.
3. Fontana L, Parente G, Tassinari G. Clinical outcomes after deep anterior lamellar keratoplasty using the big-bubble technique in patients with keratoconus. Am J Ophthalmol. 2007;143:117-24.
4. Melles GR, Remeijer L, Geerards AJ, Beekhuis WH. A quick surgical technique for deep, anterior lamellar keratoplasty using visco-dissection. Cornea. 2000;19:427-32.
5. Archila EA. Deep lamellar keratoplasty dissection of host tissue with intrastromal air injection. Cornea. 1984-1985;3:217-8.
6. Anwar M, Teichmann KD. Big-bubble technique to bare Descemet's membrane in anterior lamellar keratoplasty. J Cataract Refract Surg. 2002;28:398-403.
7. Parthasarathy A, Por YM, Tan DT. Using a "small bubble technique" to aid in success in Anwar's "big bubble technique" of deep lamellar keratoplasty with complete baring of Descemet's membrane. Br J Ophthalmol. 2008;92:422.
8. Foroutan AR, Dastjerdi MH. Shifting-bubble sign in big-bubble technique in deep anterior lamellar keratoplasty. Cornea. 2007;26:117; author reply 117-8.
9. Mannan R, Jhanji V, Sharma N, Titiyal JS, Vajpayee RB. Intracameral C(3)F(8) injection for Descemet membrane detachment after phacoemulsification in deep anterior lamellar keratoplasty. Cornea. 2007;26:636-8.
10. Sharma N, Jhanji V, Titiyal JS, Amiel H, Vajpayee RB. Use of trypan blue dye during conversion of deep anterior lamellar keratoplasty to penetrating keratoplasty. J Cataract Refract Surg. 2008;34:1242-5.

26

Large-diameter Deep Anterior Lamellar Keratoplasty

Angeli Christy Yu, Asaf Friehmann, Massimo Busin

INTRODUCTION

With refinements in the operative technique and improvements in surgical instrumentation, the turn of the 21st century saw a paradigm shift away from traditional full-thickness penetrating keratoplasty (PK) toward lamellar corneal surgery.[1] Deep anterior lamellar keratoplasty (DALK) involves targeted replacement of diseased corneal stroma while preserving healthy unaffected endothelium. Although the concept of lamellar grafting was first introduced >150 years ago, anterior lamellar keratoplasty (ALK) has recently gained popularity.

Following the pioneering works of von Walther in 1830 and Mühlbauer in 1842, the procedure was further refined with the introduction of various techniques for stromal dissection. Recent advances in corneal imaging and surgical instrumentation have driven the improvements in the DALK procedure. A variety of techniques for deep lamellar dissection such as pneumatic dissection by Archila,[2] the big-bubble technique by Anwar and Teichmann,[3] hydrodelamination by Sugita and Kondo,[4] and viscoelastic-assisted DALK by Maloney and associates have been developed.[5]

Of these various methods, big-bubble DALK has emerged as the most popular approach.[2] The original technique described by Anwar et al. involves partial thickness trephination followed by angled centripetal advancement of a needle and forceful intrastromal injection of air to obtain the so-called "big-bubble".[2] One of the main challenges with this technique is the need to reach the central cornea while relying on subjective signs of proper cannular depth.[6] However, what is most critical for successful pneumatic dissection is not the radial distance of the tip of the cannula to the center of the cornea but the depth at which air is injected within the corneal stroma.[7,8] When the tip of the cannula is inserted within 100 µm from the posterior corneal surface, big-bubble formation can exceed 90% even with minimal centripetal advancement of the cannula.[9]

Accurate measurements of the exact area of interest can be obtained through anterior segment optical coherence tomography (OCT). Using an adjustable guarded trephine calibrated within 100 µm from the thinnest pachymetry value at the 9 mm zone, deep trephination can be performed to guide subsequent insertion of the cannula.[7] Thus, instead of trying to reach the proper depth during advancement of the cannula toward the center of the cornea, the insertion of the cannula can be initiated at the base of a deep trephination with minimal centripetal advancement by approximately 2 mm.[7] Using deep trephination during large-diameter DALK, the success rate of pneumatic dissection can approach up to 85%.[10] Logistic regression analyses of consecutive DALK surgeries have likewise affirmed that both increased trephination diameter and depth positively influence successful big-bubble formation.[10-12]

INDICATIONS

The most common indication for DALK is keratoconus (KC), which accounts for more than half of cases. Other surgical indications include traumatic or infective corneal scarring, corneal stromal dystrophy, postrefractive surgery ectasia, and scarring due to various causes including severe ocular surface disease with limbal stem cell deficiency, Stevens–Johnson syndrome, ocular cicatricial pemphigoid, and chemical or thermal burns. ALK can also be performed for tectonic indications including pellucid marginal degeneration and sterile Mooren's ulcer.

Keratoconus

Keratoconus is a degenerative corneal disease characterized by progressive corneal thinning and scarring. In its early stages, KC can be managed adequately by spectacle or contact lens correction. However, in cases of reduced visual acuity secondary to corneal scarring and contact lens intolerance due to high degree irregular astigmatism, a surgical intervention would often be required. Since KC cases present with isolated anterior pathology, DALK is an ideal procedure to retain the healthy endothelium and thereby obviate the risk of endothelial graft rejection.[13] In big-bubble DALK, advanced stages of KC with high mean K values and lower pachymetry values are associated with more frequent intraoperative complications.[10] The presence of scarring and older age are also significant predictors of type 2 bubble formation which in turn confers an increased risk of complications such as conversion to full-thickness keratoplasty.[14,15]

Corneal Scarring Secondary to Trauma or Infection

In response to an injury or infection, the cornea undergoes a complex process of wound healing involving inflammation, cell proliferation, and tissue fibrosis ultimately leading to stromal scarring. For proper preoperative assessment, anterior segment optical coherence tomography (AS-OCT) is valuable for assessment of the depth and extent of scarring. When possible, the corneal endothelium should also be evaluated by specular microscopy. Given that traumatic and postinfective corneal scars are often associated with otherwise functional endothelium and that most of these patients frequently have an emmetropic fellow eye, DALK should be initially attempted (**Figs. 1A and B**). In cases with a macroperforation or unsatisfactory clearance within the optical zone because of a full-thickness opacity, DALK can be converted to full-thickness keratoplasty.

For cases of scarring due to herpes simplex virus (HSV) keratitis, DALK should be contemplated only after the eyes have remained quiescent without episodes of reactivation or inflammation for a period of 6 months or longer. Initial high dose antiviral prophylaxis with extended taper is recommended to reduce the risk of disease recurrence.[16]

Other Indications

Deep anterior lamellar keratoplasty can also be adapted for challenging cases with intracorneal ring segments,[17] previous radial keratotomy,[18] anterior lamellar keratoplasty,[19] and even previous Descemet stripping automated endothelial keratoplasty (DSAEK) surgery.[20,21]

Pneumatic dissection can also be achieved in post-PK eyes. However, it is often challenging to prevent expansion of the air bubble beyond the PK wound.[22] Alternatively, stromal exchange can be accomplished through stromal peeling along a natural plane of separation.[23] Ultrastructural alterations in the stromal microarchitecture allow stromal peeling of grafted corneas along a deep natural plane of separation without any type of dissection.[23,24] The natural plane occurs along a continuous layer of keratocytes separating the overlying anterior stroma from a thin layer of pre-Descemet's membrane stroma, which consisted of poorly organized collagen lamellae.[24]

SURGICAL TECHNIQUE

Standardization of the DALK technique has substantially simplified the procedure and allowed high success rates independent of surgical experience.[25] Initial partial thickness deep trephination is carried out by a guarded trephine calibrated within 100 mm from the thinnest AS-OCT pachymetry value at the 9 mm zone.[26] In cases with significant asymmetry in corneal thickness, peripheral intrastromal hydration with balanced salt solution (BSS) can be performed in zones with relative thinning to safely allow deep trephination.[27]

A blunt probe is then inserted 1 mm centripetally from the base of the trephination. The blunt probe is then replaced by a cannula, which is advanced 1 mm further along the same track created by the probe, before attempting pneumatic dissection. Often, significant intrastromal air accumulation in the cornea precludes visualization of the circular silvery sheen of the bubble. In such cases of extensive emphysema, one can ascertain whether big-bubble formation has been achieved based on lateral displacement of an air bubble injected intracamerally.[28]

Correct identification and management of the type of bubble achieved during pneumatic dissection is instrumental in minimizing complication rates. Depending on the movement of air injected within the corneal stroma, pneumatic dissection

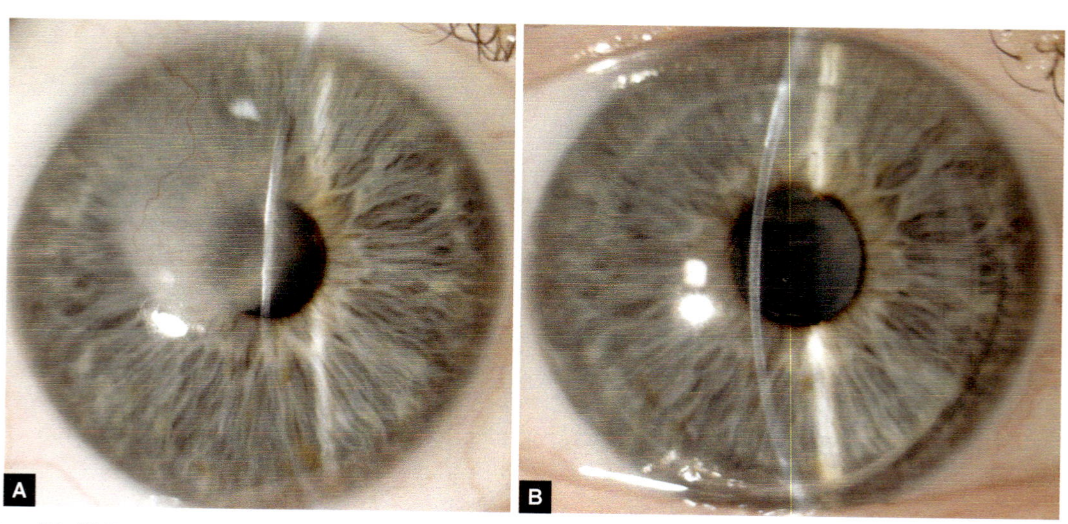

Figs. 1A and B: (A) Preoperative clinical picture of a central herpetic corneal scar with neovascularization; (B) Postoperative photo taken 5 years after deep anterior lamellar keratoplasty.

can occur along physiologic cleavage planes. A type 1 bubble is a well-circumscribed central dome-shaped elevation that results from a separation between the deep stroma from the pre-Descemet's layer while a type 2 bubble is a large, thinner-walled elevation at the level of Descemet's membrane.[29] Since the residual bed consists of a thin Descemet's membrane-endothelium complex, a type 2 bubble is associated with a lower bursting pressure and is therefore more fragile.[30]

After en bloc anterior keratectomy is performed starting from the base of deep trephination, the central 6 mm of the bubble roof is removed by baring the optical zone at the level of the pre-Descemet's layer or Descemet's membrane (DM), depending on the plane of dissection achieved.[9]

Since a type 1 bubble is often limited within 7–8 mm optical zone, we prefer to combine large-diameter keratoplasty with limited stromal clearance within the central 6 mm.[9] Several investigators have likewise employed limited stromal clearance for femtosecond laser-assisted DALK.[31,32] By respecting the anatomy of the pre-Descemet's layer, restricting the deep dissection to the central cornea has been shown to reduce the risk of DM perforation and conversion to PK.[9] The presence of a peripheral stromal shoulder also protects the recipient bed during suturing, which has been reported to cause up to 21% of intraoperative DM perforations during conventional DALK surgery.[22,33] Over time, remodeling of the corneal stromal architecture with progressive disappearance of the posterior step at the edge of the 6 mm zone has also been observed (**Fig. 2**).[13]

A 9-mm anterior lamellar graft is then prepared by means of a 400-mm microkeratome head and sutured into place. The donor cornea is initially fixed with four cardinal 10-0 nylon sutures at 3, 6, 9, and 12 o'clock. Interrupted or double-running 10-0 nylon sutures can be used depending on the primary pathology and presence of neovascularization.[9]

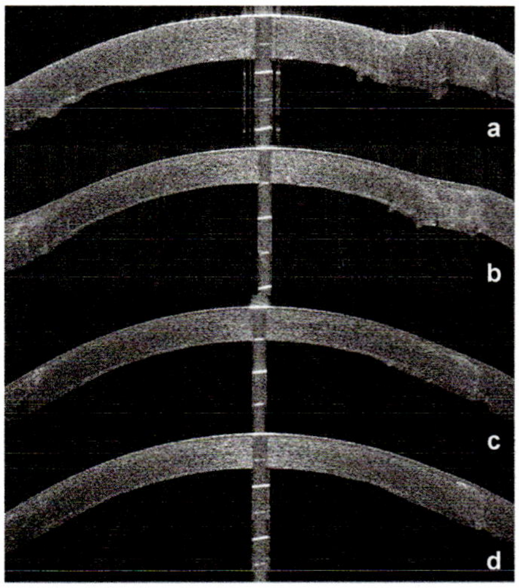

Fig. 2: Anterior segment optical coherence tomography taken 1 week postoperatively wherein a peripheral stromal shoulder is initially well-visualized (a) but eventually disappears through spontaneous stromal thinning and remodeling of posterior corneal curvature 1 year (b), 3 years (c) and 5 years (d) after deep anterior lamellar keratplasty.

Although baring of the Descemet's membrane can be attempted in cases with a type 2 bubble, manual or viscoelastic-assisted dissection techniques are often preferred in order to avoid inadvertent DM perforation.[34] Type 2 bubble formation is the strongest independent risk factor for double anterior chamber formation and conversion to PK.[14,15] A mixed type 1 and 2 bubble is typically managed as in a type 1 bubble, allowing the type 2 bubble to resorb spontaneously.[13]

Even with the current surgical technique, the overall success rate of pneumatic dissection still ranges between 60 and 85%.[1] In the event of failed big-bubble formation, other lamellar dissection techniques can be employed to salvage DALK surgery. Through the so-called microbubble incision technique, additional air can be injected into the corneal stroma. The presence of emphysematous tissue can then be used to guide layer-by-layer dissection which is aimed at achieving a smooth recipient bed while removing as much residual corneal stroma as possible.[35]

Since manual dissection is particularly tedious and is a significant risk factor for conversion to PK, we prefer sequential viscoelastic-assisted dissection in cases of failed pneumatic dissection and consider manual dissection only when all else fails.[13,36] Even in cases of failed pneumatic dissection, the success of visco-bubble formation approaches 90%.[36] Although retained viscoelastic is initially associated with visually significant interface haze, the effect on visual acuity is transient and final outcomes are comparable with those of big-bubble DALK.[37]

OPTIMIZING VISUAL OUTCOMES

In the past, success following corneal transplantation was defined by the presence of a clear corneal graft.[38] Today, however, visual acuity is considered the primary criteria for surgical success. Based on some earlier comparative studies, visual outcomes were apparently worse following DALK due to inclusion of cases, which were not reflective of the contemporary surgical technique and thus, were likely associated with irregular or incomplete lamellar dissection.[39-41] Currently used surgical techniques, which exploit physiologic cleavage planes, result in a clear graft host-interface compatible with satisfactory visual outcomes, comparable with PK.[26,42] Although prospective clinical trials are ideally required to make statistically valid comparisons, randomizing patients to PK over DALK could no longer be justified especially in view of the disproportionately higher risk for potentially severe complications following PK. Nevertheless, empiric evidence from large interventional case series has thus far validated the clinical benefits of DALK.[26,43,44]

From a refractive standpoint, the use of large-diameter grafts for DALK has been shown to provide superior visual outcomes with lower degrees of myopia and astigmatism.[36,45]

In a large series of 346 eyes, 9 mm DALK is associated with excellent outcomes with 94% of cases achieving Snellen vision ≥ 20/40 and up to 89% with refractive astigmatism <4.5 diopters.[26] Unlike PK, large-diameter DALK does not pose an increased risk of immune-mediated stromal rejection, which in any case can be manageable medically.[16] Additionally, performing large-diameter keratoplasty maximizes the removal of the diseased stroma, thereby preventing disease recurrence.[46]

MANAGING COMPLICATIONS

The most frequent complication encountered during DALK is Descemet's membrane perforation.[1] If limited to a microperforation, the surgery can still be successfully completed as per standard technique by filling the anterior chamber with air. In cases with a macroperforation or unsatisfactory clearance within the optical zone because of a full-thickness opacity, DALK can be converted to full-thickness keratoplasty. A mushroom-shaped wound configuration for full-thickness keratoplasty whether obtained through microkeratome- or femtosecond laser-assisted techniques can be considered in order to combine the advantages of a large anterior refractive surface with minimal endothelial transplantation.[9,32]

Double anterior chamber formation is another complication following DALK. Inadvertent perforation of DM, even if surgery is still successfully completed without the need for conversion to PK, has been described to lead to an increased risk of early postoperative detachment of the recipient bed and consequent double anterior chamber formation. This has been found to occur without a perforation detected intraoperatively, while, on the other hand, an intraoperative perforation does not necessarily lead to formation of a double anterior chamber. Corneal scarring, perforation and the occurrence of a type 2 bubble are known independent risk factors for double anterior formation following DALK. Although there are reports of spontaneous resolution, this complication usually requires rebubbling with air or gas to be managed successfully. Complete AC air fill is maintained for 2 hours before release of air at the slit lamp to achieve a fluid level at the height of the inferior pupillary border, thereby eliminating the risk of pupil block.[15]

One of the leading causes of limited visual recovery after DALK is high astigmatism especially when >4.5 D. With refraction after DALK stabilizing approximately 6 months after complete suture removal, refractive surgery can be subsequently performed to reduce residual postoperative astigmatism. Residual refractive errors after DALK can be managed through corneal or lens-based procedures. Astigmatic keratotomy, either manual or femtosecond laser-assisted has been found to reduce astigmatism, although generally with unpredictable results.[47] Deeper, longer, and more central incisions are often required to achieve a greater treatment effect. An advantage to DALK with limited central stromal clearance would be the ability to create deep arcuate blunt relaxing incisions within the graft-host interface which result in satisfactory outcomes with minimal risk of perforation.[48] In the presence of a cataract, lens extraction with implantation of monofocal or even toric intraocular lenses can also be contemplated.[49,50]

Other complications of DALK include persistent epithelial defect, corneal neovascularization, glaucoma, high astigmatism, cataract formation, and interface infection.[13,51]

Automated solutions have been explored to further address the technical challenges associated with DALK. Cross-sectional imaging can reduce the surgeon's dependence on subjective cues during the critical depth-dependent steps. Intraoperative OCT platform provides direct visualization and allows instantaneous quantitative analysis of acquired OCT scans for intraoperative planning based on patient-specific corneal anatomy.[52-54] Thus far, however most of the proposed applications of intraoperative OCT during DALK are primarily qualitative.[52,53] Based on our initial experience with a microscope-integrated intraoperative OCT with a built-in caliper tool, trephination depth can be used to assist decision-making on whether to proceed with pneumatic dissection or extend the trephination groove, which in turn can be used to guide subsequent placement of the air injection cannula.[54] Further work is still needed to establish and achieve the full potential of intraoperative OCT for intraoperative guidance of lamellar surgery.

Several investigators have also explored femtosecond laser-assisted DALK surgery.[55-61] As in stepped PK wounds, customized trephination patterns created using the femtosecond laser confers the advantage of an increased donor-host junction surface area, which theoretically can provide superior wound strength, induce faster wound healing, and allow earlier suture removal.[55] The femtosecond laser system can also be employed to create a deep intrastromal tunnel for the air injection cannula for pneumatic dissection.[56] However, one of the main drawbacks of femtosecond laser DALK is the poor laser penetration through opacified and neovascularized corneal tissue, which can result in incomplete or irregular dissection.[62] Although Li et al. demonstrated better visual outcomes following femtosecond laser-assisted DALK, visual performance in the manual DALK group was poorer due to greater residual bed thickness obtained in diamond knife-assisted lamellar dissection.[61] Moreover, all other published studies comparing manual and femtosecond laser-assisted DALK, thus far, consistently find no significant differences in terms of final visual acuity.[56-60] In general, the internal validity of these comparative studies is affected by the retrospective design,[57-61] heterogeneous study populations,[57,58] unequal sample sizes,[58,59,61] or varied surgical protocols for lamellar dissection,[57,60,61] graft sizing,[57,58,61] and even suture techniques.[57] Randomized controlled trials based on sufficient sample size and standard protocol would be necessary to allow direct comparison and assessment of true benefit of femtosecond laser technology for DALK.

CONCLUSION

With its superior safety profile and favorable postoperative outcomes, current evidence supports that DALK outperforms PK for the management of anterior corneal pathology sparing the endothelium. Recent advances in corneal imaging and available instrumentation have led to the standardization of the big-bubble DALK technique. Regardless of the success of big-bubble formation, other lamellar dissection techniques can be employed sequentially as an alternative to pneumatic dissection. Since the unaffected host endothelium is retained, DALK provides the opportunity to use large-diameter grafts, which can more reliably achieve maximum visual potential without an increased risk of immune-mediated stromal rejection.

REFERENCES

1. Reinhart WJ, Musch DC, Jacobs DS, Lee WB, Kaufman SC, Shtein RM. Deep anterior lamellar keratoplasty as an alternative to penetrating keratoplasty a report by the American Academy of Ophthalmology. Ophthalmology. 2011;118:209-18.
2. Archila EA. Deep lamellar keratoplasty dissection of host tissue with intrastromal air injection. Cornea. 1984;3(3):217-8.
3. Anwar M, Teichmann KD. Big-bubble technique to bare Descemet's membrane in anterior lamellar keratoplasty. J Cataract Refract Surg. 2002;28:3:398-403.
4. Sugita J, Kondo J. Deep lamellar keratoplasty with complete removal of pathological stroma for vision improvement. Br J Ophthalmol. 1997;81:184-8.
5. Manche EE, Holland GN, Maloney RK. Deep lamellar keratoplasty using viscoelastic dissection. Arch Ophthalmol. 1999;117(11):1561-5.
6. Scorcia V, Lucisano A, Pietropaolo R, Savoca Corona V, Scorcia G, Busin M, et al. Red reflex-guided big-bubble deep anterior lamellar keratoplasty: A simple technique to judge dissection depth. Cornea. 2015;34(9):1035-8.
7. Busin M, Scorcia V, Leon P, Nahum Y. Outcomes of air injection within 2 mm inside a deep trephination for deep anterior lamellar keratoplasty in eyes with keratoconus. Am J Ophthalmol. 2016;164:6-13.
8. Scorcia V, Busin M, Lucisano A, Beltz J, Carta A, Scorcia G. Anterior segment optical coherence tomography-guided big-bubble technique. Ophthalmology. 2013;120(3):471-6.
9. Busin M, Leon P, Nahum Y, Scorcia V. Large (9 mm) deep anterior lamellar keratoplasty with clearance of a 6-mm optical zone optimizes outcomes of keratoconus surgery. Ophthalmology. 2017;124(7):1072-80.
10. Scorcia V, Giannaccare G, Lucisano A, Soda M, Scalzo GC, Myerscough J, et al. Predictors of bubble formation and type obtained with pneumatic dissection during deep anterior lamellar keratoplasty in keratoconus. Am J Ophthalmol. 2020;212:127-33.
11. Borderie VM, Touhami S, Georgeon C, Sandali O. Predictive factors for successful type 1 big bubble during deep anterior lamellar keratoplasty. J Ophthalmol. 2018;2018:4685406.
12. Feizi S, Javadi MA, Daryabari SH. Factors influencing big-bubble formation during deep anterior lamellar keratoplasty in keratoconus. Br J Ophthalmol. 2016;100(5):622-5.
13. Yu AC, Mattioli L, Busin M. Optimizing outcomes for keratoplasty in ectatic corneal disease. Curr Opin Ophthalmol. 2020;21(4):268-75.
14. Myerscough J, Friehmann A, Bovone C. Evaluation of the risk factors associated with conversion of intended deep anterior lamellar keratoplasty to penetrating keratoplasty. Br J Ophthalmol. 2020;104(6):764-7.
15. Myerscough J, Bovone C, Mimouni M, Elkadim M, Rimondi E, Busin M. Factors predictive of double anterior chamber formation following deep anterior lamellar keratoplasty. Am J Ophthalmol. 2019;205:11-6.
16. Giannaccare G, Weiss JS, Sapigni L, Bovone C, Mattioli L, Campos EC, et al. Immunologic stromal rejection after deep anterior lamellar keratoplasty with grafts of a larger size (9 mm) for various stromal diseases. Cornea. 2018;37(8):967-72.
17. Ravera V, Bovone C, Scorcia V, D'Angelo S, Busin M. Deep anterior lamellar keratoplasty in eyes with intrastromal corneal ring segments. Cornea. 2019;38(5):642-4.
18. Einan-Lifshitz A, Belkin A, Sorkin N, Mednick Z, Boutin T, Kreimei M, et al. Evaluation of big bubble technique for deep anterior lamellar keratoplasty in patients with radial keratotomy. Cornea. 2019;38(2):194-7.
19. Yu AC, Myerscough J, Galante G, Furiosi L, Socea S, Bovone C, et al. Pneumatic dissection for large-diameter (9-mm) deep anterior lamellar keratoplasty in eyes with previous anterior lamellar Keratoplasty. Cornea. 2021;40(9):1098-103.
20. Gutfreund S, Leon P, Graffi S, Busin M. Deep anterior lamellar keratoplasty after Descemet stripping automated endothelial keratoplasty. Am J Ophthalmol. 2017:175:129-36.
21. Busin M, Beltz J. Deep anterior lamellar keratoplasty after descemet stripping automated endothelial keratoplasty. Cornea. 2011;30(9):1048-50.
22. Scorcia V, Beltz J, Busin M. Small-bubble deep anterior lamellar keratoplasty technique. JAMA Ophthalmol. 2014;132:1369-71.
23. Bovone C, Nahum Y, Scorcia V, Giannaccare G, Spena R, Myerscough J, et al. Stromal peeling for deep anterior lamellar keratoplasty in post-penetrating keratoplasty eyes. Br J Ophthalmol. 2020:bjophthalmol-2020-316653.
24. Busin M, Bovone C, Scorcia V, Rimondi E, Nahum Y, Myerscough J, et al. Ultrastructural alterations of grafted corneal buttons: The anatomic basis for stromal peeling along a natural plane of separation. Am J Ophthalmol. 2021;231:144-53.
25. Myerscough J, Bovone C, Scorcia V, Ricci-Filipovic B, Leon P, Mimouni M, et al. Deep trephination allows high rates of successful pneumatic dissection for DALK independent of surgical experience. Cornea. 2019;38(5):645-7.
26. Myerscough J, Roberts H, Yu AC, Elkadim M, Bovone C, Busin M. Five-year outcomes of converted mushroom keratoplasty from intended deep anterior lamellar keratoplasty (DALK) mandate 9-mm diameter DALK as the optimal approach to keratoconus. Am J Ophthalmol. 2020;220:9-18.
27. Bovone C, Myerscough J, Friehmann A, Elkadim M, Parmeggiani F, Busin M. Peripheral intrastromal hydration facilitates safe, deep trephination in corneas of irregular thickness. Cornea. 2020;39(2):207-9.
28. Parthasarathy A, Por YM, Tan DTH. Using a "small-bubble technique" to aid in success in Anwar's "big-bubble technique" of deep lamellar keratoplasty with complete baring of Descemet's membrane. Br J Ophthalmol. 2008;92(3):422.
29. Dua HS, Faraj LA, Kenawy MB. Dynamics of big bubble formation in deep anterior lamellar keratoplasty by the big bubble technique: in vitro studies. Acta Ophthalmol. 2018;96(1):69-76.

30. AlTaan SL, Mohammed I, Said DG, Dua HS. Air pressure changes in the creation and bursting of the type-1 big bubble in deep anterior lamellar keratoplasty: an ex vivo study. Eye (Lond). 2018;32(1):145-51.
31. Shehadeh-Mashor R, Chan CC, Bahar I, Lichtinger A, Yeung SN, Rootman DS. Comparison between femtosecond laser mushroom configuration and manual trephine straight-edge configuration deep anterior lamellar keratoplasty. Br J Ophthalmol. 2014;98:35-9.
32. Gadhvi KA, Romano V, Fernández-Vega Cueto L, Aiello F, Day AC, Gore DM, et al. Femtosecond laser-assisted deep anterior lamellar keratoplasty for keratoconus: Multi-surgeon results. Am J Ophthalmol. 2020;220:191-202.
33. Huang OS, Htoon HM, Chan AM, Tan D, Mehta JS. Incidence and outcomes of intraoperative Descemet membrane perforations during deep anterior lamellar keratoplasty. Am J Ophthalmol. 2019;199:9-18.
34. Myerscough J, Friehmann A, Bovone C, Mimouni M, Busin M. Management of type 2 bubble formed during big bubble deep anterior lamellar keratoplasty. Cornea. 2019;38:e20.
35. Riss S, Heindl LM, Bachmann BO, Kruse FE, Cursiefen C. Microbubble incision as a new rescue technique for big-bubble deep anterior lamellar keratoplasty with failed bubble formation. Cornea. 2013;32(2):125-9.
36. Scorcia V, De Luca V, Lucisano A, Carnevali A, Carnovale Scalzo G, Bovone C, et al. Results of viscobubble deep anterior lamellar keratoplasty after failure of pneumatic dissection. Br J Ophthalmol. 2018;102(9):1288-92.
37. Scorcia V, De Luca V, Lucisano A, Carnevali A, Carnovale Scalzo G, Bovone C, et al. Comparison of corneal densitometry between big-bubble and visco-bubble deep anterior lamellar keratoplasty. Br J Ophthalmol. 2019;104:336-40.
38. Cornea Donor Study Investigator Group. The effect of donor age on corneal transplantation outcome results of the cornea donor study. Ophthalmology. 2008;118(4):620-6.
39. Shimazaki J, Shimmura S, Ishioka M, Tsubota K. Randomized clinical trial of deep lamellar keratoplasty vs penetrating keratoplasty. Am J Ophthalmol. 2002;134:159-65.
40. Funnell CL, Ball J, Noble BA. Comparative cohort study of the outcomes of deep lamellar keratoplasty and penetrating keratoplasty for keratoconus. Eye (Lond). 2006;20:527-32.
41. Ardjomand N, Hau S, McAlister JC, Bunce C, Galaretta D, Tuft SJ, et al. Quality of vision and graft thickness in deep anterior lamellar and penetrating corneal allografts. Am J Ophthalmol. 2007;143:228-35.
42. Han DC, Mehta JS, Por YM, Htoon HM, Tan DT. Comparison of outcomes of lamellar keratoplasty and penetrating keratoplasty in keratoconus. Am J Ophthalmol. 2009;148:744-51.
43. Arundhati A, Chew MC, Lim L, Mehta JS, Lang SS, Htoon HM, et al. Comparative study of long-term graft survival between penetrating keratoplasty and deep anterior lamellar keratoplasty. Am J Ophthalmol. 2021;224:207-16. doi: 10.1016/j.ajo.2020.11.006. [epub ahead of print].
44. Borderie VM, Sandali O, Bullet J, Gaujoux T, Touzeau O, Laroche L. Long-term results of deep anterior lamellar versus penetrating keratoplasty. Ophthalmology. 2012;119(2):249-55.
45. Huang T, Hu Y, Gui M, Zhang H, Wang Y, Hou C. Large-diameter deep anterior lamellar keratoplasty for keratoconus: visual and refractive outcomes. Br J Ophthalmol. 2015;99:1196-200.
46. Yu AC, Franco E, Caruso L, Myerscough J, Spena R, Fusco F, et al. Ten-year outcomes of microkeratome-assisted lamellar keratoplasty for keratoconus. Br J Ophthalmol. 2021;105(12):1651-5.
47. Kubaloglu A, Coskun E, Sari ES, Guneş AS, Cinar Y, Piñero DP, et al. Comparison of astigmatic keratotomy results in deep anterior lamellar keratoplasty and penetrating keratoplasty in keratoconus. Am J Ophthalmol. 2011;151:637-43.e1.
48. Elkadim M, Myerscough J, Bovone C, Busin M. A novel blunt dissection technique to treat modified deep anterior lamellar keratoplasty (DALK)-associated high astigmatism. Eye (Lond). 2020;34(8):1432-7.
49. Scorcia V, Lucisano A, Savoca V, De Luca V, Carnevali A, Busin M. Deep anterior lamellar keratoplasty followed by toric lens implantation for the treatment of concomitant anterior stromal diseases and cataract. Ophthalmol Point of Care 2017;1(1):e30-e35.
50. Pellegrini M, Furiosi L, Yu AC, Giannaccare G, Scuteri G, Gardeli I, et al. Outcomes of cataract surgery with toric intraocular lens implantation after keratoplasty. J Cataract Refract Surg. 2021. doi: 10.1097/j.jcrs.0000000000000730. Online ahead of print.
51. Pellegrini M, Scorcia V, Giannaccare G, Lucisano A, Vaccaro S, Battaglia C, et al. Corneal neovascularisation following deep anterior lamellar keratoplasty for corneal ectasia: incidence, timing and risk factors. Br J Ophthalmol. 2021. doi: 10.1136/bjophthalmol-2021-319339. Online ahead of print.
52. De Benito-Llopis L, Mehta JS, Angunawela RI, Ang M, Tan DT. Intraoperative anterior segment optical coherence tomography: a novel assessment tool during deep anterior lamellar keratoplasty. Am J Ophthalmol. 2014;157(2):334-41.e3.
53. Steven P, Le Blanc C, Lankenau E, Krug M, Oelckers S, Heindl LM, et al. Optimising deep anterior lamellar keratoplasty (DALK) using intraoperative online optical coherence tomography (iOCT). Br J Ophthalmol. 2014;98(7):900-4.
54. Santorum P, Yu AC, Bertelli E, Busin M. Microscope-integrated intraoperative optical coherence tomography-guided big-bubble deep anterior lamellar keratoplasty. Cornea. 2022;41(1):125-9.
55. Farid M, Steinert RF. Deep anterior lamellar keratoplasty performed with the femtosecond laser zigzag incision for the treatment of stromal corneal pathology and ectatic disease. J Cataract Ref Surg. 2009:35(5).809-13.
56. Lucisano A, Giannaccare G, Pellegrini M, Bernabei F, Yu AC, Carnevali A, et al. Preliminary Results of a Novel Standardized Technique of Femtosecond Laser-Assisted Deep Anterior Lamellar Keratoplasty for Keratoconus. J Ophthalmol. 2020; 2020:5496162.
57. Shehadeh-Mashor R, Clan C, Yeung SN, Lichtinger A, Amiran M, Rootman DS. Long-term outcomes of femtosecond laser-assisted mushroom configuration deep anterior lamellar keratoplasty. Cornea. 2013;32(4):390-5.
58. Salouti R, Zamani M, Ghoreyshi M, Dapena I, Melles GRJ, Nowroozzadeh MH. Comparison between manual trephination versus femtosecond laser-assisted deep anterior lamellar keratoplasty for keratoconus. Br J Ophthalmol. 2019;103(12):1716-23.
59. Bleriot A, Martin E, Lebranchu P, Zimmerman K, Libeau L, Weber M, et al. Comparison of 12-month anatomic and functional results between Z6 femtosecond laser-assisted and manual trephination in deep anterior lamellar keratoplasty for advanced keratoconus. J Fr Ophthalmol. 2017:40(6):e193-e200.
60. Alio JL, Abdelghany AA, Barraquer R, Hammouda LM, Sabry AM. Femtosecond Laser assisted Deep Anterior Lamellar Keratoplasty Outcomes and Healing Patterns Compared to Manual Technique. Biomed Res Int. 2015;2015:397891.
61. Li S, Wang T, Bian J, Wang F, Han S, Shi W. Precisely Controlled Side Cut in Femtosecond Laser-assisted Deep Lamellar Keratoplasty for Advanced Keratoconus. Cornea. 2016;35(10):1289-94.
62. Yu AC, Friehmann A, Myerscough J, Socea S, Furiosi L, Giannaccare G, et al. Initial High-Dose Prophylaxis and Extended Taper for Mushroom Keratoplasty in Vascularized Herpetic Scars. Am J Ophthalmol. 2020;217:212-23.

27 Cannula-assisted Big Bubble Deep Anterior Lamellar Keratoplasty

Rajesh Fogla

INTRODUCTION

Penetrating keratoplasty is often performed in patients with advanced keratoconus, and various corneal stromal dystrophies wherein the endothelium is healthy. Full thickness grafts, however, breach the structural and immunological integrity of the eye. Ten-year cumulative risk of rejection remains at 21%.[1] Lamellar keratoplasty in comparison, eliminates the possibility of endothelial rejection and has minimal effect on endothelial cell count.[2] Other advantages being extraocular surgery, rapid wound healing, and shorter topical corticosteroid therapy.

Archila in 1984 described the use of air injection into corneal stroma to facilitate dissection down to Descemet's membrane (DM).[3] This technique although led to reduced interface haze and better postoperative visual results, had a high rate of intraoperative perforation of DM (39.2%). Anwar and Teichmann described the big bubble technique in 2002, wherein after partial thickness trephination, air is injected into the corneal stroma using a sharp 27-G needle to create a large bubble between DM and corneal stroma.[4] Success rate of achieving big bubble has been reported to be 80–90%, with 9% risk of intraoperative perforation.[4] In our experience, the success rate has been 69.2%, with 15.3% risk of intraoperative perforation.[5]

Modification of instrumentation and surgical technique of original big bubble surgery has helped improve the success rate and minimize risks of intraoperative complications.

SURGICAL TECHNIQUE

Preoperative Evaluation

It is important to assess the corneal condition prior to planning big bubble deep anterior lamellar keratoplasty (DALK). Regional pachymetry is essential to assess the overall thickness of the cornea. This can be measured from the Orbscan/Pentacam maps, regional ultrasound pachymetry measurements, or from anterior segment optical coherence tomography (AS-OCT). In the presence of corneal scars, AS-OCT is very useful to assess the corneal architecture preoperatively. If there is involvement of the DM in the scar, big bubble technique should be avoided as it leads to split in DM once the big bubble starts forming. Fleischer's cone should be identified, and its size and location noted. The trephine size on the host cornea is larger than the diameter of the cone. Health of the limbus should also be assessed, as it has an impact on postoperative epithelial recovery, especially in cases of chronic vernal conjunctivitis with advanced keratoconus.

Anesthesia

Ideally, the procedure should be performed under general anesthesia. It provides more control, minimizes positive pressure, and allows sufficient surgical time for completion of surgery. This is essential in the initial cases, however as more surgical experience is gained, surgery can be performed with equal ease under local anesthesia.

SURGICAL TECHNIQUE

Ideal trephine size is between 8 and 8.5 mm for most cases. Suction trephine such as the Barron radial vacuum trephine (Katena Products, Denville, USA) is needed to perform partial thickness trephination. Depth of initial trephination cut is at 80% of preoperative pachymetry value at the trephination site. With the Barron radial vacuum trephine, each quarter turn of radial spoke of the trephine cuts approximately 60 µm. Hence, 6–7 quarter turns are adequate to achieve a cut depth of 350–400 µm.

Anterior lamellar keratectomy is next initiated at 60% of the cut depth, using a crescent blade. The anterior stromal tissue is lifted with a tooth forceps and dissection carried out with the crescent blade to complete excision of the anterior lamella within the area of trephination.

The residual stromal tissue at the cut edge of trephination is grasped firmly using fine tooth forceps. Fogla pointed dissector is used to create a small channel at the base of the original trephination cut. This channel extends for 1.5–2 mm into the corneal stroma. Fogla pointed dissector (Storz Ophthalmics, Bausch and Lomb, USA) is a round bodied 27-G instrument with a pointed tapering tip.

Fogla air injection cannula (Storz Ophthalmics, Bausch and Lomb, USA), is a 27-G instrument, with flattened contour, closed rounded tip, and bottom port at the tip. This cannula is attached to a 5 cc air filled syringe. The residual stromal tissue at the cut edge is again grasped firmly using fine tooth forceps. Tip of the cannula is introduced into the channel created earlier using the pointed dissector (**Fig. 1**). The cannula is advanced forward toward the central cornea by applying gentle pressure and side to side motion. If the central cornea has extreme thinning, the cannula can be advanced toward paracentral cornea. Once in the desired position, air is injected with the syringe (*see* **Fig. 1**). Initial resistance is felt as the plunger is pushed forward. There is creation of small emphysema in the stroma at first, followed by appearance of the big bubble separation between DM and stroma. The bubble is outlined by a dense 1 mm band of white emphysematous stroma. Once the bubble has started forming, there is a feeling of giving way of resistance on the plunger of the syringe. Air injection is continued in a controlled manner till the bubble outline reaches the edge of trephination. Sometimes if placement of the cannula is superficial, significant amount of stromal emphysema may also occur along with formation of the big bubble. This makes it difficult to visually assess formation of the big bubble. Placement of a small air bubble in the anterior chamber has been described to confirm formation of the big bubble.[6] The small air bubble remains displaced in the periphery if there is formation of the big bubble.

At this point, the eye becomes very firm due to displacement of aqueous by the posteriorly displaced DM. Peripheral paracentesis is performed using a 15° slit knife. The tip of the knife should be directed vertically downward toward the peripheral iris rather than horizontally toward the pupil to avoid accidental perforation of the bubble. Release of aqueous helps normalize the intraocular pressure (IOP) and prevent development of anterior lenticular opacities (glaucomflecken) or fixed dilated pupil (Urrets-Zavalia syndrome).[7]

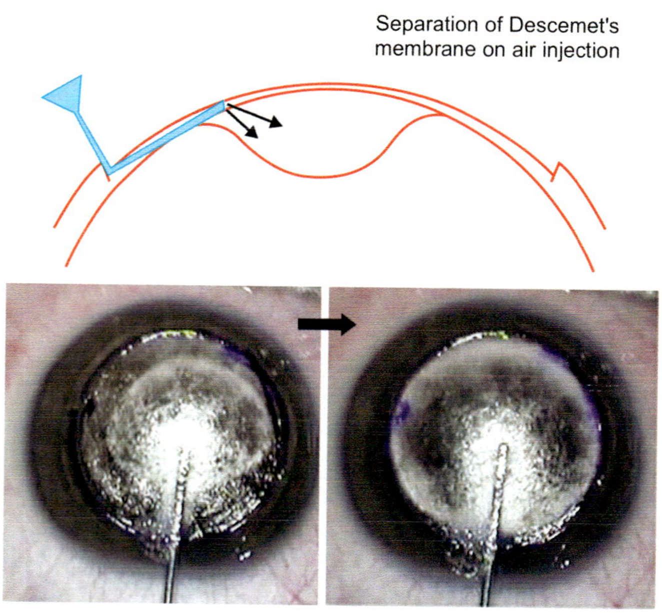

Fig. 1: Formation of big bubble following injection of air using Fogla 27-G air injection cannula.

The bubble is now deflated using a 15° slit knife. The cutting edge of the knife should be facing upward, and the point of entry should be close to the center of the cornea where the displacement of DM is maximum. The knife is introduced into the bubble and then quickly withdrawn in one smooth motion. While withdrawing the knife, forward movement of the anterior cutting edge helps enlarge the opening as well. Normalizing the IOP prior to this step allows gentle collapse of the bubble thereby preventing damage to the DM against the sharp tip of the knife. Minimizing the time between formation of bubble and deflating the bubble helps reduce damage to the endothelium, as the displaced DM is often in contact with the iris.

Fogla trifacet spatula (Storz Ophthalmics, Bausch and Lomb, USA), is then gently introduced into the space between the DM and stroma (**Fig. 2**). Using the slit knife, stromal tissue is incised over the edge of the spatula to enlarge the stromal opening.

Fogla corneal scissors (right and left) (Storz Ophthalmics, Bausch and Lomb, USA), the lower blade is 1 mm longer with rounded tip (*see* **Fig. 2**). Using these scissors, the stromal tissue is divided into four quadrants. It is important to keep the DM moist during this step to avoid drag between the instrument and DM. Each quadrant of stromal tissue is then excised one by one, to expose the DM.

Donor corneal tissue is usually of the same diameter for keratoconus cases, and 0.5 mm larger for other etiology. The peripheral cut edge of donor tissue is gently scraped on the endothelial side using a dry Merocel sponge to detach the DM. The edge of DM is grasped using fine nontooth forceps and then peeled away from the stroma. If the DM is friable, one can use the Merocel sponge to scrape DM away from the stroma. Trypan blue staining of the donor DM is also helpful to ensure complete removal.

Donor tissue is placed on the bare DM and then secured into position with 10-0 nylon sutures. Suturing technique depends on the surgeons preferred technique. I prefer initial 8 interrupted sutures followed by 16 bite continuous sutures (**Fig. 3**). Sutures can be adjusted at the end of surgery using Maloney's keratometer or intraoperative keratometer.

RESULTS

Since the instruments were developed in 2005, they have regularly been used in over 300 consecutive cases of DALK surgery using the modified big bubble technique. Success rate of achieving the big bubble has improved to 92–95%. This is a significant improvement from 69% using the original technique with sharp 27-/30-G needle. Cases,

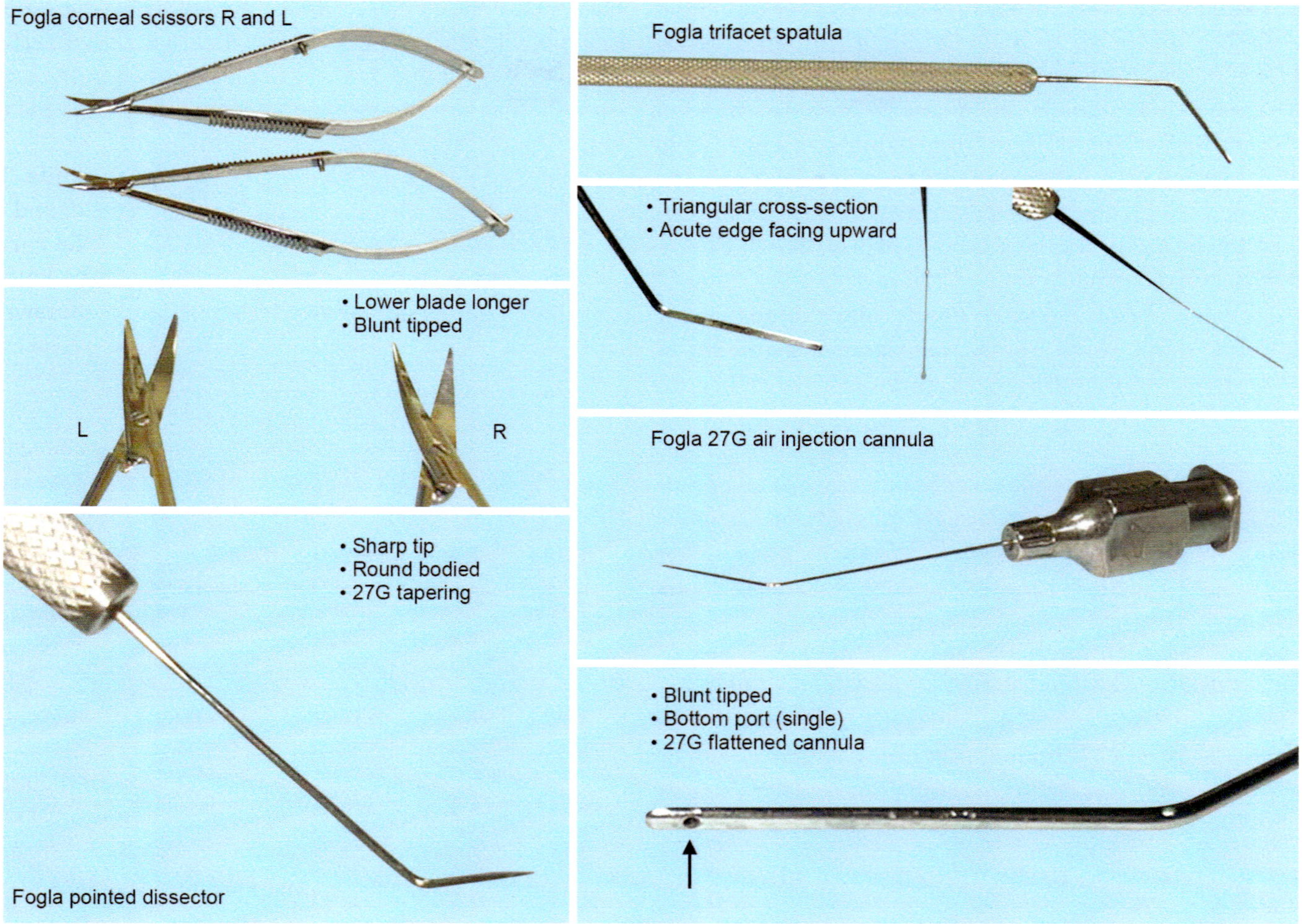

Fig. 2: Modified instruments for cannula assisted big bubble deep anterior lamellar keratoplasty surgery.

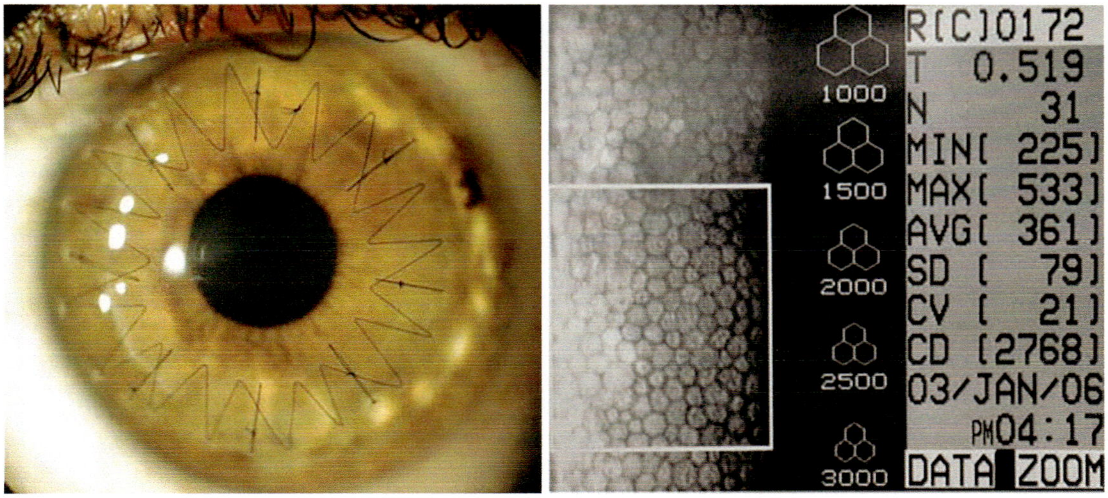

Fig. 3: Postoperative appearance at 1 month. Clear corneal graft. Note endothelial cell count of 2,768 cells/mm^2 on specular microscopy.

wherein bubble could not be achieved, were primarily due to very thin corneas. In these cases, after anterior lamellar keratectomy, minimal residual stromal tissue was noted at the thinnest point of the cornea. This led to escape of air in an anterior direction following air injection, rather than posteriorly to form the big bubble. In keratoconus cases with very thin cornea, anterior lamellar keratectomy step should be avoided, to be able to achieve the big bubble successfully. In macular stromal dystrophy, the DM seems to be friable. One case of macular stromal dystrophy had spontaneous DM rupture after successful formation of the big bubble. Microperforation was noted in 4% of cases, and usually occurred during surgical steps after formation of the big bubble. In all cases of microperforation, an air bubble filling 50% of anterior chamber was left at the end of surgery to tamponade the break and prevent formation of double anterior chamber. None of our cases needed to be converted to full thickness penetrating keratoplasty. Average best spectacle corrected visual acuity was noted to be 6/12 (20/40) (ranging from 6/24–6/6, 20/80–20/20). In 80% eyes, astigmatism was <4 diopters. Suture removal was usually performed after 1 year. Interrupted sutures were removed earlier if there was significant amount of astigmatism (>4 diopters). Average endothelial cell count was 2,800 cells/mm^2, with normal morphology. Thirty-five of our cases successfully underwent laser refractive surgery [laser in situ keratomileusis (LASIK) or surface ablation] for correction of residual astigmatism or refractive errors. Laser procedure was performed 6 months post-complete suture removal, with stable corneal topography. No complications were noted post-laser refractive surgery.

Modified technique of DALK using Fogla set of instruments, makes it possible to achieve the big bubble in a more consistent manner. Replacing the sharp needle with a flattened blunt 27-G bottom port cannula reduces risk of perforation, and simplifies the learning curve of this surgical technique. Initial anterior lamellar keratectomy ensures deeper placement of the cannula, thereby increasing success rate of achieving the big bubble. The original technique of Anwar's big bubble DALK surgery, with modifications described in this chapter, will become easier for corneal surgeons to incorporate in the management of corneal disorders.

REFERENCES

1. Ing JJ, Ing H, Nelson LR, Hodge DO, Bourne WM. Ten-year postoperative results of penetrating keratoplasty. Ophthalmology. 1998;105:1855-65.
2. Shimazaki J, Shimmura S, Ishioka M, Tsubota K. Randomized clinical trial of deep lamellar keratoplasty vs penetrating keratoplasty. Am J Ophthalmol. 2002;134:159-65.
3. Archila EA. Deep lamellar keratoplasty for dissection of host tissue with intrastromal air injection. Cornea. 1984-1985;3:217-8.
4. Anwar M, Teichmann KD. Big-bubble technique to bare Descemet's membrane in anterior lamellar keratoplasty. J Cataract Refract Surg. 2002;28:398-403.
5. Fogla R, Padmanabhan P. Results of deep lamellar keratoplasty using the big bubble technique in patients with keratoconus. Am J Ophthalmol. 2006;141:254-9.
6. Fontana L, Parente G, Tassinari G. Simple test to confirm cleavage with air between Descemet's membrane and stroma during big bubble deep anterior lamellar keratoplasty. J Cataract Refract Surg. 2007;33:570-2.
7. Niknam S, Rajabi MT. Fixed dilated pupil (urrets-zavalia syndrome) after deep anterior lamellar keratoplasty. Cornea. 2009;28:1187-90.

28 "Groove and Peel" Deep Anterior Lamellar Keratoplasty

Rishi Swarup

INTRODUCTION

For a good part of the last decade, deep anterior lamellar keratoplasty (DALK) has gained wide acceptance as the preferred surgical modality for treatment of corneal stromal opacities and ectasias, where the underlying endothelium is healthy.

Unlike the conventional penetrating keratoplasty, deep lamellar keratoplasty offers the distinct advantage of retaining the host endothelium and hence virtually eliminating the possibility of endothelial rejection—the most common cause of graft failure.[1,2] In countries where optical grade corneal tissue is a scarce commodity, one can ever use poor grade corneal tissue and get excellent optical results with DALK.[1]

CONVENTIONAL TECHNIQUES OF DEEP ANTERIOR LAMELLAR KERATOPLASTY

Deep lamellar keratoplasty involves excision of diseased corneal stroma by dissection, deep down to the level of Descemet's membrane or near-Descemet's. The technical challenge in DALK is to achieve Descemet's level dissection without compromising the integrity of the delicate Descemet's membrane. Several different techniques have to be devised to circumvent this challenge. Conventional manual (Cut and Peel) DALK which involves layer by layer excision of the stroma till the desired depth is reached, carries a high-risk of Descemet's perforation due to need for introduction of sharp dissectors in the deep stromal layers. Melles technique of DALK, which involves introduction of curved dissectors in the deep stroma, although safer gives suboptimal results due to higher possibility of interface scarring between host stromal bed and donor stromal button.[3,4] Other techniques such as intrastromal air[5,6] and fluid injection have attempted in thickening and opacifying the stroma to provide a better visualization of Descemet's on reaching the desired plane.

The most accepted technique currently is the "big bubble" technique, invented by Anwar and Teichmann.[7] This technique involved injection of air using a 27-gauge needle, introduced bevel-down in the deep stroma. The air finds its way through the deep stromal fibers to the pre-Descemet's space and induces detachment of the Descemet's membrane by a "big bubble" of air. This technique too carries a risk of inadvertent Descemet's rupture due to accidental full thickness puncture by the needle or due to rupture of Descemet's membrane induced by pressure of air. Rarely, the air may find its way between the banded and nonbanded layers of the Descemet's membrane. While attempting air injection, if the needle is not deep enough, the air enters intrastromally (corneal emphysema), creating feathery opacification of the stroma without achieving the objective of separating the Descemet's membrane from the stroma. Some authors have modified the original Anwar's big bubble to make the technique more reliable and predictable, but the technique still carries its inherent risks.

The "Groove and Peel" technique, overcomes many of these difficulties without the need for expensive instrumentation or tremendous surgical skill—making it the ideal technique for the novice lamellar surgeon.

SURGICAL TECHNIQUE

The Groove and Peel technique involves partial thickness trephination of the corneal using a simple or guarded trephine till about 50–75% depth (**Figs. 1A and 2A**). At one point in the trephination groove, the groove is slightly deepened using a Bard Parker blade to create a stromal pocket (**Fig. 1B**). Blunt tipped curved corneal scissors are introduced into this pocket with the blades of the scissor oriented horizontally and the tips closed. Once, the tips are intrastromal, the blades are slowly opened to separate the collagen lamellae and hence, widen the intrastromal pocket. The anterior layer of this pocket is cut with the scissor and the dissection is advanced in a similar manner along the trephination groove (**Fig. 1C**). This blunt dissection is slowly progressed along the entire length of the trephination mark till a circular stromal gutter is created. As the dissection proceeds from one end to the other the plane of separation gradually advances closer the stromal in a spiraling fashion with each pass such that one may complete two or

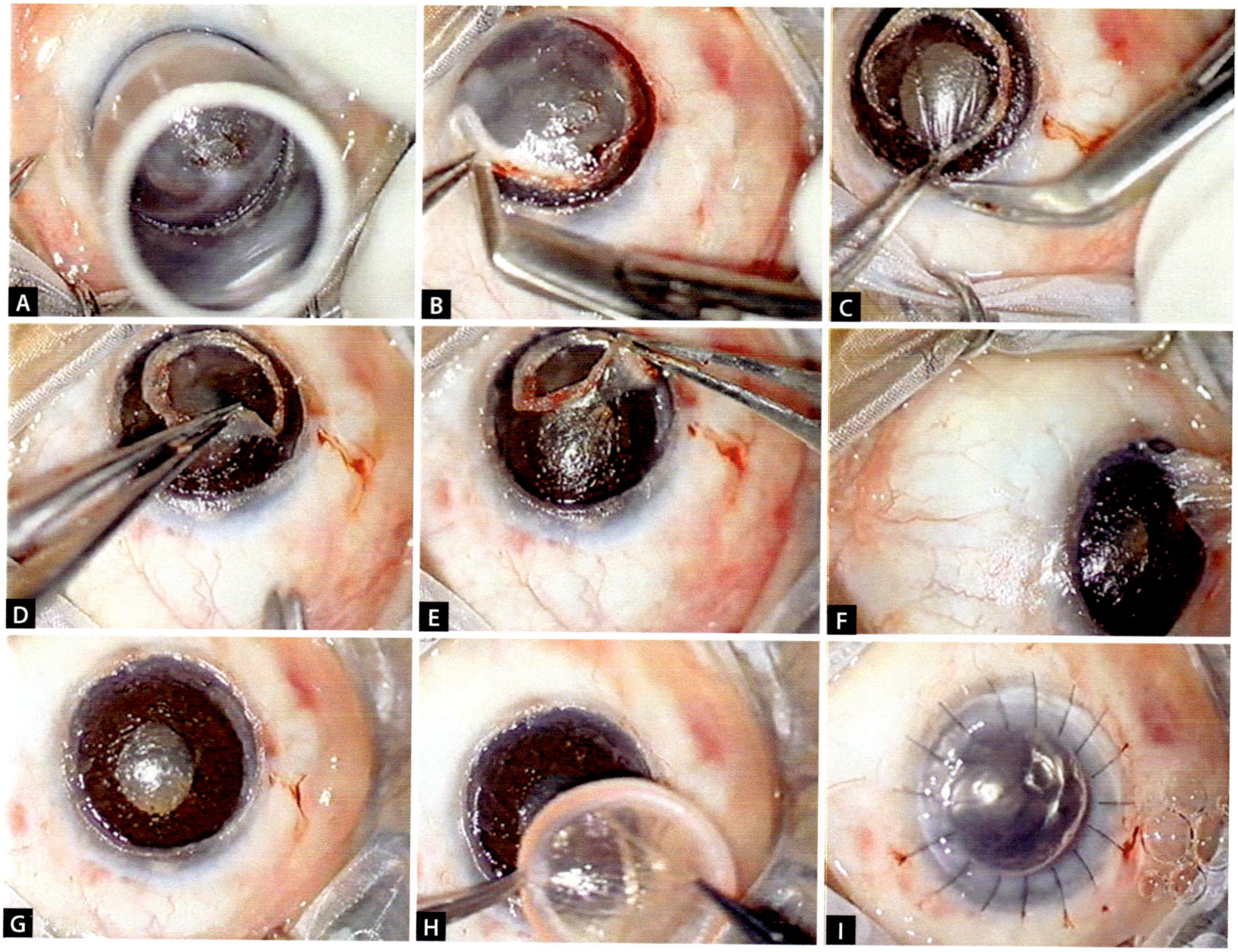

Figs. 1A to I: Surgical steps—Groove and Peel technique of deep lamellar keratoplasty. (A) Partial thickness trephination; (B) Creation of initial gutter; (C) Spiral groove till Descemet's membrane is reached; (D) Stromal tissue grasped and tented up under traction; (E) Stretch forces are distributed over a large surface area of the Descemet's membrane; (F) Entire stroma is peeled off in one smooth sweeping motion; (G) Prepared host bed with bare Descemet's membrane; (H) Donor corneal button is denuded of Descemet's membrane and endothelium; (I) Stromal button sutured in place with interrupted 10-0 nylon sutures.

three turns of the spiral before the desired depth is achieved (**Figs. 1D and E, 2B and C**). This spiraling dissection is to be halted once, the Descemet's membrane is visualized, seen a glistening clear membrane devoid of any significant overlying stromal attachments (**Fig. 1F**). At this point making a paracentesis, help to decompress the anterior chamber and reduces the chances of Descemet's membrane perforation. Once, the correct plane is reached the dissection is free of any resistance and the iatrogenic descemetocele is slowly enlarged till 3–4 clock hours. The stromal edge is then grasped and tented up (**Figs. 1F and 2D**). Stretch forces, thus created help cleave the microscopic adhesions between the deep stroma and Descemet's membrane. In one continuous motion, the entire stroma within the trephination groove is easily peeled away using traction forces distributed over a large surface area of the Descemet's membrane. Countertraction may be provided by means of a fixation forceps at the limbus opposite to the direction of the applied force.

Once, the host dissection has been completed (**Figs. 1G and 2E**), the donor corneal button is trephined to appropriate size. The anterior edge of this button is then grasped with a toothed forced and the endothelial edge dried with a surgical sponge gently rubbing the inner edge of the button with the tip of the sponge. This maneuver makes the Descemet's membrane edge stand up distinctly. This edge is then grasped with a nontoothed forceps such as a suture tying forceps and slowly peeled away from the underside of the corneal button (**Fig. 1H**).

The stromal button is then placed in the host bed and sutured with interrupted/continuous 10-0 nylon sutures (**Figs. 1I and 2F**).

DISCUSSION

An ideal technique of DALK is one which is technically easy, repeatable, safe, and is able to achieve Descemet's level dissection with minimal chances of perforation.

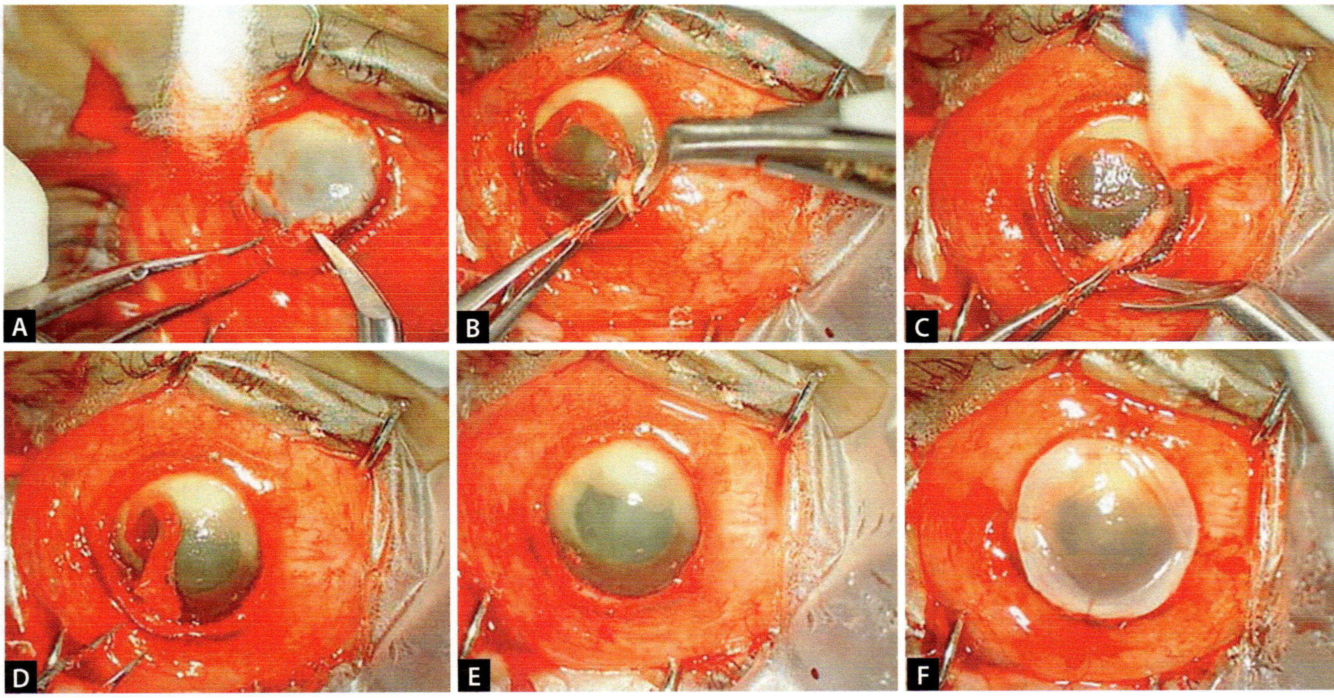

Figs. 2A to F: Groove and Peel deep anterior lamellar keratoplasty (DALK) in Acanthamoeba keratitis. (A) Partial thickness trephination encompassing the entire infiltrated stroma; (B) Creation of a spiralling groove all around after excising a layer of stroma to facilitate visualization; (C) The spiral dissection proceed deeper till the pre-Descemet's space is reached; (D) Stromal tissue is grasped and peeled away under traction; (E) Bare Descemet's with an underlying fixed hypopyon in the anterior chamber; (F) Stromal bed placed in host bed and sutured with 10-0 nylon.

Although the big bubble technique is able to provide very clean Descemet's dissection and excellent optical and visual results, it has a steep learning curve and is not easily reproducible.

The Groove and Peel technique, addresses many of these issues and makes the surgery simpler and safer. Although it is a manual technique, it avoids introduction of sharp instruments in the deeper stromal layers. Microperforation of the Descemet's membrane usually occur during excision of the stroma with a sharp blade or scissor. Macroperforations usually occur when extraneous fluid or gas is injected under pressure to separate the Descemet's membrane from the stroma. Both these situations are avoided in the Groove and Peel technique, where the stroma and Descemet's are separated by traction forces distributed over a large surface area, without the need for any sharp instrumentation or injection in the deep stromal layers.

Although microperforations can still occur during the creation of the initial gutter (3% as per the author's unpublished data of first 100 cases), the incidence is much lesser than other techniques of DALK. Also, the microperforation in this situation is the trephine groove and hence can easily sealed with air, fibrin glue or a suture. The dissection can then be completed from the opposite direction leaving behind a small sliver of stromal tissue to plug the microperforation.

The Groove and Peel technique also serves as a useful salvage manual technique in case of a failed big bubble attempt and is hence a useful technique in the armamentarium of even the skilled lamellar surgeon.

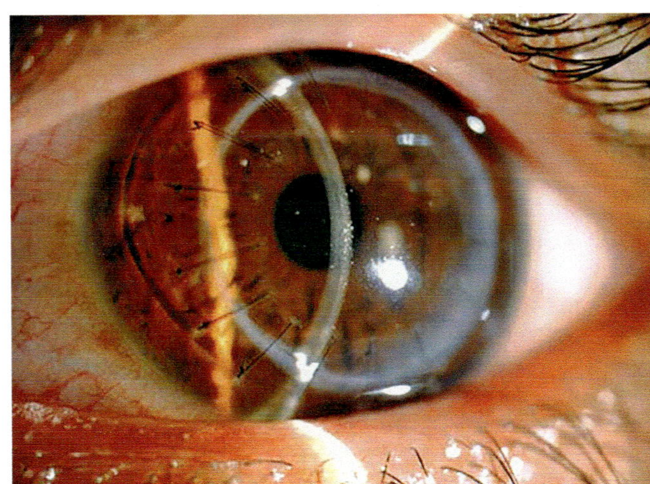

Fig. 3: Six months after Groove and Peel deep anterior lamellar keratoplasty (DALK) done for keratoconus—clear graft with best-spectacle corrected visual acuity (BSCVA) 20/20.

Other complications, optical and visual results with this surgery are comparable to big bubble technique of DALK (**Figs. 3 to 5**).

Thus, the Groove and Peel technique provides a simple, safe, effective, and reliable technique of deep lamellar keratoplasty. It is the ideal technique for the learning surgeon and may, in time, become the preferred technique for deep lamellar keratoplasty.

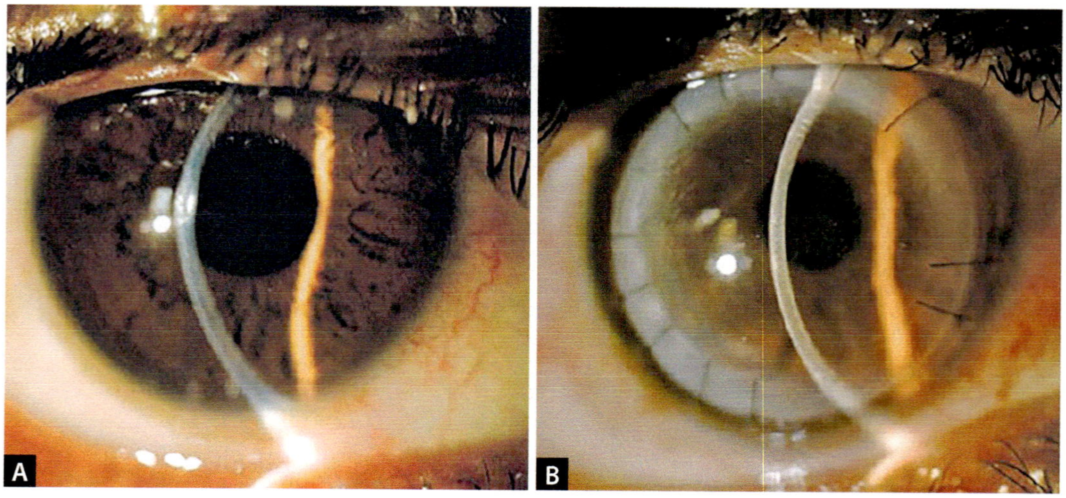

Figs. 4A and B: (A) Keratoconus prior to surgery; (B) Four months after Groove and Peel deep anterior lamellar keratoplasty (DALK).

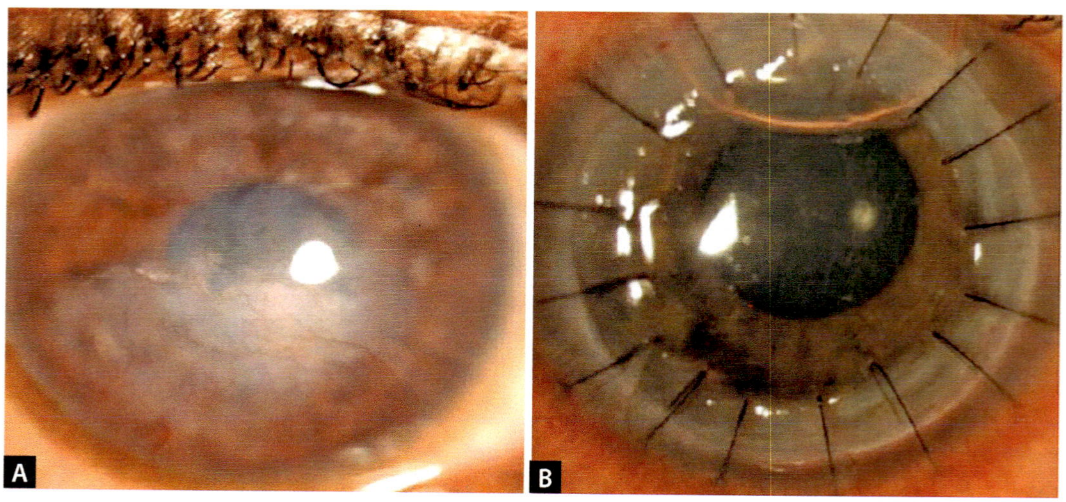

Figs. 5A and B: Before and after Groove and Peel deep anterior lamellar keratoplasty (DALK). (A) Preoperative: Stromal scar with vascularization; (B) Postoperative day 1: Clear and compact graft.

REFERENCES

1. Reinhart WJ, Musch DC, Jacobs DS, Lee WB, Kaufman SC, Shtein RM. Deep anterior lamellar keratoplasty as an alternative to penetrating keratoplasty, a report by the American Academy of Ophthalmology. Ophthalmology. 2011;118(1):209-18.
2. Price MO, Price FW Jr. Deep anterior lamellar keratoplasty: coming of age. Br J Ophthalmol. 2010;94(10):1275-6.
3. Melles GR, Remeijer L, Geerards AJ, Beekhuis WH. The future of lamellar keratoplasty. Curr Opin Ophthalmol. 1999;10(4):253-9.
4. Saw VP, Ng T, Crouch R, Maloof AJ. Deep anterior lamellar keratoplasty using the manual dissection technique of Melles: A histopathologic correlation. Cornea. 2006;25(8):882-5.
5. Archila EA. Deep lamellar keratoplasty dissection of host tissue with intrastromal air injection. Cornea. 1984-1985;3(3):217-8.
6. Price FW Jr. Air lamellar keratoplasty. Refract Corneal Surg. 1989;5(4):240-3.
7. Anwar M, Teichmann KD. Deep lamellar keratoplasty: surgical techniques for anterior lamellar keratoplasty with and without baring of Descemet's membrane. Cornea. 2002;21(4):374-83.

29 Diamond Knife-assisted Deep Anterior Lamellar Keratoplasty

Sri Vatsa Sehra, Prafulla K Maharana, Elsie Chan, Namrata Sharma, Rasik B Vajpayee

INTRODUCTION

The technique of deep anterior lamellar keratoplasty (DALK) has been developed to treat corneal pathologies, which involve only the stromal layers and spare the Descemet's membrane. In this, only a thin layer of host stromal bed or just the Descemet's membrane is left and it thus circumvents the major problems of interface haze, poor visual acuity, and contrast sensitivity found in earlier techniques of lamellar keratoplasty. The technique of DALK has evolved over time; in the mid-1980s Archila[1] popularized host stromal dissection with the aid of intrastromal air injection and spatula dissection. Sujita and Kundo[2] described a technique of hydrodelamination of the stroma from the Descemet's membrane in 1997. In 1999, Melles et al.[3] described a new technique of manual deep stromal, anterior keratoplasty with the use of semi-sharp spatula and mirror reflection from air injected in the anterior chamber, deeper dissection was done with the help of viscoelastic injection from the lamellar stromal pocket. Anwar and Teichmann[4] subsequently described the "big-bubble" technique in 2002 in which air injection was used to separate deeper stromal layers from the Descemet's membrane. While the big-bubble technique has shown good visual outcomes there is a steep learning curve and there are issues regarding repeatability of the results in the hands of different corneal surgeons. In some cases, even in the most experienced hands, the big bubble does not form; when the big bubble does form it is not always easily identifiable. For the purpose of identification, Parathasarthy et al.[5] have described a "small bubble technique", Foroutan et al.[6] have described the shifting bubble sign and Vajpayee et al.[7] have described a technique of "double bubble" DALK in which the visualization of movement of a bubble of intracameral air from the center to the periphery helps to determine the formation of the intrastromal "big bubble". Also, no standardized guidelines exist as to the volume of air to be injected, which is left to the subjective decision of the operating surgeon. Injection of excessive air is known to cause perforations of the Descemet's membrane.[8] As such, there is a high risk of perforation in the big-bubble technique that may range from 2 to 23%, especially in cases where the formation of an adequate big bubble is not achieved.[8-10] As compared to the big-bubble technique, earlier techniques do not have such a high rate of perforation, but they are associated with poorer outcome in terms of final visual acuity and quality of vision. This has been attributed to interface haze on account of a thicker residual stromal bed.

We have developed a new technique of micrometer-guided diamond knife-assisted deep anterior lamellar keratoplasty (Dia-DALK) which is safer than big-bubble DALK and offers comparable visual results. All the steps are under the control of the surgeon with minimal chance of Descemet's membrane perforation. Also, since a very thin layer of posterior stroma is left, the interface haze is negligible and visual outcomes are good.

INDICATIONS

We have used this technique to treat corneal ectatic disorders including keratoconus, pellucidal marginal degeneration (PMD), PMD with keratoconus, and keratoglobus. Dia-DALK has the added advantage of successful outcomes in very thin corneas where other techniques of DALK carry a high risk of perforation. Whereas the outcomes of Dia-DALK are better in patients of keratoconus with no past evidence of hydrops, we have also successfully treated cases of healed hydrops where the Descemet's scar is paracentral.

PREOPERATIVE WORK-UP

Preoperative investigations include assessment of corneal topography using Orbscan or a Pentacam. An anterior segment optical coherence tomography (OCT) is helpful to document level of pathological involvement as well as to get an estimate of the corneal thickness and the angle. Schirmer's test and a Tear break-up time (TBUT) are required to assess the ocular surface, which has an important bearing on the postoperative outcome. An ultrasonic nine point pachymetry is performed to determine the thinnest corneal thickness, which is required to plan surgery. A specular microscopy and Confoscan is optional to assess the status of corneal endothelium.

INSTRUMENTS REQUIRED

Wire speculum, calipers, Pierce–Hoskins forceps, trephine blade of desired diameter, ultrasonic intraoperative pachymeter, diamond knife with micrometer, curved Vannas scissors, lamellar dissectors, needle holder, paraffin block, and McPherson's forceps.

SURGICAL TECHNIQUE

Patient Preparation

The surgery should preferably be undertaken under general anesthesia but can be done under peribulbar anesthesia in cooperative adult patients. Povidone-iodine 0.5% is used to clean lids and irrigate the fornices; a sterile surgical opsite is placed such that all the eyelashes are covered. A wire speculum should preferably be used as it does not apply pressure on the globe, which may cause bulging and inadvertent perforation of the exposed Descemet's membrane intraoperatively.

Marking

The vertical and horizontal corneal diameters are measured with the help of callipers and the center of the cornea is marked with the help of gentian violet dye. Subsequently, the planned corneal area to be dissected is marked with the help of a manual corneal trephine centered on the premarked central point, whose edge has been marked with gentian violet (**Fig. 1**).

Intraoperative Pachymetry

Intraoperative ultrasonic pachymetry is done to determine the corneal thickness at a point between 11 and 1 o'clock to adjust the diamond blade micrometer accordingly (**Fig. 2**).

Diamond Knife-assisted Incision

The micrometer of the diamond knife is adjusted so that it cuts around 90% of the corneal stromal depth (**Fig. 3**) and an incision is made superiorly along the marking (**Fig. 4**). Curved Vannas scissors are used to extend the incision on either side (**Fig. 5**).

Lamellar Dissection

Lamellar dissection is completed in the resultant corneal plane by a combination of radial and centrifugal dissection using the open technique. Dissection is done under visualization using lamellar dissectors, Vannas scissors and crescent knife (**Fig. 6**) and a very thin layer of posterior stroma is left (**Fig. 7**). For cases of keratoglobus and PMD, we prepare a stromal pocket in the peripheral part of host cornea for tuck in lamellar keratoplasty (TILK)[11,12] (**Fig. 8**).

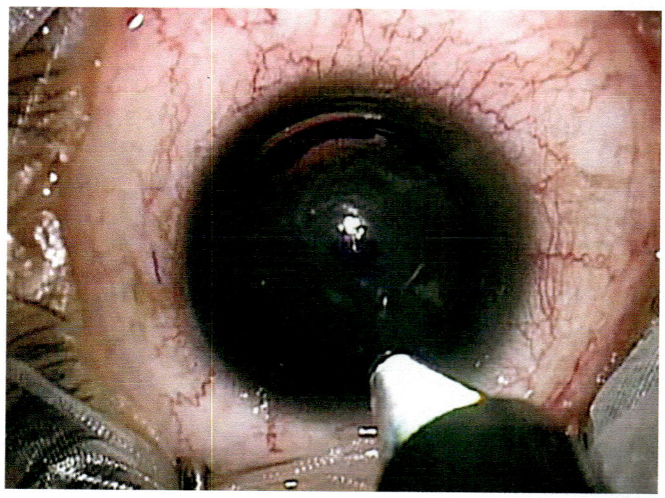

Fig. 2: Intraoperative pachymeter is used to determine the corneal thickness at a point between 11 and 1 o'clock.

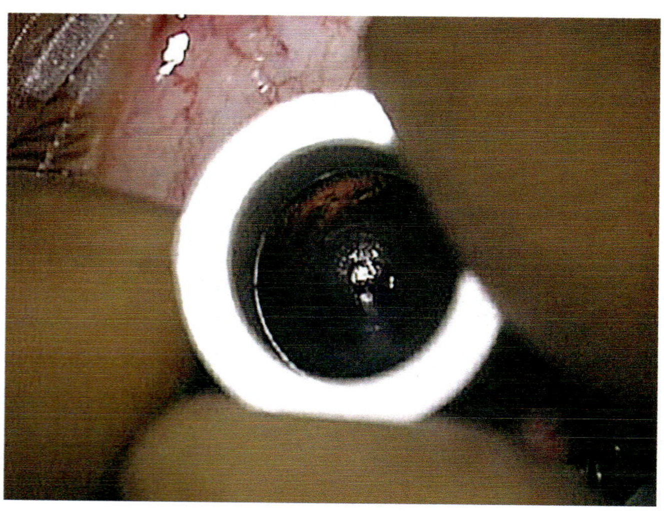

Fig. 1: After marking center of the cornea, a manual trephine is used to mark the desired size of host tissue to be cut.

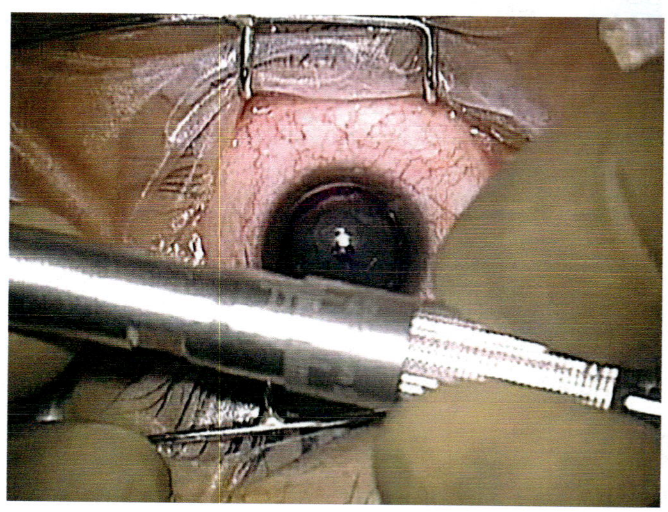

Fig. 3: Diamond knife micrometer is adjusted to 90% of the measured corneal thickness.

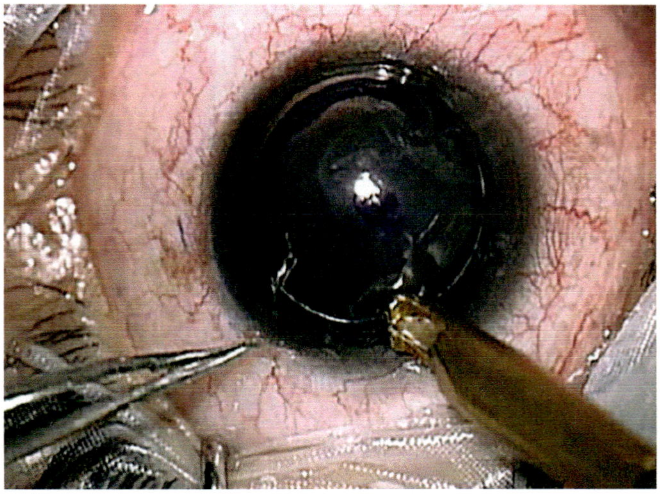

Fig. 4: An incision is made at 12 o'clock using the diamond knife micrometer along the mark made previously.

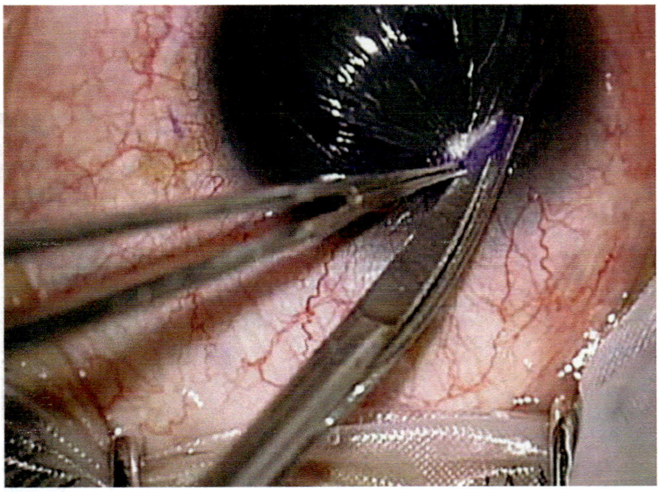

Fig. 5: Curved Vannas scissors are used to extend the incision on either side to create space for subsequent dissection.

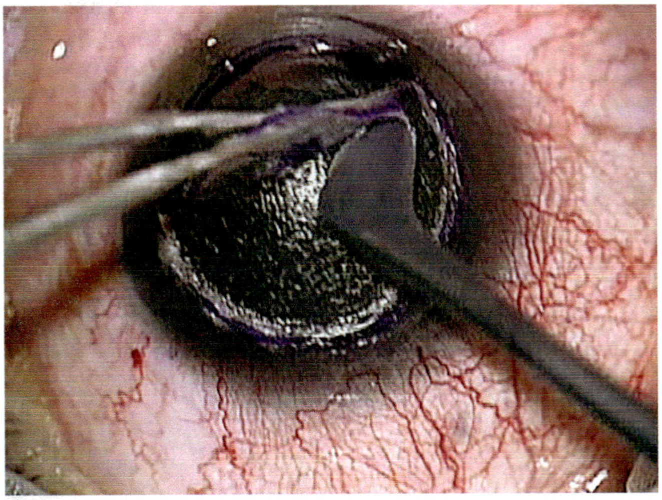

Fig. 6: Lamellar dissection is done using lamellar dissector.

Donor Preparation

A poor endothelial quality donor tissue is used. The donor button is placed endothelial side up on a wet teflon block and the appropriate size is punched using a manual trephine. We prefer to oversize the graft by 0.25 mm. The graft Descemet's membrane is then stained with 0.06% trypan blue dye and is scraped off (**Fig. 9**). For TILK, a donor tissue with a flange is fashioned using an artificial anterior chamber (**Fig. 10**).[11,12]

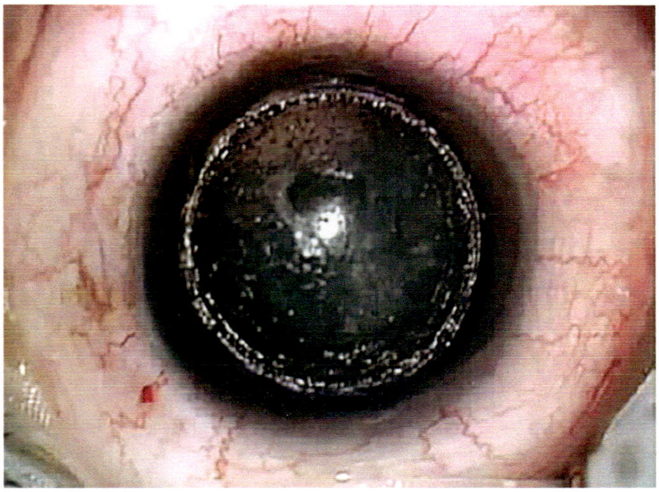

Fig. 7: A very thin layer of posterior stroma left after the completion of lamellar dissection.

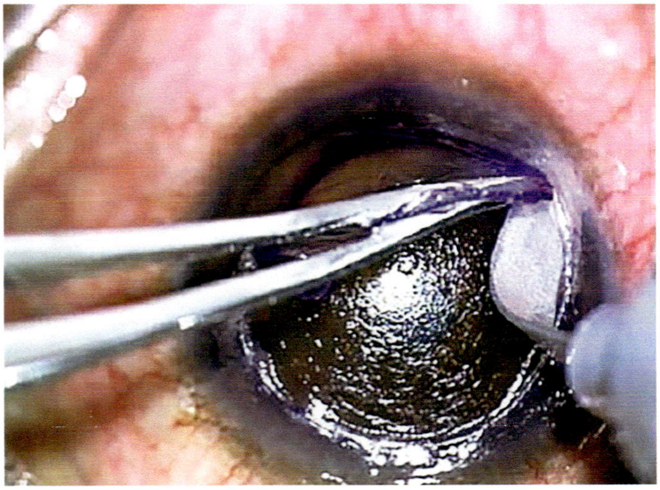

Fig. 8: Stromal pocket is created in the periphery in a case of keratoconus with pellucid marginal degeneration for "tuck in keratoplasty".

Cone Decompressing Incisions

Paracentral stab incisions are made using a microvitreoretinal (MVR) blade (Alcon Surgical, Fort Worth, Texas, USA) or a 15 degree blade (BD Pharmaceuticals, Becton Drive, Franklin Lakes, NJ, USA) (**Fig. 11**). We generally prefer to make two or three in number, preferably close to the site of ectasia. These incisions help to flatten the cone in keratoconus and take care of the posterior ectasia. It may also improve postoperative refractive outcome and make suturing easier.

Suturing

The prepared donor lenticule is placed on the host bed. Standard suturing techniques can be applied as in penetrating keratoplasty including intermittent, running or combined intermittent-running technique (**Figs. 12 to 15**).

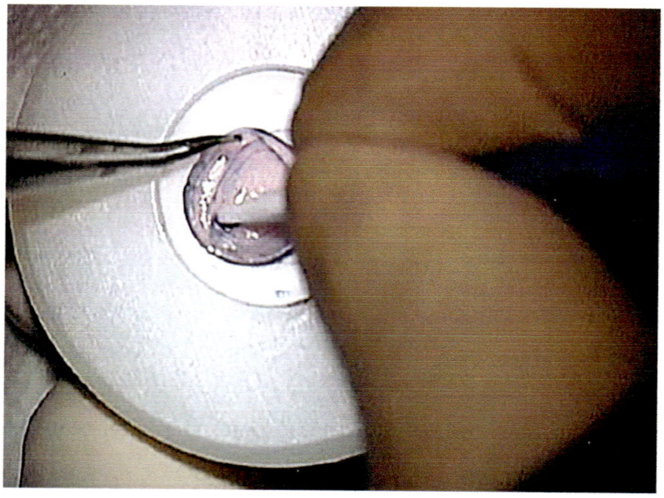

Fig. 9: Same sized or 0.25 mm oversized donor button is used, the Descemet's of which is stained with 0.06% trypan blue dye and scraped off.

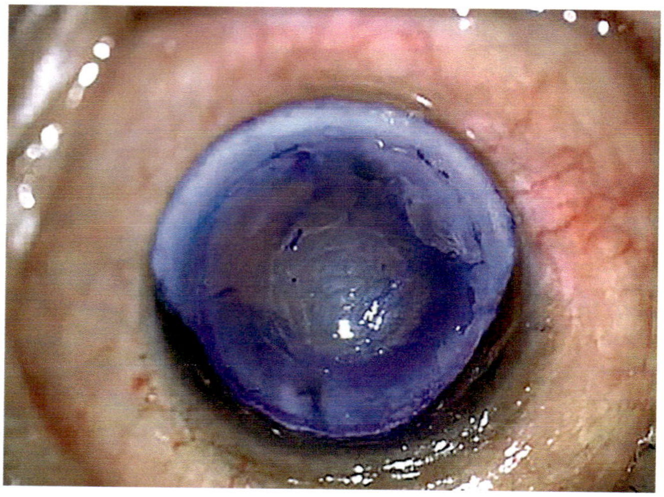

Fig. 10: A donor button with an inferior flange, fashioned by dissection done in an artificial anterior chamber, for "tuck in keratoplasty" in a case of keratoconus with pellucid marginal degeneration.

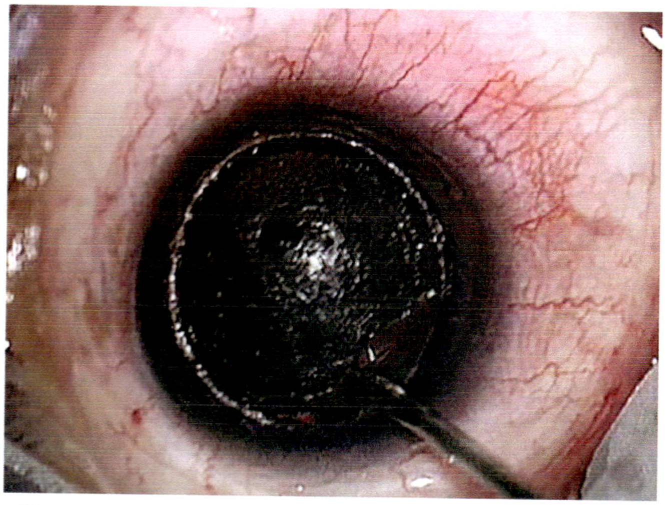

Fig. 11: Paracentral cone decompressing incisions are made using 15 degree blades to flatten the cone.

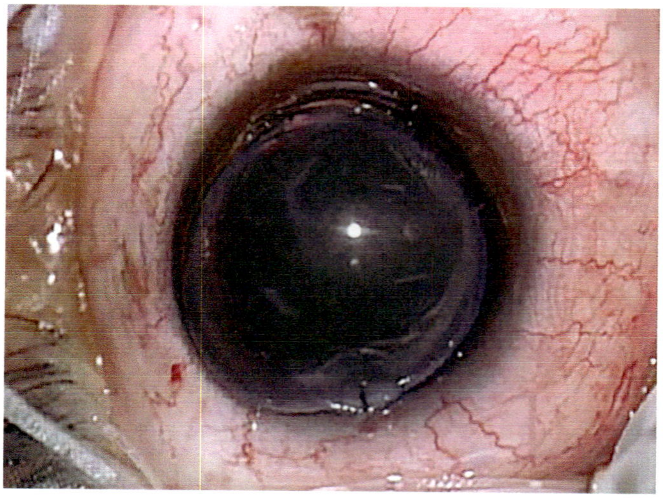

Fig. 12: The donor lenticule is sutured with intermittent 10-0 monofilament nylon suture. First cardinal suture passed.

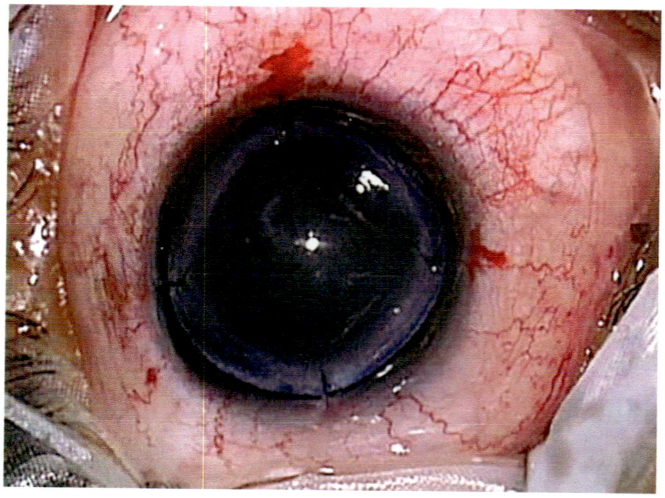

Fig. 13: Four cardinal sutures passed.

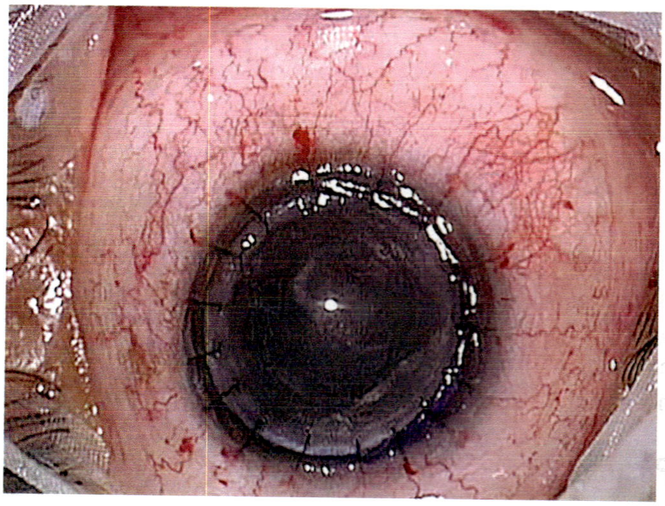

Fig. 14: Sixteen interrupted sutures.

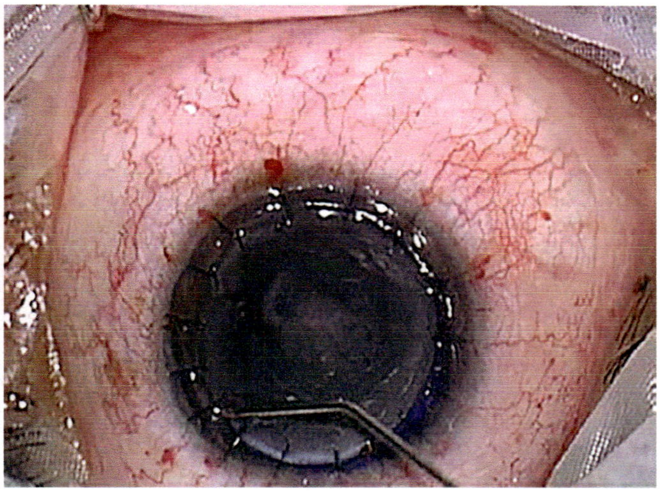

Fig. 15: The graft is tucked into host tissue and the suture knots are buried.

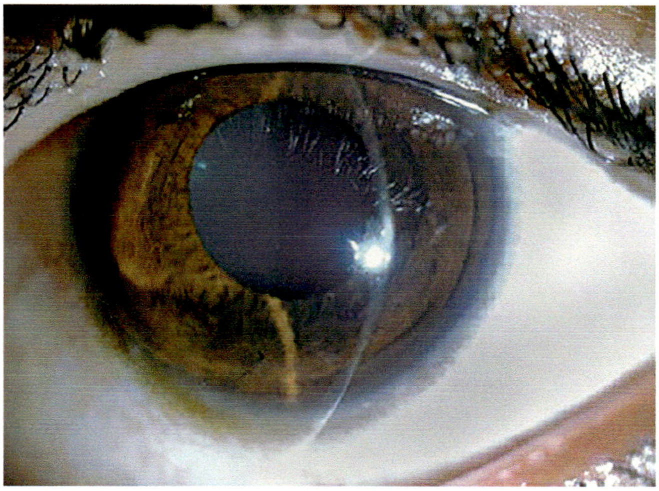

Fig. 16: Preoperative slit-lamp photograph of a patient of keratoconus with pellucid marginal degeneration. There is central corneal thinning and ectasia and peripheral corneal thinning between 4 and 8 o'clock with an area of normal corneal thickness between the limbus and the area of peripheral thinning.

POSTOPERATIVE MANAGEMENT

Postoperatively, the patients receive 0.5% antibiotic drops 3 times a day for 4 weeks. Prednisolone acetate 1% eye drops 4 times per day, which are subsequently tapered off over the next year. Lubricating eye drops, 4–6 times per day are also given.

Suture Removal

Selective suture removal is done for control of postoperative astigmatism and for any suture-related complications. All the sutures are removed by 1 year postoperatively.

Postoperative Follow-up

Follow-up visits are scheduled at 1 week and 2 weeks, 1 month, 2 months, 3 months, 6 months, 1 year, and then annually. At every follow-up, it is essential to perform a detailed examination and document the uncorrected visual acuity (UCVA) and best-corrected visual acuity (BCVA), graft status and clarity, graft-host junction, the interface, and the anterior chamber. Fundus examination should be performed regularly and the intraocular pressure (IOP) should be recorded at every visit.

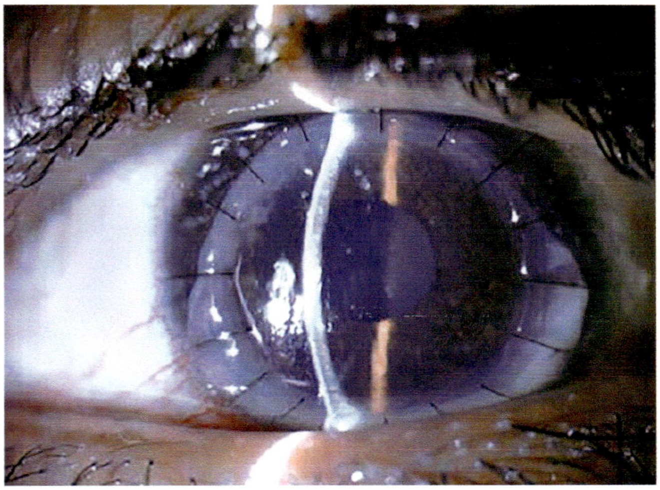

Fig. 17: Postoperative day 1 clinical photograph of the same patient. The patient underwent a diamond knife-assisted deep anterior lamellar keratoplasty with inferior intrastromal tuck.

COMPLICATIONS

Intraoperative

Perforation may occur at any time during the lamellar dissection. An inadvertent perforation, if small, can generally be managed by leaving a small amount of residual stroma over it, which will seal it and using air tamponade in the anterior chamber. However, a large perforation will require conversion to a penetrating graft. Usually, perforations do not take place with this technique.

Postoperative

The postoperative complications are expected to be similar to other forms of DALK,[1-3] however, since only a very thin layer of stroma is left, interface haze is less although further studies are required to confirm this. In our experience, we did not encounter any postoperative complications.

RESULTS

In our case series of six eyes (unpublished) that underwent Dia-DALK for keratoconus in our center, none of the cases had an intraoperative perforation. On the first postoperative day all grafts were clear (**Figs. 16 and 17**). In all the cases ≤70 µ of host stroma was left as determined on anterior segment optical coherence tomography (AS-OCT) (**Figs. 18A to C**). The median preoperative BCVA was 2/60, which improved to a median postoperative BCVA of 6/12 at the last follow-up of 1 month. The median central corneal keratometry reduced

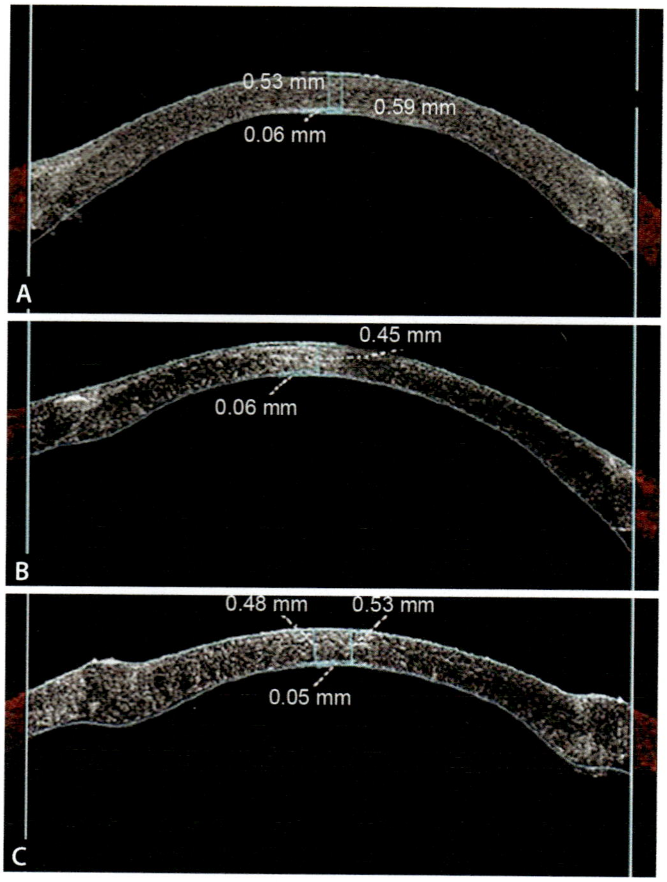

Figs. 18A to C: Postoperative diamond knife-assisted deep anterior lamellar keratoplasty anterior segment optical coherence tomography photographs showing residual stromal thickness of 60 µm, 60 µm, and 50 µm, respectively.

from 59.9 to 43.4 D. None of the eyes had a raised IOP or any suture-related complications at last follow-up.

REFERENCES

1. Archila EA. Deep lamellar keratoplasty dissection of host tissue with intrastromal air injection. Cornea. 1984-1985;3(3):217-8.
2. Sugita J, Kundo J. Deep anterior lamellar keratoplasty with complete removal of pathological stroma for visual improvement. Br J Ophthalmol. 1997;81:184-8.
3. Melles GR, Lander F, Rietveld FJ, Remeijer L, Beekhuis WH, Binder PS. A new surgical technique for deep stromal, anterior lamellar keratoplasty. Br J Ophthalmol. 1999;83(3):323-33.
4. Anwar M, Teichmann KD. Big-bubble technique to bare Descemet's membrane in anterior lamellar keratoplasty. J Cataract Refract Surg. 2002;28(3):398-403.
5. Parthasarathy A, Por YM, Tan DT. Using a "small bubble technique" to aid in success in Anwar's "big bubble technique" of deep lamellar keratoplasty with complete baring of Descemet's membrane. Br J Ophthalmol. 2008;92:422.
6. Foroutan AR, Dastjerdi MH. Shifting-bubble sign in big-bubble technique in deep anterior lamellar keratoplasty. Cornea. 2007;26:117; author reply 117-8.
7. Jhanji V, Beltz J, Sharma N, Graue E, Vajpayee RB. "Double bubble" deep anterior lamellar keratoplasty for management of corneal stromal pathologies. Int Ophthalmol. 2011;31(4): 257-62.
8. Jhanji V, Sharma N, Vajpayee RB. Intraoperative perforation of Descemet's membrane during "big bubble" deep anterior lamellar keratoplasty. Int Ophthalmol. 2010;30(3):291-5.
9. Leccisotti A. Descemet's membrane perforation during deep anterior lamellar keratoplasty: prognosis. J Cataract Refract Surg. 2007;33(5):825-9.
10. Feizi S, Javadi MA, Jamali H, Mirbabaee F. Deep anterior lamellar keratoplasty in patients with keratoconus: big bubble technique. Cornea. 2010;29(2):177-82.
11. Vajpayee RB, Bharatiya P, Sharma N. Central lamellar keratoplasty with peripheral intralamellar tuck: a new surgical technique for keratoglobus. Cornea. 2002;21:657-60.
12. Kaushal S, Jhanji V, Sharma N, Tandon R, Titiyal JS, Vajpayee RB. "Tuck in" lamellar keratoplasty (TILK) for corneal ectasias involving corneal periphery. Br J Ophthalmol. 2008;92:286-90.

30 "Tuck in" Lamellar Keratoplasty

Namrata Sharma, Vishal Jhanji, Sohini Mandal, Rahul Kumar Bafna, Rasik B Vajpayee

INTRODUCTION

Tuck in lamellar keratoplasty (TILK) is a surgical technique useful for the treatment of peripheral corneal thinning disorders. Peripheral corneal thinning is seen in cases of keratoglobus, advanced keratoconus, combined keratoconus and pellucid marginal degeneration (PMD), and post-penetrating keratoplasty corneal ectasia.

These cases may not be best treated with standard surgical techniques, as there is no tectonically stable host margin to fix the graft. Discrepancy between host and donor corneal thickness makes the procedure technically difficult with, often, poor visual results. Larger diameter grafts may be considered, but graft survival is poor in these cases, with up to 100% graft rejection rates reported.[1] Success has been variable with other surgical techniques employed for these cases.[2-6]

Tuck in lamellar keratoplasty is a technique designed for the treatment of advanced corneal ectasias.[7,8] This technique provides better support to both the central as well as the peripheral cornea, besides avoiding damage to the limbal stem cells or the angles.

In this technique, the donor lenticule has a peripheral partial thickness flange of posterior stromal tissue. Support for the central cornea is provided by the central 8.5 mm of donor, while the peripheral flange integrates into the host, providing tectonic support to the peripheral cornea.[7,8] The peripheral flange can extend circumferentially,[7] or just across the inferior aspect of the donor lenticule,[8] depending upon the circumferential extent of peripheral thinning.

INDICATIONS

- Keratoglobus
- Advanced keratoconus with involvement of the peripheral cornea
- Pellucid marginal corneal degeneration (PMCD)
- Terrien's marginal degeneration (TMD)
- Keratoconus occurring concurrently with pellucid marginal degeneration
- Peripheral progression of keratoconus post-penetrating keratoplasty
- Post-refractive surgery corneal ectasia (PRCE)

TECHNIQUE

Tuck in lamellar keratoplasty can be performed under either local or general anesthesia. The host bed should be prepared first.

Preparation of the Host Bed

- Bridle the vertical recti
- Mark the center of the pupil
- Perform 8.5–9.0 mm partial thickness trephination of the host cornea up to a depth of 50% of the host corneal thickness.
- Perform centripetal dissection using lamellar dissectors to excise central anterior stromal disk (**Fig. 1A**).
- Perform centrifugal lamellar dissection with a crescent knife to create a peripheral intrastromal pocket extending 0.5 mm posterior to the limbus (**Fig. 1B**).
- Pocket can be made circumferentially in the corneal periphery, or just inferiorly, depending on the host pathology.

Preparation of the Graft

The graft can be prepared by either of the following two methods.

Anterior Approach

- Fix the donor button on an artificial anterior chamber (Moria, Antony, France)
- Remove the epithelium
- Make a partial thickness 8.5–9.0 mm diameter incision up to a depth of 300 μm using a Hessburg–Barron vacuum trephine (Jedmed Instruments, St. Louis, MO).
- Perform lamellar dissection peripheral to the trephine cut, extending out to the limbus circumferentially.

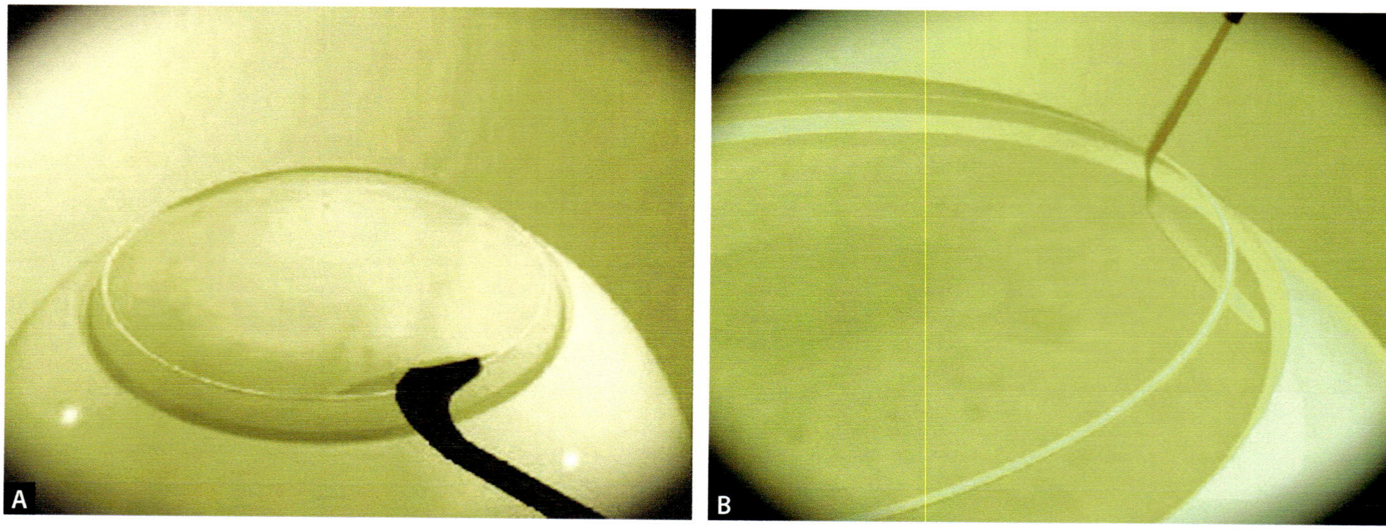

Figs. 1A and B: (A) Centripetal lamellar dissection; (B) Centrifugal lamellar dissection.

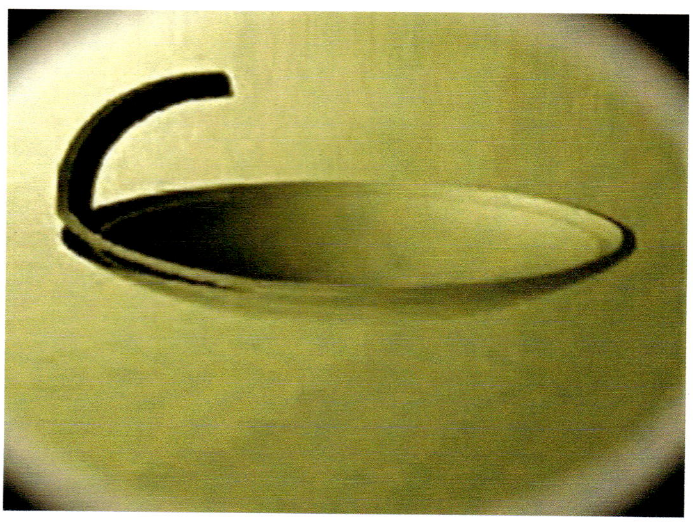

Fig. 2: Endothelium and posterior stroma are removed from peripheral flange using Vannas scissors, via posterior approach.

- Excise the superficial corneal tissue extending from the trephine mark till the limbus. This leaves a central 8.5–9.0 mm of full thickness graft with a peripheral partial thickness flange of approximately 2.5–3.0 mm.
- Punch the tissue from the endothelial side with an 11 or 12 mm trephine.
- If using just an inferior tuck, excise the 180° excess donor tissue flange with Vannas scissors.
- Stain the Descemet membrane of the donor using trypan blue dye and strip it using a cellulose sponge.

Posterior Approach

- Punch the tissue from the endothelial side with an 11 or 12 mm trephine
- Remove epithelium
- From the posterior side, using Vannas scissors, remove an approximately 3 mm ellipse of tissue circumferentially (**Fig. 2**)
- This leaves an 8 or 9 mm central full thickness graft with a peripheral partial thickness flange of 2–3 mm
- If an inferior is planned, excise the 180° excess donor tissue flange
- Stain the Descemet membrane of the donor using trypan blue dye and strip it using a cellulose sponge.

Fixation of Graft

- Perform paracentesis to decompress the eye
- Tuck the peripheral flange of the donor into the peripheral intrastromal pocket of the host (**Figs. 3A and B**)
- Secure the graft using 16 interrupted 10-0 nylon sutures, using a sharp point needle (Alcon Surgical, Fort Worth, TX). Pass the needle partial thickness through the donor and then into the peripheral pocket up to the limbus (**Fig. 4**). If using just an inferior tuck, the superior half can be sutured as per the normal technique of PK.
- **Figures 5 and 6** reveal the postoperative appearance.
- **Figures 7A to F** highlights the difference between a standard deep anterior lamellar keratoplasty and the tuck-in keratoplasty procedure.

MODIFICATIONS

As with all surgical techniques, many modifications are possible, and may be beneficial when considering individual patient needs. We have had good results performing intralase-enabled TILK. In these cases, intralase was used to create a central 200 µm flap prior to the scheduled date of surgery. This flap was then excised on the day of surgery, and centrifugal dissection performed as per the standard technique. Unfortunately, these ectatic corneas tend to be too thin for an automated microkeratome to be used for making the initial host cut. We have had success with the application of mitomycin C (0.02% for 10 seconds) to the host bed prior to fixation of the donor lenticule, in order to reduce interface haze. It is also possible to perform full thickness penetrating

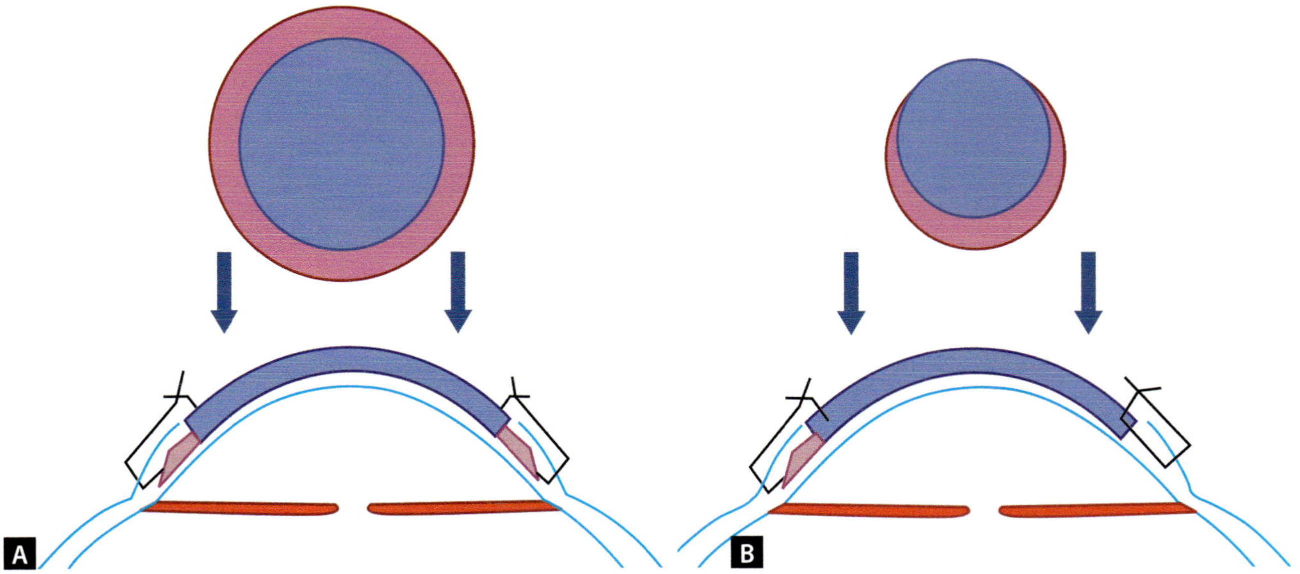

Figs. 3A and B: Schematic representation of a 360° tuck for keratoglobus (A), and an inferior tuck for pellucid marginal degeneration (B).

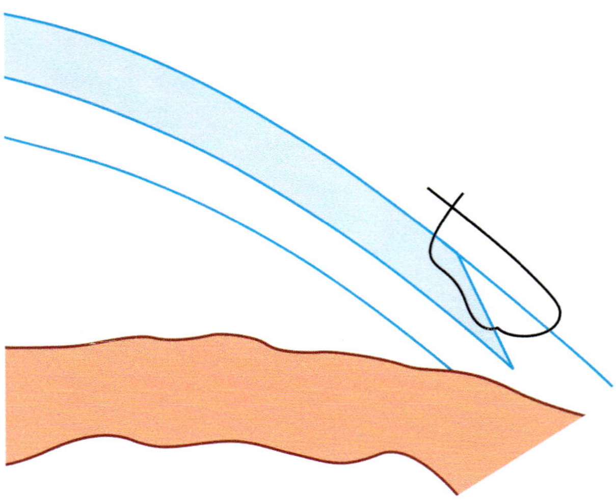

Fig. 4: Suture is passed partial thickness through the donor and then into the peripheral pocket up to the limbus.

keratoplasty with a 360° peripheral flange to improve the peripheral tectonic support of the graft.[9]

TUCK IN LAMELLAR KERATOPLASTY WITH LENTICULE OBTAINED BY SMALL INCISION LENTICULE EXTRACTION FOR TREATMENT OF POST-LASER-ASSISTED IN SITU KERATOMILEUSIS ECTASIA

Post-LASIK ectasia has been successfully treated with small incision lenticule extraction (SMILE) lenticule in three post-LASIK cornea ectasia patients with significant increase in corneal thickness postoperatively making TILK a safe and alternative surgical approach for the treatment of post-LASIK cornea ectasia, especially for severe cases with cornea thickness <400 µm.

EVALUATION OF TUCK IN LAMELLAR KERATOPLASTY FOR POSTKERATOPLASTY CORNEAL ECTASIA WITH PERIPHERAL CORNEAL INVOLVEMENT

Four eyes of 3 patients with post-penetrating keratoplasty corneal ectasia and contact lens intolerance underwent TILK that included a central lamellar keratoplasty with intrastromal tucking of the peripheral flange. Mean keratometry decreased from 59.67 to 43.50 D postoperatively. Mean endothelial cell loss after TILK was 5.93%. All grafts were clear at the last follow-up, and no cases of stromal or endothelial graft rejection were encountered.[10]

TUCK IN FEMTOSECOND LASER-ASSISTED ANTERIOR LAMELLAR KERATOPLASTY FOR THE MANAGEMENT OF SUPERFICIAL ANTERIOR CORNEAL SCARS

A modified sutureless and glueless technique, termed tuck in femtosecond laser-assisted anterior lamellar keratoplasty (T-FALK) was done in 15 eyes of 15 patients. The donor and recipient lenticules were prepared using femtosecond laser. After removing the anterior scarred lenticule of the recipient, the transparent donor lenticule was positioned on the recipient bed and margins tucked in under the recipient cornea. All patients had good graft-host junction apposition with a good visual outcome postoperatively.[11]

POSTOPERATIVE CARE

- Topical steroids and antibiotics, tapered over 3–4 months
- Topical unpreserved lubricants for 6 months
- Follow-up, weekly for 1 month, monthly until 6 months, and 6 monthly thereafter
- All sutures are removed at 6–12 months.

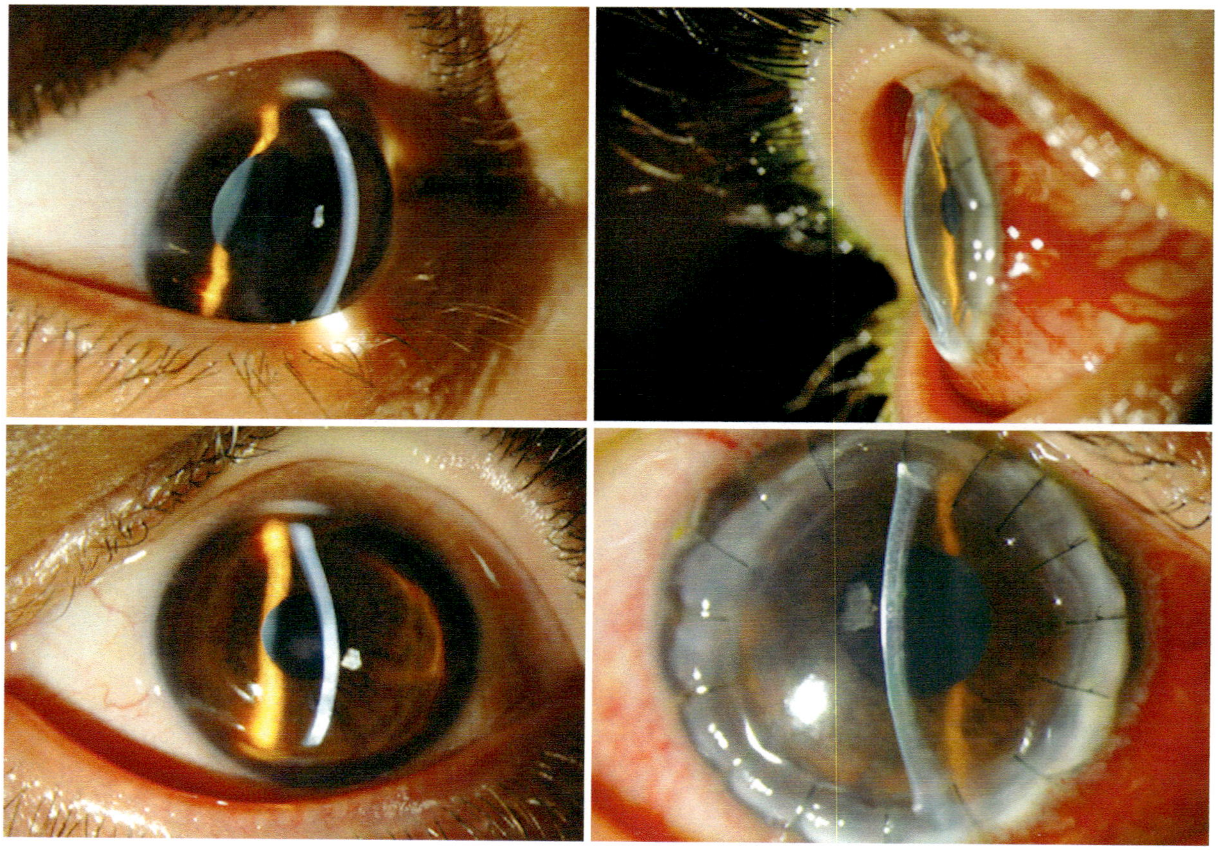

Fig. 5: Pre- and postoperative appearance of an intralase-enabled tuck in lamellar keratoplasty (TILK) procedure performed for post-penetrating keratoplasty ectasia in a keratoconic patient.

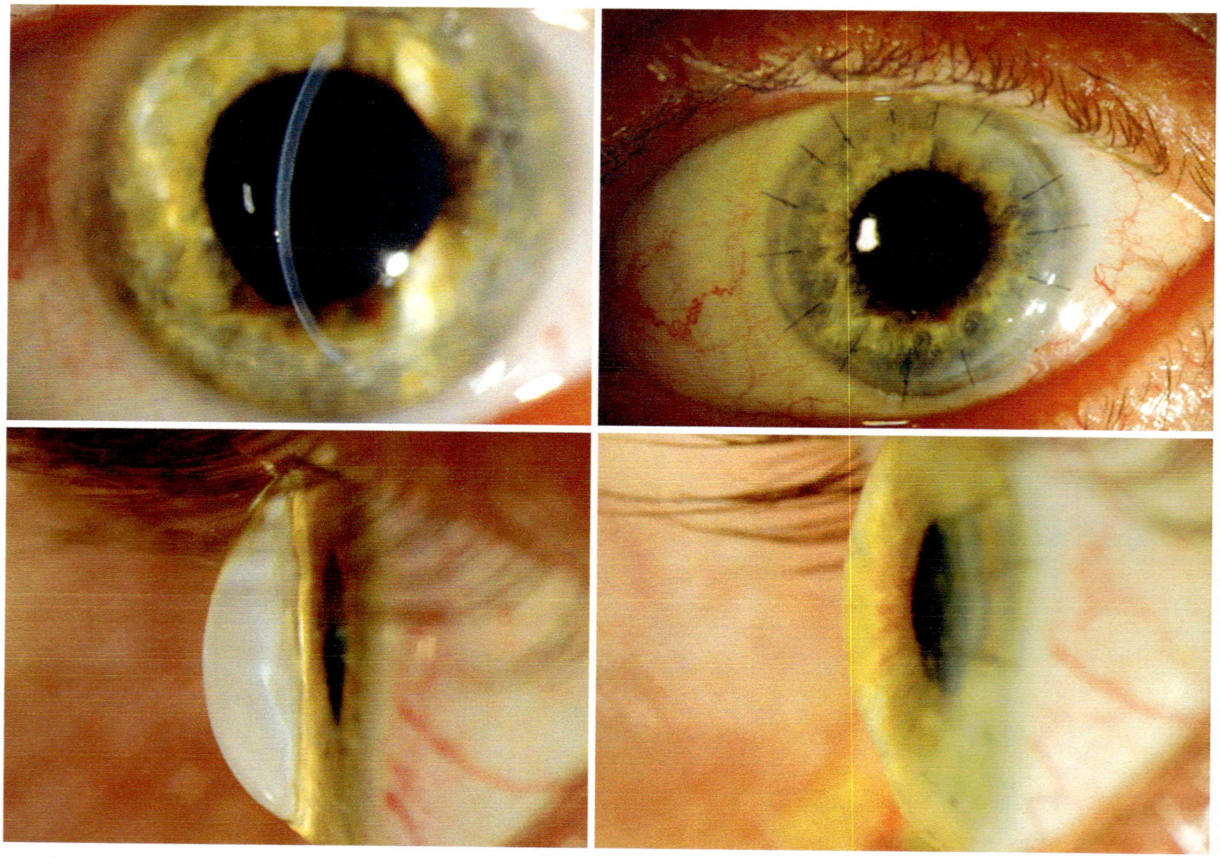

Fig. 6: Pre- and postoperative slit-lamp photographs of patient with progression of keratoconus post-penetrating keratoplasty. Treated with tuck in lamellar keratoplasty (TILK) with short application of mitomycin C.

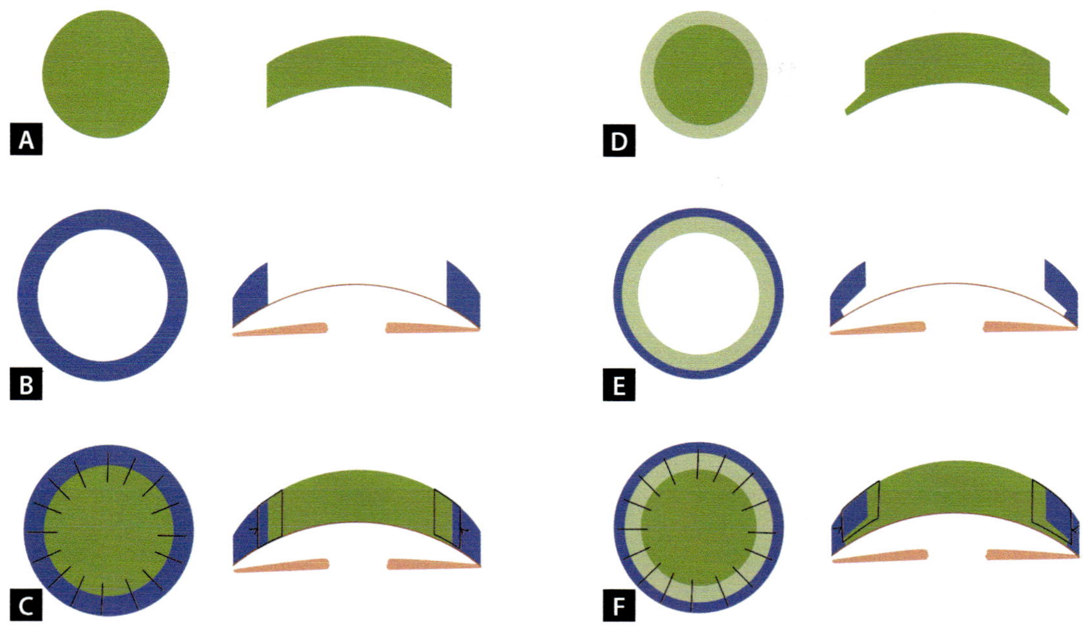

Figs. 7A to F: Schematic diagram depicting the difference between a standard deep anterior lamellar keratoplasty (DALK) technique and the tuck-in DALK procedure. (A to C) Cross-sectional view of the donor button (A), post dissection host bed (B) and apposition between donor and host (C) for a standard DALK procedure. (D to F) Cross-sectional view of the mushroom shaped donor button (D), host bed (E) and apposition between donor and host tissue for tuck-in DALK technique.

OUTCOMES

Advanced PMCD has been reported to be surgically treated with crescentic TILK by Arora et al.[12] Peripheral crescent-shaped lamellar corneal dissection of 3.5 mm width was performed, and an intrastromal pocket was fashioned from 4 to 8 o'clock, extending beyond the limbus. A crescent-shaped donor corneal button of 3.5 mm width was denuded of its endothelium and beveled in inferior periphery to create a flange which was tucked into the peripheral scleral pocket. Best spectacle-corrected visual acuity at 1 year improved to 6/9 and astigmatism reduced from 14.6 to 5.5 D.[12]

SUMMARY

Advanced corneal ectasias have been successfully treated with TILK.[7,8] In a series of 12 cases reported in 2008,[8] all grafts were clear at last follow-up (mean 1.7 years), and there was no significant interface haze or corneal vascularization seen. All of these patients had best-corrected visual acuity (BCVA) of <20/200 preoperatively, improving to 20/80, post TILK. Spherical equivalent decreased from a mean value of –7.8 D to –1.23 D at last follow-up. The mean keratometry decreased from 57.54 D preoperatively to 46.36 D, postoperatively. A significant decrease was also seen in mean refractive astigmatism which decreased from 5.93 D preoperatively to 3.23 D, after surgery.

Tuck in lamellar keratoplasty provides a single-stage technique for the management of extreme corneal ectasias. It helps to stabilize the peripheral cornea, besides providing optimal visual outcomes, and preserving the integrity of host limbal stem cells.

REFERENCES

1. Speaker MG, Arentsen JJ, Laibson PR. Long-term survival of large diameter penetrating keratoplasties for keratoconus and pellucid marginal degeneration. Acta Ophthalmol Suppl. 1989;192:17-9.
2. Cameron JA. Keratoglobus. Cornea. 1993;12:124-30.
3. Burk RO, Joussen AM. Corneoscleroplasty with maintenance of the angle in two cases of extensive corneoscleral disease. Eye. 2000;14:196-200.
4. Cameron JA, Cotter JB, Risco JM, Alvarez H. Epikeratoplasty for keratoglobus associated with blue sclera. Ophthalmology. 1991;98:446-52.
5. Dubroff S. Pellucid marginal corneal degeneration: report on corrective surgery. J Cataract Refract Surg. 1989;15:89-93.
6. Tan BU, Purcell TL, Torres LF, Schanzlin DJ. New surgical approaches to the management of keratoconus and post-LASIK ectasia. Trans Am Ophthalmol Soc. 2006;104:212-20.
7. Vajpayee RB, Bhartiya P, Sharma N. Central lamellar keratoplasty with peripheral intralamellar tuck – A new technique for keratoglobus. Cornea. 2002;21:657-60.
8. Kaushal S, Jhanji V, Sharma N, Tandon R, Titiyal JS, Vajpayee RB. "Tuck In" Lamellar Keratoplasty (TILK) for corneal ectasias involving corneal periphery. Br J Ophthalmol. 2008;92:286-90.
9. Vajpayee RB, Sharma N, Bhartiya P, Agarwal T, Tandon R, Titiyal JS. Central penetrating keratoplasty with peripheral intrastromal tuck. Cornea. 2005;24(8):947-50.
10. Vajpayee RB, Jhanji V, Beltz J, Moorthy S. "Tuck in" lamellar keratoplasty for tectonic management of postkeratoplasty corneal ectasia with peripheral corneal involvement. Cornea. 2011;30(2):171-4.
11. Sharma VK, Sati A, Kaushik J, Kumar S, Agarwal M. Tuck In Femtosecond Laser Assisted Anterior Lamellar Keratoplasty (T-FALK) for the Management of Superficial Anterior Corneal Scars—A Modified Technique. Cornea. 2021;40(1):125-30.
12. Arora R, Manudhane A, Jain P, Goyal JL. Crescentic Tuck in Lamellar Keratoplasty—A Novel Technique in a Case of Advanced Pellucid Marginal Corneal Degeneration. Eye Contact Lens. 2018;44(Suppl 1):S345-S7.

B: Endothelial Keratoplasty Techniques

31 Surgical Instruments for Endothelial Keratoplasty

Priyadarshini K, Ritu Nagpal, Namrata Sharma, Rasik B Vajpayee

INTRODUCTION

The selective replacement of Descemet's membrane and endothelium complex in patients with endothelial pathologies has revolutionized the field of corneal transplantation in terms of improvement in surgical and postoperative care, following an endothelial keratoplasty (EK), compared to a full-thickness graft. The various advantages of EK such as introduction of minimal astigmatism, early tapering of corticosteroids in the postoperative period and containment of the risks associated with an open-sky procedure, all have contributed to the preferential of EK by the corneal surgeons worldwide. Advancements in the field of instrumentation and the introduction of automated microkeratomes for donor corneal tissue dissection have been a key contributory factor in the attainment of desirable outcomes, following an endothelial transplant.

The various instruments required for an EK can be categorized under two broad groups:

1. Instruments which assist in the preparation of donor corneal tissue
2. Instruments which help in graft insertion and its appropriate placement

INSTRUMENTS REQUIRED FOR THE PREPARATION OF DONOR CORNEAL TISSUE

Moria Automated Lamellar Therapeutic Keratoplasty System

The donor corneal tissue for Descemet's stripping automated endothelial keratoplasty (DSAEK) is prepared using the Moria Automated Lamellar Therapeutic Keratoplasty (ALTK) system (Moria SA, Antony, France). This system comprises of an artificial anterior chamber (AAC) which has a central post on which the donor corneoscleral button is positioned with the endothelial surface down (**Fig. 1**). The artificial chamber cover (ACC) is a cylindrical unit which has three posts which fit onto the corresponding slots at the base of the AAC and has a central opening for the donor cornea (**Fig. 2**). The ACC ensures that the donor corneoscleral button is positioned centrally with uniform pressure being applied to the entire scleral rim. The locking ring helps to secure the donor tissue during the process of tissue dissection. Donor preparation is done using the Moria Carriazo-Barraquer (CBm) microkeratome. A microkeratome head of required size, (available sizes range from 130–350 µm—130,

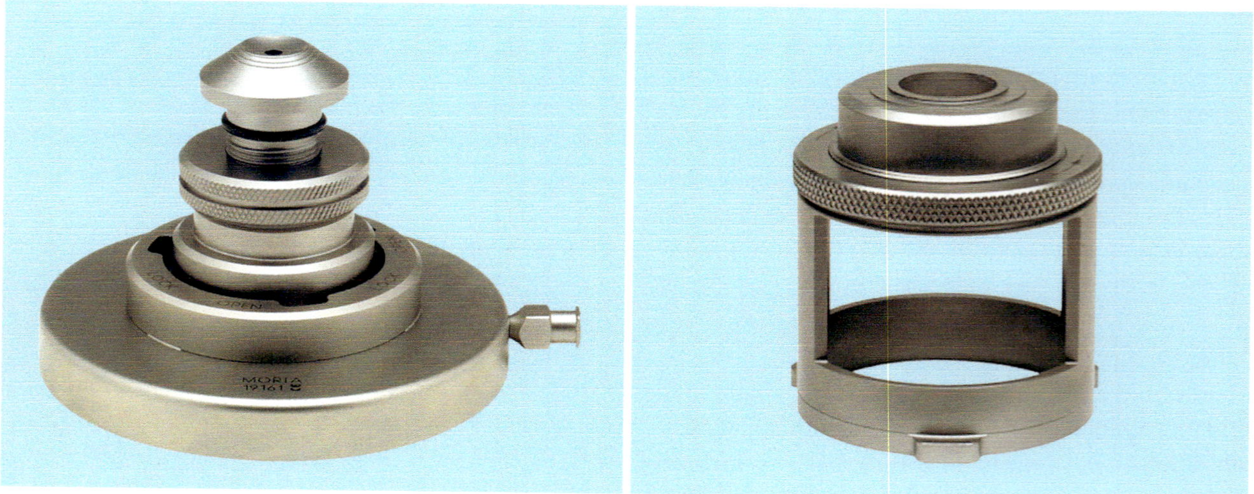

Fig. 1: Automated lamellar therapeutic keratoplasty (ALTK) artificial anterior chamber base and cover.

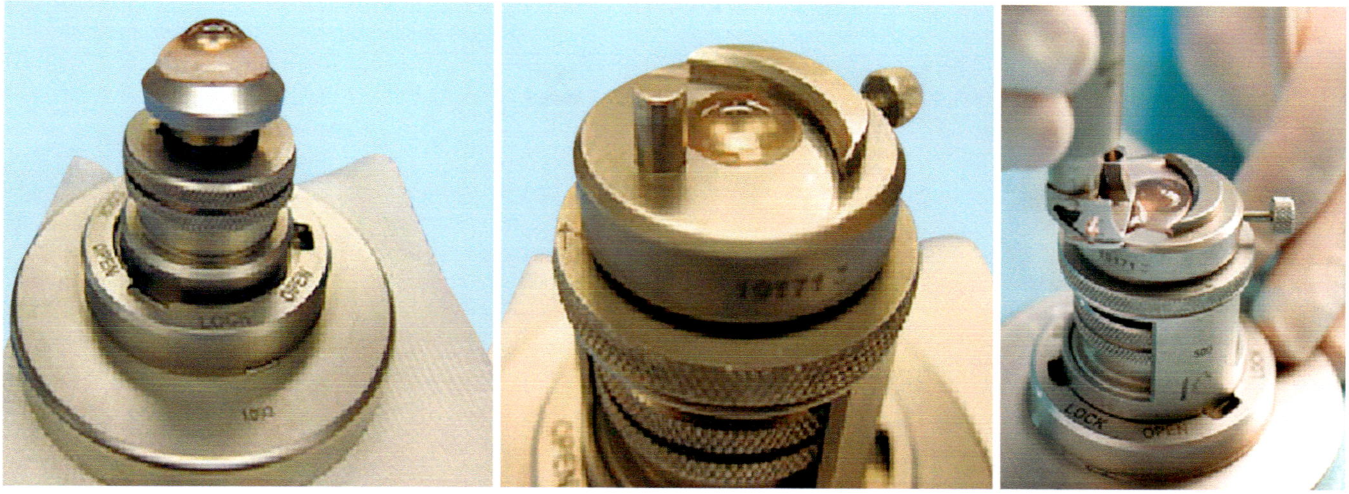

Fig. 2: Automated lamellar therapeutic keratoplasty (ALTK) artificial anterior chamber assembly with corneoscleral rim mounted over the artificial anterior chamber base, secured in place by anterior chamber cover and the guide ring before being dissected by the microkeratome blade.

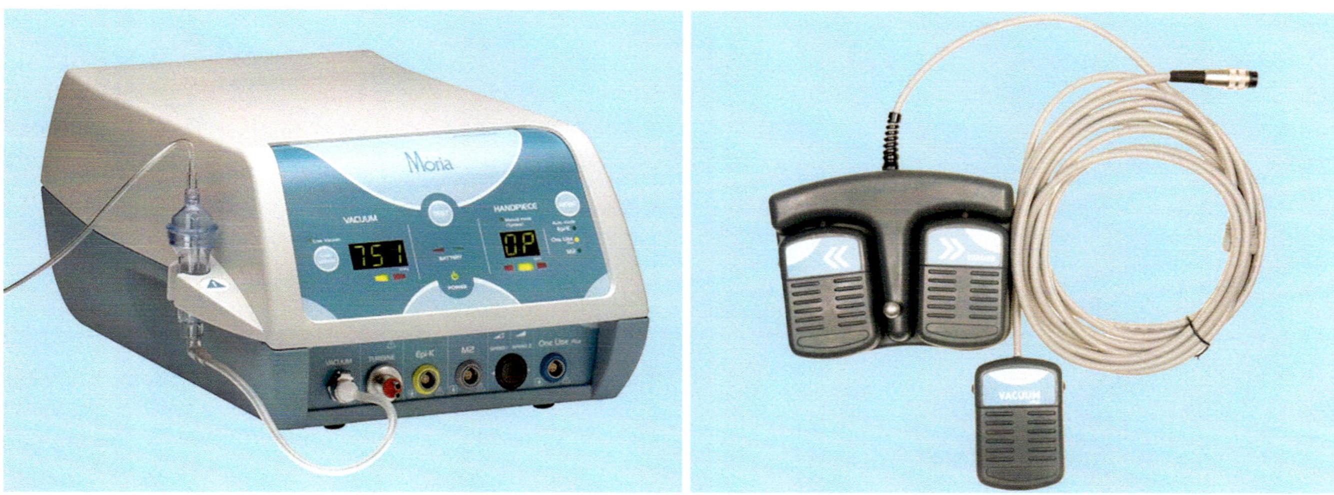

Fig. 3: Evolution 3E console and footswitch.

150, 250, 300, and 350 μm) mounted over a microkeratome blade holder, is passed over the donor corneal tissue, to dissect out the superior lamellar part of the required thickness (**Fig. 3**). A donor scleral rim of at least 16 mm, ensures adequate securing of the tissue and building of vacuum while the microkeratome is passed.[1,2]

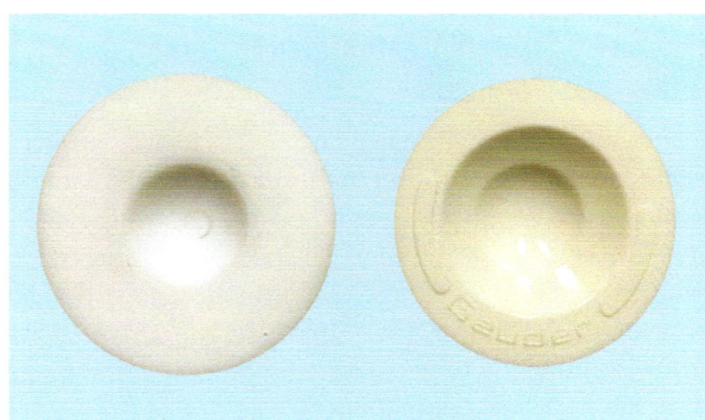

Fig. 4: Teflon blocks.

Teflon Block

Teflon blocks help to adequately secure the donor corneal tissue while preparing the Descemet's membrane-endothelium graft for Descemet's membrane endothelial keratoplasty (DMEK) surgery as well as to punch out the desired size of DSAEK graft tissue (**Fig. 4**).

Disposable Trephines

Disposable trephines of various diameter are available to cut the harvested graft tissue into the preferred diametric size (**Fig. 5**).

Busin Glide

Insertion of the harvested DSAEK lenticule can be done by adapting the pull through technique using a specially designed glide known as the Busin glide, which allows insertion of the folded graft via a 3.2-mm incision (**Fig. 6**).

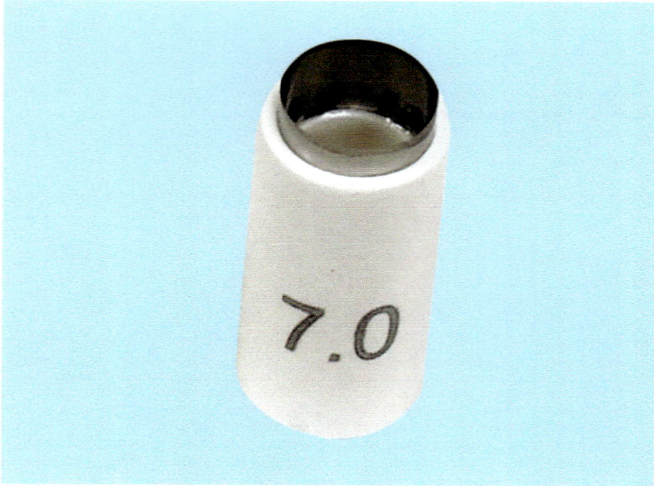

Fig. 5: Disposable trephine.

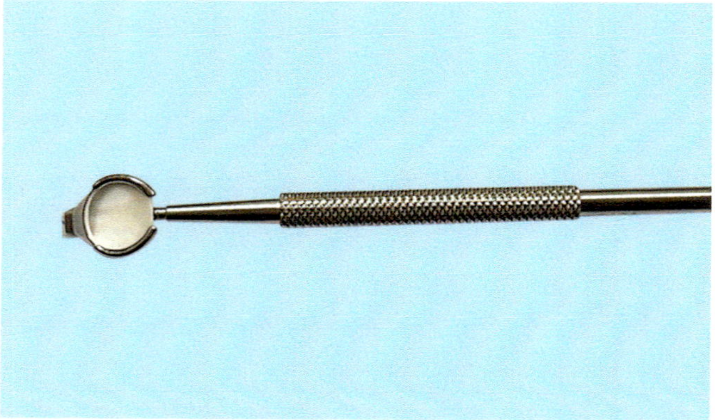

Fig. 6: Busin glide used to load the Descemet's stripping automated endothelial keratoplasty (DSAEK) graft for insertion.

It then facilitates the unfolding of the graft and simplifies centration of the donor lenticule in the anterior chamber. It helps to minimize intraoperative manipulation of the graft and subsequently possibility of endothelial loss.[3]

Descemet's Stripping Automated Endothelial Keratoplasty Forceps

It is a microincision forceps with 20-G diameter, which is designed to position the graft in the glide and to pull it from the glide into the anterior chamber. The periphery of the graft is held using its tip, which are specifically designed for it, so that the endothelial and the stromal surfaces remain untouched in the optical zone. The size of the tip is perfectly adapted to the glide to avoid any endothelial cell damage during the pull-through maneuver. The tips of the forceps remain separated when the handles are closed, to minimize injury to the folded donor tissue (**Fig. 7**).

Petri Dish

The graft tissue consisting of Descemet's membrane-endothelium complex, prepared for the DMEK procedure is floated in balanced salt solution placed in a petri dish, after its complete separation from the donor corneoscleral rim (**Fig. 8**).

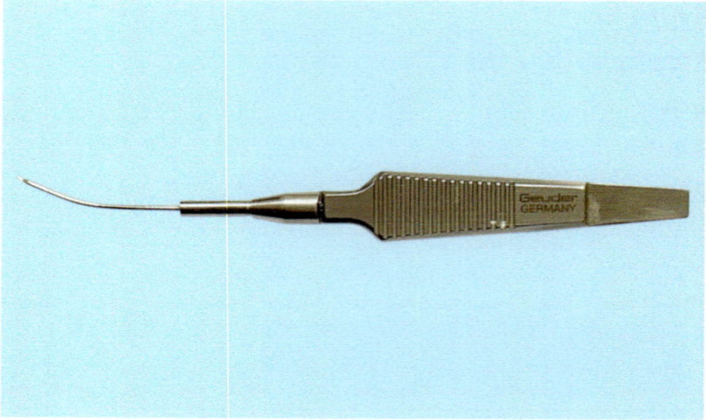

Fig. 7: Descemet's stripping automated endothelial keratoplasty (DSAEK) forceps.

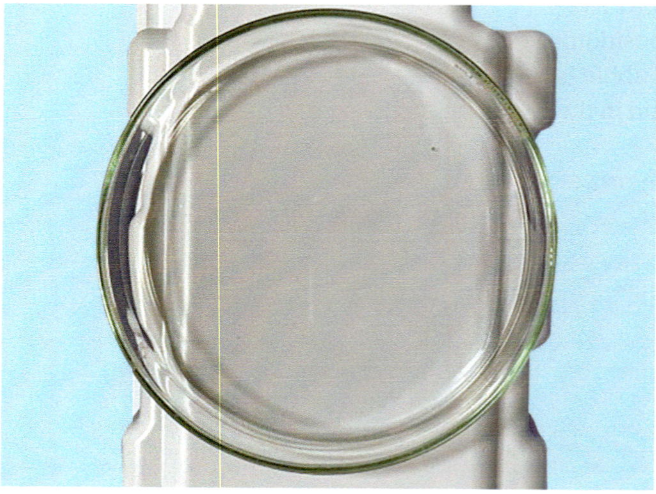

Fig. 8: Glass petri dish used to submerge the Descemet's membrane endothelial keratoplasty (DMEK) graft tissue after stripping from the donor corneal tissue.

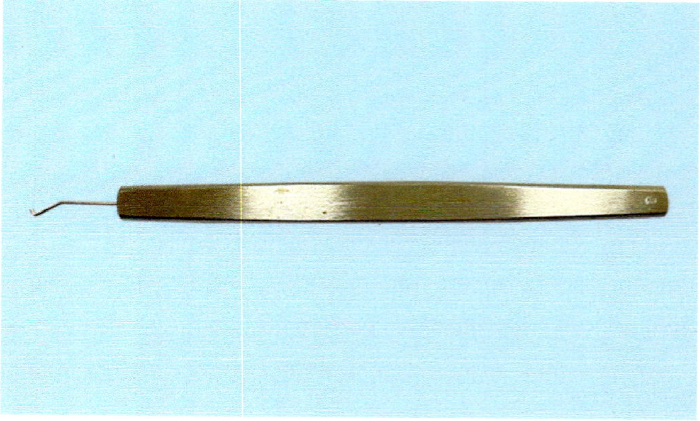

Fig. 9: Szurman Descemet's membrane endothelial keratoplasty (DMEK) marker.

Szurman Descemet's Membrane Endothelial Keratoplasty Marker

It is used to mark the Descemet's membrane of the donor tissue during preparation (**Fig. 9**).

Szurman Descemet's Membrane Endothelial Keratoplasty Preparation Spatula

It is made of stainless steel and is a blunt, disk-shaped spatula of 2.5 mm diameter with a flat handle. Trypan blue dye is injected beneath the Descemet's membrane, staying cautious not to damage the endothelial cells and the Descemet's membrane is scraped off from the donor tissue using the spatula (**Fig. 10**).

Descemet's Membrane Endothelial Keratoplasty Graft Injector

It consists of a transparent glass cartridge with a double irrigation set for controlled injection of the DMEK scroll and its spontaneous touch-free aspiration, unfolding and positioning toward the posterior stroma of the host.[4] An air bubble is injected into the anterior chamber of the host to aid in the adherence of the graft-host interface (**Fig. 11**).

Syringe

The DMEK graft loaded in the cartridge is connected to the syringe to aid in smooth release and unfolding of the graft in the host anterior chamber (**Fig. 12**).

INSTRUMENTS FOR HOST CORNEA DISSECTION AND MANIPULATION

Corneal Marker

An 8.0–9.0-mm marker is available to mark the area of the recipient's cornea to be stripped. The anterior surface of this marker can be marked using gentian violet blue or a surgical marker pen (**Fig. 13**).

Descemet's Stripping Automated Endothelial Keratoplasty Spatula/Stripper

The recipient's Descemet's membrane is stripped using this spatula during the DSAEK and DMEK procedure (**Figs. 14 and 15**). These are available in 45° and 90° angled models, in both irrigating and nonirrigating versions and are made of surgical steel. The efficient dissection and removal of Descemet's membrane without inadvertent damage to the stroma is facilitated by the angled tips.

Anterior Chamber Maintainer

Descemet's stripping automated endothelial keratoplasty anterior chamber maintainer has a 20-G threaded tip and is

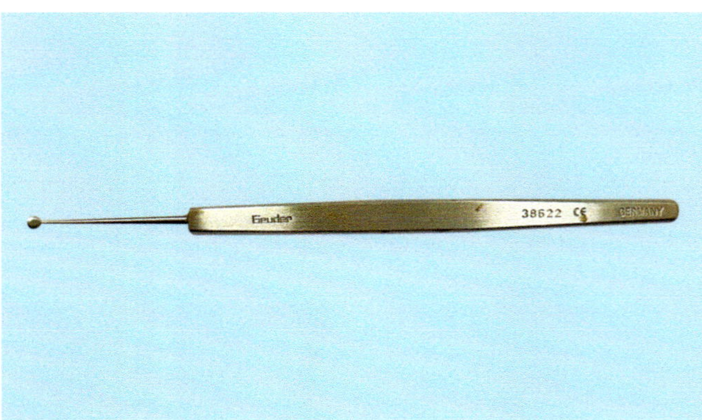

Fig. 10: Szurman Descemet's membrane endothelial keratoplasty (DMEK) preparation spatula.

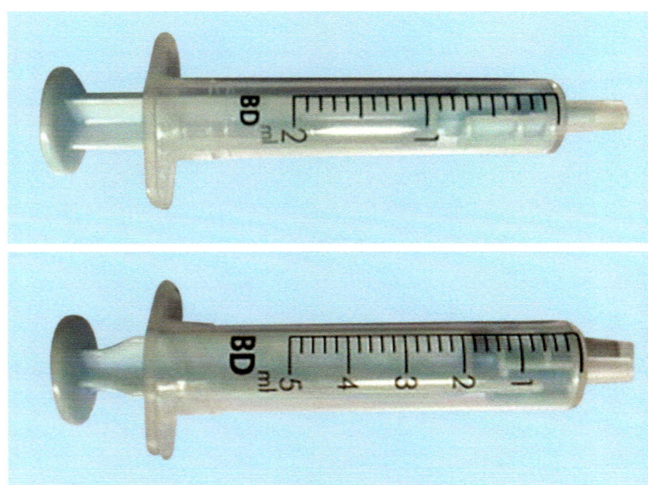

Fig. 12: 2 mL and 5 mL syringes to connect with the cartridge of the Descemet's membrane endothelial keratoplasty (DMEK) graft injector.

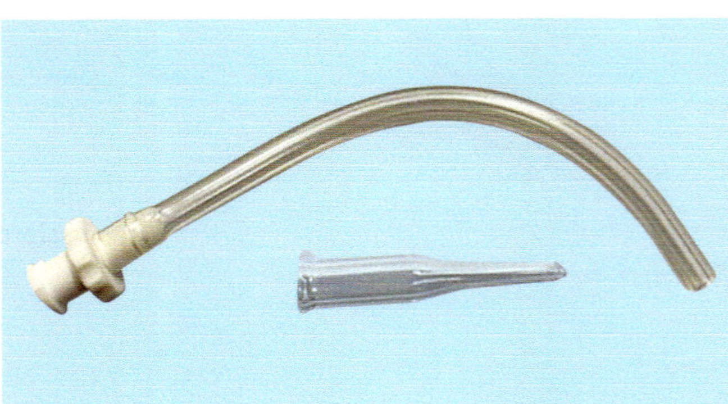

Fig. 11: Descemet's membrane endothelial keratoplasty (DMEK) graft injector.

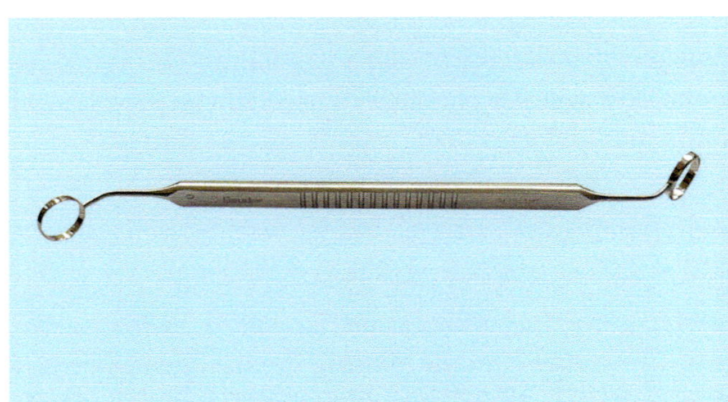

Fig. 13: Corneal marker.

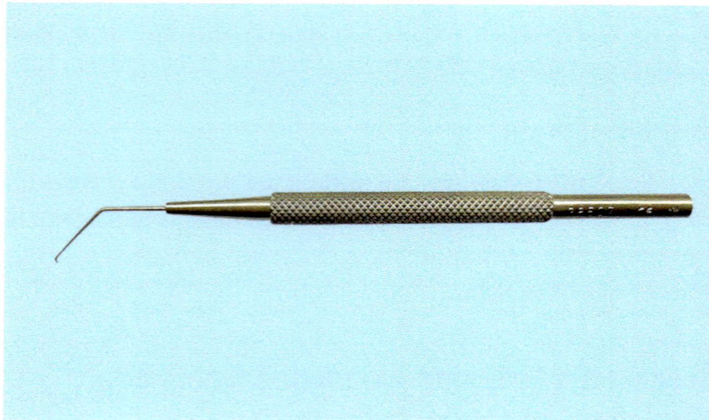

Fig. 14: Descemet's spatula.

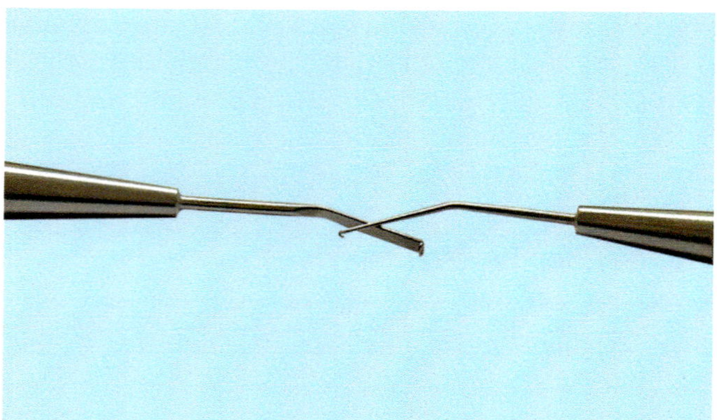

Fig. 15: Descemet's spatula with a thinner tip compared to Descemet's stripper which has a comparatively braoder end.

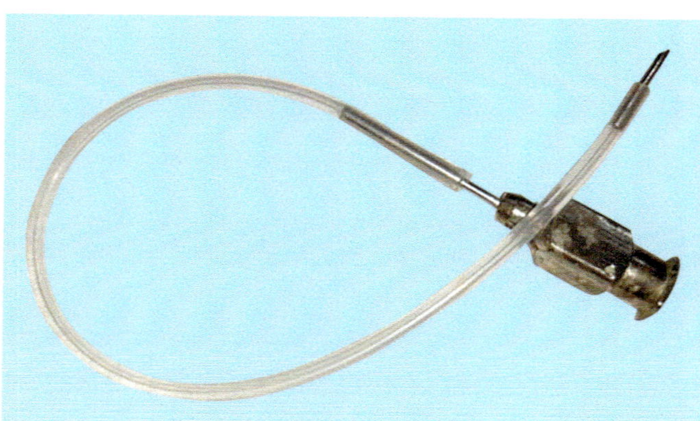

Fig. 16A: Anterior chamber maintainer.

supplied with a silicone tubing and adaptor. This is inserted into the host anterior chamber to maintain its depth during surgical manipulation of the graft (**Figs. 16A and B**).

Colibri Forceps

Derived from the Italian word, which means bird, this forceps is used to grasp the corneal and scleral tissues while passing sutures. It can also aid in holding the iris during surgical manipulations. It can fit into narrow incisions and provides and elevated tying platform (**Fig. 17**).

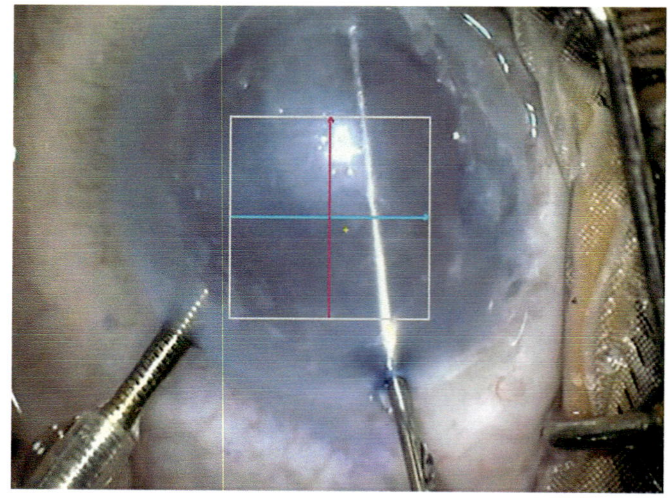

Fig. 16B: Intraoperative image, showing 20-G tip of the anterior chamber maintainer, threaded into the side port, while the Descemet's membrane is being stripped, during DSAEK procedure.

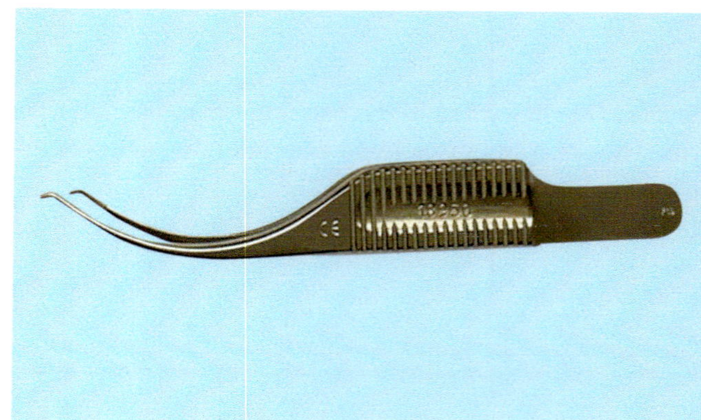

Fig. 17: Colibri forceps with tying platform.

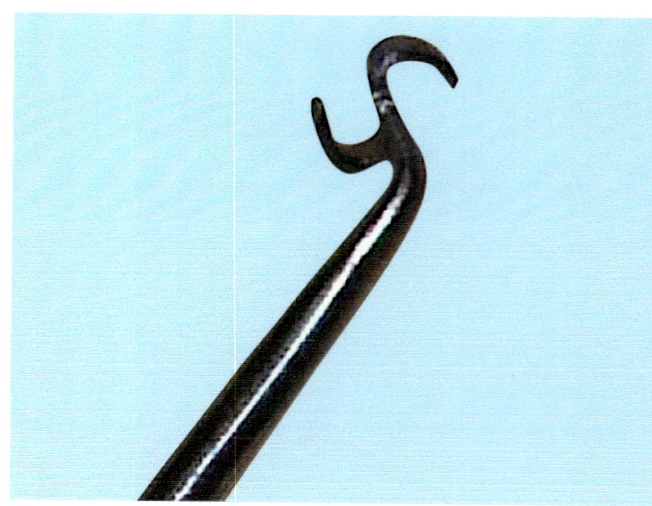

Fig. 18: The "S" stamp.

S Stamp (Fig. 18)

Application of a "S" or "F" mark, using gentian violet stain during the process of DMEK graft preparation is really helpful for the surgeon, once the graft has been injected into the anterior chamber.

By recognizing the orientation of the mark, correct orientation of the DMEK graft can be made out, after it is completely unfolded into the anterior chamber.

REFERENCES

1. Lichtinger A, Yeung SN, Kim P, Amiran MD, Rootman DS. The era of lamellar keratoplasty, evolving surgical techniques in corneal transplantation: the University of Toronto experience. Can J Ophthalmol. 2012;47(3):287-90.
2. Shekhar H, Sharma N, Vajpayee RB. Future of Endothelial Keratoplasty. In: Cassidy D, Sharma N, Jhanji V, Vajpayee RB (Eds). Descemet's Stripping Automated Endothelial Keratoplasty: Different Strokes, 1st edition. New Delhi, India: Jaypee Brothers Medical Publisher (P) Ltd.; 2013. p. 174.
3. Busin M, Bhatt PR, Scorcia V. A modified technique for Descemet's membrane stripping automated endothelial keratoplasty to minimize endothelial cell loss. Arch Ophthalmol. 2008;126(8):1133-7.
4. Rickmann A, Wahl S, Katsen-Globa A, Szurman P. Safety analysis and results of a borosilicate glass cartridge for no-touch graft loading and injection in Descemet's membrane endothelial keratoplasty. International ophthalmology. 2019;39(10):2295-301.

32 Descemet's Stripping Automated Endothelial Keratoplasty

Marianne O Price, Sohini Mandal, Francis W Price Jr

INTRODUCTION AND BACKGROUND

Endothelial keratoplasty (EK) selectively replaces dysfunctional corneal endothelium without significantly altering the refractive status of the eye, and it is rapidly replacing standard penetrating keratoplasty (PK) as the treatment of choice for endothelial disorders.[1-4] Among the drawbacks of a standard PK are the prolonged recovery period, frequent increase in astigmatic error, and permanent weakening of the eye, which increases the risk of subsequent loss from traumatic injury.[5-10] In contrast, EK can be performed through a relatively small incision without any sutures, so visual recovery is rapid, the procedure is essentially refractive-neutral, and most of the structural integrity of the eye is retained.[11,12]

EVOLUTION OF ENDOTHELIAL KERATOPLASTY

Endothelial keratoplasty techniques were initially proposed over 40 years ago but only recently have become widely adopted. Early techniques entailed creating an anterior flap prior to replacing the posterior portion of the recipient cornea, and sutures were still required to secure the donor graft. This approach suffered from many of the same limitations as standard PK, including unpredictable corneal topography and induced irregular astigmatism.[13-17] In 1993, Ko et al. pioneered a limbal approach in a rabbit model, but still used sutures to secure the posterior donor graft.[18]

The current success of EK is largely attributable to a series of key breakthroughs by Melles, who demonstrated that air could be used to press the posterior portion of a dissected donor graft against the anterior portion of a dissected recipient cornea, and the graft would adhere without any sutures, a technique he called posterior lamellar keratoplasty (PLK) (**Fig. 1A**).[19,20] Melles further showed that lamellar dissection of the donor and recipient corneas could be facilitated if the anterior chamber (AC) was filled with air, because air creates a light reflection that helps the surgeon estimate the dissection depth.[21]

Melles originally laid the dissected donor tissue out flat with the endothelial side downward on a viscoelastic-coated spatula for insertion through a 9-mm incision.[20] He subsequently demonstrated that the donor tissue could be folded in half, allowing a 9-mm diameter donor graft to be inserted through a 5-mm scleral tunnel incision, in a completely sutureless procedure.[11] Melles used a superior approach, whereas we pioneered a temporal approach because it facilitates donor insertion, makes the procedure less sensitive to orbital anatomy, and spares the trabecular meshwork should future glaucoma surgery ever be required (Ocular Surgery News, August 2003). Terry organized a prospective clinical study of the large incision and small incision procedures, which he renamed deep lamellar endothelial keratoplasty (DLEK).[4,22]

The most difficult aspect of the PLK/DLEK technique was lamellar dissection of the recipient cornea and excision of posterior recipient tissue using small curved scissors, with or without the aid of a trephine. Melles made yet another breakthrough when he showed that Descemet's membrane with dysfunctional endothelium could simply be stripped from the recipient cornea prior to implanting the donor graft (**Fig. 1B**), a technique he called descemetorhexis.[1] We found that lightly scoring Descemet's membrane with a modified Sinskey hook along the perimeter of the area to be stripped could facilitate removal of the membrane, and we called the procedure Descemet's stripping endothelial keratoplasty (DSEK), to help distinguish it from Melles original PLK technique.[2] Donor detachment is the most frequent complication after DSEK, so a number of techniques have been developed to help promote graft attachment to the exquisitely smooth stromal interface exposed after Descemet's membrane removal.[23]

Gorovoy found that DSEK could be facilitated by using a microkeratome to dissect the donor tissue and named this technique variation Descemet's stripping automated endothelial keratoplasty (DSAEK).[24] Subsequently, a number of eye banks have begun to provide microkeratome-dissected donor tissue to surgeons.

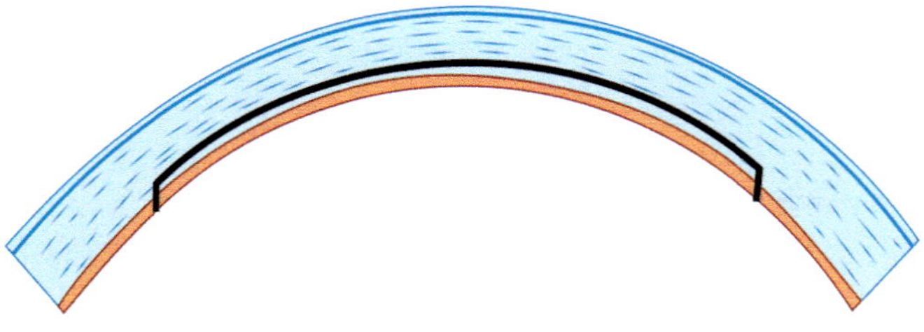

Fig. 1A: In posterior lamellar keratoplasty and deep lamellar endothelial keratoplasty, a posterior lenticule of recipient stroma with diseased endothelium is removed and replaced with a comparable lenticule of posterior donor stroma and healthy endothelium.

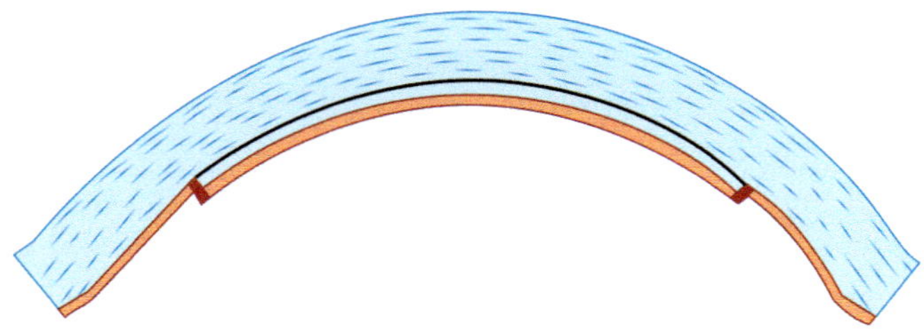

Fig. 1B: In Descemet's stripping endothelial keratoplasty or Descemet's stripping automated endothelial keratoplasty, Descemet's membrane and diseased endothelium are removed from the recipient cornea and a lenticule of posterior donor stroma and healthy endothelium is implanted.

INDICATIONS

Favorable clinical outcomes have made EK the treatment of choice for various types of endothelial dysfunction.[4,12,24] While Fuchs' dystrophy and bullous keratopathy are the most common indications, EK can also successfully treat corneal edema associated with iridocorneal endothelial (ICE) syndrome.[25]

Endothelial keratoplasty can also restore clarity to a failed prior penetrating graft and provide the patient with an easier postoperative course compared with a PK regraft.[26] However, visual recovery and clearing of a failed PK often takes longer than in a virgin eye, and we have noticed that failed PK eyes that also have hypotony do not seem to clear well after the EK. Since EK does not significantly alter the topography of the prior PK, it is preferable to reserve this treatment for PKs that have achieved a reasonably acceptable topography and refractive outcome prior to endothelial failure.

INSTRUMENTATION

Several companies provide specially designed instruments to facilitate EK, including Moria (Antony, France), DORC International (Zuidland, the Netherlands), and Bausch and Lomb Surgical (St. Louis, MO).

Instruments for donor preparation:

- Artificial anterior chamber (AAC)
- Dissecting blades, microkeratome, or femtosecond laser that can perform deep dissections
- Trephine

Instruments for recipient preparation:

- Anterior chamber maintainer, or 23-gauge needle to provide continuous infusion of balanced salt solution, or cohesive viscoelastic to maintain chamber.
- Modified Sinskey hook to score Descemet's membrane.
- Trypan blue to improve visualization of Descemet's membrane.
- Stripping instrument, or inspiration/aspiration device to strip Descemet's membrane.

Instruments for graft insertion and positioning:

- Spatula—if inserting open donor lenticule
- Single point fixation forceps—if inserting folded donor lenticule
- Micro-forceps—if pulling the donor lenticule into the eye
- Injector
- LASIK flap roller

SURGICAL TECHNIQUES

The donor tissue should be prepared and determined suitable for transplantation prior to opening the recipient eye. Donor preparation entails lamellar dissection and sizing to the appropriate diameter with a trephine. The donor lamellar dissection can be performed manually, using specially designed blades, or with the aid of a microkeratome, or a predissected donor graft can be obtained from an eye bank. Femtosecond lasers also hold great promise for creating precise donor tissue dissections that could be custom-designed to match recipient corneal dimensions.[29-31] However, at the time of this writing, efforts are still underway to optimize donor contour and smoothness.

Manual Donor Dissection

Manual dissection can be done either on whole donor globes or on a donor corneal/scleral rim that has been mounted on an AAC. Whole donor globes are not readily available from US eye banks because of the length of time required for serology. A number of companies provide AACs that are suitable for manual donor dissection. To ensure firm and air tight fixation on the AAC, donor corneal/scleral rims should have a diameter of 16–17 mm and not have any edge defects that might allow the tissue to depressurize or slip during dissection.

The AAC should be pressurized with air, balanced salt solution, or tissue storage solution so that the donor cornea is firm. Melles showed that air creates a reflection from the posterior surface of the cornea that can help the surgeon estimate the dissection depth.[21] However, some surgeons prefer to use viscoelastic on the donor cornea with tissue storage solution or balanced salt solution in the AAC to help protect the donor corneal endothelium, even though this makes it much harder to judge the dissection depth.[32]

Also, if viscoelastic is used on a reuseable AAC, it must be thoroughly cleaned off prior to autoclaving, otherwise it will form toxic by-products that could lead to toxic anterior segment syndrome (TASS) in subsequent cases.

A manual dissection can begin with a small one-third depth incision in the peripheral cornea and then the dissection plane can be extended across the cornea using curved dissecting blades of increasing length (**Fig. 2**).[19] As another option, a Barron suction recipient trephine can be used to cut the donor cornea to 60% depth and then a dissection plane can be extended across the cornea. The surgeon should aim for approximately 80% dissection depth and care should be taken to maintain a single dissection plane. Extremely deep dissections should be avoided because they may cause endothelial damage. Also, very thin donor tissue is more difficult to handle and more likely to develop wrinkles that can be difficult to remove when placed against the recipient cornea.

Microkeratome Donor Dissection

The Moria CB is one of only a few microkeratomes that provide a sufficiently deep dissection for EK and are compatible for use with an AAC on which to mount the donor tissue (**Fig. 3**). Donor cornea thicknesses can vary substantially. Donor corneas stored in Optisol tissue storage solution, which is how corneas are usually supplied by US eye banks, typically range from 0.45 to 0.70 mm after epithelial removal. If the AAC is pressurized with balanced salt solution or tissue storage solution, the donor thickness can be measured with ultrasonic pachymetry after epithelial removal to help the surgeon select an appropriate microkeratome depth plate to achieve a posterior thickness of 100–200 μm. The amount of AAC pressurization and the speed of the microkeratome pass influence the actual depth of cut achieved. A gentian violet mark placed on one edge of the donor cornea prior to making the cut can help the surgeon correctly realign the anterior cap prior to transferring the donor tissue to a trephine.

After the microkeratome pass, the anterior cap is carefully replaced in its original position and the exact center of the resection is marked with gentian violet. The AAC is disassembled and the donor tissue is carefully removed without touching the endothelial surface on metal. The donor tissue is placed endothelial side upward on a trephine, taking care to match the center of the resection with the center of the trephine (**Fig. 4**). Usually, an 8, 8.5, or 9-mm diameter is used for EK. The choice of trephine diameter is usually determined after measuring the recipient's horizontal white-to-white corneal diameter with calipers while the patient is in a supine position. We usually use a 9-mm donor diameter if the recipient horizontal white-to-white diameter is 11.75 mm or longer; otherwise we usually use an 8.5-mm diameter. However, a smaller EK donor diameter may be indicated if there are peripheral anterior synechiae (PAS) or the AC is relatively shallow. Once donor preparation is complete, the

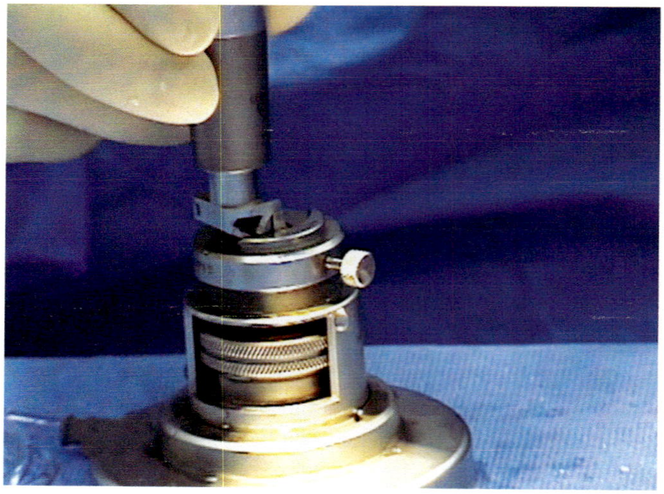

Fig. 3: Automated lamellar dissection of a donor graft with a microkeratome.

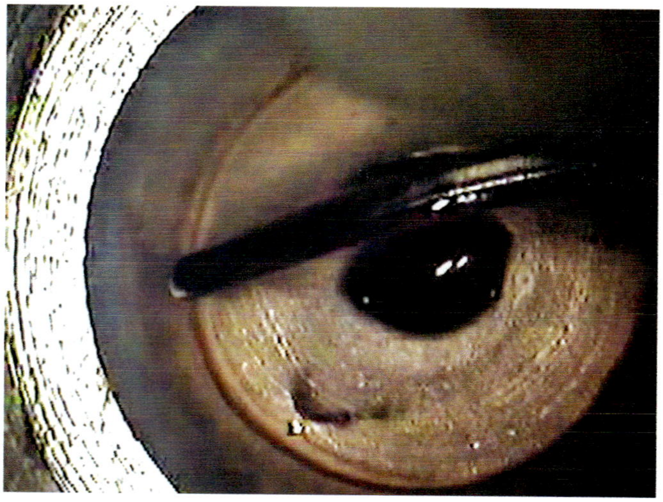

Fig. 2: Manual lamellar dissection of a donor corneal/scleral rim mounted on an artificial anterior chamber.

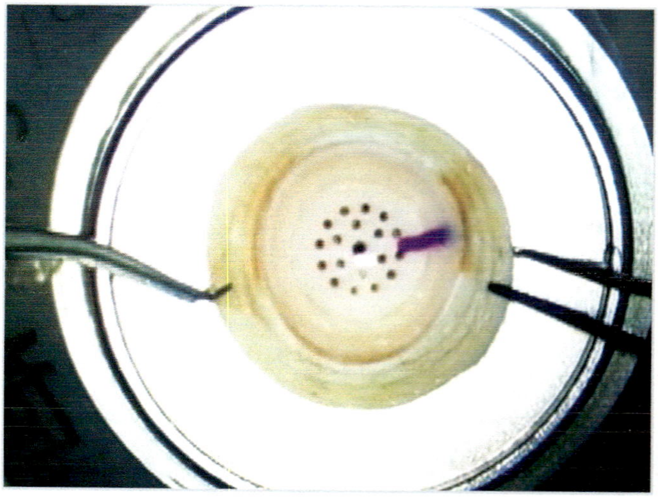

Fig. 4: Centering the resected donor tissue with the endothelial side facing upward on a suction trephine block.

donor tissue can be covered with tissue storage solution while the recipient cornea is prepared.

Gebauer SLc Original and SLc Expert Microkeratomes offer to provide ultrathin lenticules (<100 μm) with a single-pass or double-pass technique.

Single-pass Technique

Vajpayee et al. using a 400-μm microkeratome head slowed the speed of the pass to achieve a thinner donor lenticule without any complications during the donor preparation.[33] A single, slow pass of 400 μm microkeratome yielded thin donor lenticules in all the cases, and the mean graft thickness achieved at the end of 6 months was 111 ± 17.62 μm (range 70–134 μm). Excellent visual outcomes were obtained in the majority of the patients. Nahum et al. have described a nomogram for choosing the appropriate microkeratome head size in single pass microkeratome-assisted dissection of donor tissue.[34] The authors reported mean postoperative donor graft central thickness of 63 ± 29 μm in 42 eyes using this nomogram. Thus, creation of ultrathin DSAEK lenticules has been made possible with a single microkeratome pass.

Double-pass Technique

In this technique, an initial debulking cut is performed using a microkeratome with a 300-μm head. A second cut (refinement cut) is carried out from the direction opposite to the one of the first cut.[35] The size of the head used for this step is selected such that a residual bed with a central thickness of approximately 100 μm is left. Intraoperative pachymetry or anterior segment optical coherence tomography helps in deciding the residual stromal thickness during the procedure.

The double-pass technique, in experienced hands and when successful, results in excellent outcome.[35] However, it has some issues such as the potential higher risk of donor tissue perforation, difficult manipulation of a thinner graft which may lead to increased endothelial loss, prolonged time for second cut, chances of second pass creating a smaller diameter cut, and unpredictability when donor thickness exceeds 600 μm.

Precut Tissue

Tissue preparation is done in advance either by the operating surgeon or by an eye bank technician before surgery.[36,37] This has the advantage of reducing the cost as well as the time of surgery. Moreover, in countries like India where every corneal surgeon does not have the microkeratome, it is extremely useful.

Femtosecond Laser-assisted Endothelial Keratoplasty

Femtosecond laser-assisted EK is another addition to the existing techniques of EK donor lenticule preparation. In this technique, the donor cornea undergoes a lamellar cut from the endothelial side with the femtosecond laser at the desired depth. This may be followed by excimer laser photoablation of the stromal tissue to achieve a smooth surface. While femtosecond laser dissection yields a thin and reproducible endothelial graft cut with a high level of safety and accuracy, excimer photoablation provides a smooth and high-quality interface.[38,39]

One of the major concerns with this technique is the endothelial cell loss attributed to direct applanation of the endothelial side. This can be minimized by the use of viscodispersive agent (Viscoat) as the interface fluid.[40]

Recipient Preparation

Descemet's stripping endothelial keratoplasty/Descemet's stripping automated endothelial keratoplasty can readily be performed with topical or local anesthesia, thereby avoiding the risks and cost associated with general anesthesia.[12,24,41] We have found that most patients who have experienced topical anesthesia in one eye and local anesthesia in the other, prefer the topical anesthesia. However, surgeons who are not experienced with EK procedures may feel more comfortable performing their early cases with local anesthesia. With use of a local retrobulbar or peribulbar block, it is important to ensure there is no back pressure from periorbital swelling, because that could cause forceful shallowing of the AC while the donor graft is being inserted and it could even push the graft back out of the eye. A Honan balloon (the Lebanon Corporation, Lebanon, IN), or similar device, can be applied for 1 hour after injecting the block to ensure the eye is soft before beginning the procedure.

Traction sutures can be placed in the sclera peripheral to the limbus at 6 and 12 o'clock positions to help stabilize the eye during the procedure. These can be used with any anesthesia method.

A 5-mm temporal clear corneal or scleral tunnel incision is made (**Fig. 5**). A clear corneal incision can facilitate performing phacoemulsification and intraocular lens (IOL) implantation as a combined procedure with EK. However, a properly constructed scleral tunnel incision allows the entire procedure to be performed without any sutures. Also, a scleral tunnel incision can be closed very quickly if the patient coughs or develops a suprachoroidal hemorrhage, thereby providing a greater margin of safety. Temporal placement of the incision facilitates donor insertion because the corneal diameter is longest horizontally and it preserves the superior conjunctiva should future glaucoma surgery ever be needed. If the recipient epithelium is hazy or scarred, it can be removed and this generally improves the view into the eye.

The trephine used on the donor graft can be used to lightly mark the recipient epithelium to indicate the area that will be covered with the donor tissue. An AC maintainer or 23-gauge needle can be used to provide a continuous infusion

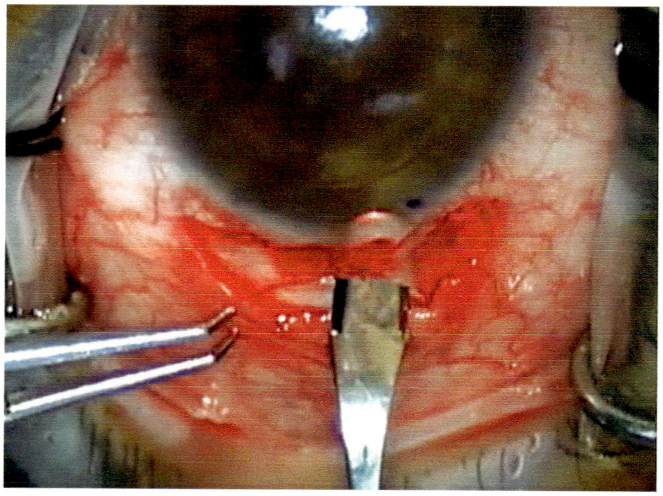

Fig. 5: Extension of a 5-mm scleral tunnel incision with a diamond crescent blade.

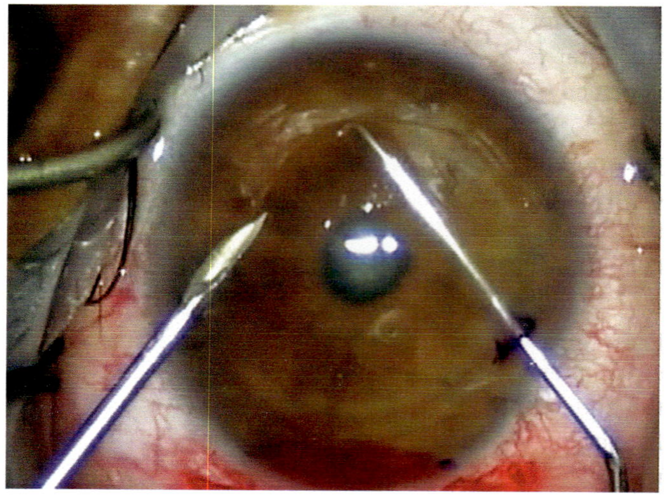

Fig. 6: Scoring Descemet's membrane with a modified Sinskey hook along the perimeter of the area to be stripped.

of balanced salt solution while Descemet's membrane is scored and stripped, or the AC can be filled with a cohesive viscoelastic. However, if viscoelastic is used, great care must be taken to completely remove it from the AC and back of the recipient cornea prior to implanting the donor tissue, because any residual viscoelastic will impair donor attachment.

A modified Sinskey hook is introduced through a stab incision and used to score Descemet's membrane in a circular pattern, outlining the area from which the membrane will be stripped (**Fig. 6**). The scoring should be done slightly inside the trephine reference mark on the epithelium to ensure that Descemet's membrane will only be stripped from areas that will be covered by the donor graft, because any areas not covered by either donor or recipient endothelium will become edematous. Also, a gentle touch should be used to avoid penetrating into the stroma. Trypan blue can be injected into the eye to help improve visualization of Descemet's membrane during the subsequent stripping procedure. This is particularly helpful if the membrane fragments while being stripped.

The far edge of Descemet's membrane is grasped with a stripping instrument or infusion/aspiration tip and carefully peeled off and removed from the eye (**Fig. 7**). The surgeon should avoid penetrating into the stroma, especially in the visual axis, and should usually be able to strip Descemet's membrane without ever passing the stripping instrument directly across the center of the pupil. The membrane can be spread out on the surface of the eye and examined to determine whether removal is complete. To facilitate subsequent donor attachment, some surgeons gently scrape the peripheral recipient stroma to roughen it, while other surgeons make a small fenestration in each quadrant of the peripheral recipient corneal to provide pathways for interface fluid to exit after the donor graft is inserted. After the recipient cornea is prepared, the continuous infusion or viscoelastic is removed from the eye.

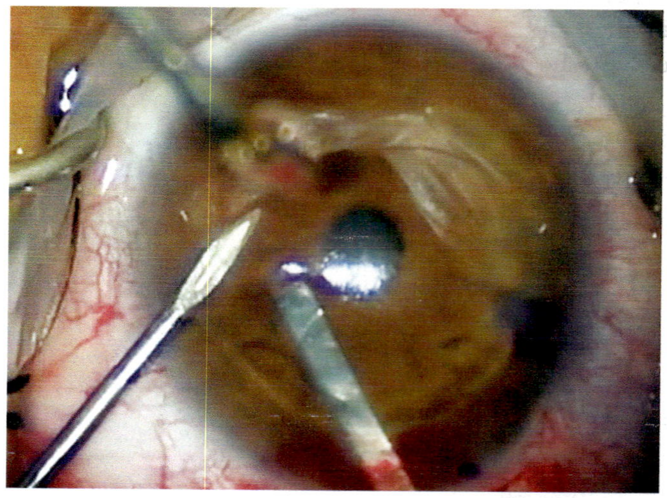

Fig. 7: Stripping Descemet's membrane. The stripping instrument was introduced through the scleral tunnel incision at the bottom of the image, and continuous infusion of the anterior chamber was provided through a stab incision at the lower left, while irrigation of the corneal surface was being provided from the upper left.

When treating a failed PK, the donor tissue can be implanted without stripping Descemet's membrane from the prior graft, if the membrane did not exhibit any guttata or other light-scattering abnormalities. Retaining Descemet's membrane may help maintain the strength of the healed PK incision and does not seem to impair graft attachment.[26]

Graft Insertion and Attachment

The donor tissue is brought into the operative field and one of several methods can be utilized for graft insertion. In Melles original PLK technique, the graft was laid endothelial side downward on a spatula coated with viscoelastic for insertion through an incision somewhat larger than the graft diameter.[20] Some surgeons lay the graft on a cushion of viscoelastic on the conjunctiva and pull the graft into the eye using either small forceps or a suture tied to the leading edge of the graft. The graft can be folded for insertion through a

3–5 mm incision, as originally described by Melles.[11] With the latter technique, a small drop of cohesive viscoelastic is placed on the center of the endothelial surface, and the posterior donor button is gently separated from the anterior portion and folded over on itself like a taco, with a slight over-folding of the top surface (**Fig. 8**). The folded graft is then gently grasped with forceps and inserted into the eye (**Fig. 9**). Although the over-folding allows some peripheral endothelium to be exposed during insertion, keeping the posterior flap somewhat smaller makes it easier for it to swing open, keeping the endothelial side facing the AC, after the folded graft is inserted into the eye. Use of single point fixation forceps, that only apply compression at the tip, helps minimize endothelial damage during graft insertion.

"Pull-through" Techniques

In pull-through techniques, the donor is docked into the main incision and pulled within the eye from the opposite small clear corneal incision with the help of forceps/suture. One of the most commonly performed pull-through techniques is the use of Busin glide (Asico, Westmont, IL, USA). The glide with the donor tissue is docked into the scleral tunnel/ clear corneal incision. The donor lenticule is pulled into the AC by grasping the edge of the donor lenticule with a bent disposable 23-gauge vitreous forceps from the opposite side port.

Another pull-through technique is the "suture pull-through" technique, in which a prolene suture is passed through the graft before inserting it and pulling it within the eye. The suture is then hitched on to the recipient cornea.

Endoglide is based on pull-in and pull-out technique. It requires 4–5.0 mm incision size and an AC maintainer.

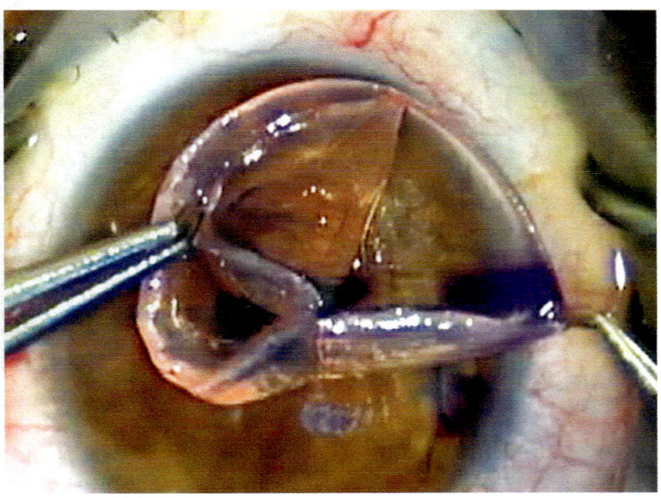

Fig. 8: Folding the posterior donor lenticule with the endothelial side facing inward, protected with a drop of cohesive viscoelastic.

Push-in Techniques

In push-in techniques, the donor is pushed in through the main incision with forceps/glides and injectors. The various donor insertion techniques include forceps: Taco with 60/40 overfold, trifold, 40/60 underfold; glides: Busin glide, sheets glide, Tan EndoGlide; and inserters: Endoserter (Winston-Salem, NC, USA), Endoshield/Endoinjector (Keramed, San Jose, CA, USA), and Neusidl Corneal Inserter (Fischer Surgical, Arnold, MO, USA).[42-46] In general, the inserters facilitate maintenance of the AC and unfolding of the donor tissue during insertion.[47-49] Endoserter requires 4–5.5 mm incision size and no AC maintainer is needed.

To unfold donor tissue folded into a taco configuration, the AC is inflated with balanced salt solution or air directed toward the open side of the taco allowing the underside of the folded tissue to sweep across and unfold stromal side up (**Fig. 10**). Unfolding the graft in the correct orientation is one of the most challenging steps, particularly for surgeons who are new to the procedure, so several techniques have been developed to facilitate this step. Vajpayee et al. insert a "hitch suture" through the peripheral edge of the donor lenticule prior to folding it for insertion. After inserting the

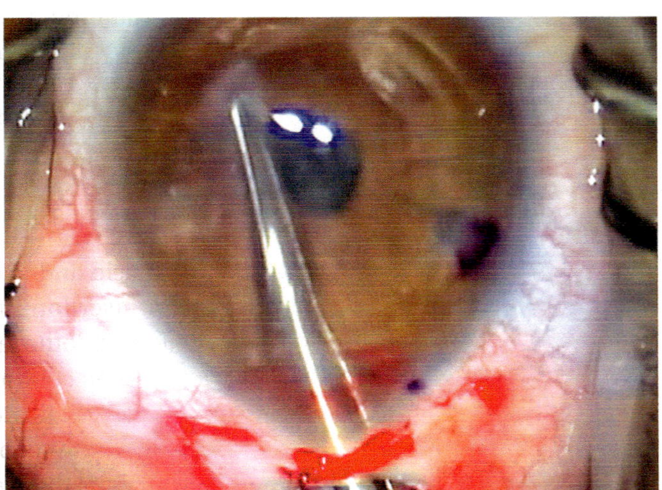

Fig. 9: Inserting the donor lenticule into the anterior chamber.

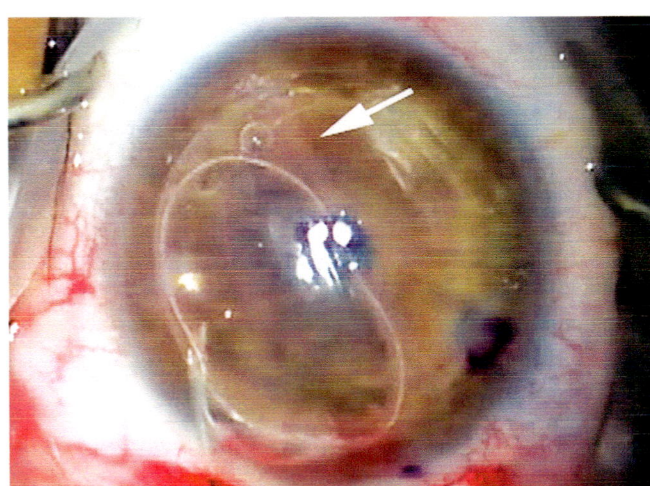

Fig. 10: Unfolding the donor lenticule with air. An arrow indicates the folded edge of the donor lenticule.

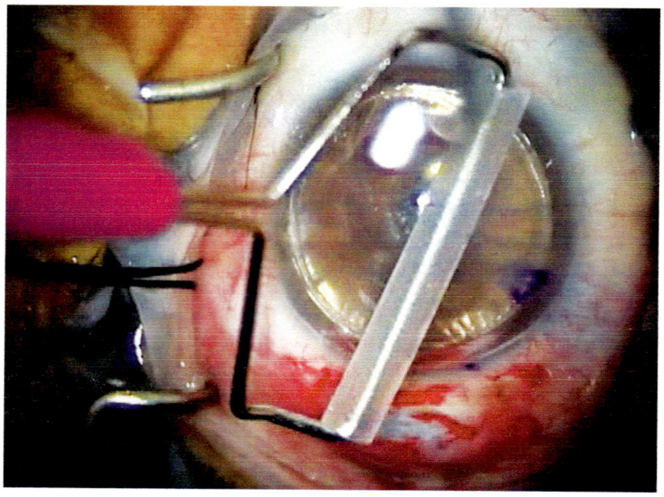

Fig. 11: Massaging the corneal surface while the anterior chamber is completely filled with air to remove any fluid entrapped at the graft interface.

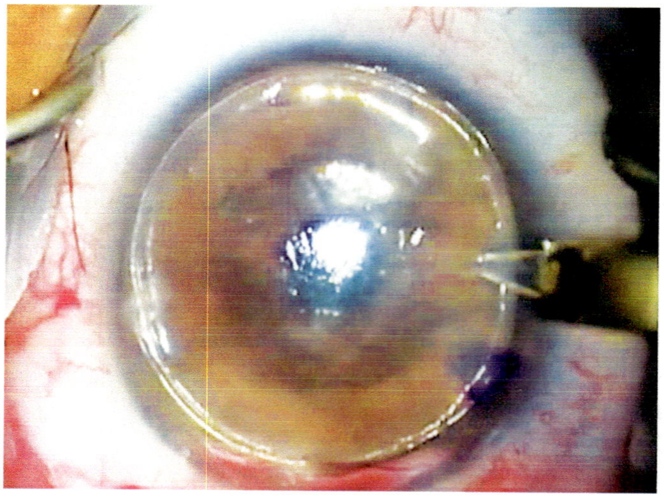

Fig. 12: Placing small fenestrations in four quadrants of the peripheral cornea.

folded graft, they introduce a Sinskey hook through a limbal stab incision and grab the suture loop to unfold the donor.[50] Koenig et al. use a bent 30-gauge needle on a 3 cc air syringe to engage the posterior edge of the anterior flap of the folded donor lenticule and fixate it against the host corneal stroma, then they inject an air bubble posterior to the graft to unfold it.[51] Each of these procedures may cause some peripheral endothelial cell loss.

If the graft is not well centered, the corneal surface can be massaged with a LASIK roller to help nudge the graft into position, or a bent needle can be used to gently grab the edge of the graft and pull it into position. Sometimes, there are folds or undulations in the graft and these can degrade visual acuity if they cross the visual axis.[52] Techniques to remove folds include massaging the corneal surface, or grabbing the edge of the graft with a bent needle to pull it flat. Care should be exercised to minimize endothelial damage when using any technique that involves touching the endothelium.

Once the graft is properly positioned, the AC is completely filled with air to press the graft up against the recipient cornea. It is essential to remove all fluid from the graft interface to ensure firm attachment. With the AC completely filled with air, the corneal surface can be gently massaged to help move fluid out of the graft interface into the AC (**Fig. 11**).[23] A cannula or other instrument could be used for this, but a Lindstrom LASIK roller (BD Medical) causes the least damage to the recipient epithelium. If fenestrations were not made during recipient cornea preparation, they can be made at this time (**Fig. 12**). Essentially, a small incision is made in each quadrant of the peripheral recipient cornea going down just to the graft interface to help drain any fluid entrapped between the donor and recipient tissue.[23]

Many surgeons leave the eye completely filled with air for 8–10 minutes and then remove most of the air to prevent pupillary block, just leaving a residual air bubble approximately the diameter of the donor graft. Other surgeons leave the AC completely filled with air for 1–2 hours. If the recipient has a glaucoma filtration device, the eye can be left completely filled with air and the air will escape through the glaucoma filter.

At the completion of surgery, dilating agents are applied to the treated eye to prevent pupillary block, antibiotics are given to prevent infection, and steroids and nonsteroidal anti-inflammatory drugs (NSAIDs) medications are given to minimize inflammation.

Combined Procedures

Endothelial keratoplasty can be combined with a variety of other intraocular procedures such as phacoemulsification, IOL implantation or exchange, secondary lens implantation, pars plana vitrectomy or anterior vitrectomy. However, it is often preferable to perform the other procedures first and then schedule the EK as a separate procedure.

In particular, performing cataract extraction and IOL implantation prior to EK is particularly advantageous because it helps deepen the AC and facilitates unfolding the EK donor graft. This represents a paradigm shift from how cataract surgery is staged relative to standard PK. Refractive outcomes are so unpredictable after PK that cataract surgery is usually postponed, so that it can be used to help correct the final refractive error after the PK sutures are removed. This is much less of a concern with EK because it is essentially refractive-neutral. Performing cataract surgery beforehand both facilitates the EK surgery and avoids subsequent surgical trauma to the graft endothelium.

POSTOPERATIVE CARE AND COMPLICATIONS

Graft detachment and dislocation: The most frequent complication with EK is donor detachment in the first 1–7 days after surgery.[23,24,32] It manifests as interface fluid, significant graft displacement, or a graft that is completely dislocated into the AC. The reported average dislocation rate is around 14.5%.[53] If this happens, air can be reinjected into the AC to once again press the donor graft firmly against the recipient cornea. Usually, the graft reattaches without any problem. Patients should be cautioned not to rub their treated eye, because eye rubbing can dislodge the donor tissue in the early postoperative period.[23]

Graft rejection: Graft rejection is a potential complication after any type of transplant. A multicenter, retrospective analysis of rejection episodes post-EK found that 15 of 199 grafts (7.5%) experienced a graft rejection episode within 2 years of an EK procedure (either DLEK or DSEK).[54] This rejection rate was significantly lower ($P = 0.035$) than the 13% incidence of graft rejection episodes experienced in the first 2 years after a PK by a comparator group of patients treated for Fuchs' dystrophy or bullous keratopathy as part of the Swedish Corneal Graft Registry.[54] Interestingly, the use of topical steroids differed considerably between the EK and PK groups. Whereas 80% of the EK patients were still using topical steroids 2 years after surgery, almost all PK patients in the comparator group were completely off steroids within 1 year of surgery.[54] PK patients are often taken off steroids within a year to accelerate wound healing and suture removal, but these are not significant concerns with EK. Also, EK is essentially refractive neutral so cataracts can be removed ahead of time—this eliminates the concern that prolonged use of topical corticosteroids might induce a cataract. Consequently, some surgeons keep EK patients on once daily topical steroids indefinitely to help prevent graft rejection.

While ocular surface complications are relatively common after standard PK,[55] they are rarely encountered after EK procedures because EK retains corneal innervation and requires no corneal sutures.[23]

Endothelial Cell Loss

Endothelial cell loss is still a major concern in DSAEK. Surgical trauma related to graft insertion appears to be the primary cause for this loss. The endothelial loss reported from larger series ranges from 14.9 to 59% with follow-up ranging from 6 months to 3 years.[56,57]

Raised Intraocular Pressure and Glaucoma

Glaucoma following DSAEK can occur due to pupillary block, inflammation, or steroid use. The reported incidence of glaucoma after DSAEK ranges from 0 to 15%, with an average rate of 3.0%.[53] Pupillary block is a rare but serious immediate postoperative complication after DSAEK, with a reported incidence of 0–10%.[58]

Epithelial Ingrowth

Epithelial ingrowth is a rare complication of DSAEK. The source of these epithelial cells can be host epithelial cells transported during donor insertion, donor epithelial cells transferred after eccentric trephination that has included full-thickness tissue beyond the microkeratome dissection and epithelial ingrowth related to the use of midperipheral full-thickness venting incisions.

Infectious Keratitis

Bacterial, fungal, and herpetic, all forms of keratitis have been reported following DSAEK. The most commonly isolated causative organism is *Candida albicans*.[42] Source of infection is often the donor tissue and rarely from late inoculation from conjunctiva and adnexa microflora. The infiltrate at the onset is often small and involves the donor lenticule or the interface. In addition, the effectiveness of topical antifungal agents may be reduced by posterior lamellar location of infiltrate. All these factors result in a poor prognosis of such cases. Majority of cases may require the removal of the lenticule with a therapeutic PK.[59]

Interface Haze

Interface abnormalities can occur in any form of lamellar keratoplasty, including DSAEK. The source of interface haze may include blood, retained ophthalmic viscoelastic, inflammatory cells, debris, and irregular cut of the donor tissue by the microkeratome, retained fragments of Descemet's membrane, microkeratome-generated plastic particles, and epithelial cells.

Other Less Common Complications

Other less frequent complications of DSAEK include endophthalmitis and folds in donor tissue.[60]

OUTCOMES

Refractive Outcomes

Favorable visual and refractive outcomes have made EK the treatment of choice for endothelial dysfunction. Whereas PK typically causes a 3–4 D increase in mean refractive cylinder, EK causes little to no change from the preoperative mean (**Table 1**).[4,12,24,27,28,61] However, a transient increase in manifest cylinder may occur if sutures are used to close the incision, and individual patients may experience a mild increase or decrease in manifest cylinder even though there is no significant change in the population mean as a result of the procedure.[2]

On average, DSEK results in a mild hyperopic shift in spherical equivalent refraction, although individual patients may experience a mild hyperopic or myopic shift.[4,12,24,27] Spherical equivalent outcomes can be influenced by donor dissection technique. For example, manual donor dissection on an AAC tends to produce a shallower depth in the periphery, resulting in a meniscus-shaped donor lenticule, which can cause a hyperopic shift. Many microkeratomes

Table 1: Comparative manifest cylinder outcomes with endothelial or penetrating keratoplasty procedures.

Keratoplasty technique and investigator	Preoperative cylinder diopters (mean ± SD)	Postoperative cylinder diopters (mean ± SD)
DSAEK		
Price[12]	1.5 ± **1.2**	1.5 ± **1.2**
Gorovoy[24]	0.96 ± **.8**	1.5 ± **1.2**
Koenig[27]	2.0 ± **1.2**	2.1 ± **1.3**
DSEK		
Price[12]	1.5 ± **1.3**	1.5 ± **1.0**
DLEK		
Terry[4]	1.1 ± **0.8**	1.3 ± **0.9**
Fogla[28]		1.5 ± **1.2**
PLK		
Melles		1.5 ± **0.8**
PK (for Fuchs')		
Claesson[7]		4.2 ± **2.9**
Pineros[9]		3.9 ± **1.9**

(DSAEK: Descemet's stripping automated endothelial keratoplasty; DSEK: Descemet's stripping endothelial keratoplasty; DLEK: deep lamellar endothelial keratoplasty; PLK: posterior lamellar keratoplasty; PK: penetrating keratoplasty; SD: standard deviation)

tend to cut deeper in the periphery, and since the cornea is deeper in the periphery, this can result in a relatively planar central donor lenticule. However, some surgeons have seen a mild hyperopic shift with microkeratome-dissected donor tissue. By tracking their own EK refractive outcomes, individual surgeons can help compensate for any systematic shift they experience in spherical equivalent refraction by factoring it into their IOL calculation nomogram.

Hyperopia

The induced hyperopia ranges from 0.7 to 1.5 D with an average induced hyperopia of 1 D.[62,63] The induced hyperopia is primarily due to nonuniform thickness profiles of donor lenticules.[64] Donor lenticules prepared with the microkeratome are thinner centrally and thicker in the periphery, resulting in a reduced radius of curvature of the posterior corneal surface and reduced effective corneal power.[63] The hyperopic shift from DSAEK must be considered while calculating IOLs power in cases undergoing triple procedure. Target refraction should be aimed at about 1.0 D of myopia in these cases.

Astigmatism

The average postoperative astigmatism after DSAEK is 1.5 D.[53] The amount of astigmatism often depends on the type of incision.

Higher Order Aberration

Descemet's stripping automated endothelial keratoplasty does not change the anterior corneal curvature but the posterior corneal curvature is altered due to differences in curvatures between the host and the donor lenticule as well as an uneven thickness of donor lenticule. These changes can induce posterior corneal higher order aberrations after DSAEK.[65]

Visual Outcomes

Current EK techniques provide rapid visual recovery and an easier postoperative course compared with PK. After PK, 10–15% of treated eyes typically require a hard contact lens to normalize the anterior corneal surface in order to achieve best visual acuity, and a small but significant percentage of PK patients require subsequent refractive procedures, such as limbal relaxing incisions or laser-assisted in situ keratomileusis (LASIK) to help reduce high astigmatic errors.[7-9,66] In contrast, hard lenses or subsequent refractive procedures are not required for best vision after EK because corneal topography is not significantly altered.[4,12,24]

Retinal disease or amblyopia in the treated eye are the most significant factors that may limit visual acuity after EK.[12] Interestingly, we have found that the visual prognosis is somewhat better for younger patients than older patients even after patients with preexisting retinal disease are excluded.[12] Also, since EK does not replace the anterior stroma, patients are likely to recover better vision if EK is performed before long-standing corneal edema has caused significant anterior stromal scarring, which can scatter light and degrade vision.

Descemet's stripping endothelial keratoplasty and DSAEK increase corneal thickness because posterior donor stroma is added without removal of any recipient stroma. Use of ultra-thin DSAEK donor lenticules is associated with better visual outcomes.[12]

Endothelial keratoplasty visual outcomes are more predictable than PK outcomes, and the majority of patients without retinal disease recover 20/25 to 20/40 visual acuity.[4,12,24]

It is important to keep in mind that visual acuity measurements taken in a darkened room do not really indicate the degree of visual impairment many Fuchs' patients experience in their daily lives. Often Fuchs' patients have difficulty driving on sunny days or reading under fluorescent lights, even when their Snellen acuity measures 20/30 in a darkened room, because their guttate cause significant light-scattering and glare. At the 1-month postoperative examination after EK, most Fuchs' patients report a significant improvement in visual quality, including fewer problems with glare and a renewed appreciation of colors. Many request surgery on their second eye within 6 months of having the first eye treated, even when their Snellen acuity is the same in the treated and untreated eyes!

DESCEMET STRIPPING AUTOMATED ENDOTHELIAL KERATOPLASTY IN SPECIAL SITUATIONS

Descemet's Stripping Automated Endothelial Keratoplasty in the Presence of Anterior Chamber Intraocular Lens

The primary concerns of performing DSAEK in the presence of an anterior chamber intraocular lens (ACIOL) are increased tissue manipulation, reduced AC depth (ACD), difficulty in graft manipulation, more difficult air-bubble management, and intermittent postoperative IOL touch.[68] In the presence of a well-centered ACIOL and an ACD > 3 mm, DSAEK can be performed successfully in such cases.[68]

Descemet's Stripping Automated Endothelial Keratoplasty in Aphakia

The difficulties in performing DSAEK in aphakic eyes are difficulty of air retention in the AC, migration of air posteriorly, chances of graft dislocation into vitreous cavity, and chances of host Descemet's membrane dislocation posteriorly. The various modifications that can be employed to address these difficulties are implantation of an IOL before DSAEK,[69] insertion of an infusion cannula through pars plana route,[70] or placement of temporary anchor sutures to prevent donor dislodgement and improve graft adherence.[71]

Descemet's Stripping Automated Endothelial Keratoplasty in Aniridia

Congenital aniridia or aniridia associated with trauma along with aphakia carries a risk of posterior migration of air into vitreous cavity. This problem can be overcome by performing an aniridia IOL implantation followed by DSAEK in stepwise manner or placing an anchor suture in the peripheral edge of the donor tissue and securing it to the overlying recipient cornea.[72]

Descemet's Stripping Automated Endothelial Keratoplasty with Previous Trabeculectomy or Tube Shunt Implantation

The problems encountered in such cases include loss of the remaining field of vision due to the transient intraocular pressure (IOP) rise, difficulty in surgery due to presence of tube of the glaucoma valve, tube position contributing to corneal decompensation, and possibility of air escaping through the sclerostomy or tube or large iridotomy. The various technical modifications that can be helpful in such cases include trimming of the tube if it extends centrally, placement of viscoelastic between the graft and the iris to block the escape of air from the AC, suture closure of the iridotomy opening, and meticulous monitoring of IOP.[73,74]

FUTURE DIRECTIONS

The next EK iteration, Descemet membrane endothelial keratoplasty (DMEK) utilizes only Descemet membrane and endothelium from the donor cornea in contrast to DSEK and DSAEK, which also include donor stromal tissue.[75–78] Compared with DSEK and DSAEK, DMEK produces better visual acuity outcomes and has a lower risk of rejection. However, DMEK can be more difficult to perform in eyes with anatomical challenges. DMEK is discussed in detail in Chapter 39.

Overall, EK has significantly improved the risk/benefit ratio of having a corneal transplant and this is causing more patients with endothelial dysfunction to choose transplantation at an earlier age, increasing the demand for donor corneas. Many groups are developing cultured endothelial cell sheets for use with EK, and these efforts may ultimately help alleviate the chronic worldwide shortage of donor corneas suitable for transplantation.

Descemet Stripping only/Descemetorhexis without Endothelial Keratoplasty

Use of donor tissue may not be necessary for patients in the early stages of Fuchs dystrophy, when the guttae are primarily within the central 4–5 mm of the cornea and the peripheral endothelium is relatively healthy. In such cases a 4–5-mm diameter of Descemet membrane and endothelium can be removed from the recipient cornea using techniques similar to those used with DSEK, and over the next few weeks to months, the patient's healthy peripheral endothelial cells will usually migrate and cover the denuded area, resolving the corneal edema. This technique has been called Descemetorhexis without Endothelial Keratoplasty (DWEK) or Descemet Stripping Only (DSO).[79,80] It is extremely important not to roughen the stroma during the descemetorhexis because any rough areas will impede migration of the endothelial cells and may result in a persistently edematous area. Also, it is important to limit the diameter of the descemetorhexis to about 5 mm or less.

ROLE OF ADDITIONAL RHO-ASSOCIATED KINASE INHIBITOR

It has been shown that use of the Rho-associated kinase inhibitor (ROCK inhibitor), ripasudil, can facilitate corneal clearance after DSO. Ripasudil is approved in Japan for the treatment of glaucoma and is being evaluated in a clinical trial for use with DSO. The primary effects of Rho proteins are to induce structural change in the internal cell cytoskeleton, inhibiting smooth muscle vasodilation, cellular delamination and migration.[81] An in vitro study of Ripasudil's effect on the trabecular meshwork and Schlemm's canal endothelial cells also showed cytoskeletal rearrangement (cell rounding and reduced actin bundles). It also decreases ZO-1 cell junctional complex proteins.[82] The first double-armed prospective study of ROCK inhibitor as an adjuvant to DSO has recently been published by Macsai et al. They found that DSO patients who used ripasudil postoperatively had significantly faster recovery and higher central endothelial cell density than those who did not use it.[83]

CONCLUSION

Endothelial keratoplasty has become the preferred method for treating endothelial dysfunction because it provides more rapid visual rehabilitation and an improved safety profile compared with standard PK. To address the worldwide donor tissue shortage, techniques are being developed to allow one donor cornea to be used for multiple recipients and to treat Fuchs dystrophy without use of any donor tissue.

REFERENCES

1. Melles GR, Wijdh RH, Nieuwendaal CP. A technique to excise the descemet membrane from a recipient cornea (descemetorhexis). Cornea. 2004;23:286-8.
2. Price FW Jr, Price MO. Descemet's stripping with endothelial keratoplasty in 50 eyes: A refractive neutral corneal transplant. J Refract Surg. 2005;21:339-45.
3. Price FW Jr. Corneal transplantation as a refractive surgical procedure. J Refract Surg. 2005;21:216-7.
4. Terry MA, Ousley PJ. Deep lamellar endothelial keratoplasty visual acuity, astigmatism, and endothelial survival in a large prospective series. Ophthalmology. 2005;112:1541-8.
5. Riddle HK Jr, Parker DA, Price FW Jr. Management of postkeratoplasty astigmatism. Curr Opin Ophthalmol. 1998;9:15-28.
6. Binder PS, Waring GO. Keratotomy for astigmatism. In: Waring GO (Ed). Refractive Keratotomy for Myopia and Astigmatism. St. Louis, MO: Mosby; 1992. pp. 1157-86.
7. Claesson M, Armitage WJ, Fagerholm P, Stenevi U. Visual outcome in corneal grafts: a preliminary analysis of the Swedish Corneal Transplant Register. Br J Ophthalmol. 2002;86:174-80.
8. Price FW Jr, Whitson WE, Marks RG. Progression of visual acuity after penetrating keratoplasty. Ophthalmology. 1991;98:1177-85.
9. Pineros O, Cohen EJ, Rapuano CJ, Laibson PR. Long-term results after penetrating keratoplasty for Fuchs' endothelial dystrophy. Arch Ophthalmol. 1996;114:15-8.
10. Elder MJ, Stack RR. Globe rupture following penetrating keratoplasty: how often, why, and what can we do to prevent it? Cornea. 2004;23:776-80.
11. Melles GR, Lander F, Nieuwendaal C. Sutureless, posterior lamellar keratoplasty: A case report of a modified technique. Cornea. 2002;21:325-7.
12. Price MO, Price FW Jr. Descemet's Stripping with Endothelial Keratoplasty Comparative Outcomes with Microkeratome-Dissected and Manually Dissected Donor Tissue. Ophthalmology. 2006;113:1936-42.
13. Barraquer J. Special methods in corneal surgery. In: King JH, McTigue JW (Eds). The Comea World Congress. Washington, DC: Rutterworths; 1965. pp. 586-604.
14. Busin M, Arffa RC, Sebastiani A. Endokeratoplasty as an alternative to penetrating keratoplasty for the surgical treatment of diseased endothelium: initial results. Ophthalmology. 2000;107:2077-82.
15. Ehlers N, Ehlers H, Hjortdal J, Moller-Pedersen T. Grafting of the posterior cornea. Description of a new technique with 12-month clinical results. Acta Ophthalmol Scand. 2000;78:543-6.
16. Güell JL, Velasco F, Guerrero E, Gris O, Calatayud M. Preliminary results with posterior lamellar keratoplasty for endothelial failure. Br J Ophthalmol. 2003;87:241-3.
17. Azar DT, Jain S. Microkeratome-assisted posterior keratoplasty. J Cataract Refract Surg. 2002;28:732-3.
18. Ko WW, Freuh B, Shields C, Costello M, Feldman ST. Experimental posterior lamellar transplantation of the rabbit cornea. Invest Ophthalmol Vis Sci. 1993;34:1102.
19. Melles GR, Eggink FA, Lander F, Pels E, Rietveld FJ, Beekhuis WH, et al. A surgical technique for posterior lamellar keratoplasty. Cornea. 1998;17:618-26.
20. Melles GR, Lander F, Beekhuis WH, Remeijer L, Binder PS. Posterior lamellar keratoplasty for a case of pseudophakic bullous keratopathy. Am J Ophthalmol. 1999;127:340-1.
21. Melles GR, Rietveld FJ, Beekhuis WH, Binder PS. A technique to visualize corneal incision and lamellar dissection depth during surgery. Cornea. 1999;18:80-6.
22. Terry MA, Ousley PJ. Deep lamellar endothelial keratoplasty in the first United States patients: early clinical results. Cornea. 2001;20:239-43.
23. Price FW Jr, Price MO. Descemet's stripping with endothelial keratoplasty in 200 eyes: Early challenges and techniques to enhance donor adherence. J Cataract Refract Surg. 2006;32:411-8.
24. Gorovoy MS. Descemet-stripping automated endothelial keratoplasty. Cornea. 2006;25:886-9.
25. Price MO, Price FW Jr. Descemet's stripping endothelial keratoplasty for treatment of iridocorneal endothelial syndrome. Cornea. 2007;26(4):493-7.
26. Price F, Price M. Endothelial keratoplasty to restore clarity to a failed penetrating graft. Cornea. 2006;25:895-9.
27. Koenig SB, Covert DJ. Early results of small-incision Descemet's stripping and automated endothelial keratoplasty. Ophthalmology. 2007;114:221-6.
28. Fogla R, Padmanabhan P. Initial results of small incision deep lamellar endothelial keratoplasty (DLEK). Am J Ophthalmol. 2006;141:346-51.
29. Sarayba MA, Juhasz T, Chuck RS, Ignacio TS, Nguyen TB, Sweet P, et al. Femtosecond laser posterior lamellar keratoplasty: A laboratory model. Cornea. 2005;24:328-33.
30. Suwan-Apichon O, Reyes JM, Griffin NB, Barker J, Gore P, Chuck RS. Microkeratome versus femtosecond laser predissection of corneal grafts for anterior and posterior lamellar keratoplasty. Cornea. 2006;25:966-8.
31. Cheng YY, Pels E, Nuijts RM. Femtosecond-laser-assisted Descemet's stripping endothelial keratoplasty. J Cataract Refract Surg. 2007;33:152-5.
32. Terry MA, Hoar KL, Wall J, Ousley P. Histology of dislocations in endothelial keratoplasty (DSEK and DLEK): A laboratory-based, surgical solution to dislocation in 100 consecutive DSEK cases. Cornea. 2006;25:926-32.
33. Vajpayee RB, Maharana PK, Jain S, Sharma N, Jhanji V. Thin lenticule Descemet's stripping automated endothelial keratoplasty: Single, slow pass technique. Clin Exp Ophthalmol. 2014;42:411-6.
34. Nahum Y, Leon P, Busin M. Postoperative graft thickness obtained with single-pass microkeratome-assisted ultrathin Descemet stripping automated endothelial keratoplasty. Cornea. 2015;34:1362-4.
35. Busin M, Madi S, Santorum P, Scorcia V, Beltz J. Ultrathin Descemet's stripping automated endothelial keratoplasty with the microkeratome double-pass technique: Two-year outcomes. Ophthalmology. 2013;120:1186-94.
36. Terry MA, Shamie N, Chen ES, Phillips PM, Hoar KL, Friend DJ. Precut tissue for Descemet's stripping automated endothelial keratoplasty: Vision, astigmatism, and endothelial survival. Ophthalmology. 2009;116:248-56.

37. Chen ES, Terry MA, Shamie N, Hoar KL, Friend DJ. Precut tissue in Descemet's stripping automated endothelial keratoplasty donor characteristics and early postoperative complications. Ophthalmology. 2008;115:497-502.
38. Vetter JM, Holtz C, Vossmerbaeumer U, Pfeiffer N. Irregularity of the posterior corneal surface during applanation using a curved femtosecond laser interface and microkeratome cutting head. J Refract Surg. 2012;28:209-14.
39. Trinh L, Saubaméa B, Auclin F, Denoyer A, Lai-Kuen R, El Hamdaoui M, et al. Femtosecond and excimer laser-assisted endothelial keratoplasty (FELEK): A new technique of endothelial transplantation. J Fr Ophtalmol. 2014;37:211-9.
40. Liu YC, Teo EP, Adnan KB, Yam GH, Peh GS, Tan DT, et al. Endothelial approach ultrathin corneal grafts prepared by femtosecond laser for descemet stripping endothelial keratoplasty. Invest Ophthalmol Vis Sci. 2014;55:8393-401.
41. Fang JP, Hamill MB. Descemet's stripping endothelial keratoplasty under topical anesthesia. J Cataract Refract Surg. 2007;33:187-8.
42. Anshu A, Price MO, Tan DT, Price FW Jr. Endothelial keratoplasty: A revolution in evolution. Surv Ophthalmol. 2012;57:236-52.
43. Terry MA, Shamie N, Chen ES, Hoar KL, Friend DJ. Endothelial keratoplasty a simplified technique to minimize graft dislocation, iatrogenic graft failure, and pupillary block. Ophthalmology. 2008;115:1179-86.
44. Elbaz U, Yeung SN, Lichtinger A, Zauberman NA, Goldich Y, Ziai S, et al. EndoGlide versus EndoSerter for the insertion of donor graft in descemet stripping automated endothelial keratoplasty. Am J Ophthalmol. 2014;158:257-62.e1.
45. Letko E, Price DA, Lindoso EM, Price MO, Price FW Jr. Secondary graft failure and repeat endothelial keratoplasty after Descemet's stripping automated endothelial keratoplasty. Ophthalmology. 2011;118:310-4.
46. Mehta JS, Por YM, Beuerman RW, Tan DT. Glide insertion technique for donor cornea lenticule during Descemet's stripping automated endothelial keratoplasty. J Cataract Refract Surg. 2007;33:1846-50.
47. Ang M, Saroj L, Htoon HM, Kiew S, Mehta JS, Tan D. Comparison of a donor insertion device to sheets glide in Descemet stripping endothelial keratoplasty: 3-year outcomes. Am J Ophthalmol. 2014;157:1163-9.e3.
48. Toyama T, Honda N, Usui T, Amano S. New graft inserter for descemet stripping automated endothelial keratoplasty. Cornea. 2014;33:432-5.
49. Kobayashi A, Yokogawa H, Sugiyama K. Clinical results of the Neusidl Corneal Inserter®, a new donor inserter for Descemet's stripping automated endothelial keratoplasty, for small Asian eyes. Ophthalmic Surg Lasers Imaging. 2012;43:311-8.
50. Vajpayee RB, Agarwal T, Jhanji V, Sharma N. Modification in descemet-stripping automated endothelial keratoplasty: "Hitch suture" technique. Cornea. 2006;25:1060-2.
51. Koenig SB, Dupps WJ Jr, Covert DJ, Meisler DM. Simple technique to unfold the donor corneal lenticule during Descemet's stripping and automated endothelial keratoplasty. J Cataract Refract Surg. 2007;33:189-90.
52. Faia LJ, Baratz KH, Bourne WM. Corneal graft folds: a complication of deep lamellar endothelial keratoplasty. Arch Ophthalmol. 2006;124:593-5.
53. Lee WB, Jacobs DS, Musch DC, Kaufman SC, Reinhart WJ, Shtein RM. Descemet's stripping endothelial keratoplasty: Safety and outcomes: A report by the American Academy of Ophthalmology. Ophthalmology. 2009;116:1818-30.
54. Allan BD, Terry MA, Price FW Jr, Price MO, Griffin NB, Claesson M. Corneal transplant rejection rate and severity after endothelial keratoplasty. Cornea. 2007;26(9):1039-42.
55. Price MO, Thompson RW Jr, Price FW Jr. Risk factors for various causes of failure in initial corneal grafts. Arch Ophthalmol. 2003;121(8):1087-92.
56. Wu EI, Ritterband DC, Yu G, Shields RA, Seedor JA. Graft rejection following descemet stripping automated endothelial keratoplasty: Features, risk factors, and outcomes. Am J Ophthalmol. 2012;153:949-57.e1.
57. Terry MA, Straiko MD, Goshe JM, Shamie N, Shah A, Alqudah AA, et al. Endothelial keratoplasty: Prospective, randomized, masked clinical trial comparing an injector with forceps for tissue insertion. Am J Ophthalmol. 2013;156:61-8.e3.
58. Koenig SB. Descemet stripping automated endothelial keratoplasty in the phakic eye. Cornea. 2010;29:531-3.
59. Araki-Sasaki K, Fukumoto A, Osakabe Y, Kimura H, Kuroda S. The clinical characteristics of fungal keratitis in eyes after Descemet's stripping and automated endothelial keratoplasty. Clin Ophthalmol. 2014;8:1757-60.
60. Chew AC, Mehta JS, Li L, Busmanis I, Tan DT. Fungal endophthalmitis after descemet stripping automated endothelial keratoplasty—a case report. Cornea. 2010;29:346-9.
61. Baratz KH, Nau CB, Hodge DO, Bourne WM. A prospective, randomized study of deep lamellar endothelial keratoplasty versus penetrating keratoplasty: Early results. Invest Ophthalmol Vis Sci. 2005;46:2703.
62. Nakatani S, Murakami A. Three-year outcome of Descemet stripping automated endothelial keratoplasty for bullous keratopathy after argon laser iridotomy. Cornea. 2014;33:780-4.
63. Dupps WJ Jr, Qian Y, Meisler DM. Multivariate model of refractive shift in Descemet-stripping automated endothelial keratoplasty. J Cataract Refract Surg. 2008;34:578-84.
64. Tsui JY, Goins KM, Sutphin JE, Wagoner MD. Phakic descemet stripping automated endothelial keratoplasty: Prevalence and prognostic impact of postoperative cataracts. Cornea. 2011;30:291-5.
65. Muftuoglu O, Prasher P, Bowman RW, McCulley JP, Mootha VV. Corneal higher-order aberrations after Descemet's stripping automated endothelial keratoplasty. Ophthalmology. 2010;117:878-84.e6.
66. Davis EA, Azar DT, Jakobs FM, Stark WJ. Refractive and keratometric results after the triple procedure: Experience with early and late suture removal. Ophthalmology. 1998;105:624-30.
67. Williams KA, Hornsby NB, Bartlett CM, Holland HK, Esterman A, Coster DJ (Eds). The Australian Corneal Graft Registry 2004 Report. Adelaide: Snap Printing; 2004.
68. Allen MB, Lieu P, Mootha VV, Bowman RW, Petroll WM, Tong L, et al. Risk factors for intraocular pressure elevation after descemet stripping automated endothelial keratoplasty. Eye Contact Lens. 2010;36:223-7.
69. Sinha R, Shekhar H, Sharma N, Tandon R, Titiyal JS, Vajpayee RB. Intrascleral fibrin glue intraocular lens fixation combined with Descemet-stripping automated endothelial keratoplasty or penetrating keratoplasty. J Cataract Refract Surg. 2012; 38:1240-5.
70. Titiyal JS, Sachdev R, Sinha R, Tandon R, Sharma N. Modified surgical technique for improving donor adherence in DSAEK in the aphakic vitrectomized eye. Cornea. 2012;31:462-4.
71. Huang T, Wang YJ, Luo Y, Huan DN, Chen JQ. Effect of temporary anchor sutures on Descemet stripping endothelial keratoplasty in aphakic eyes. Zhonghua Yan Ke Za Zhi. 2010;46:233-7.
72. Price MO, Price FW Jr, Trespalacios R. Endothelial keratoplasty technique for aniridic aphakic eyes. J Cataract Refract Surg. 2007;33:376-9.
73. Sansanayudh W, Bahar I, Rootman D. Novel technique in preparing a donor DSAEK lenticule in a patient with a glaucoma drainage device. Br J Ophthalmol. 2009;93:1267-9.
74. Peng RM, Hao YS, Chen HJ, Sun YX, Hong J. Endothelial keratoplasty: The use of viscoelastic as an aid in reattaching the dislocated graft in abnormally structured eyes. Ophthalmology. 2009;116:1897-900.

75. Melles GR, Lander F, Rietveld FJ. Transplantation of Descemet's membrane carrying viable endothelium through a small scleral incision. Cornea. 2002;21:415-8.
76. Melles GR, Ong TS, Ververs B, van der Wees J. Descemet membrane endothelial keratoplasty (DMEK). Cornea. 2006;25:987-90.
77. Tappin M. A method for true endothelial cell (Tencell) transplantation using a custom-made cannula for the treatment of endothelial cell failure. Eye (Lond). 2007;21(6):775-9.
78. Melles GR, Lander F, van Dooren BT, Pels E, Beekhuis WH. Preliminary clinical results of posterior lamellar keratoplasty through a sclerocorneal pocket incision. Ophthalmology. 2000;107:1850-6.
79. Kaufman AR, Nosé RM, Pineda R 2nd. Descemetorhexis without endothelial keratoplasty (DWEK): proposal for nomenclature standardization. Cornea. 2018;37:e20-e21.
80. Moshirfar M, Ding Y, Shah TJ. A historical perspective on treatment of Fuchs' endothelial dystrophy: we have come a long way. J Ophthalmic Vis Res. 2018;13:339-43.
81. Nakagawa H, Koizumi N, Okumura N, Suganami H, Kinoshita S. Morphological changes of human corneal endothelial cells after Rho-associated kinase inhibitor eye drop (Ripasudil) administration: a prospective open-label clinical study. PLoS One. 2015;10:e0136802.
82. Kaneko Y, Ohta M, Inoue T, Mizuno K, Isobe T, Tanabe S, et al. Effects of K-115 (Ripasudil), a novel ROCK inhibitor, on trabecular meshwork and Schlemm's canal endothelial cells. Sci Rep. 2016;6:19640.
83. Macsai MS, Shiloach M. Use of topical Rho kinase inhibitors in the treatment of Fuchs dystrophy after descemet stripping only. Cornea. 2019;38:529-34.

33 Thin Lenticule Descemet's Stripping Automated Endothelial Keratoplasty

Prabhakar Singh, Sohini Mandal, Namrata Sharma

INTRODUCTION

Keratoplasty has evolved over time from full thickness graft to isolated endothelial cell transplantation. The endothelial keratoplasty initially started with posterior lamellar keratoplasty (PLK), with incision for graft insertion to be as large as 9 mm. With time, modifications were made in the surgical steps to make it simpler and reproducible in the hands of different surgeons worldwide.

WHY THIN LENTICULE DESCEMET'S STRIPPING AUTOMATED ENDOTHELIAL KERATOPLASTY OVER DESCEMET'S MEMBRANE ENDOTHELIAL KERATOPLASTY?

Though, in Descemet's membrane endothelial keratoplasty (DMEK), there is actual replacement of Descemet's membrane (DM) and the endothelium of host cornea with DM and the endothelium of donor cornea, and is the most physiological option; however, it is surgically challenging and the learning curve is steep. In a randomized controlled trial (RCT), comparing DMEK with ultrathin Descemet's stripping automated endothelial keratoplasty (UT-DSAEK) by Dunker et al., they found that the mean best spectacle corrected visual acuity, hyperopic shift, and endothelial cell loss did not differ significantly between the two groups. However, adverse events were more in the DMEK group.[1] So, one can achieve nearly similar results with thinner grafts with relatively easier surgical steps and easier graft handling. Endothelial keratoplasty involves fashioning of a donor lenticule to replace the diseased Descemet's membrane-endothelial cell complex. Various methods have been discussed in literature to fashion thinner lenticules. Manual dissection, single- and double-pass automated microkeratomes have been described in creating thinner lenticules. Reproducibility in creating thinner grafts is not always feasible in manual dissection. Here comes the role of automated microkeratomes in creating similar grafts with reproducible results. Busin et al. in their study published that the UT-DSAEK grafts (<131 μm) could be harvested using double-pass technique, even by relatively naive eye bank technicians.[2] Thinner the DSAEK graft, better is the visual outcome and reduced observed postoperative hyperopic shift. Literature suggests that DSAEK grafts ≤131 μm showed better postoperative visual outcome compared to thicker >131 μm DSAEK grafts.[3] However, there are studies with conflicting results on relationship between thickness of graft and visual outcome.[3-8]

TECHNIQUES

Initially, Busin described the double-pass microkeratome technique at American Society of Cataract and Refractive Surgery (ASCRS) 2011 annual symposium. In 2012, modifications of Busin's surgical steps were published by Maylon H et al; in which they had first chosen 200 μm head for first pass in a patient with 400–500 μm thick cornea. The second pass was decided again with a head of 130, 110, or 90 μm based on residual stromal bed thickness of >235, 216–235, 190–215, respectively. The second pass was done such that the reference dot was placed 180° away from the alignment mark. This helped in achieving a residual stromal bed of approximately 100 μm or less.[9] However, Waite et al. demonstrated an increased endothelial cell loss during double-pass technique.[10] Apart from this, there is a potential risk of corneal perforation.[9] In contrast to the results obtained in the previous study, in a RCT on single-pass versus double-pass UT-DSAEK by Sharma N et al., comparable endothelial cell loss between two groups were noted at final follow-up visit. Considering the problems associated with grafts from double-pass technique, clinicians devised single-pass techniques with relative high safety margin but comparable visual outcome. In study by Vajpayee et al., single, slow pass technique using 400 μm microkeratome head was safely used to harvest the thin DSAEK graft.[11] Another technique described as NT-DSAEK (Nanothin DSAEK) to obtain nanothin grafts up to ≤50 μm, used nomograms for standardized creation of grafts by single-pass technique. The authors found the technique safe with minimal endothelial cell loss compared to UT-DSAEK and DMEK grafts.[12] In an attempt to obtain a thinner DSAEK graft, it is preferable to use thinner corneas <550 μm thick centrally. Deep microkeratome cuts often lead to variable depth cuts due to inherent elastic property of corneal stroma. Considering, the fact that thinner corneas require less removal of corneal tissue, they are preferred when trying to achieve thinner grafts.[13] Literature search reveals use of Thin-C media for osmotic deswelling of cornea prior to UT-DSAEK graft preparation. Deswelling with Thin-C media before graft preparation results in better quality of cut surface and more consistent deeper cuts; and this was termed as "OSMO-UT-DSAEK".[14] Apart from these, high pressures in AAC, drying the corneal stroma with sponge soaked in polyvinyl alcohol, and directing sterile airflow over stroma before microkeratome cut have been discussed to dehydrate corneal stroma.[14-16] In contrast to the OSMO-UT-DSAEK, a new concept was introduced by NH Farbman et al., wherein they had devised a technique of 60 second swelling for consistent UT-DSAEK graft preparation. Here, after the epithelial removal and before the microkeratome cut, anterior corneal surface is soaked with BSS for 60 seconds, meanwhile Jameson muscle hook is used to agitate the anterior stroma. Rest of the procedures are like any other single-pass technique. Author used a nomogram-based technique to select microkeratome head size depending on corneal thickness. Corneas were swollen to a size in the range of larger cutting head, allowing safer deeper cuts. The artificial anterior chamber pressures were also modified depending on thickness of cornea.

In 2015, another paper published by Agarwal A et al. introduced a newer technique of endothelial keratoplasty and termed it "pre-Descemet's endothelial keratoplasty (PDEK)". Here, donor endothelial graft was created using pneumatic dissection and attaining type 1 bubble. The grafts so obtained had a mean thickness of 28 ± 5.6 μm with good postoperative outcome.[17]

Apart from these, femtosecond laser may be used to create thinner grafts. In FS-DSEK, the results are consistent in terms of graft thickness; however, the visual outcome is limited compared to PK and DSAEK.[18,19] Femtosecond and excimer laser-assisted EK (FELEK) is another technique which combined thin graft dissection followed by smoothening of graft with excimer laser.[20] Another promising technique using femtolaser is femtosecond laser-enabled descemetorhexis DMEK (F-DMEK) and the outcomes seem to be better with lesser rates of graft detachment.[21-23]

OUTCOME

Various studies suggest that thinner DSAEK grafts have comparable visual outcome to DMEK.[24] Dunker et al. also found that the mean best spectacle corrected visual acuity, hyperopic shift, and endothelial cell loss did not differ significantly between the two groups. However, adverse events were more in the DMEK group. However, the percentage of eyes achieving 20/25 vision was significantly higher in DMEK group.[1,25] Another study by Hirabayashi et al. suggested that, both the procedures (UT-DSAEK and DMEK) result in improved light scattering.[26] DMEK is associated with relatively lesser posterior corneal higher order aberration compared to UT-DSAEK.[27]

In future, different techniques with relatively easier and reproducible surgical steps with reasonable surgical outcome are likely to evolve.

REFERENCES

1. Dunker SL, Dickman MM, Wisse RPL, Nobacht S, Wijdh RHJ, Bartels MC, et al. Descemet membrane endothelial keratoplasty versus ultrathin Descemet stripping automated endothelial keratoplasty: A multicenter randomized controlled clinical trial. Ophthalmology. 2020;127(9):1152-9.
2. Busin M, Patel AK, Scorcia V, Ponzin D. Microkeratome-assisted preparation of ultrathin grafts for descemet stripping automated endothelial keratoplasty. Invest Ophthalmol Vis Sci. 2012;53:521-4.
3. Neff KD, Biber JM, Holland EJ. Comparison of central corneal graft thickness to visual acuity outcomes in endothelial keratoplasty. Cornea. 2011;30:388-91.
4. Van Cleynenbreugel H, Remeijer L, Hillenaar T. Descemet stripping automated endothelial keratoplasty: effect of intraoperative lenticule thickness on visual outcome and endothelial cell density. Cornea. 2011;30:1195-200.
5. Terry MA, Straiko MD, Goshe JM, Li JY, Davis-Boozer D. Descemet's stripping automated endothelial keratoplasty: the tenuous relationship between donor thickness and postoperative vision. Ophthalmology. 2012;119:1988-996.
6. Maier AK, Gundlach E, Klamann MK, Gonnermann J, Bertelmann E, Joussen AM, et al. Influence of donor lamella thickness on visual acuity after Descemet's stripping automated endothelial keratoplasty (DSAEK). Ophthalmologe. 2014;111:128-34.
7. Busin M, Madi S, Santorum P, Scorcia V, Beltz J. Ultrathin Descemet's stripping automated endothelial keratoplasty with the microkeratome double-pass technique: two-year outcomes. Ophthalmology. 2013;120:1186-94.
8. Wisse RP, Achterberg JA, Van der Lelij A. DSAEK: practical approach to choose the microkeratome head on the basis of donor cornea pachymetry. Cornea. 2014;33:230-4.
9. Hsu M, Hereth WL, Moshirfar M. Double-pass microkeratome technique for ultra-thin graft preparation in Descemet's stripping automated endothelial keratoplasty. Clin Ophthalmol. 2012;6:425-32.
10. Waite A, Davidson R, Taravella MJ. Descemet-stripping automated endothelial keratoplasty donor tissue preparation using the double-pass microkeratome technique. J Cataract Refract Surg. 2013;39:446-50.
11. Vajpayee RB, Maharana PK, Jain S, Sharma N, Jhanji V. Thin lenticule Descemet's stripping automated endothelial keratoplasty: single, slow pass technique. Clin Exp Ophthalmol. 2014;42:411-6.
12. Cheung AY, Hou JH, Bedard P, Grimes V, Buckman N, Eslani M, et al. Technique for preparing ultrathin and nanothin Descemet stripping automated endothelial keratoplasty tissue. Cornea. 2018;37(5):661-6.
13. Dapena I, Ham L, Melles GR. Endothelial keratoplasty: DSEK/DSAEK or DMEK—the thinner the better? Curr Opin Ophthalmol. 2009;20:299-307.
14. Bucher F, Roters S, Mellein A, Hos D, Heindl LM, Cursiefen C, et al. "OSMO-UT-DSAEK" using THIN-C medium. Graefes Arch Clin Exp Ophthalmol. 2013;251(9):2181-5.

15. Romano V, Steger B, Chen JY, Hassaan S, Batterbury M, Willoughby CE, et al. Reliability of the effect of artificial anterior chamber pressure and corneal drying on corneal graft thickness. Cornea. 2015;34:866-9.
16. Romano V, Steger B, Myneni J, Stappler T, Wong D. Preparation of ultrathin grafts for Descemet-stripping endothelial keratoplasty with a single microkeratome pass. J Cataract Refract Surg. 2017;43:12-15.
17. Agarwal A, Dua HS, Narang P, Kumar DA, Agarwal A, Jacob S, et al. Pre-Descemet's endothelial keratoplasty (PDEK). Br J Ophthalmol. 2014;98(9):1181-5.
18. Cheng YY, van den Berg TJ, Schouten JS, Pels E, Wijdh RJ, van Cleynenbreugel H, et al. Quality of vision after femtosecond laser-assisted Descemet stripping endothelial keratoplasty and penetrating keratoplasty: a randomized, multicenter clinical trial. Am J Ophthalmol. 2011;152(4):556-66.e1.
19. Chen H, Tian L, Le Q, Zhao F, Zhao Y, Chen Y, et al. Femtosecond laser-assisted Descemet's stripping endothelial keratoplasty: a prospective study of 6-month visual outcomes, corneal thickness and endothelial cell loss. Int Ophthalmol. 2020;40(8):2065-75.
20. Trinh L, Saubaméa B, Auclin F, Denoyer A, Lai-Kuen R, El Hamdaoui M, et al. Femtosecond and excimer laser-assisted endothelial keratoplasty (FELEK): a new technique of endothelial transplantation. J Fr Ophtalmol. 2014;37(3):211-9.
21. Einan-Lifshitz A, Sorkin N, Boutin T, Showail M, Borovik A, Alobthani M, et al. Comparison of femtosecond laser-enabled descemetorhexis and manual descemetorhexis in Descemet membrane endothelial keratoplasty. Cornea. 2017;36(7):767-70.
22. Pilger D, von Sonnleithner C, Bertelmann E, Maier AB, Joussen AM, Torun N. Exploring the precision of femtosecond laser-assisted descemetorhexis in Descemet membrane endothelial keratoplasty. BMJ Open Ophthalmol. 2018;3(1):e000148.
23. Sorkin N, Mednick Z, Einan-Lifshitz A, Trinh T, Santaella G, Telli A, et al. Three-year outcome comparison between femtosecond laser-assisted and manual Descemet membrane endothelial keratoplasty. Cornea. 2019;38(7):812-6.
24. Taravella MJ, Shah V, Davidson R. Ultrathin DSAEK. Int Ophthalmol Clin. 2013;53(2):21-30.
25. Turnbull AM, Tsatsos M, Hossain PN, Anderson DF. Determinants of visual quality after endothelial keratoplasty. Surv Ophthalmol. 2016; 61(3):257-71.
26. Hirabayashi KE, Chamberlain W, Rose-Nussbaumer J, Austin A, Stell L, Lin CC. Corneal light scatter after ultrathin Descemet stripping automated endothelial keratoplasty versus Descemet membrane endothelial keratoplasty in Descemet endothelial thickness comparison trial: A randomized controlled trial. Cornea. 2020;39(6):691-6.
27. Duggan MJ, Rose-Nussbaumer J, Lin CC, Austin A, Labadzinzki PC, Chamberlain WD. Corneal higher-order aberrations in Descemet membrane endothelial keratoplasty versus ultrathin DSAEK in the Descemet endothelial thickness comparison trial: A randomized clinical trial. Ophthalmology. 2019;126(7):946-57.

34 Ultrathin Descemet Stripping Automated Endothelial Keratoplasty

Angeli Christy Yu, Asaf Friehmann, Massimo Busin

INTRODUCTION

Over the last two decades, endothelial keratoplasty (EK) has become the gold standard for the surgical management of endothelial decompensation.[1] Its advantages over conventional penetrating keratoplasty (PK) include an improved safety profile, faster visual rehabilitation, and lower rates of immunologic rejection.

Modern EK procedures can broadly be divided into Descemet stripping automated endothelial keratoplasty (DSAEK) and Descemet membrane endothelial keratoplasty (DMEK).[1] While DMEK provides faster visual rehabilitation and lower rate of immune rejection in comparison to DSAEK, adoption of DMEK has been relatively slow,[2] mainly because of challenges in graft preparation and delivery and increased frequency of postoperative complications both during and after surgery.[3] Moreover, the learning curve of DMEK is accompanied by a high rate of tissue loss of up to 16%, a high graft detachment rate of up to 63%, and a graft failure rate of up to 8%.[4-6] Additionally, in eyes with complex anterior segment anatomy such as abnormalities of the iris-lens diaphragm or in eyes with previous glaucoma surgery or pars plana vitrectomy, poor control of the DMEK graft within the anterior chamber during unfolding increases the technical complexity of the procedure and often results in excess graft manipulation.[7-10] Currently, DSAEK is still the most popular EK technique performed worldwide.[2,11]

Descemet stripping automated endothelial keratoplasty involves replacement of Descemet membrane and the diseased endothelium with donor tissue composed of a thin layer of posterior stroma, Descemet membrane, and endothelium.[1] In 2006, Holland reported that the postoperative best-corrected visual acuity of DSAEK grafts thinner 131 µm compared favorably to that of thicker grafts and even those DMEK. This data supported the correlation of postoperative vision to the morphologic characteristics of the DSAEK graft. Since then, there has been conflicting evidence on the role of central graft thickness on the postoperative visual performance following DSAEK.[12,13] However, all these studies were retrospective in design and did not account for other parameters of graft morphology other than central graft thickness. Graft regularity has increasingly been recognized as a key determinant of the quality of DSAEK grafts.[14] Aberrations derived from substantial irregularities in lenticule shape and graft thickness have been also found to play a significant role in determining the final visual outcome.[15,16]

In an attempt to improve the postoperative outcomes of DSAEK, Busin introduced the concept of ultrathin DSAEK (UT-DSAEK) in 2009. UT-DSAEK employed grafts within 100 µm in thickness, thereby, combining the visual outcomes of DMEK with the technical ease of DSAEK. UT-DSAEK employed grafts within 100 µm in thickness. Since then, double and single pass techniques have been used by surgeons and eye banks to reproducibly obtain DSAEK grafts of a predetermined thickness and planar profile, which have substantially improved the outcomes of DSAEK.[17,18]

INDICATIONS

Ultrathin-DSAEK shares the same indications of conventional DSAEK. Conditions requiring the procedure include patients with any type of endothelial dysfunction such as endothelial dystrophies including Fuchs endothelial dystrophy or posterior polymorphous dystrophy, pseudophakic or aphakic bullous keratopathy, iridocorneal endothelial syndrome and endothelial decompensation secondary to previous trauma, intraocular surgery, or failed previous grafts.[19] Like conventional DSAEK, UT-DSAEK can be performed in phakic eyes as well as in the presence of ocular comorbidities such as aniridia, aphakia, extensive iris trauma, anterior chamber intraocular lenses (ACIOLs), and previous glaucoma surgery. However, when subsequent surgery of the host cornea can be anticipated, either because of stromal ulceration or fibrosis or because of high-degree refractive errors, a thicker DSAEK graft may preferred to avoid inadvertent penetration into the anterior chamber while performing the secondary anterior procedure.

PREOPERATIVE PLANNING

The first step of the preoperative evaluation involves eliciting a careful and detailed general and ophthalmic history. The presence of concomitant eye diseases such as amblyopia, glaucoma, optic neuropathy, and retinal disease must be explored. A history of previous operations or prior infections may require modifications of the surgical technique and perioperative management.

Complete ophthalmologic examination including slit-lamp examination, best spectacle-corrected visual acuity (BSCVA), manifest refraction, applanation tonometry, and funduscopy must also be performed. Endothelial cell function is assessed by specular or confocal microscopy of the central and peripheral cornea. Additionally, anterior segment optical coherence tomography (OCT) is useful to assess corneal curvature and pachymetry.

The decision to perform either combined or sequential EK and cataract surgery is dependent on several preoperative factors. A combined procedure is often considered in patients aged 50 years and older with signs of corneal decompensation, as the retained crystalline lens will otherwise invariably develop a cataract as a consequence of both surgical trauma and postoperative topical steroid treatment.[20] Phakic UT-DSAEK may be alternatively performed in younger patients with otherwise clear crystalline lens.

If a modern flexible open loop ACIOL or an iris fixated IOL is well-positioned and of appropriate size, it may be left in place.[21,22] Otherwise, poorly positioned IOLs can be exchanged for a posterior chamber IOL (PCIOL) using transscleral suture fixation.

Finally, phakic IOLs causing progressive endothelial cell loss (ECL) may be removed at the time of a combined UT-DSAEK. Phacoemulsification and PCIOL implantation can then be sequentially performed to minimize the time required for visual rehabilitation.[23]

ANESTHESIA CONSIDERATIONS

Selection of anesthesia should be individualized for every patient. In most cases, DMEK can be performed under local anesthesia such as peribulbar or retrobulbar anesthesia. Adjunct intravenous sedation can also be considered. Decompression with a Honan balloon or similar devices for at least 10 minutes allows vitreous dehydration and softening of the eye, thereby reducing the risk of excessive posterior pressure and anterior chamber shallowing.

SURGICAL TECHNIQUE

Donor preparation is a crucial step of UT-DSAEK surgery. The donor cornea is mounted on an artificial anterior chamber (AAC) of the ALTK system (Moria, Antony, France). The central corneal thickness of the donor is measured during surgery using ultrasound pachymetry (SP-3000; Tomey GmbH).

The first attempts at standardizing UT-DSAEK graft preparation by means of a pivoting microkeratome (Carriazo-Barraquer, Moria SA, Antony, France) have led to the development of the "double-pass" technique. The technique is based on the observation that the predictability of the dissection depth is inversely proportional to the width of the microkeratome head slit.

In the double-pass technique, an initial debulking step is performed using 300 µm microkeratome head which would debulk the donor tissue to around 180–250 µm in thickness. After turning the dovetail of the AAC by 180°, a second microkeratome-assisted dissection (refinement cut) is carried out from the direction opposite to the first cut. As microkeratome dissection is deepest at the beginning of the cut, dissecting twice from opposite directions not only prevents perforation, but also equalizes peripheral graft thickness, thereby producing a regular lenticule with planar configuration and less optical aberrations. A thinner microkeratome head (90, 110, or 130 µm) is used in the refinement cut based on the Busin nomogram which has been optimized to obtain a final central graft thickness within 100 µm. The pressure of the system is standardized to an ideal level of 80–90 mm Hg by raising the infusion bottle to a height of 120 cm above the level of the AAC and then clamping the tubing at 50 cm from the entrance into the AAC. In order to obtain regular graft thickness, care must be taken in maintaining a slow uniform movement during manual microkeratome dissection.

More recently, linear microkeratomes have been used for the creation of UT-DSAEK grafts. The improved predictability of the current ALTK systems has allowed the use of single pass techniques with microkeratome heads even up to 450 µm cutting depth. An additional advantage of the single pass technique is that the dissection yields an anterior lamella thicker than that the resulting anterior lamella of the first dissection of the double-pass technique and can be more properly used for tectonic keratoplasty or deep anterior lamellar keratoplasty (DALK).

Before removing the tissue from the AAC, the stromal side is marked to facilitate correct intraoperative orientation of the graft. The posterior donor lamella is then placed on a punch with the endothelial side up and cut to the desired diameter (8.0–9.0 mm).

Recipient Preparation and Graft Delivery

The initial steps of UT-DSAEK (**Figs. 1A to D**) do not differ from those of conventional DSAEK. Prior to commencing surgery, loose, and edematous epithelium is removed from the recipient cornea to allow better intraoperative visualization and postoperative epithelialization. A small aliquot of aqueous is aspirated and air is injected intracamerally. Descemet membrane-endothelium complex is scored and stripped using a 25-gauge needle

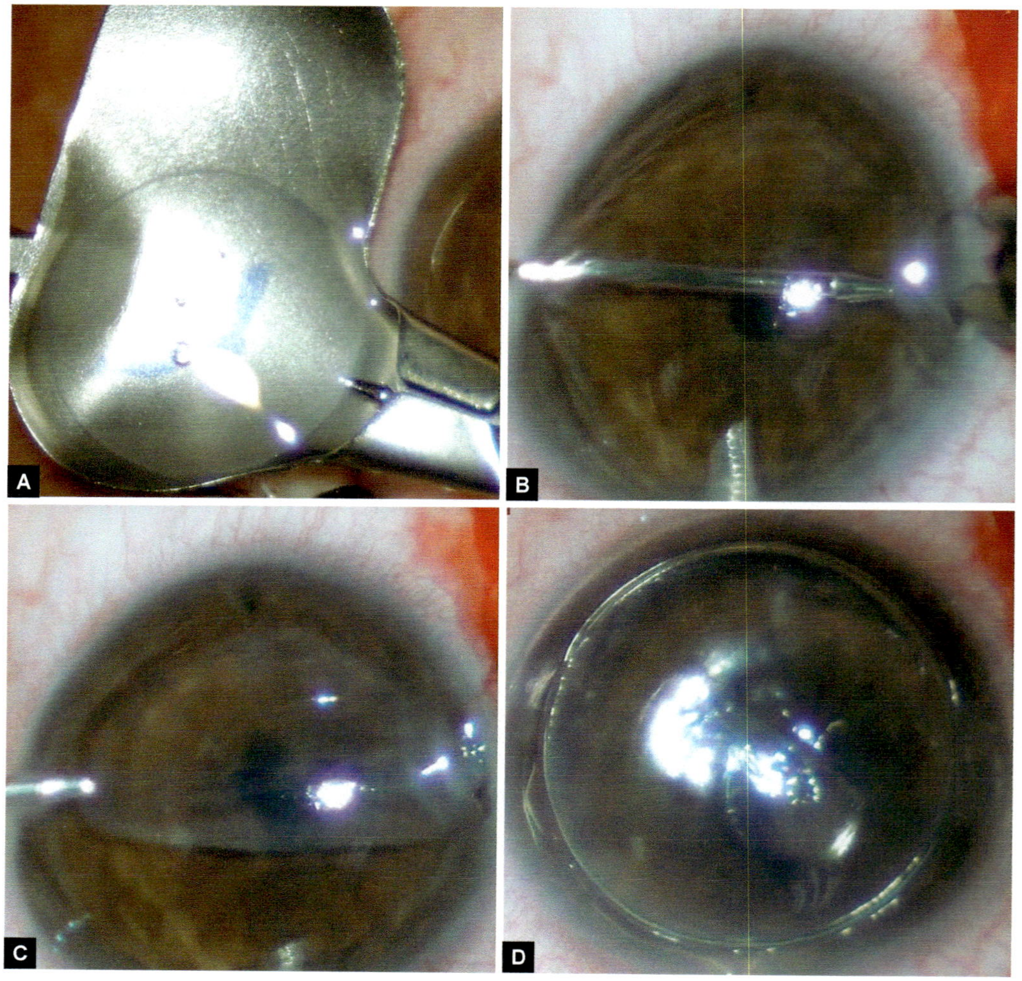

Figs. 1A to D: Intraoperative steps of ultrathin Descemet stripping automated endothelial keratoplasty.

or cannula, Descemet stripper, or reverse Sinskey hook. Gentle pressure is applied, taking care not to press into corneal stroma in order to avoid creation of stromal tissue strands. Descemetorhexis under air improves visualization and obviates the need for viscoelastic or trypan blue. In cases with poor anterior chamber visualization, Descemet membrane may be left in situ.

If not present, a peripheral iridotomy (PI) is created to avoid postoperative pupillary block. The authors prefer to perform a surgical inferior PI using guillotine micro-incision scissors under continuous irrigation from an anterior chamber maintainer.

While several glides have been developed, our preferred delivery device for UT-DSAEK is the modified Busin glide (mini-glide or mini Busin Spatula, Moria SA, Antony, France). The modified Busin glide ensures proper graft delivery with correct orientation. The graft can also be trifolded before pulling it into the glide funnel. No viscoelastic substance is required during insertion. Using micro-incision forceps inserted in the temporal paracentesis, the UT-DSAEK graft is delivered bimanually under continuous, low-flow irrigation through an anterior chamber maintainer. Delivering the graft using the pull through technique provides total control throughout the procedure and allows spontaneous unfolding of the graft with minimal graft manipulation. Gentle tapping onto the surface of the anterior cornea allows spontaneous unfolding and centration of the UT-DSAEK graft.

Both the clear cornea tunnel and the side entry are sutured watertight with interrupted 10-0 nylon sutures. The graft is attached to the posterior corneal surface by filling the anterior chamber with air. The authors prefer intracameral injection of air due to concerns of potential endothelial toxicity with SF_6 and conflicting evidence of the latter's efficacy. Triamcinolone acetonide and gentamicin sulfate, 0.3%, are injected subconjunctivally at the end of the procedure.

Combined Surgeries

Ultrathin-DSAEK can be combined with other intraocular procedures such as phacoemulsification, IOL implantation, IOL exchange, secondary IOL implantation, pupilloplasty, and vitrectomy. These procedures are often performed immediately before insertion of the UT-DSAEK graft. Viscoelastic is also preferably avoided even in combined procedures. Continuous curvilinear capsulorhexis can be performed using a bent needle mounted on a syringe filled with saline to maintain a closed system, while a foldable IOL can be injected under continuous irrigation from an anterior chamber maintainer. IOLs should be of the hydrophobic type, as recent reports have pointed out the possibility of opacification of hydrophilic IOLs after DSAEK.[24,25] Intracameral acetylcholine chloride is used to constrict the pupil after IOL implantation and prior to UT-DSAEK.

If use of viscoelastic is preferred, careful removal from the anterior chamber must be performed because retained material may hinder graft attachment or may result in interface opacities that can interfere with vision months after surgery. Intracameral acetylcholine is used to constrict the pupil after IOL implantation and prior to UT-DSAEK surgery.

Postoperative Care

Subconjunctival antibiotic and corticosteroid injections may be administered immediately after completion of surgery. A fixed combination of topical antibiotic and steroid drops are initiated every 2 hours daily and tapered off to four times daily over the first postoperative month. Subsequently, topical antibiotics is discontinued while topical steroid is slowly tapered to once daily indefinitely. Steroid-induced ocular hypertension is treated with intraocular pressure lowering agents.

After the surgery, patients are instructed to lie supine for at least 2 hours. Slit-lamp examination is then performed to check for graft attachment. Air can be removed from one of the side entries using a blunt cannula, in order to avoid pupillary block. When the graft is detached, a rebubbling procedure is performed.

RESULTS

Visual Outcomes

Comparing DMEK with UT-DSAEK (**Figs. 2A and B**), recently published randomized controlled trials comparing provide discordant results with regards to visual outcomes. Unlike the DETECT study, Dunker et al. found no significant differences in visual acuity between DMEK and UT-DSAEK as early as 3 months and up to 1 year after surgery.[19,26] No significant differences were also observed in terms of combined higher order aberrations, contrast sensitivity, straylight, and vision-related quality of life.[27-29] Although 2-year results of DETECT seemed to suggest that DMEK provides superior visual outcomes, the results were inconclusive as the loss to follow-up may have affected the study findings.[30] A larger randomized clinical trial is warranted to further clarify differences in visual acuity after DMEK and UT-DSAEK.

Refractive Outcomes

Similar to DMEK, no significant change in astigmatism is seen after UT-DSAEK.[17] While a significant-induced cylinder (up to 0.6 D) has been reported by several authors after conventional DSAEK, this is probably due to differences in incision length employed for graft delivery.[31] UT-DSAEK grafts can be delivered through a 3-mm incision using the modified Busin glide.

Mild hyperopic shifts (0.78 ± 0.59 D) commonly occur after UT-DSAEK procedures. Reversal of corneal edema after surgery can result in significant alterations in corneal curvature. Taking into account this shift during (IOL) calculations can minimize refractive surprises.

Endothelial Cell Density

Five years after UT-DSAEK, an average of 52% ECL has been observed. This is similar to the values reported after conventional DSAEK by Price et al. (53%),[32] Wacker et al. (55%),[33] and Ang et al. (48.7%),[34] and with that of DMEK by Ham et al. (55%),[35] and by Vasiliauskaite et al. (59%).[36] Randomized controlled trials comparing UT-DSAEK and DMEK likewise did not find significant differences in ECD and ECL.[19,26]

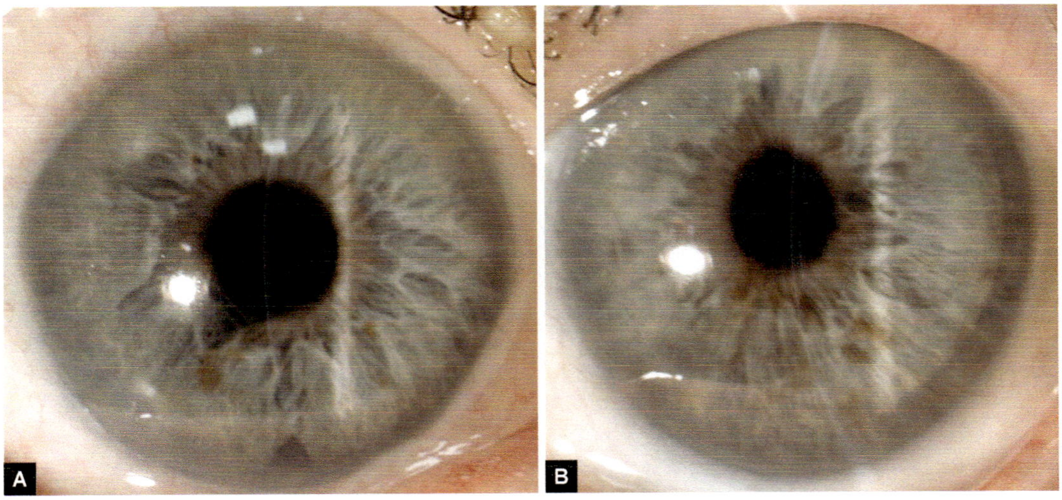

Figs. 2A and B: Postoperative images from the same patient who underwent Descemet membrane endothelial keratoplasty on the right eye (A) and ultrathin Descemet stripping automated endothelial keratoplasty on the left eye (B). Snellen visual acuity is 20/20 on both eyes.

At 1 year, the ECL was comparable with that of conventional DSAEK, despite the fact that the use of smaller (3.0-mm) incisions. After UT-DSAEK, ECD is significantly higher in glaucoma patients, as was previously reported after DSAEK.[37]

Graft Survival

One-year graft survival for conventional DSAEK in series excluding the initial learning curve has been reported to vary between 94 and 100%.[38,39] In our recent study on UT-DSAEK, Kaplan–Meier graft survival probability at 1, 2, 3, and 5 years was 99.1% (212/214 eyes), 96.2% (167/172 eyes), 94.2% (144/147 eyes), and 94.2% (105/105 eyes), respectively.[40] This compares favorably to the rates of graft survival following conventional DSAEK (93%) at 5 years with a significantly higher value for Fuchs patients (95%) than for patients with pseudophakic bullous keratopathy (76%) or previous glaucoma surgery (40%).[35] Vasiliauskaite et al. reported a cumulative survival probability of 83% [95% confidence interval (CI), 0.75–0.92] 5 years following DMEK.

COMPLICATIONS

Immunologic rejection occurs less frequently after UT-DSAEK than after DSAEK, but still occurs more frequently over DMEK.

The most common complication following UT-DSAEK is transient cystoid macular edema, which responds well to conservative treatment. Graft detachment is much less frequent than after conventional DSAEK or DMEK. In particular, the rate of rebubbling following UT-DSAEK is within 4%, which is lower than any DMEK statistic published to date. Total detachment is seen in most cases and generally successfully managed by rebubbling. Recent randomized controlled trials have shown higher rebubbling rates for DMEK compared to UT-DSAEK.[19,26] Both clinical trials report markedly similar rates of graft detachment (24%) in DMEK versus 4% in UT-DSAEK. Considering their absolute differences, the graft detachment rates after DMEK is appreciably higher than after UT-DSAEK.

Other complications of the procedure including pupillary block, persistent epithelial defect, persistent interface haze, interface infections, and cataract formation. Such adverse events do not seem to occur more or less frequently than after conventional DSAEK.

CONCLUSIONS

Ultrathin-DSAEK offers the potential to achieve the visual results of DMEK with the ease of handling and tissue preparation of conventional DSAEK. Visual recovery is faster and the proportion of eyes with final acuity of 20/20 is higher after UT-DSAEK than after conventional DSAEK, while no substantial difference is found with post-DMEK outcomes. In addition, similar to conventional DSAEK and unlike DMEK, UT-DSAEK can be performed in all types of eyes, even those with complex anatomy or poor anterior chamber visualization.

Quality control of donor tissue is mandatory in order to optimize postoperative outcomes. Although highly functional vision can still be achieved in conventional DSAEK, raising the bar must also involve standardized graft preparation that yields consistent graft quality, regularity, and thickness for UT-DSAEK.

Currently, the ability to perform DMEK is widely perceived as the hallmark of superior technical prowess in the field of corneal surgery, thereby unduly driving many novice surgeons to solely perform DMEK. Beyond the analysis of empirical evidence from published data, surgical decision making must be informed by pragmatic and prudent determination of the right procedure for the right patient by the right surgeon. Ultimately, both DMEK and UT-DSAEK represent valuable tools in the surgical armamentarium of any corneal specialist.

REFERENCES

1. Deng SX, Lee WB, Hammersmith KM, Kuo AN, Li JY, Shen JF, et al. Descemet Membrane Endothelial Keratoplasty: Safety and Outcomes. Ophthalmology. 2018;125(2):295-310.
2. Eye Bank Association of America. (2020). 2019 Eye Banking Statistical Report. [online]. Available from: https://restoresight.org/wp-content/uploads/2020/04/2019-EBAA-Stat-Report-FINAL.pdf [Last accessed December, 2021].
3. Zafar S, Parker JS, de Kort C, Melles G, Sikder S. Perceived difficulties and barriers to uptake of Descemet's membrane endothelial keratoplasty among surgeons. Clin Ophthalmol. 2019;13:1055-61.
4. Dapena I, Ham L, Droutsas K, van Dijk K, Moutsouris K, Melles GR. Learning Curve in Descemet's Membrane Endothelial Keratoplasty: First Series of 135 Consecutive Cases. Ophthalmology. 2011;118(11):2147-54.
5. Rodríguez-Calvo-de-Mora M, Quilendrino R, Ham L, Liarakos VS, van Dijk K, Baydoun L, et al. Clinical outcome of 500 consecutive cases undergoing Descemet's membrane endothelial keratoplasty. Ophthalmology. 2015;122(3):464-70.
6. Gorovoy MS. DMEK Complications. Cornea. 2014;33(1):101-4.
7. Aravena C, Yu F, Deng SX. Outcomes of Descemet membrane endothelial keratoplasty in patients with prior glaucoma surgery. Cornea. 2017;36(3):284-9.
8. Sorkin N, Mimouni M, Kisilevsky E, Boutin T, Cohen E, Trinh T, et al. Four-Year Survival of Descemet Membrane Endothelial Keratoplasty in Patients With Previous Glaucoma Surgery. Am J Ophthalmol. 2020;218:7-16.
9. Santaella G, Sorkin N, Mimouni M. Outcomes of Descemet Membrane Endothelial Keratoplasty in Aphakic and Aniridic Patients. Cornea. 2020;39(11):1389-93.
10. Spaniol K, Holtmann C, Schwinde JH, Deffaa S, Guthoff R, Geerling G. Descemet-membrane endothelial keratoplasty in patients with retinal comorbidity-a prospective cohort study. Int J Ophthalmol. 2016;9(3):390-4.
11. Dunker SL, Armitage WJ, Armitage M, Brocato L, Figueiredo FC, Heemskerk MBA, et al. Outcomes of corneal transplantation in Europe: report by the European Cornea and Cell Transplantation Registry. J Cataract Ref Surg. 2021;47(6):780-5.
12. Busin M, Albé E. Does thickness matter: ultrathin Descemet stripping automated endothelial keratoplasty. Curr Opin Ophthalmol. 2014;25(4):312-8.

13. Phillips PM, Phillips LJ, Maloney CM. Preoperative graft thickness measurements do not influence final BSCVA or speed of vision recovery after descemet stripping automated endothelial keratoplasty. Cornea. 2013;32(11):1423-7.
14. Dickman MM, Cheng YY, Berendschot TT, van den Biggelaar FJ, Nuijts RM. Effects of graft thickness and asymmetry on visual gain and aberrations after Descemet stripping automated endothelial keratoplasty. JAMA Ophthalmol. 2013;131:737-44.
15. Rudolph M, Laaser K, Bachmann BO, Cursiefen C, Epstein D, Kruse FE. Corneal higher-order aberrations after Descemet's membrane endothelial keratoplasty. Ophthalmology. 2012;119(3):528-35.
16. Ruzza A, Parekh M, Ferrari S, Salvalaio G, Nahum Y, Bovone C, et al. Preloaded donor corneal lenticules in a new validated 3D printed smart storage glide for Descemet stripping automated endothelial keratoplasty. Br J Ophthalmol. 2015;99(10):1388-95.
17. Busin M, Madi S, Santorum P, Scorcia V, Beltz J. Ultrathin descemet's stripping automated endothelial keratoplasty with the microkeratome double-pass technique: two-year outcomes. Ophthalmology. 2013;120(6):1186-94.
18. Villarrubia A, Cano-Ortiz A. Development of a nomogram to achieve ultrathin donor corneal disks for Descemet-stripping automated endothelial keratoplasty. J Cataract Refract Surg. 2015;41(1):146-51.
19. Dunker SL, Dickman MM, Wisse RPL, Nobacht S, Wijdh RHJ, Bartels MC, et al. DMEK versus ultrathin DSAEK: a multicenter randomized controlled clinical trial. Ophthalmology. 2020;127(9):1152-9.
20. Burkhart ZN, Feng MT, Price FW Jr, Price MO. One-year outcomes in eyes remaining phakic after Descemet membrane endothelial keratoplasty. J Cataract Refract Surg. 2014;40(3):430-4.
21. Elderkin S, Tu E, Sugar J, Reddy S, Kadakia A, Ramaswamy R, et al. Outcome of descemet stripping automated endothelial keratoplasty in patients with an anterior chamber intraocular lens. Cornea. 2010;29(11):1273-7.
22. Beltz J, Busin M. Descemet stripping automated endothelial keratoplasty in a case with a posteriorly fixated iris-claw intraocular lens. Cornea. 2012;31(1):96-7.
23. Nahum Y, Busin M. Quadruple procedure for visual rehabilitation of endothelial decompensation following phakic intraocular lens implantation. Am J Ophthalmol. 2014;158(6):1330-4.
24. Ahad MA, Darcy K, Cook SD, Tole DM. Intraocular lens opacification after descemet stripping automated endothelial keratoplasty. Cornea. 2014;33(12):1307-11.
25. Werner L, Wilbanks G, Nieuwendaal CP, Dhital A, Waite A, Schmidinger G, et al. Localized opacification of hydrophilic acrylic intraocular lenses after procedures using intracameral injection of air or gas. J Cataract Refract Surg. 2015;41(1):199-207.
26. Chamberlain W, Lin CC, Austin A, Schubach N, Clover J, McLeod SD, et al. Descemet endothelial thickness comparison trial: a randomized trial comparing ultrathin Descemet stripping automated endothelial keratoplasty with Descemet membrane endothelial keratoplasty. Ophthalmology. 2019;126:19-26.
27. Duggan MJ, Rose-Nussbaumer J, Lin CC, Austin A, Labadzinzki PC, Chamberlain WD. Corneal Higher-Order Aberrations in Descemet Membrane Endothelial Keratoplasty versus Ultrathin DSAEK in the Descemet Endothelial Thickness Comparison Trial: A Randomized Clinical Trial. Ophthalmology. 2019;126(7):946-57.
28. Ang MJ, Chamberlain W, Lin CC, Pickel J, Austin A, Rose-Nussbaumer J. Effect of Unilateral Endothelial Keratoplasty on Vision-Related Quality-of-Life Outcomes in the Descemet Endothelial Thickness Comparison Trial (DETECT): A Secondary Analysis of a Randomized Clinical Trial. JAMA Ophthalmol. 2019;137(7):747-54.
29. Dunker SL, Dickman MM, Wisse RPL, Nobacht S, Wijdh RHJ, Bartels MC, et al. Quality of vision and vision-related quality of life after Descemet membrane endothelial keratoplasty: a randomized clinical trial. Acta Ophthalmol. 2021;99(7):e1127-e1134.
30. Rose-Nussbaumer J, Lin CC, Austin A, Liu Z, Clover J, McLeod SD, et al. Descemet Endothelial Thickness Comparison Trial: Two-Year Results from a Randomized Trial Comparing Ultrathin Descemet Stripping Automated Endothelial Keratoplasty with Descemet Membrane Endothelial Keratoplasty. Ophthalmology. 2021;128(8):1238-40.
31. Koenig SB, Covert DJ. Early results of small-incision Descemet's stripping and automated endothelial keratoplasty. Ophthalmology. 2007;114(2):221-6.
32. Price MO, Fairchild KM, Price DA. Descemet's stripping endothelial keratoplasty: five-year graft survival and endothelial cell loss. Ophthalmology. 2011;118:725-9.
33. Wacker K, Baratz KH, Maguire LJ, McLaren JW, Patel SV. Descemet stripping endothelial keratoplasty for Fuchs' endothelial corneal dystrophy: five-year results of a prospective study. Ophthalmology. 2016;123:154-60.
34. Ang M, Soh Y, Htoon HM, Mehta JS, Tan D. Five-year graft survival comparing Descemet stripping automated endothelial keratoplasty and penetrating keratoplasty. Ophthalmology. 2016;123:1646-52.
35. Ham L, Dapena I, Liarakos VS, Baydoun L, van Dijk K, Ilyas A, et al. Midterm results of Descemet membrane endothelial keratoplasty: 4 to 7 years clinical outcome. Am J Ophthalmol. 2016;171:113-21.
36. Vasiliauskaite I, Oellerich S, Ham L, Dapena I, Baydoun L, van Dijk K, et al. Descemet Membrane Endothelial Keratoplasty: Ten-Year Graft Survival and Clinical Outcomes. Am J Ophthalmol. 2020;217:114-20.
37. Quek DT, Wong T, Tan D, Mehta JS. Corneal graft survival and intraocular pressure control after descemet stripping automated endothelial keratoplasty in eyes with pre-existing glaucoma. Am J Ophthalmol. 2011;152(1):48-54.
38. Busin M, Bhatt PR, Scorcia V. A modified technique for descemet membrane stripping automated endothelial keratoplasty to minimize endothelial cell loss. Arch Ophthalmol. 2008;126(8):1133-7.
39. Price MO, Gorovoy M, Benetz BA, Price FW Jr, Menegay HJ, Debanne SM, et al. Descemet's stripping automated endothelial keratoplasty outcomes compared with penetrating keratoplasty from the Cornea Donor Study. Ophthalmology. 2010;117(3):438-44.
40. Madi S, Leon P, Nahum Y, D'Angelo S, Giannaccare G, Beltz J, et al. Five-Year Outcomes of Ultrathin Descemet Stripping Automated Endothelial Keratoplasty. Cornea. 2019;38:1192-7.

35 Manual DSEK: "Manual Dissection" Technique of Descemet Stripping Endothelial Keratoplasty

Samar K Basak, Soham Basak

INTRODUCTION

Endothelial dysfunction from surgery or diseases is one of the leading indications for corneal transplantation. The only solution for this dysfunction over the past 100 years has been penetrating keratoplasty (PK) which was considered as the gold standard for treating this disorder.[1] But its disadvantages are well known: they are delayed rehabilitation, long visual recovery time, and poor visual quality due to high and irregular astigmatism. Furthermore, there are surface and suture-related problems, more chance of graft rejection or infection, greatest risk of trauma and wound dehiscence, frequent and long follow-up visits, and problems of long-term use of topical steroids.[2]

Descemet stripping endothelial keratoplasty (DSEK) represents the one of the preferred types of posterior lamellar keratoplasty for endothelial dysfunctions for the past 15 years. It allows selective replacement of diseased host endothelium with a suitable and healthy donor posterior lamella (endothelium, Descemet membrane, and about 100–150 μm of the posterior stroma).

The advantages of DSEK are: Faster visual recovery, better uncorrected visual acuity because of less astigmatism and without any irregular astigmatism. Furthermore, there are no suture- and surface-related problems, no infection, no chance of graft dehiscence, and less incidence of graft rejection. It also minimizes the follow-up visits and use of corticosteroids to softer steroids. But it has its own disadvantages—such as, donor dislocation, higher iatrogenic primary graft failure, longer operating time (for beginners), and a relatively steeper learning curve.[3]

Lamellar dissection of donor tissue mounted on an artificial anterior chamber (AC) was initially started manually using different types of keratome. Later with the introduction of automated microkeratome [Descemet stripping automated endothelial keratoplasty (DASEK)], the dissection is much easier with smooth interface compared to manual dissection. However, this microkeratome is hugely expensive and may not be available to all corneal surgeons, especially in the developing countries. Moreover, there is involvement of certain consumables which add to the cost.

We are doing manual dissection of donor tissue and DSEK since July, 2006. It is relatively easy with much less costly instruments, which is accessible to every corneal surgeon across the world. The results are equally comparable.[4] Till date I have completed >1,200 DSEK surgeries with similar technique and instrumentation. The other surgeons (including the junior surgeons) are regularly performing manual DSEK and in total we have done >2,500 DSEK procedures over last 14 years. This technique is easily reproducible as evident by "DSEK surgical skill transfer workshop" organized at our hospital every year which focuses on training junior surgeons across the country.

DESCEMET STRIPPING ENDOTHELIAL KERATOPLASTY: DONOR TISSUE PREREQUISITES

- Healthy young donor tissue ≤65 years
- McCarey-Kaufman (MK) medium/Cornisol (Aurolab, India)/Optisol-GS (Bausch and Lomb) preserved cornea
- Scleral rim must be 2–2.5 mm all around during corneoscleral button preparation (or overall diameter is 15.5–16.0 mm).
- The corneoscleral button should be free from loose conjunctiva or iris tissue.
- Donor endothelial cell count must be ≥2,500/mm^2.
- It is wise to keep stand by 2nd optical quality tissue—for the first few cases.

DESCEMET STRIPPING ENDOTHELIAL KERATOPLASTY: RECIPIENT PREOPERATIVE PREPARATION

- Moxifloxacin (0.5%) eye drop—four times at 5 minutes interval—30 minutes before surgery
- Constrict pupil by pilocarpine (2%) eye drop—three times at 5 minutes interval—30 minutes before surgery (for only DSEK cases)

- Dilate pupil for combined cataract surgery [DSEK with phaco or with manual small incision cataract surgery (SICS) with posterior chamber intraocular lens (PCIOL) implantation: DSEK-triple]
- Povidone iodine antiseptic
- Routine peribulbar block
- Patient should go to the toilet before surgery

DESCEMET STRIPPING ENDOTHELIAL KERATOPLASTY: SPECIAL INSTRUMENTATION

- Artificial anterior chamber (**Fig. 1**)
- Guarded depth blades—disposable, or diamond (500 μm, 450 μm, or variable depth), or No 11 blade
- 8.0/8.5/9.0 mm marker/marker Pen
- Special lamellar dissector (**Fig. 2**)
- Fine toothed forceps
- Viscoelastic—sodium hyaluronate (1%)
- Reverse Sinskey's hook
- Utrata forceps

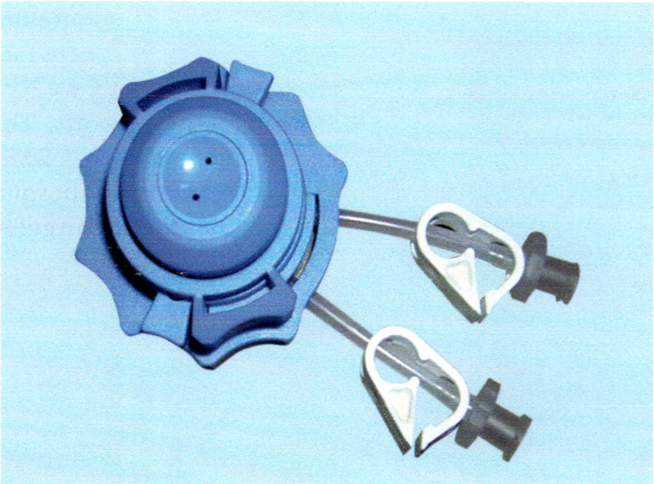

Fig. 1: Barron's artificial anterior chamber.

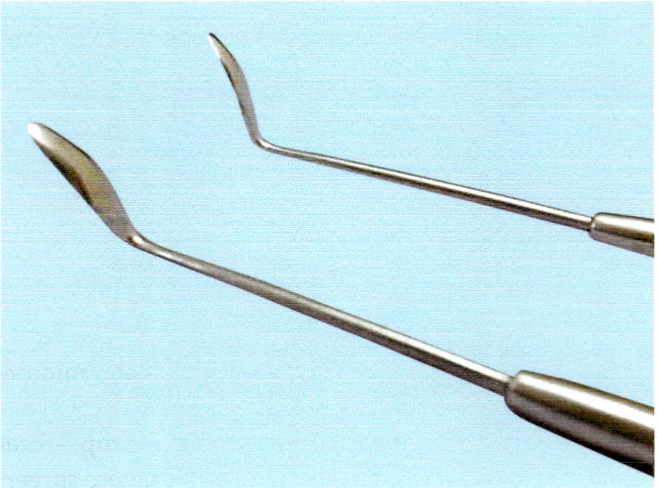

Fig. 2: Lamellar dissector.

DESCEMET STRIPPING ENDOTHELIAL KERATOPLASTY: RECIPIENT VERSUS DONOR DISK DIAMETER

- Donor size and host Descemet stripping area is the same (7.0–9.0 mm)
- Determined by diameter of the recipient's cornea
- Must have 1 mm working space—on either side for donor manipulation through the side ports
- During measurement, always try to give more (**Table 1**)
- So, it may be unconventional size, e.g., 7.25, 7.75, and 8.25, etc.

Anesthesia

Routine peribulbar block using a mixture of 2% lignocaine and 0.75% bupivacaine or 0.5% ropivacaine (1:1) and hyaluronidase. General anesthesia may be required rarely.

Surgical Technique Step-by-step

Mounting the Sclerocorneal Button on Barron's Artificial Anterior Chamber[5]

The Barron's artificial anterior chamber (Katena Products, Inc., NJ, USA) is comprised of three parts:

1. Base with tissue pedestal
2. Tissue retainer
3. Locking ring

The base has two ports with silicone tubing, in-line pinch clamps, and female Luer-lock connectors. Either port may be used to inject balanced salt solution (BSS) or air beneath the donor cornea to form artificial AC (**Fig. 3**). For mounting the donor cornea, and for best results, the overall diameter should be between 15 and 17 mm.

- Balanced salt solution is injected into one of the tubing ports and then lock this tubing. Remove the excess BSS from the well in the tissue pedestal.

Table 1: Difference in number of endothelial cells transferred during DSEK with different trephine sizes (assuming endothelial cell count@2,000/mm^2).

Diameter	*Area = πr^2*	*Cells transferred*
7.50 mm	44.2 mm^2	88,400
8.00 mm	50.3 mm^2	100,600
8.50 mm	56.8 mm^2	113,535
9.0 mm	63.6 mm^2	127,285
7.75 mm	46.6 mm^2	93,200
8.25 mm	52.8 mm^2	105,660
8.75 mm	59.5 mm^2	118,941

(DSEK: Descemet stripping endothelial keratoplasty)

Note: When the difference is *conventional* (i.e., 0.50 mm) = we are adding 12,000–14,000 cells. But, when it is *unconventional* (i.e., 0.25 mm) = we are still transferring 5,000–6,000 cells more.

- Put a drop of sodium hyaluronate (Healon, Advanced Medical Optics, Inc., Uppsala, Sweden) into the well prior to placement of the donor tissue.
- Tissue is placed carefully so that the cornea is well centered in the well and the scleral rim is covering the concentric rings around the well equally on all sides.
- With the tissue in place, carefully align the two holes of the tissue retainer with two pegs projected from the base and press down firmly.
- Now place the locking ring over the tissue retainer and turn clockwise until the ring is locked firmly in place.
- Additional air is now injected via the other tubing ports to obtain the desired pressure, then again lock the pinch clamp. Check the pressure by index finger or by any flat instrument. If required further tighten the locking ring. During the dissection process, both pinch clamps are to be locked to maintain the desired AC pressure.
- After complete dissection of the donor tissue, first unlock the locking ring, release the two pinch clamps, then withdraw the tissue retainer and now the tissue is ready for transfer.

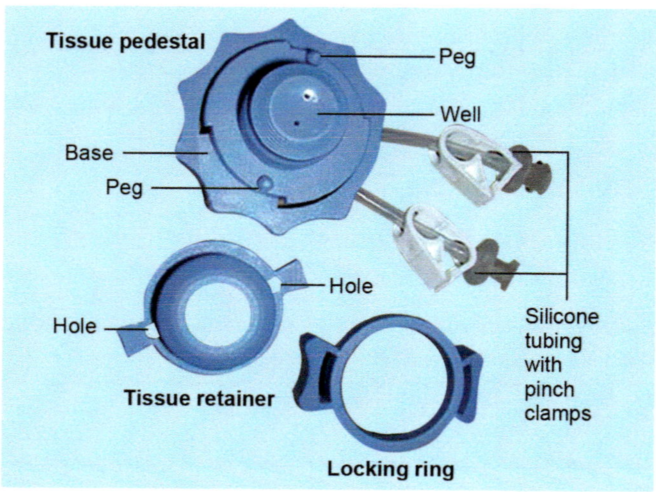

Fig. 3: Barron's artificial anterior chamber.

Donor Lamellar Tissue Preparation (Figs. 4 and 5)

- The donor cornea with its scleral rim is mounted on a disposable artificial AC.
- The central point and 8.0–9.0 mm trephination site are marked with gentian violet. Initial 5 mm corneal incision is first made at the limbus with a guarded depth blade.
- Choosing the depth of initial incision—depends on the storage media. With MK media the tissue is more edematous so 450- or 500-µm depth is ideal. Whereas with Cornisol or Optisol-GS, the tissue is more compact—here a 380- or 400-µm depth incision is preferred. If handheld pachymetry is available, then this depth can further be titrated and customized with variable guarded blade.
- Manual lamellar dissection is then carried out at approximately two-thirds depth with a crescent blade and innovative spatula by close method.
- After complete lamellar dissection of whole cornea, the donor tissue is transferred on a Teflon block with endothelial side up, filled up with storage medium or BSS

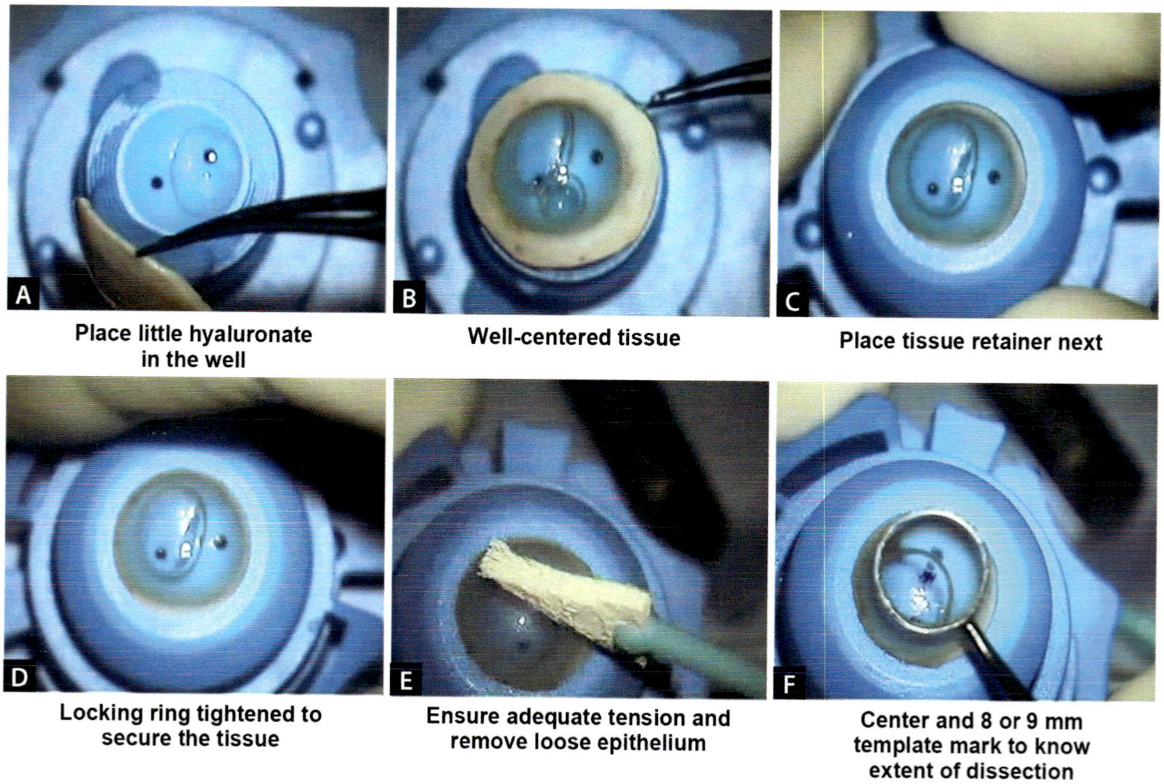

Figs. 4A to F: *Step-by-step*: Donor cornea mounting in artificial anterior chamber.

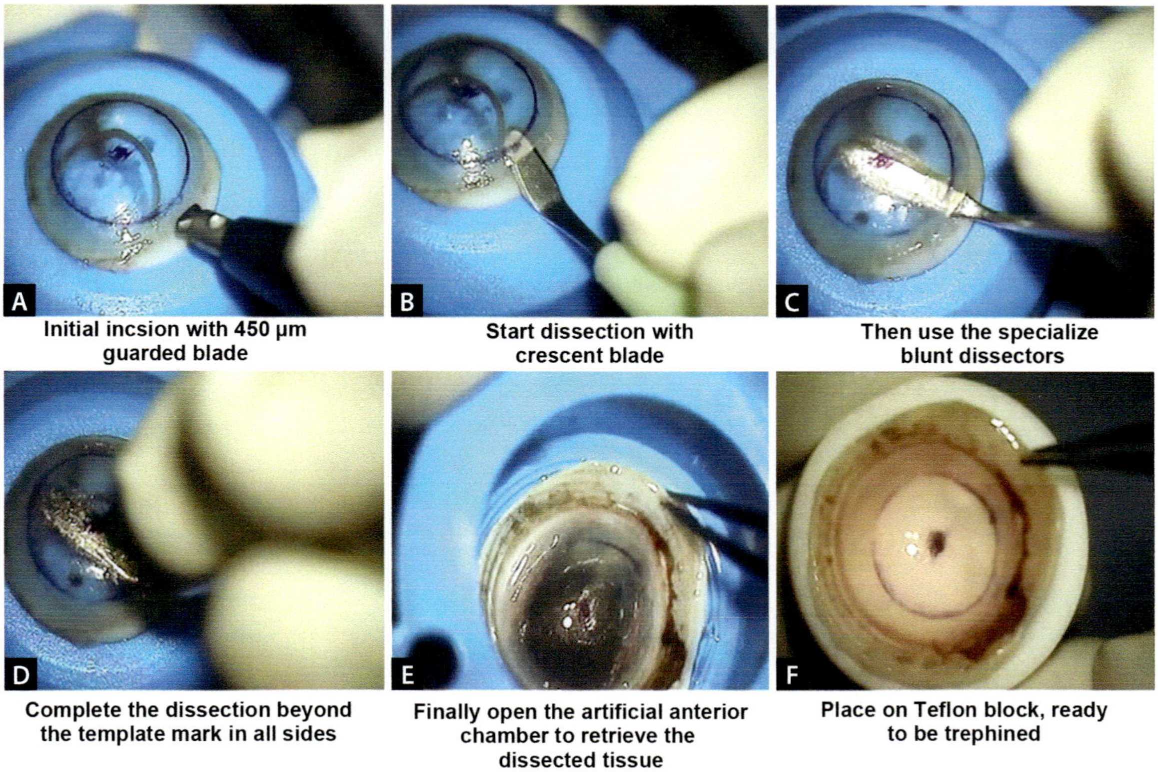

Figs. 5A to F: *Step-by-step* "manual dissection" technique.

and is covered for further preparation of appropriate size donor lenticule later on.

Recipient Bed Preparation

- A circular template mark (with a diameter of 7.5, 8.0, 8.5, or 9.0 mm) with gentian violet is made on the corneal epithelial surface which serves as a reference mark for Descemet stripping. In some cases, loose, edematous, and hypertrophied epithelium is removed before marking.
- After making a conjunctival flap and applying wet field cautery, a 5–5.5-mm sclerocorneal tunnel is prepared just like making a tunnel in manual small incision cataract surgery.
- Two 1-mm side ports are made on either side of the main incision at 10 and 2 o'clock positions. These are to manipulate and unfold the donor lenticule within AC.
- Cohesive viscoelastic agent, 1% sodium hyaluronate (Healon, Advanced Medical Optics, Inc, Uppsala, Sweden) is injected through the side port. Dispersive viscoelastic agent should not be used during any step of the procedure.
- The AC is entered with a 2.8-mm angular keratome in such a way that the internal incision is at or posterior to the template line. It is enlarged on either side to the same length as the external incision.
- In patients who undergo a combined procedure (DSEK and manual SICS with PCIOL), the cataract surgery is performed through a 6.0-mm tunnel and irrigating vectis technique is used to remove the nucleus. After cortical cleaning, a 6.0-mm single-piece PCIOL is placed in the bag. Every attempt is made to overlap the capsulorrhexis margin by 1 mm on the optic of the IOL. The IOL power is calculated from the spectacle history or from the biometry of the same or the other eye. The pupil is then constricted with intracameral pilocarpine (0.5%) injection.
- Circular dissection of the Descemet membrane (or Descemet scoring) is carried out with a reverse Sinskey's hook which corresponds to the 8.0–9.0 mm epithelial template mark. Descemet membrane is completely stripped off with the help of the hook, and the diseased tissue is removed. In some cases, with severe corneal edema, trypan blue (0.06%) solution is used to stain the diseased endothelium and it is also useful to stain the anterior capsule in the combined procedure.
- Viscoelastic agent is then washed out thoroughly and carefully with BSS using an irrigation/aspiration cannula, and AC was then well formed with BSS.

Transplantation of Donor Lenticule

- The posterior lamellar donor lenticule is punched from the endothelial side on the Teflon block using a same-size disposable trephine (8.0, 8.2, 8.5, 8.7, or 9.0 mm). It was then transferred on the recipient's corneal surface with the endothelial side up.
- The endothelial side is coated and protected by a thin layer of Healon. The posterior lamella of the donor tissue

is then folded into an asymmetric "taco-shape", in a 60:40% ratio with a fine (0.12 mm) forceps grasping only the edge of the donor lenticule. This "taco" is gently held at the leading edge with an Utrata forceps with 60%-side up and is inserted through the tunnel into the AC like a foldable IOL. The platforms of the Utrata forceps do not oppose (noncoapting) thereby minimizing the crush injury to the donor endothelium.

- The AC is filled up by BSS and one could notice the tissue is unfolding to 60–80°. Air is then injected carefully through a 30-gauze cannula from the left-side port to unfold the donor lenticule completely.
- Centering of the donor lenticule is done by massaging over the cornea with an iris repositor or round cannula. More air is injected until a "golden ring" was observed around the edge of the donor lenticule. Interface fluid is removed by gentle massage and stroking the corneal epithelial surface with a flat cannula.
- The microscope light is turned off and the eye is left undisturbed for 10 minutes.
- After 10 minutes, 30–40% of the AC air bubble is replaced with BSS. The intraocular tension is checked digitally. The conjunctiva is closed by wet field cautery. Patient receives subconjunctival injection of dexamethasone and gentamycin, and one drop of atropine is put at the end of the procedure. A bandage contact lens is given in selective cases when more than two-thirds of the recipient's corneal epithelium is removed during the procedure.
- The eye is patched, and the patient was instructed to lie supine for at least 4–6 hours.

Postoperative Management

The patient is instructed to lie supine for at least 4–6 hours. The topical medication is started after that. The patients are discharged after 24–48 hours. Special instruction is given not to rub the operated eye. Postoperatively, the patients receive topical antibiotics four times, timolol maleate (0.5%) twice, and mydriatic eye drop twice daily for the first 10 days. In addition, they also receive topical prednisolone eight times daily for 1 week and then six times daily for the next 3 weeks. After 1 month, the dose of topical prednisolone is gradually tapered over 6 months and finally maintained on topical fluorometholone—once daily dose and continued. The same regimen is employed in patients with DSEK triple procedure.

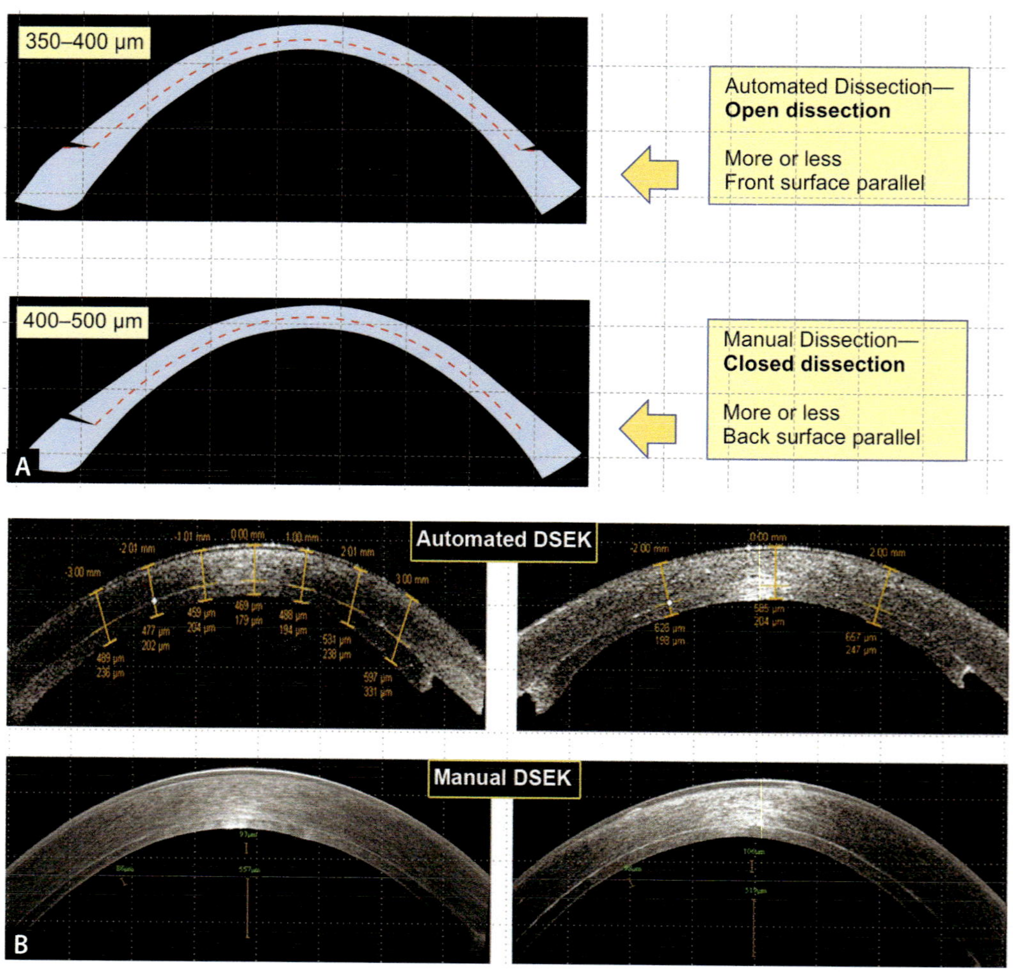

Figs. 6A and B: Graft thickness in automated versus manual dissection.[6]
(DSEK: Descemet stripping endothelial keratoplasty)

DIFFERENCE WITH AUTOMATED DESCEMET STRIPPING ENDOTHELIAL KERATOPLASTY

- The dissection in manual techniques is a closed method, whereas in automated process it is an open method. In other words, the lamellar dissection is accessible only through an incision in the manual method, but the automated technique creates a separate tissue cap after the microkeratome pass (**Fig. 6A**).
- The thickness of the lenticule in manual DSEK is planar—the thickness is equal at the center and periphery. Conversely, the automated DSEK lenticule has a concave profile, thinner in the center and thicker at the periphery. Because of this, the manual DSEK lenticule by itself causes minimal spherical power change (**Fig. 6B**).

Complications of Manual Descemet Stripping Endothelial Keratoplasty Graft Preparation

Various complications may arise while preparing the graft such as button-holing or perforation. Sometimes, if these happen in the peripherally, the same tissue can be rescued and prepared from a different deeper or superficial plane. If the damage is central or large in area, the tissue unfortunately must be replaced.

Table 2 shows the various donor preparation complications from a large series of 430 DSEK surgeries published by the author.[7] Thinner grafts are difficult to unfold and needs more manipulation, while thicker grafts take longer time to get optically clear and compact.

Manual dissection in DSEK is the least expensive and may be the more appropriate procedure in the Indian scenario. It is simple, requires less costly instrumentation, with short learning curve and easily reproducible.

Table 2: Complications of various donor preparation.

Complications	*No.*	*Percentage*
Descemet's perforation of the donor cornea*	1	0.2
Excessive thick donor preparation*	2	0.5
Buttonholing of the donor cornea#	2	0.2
Too thin donor preparation^	8	1.9
Total	13	3.0

*Change with a new donor button in 3 cases (0.7%)
#New area was selected and donor dissection completed
^Handled the lamellar tissue delicately and used

Proprietary/Financial interest: None
Conflict of interest: None

REFERENCES

1. Sugar A, Sugar J. Techniques in penetrating keratoplasty: A quarter century of development. Cornea. 2000;19:603-10.
2. Patel SV. Keratoplasty for endothelial dysfunction. Ophthalmology. 2007;114:627-8.
3. Lee WB, Jacobs DS, Musch DC, Kaufman SC, Reinhart WJ, Shtein RM. Descemet's stripping endothelial keratoplasty: safety and outcomes: a report by the American Academy of Ophthalmology. Ophthalmology. 2009;116:1818-30.
4. Basak SK. Descemet stripping and endothelial keratoplasty in endothelial dysfunctions: three-month results in 75 eyes. Indian J Ophthalmol. 2008;56:291-6.
5. Barron Artificial Anterior Chamber; Katena Products, Inc., Denville, NJ, USA. www.katena.com.
6. Price MO, Price FW. Descemet's stripping with endothelial keratoplasty: comparative outcomes with microkeratome-dissected and manually dissected donor tissue. Ophthalmology. 2006;113:1936-42.
7. Basak SK, Basak S. Complications and management in Descemet's stripping endothelial keratoplasty: analysis of consecutive 430 cases. Indian J Ophthalmol. 2014;62:209-18.

36 Pre-Descemet's Endothelial Keratoplasty

Amar Agarwal

INTRODUCTION

Endothelial keratoplasty (EK) comprises Descemet's membrane endothelial keratoplasty (DMEK) and Descemet's stripping endothelial keratoplasty (DSEK) as the major variants whereas many surgeons have also employed their automated version of Descemet's membrane automated endothelial keratoplasty (DMAEK) and Descemet's stripping automated endothelial keratoplasty (DSAEK) across the globe. In terms of visual output, DMEK as an EK procedure has always scored inspite of it being technically challenging as compared to other subtypes. Melles et al. described DMEK that represents the perfect anatomic replacement of the diseased Descemet's membrane (DM)-endothelium complex with a healthy donor DM-endothelium.[1,2]

Pre-Descemet's endothelial keratoplasty (PDEK)[3] being a new variant in the field of EK further extends the lexicon of EK that mainly comprises of the separation of pre-Descemet's membrane (PDL) along with DM-endothelium complex from the residual donor stroma by the formation a type-1 bubble (bb).[4] The feasibility of the PDEK procedure with both an adult and infant donor tissue[3,5] makes it highly acceptable in the era of shortage of donor tissue.

IMPORTANCE OF AIR DISSECTION AND TYPES OF BUBBLES

Air dissection is a well-established entity that relegates the use of micro forceps or a micro keratome for dissection of the corneal stroma. An air-filled syringe is used to inject air into the stroma with the endothelial side up and is advanced under direct observation at a required depth beneath the endothelium. The advantage with air dissection is that it is cost effective as it is done manually by the surgeon and the major drawback with it is that it requires a certain amount of surgical skill set on behalf of the surgeon as the needle that is employed to inject air must be introduced at the correct depth below the DM-endothelium complex.

Type-1 Bubble

Type-1 bubble is the kind of bb that is essential to obtain for performing a PDEK procedure. This bb typically spreads from center to periphery and is dome shaped. The diameter of the bb usually varies from 7.5 to 8.5 mm; this bb never extends to extreme periphery due to adhesions between the PDL and the residual stroma. Injection of air leads to separation of the PDL-DM-endothelium complex in to from the residual stromal bed (**Figs. 1A to D**).

Type-2 Bubble

Type-2 bubble is typically formed when the air enters the plane between the PDL and the DM-endothelium complex. Type-2 bb typically spreads from periphery to center and is around 10–11 mm in diameter. It extends up to extreme periphery as there are no adhesions between the PDL and the DM (**Figs. 2A to D**). With the formation of this bb, it becomes essential to perform a DMEK instead of a PDEK procedure. Immense care should be taken when a type-2 bb is formed as it has a thin wall and if it is subjected to excessive air push then the bb can rupture leading to perforation of graft and eventually transcending into donor tissue wastage.

Mixed Bubble

When both type-1 and type-2 bubbles are formed and they coexist; mixed bubble is said to have been achieved. These types of bubbles pose a surgical challenge to the surgeon, as it requires delicate handling and manipulation to avoid the rupture of the bubble.

During the process of bb formation, the tip of the needle may rupture the endothelium (**Figs. 3A and B**), which is completely an undesirable event as it may often lead to a situation where the corneal tissue can no longer be used and needs to be discarded as neither a type-1 nor a type-2 bubble can be created either for a PDEK or a DMEK procedure, respectively. However, if the DM perforation occurs and if it is recognized the surgeon can withhold the injection of air. The surgeon can again withdraw and re-enter at a deeper plane as

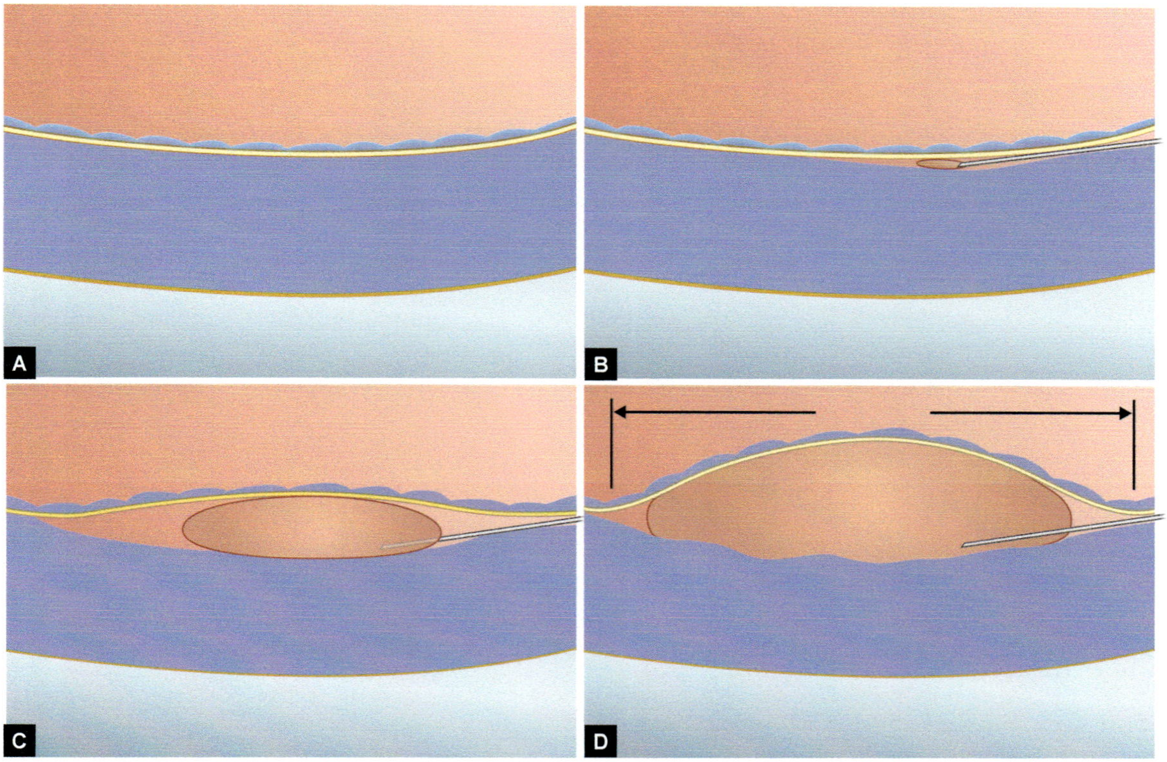

Figs. 1A to D: Graphical display of creation of Type-1 bubble (bb). (A) All the layers of cornea with graft placed with endothelial side up; (B) An air filled 30 G needle introduced from the periphery beneath the pre-Descemet's layer (PDL). The PDL-Descemet's membrane (DM)-endothelium complex is seen lying above the bevel of the needle; (C) Further injection of air lifts the entire PDL-DM-endothelium complex that comprises of pre-Descemet's endothelial keratoplasty (PDEK) graft above the residual stroma; (D) Fully formed type-1 bb formed (Yellow color-PDL).

compared to the previous one and again attempt at making a bb. Alternatively, a cannula attached to a syringe filled with viscoelastic can also be taken and can be reintroduced to make a bb, although the use of viscoelastic is not recommended. The advantage with the use of viscoelastic is that it seems to plug the small hole in the DM and facilitates the creation of the type-1 bb (**Figs. 3A to D**). Eventually, if the hole in the DM is big enough then one should discard the graft.

Occasionally, a very small bb is formed after injection of air. In such a scenario, viscoelastic can come to the rescue of the surgeon as injection of viscoelastic facilitates the breakdown of superficial adhesions between the PDL and the stromal layer, as it tends to overcome resistance offered by the collagenous layer better than air.

Despite all the surgical challenges that a surgeon comes across in the creation of a bubble, the surgical competence and the correct art of handling the corneal tissue effectively saves the loss of corneal tissue, renders economic practicality, and enhances the productivity by retaining the clinical merits of the PDEK procedure.

SURGICAL TECHNIQUE

Donor-graft Preparation

Bubble Creation

The donor button with the corneoscleral rim is dissected from the whole cornea and is placed with the endothelial side up. For the process of bb creation, a 30 G needle is used that is attached to an air filled 5 mL syringe. The needle is introduced with a bevel up position from the periphery up to the mid peripheral area at a considerable depth from the DM so as to create a plane of separation between the PDL and the residual stroma (**Fig. 4A**). Air is injected and a type-1 bb is formed that is dome-shaped and is around 8 mm in diameter.

Graft Staining

Staining of the graft is done with trypan blue that allows a considerable clear visualization of the graft. The bb is penetrated with a side port blade at the extreme periphery (**Fig. 4B**) and trypan blue is injected inside (**Fig. 4C**). The bb is then cut all across the periphery with a corneoscleral scissors (**Fig. 4D**) and is placed in the storage media.

Recipient Bed Preparation

The procedure is performed under local anesthesia; supplemental anesthesia is administered as necessary.

In cases of bullous keratopathy, the initial step comprises of scrapping and debridement of epithelium. This facilitates enhanced intraoperative view during the surgical procedure. An anterior chamber maintainer (ACM) or a Trocar ACM (T-ACM)[6] is introduced in to the eye that is connected to the air pump. This helps to maintain adequate depth of anterior chamber (AC) at all times and it also

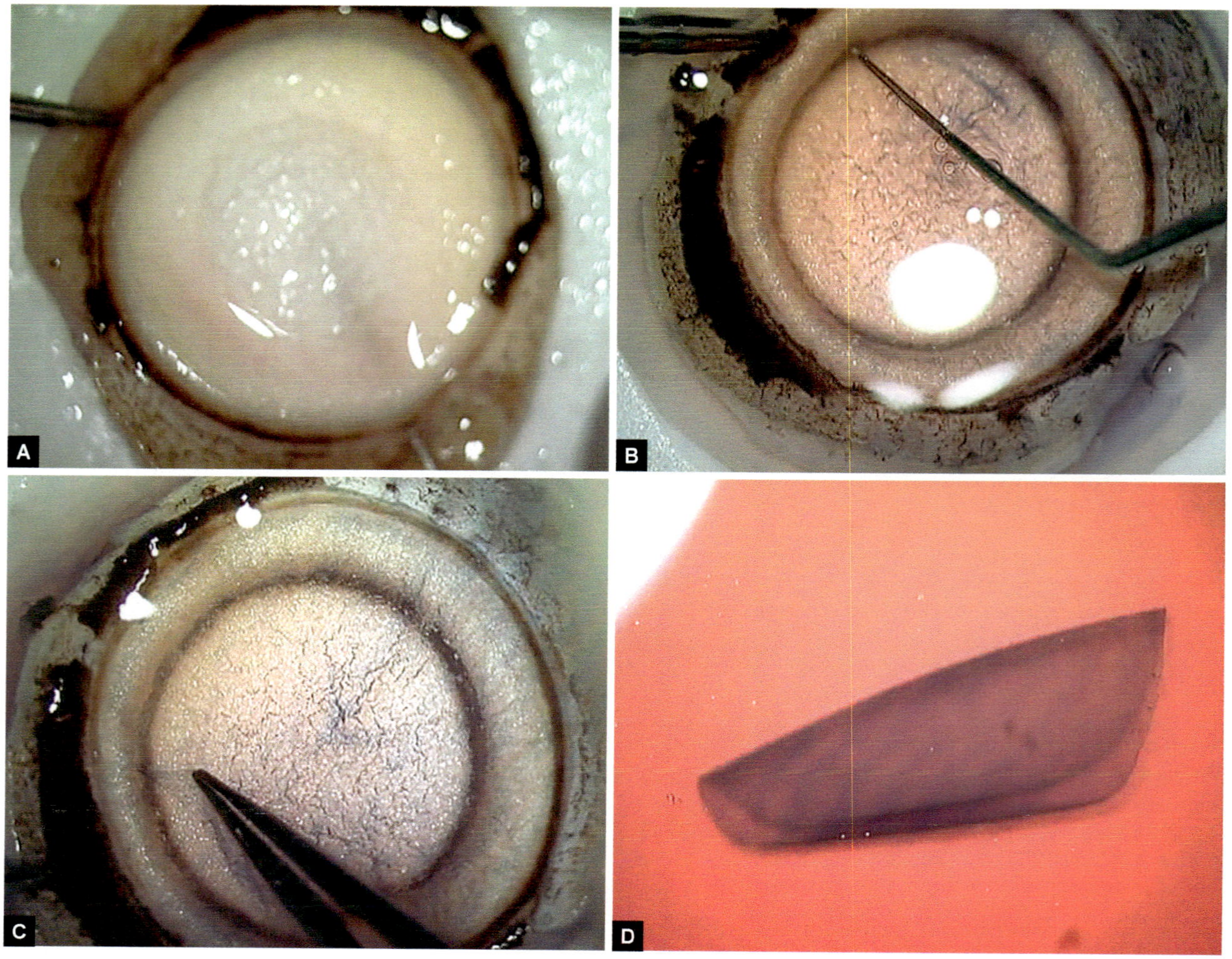

Figs. 2A to D: Accidental creation of type-2 bb. (A) Air being injected to form a type-1 bb; (B) Type-2 bb is formed that extends up to extreme periphery; (C) Descemet's membrane-endothelium complex being separated from above the surface of the bb; (D) Descemet's membrane endothelial keratoplasty (DMEK) graft placed in the storage media.

ensures appropriate shift between air and fluid infusion as and when required (**Figs. 5A to F**). A 2.8 mm corneal tunnel is made and two side port incisions are framed. With the AC completely inflated with air, DM is scored and stripped using a reverse Sinskey hook (**Figs. 6A to D**). Inferior iridectomy is performed with a vitrectomy probe introduced from the corneal incision (**Fig. 6E**). This maneuver ensures prevention of pupillary block at a later stage.

Donor-graft Insertion

The graft is held gently with a nontoothed forceps and is placed in to the cartridge of a foldable intraocular lens (IOL) that is filled with balanced salt solution (**Fig. 6F**).[7] Air infusion is stopped and the graft is gently injected into the AC through a clear corneal incision, avoiding wound-assisted implantation (**Fig. 7A**). Graft orientation is verified and the graft is gently unfolded using air and fluidics. Corneal indentation and massaging is also performed to facilitate the graft unrolling. Once the graft has partly unrolled, a small air bb is injected beneath the graft that helps it to adhere to the corneal surface (**Figs. 7B and C**). The peripheral edges of the graft can be unrolled by gently manipulating it with reverse Sinskey hook (**Fig. 7D**). Once the graft has fully unrolled, air infusion is started (**Figs. 7E and F**). This facilitates total adherence of the graft to the recipient bed. Corneal sutures are taken and a complete closure of all wounds is achieved to get the well-formed AC in the postoperative period (**Figs. 8A and B**).

POSTOPERATIVE CARE

In the immediate postoperative period, the patient is advised to lie in supine position for approximately 3 hours and continue doing so for most part of the day. Slit-lamp examination is done to confirm the graft centration and location. On the second postoperative day, intraocular pressure is checked and the patency of inferior iridectomy is confirmed. Topical antibiotics and steroids are prescribed that are slowly tapered over a period of 4 months (**Figs. 9 to 14**).

PRE-DESCEMET'S ENDOTHELIAL KERATOPLASTY DISCUSSION

Endothelial keratoplasty as a technique has evolved from deep lamellar endothelial keratoplasty (DLEK) and

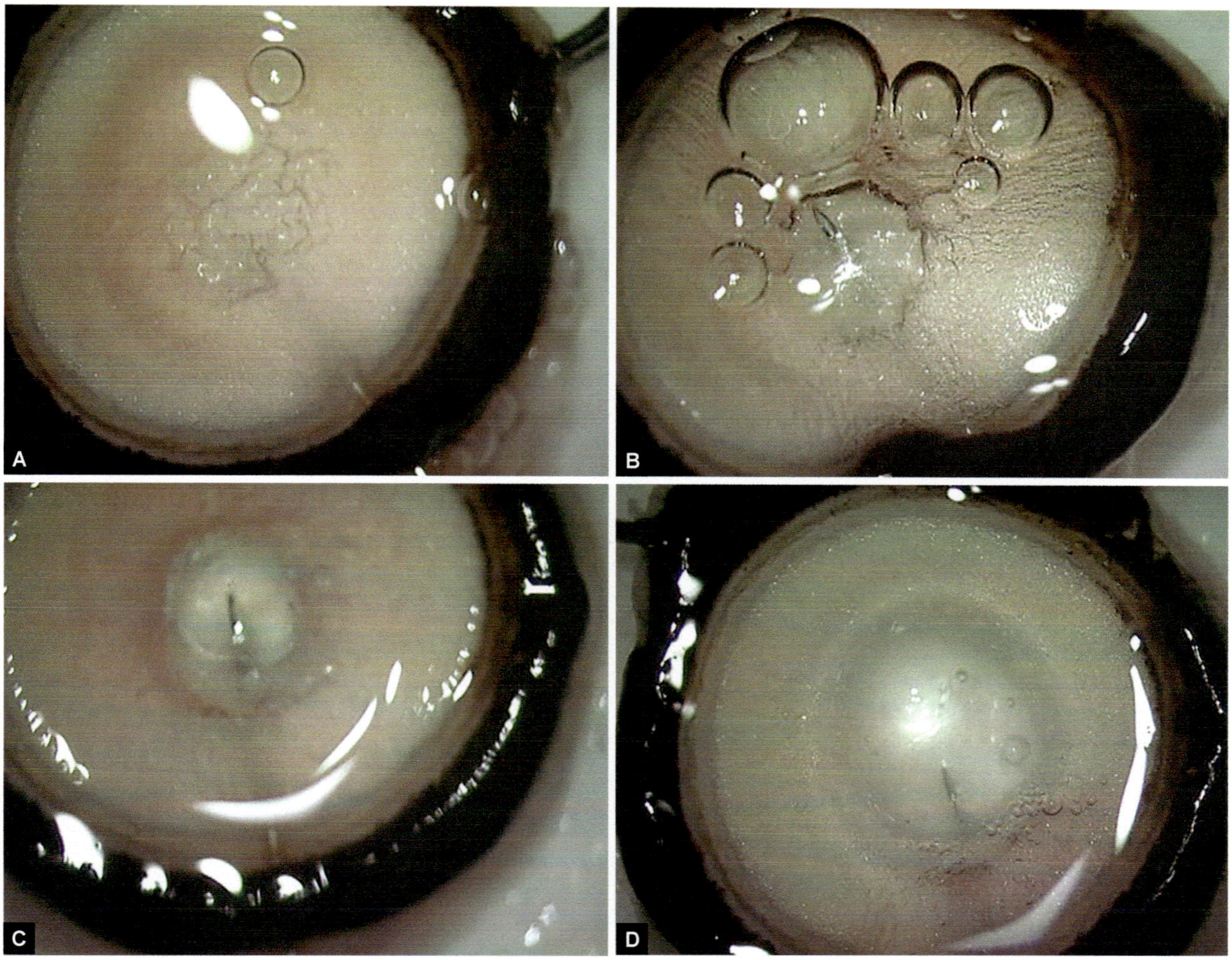

Figs. 3A to D: Plugging the Descemet's membrane (DM)-endothelium hole with viscoelastic. (A) Air being injected in to the donor tissue to create a type-1 bb; (B) Perforation of the DM is noted with leakage of small air bubbles from the endothelium side; (C) Further injection of air is withheld. The needle is withdrawn and 30 G needle attached to a syringe filled with viscoelastic is introduced. Viscoelastic is injected as it helps to plug the small perforation; (D) Type-1 bb created with the help of viscoelastic.

transitioned to DSEK/DSAEK and further to DMEK (**Table 1**). PDEK being a latest entry into this horizon is expected to have a broad acceptance due to its similar characteristics of rapid visual recovery, predictable wound strength, and a significant greater optical predictability similar to a DMEK procedure with an added advantage of less chances of donor tissue loss due to tearing away of the DM and also of better graft maneuverability due to extra strength and splinting effect of the PDL to the DM-endothelium complex. Like DMEK, preparation of PDEK graft does not require large investment in addition to all the other benefits of a DMEK procedure. PDEK involves the addition of the PDL in the donor graft that increases the thickness of the graft to approximately 30–35 µm as measured with an optical coherence tomography (OCT). The graft is comparatively thicker than that of the DMEK but is thinner as compared to DSEK/ DSAEK or an ultra-thin DSAEK (UT-DSAEK). Visual rehabilitation after PDEK is comparatively faster as compared to other EK techniques except DMEK that involves pure DM transplantation.

Clinically, in our series we have observed that the incidence of graft dislocation and rebubbling rate are comparatively less in PDEK as compared to DMEK and that can probably be attributed to the addition of the PDL to the donor graft that enhances the graft sustainability. Although validation of the PDEK procedure by other surgeons would enhance the acceptability of the technique before it is widely emulated and performed across the globe taking in to consideration the complications and feasibility of the technique. The risk of donor tissue loss can be minimized by the eye banks, if they supply premade ready to use donor graft tissue.

INFANT DONOR CORNEA FOR PDEK

There is a substantial shortage of donor tissue for EK worldwide. The feasibility of using infant donor graft for PDEK (**Figs. 10 and 11**) has been highlighted before and doing so potentially increase the pool of suitable donor tissue for (PDEK).[5]

The upper age limit for donor tissue usage is considered to be around 75 years but there is still not a clear-cut consensus

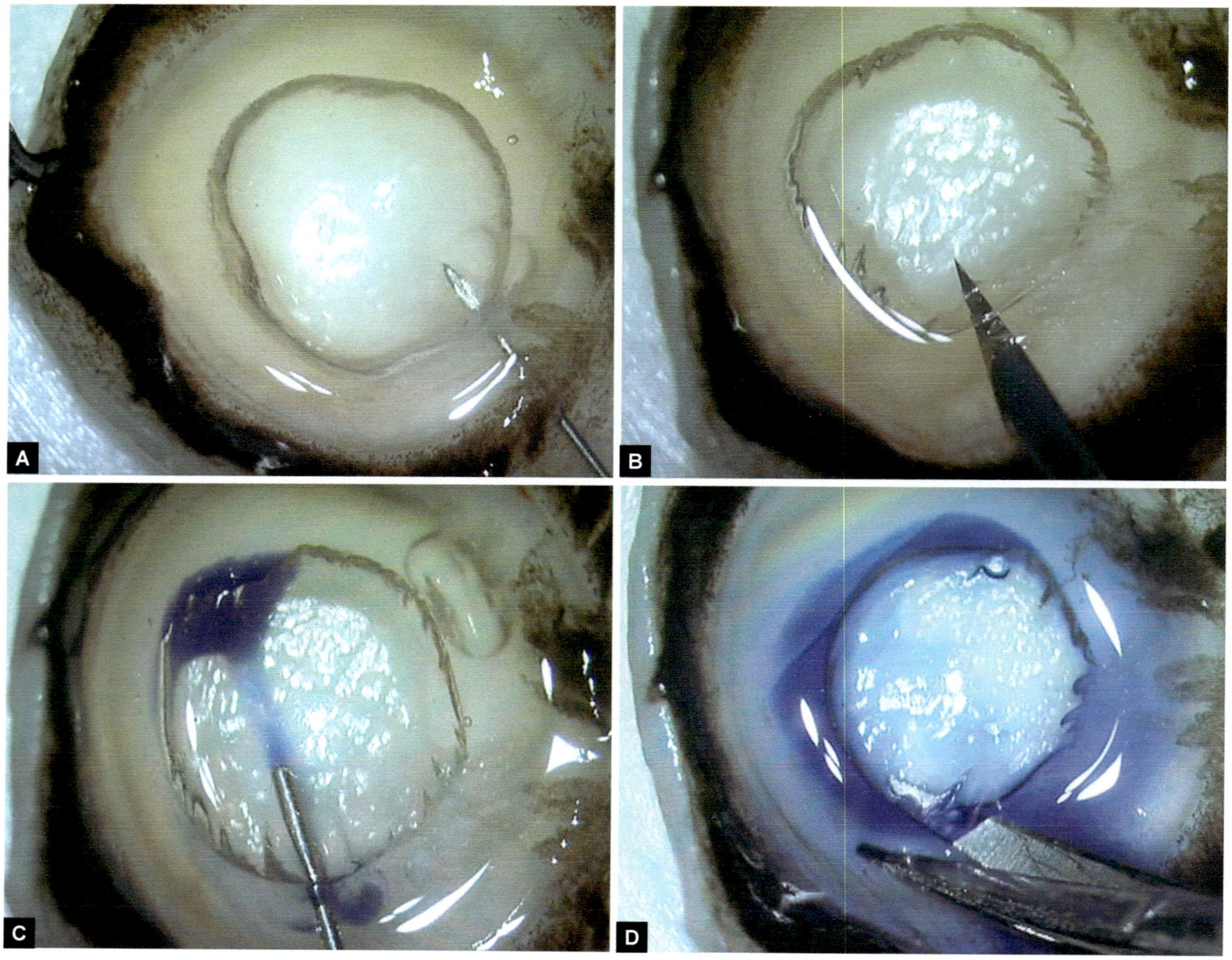

Figs. 4A to D: Donor graft preparation. (A) An air filled 30 G needle is introduced from the corneo-scleral rim up to the mid-periphery and air is injected to create a type-1 bb PDEK; (B) The bb is punctured at the extreme periphery with the help of a side port blade; (C) Trypan blue is injected to stain the bb; (D) The graft is cut along the peripheral edge of the bb with the corneo-scleral scissor.

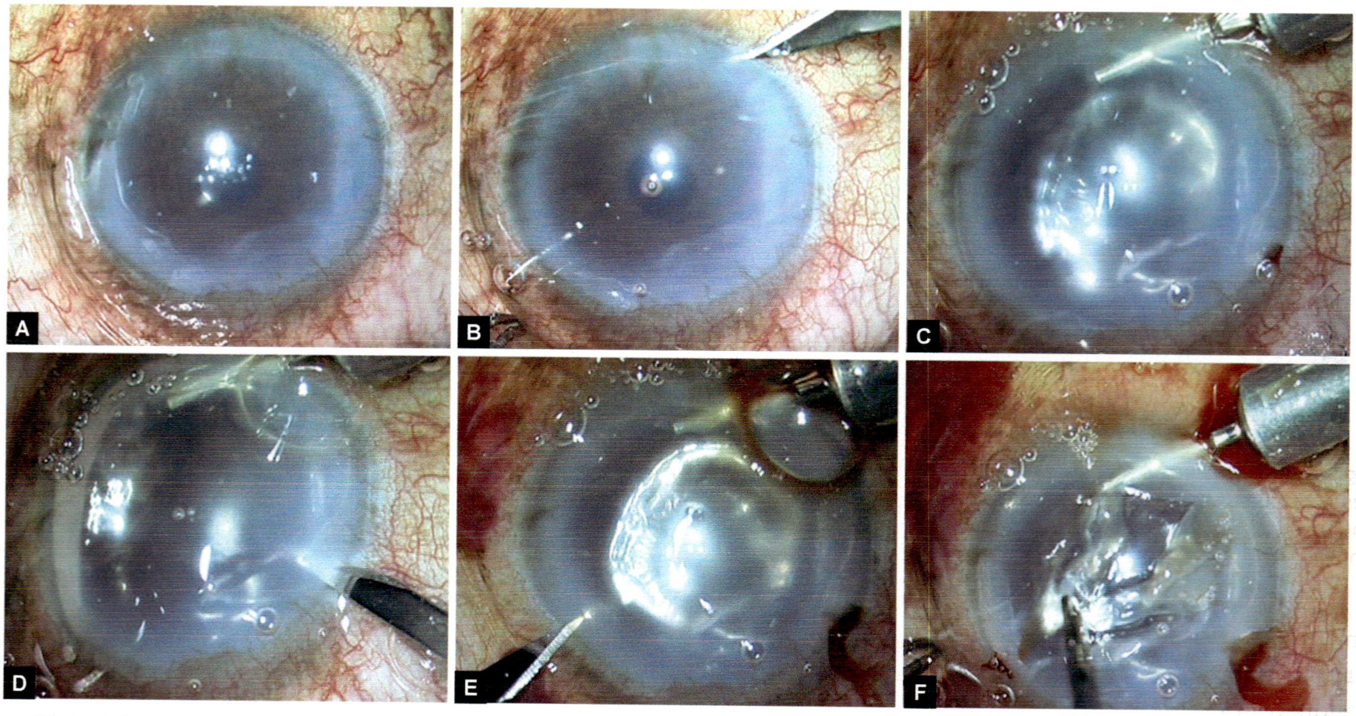

Figs. 5A to F: Patient surgery. (A) Preoperative status of the recipient eye; (B) Side-port incision being made to introduce an anterior chamber maintainer (ACM); (C) ACM is placed in position and is connected to an air pump for continuous air infusion; (D) Superotemporal side port incision being made; (E) Superonasal side port incision made; (F) Epithelium debridement done to facilitate intraoperative view.

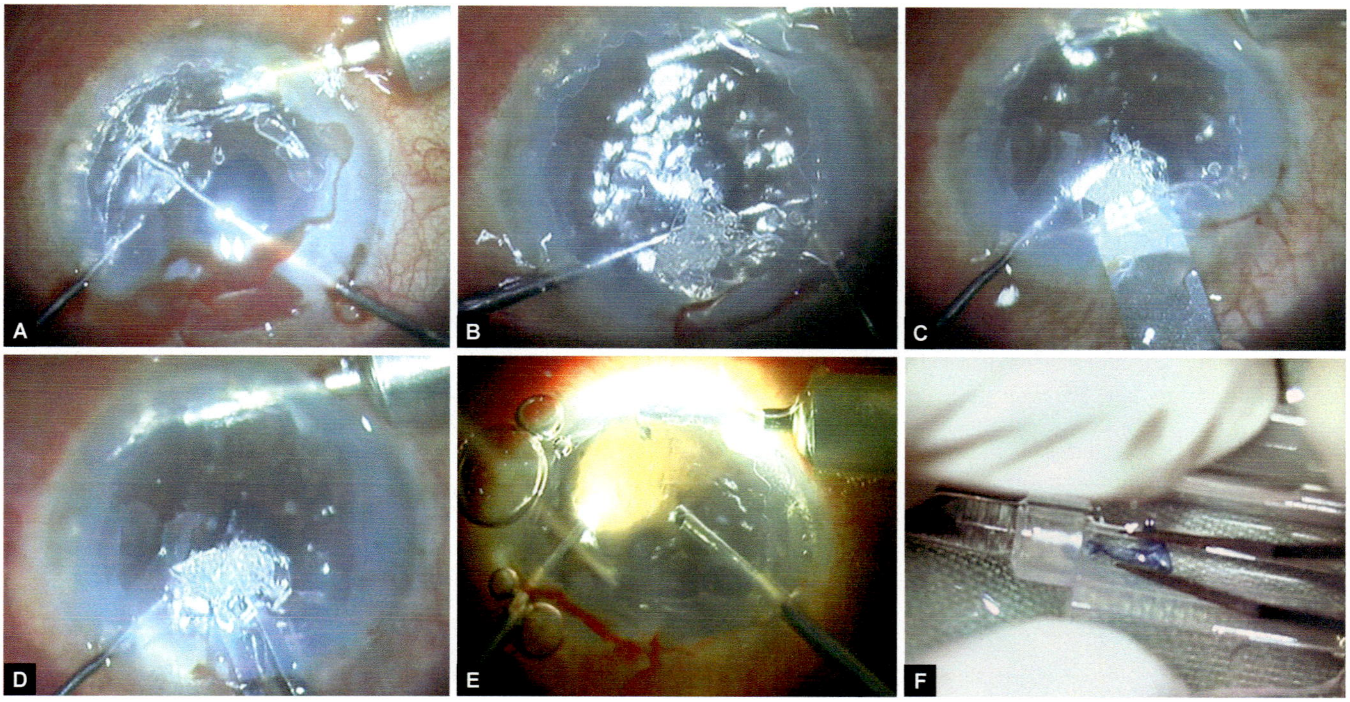

Figs. 6A to F: Patient surgery. (A) Descemetorhexis initiated with reverse Sinskey hook; (B) Descemetorhexis is completely performed 360 degrees; (C) 2.8 mm corneal tunnel incision is made; (D) The recipient's diseased Descemet's membrane complex being removed; (E) Inferior iridectomy being performed with vitrectomy probe; (F) Donor graft is loaded on to the cartridge of the foldable intraocular lens.

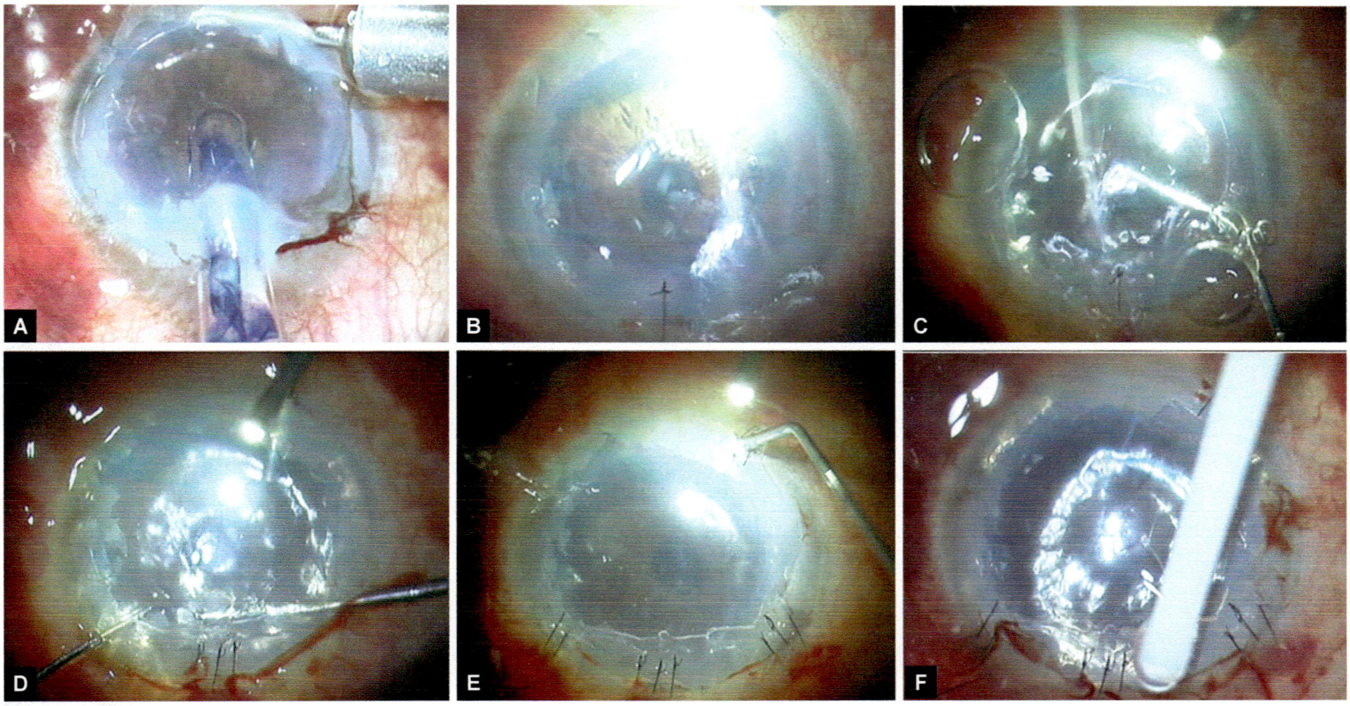

Figs. 7A to F: Donor-graft insertion. (A) Donor graft is inserted in to the anterior chamber. Wound-assisted graft insertion is avoided; (B) Donor graft lies in the anterior chamber; (C) Graft unrolling is attempted with air and fluidics. Endoilluminator is used to enhance the graft visualization and also to check the correct orientation; (D) The periphery of the unrolled graft is gently manipulated with reverse Sinskey hook; (E) After proper centration and unrolling of the graft, air is injected beneath and all the corneal wounds are sutured; (F) The tautness of the globe is confirmed.

on the lower age limit of donor tissue usage. Under such circumstances, most centers accept tissue from pediatric donors over 6 months of age. Infant donor tissue has not been used in the past due to various reasons involved with the fear of implanting an immature tissue although it runs high on endothelial cell density (ECD) count along with the technical reason of implanting a tissue with greater corneal curvature and also increased antigenicity that would increase the risk of immune reaction. Increased steepness, elasticity, and flexibility of the infant donor tissue have limited its

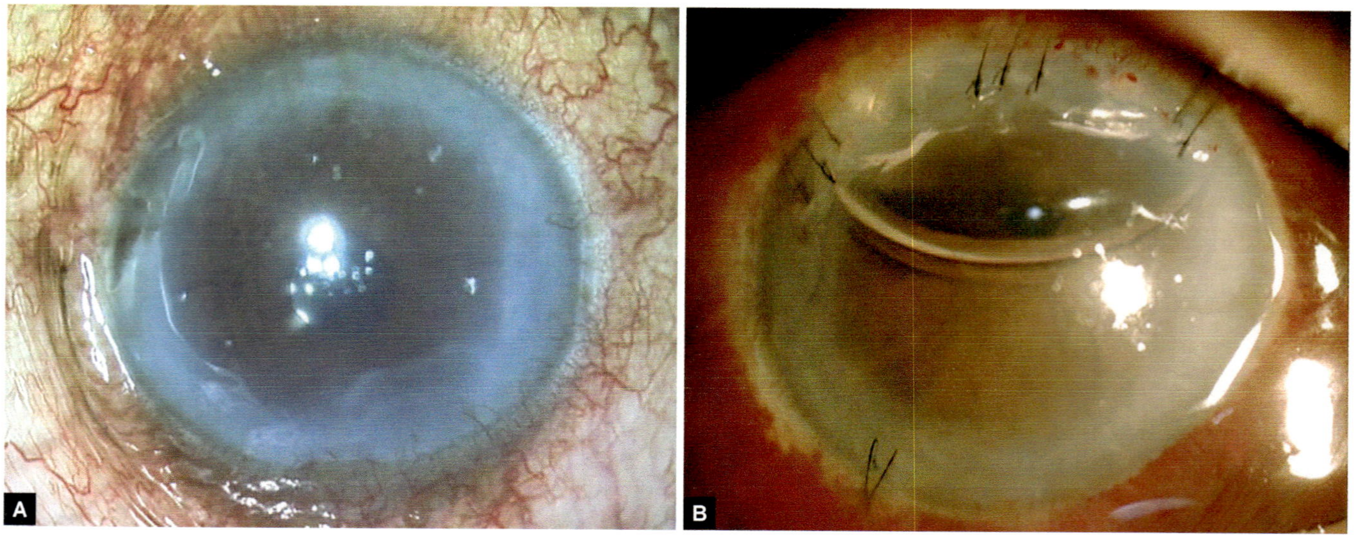

Figs. 8A and B: Preoperative and postoperative image. (A) Preoperative image of the patient; (B) 1 week postoperative image of the patient.

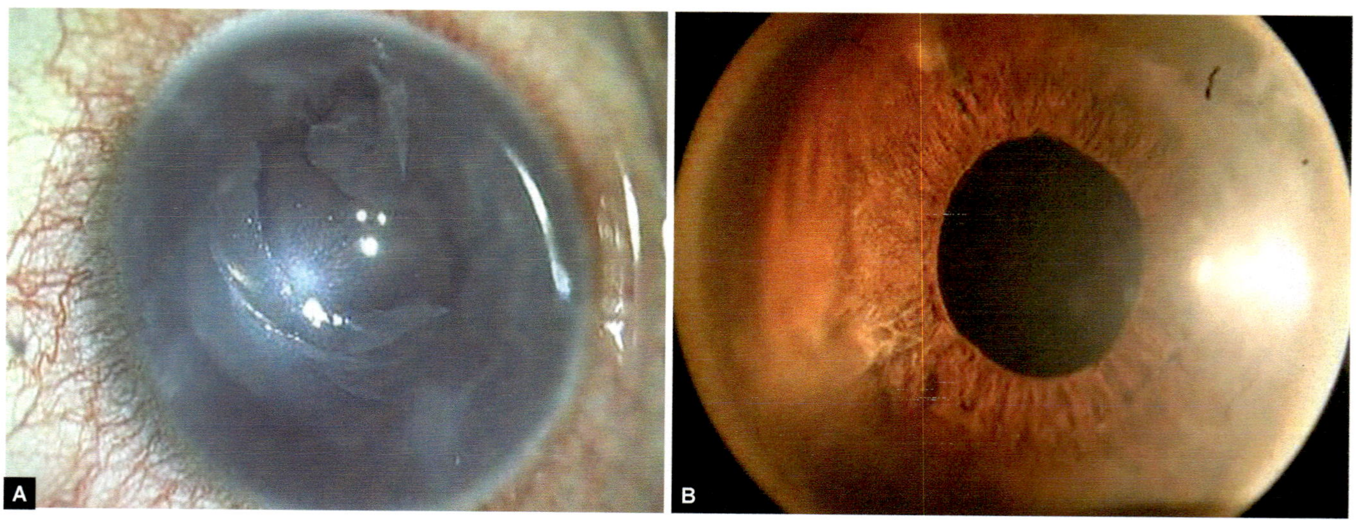

Figs. 9A and B: Preoperative and postoperative image. (A) Preoperative pseudophakic bullous keratopathy; (B) 3-month postoperative vision 20/20.

application for graft replacement especially for a penetrating keratoplasty (PK). The same criteria also applies for EK where difficulty in unrolling the graft is observed more so in a DMEK. Harvesting a donor tissue for DMEK with young donors below 40 years of age is believed and considered to be difficult and should be avoided due to presumed strong adhesions between the DM and stroma that can lead to tearing of the DM during harvesting of donor tissue.

Utilization of young donor tissue with favorable outcomes has been reported for DSEK[8] and of an infant donor tissue for DSAEK.[9] Sun et al., have reported conflicting results with neonate corneas in DSEK procedure[10] whereas in our study, we reported the feasibility of an infant donor tissue in PDEK.[5]

PRINCIPLES OF COMBINING GLUED INTRAOCCULAR LENS WITH PDEK

In aphakic eyes, a loss of bicamerality of the eye occurs that leads to posterior migration of the air bb used for attaching the PDEK graft. This increases the risk for a consequent postoperative partial or total graft detachment, forward bowing of the iris, iris-graft touch, graft dislocation into the vitreous, and so on, all of which can necessitate secondary procedures such as refloating, rebubbling, vitrectomy, AC formation, and so on in turn increasing graft endothelial cell loss. An effective compartmentalization of the eye can be obtained through the glued IOL technique. The glued IOL offers advantages of posterior chamber IOL placement, ease of centration, scleral fixation as well as stable and sturdy fixation without pseudophakodonesis. It is therefore our preferred technique when combining with PDEK unlike AC IOL, which has disadvantages of decreased AC space, iris fixated IOLs, which require intact iris all around as well as sutured scleral fixated IOL, which has disadvantages of greater pseudophakodonesis and greater difficulty in centration (**Figs. 15 to 17**).

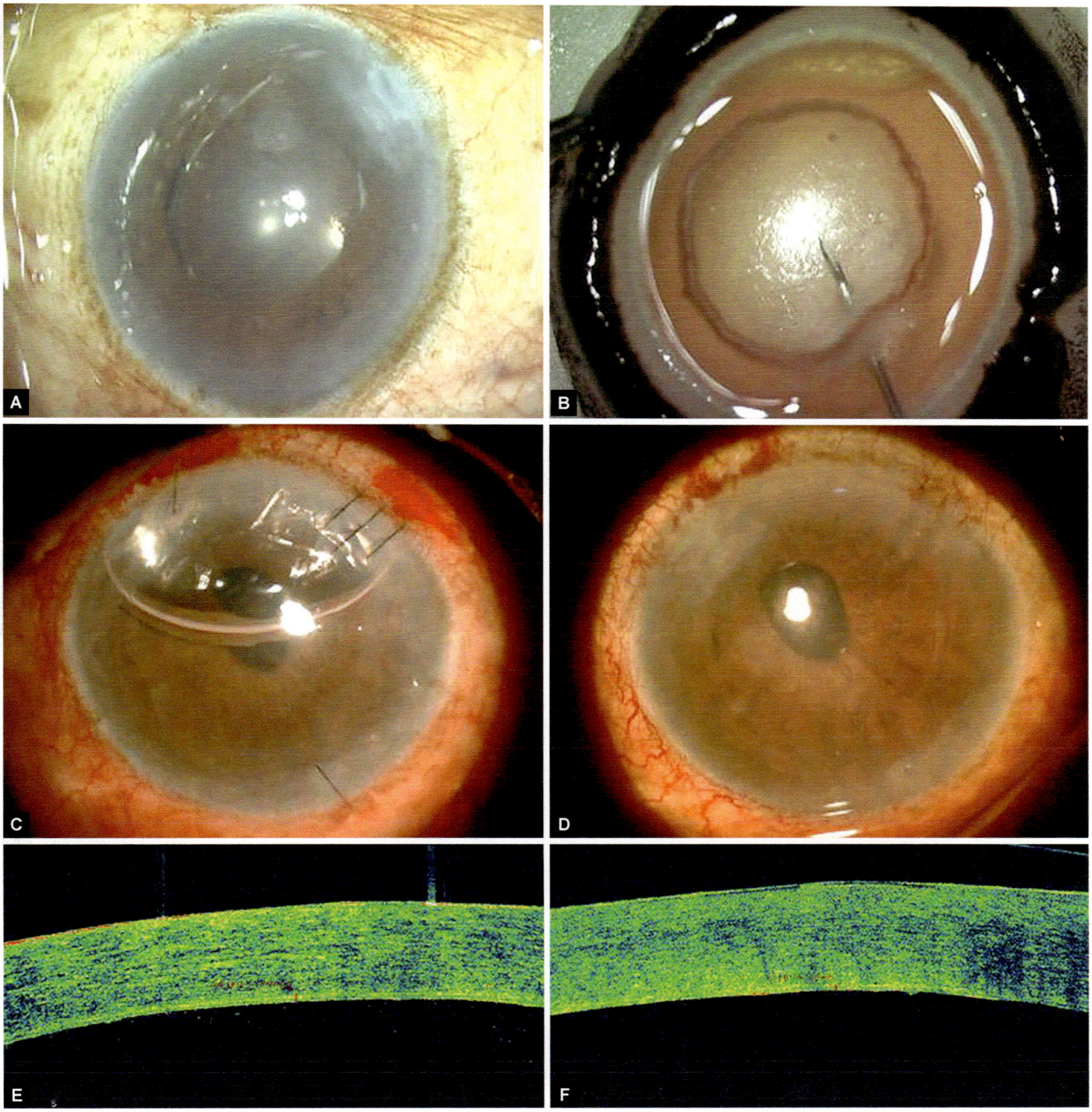

Figs. 10A to F: Pre-Descemet's endothelial keratoplasty (PDEK) using a 1-year-old donor. (A) Pseudophakic bullous keratopathy; (B) Type 1 big bubble prepared for PDEK graft; (C) Postoperative day 1 after PDEK; (D) Postoperative 1 week after PDEK vision 20/20; (E) Anterior segment optical coherence tomography (OCT) postoperative day 1; (F) Anterior segment OCT postoperative 1 week.

The procedure is started as a conventional glued IOL. An ACM or a T-ACM is inserted. Conjunctival flaps and lamellar scleral flaps are made 180 degrees apart as explained earlier. 22 gauge sclerotomies are made under the scleral flap about 1 mm from the limbus. This is followed by limited 23 G vitrectomy through the sclerotomies followed by glued IOL implantation. The haptics are tucked in the Scharioth pockets and the flaps may be glued down. As the posterior capsule is unlikely to be intact, there is still a chance of posterior migration of air that is injected into the AC for graft support. Migration of air behind the IOL leads to insufficient support for the graft with consequent graft detachment. It is therefore imperative to have a good iris- IOL diaphragm separating the AC from the vitreous cavity. Therefore, when combining a glued IOL with PDEK, the sclerotomy should be made slightly closer to the limbus than usual in order to decrease the potential gap between the iris and the IOL. At the same time, a single pass four throw pupilloplasty should be done to obtain a round pupil that overlaps the

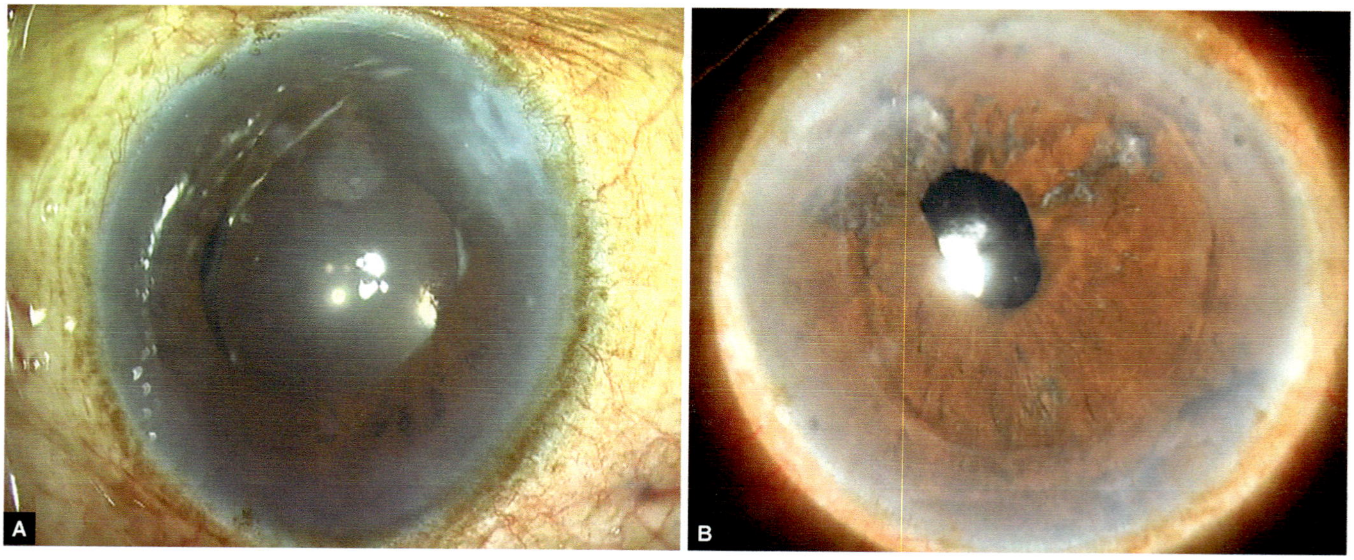

Figs. 11A and B: Preoperative and postoperative follow-up images of pre-Descemet's endothelial keratoplasty using a 1 year donor. (A) Preoperative clinical photograph showing the corneal decompensation; (B) Postoperative image of the same case at 15-month follow-up. Vision 20/20.

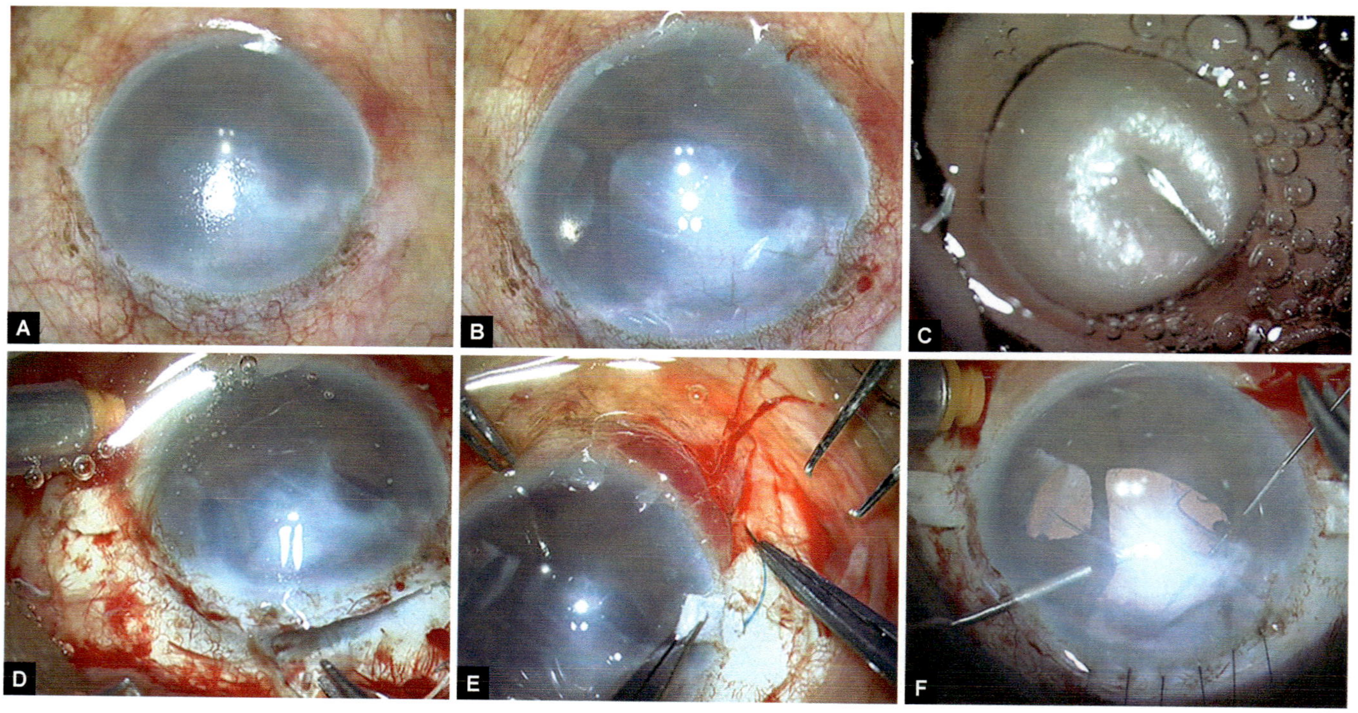

Figs. 12A to F: Surgical procedure of pre-Descemet's endothelial keratoplasty (PDEK) with an infant 9-month-old donor cornea–Step 1. (A) Pseudophakic bullous keratopathy with decentered intraocular lens intraocular lens (IOL); (B) Epithelium removed. Note corneal vascularization and corneal haze; (C) Type 1 big bubble prepared for PDEK graft; (D) IOL explanted; (E) Glued IOL; (F) Single pass four throw pupilloplasty.

IOL optic all around. Once this is done the adequacy of air fill is checked by turning off the infusion and checking for the air fill. If inadequate, the pupil may need to become smaller or the IOL may need to come closer to the iris. A well-formed iris-IOL diaphragm prevents air from going back into the vitreous cavity and allows good postoperative support for the graft. Once the air fill is found to be adequate, air is attached to the ACM through an air-pump and host descemetorhexis is performed. The PDEK graft is then injected into the AC, unfolded and floated up using air. In cases with subluxated or dislocated three piece IOL needing PDEK, a closed chamber translocation of the subluxated IOL into a glued IOL may be done using the handshake technique. This is followed by iridoplasty, if required and PDEK.

Cases with malpositioned single piece IOL requiring explantation or AC IOL need an enlargement of the wound followed by explantation of the IOL. This is followed by the technique described above. Construction of a scleral tunnel for IOL explantation or a 3 mm L-shaped sclera tunnel incision gives very good wound closure and excellent AC stability.

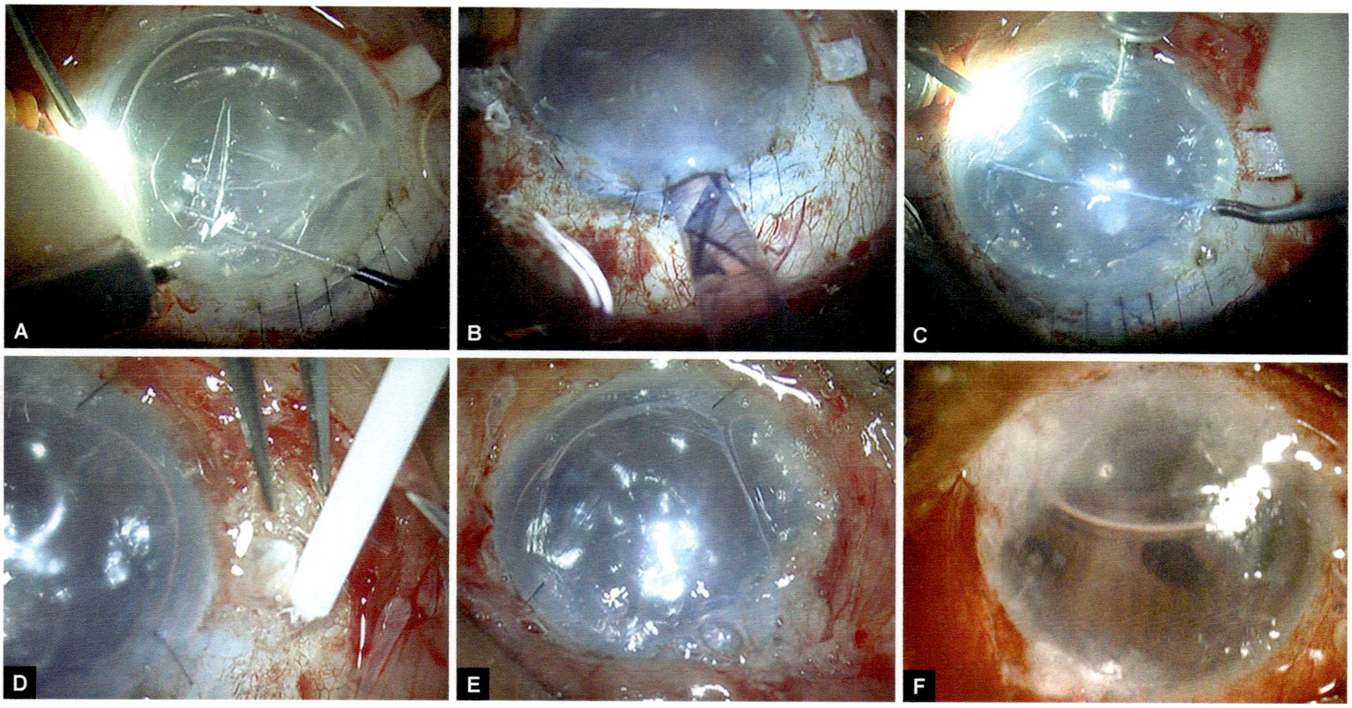

Figs. 13A to F: Surgical procedure of pre-Descemet's endothelial keratoplasty with an infant 9-month-old donor cornea–Step 2. (A) Descemetorhexis being performed under air. The endoilluminator helps to enhance the visualization; (B) The infant donor graft is loaded onto the cartridge of a foldable intraocular lens injector (the spring is removed to prevent any damage to the graft), and is slowly injected into the eye; (C) The donor graft is unrolled, and the endoilluminator helps to identify the correct graft orientation; (D) Fibrin glue being applied beneath the scleral flaps; (E) Corneal incisions closed with 10-0 nylon suture and the anterior chamber is filled with air; (F) Postoperative image of the case on the fourth postoperative day.

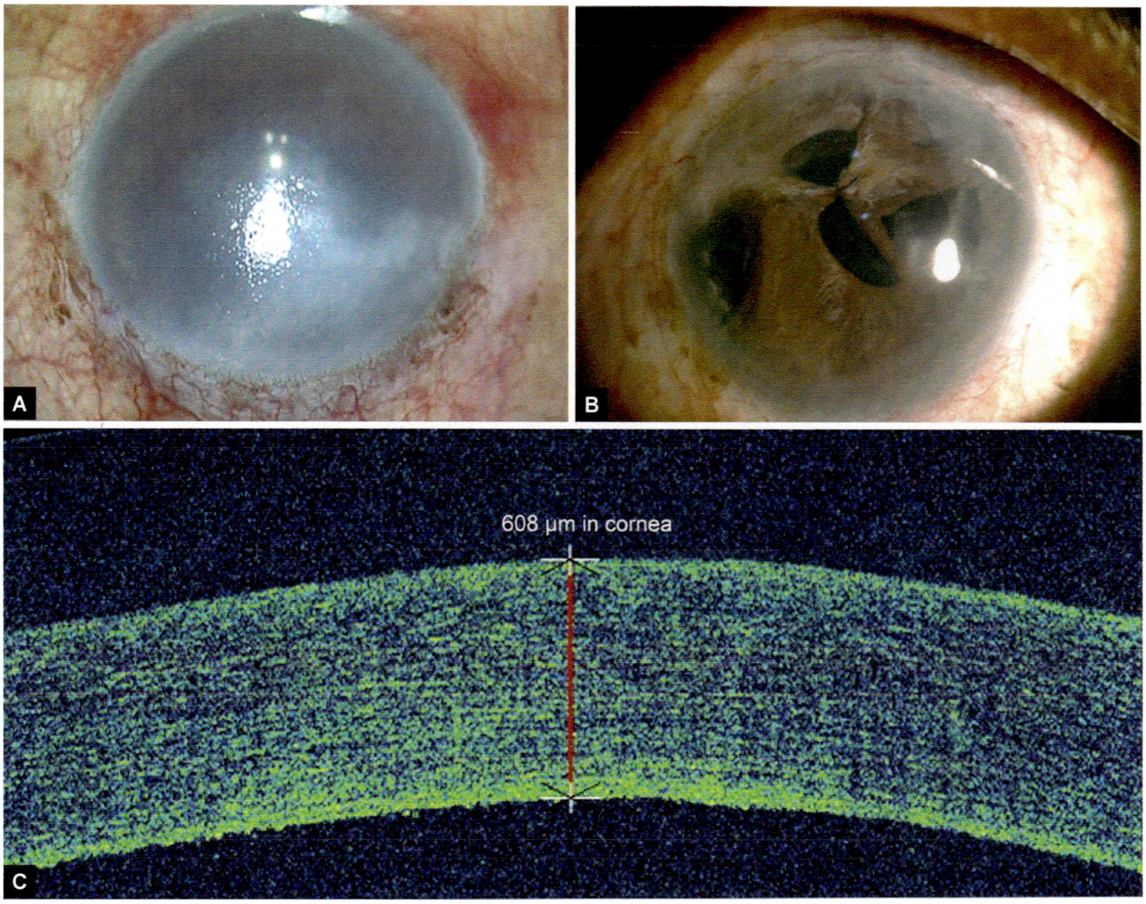

Figs. 14A to C: Preoperative and postoperative follow-up images using a 9-month-old donor. (A) Preoperative image of decentered. Intraocular lens with bullous keratopathy with anterior stromal haze; (B) Postoperative image of at 6-month follow-up. Vision 20/30; (C) Anterior segment optical coherence tomography showing attached graft.

Table 1: Comparison of different endothelial keratoplasty techniques.

	DSEK	***DMEK***	***PDEK***
Surgical layers	Stroma + DM + Endo	DM + Endo	Pre-Descemet's + DM + Endo
Technical difficulty	Easy	Difficult	Moderate
Type of procedure	Tissue additive	Tissue neutral	Minimal tissue additive
Artificial anterior chamber	Required	NR	NR
Microkeratome	Required (DSAEK)	NR	NR
Induced hyperopia	Yes	No	No
Corneal thickness	Increased	Normal	Minimal
Intrastromal interface	Yes	No	Minimal
Cost	Costly	Cost effective	Cost effective
Eye bank prepared donor tissue	Available	Available	Available
Graft unrolling	Easy	Difficult	Easy
Tissue handling	Good	Difficult	Good
Visual recovery	Slow	Fast	Fast

(DM: Descemet's membrane; DSAEK: Descemet's stripping automated endothelial keratoplasty; Endo: endothelium; NR: not required; PDEK: pre-Descemet's endothelial keratoplasty)

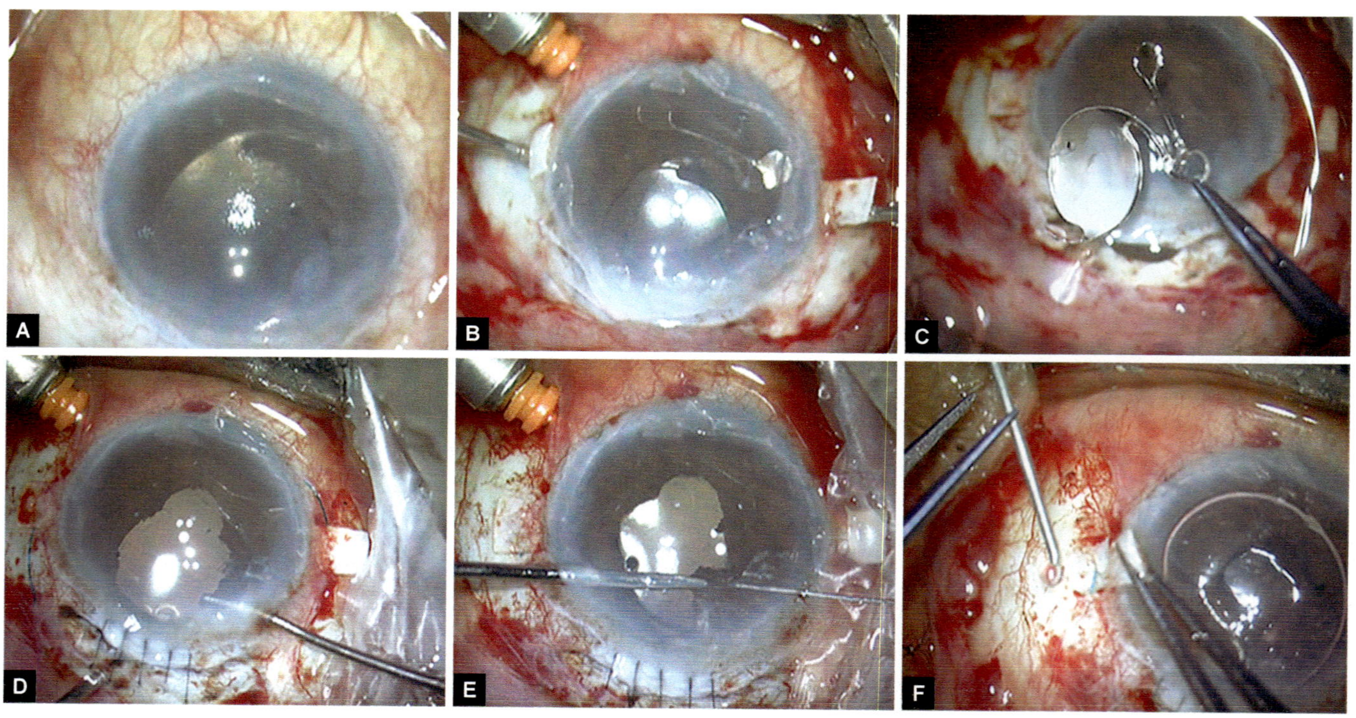

Figs. 15A to F: Pre-Descemet's endothelial keratoplasty (PDEK) with glued intraocular lens (IOL) (Part 1). (A) Pseudophakic bullous keratopathy. Note the corneal haze and an anterior chamber intraocular lens (ACIOL) in the eye; (B) Trocar cannula fixed. Two scleral flaps created 180 degrees apart and a 22 G sclerotomy created with a needle 1 mm from the limbus; (C) After vitrectomy, the haptics are grasped with glued IOL forceps and ACIOL explanted; (D) Glued IOL in place. Note the haptics externalized under the scleral flaps. Suturing of the scleral tunnel done; (E) Single pass four throw pupilloplasty (SFT) done to make the pupil smaller so that air remains in the AC and does not go into the vitreous cavity when PDEK will be done; (F) Fibrin glue applied.

A potential complication that may occur on combining glued IOL with PDEK is the risk for hypotonous and subsequent graft detachment in the postoperative period. Hypotony can lead to detachment of the PDEK graft from the eye lids pushing on the cornea with normal lid movements. This risk can be decreased by making sure that the globe is adequately pressurized at the end of surgery. As noted, this is done by achieving an adequately tight air bubble in the AC. If the globe still feels hypotonic, air is injected through the pars plicata into the vitreous cavity with a 30 G needle under

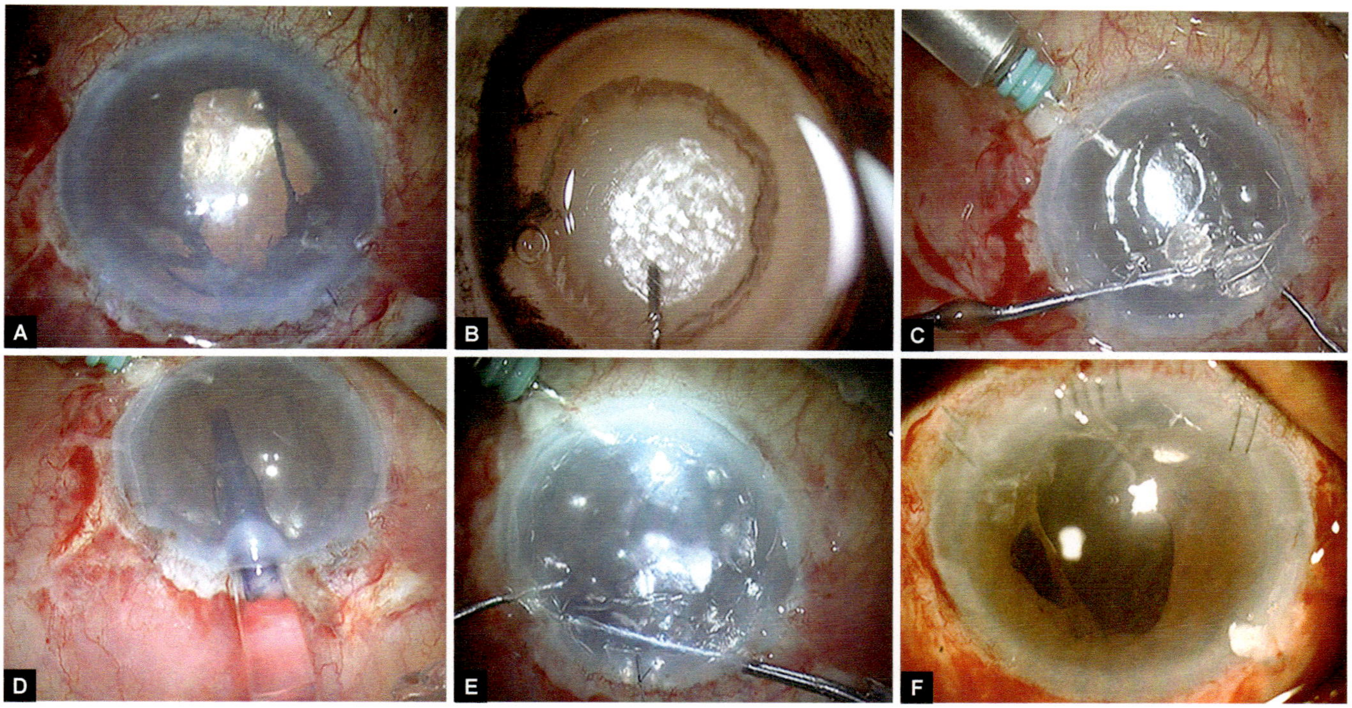

Figs. 16A to F: Pre-Descemet's endothelial keratoplasty (PDEK) with glued intraocular lens (IOL) (Part 2). (A) 1 month after glued IOL. Note the corneal haze; (B) Type 1 big bubble created. One can do the PDEK in one sitting with the glued IOL; (C) Descemetorhexis being performed. Air pump assisted PDEK. In this the air pump is connected to the trocar anterior chamber (AC) maintainer or AC maintainer, so that air is continuously flowing inside the AC. If one is doing PDEK with glued IOL in one sitting it is better to have a trocar cannula in the pars plana with fluid being passed inside and an AC maintainer or a trocar AC maintainer in the AC passing air. This way there will not be any hypotony and one can control the amount of fluid being passed inside the eye; (D) PDEK graft injected inside the AC; (E) PDEK graft unrolled with the help of endoilluminator-assisted PDEK; (F) 1-week postoperative.

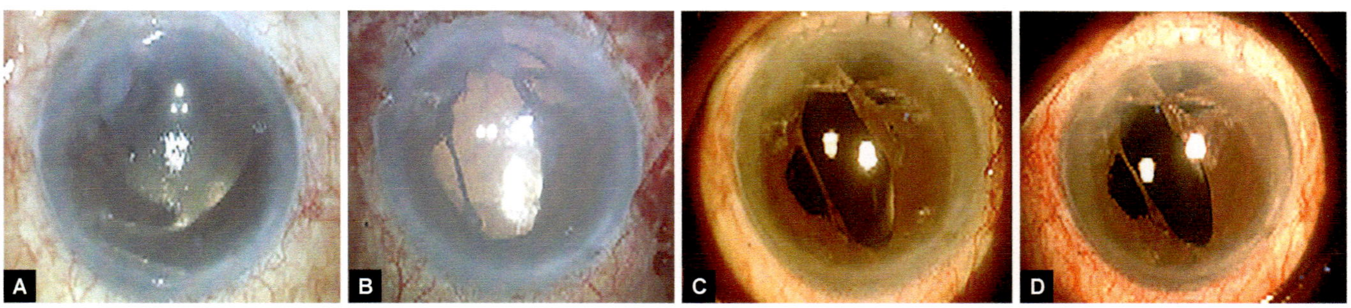

Figs. 17A to D: Pre-Descemet's endothelial keratoplasty (PDEK) with glued intraocular lens (IOL); (Part 3). (A) Preoperative; (B) 1 month after glued IOL; (C) 2 months postoperative after PDEK- Vision 6/12; (D) 4 months postoperative after PDEK- Vision 6/6.

direct visualizing of the needle tip in the vitreous cavity. At the conclusion of surgery, it should also be made sure that the sclerotomies are well-sealed by the scleral flaps using fibrin glue. All corneal incisions should be leak proof and may also be sealed using fibrin glue to avoid any postoperative leak of aqueous or escape of air, which could increase the risk of detachment. Patients undergoing the procedure therefore need to be watched more closely after surgery to look for any evidence of partial or total graft detachments and taken for rebubbling, if required.

A properly positioned IOL and a good iridoplasty decrease the chances of the graft slipping into the vitreous cavity during surgery. However, this possibility should be kept in mind and care should be taken to avoid any inappropriate fluidics, which may cause a graft drop (**Figs. 18 to 20**).

DISCUSSION

Posterior lamellar keratoplasty has the benefit of transferring the healthy endothelium from the donors with or without the addition of the stromal tissue.

Surgeons have performed DSEK with neonate corneas where they have reported achieving the maximum size of lenticule as 8 mm along with the thinner central lenticule as compared to a thicker peripheral rim of the lenticule.

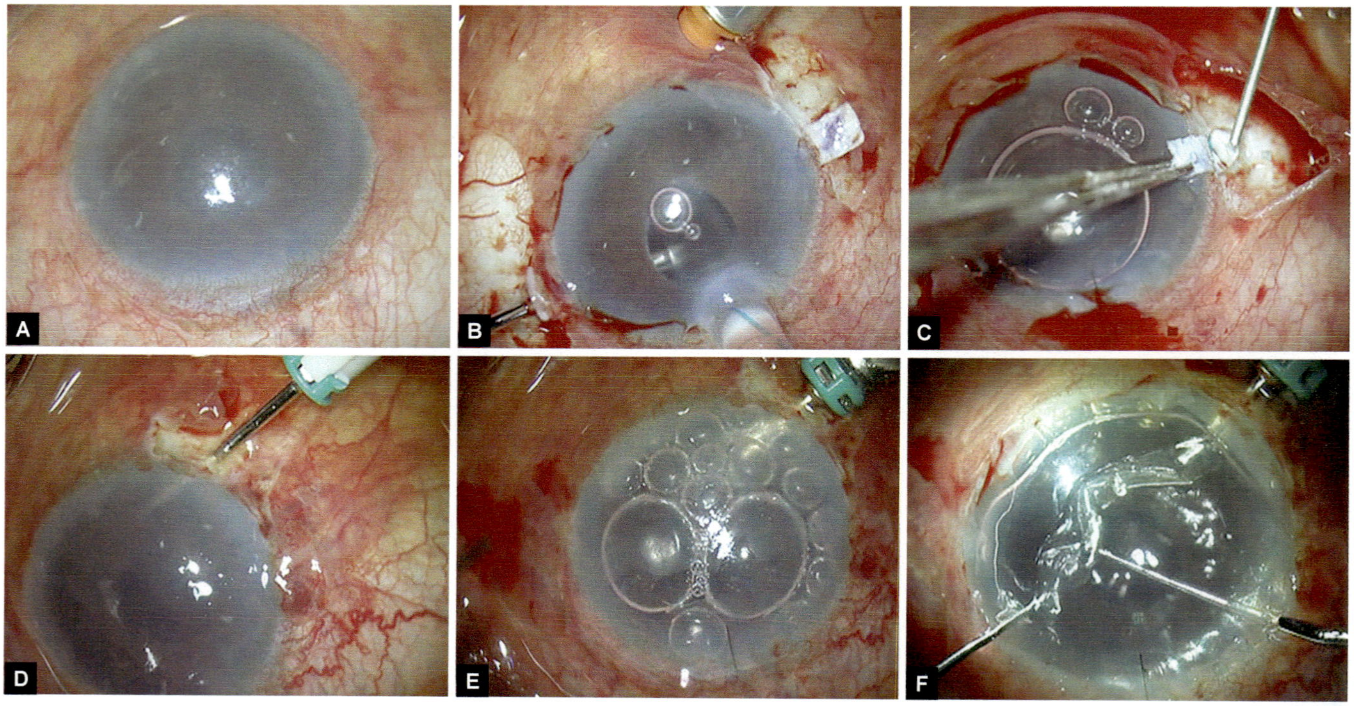

Figs. 18A to F: Pre-Descemet's endothelial keratoplasty (PDEK) with glued intraocular lens (IOL) in a one eyed patient (Part 1). (A) Aphakic bullous keratopathy; (B) Two partial scleral thickness limbal-based scleral flaps of 2.5 mm × 2.5 mm are created 180 degrees opposite to each other followed by placement of infusion cannula. Glued IOL performed; (C) Fibrin glue applied; (D) 1 week after glued IOL-Trocar AC maintainer fixed; (E) Air pump connected to the trocar anterior chamber maintainer; (F) Descemetorhexis.

This can be attributed to the increased corneal curvature in newborns as compared to adults. They also observed that due to increased flexibility of the cornea, the unrolling of the graft was bit difficult and that due to this there were increased chances of graft dislocation and lenticule contraction in the postoperative period.[10]

Other group of surgeons have performed DSEK with pediatric donor tissue and have reported good outcomes. The employment of young donor tissue for EK has a theoretical advantage of transferring a donor lenticule with high ECD that could compensate the issue of ECD loss that eventually occurs in postsurgery. In EK, a frequent concern among surgeons is potential tissue loss as a result of DM graft preparation failure, which is minimized with the PDEK procedure, as failure to get a type-1 bb may be associated with the formation of type-2 bb. Under such a scenario the surgeon can perform a DMEK instead of PDEK procedure.

In conclusion, a stepwise approach to donor preparation and donor insertion makes PDEK a standardized and reproducible procedure with a successful outcome in terms of usage of young donor corneas with high-endothelial cell density. The procedure of PDEK also involves skill set on behalf of the surgeon to create a type-1 bb but this limitation is totally circumvented by the fact that PDEK does not require the employment of costly microkeratome as in a DSAEK, DMAEK, or UT-DSEK thereby cutting the cost of surgical procedure and also inculcating the procedure of use of infant donor cornea with a graft thickness of around 35 μm, i.e., eventually less as compared to DSAEK or UT-DSEK tissue.

COMPLICATIONS OF PDEK

Complications are an inherent and an integral part of any intraocular surgery and they act as a source of continuous refinement in the surgical procedure taking into consideration the technicality of the surgery and also of the surgical skill of the surgeon.

Tissue loss in graft preparation: This complication can occur when the surgeon dissects in a wrong plane creating either a type-2 bb or perforation of the DM-endothelium complex. In the previously mentioned situation, the surgeon can switch over from PDEK to DMEK whereas in case of latter situation the donor tissue is totally lost and is rendered useless. A fresh donor tissue is then needed to complete the surgical procedure.

Air reinjection and rebubbling: In cases of partial graft detachment where there is an inadequate air fill, rebubbling is often needed to place the graft back in position. Air leakage can occur due to either inappropriate wound closure or due to loss of air in the posterior chamber in pseudophakic and aphakic eyes. In such cases performing pupilloplasty helps to adequately maintain the anterior chamber air fill. Graft repositioning and centration needs to be done properly and the patient should be regularly followed up at periodic intervals to detect any incidence of reoccurrence.

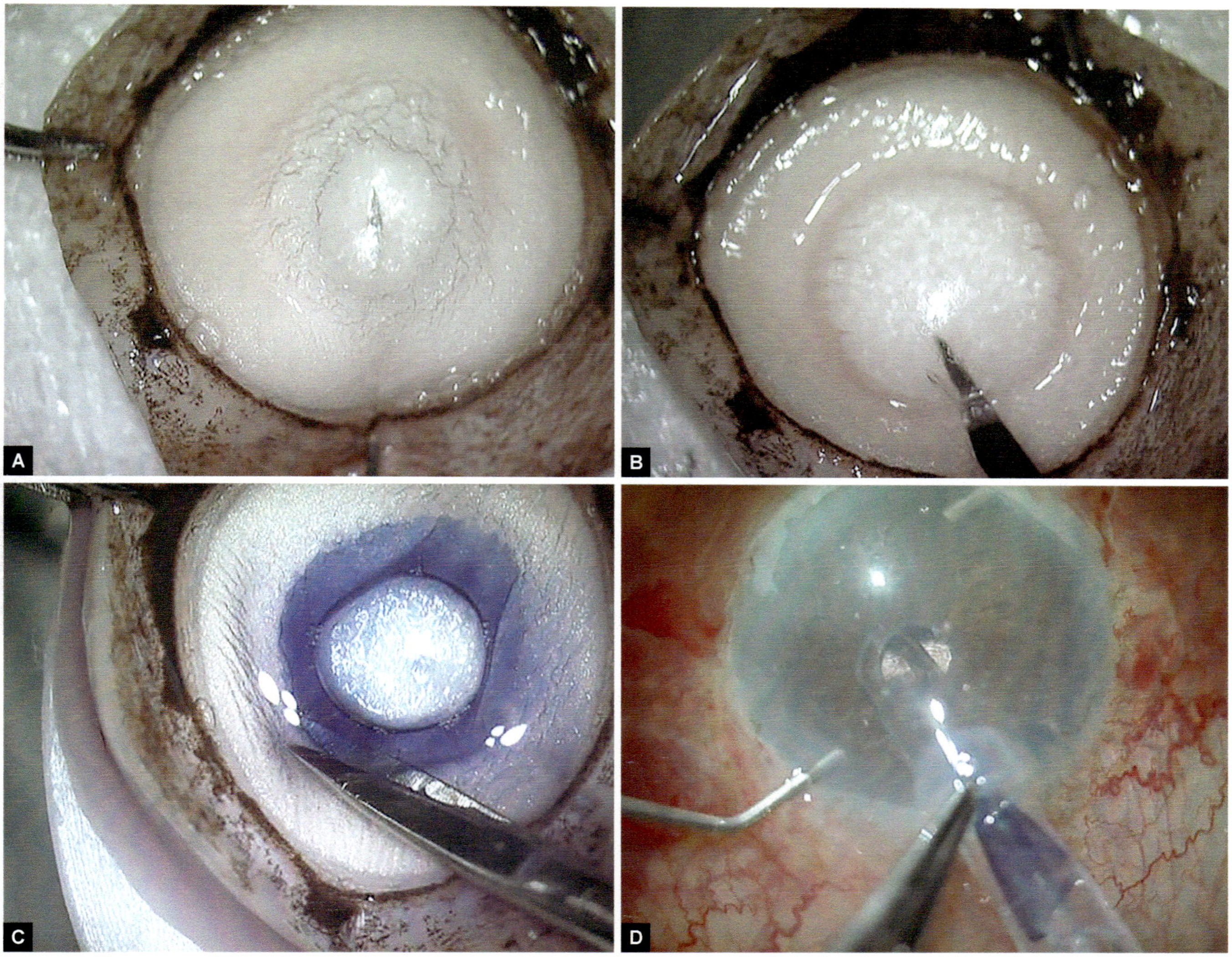

Figs. 19A to D: Pre-Descemet's endothelial keratoplasty (PDEK) with glued intraocular lens in a one-eyed patient (Part 2). (A) 30 G needle injecting air into the stroma to create a type 1 big bubble; (B)Type 1 big bubble created; (C) PDEK graft stained with trypan blue and dissected; (D) PDEK graft injected into the anterior chamber.

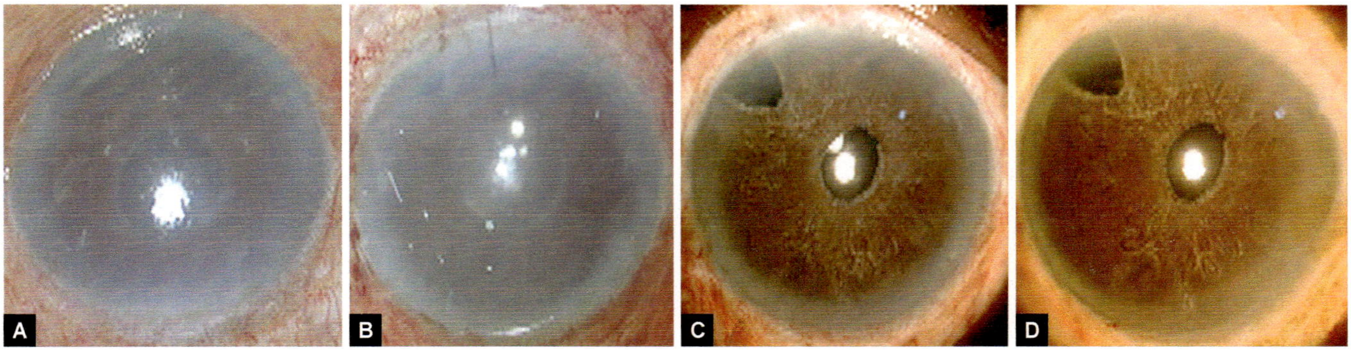

Figs. 20A to D: Pre-Descemet's endothelial keratoplasty (PDEK) with glued intraocular lens (IOL) in a one-eyed patient (Part 3). (A) Preoperative; (B) 1 week after glued IOL; (C) 2 months postoperative after PDEK-vision 6/9; (D) 7 months postoperative after PDEK- vision 6/6.

Graft failure and resurgery: Graft failure can occur following a complete graft detachment from the recipient bed. Relocation of the same graft is attempted initially and in case if it is extremely reticent then resurgery is preferred.

Pupillary block: This can occur due to blockage of the iridectomy leading to rise in intraocular pressure. If the AC is overfilled with air then slight decompression should be attempted by pressing the corneal tunnel.

REFERENCES

1. Melles GR, Eggink FA, Lander F, Pels E, Rietveld FJ, Beekhuis WH, et al. A surgical technique for posterior lamellar keratoplasty. Cornea. 1998;17:618-26.
2. Melles GR, Ong TS, Ververs B, van der Wees J. Descemet's membrane endothelial keratoplasty (DMEK). Cornea. 2006;25:987-90.
3. Agarwal A, Dua HS, Narang P, Kumar DA, Agarwal A, Jacob S, et al. Pre-Descemet's endothelial keratoplasty (PDEK). Br J Ophthalmol. 2014; 98:1181-5.
4. Dua HS, Faraj LA, Said DG, Gray T, Lowe J. Human corneal anatomy redefined: A novel pre-Descemet's layer (Dua's layer). Ophthalmology. 2013;120:1778-5.
5. Agarwal A, Agarwal A, Narang P, Kumar DA, Jacob S. Pre-Descemet's endothelial keratoplasty with infant donor corneas: a prospective analysis. Cornea. 2015;34:859-65.
6. Agarwal A, Narang P, Kumar DA, Agarwal A. Trocar anterior chamber maintainer (T-ACM): improvised technique of infusion. J Cataract Refract Surg. 2016;42(2):185-9.
7. Price FW Jr, Price MO. Descemet's stripping with endothelial keratoplasty in 200 eyes: early challenges and technique to enhance donor adherence. J Cataract Refract Surg. 2006; 32:411-8.
8. Huang T, Wang Y, Hu A, Luo Y, Chen J. Use of pediatric donor tissue in Descemet's stripping endothelial keratoplasty. Br J Ophthalmol. 2009; 93:1625-8.
9. Kim P, Yeung SN, Lichtinger A, Amiran MD, Rootman DS. Descemet's stripping automated endothelial keratoplasty using infant donor tissue. Cornea. 2012;31:52-4.
10. Sun YX, Hao YS, Hong J. Descemet's membrane stripping endothelial keratoplasty with neonate donors in two cases. Br J Ophthalmol. 2009;93:1692-3.

37 Tectonic Descemet Stripping Automated Endothelial Keratoplasty

Vincenzo Scorcia, Angeli Christy Yu, Massimo Busin

INTRODUCTION

Corneal perforation is an ophthalmic emergency that can occur secondary to various causes such as infection, trauma, collagen vascular disorders, or severe ocular surface disease. The primary goal of management is the immediate restoration of the structural integrity of the globe for the preservation of functional vision. Treatment options include application of cyanoacrylate glue or fibrin tissue adhesive; amniotic membrane grafting; and corneal transplantation.[1]

Tectonic keratoplasty, either using full-thickness or lamellar patch grafts is often employed as a temporary measure prior to performing definitive penetrating keratoplasty (PK). But localized corneal patch grafts and conventional PK often induce high and irregular corneal astigmatism and result in a delayed recovery of stable postoperative vision. Alternatively, Descemet stripping automated endothelial keratoplasty (DSAEK) has been demonstrated as a safe and effective surgical approach for sterile ulcers with impending or frank corneal perforation.[2,3]

SURGICAL TECHNIQUE

Tectonic DSAEK may be performed using the standard DSAEK technique.[4,5] The donor cornea is mounted on an artificial anterior chamber of a microkeratome system. After measurement of the central corneal thickness through ultrasound pachymetry, microkeratome-assisted lamellar dissection is performed. To achieve successful closure of the perforation and a stable corneal architecture, conventional DSAEK grafts >100 μm in thickness are used rather than ultrathin grafts (<100 μm). The size of the DSAEK graft is kept at a minimum with the aim of simply sealing the perforation, while leaving as much of the recipient endothelium untouched. After the graft is punched to the appropriate size, it is transferred from the cutting block to the side platform of a modified Busin glide. The graft is then advanced through the mouth of the glide until the tissue just slightly protrudes beyond the edge of the glide.

In the recipient cornea, descemetorrhexis is performed under air. Continuous air infusion either manually or from a vitrectomy system may be used to maintain the chamber during descemetorrhexis. If safe removal of Descemet membrane cannot be accomplished, it can simply be retained. Under continuous low flow irrigation with balanced salt solution, the graft is delivered through a 3-mm clear-corneal incision into the anterior chamber by means of the pull-through technique with the Busin forceps.

As in conventional DSAEK, maintaining the anterior chamber deep and stable throughout the procedure is essential. To avoid chamber collapse and iatrogenic trauma to the intraocular structures, the use of the anterior chamber maintainer is advised until the graft is well-positioned. If cyanoacrylate glue or tissue adhesives have been used as a temporizing measure, these should be left in place until the graft has been properly positioned to seal off the perforation.

For proper graft attachment and positioning, a 27-gauge cannula is inserted through the 12-o'clock side port and is advanced under the donor tissue up to approximately the center of the pupil to fill the anterior chamber with air. It is important to note that the graft may prolapse through the perforation site creating star-shaped folds which may interfere with postoperative vision or result in graft detachment. To reduce this possibility, overinflation of the anterior chamber should be avoided. In cases in which the perforation site is peripheral, the graft could be slightly decentered to properly seal the perforation. The perforation can also act as a venting incision, which can be used to reach the graft and move it across the posterior surface of the host cornea. Graft positioning can be easily performed through the perforation site using a Sinskey hook or a 27-gauge bent needle. In cases with relatively large perforations, the DSAEK graft could be delivered through the opening and into the anterior chamber, thereby eliminating the need to create a main corneal incision. The surgery is completed by air-tight suturing of the main wound and side ports with 10-0 nylon. **Figures 1 and 2** show preoperative and postoperative clinical photos of two eyes that underwent tectonic DSAEK for sterile corneal ulcers.

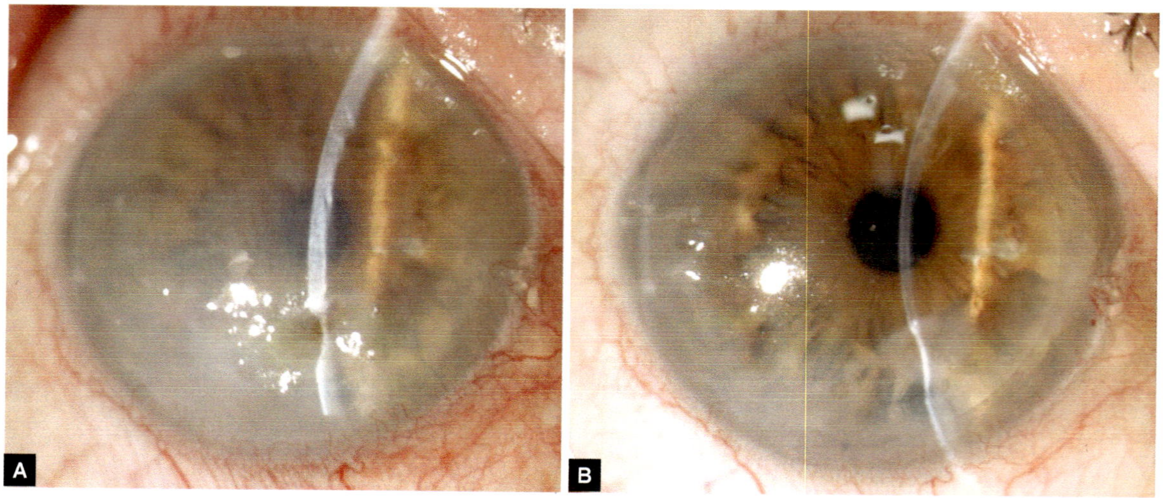

Figs. 1A and B: Preoperative (A) and postoperative (B) clinical photo of a patient who underwent tectonic DSAEK for a corneal perforation associated with endothelial decompensation.

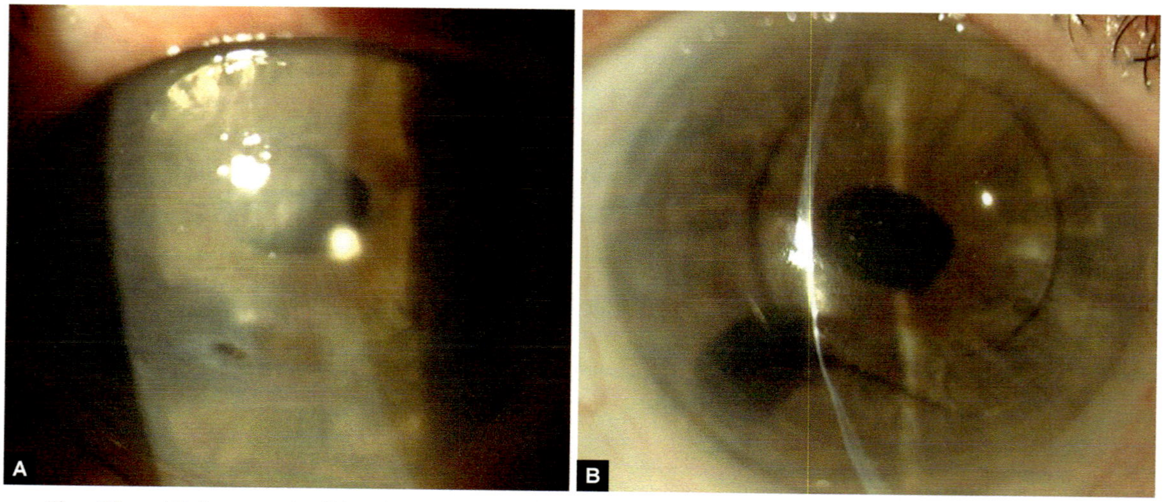

Figs. 2A and B: Preoperative (A) and postoperative (B) clinical photo of a second patient who underwent tectonic DSAEK for a corneal perforation associated with endothelial decompensation.

POSTOPERATIVE MANAGEMENT

Postoperatively, the patient is instructed to lie supine for at least 2 hours. If no air-fluid level is observed thereafter, air is removed at the slit lamp. Topical antibiotics with corticosteroids is started every 2 hours daily and tapered to 4 times daily over the first postoperative month. Subsequently, topical antibiotic treatment is discontinued while topical corticosteroids are slowly tapered to once daily indefinitely. All sutures may be removed between 4 and 6 weeks after surgery.

Although this technique does not substantially alter the anterior corneal curvature, a central/paracentral location of the corneal ulcer may limit improvement of postoperative visual acuity. In these cases, irregular astigmatism can be managed using a rigid contact lens or may require additional surgery. There is a potential risk of epithelial downgrowth because of the presence of epithelium in the perforation bed with an overlying graft. As previously reported, deep anterior lamellar keratoplasty (DALK) may be performed as early as 2 months after DSAEK.[6]

DISCUSSION

Descemet stripping automated endothelial keratoplasty is a feasible surgical option for small sterile ulcers with associated endothelial decompensation. Even in the presence of a frank perforation, DSAEK achieves successful closure of the perforation and restores both ocular integrity and corneal clarity. When extending the use of tectonic DSAEK to perforated corneas with healthy endothelium, the risk of allograft transplantation must be considered. In such cases, tectonic DSAEK should only be performed when conventional treatment with tissue adhesive or tectonic patch has failed.

Compared to PK à chaud, DSAEK avoids the complications of an open-sky surgery and confers better tectonic stability. As the DSAEK graft is not sutured onto the recipient cornea, DSAEK allows faster visual rehabilitation and minimizes postoperative refractive errors, while eliminating graft suture-related complications such as "cheese-wiring" through macerated tissue, irregular astigmatism, corneal neovascularization, infection or loose stitches. More importantly, DSAEK is associated with lower rates of immunologic rejection and graft failure. Although tectonic DSAEK is primarily considered a temporizing measure, it may obviate the need for a subsequent corneal transplantation in a few cases.[3]

Tectonic DSAEK can facilitate healing of a perforated ulcer by stopping aqueous flow through it, but for complete healing to occur, it is of outmost importance to identify and address the underlying disease process that caused the perforation.

REFERENCES

1. Jhanji V, Young AL, Mehta JS, Sharma N, Agarwal T, Vajpayee RB. Management of corneal perforation. Surv Ophthalmol. 2011;56(6):522-38.
2. Graue-Hernandez EO, Zuñiga-Gonzalez I, Hernandez-Camarena JC, Jaimes M, Chirinos-Saldaña P, Navas A, et al. Tectonic DSAEK for the management of impending corneal perforation. Case Rep Ophthalmol Med. 2012;2012:916528.
3. Nahum Y, Bahar I, Busin M. Tectonic Descemet stripping automated endothelial keratoplasty for the management of sterile corneal perforations in decompensated corneas. Cornea. 2016;35(12):1516-9.
4. Aralikatti A, Dean S, Busin M, Shah S. Pull-through technique for graft insertion in DSAEK. J Cataract Refract Surg. 2008;34(3):341; author reply 341-2.
5. Busin M, Madi S, Santorum P, Scorcia V, Beltz J. Ultrathin Descemet's stripping automated endothelial keratoplasty with the microkeratome double-pass technique two year outcomes. Ophthalmology. 2013;120:1186-94.
6. Busin M, Beltz J. Deep anterior lamellar keratoplasty after Descemet stripping automated endothelial keratoplasty. Cornea. 2011;30:1048-50.

38 Descemet's Stripping Automated Endothelial Keratoplasty: Triple Procedure

Vishal Jhanji, Sarath S, Ritu Nagpal, Rasik B Vajpayee

INTRODUCTION

Presence of cataract in an eye with corneal pathology is not an uncommon phenomena and such a situation often warrants a simultaneous corneal transplantation surgery and cataract removal with intraocular lens (IOL) implantation. Such a procedure is called as a triple procedure and corneal surgeons all over the world are well conversant with the nuances of this procedure. Usually, cataract surgery is performed simultaneously with a corneal transplantation surgery using an open-sky method. However, some surgeons prefer to perform these surgeries in a sequential manner which entails carrying out cataract surgery as a first procedure followed by corneal transplantation couple of months later. Both approaches have their own benefits and limitations. Cataract removal in eyes undergoing Descemet's stripping automated endothelial keratoplasty (DSAEK) surgery adds a new dimension in the procedure and certain modifications are required in the standard technique if both the surgeries are to be undertaken simultaneously.[1] Like with penetrating keratoplasty (PKP), it is possible to perform a cataract surgery and DSAEK in a sequential manner. However, we prefer to perform these procedures at the same sitting as the DSAEK procedure. Triple-procedure provides rapid visual recovery and allows selection of an appropriate intraocular lens.[2] Combined surgery may however be deferred in eyes with early incipient cataract, poor visualization of anterior chamber details due to significant corneal haze and in young patients in order to preserve accommodation.[3]

INDICATIONS

Descemet's stripping automated endothelial keratoplasty triple procedure is indicated in eyes which have coexisting endothelial decompensation and cataract, with a relatively clear stroma.

- *Fuchs' endothelial dystrophy*: Fuchs' endothelial corneal dystrophy is characterized by gradual loss of endothelial cells, thickening of Descemet's membrane and the formation of corneal guttata. The endothelial cell loss gets aggravated by any kind of intraocular intervention. Most cases of Fuchs' endothelial dystrophy have an associated cataract and require a triple procedure.
- *Failed graft*: A previously performed full thickness corneal graft may fail due to depletion of endothelial cells over a period of time or due to episodes of graft rejection. In such instances a co-occurrence of cataract warrants a triple procedure. However, it should be ensured that the previous graft does not have any kind of stromal scarring and has a regular anterior surface. Presence of stromal scarring or high astigmatism require a standard full-thickness graft with cataract surgery.
- *Viral endotheliitis*: Persistent corneal edema may also occur due to the destruction of corneal endothelium caused by an episode of viral keratitis. If cataract is also present, a DSAEK triple procedure can successfully be performed in a single sitting under the cover of oral antivirals.

PREOPERATIVE WORKUP

Ocular examination: Patients undergoing DSAEK triple procedure should undergo a comprehensive ophthalmic examination including a record of visual acuity, estimation of potential acuity, slit-lamp biomicroscopy, and estimation of intraocular pressure.

Ocular surface should be examined for any evidence of dry eye, corneal or scleral thinning, and evidence of past ocular surgeries. All these factors play a major role in determining a successful outcome after DSAEK surgery.

Corneal topography should be performed using Oculus Pentacam to document any astigmatism particularly in cases of previous failed grafts.

Special investigations such as anterior segment optical coherence tomography (AS-OCT) should be performed when the cornea is not very clear preoperatively. In cases with previously operated corneal grafts, AS-OCT helps in the evaluation of posterior graft host junction.[4] This helps to facilitate the decision regarding the size of the donor lenticule to be chosen in order to avoid overlap between the graft edge and the previous graft host junction.

CONSIDERATIONS FOR SELECTION OF INTRAOCULAR LENS

While DSAEK was initially presumed to be a refractively neutral procedure, corneal surgeons have come to realize that some degree of hyperopic shift is expected to occur following DSAEK.[1,5] This should be taken into account while selecting an IOL for a DSAEK triple procedure, or, while selecting an IOL for a patient with Fuchs' endothelial dystrophy planned for cataract surgery.

Evidence is beginning to emerge in the ophthalmic literature outlining the optical explanation for this hyperopic shift.[6,7] Anterior segment OCT, and Pentacam evidence, point toward the negative, or a minus lens effect of the lenticule, as the most significant factor.[6,7] Corneal thickness is not considered to be as relevant for determining the final refractive outcome.[8,9] The concave nature of the lenticule, with increased thickness in the periphery compared to the center occurs for two reasons. Firstly, an automated keratome will naturally cut thinner in the periphery, as the blade takes hold and eventually cuts toward the expected (predetermined) depth as it reaches the center, thus, leaving a posterior lenticule that is thicker around the edges. Secondly, exposure of the peripheral stroma of the lenticule to the aqueous humor, leads to its differential swelling.[6,7] The second mechanism reduces with time, possibly due to the migration of the endothelial cells across the graft host junction, and has been proposed as a reason for the hypermetropic shift gradually reducing through the first 6 months postoperatively.[6]

The actual predicted amount of hyperopic shift ranges from –0.66 to –1.19 D as reported in the literature.[5,7,10,11] One group did report DSAEK as a refractively neutral procedure[12] but this has not been reproduced by other groups. As with many surgical procedures, each individual surgeon should perform an individual audit to quantify expected refractive outcome for his or her own patients. Until this time, we recommend selection of an IOL expected, from A scan results, to yield a refractive outcome of approximately –1.0 D. In this way, post triple procedure, approximately emmetropic outcome may be expected. For a patient with endothelial disease who is at high risk of corneal decompensation, should decompensation fail to occur, a 1-D myopic outcome is relatively well tolerated.

Usually, A-scan measurements using regular methods, e.g., IOLMaster (Zeiss, Germany) should be possible preoperatively. In some cases, particularly if corneal edema is significant, accurate keratometry readings may not be possible. In such cases, keratometry readings from the other eye should be used. We usually choose a single piece foldable IOL for insertion during the DSAEK triple procedure. Both open loop as well as plate-haptic designs may be used with equal ease. In cases of capsular compromise a multipiece IOL in sulcus or an iris supported lens[13] or an anterior chamber IOL can be placed.

Limited data is available to quantify possible changes in the keratometric readings post-DSAEK. There may be a small trend towards flattening. This may be explained by the reduction in corneal edema, which is often most pronounced in the central cornea. No data is available regarding the accuracy of prediction of postoperative results using toric IOLs in eyes with preexisting corneal astigmatism. Postoperative prediction of refraction is not considered accurate enough to successfully implant a multifocal IOL, although, this has also not been quantified in the literature. For these reasons, we recommend, whenever possible, the implantation of a spherical IOL within the capsular bag. Individual lens type may be determined according to the surgeon's choice, however, it is important that the lens is secured well within the capsular bag, as protrusion of the lens through the capsulorhexis during implantation of the DSAEK lenticule may result in damage to the endothelium.

If vitreous loss occurs during cataract surgery, we suggest anterior vitrectomy and placement of IOL in the best possible position, whether in the bag, in the sulcus, or in the AC. In these cases, DSAEK may be planned as a second stage procedure.

Preparation of Donor Lenticule

The donor tissue can be prepared intraoperatively or before the surgery. When prepared before the surgery, it is termed as "precut tissue". The preparation of precut tissue can be accomplished either in the operating theater or in the eye bank depending upon the facilities available. In many parts of the world, the eye banks supply precut tissues for DSAEK to the corneal surgeons. This has the advantage of reducing the cost as well as the time of surgery.[14,15] Precut tissues have been reported to be comparable in terms of complication rates and endothelial loss with tissues prepared by the surgeons themselves in the operating room.[16] We prepare donor lenticule using the Moria automated lamellar therapeutic keratoplasty (ALTK) system (Moria, Antony, France). An appropriate microkeratome head is chosen depending upon the thickness of the donor corneal tissue. The donor button is trephined using 7.75–8.5 mm diameter trephine (depending upon the diameter of the recipient cornea) and covered with a layer of transport medium. In cases of regraft it is advisable to use a graft smaller than the diameter of the previous graft so that it does not overlap with the graft-host junction, potentially reducing the chances of postoperative graft detachment.[4]

PRESURGICAL PREPARATION

It is desirable to have a low intraocular pressure during the surgery. Intravenous mannitol (20%, 1 g/kg body weight) can be given to the patient about 1 hour before surgery. The pupil should be well dilated in order to have maximum possible view through a hazy cornea.

Anesthesia

The surgery can be performed either under general anesthesia or under a peribulbar block, depending upon the comfort of the operating surgeon. The most common indication of DSAEK triple in our hospital is Fuchs' endothelial corneal dystrophy. General anesthesia provides an optimal environment for the surgeon to go about performing this complex surgery in a calm manner.

Patient Preparation

A good ocular exposure makes it easy to create optimal sutureless wounds and insertion of the donor lenticule through the main wound. A wire speculum should preferably be used in these cases. A Lieberman speculum can cause too much pressure on the globe and lead to repeated iris prolapse intraoperatively. However, if the eye is deep set and has small palpebral aperture, it is imperative to use a Lieberman speculum to achieve optimal exposure of the globe.

SURGICAL STEPS[17]

1. *Creation of wound:* We prefer to perform DSAEK triple surgery through a superior approach because of easy maneuverability and the protection offered by the upper eyelid, by covering the main wound. A temporal surgery may be planned in very deep-set eyes but it may be difficult to pull the graft into the AC due to the obstruction presented by the nose.

   When planned superiorly, the main wound is fashioned slightly superonasally, i.e., at about 12:30 o'clock in the right eye and 11:30 o'clock in the left eye. This positioning aids in easy insertion of the donor lenticule. A limited peritomy is fashioned in the superior quadrant for creating a fornix-based conjunctival flap. A perpendicularly held 15-degree blade (Alcon, Fort Worth, Texas) is used to fashion a 4.75-mm long, partial thickness "reverse smile" scleral incision positioned 1.5 mm from the limbus centrally and 3 mm from the limbus at the edges. Subsequently, a crescent blade is used to construct the scleral tunnel extending approximately 1 mm into the clear cornea. Subsequently, a 3-mm keratome is passed through the tunnel and the anterior chamber is entered. Three side port incisions are created using a 15-degree blade:
   i. *10 o'clock incision*: For scoring and stripping of DM
   ii. *2 o'clock incision*: For inserting chopper during the process of nucleus emulsification and subsequently for the insertion of AC maintainer
   iii. *7–8 o'clock for right eye and 4–5 o'clock for left eye*: A 1.5 mm self-sealing side port is created at the inferotemporal limbus. This incision is required for inserting the Busin's forceps to pull the graft into the anterior chamber.
2. *Phacoemulsification*: A dye-assisted phacoemulsification surgery is performed using the standard technique. After creation of a scleral tunnel wound as described above 0.2 mL of 0.06% trypan blue dye (VisionBlue, DORC International, the Netherlands) is injected under air in the AC to stain the anterior capsule. We use trypan blue dye to increase the visibility of anterior capsule as most of these cases have hazy corneas.

   Anterior capsulorhexis is performed using a visco-cohesive viscoelastic (**Fig. 1**).

   A dispersive viscoelastic should not be used as it is difficult to aspirate. Even a small remnant of viscoelastic can cause dislocation of the lenticule in the postoperative period. We use chopping technique to emulsify the nucleus. After cortical lens matter aspiration, a single piece IOL is implanted taking care to remove all the viscoelastic including the one trapped behind the IOL.
3. *Removal of the host DM*: The anterior corneal surface of the recipient eye is marked using gentian violet applied using a 9-mm diameter circular marking instrument (Moria, Antony, France). An anterior chamber maintainer is inserted to have a well formed AC throughout the surgical procedure. The Descemet's membrane is scored using the external epithelial mark as a guide. After completing the scoring, the anterior chamber is turned off and trypan blue dye (0.06%) is then injected to stain the host DM. Subsequently, the AC maintainer is opened again and the DM is stripped.
4. *Constriction of pupil*: A small pupil precludes the occurrence of iris prolapse during the insertion of donor lenticule. Since, in DSAEK triple procedure, the pupil is dilated preoperatively for cataract surgery, it is imperative that pupil should be re-constricted using

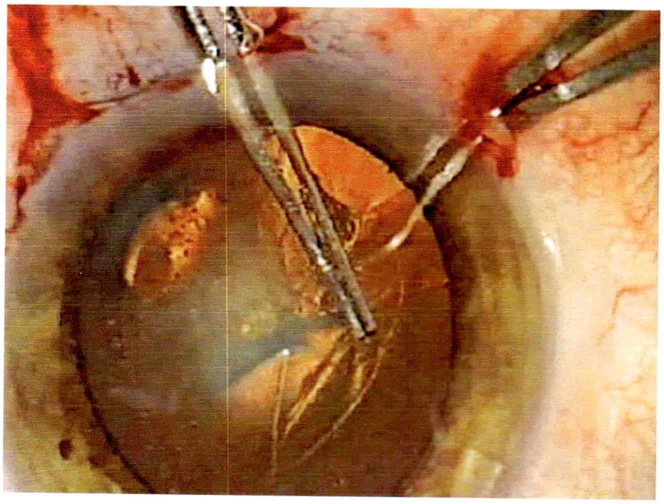

Fig. 1: Capsulorhexis being performed through a scleral tunnel incision.

intraocular Miochol and/or preservative-free topical 2% pilocarpine.

5. *Creation of stab wounds*: Four full-thickness stab wounds are made in each of the four quadrants of the host cornea in the midperipheral area using a microvitreoretinal blade after staining the tip of the blade with gentian violet. These incisions should be made at a distance of about 6.5 mm from the center of the cornea by using the blade held in an oblique fashion in order to make them self-sealing. The stab wounds facilitate drainage of fluid from the donor-graft interface.
6. *Donor lenticule transplantation*: The main wound is enlarged to 4.75 mm internally. The donor button is transferred onto the Busin's glide. A pair of Busin's forceps or crocodile vitreous forceps is utilized to engage the donor lenticule within the glide. Subsequently, the glide is placed close to the scleral wound. Using the other hand, the forceps are passed via the inferotemporal side port (5 o'clock left eye, 7 o'clock right eye) out of the scleral tunnel to grasp the edge of donor lenticule. Subsequently, in one motion, both the glide and forceps are moved in the AC through the scleral tunnel (**Fig. 2**).

All this time the edge of the lenticule is held by the forceps. After achieving a partial docking in of the glide, the donor lenticule is pulled in the AC. It is important that during this maneuver, the AC is maintained under low flow with the help of an AC maintainer infusion line. Once the lenticule is drawn into the AC, the Busin glide and the forceps are gently drawn out of their respective entry wounds. As soon as the lenticule is inserted, it unfolds itself due to the jet of BSS from the AC maintainer. In case the donor lenticule does not unfold itself, it is unfolded using gentle hydraulic pressure by injecting BSS using a Rycroft cannula inserted through the side port. The AC maintainer is removed from the eye and AC is filled with filtered air slowly taking care, that the air does not enter the graft-host interface. The donor button is gently manipulated towards the center of cornea, by stroking motions given across the anterior corneal surface, using a blunt cannula. A microvitreoretinal blade is utilized to gently open the previously fashioned anterior corneal stab wounds, expressing out the fluid trapped between the host cornea and the donor button. A small air bubble of about 6–8 mm diameter is left inside the AC. The wounds are checked for any leak at the end of surgery. The air tamponade is maintained for a period of 10 minutes and the patient is advised to be in a supine position for the next 24 hours.

POSTOPERATIVE TREATMENT

The postoperative treatment in a case of DSAEK triple procedure is the same as after a DSAEK procedure performed without cataract surgery (**Figs. 3 and 4**). Postoperatively antibiotic and corticosteroid eye drops are administered on a 4 hourly basis. The antibiotic drops are continued for the initial 1 month and the corticosteroid eye drops are tapered off by one drop every month starting 3 months after the surgery. Patients of DSAEK triple are required to be maintained on low dose corticosteroids at a frequency of one drop a day for a longer period. Antiglaucoma drops are used whenever indicated.

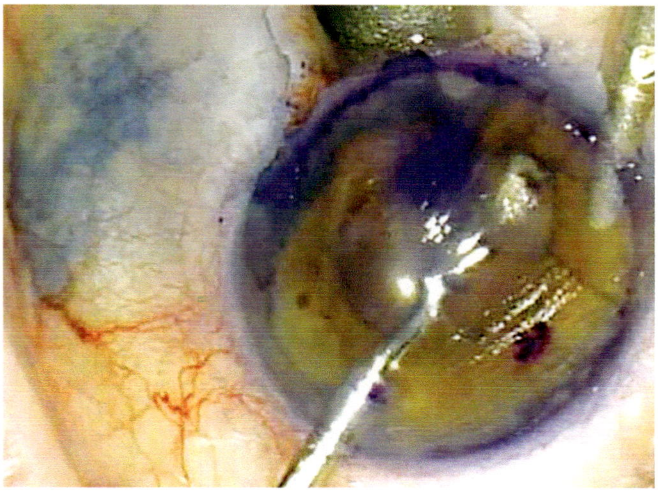

Fig. 2: Insertion of the donor lenticule using Busin's glide and forceps after phacoemulsification during Descemet's stripping automated endothelial keratoplasty triple procedure.

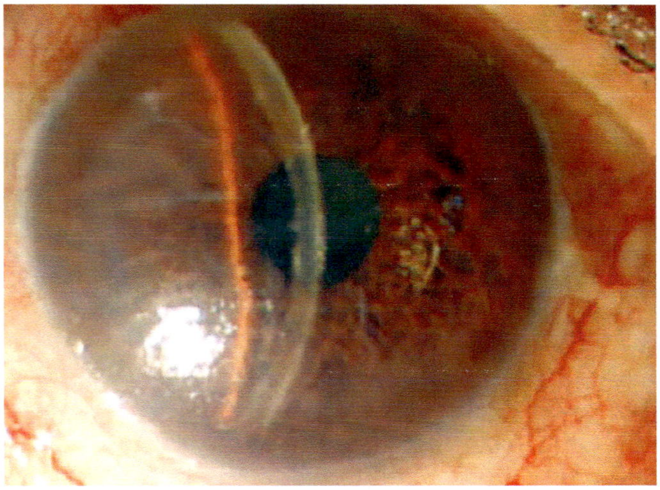

Fig. 3: Preoperative slit-lamp photograph of the right eye of a patient with Fuchs' dystrophy and concomitant cataract.

COMPLICATIONS AND THEIR MANAGEMENT

Complications related to DSAEK surgery have been described in the previous chapter. Other complications related to cataract surgery may occur like rupture of posterior capsule with vitreous prolapse. It is best to abort the DSAEK surgery in such a situation and plan it at a later date. Posterior capsule opacification and cystoid macular

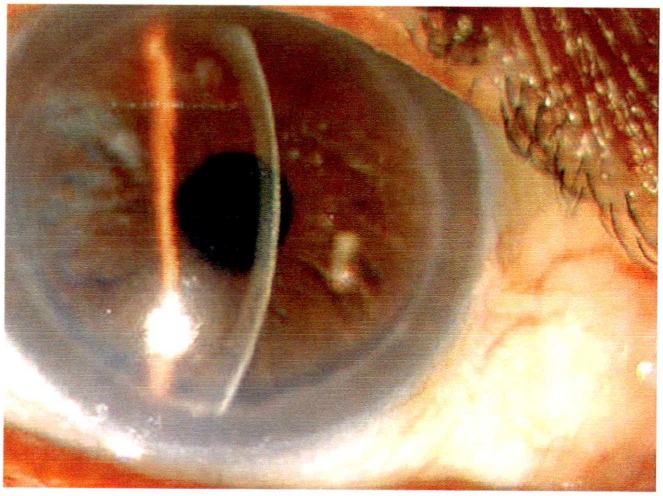

Fig. 4: Postoperative slit-lamp photograph of the same patient as shown in **Figure 3**, following Descemet's stripping and automated endothelial keratoplasty triple procedure.

edema can occur 5.7 and 1.8% cases respectively.[18] IOL opacification may result from a direct contact between the IOL surface and exogenous air, particularly in association with hydrophilic IOLs. Clinicians should consider the composition of the IOL, the amount of intracameral air injected, duration of air fill, and the intraocular pressure, while planning a DSAEK surgery.[19]

OUTCOMES

There are very few studies in the literature that have discussed the outcomes of DSAEK triple procedure specifically. In a study by Covert et al., the authors reported the use of "new triple procedure" that combines DSAEK with concurrent cataract surgery.[1] In this study, the DSAEK triple surgery was performed in 21 eyes of 21 patients. The average best spectacle-corrected visual acuity (BSCVA) improved from 20/68 ± 1.7 lines preoperatively to 20/34 ± 1.1 lines at the end of 6 months. The average preoperative spherical equivalent refractive error changed from "0.53 ± 3.2 D to 0.45 ± 1.1 D" postoperatively (6 months follow-up).

In another study by Terry et al., the results of simultaneous DSAEK and cataract surgery were analyzed in 135 eyes.[2] Preoperative BSCVA improved from an average of 20/28 to 20/31 postoperatively (6 months follow-up). The mean refractive spherical equivalent of eyes was 0.09 ± 2.32 D before surgery and 0.11 ± 1.08 D at 6 months follow-up. Mean endothelial cell loss was found to be 32 ± 14% in this series. The study did not find any difference between a staged and a triple procedure, therefore recommending a triple procedure whenever indicated.

In a study by Alqudah et al., 5 years postoperative endothelial cell density, following both DSAEK as well as DSAEK triple procedure was found to correlate significantly with preoperative endothelial cell density.[20] At 5-year follow-up, the endothelial cell loss was comparable among DSAEK (44.4% ± 21.7%) and DSAEK triple eyes (44.4% ± 22.0%) (P = 0.99). The study concluded that a higher preoperative donor endothelial cell density was correlated with a higher postoperative endothelial density at 5 year follow-up and the concomitant performance of phacoemulsification does not affect the final cell density.

SUMMARY

A suture less DSAEK triple procedure offers the advantages of faster visual rehabilitation compared to a staged approach. The application of this surgical technique might reduce the overall healthcare costs and is also more convenient to the patient.

REFERENCES

1. Covert DJ, Koenig SB. New triple procedure: Descemet's stripping and automated endothelial keratoplasty combined with phacoemulsification and intraocular lens implantation. Ophthalmology. 2007;114:1272-7.
2. Terry MA, Shamie N, Chen ES, Phillips PM, Shah AK, Hoar KL, et al. Endothelial keratoplasty for Fuch's dystrophy with cataract. Complications and clinical results with the new triple procedure. Ophthalmology. 2009;116:631-9.
3. Chaurasia S, Ramappa M, Sangwan V. Cataract surgery after Descemet's stripping endothelial keratoplasty. Indian J Ophthalmol. 2012;60(6):572-4.
4. Jhanji V, Greenrod E, Vajpayee RB. Donor dislocation after DSAEK for a failed corneal graft. Br J Ophthalmol. 2008;92:1185-1292.
5. Koenig SB, Covert DJ, Dupps WJ, Meisler DM. Visual acuity, refractive error and endothelial cell density six months after Descemet's stripping and automated endothelial keratoplasty (DSAEK). Cornea. 2007;26:670-4.
6. Scorcia V, Matteoni S, Scorcia GB, Scorcia G, Busin M. Pentacam assessment of posterior lamellar grafts to explain hyperopization after Descemet's stripping automated endothelial keratoplasty. Ophthalmology. 2009;116:1651-5.
7. Holz HA, Meyer JJ, Espandar L, Tabin GC, Mifflin MD, Moshirfar M. Corneal profile analysis after Descemet's stripping endothelial keratoplasty and its relationship to postoperative hyperopic shift. J Cataract Refract Surg. 2008;34:211-4.
8. Marcon AS, Terry MA, Kara-Jose N, Wall J, Ousley PJ, Hoar K. Influence of final corneal thickness in visual acuity after deep lamellar endothelial keratoplasty. Cornea. 2007;26:543-5.
9. Rao SK, Leung CK, Cheung CY, Li EY, Cheng AC, Lam PT, et al. Descemet's stripping endothelial keratoplasty: effect of the surgical procedure on corneal optics. Am J Ophthalmol. 2008;145:991-6.
10. Dupps WJ Jr, Qian Y, Meisler DM. Multivariate model of refractive shift in Descemet's-stripping automated endothelial keratoplasty. J Cataract Refract Surg. 2008;34:578-84.
11. Jun B, Kuo AN, Afshari NA, Carlson AN, Kim T. Refractive change after Descemet's stripping automated endothelial keratoplasty surgery and its correlation with graft thickness and diameter. Cornea. 2009;28(1):19-23.
12. Price PO, Price FW Jr. Descemet's stripping with endothelial keratoplasty: comparative outcomes with microkeratome-dissected and manually dissected donor tissue. Ophthalmology. 2006;113:1936-42.
13. Mikropoulos DG, Kymionis GD, Grentzelos MA, Voulgari N, Katsanos A, Konstas AG. Combined pupilloplasty and

retropupillary Iris-Claw intraocular lens implantation with DSAEK in a patient with traumatic Iridoplegia, Aphakia and Corneal Decompensation. Ophthalmol Ther. 2019;8(3):497-500.

14. Terry MA, Shamie N, Chen ES, Phillips PM, Hoar KL, Friend DJ. Precut tissue for Descemet's stripping automated endothelial keratoplasty: vision, astigmatism, and endothelial survival. Ophthalmology. 2009;116(2):248-56.
15. Sharma N, Maharana PK, Singhi S, Aron N, Patil M. Descemet's stripping automated endothelial keratoplasty. Indian J Ophthalmol. 2017;65(3):198-209.
16. Terry MA. Endothelial keratoplasty: a comparison of complication rates and endothelial survival between precut tissue and surgeon-cut tissue by a single DSAEK surgeon. Trans Am Ophthalmol Soc. 2009;107:184-91.
17. Jhanji V, Greenrod E, Sharma N, Vajpayee RB. Modifications in the surgical technique of Descemet's stripping automated endothelial keratoplasty. Br J Ophthalmol. 2008;92:1311-68.
18. Lanza M, Boccia R, Ruggiero A, Melillo P, Bifani Sconocchia M, Simonelli F, et al. Evaluation of donor and recipient characteristics involved in Descemet's stripping automated endothelial keratoplasty outcomes. Front Med (Lausanne). 2021;8:605160.
19. Lee MS, Tsai IL, Tsai CY, Kuo LL, Liou SW, Woung LC. Intraocular lens opacification after Descemet's stripping automated endothelial keratoplasty. Taiwan J Ophthalmol. 2017;7(3):160-3.
20. Alqudah AA, Bauer AJ, Straiko MD, Sanchez PJ, Terry MA. Descemet's stripping automated endothelial keratoplasty: The influence of preoperative endothelial cell density and triple procedures on grafts at 5 years postoperative. Medicine (Baltimore). 2020;99(45):e23139.

39 Descemet's Membrane Endothelial Keratoplasty

Denisse Pinkus, Marianne O Price, Francis W Price Jr

INTRODUCTION

Endothelial keratoplasty is a breakthrough in corneal transplantation; it has evolved to a less invasive procedure since 1998, when Melles et al. introduced the first successful approach for posterior lamellar keratoplasty (PLK) in humans.[1,2] In 2001, Terry and Ousley performed a similar procedure calling it "deep lamellar endothelial keratoplasty" (DLEK) in the United States.[3] In 2004, Melles et al. introduced a technique for removing Descemet membrane (DM) called "descemetorhexis",[4] this step is followed by the insertion of a posterior lamellar disk positioned onto the denuded host posterior stroma and was popularized as "Descemet stripping endothelial keratoplasty" (DSEK) by Price et al.[5] Gorovoy introduced an automated microkeratome for the preparation of the donor tissue; this procedure was known as "Descemet stripping automated endothelial keratoplasty" (DSAEK).[6] It was in 2006 when "Descemet membrane endothelial keratoplasty" (DMEK) was first performed by Melles; since then, it is the endothelial keratoplasty technique with the best visual results.[7]

Descemet membrane endothelial keratoplasty replaces the diseased endothelium and DM with healthy donor tissue without any posterior donor stroma, allowing preservation of a true anatomical structure.[7] These properties confer advantages over DSAEK, but preparation and handling of the thin DMEK tissue was initially more challenging. Subsequent improvements in the technique and increasing availability of eye bank prepared tissue have increased the popularity of DMEK among cornea surgeons.[8-15]

Some advantages of DMEK over DSEK/DSAEK include minimal expense for donor preparation because expensive instrumentation is not required, faster visual recovery, better visual outcomes, less refractive error, and reduced risk of immunologic rejection, which allows earlier topical corticosteroid reduction resulting in reduced risk of steroid-associated side effects.[16-20]

INDICATIONS AND SPECIAL CONSIDERATIONS

Indications

In general, endothelial keratoplasty is indicated for patients with corneal endothelial dysfunction that causes ocular symptoms and/or visual disability. The most frequent indications for DMEK are Fuchs' endothelial corneal dystrophy (FECD), pseudophakic or aphakic bullous keratopathy, failed penetrating corneal graft and failed endothelial corneal graft (DMEK and DSAEK).[21-27] Other indications include posterior polymorphous dystrophy, iridocorneal endothelial syndrome, endothelial failure from trauma and corneal decompensation caused by herpetic endotheliitis.[28,29]

Contraindications

In eyes with significant stromal scarring or opacification, relative to the retinal potential, DMEK surgery may not be desirable unless just relief of the edema is needed.[28,30] For dislocated intraocular lens (IOL) or anterior chamber (AC) IOL we do not recommend DMEK surgery unless the lens abnormality is fixed first, as either a combined procedure or a staged surgery. In eyes with aniridia, significant iris abnormalities or aphakia, DSEK/DSAEK is preferable to DMEK because the thicker graft can be more easily suture fixated to the recipient to prevent dislocation of the graft to the posterior chamber.

Special Considerations

In addition to the ophthalmological examination, pre-operative assessment is important to detect patient characteristics that could interfere with the surgery. These factors include—conditions that interfere with supine positioning; conditions that interfere with graft attachment such as essential blepharospasm and chronic rubbing of the eyes; conditions that can increase the posterior pressure during surgery such as obesity or thyroid orbitopathy; and conditions that may reduce adequate postoperative care such as mental disorders or in very young or very old patients.[31]

Crystalline Lens Status

If visually significant lens opacity is present, DMEK can be combined with cataract extraction or it can be performed before or afterward. In our practice, many patients prefer to undergo a single combined procedure, but we are currently recommending staged cataract surgery after DMEK for patients who desire a multifocal and/or toric intraocular lens with a more predictable refractive result.

It may be preferable to perform DMEK alone in patients under 50 years of age in cases with little or no lens opacity. DMEK or any other intraocular surgery increases the risk of cataract formation and progression, so the pros and cons of each approach should be discussed with an older patient to help make an informed choice.[32]

Anterior Chamber Abnormalities

Eyes with a shallow AC and associated increased posterior pressure (such as in hyperopic eyes, Asian eyes, and nanophthalmic eyes) are at increased risk of donor endothelial cell loss. Technique modifications include—performing Descemetorhexis under viscoelastic to improve AC stability or an air-assisted Descemetorhexis to improve visibility; using an AC maintainer during graft insertion to stabilize the AC; and using a glide method of donor insertion to hold back the iris. A more invasive strategy is the use of a core vitrectomy to deepen the AC. If anterior synechiae are present, they should be lysed before inserting the graft because they decrease the effective recipient corneal diameter. Prolapsed vitreous in the AC should be addressed before insertion of the graft.[28,31]

An excessively deep AC can make the surgery more difficult because the graft tends to scroll and it is easier to uncurl it and hold it open between the cornea and iris when the AC can be shallowed. A deep AC can be addressed by choosing older donors who have less scrolling tendency and using a larger graft so it is easier to unfold it and hold it open. In eyes with previous pars plana vitrectomy and scleral fixated lens we prefer to fold the DMEK tissue endothelium-inward, pull it into the eye with forceps and hold onto it until it is supported with an air bubble in the correct orientation.[33]

Previous Glaucoma Surgery

Achieving and maintaining a firm air fill may be difficult in eyes with previous glaucoma surgery because air tends to escape out of the AC via filters or tubes. To promote graft attachment, full or nearly full air fills may be safely left. If a firm fill cannot be achieved intraoperatively, it may be necessary to inject cohesive viscoelastic after the graft is in place at the tube tip or filter ostium to prevent air escape. If a tube is at risk of having contact with the graft, it should be trimmed or repositioned. If the latter is needed, it is recommended to stage it about 1 month before the DMEK procedure.

Previous Failed Penetrating Keratoplasty

Descemet membrane endothelial keratoplasty can be done in an eye with a failed penetrating keratoplasty (PK) that was acceptable refractively to the patient before failure (**Fig. 1**). It is recommended to score and strip within the previous PK margin very carefully to avoid wound dehiscence.

When the PK graft diameter measures 8 mm or more, we prefer to use a DMEK of the same size or slightly smaller. If the PK graft diameter measures less than 8 mm, we prefer to use a 9-mm graft to provide more healthy donor endothelial cells, although adherence is more challenging if the DMEK diameter exceeds the diameter of the prior PK.[26] Preoperative imaging of the posterior corneal surface can show the extent of irregularity and help when choosing the size and location of the DMEK graft.[26,27,31] In eyes with a failed PK, repeated air injections or use of long-acting gases rather than air may be needed to achieve good DMEK attachment.

DONOR PREPARATION

Choosing the Donor Tissue

Descemet membrane thickness increases and elasticity decreases with age. These characteristics are believed to be the reason why DM from a younger donor is more likely to roll up tightly when peeled off from the stroma, as well as why it can be more difficult to peel off Descemet membrane with younger corneas. Younger grafts generally take longer to unfold in the AC, and the endothelial cell loss may increase with more manipulation. Therefore, when surgeons are first learning DMEK it can be easier to use grafts from donors older than 60 years of age, whereas experienced surgeons may accept donors as young as 45 years old.[34]

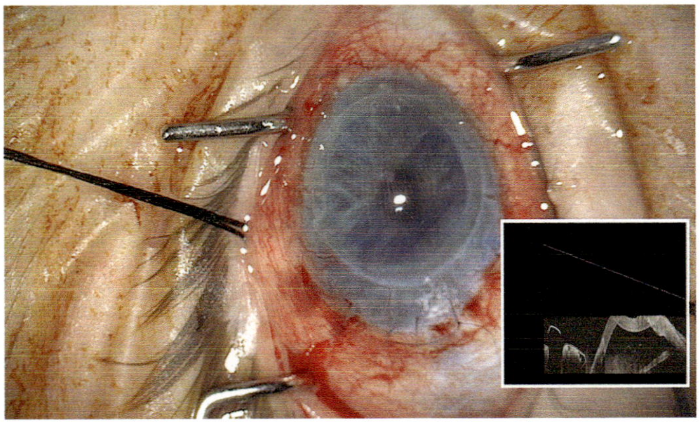

Fig. 1: Intraoperative image of Descemet membrane endothelial keratoplasty (DMEK) after failed penetrating keratoplasty (PK) showing Descemetorhexis inside the previous PK graft; the new graft is in a double scroll configuration before unfolding and orientation can be confirmed by intraoperative optical coherence tomography (OCT).

Another factor to consider is a positive history of donor diabetes because the adhesion between DM and stroma tends to be stronger in donors with diabetes, and this is associated with an increased risk of DMEK tissue preparation failure. An eye bank developed a donor risk rating scale that assigned greater risk to donors with more than 10 years history of diabetes or who had diabetes-related complications, such as neuropathy. They found that the risk of donor tissue preparation failure was higher with corneas from donors rated 4 or 5 on the 5-point rating scale.[35-39]

The donor tissue can be prepared ahead of time by the surgeon or by the eye bank, or on the day of the surgery by the surgeon.[40] Multiple techniques have been previously described; they can be classified into those based on manual peeling and those based in an air or liquid injection to detach DM.[41] Currently, most eye banks and surgeons use manual peeling.

Technique

Here we describe the current technique used in our practice which is the modified submerged cornea using backgrounds away (SCUBA) technique (**Figs. 2 and 3**).[11,42,43] The first step is marking the periphery of the DM with a blunt instrument. This process is called "scoring" and is done with the corneoscleral tissue submerged in a viewing chamber (Krolman viewing chamber, K55-57007-23, Bausch and Lomb, Rochester, NY). It can also be done on a cutting block. The donor is fixated with a toothed forceps holding the scleral rim with the left hand (if right handed) while a peripheral break or "score" in the DM is created with a blunt Y-hook (9217E, Ambler Surgical, Exton, PA, 17157 Moria, Antony, France) positioned at 12 o'clock and 0.5–1 mm central to the trabecular meshwork with the right hand (counter pressure can be made on a protruding viewing chamber pillar). Then the donor is rotated counterclockwise, grabbing it with toothed forceps at 10–11 o'clock and rotating it approximately 2 clock hours each time until completing 360° of scoring.

After excess storage solution is dripped away, the donor graft is stained with trypan blue (Vision Blue; DORC, Zuidland, the Netherlands) for 10 seconds, then excess of stain is dripped away and the tissue is submerged again in the viewing chamber. Incomplete blue lines may represent incomplete scoring or incomplete staining. Scars, insufficient scoring strokes that only denuded endothelial

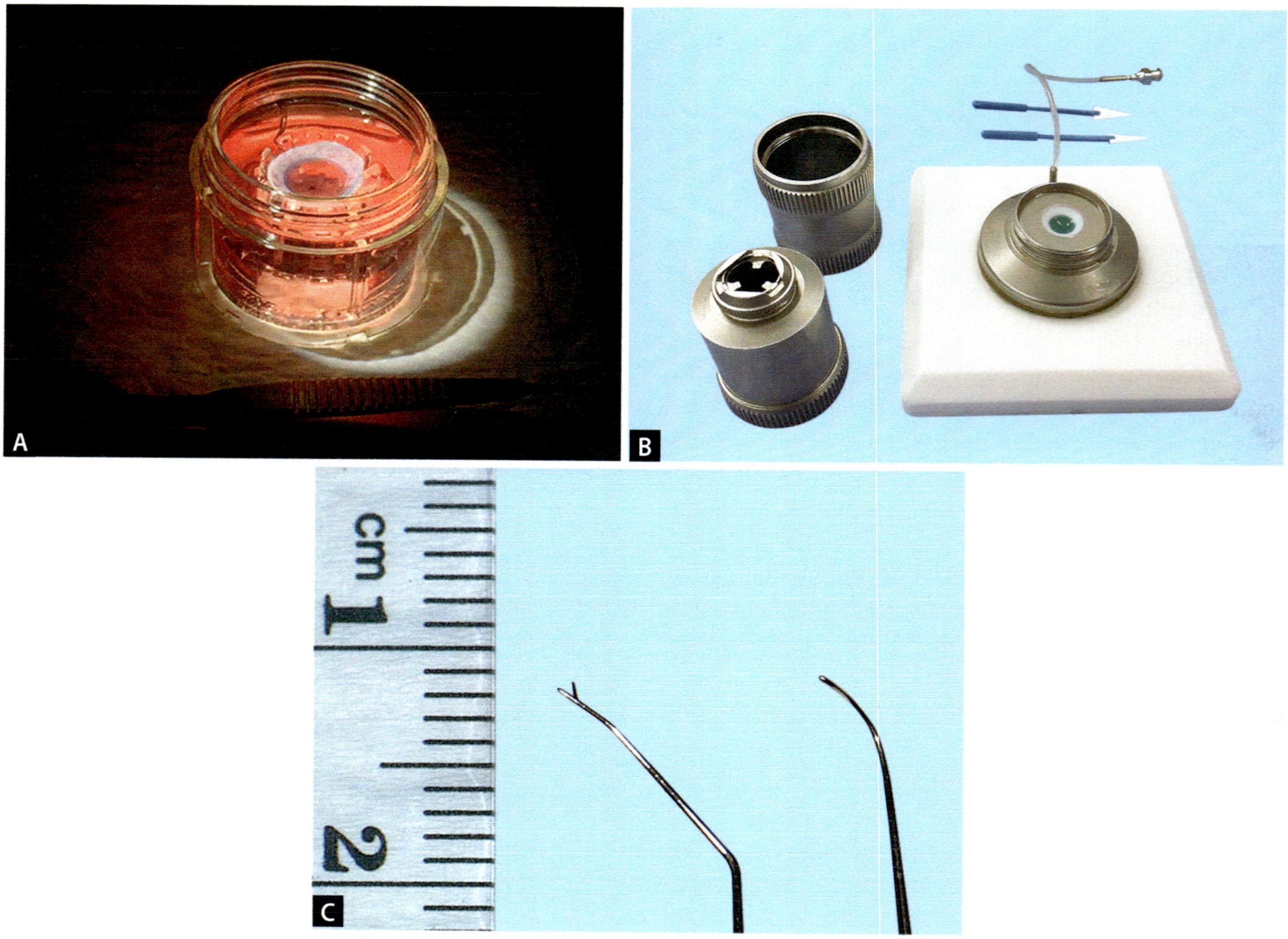

Figs. 2A to C: Instruments needed for donor graft preparation. (A) Krolman viewing chamber; (B) Punch and cutting block; (C) Blunt Y-hook and microfinger.

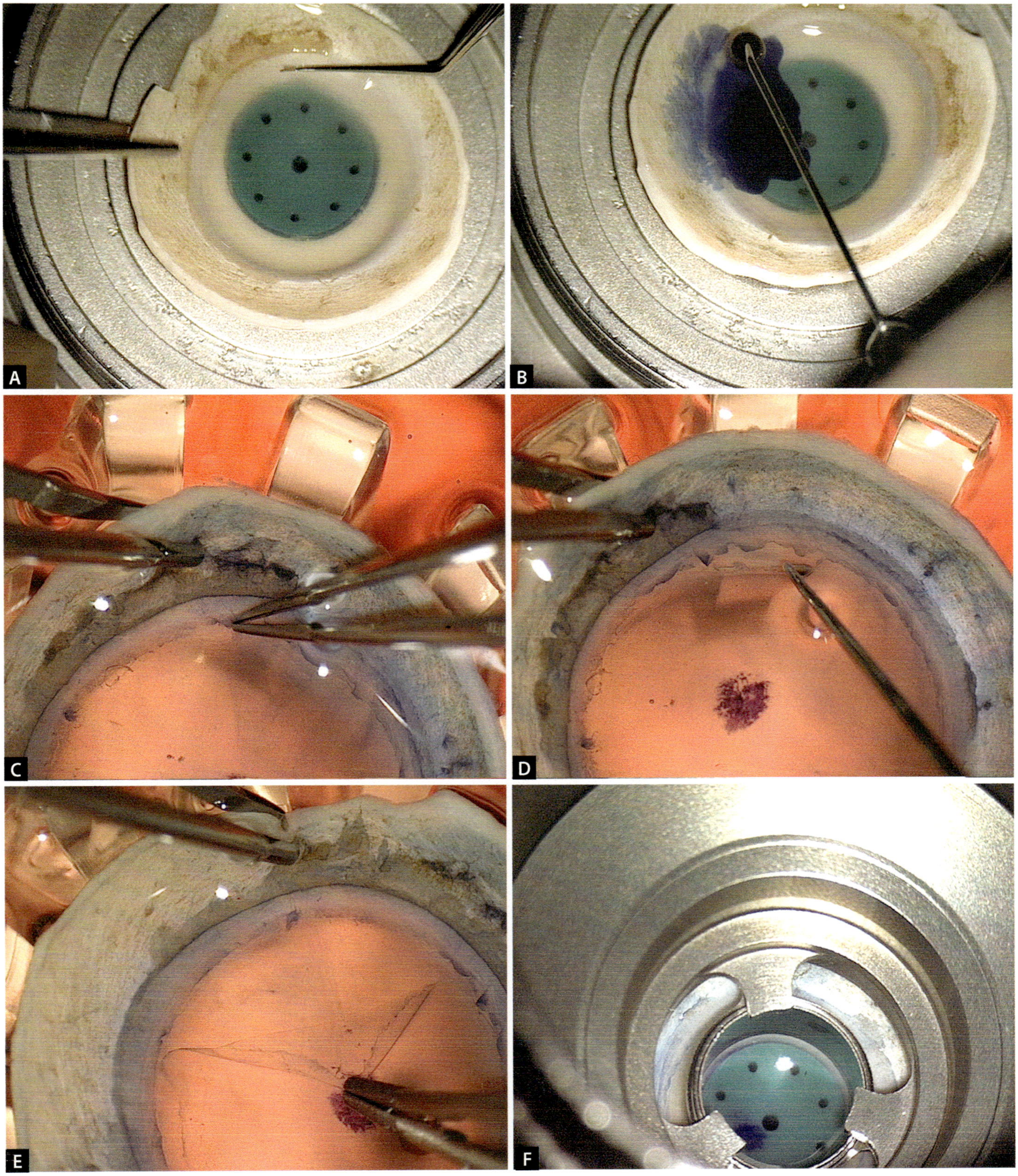

Figs. 3A to F: Donor preparation technique. (A) Scoring DM with a blunt Y-hook; (B) Staining the graft with trypan blue; (C) Removing irregular DM tags outside the area of scoring; (D) Lifting the scored edge with a blunt microfinger; (E) Peeling of the DM by quadrants; (F) Trephining the DM.

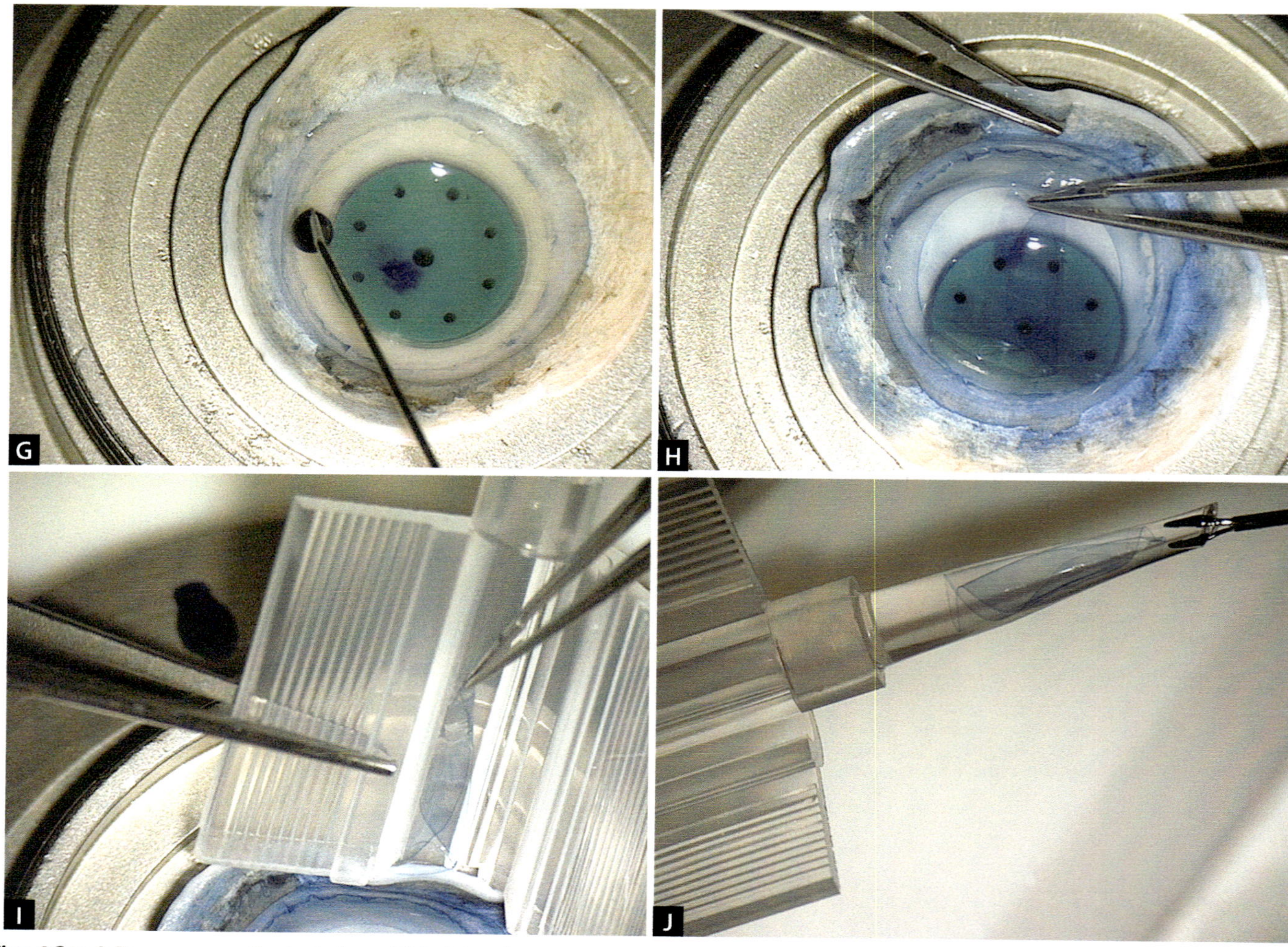

Figs. 3G to J: Donor preparation technique. (G) Staining the trephined DM with trypan blue; (H) Graft in a trifold configuration ready for loading to the cartridge; (I) Loading the graft into the cartridge; (J) Pulling the graft through the tip filled with balanced salt solution (BSS) with Tan forceps.

cells, and endothelial damage such as snail tracks or stress lines also stain blue. The next step is to remove irregular DM tags outside the area of scoring to improve the view of the DM edge and detect if unsuccessful score zones or radial tears are present.

The scored edge is lifted 360° with a blunt microfinger (Moria, Antony, France). The microfinger is placed 0.5 mm under the DM edge in an area with loose DM attachment and held against the stroma. The microfinger is advanced away from fixation gently gliding it from an area of minimal tension toward an area of maximum tension. If a radial tear develops, it needs to be rescued to prevent central extension; the loose edges must be torn off leaving a new continuous edge. This leaves an irregularity on the edge with "peaks" and "craters". Edge lifting should be initiated from areas of minimal tension at the "peaks", gliding the microfinger downhill to the depth of the "crater" where tension is maximal.

Partially peeling DM before final trephination allows any zones of strong adhesions that can develop tears to be discovered. The DM is peeled by quadrants ("Corridor Method") to help minimize tension by minimizing the width of the peel zone.[11] The DM edge is grabbed with a Tubingen forceps (2457E, Ambler Surgical) central to fixation without twisting the forceps or elevating away from the cornea. Each pull should be straight across. The first quadrant is taken about halfway to the center of the cornea; the second quadrant is started 180° away and taken halfway to the center; the third quadrant is started 90° away from second quadrant; the fourth quadrant is made 180° away halfway to the center. The meridian of peel 4 is marked as the intended start site for the final peel after trephination. When separation resistance is encountered, it can be felt as tension or seen as a "smile configuration" of the leading edge of the peel with stress lines, and a horseshoe tear (HST) may form. In this scenario, peeling at 45° to both sides of the smile configuration and then continuing from the original site is helpful.

If an HST is suspected, stop and apply focal trypan blue staining. If an HST is confirmed, one can partially peel all other quadrants, trephine, and then start the final donor peel 180° away from the HST. If two or more HSTs develop, the tongues of the HSTs have to be lifted so that the peel can be continued through those HSTs. The centrally protruding viewing chamber pillar can be used for counterpressure to lift the tongues.[11]

The next step is to trephine the DM. A graft diameter of 8–9 mm is suitable in most cases. The size should be selected based on the white-to-white diameter of the host cornea, considering the main and paracentesis incisions so they do not overlap with the graft.

If the surgeon would like to have an "S" stamp on the donor tissue to aid in discerning graft orientation after it is inside the recipient eye, this is the time to add it.[44]

The excess storage solution is dripped away from the donor, and a cellulose sponge is used to drain the storage solution under the DM and make it lay flat. Then the donor is placed on the cutting block and aligned as needed to keep any imperfections such as HSTs outside the trephine zone to the extent possible. A cutting block with a marked central 8 mm area can facilitate alignment [Hanna punch with a Price cutting block (17169 and 630/660-7540, Moria)]. Suction is activated on the cutting block and the DM is checked to ensure that it is not curled.

The guide cylinder is attached; then the trephine punch cylinder is advanced into the guide until the blade makes contact with the cornea without rotating. The corneal thickness holds the punch cylinder up so that a small gap remains present between the guide and punch rims. The thumb and index finger of one hand is placed in this gap to hold the circumference of both rims while the other hand is used to lightly tap the punch in all four quadrants. When the gap is lessened, tapping is stopped so that the cornea is only penetrated but not perforated and both cylinders are removed.

With the suction still on, the donor is stained again with trypan blue to make sure a 360 trephination was made. Suction is turned off, and the peripheral rim of the DM beyond the trephination is removed. The final peel should be done at the same meridian where the peel of the fourth quadrant was made.

The graft is stained with trypan blue for 60 seconds to make it more visible during the process of insertion and orientation inside the recipient AC, then it is submerged in balanced salt solution (BSS) where it will curl with the endothelium side out. The graft is loaded in an IOL cartridge (Viscoject cartridge #2.2) also submerged in BSS and the cartridge is assembled in the Viscoject IOL injector (Viscoject, Medicel AG, Switzerland).

Another option is to load the graft with the endothelium side in, folded into a trifold configuration. This method facilitates tissue unfolding inside the recipient eye.[45] After the peripheral rim of the DM beyond the trephination is removed at the cutting block, the graft is folded by grabbing one edge of the tissue with either a small tying or jeweler forceps and folding it approximately one-third of way across the tissue. Then, the opposite edge is grabbed and folded over the first fold, making a trifold or burrito configuration. Tapping maneuvers on the Descemet membrane side during folding can help with getting the edges to fold over completely. To load a trifold graft into the IOL cartridge (Viscoject cartridge #1.8) we hold the tissue at one of the unfolded ends and slide it onto the cartridge, then with the tip filled with BSS the tissue is pulled through with a Tan loading forceps (Tan EndoGlide Loading Forceps, Network Medical Products Ltd, UK or Asico, Westmont, IL).

RECIPIENT PREPARATION

The patients are instructed to use topical nonsteroidal anti-inflammatory drugs (NSAIDs) such as bromfenac 0.07% for 3 days prior to surgery. Prior to surgery, pilocarpine nitrate 2% drops are instilled to constrict the pupil (or carbachol 0.01% is used when doing triple procedures, i.e., DMEK combined with cataract surgery).

Topical anesthesia supplemented by intravenous sedation and intracameral lidocaine is used in the majority of our DMEK procedures to eliminate the risks associated with general anesthesia or a local block. We place 4-0 silk scleral traction sutures inferiorly and superiorly to facilitate eye positioning. If a peribulbar or retrobulbar block is used, a Honan balloon (The Lebanon Corporation, Lebanon, IN) should be placed for 30 minutes to eliminate back pressure.

Technique

Figures 4A to H illustrate key aspects of the DMEK technique performed in a phakic eye. We first use the trephine that was used to punch the donor tissue to indent the epithelium on the corneal surface to provide a reference for later removal of DM and placement of the donor tissue. A temporal peritomy is made with Westcott scissors removing the conjunctival and Tenon's tissue from the temporal quadrant of the limbus and adjacent sclera. Mild cautery is used to control any bleeding. The limbus is marked with Gentian violet using the calipers to measure a 2-mm length. At 1.5 mm posterior to the limbus, a curved incision is made with a calibrated diamond blade to 200 microns depth. A crescent blade is used to extend this incision in a lamellar dissection into clear cornea creating a scleral tunnel. We then make two short self-sealing paracenteses 45° away from the main incision (one superior temporal and one inferior temporal) with 15° super sharp paracentesis blades.

Scoring and stripping of the DM can be done under viscoelastic (**Figs. 5A and B**), air, or BSS infusion. Air or viscoelastic provide better visualization than BSS and prevent increasing corneal edema during the stripping process. A specially modified Price-Sinskey hook (Price Endothelial Keratoplasty Hook; Moria SA or reverse Sinskey hook, DORC. International, Zuidland, the Netherlands) is introduced through a paracentesis to score DM just along or slightly larger than the previously made reference mark

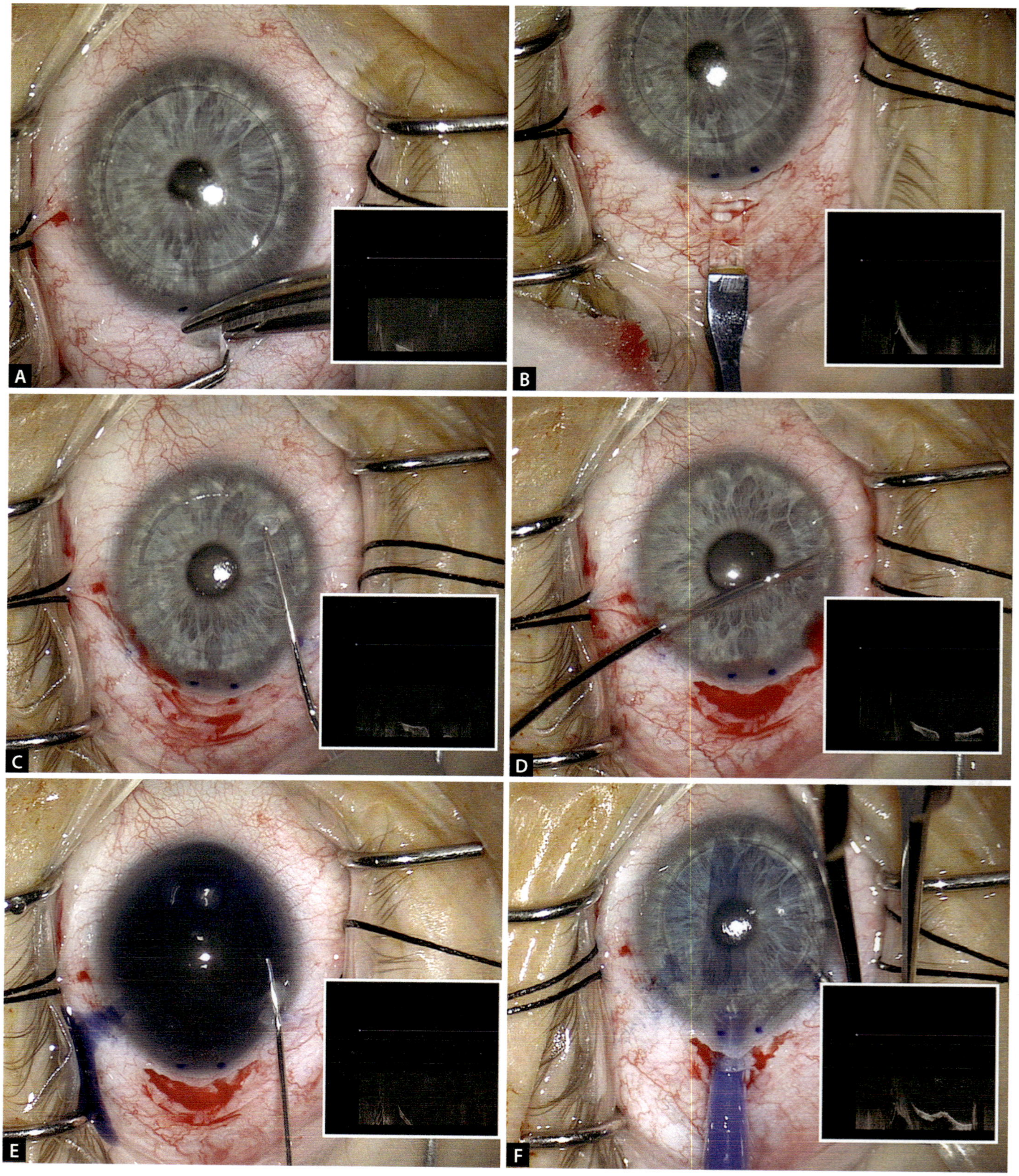

Figs. 4A to F: Descemet membrane endothelial keratoplasty in a phakic eye. (A) Temporal peritomy with Wescott scissors; (B) Extending the scleral tunnel incision with a crescent blade; (C) Stripping DM with a Price-Sinskey hook under viscoelastic; (D) Peripheral inferior iridotomy with microscissors; (E) Injecting trypan blue into the anterior chamber (AC); (F) Injection of the donor graft in a trifold configuration.

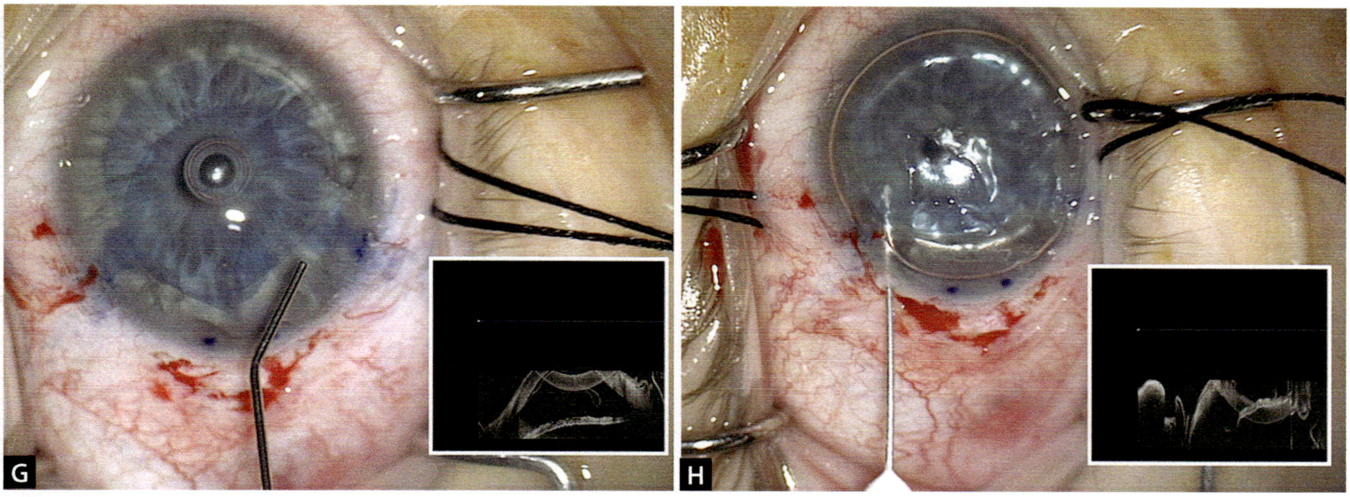

Figs. 4G and H: Descemet membrane endothelial keratoplasty in a phakic eye. (G) Positioning the graft with a no-touch technique; (H) Injecting air to attach the graft to the recipient cornea.

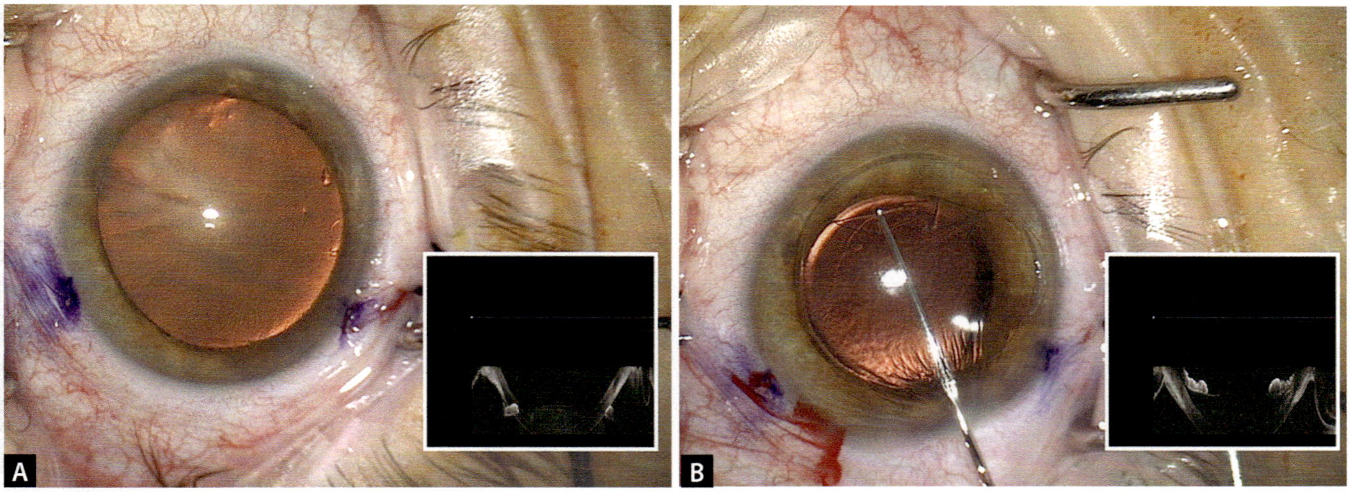

Figs. 5A and B: (A) Intraoperative image of an eye that underwent cataract extraction and Descemet membrane endothelial keratoplasty, you can see the guttae through the red reflex; (B) Stripping DM under viscoelastic in the same eye.

on the epithelium and then to strip the delineated inner portion of DM and remove it from the eye. The bi-manuals are used to completely remove viscoelastic from the AC, if used. Trypan blue is injected into the AC and allowed to remain for about 30 seconds and then irrigated out with BSS, this helps identify any loose strands of DM or areas which were not stripped enough. Areas of exposed DM will stain dense blue, those with exposed stroma will stain light blue, and those with attached DM will have minimal or no staining.

The main incision is finished by introducing a 2.8-mm keratome through the scleral tunnel. Loose residual tags of DM are removed with the bi-manuals or micro-scissors.

Intraocular micro-scissors are introduced into the eye and used to make an inferior peripheral iridotomy (PI) at about 6 o'clock; the aspiration tip of the bi-manuals is used to aspirate any residual posterior iris pigment from behind the iridotomy and ensure the PI is patent. The paracenteses are now sealed with hydration.

TRANSPLANTATION OF DONOR TISSUE

The DMEK graft can be inserted into the eye with a glass pipette, an intraocular lens cartridge or a custom injector. We prefer using an IOL cartridge (Viscoject, Medicel AG, Switzerland) because it provides a more controlled delivery. The IOL injector needs to be modified by removing the plunger and spring and reattaching the plunger alone in the cartridge after loading the graft into the barrel tip to prevent inadvertent damage of the graft. After this, the cartridge can be assembled to the injector, making sure the donor tissue moves without getting stuck in the plunger.

An AC maintainer can be used for insertion of the graft. The graft is inserted in the AC by placing the cartridge into the main wound with the bevel facing downward, pushing and rotating it so the cartridge is inserted into the AC, then injecting the graft. Before removing the cartridge, decompression of the AC and removal of the AC maintainer should be done. Also, the main incision should be secured by pushing on the cornea central to the wound to prevent graft ejection from the AC. If the scleral tunnel is self-sealing no suture is necessary, but if it is not self-sealing or if a clear corneal incision was used then the wound must be sutured with 10-0 nylon.

After the graft has been inserted, small intermittent bursts of BSS from a 10-cc syringe can be used to move and rotate the donor tissue. Fluid can also be directed to unwrap the donor. It is very important to confirm the orientation of the graft before fully unfolding it. We prefer to use a handheld slit beam (510L, Eidolon Optical LLC, Natick, MA) or an intraoperative OCT (iOCT; Haag-Streit, Bern, Switzerland) to confirm the graft orientation (**Figs. 6A to C**).

The handheld slit beam is used with the operating room and microscope lights off. The slit beam light is directed into the AC and onto the graft. If the graft is properly positioned with the endothelium facing downward, it appears in the slit beam as two adjacent arcs representing the two scrolls, with the "connector" between them as a short beam segment posterior to the arcs. If the graft is upside down, the slit beam shines on the "connector," which appears to the surgeon as a single broad arc in the AC just below the recipient cornea.[8]

After the orientation of the graft is confirmed, a small air bubble (0.02 cc) is placed with a 1-cc syringe on 30-gauge cannula under the partially unfolded graft. A small amount of BSS is then injected to allow easier manipulation. While the small bubble is helping to maintain the graft orientation, tapping on the cornea and directing the bubble helps unfold the graft. To help position the graft under the scored and stripped area, a quick stroke of the cannula over the anterior corneal surface induces fluid waves in the interface that shifts the donor in the direction of the sweep.

Once the donor is correctly centered and totally unfolded, the AC is filled 90–95% full with air. The air pressure should be enough to keep the graft in position but not so high to compromise the optic nerve and its blood supply. This is confirmed by asking the patient if he or she can see the lights of the microscope go off and on. Air and fluid levels in the AC can be adjusted as needed. Finally the peritomy is closed with cautery and traction sutures are removed. Some surgeons prefer to fill the AC with a long-acting gas such as 20% sulfur hexafluoride (SF6) instead of air to promote graft attachment.

The following medications are immediately administered—topical antibiotic, timolol maleate 0.5%, cyclopentolate hydrochloride 1%, antibiotic/steroid ointment and intravenous 125 mg methylprednisolone.

POSTOPERATIVE MANAGEMENT

One of the advantages of DMEK is that the recovery time is usually so fast that patients can have the second eye treated within 1 week of the first eye.[28,46]

In the immediate postoperative period patients are instructed to remain in a supine position looking at the ceiling for 60 minutes to allow the graft to adhere. Rubbing or pushing of the eyes should be avoided because this can affect the graft adherence. The patients undergo a slit-lamp and intraocular pressure (IOP) examination before they are released. If the IOP is normal and fluid is present over a patent PI the patient is sent home and instructed to remain in a supine position as much as possible until the next day appointment. If a patent PI cannot be visualized or a total air fill is suspected without elevated IOP, the patient is instructed to return to the clinic after 1 hour to make sure the IOP is not elevated from an air block of the pupil and PI. If the IOP is elevated and a patent PI with a fluid meniscus over it is present, then topical glaucoma drops are administered and IOP is rechecked after 30 minutes.[13] If the IOP is elevated and a total air fill is seen, then a paracentesis should be done to remove some air and allow fluid to cover the PI, and the patient is instructed to return after 1 hour for a recheck.[13] If the IOP remains elevated, air should be removed so it does not block the pupil and dilating drops are administered.[13] For air removal we use a 30-gauge needle on

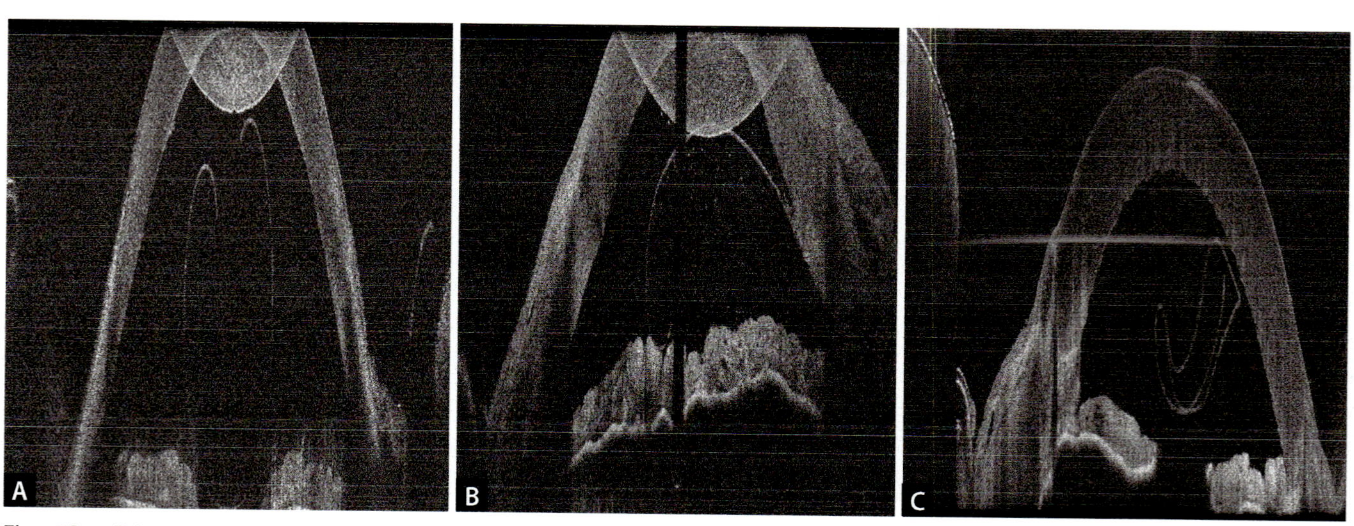

Figs. 6A to C: Intraoperative optical coherence tomography to confirm orientation of the donor graft. (A) Correct orientation of the donor graft; (B) Upside-down orientation of the donor graft; (C) Upside-down orientation of a graft in a trifold configuration.

a 1-mL syringe; sometimes BSS or additional air needs to be injected to achieve the desired bubble size.[13]

The patient is usually examined on day 1, day 2, and week 1 after surgery to assess graft adherence, bubble size, and IOP. If the graft is attached and the IOP is normal then subsequent follow-up visits are typically scheduled at 1, 3, 6, and 12 months after surgery.

If a partial graft detachment is seen or suspected, it can be confirmed by doing an anterior segment optical coherence tomography (OCT). If the detached areas of the graft are increasing in size or seem to affect vision, then air should be injected and this is easier if a partial bubble is still in the AC. A 30-gauge needle on a 1-mL syringe is used to inject air; the needle is inserted parallel to the iris with the bevel facing up, reaching up to the area of the residual air bubble. Slit lamp examination and IOP measurement should be performed 1 hour after the procedure.

Antibiotic eye drops are used four times daily for 1 week. Topical corticosteroids are indicated as follows—prednisolone acetate 1% four times daily for 1–2 months followed by fluorometholone 0.1% or loteprednol 0.5% four times daily during the third month after DMEK, three times daily in month 4, twice daily in month 5, and then once daily until the 1-year examination. For non-Caucasian patients we start with 6–8 times daily dosing and taper more slowly, because increased pigment seems to be associated with increased AC reaction.[19,20,47]

COMPLICATIONS

For a successful DMEK surgery and outcome, the surgeon should know how to recognize and treat intraoperative and postoperative complications.

Intraoperative Complications

Visualizing and Orienting the Graft

To prevent poor visualization of donor tissue, sufficient staining should be done before injecting the graft. The graft can also be re-stained in the AC by injecting trypan blue and gently irrigating with BSS. If the recipient cornea is too edematous and interferes with good visualization, one may consider doing DSAEK instead of DMEK.

Different options are available to verify correct graft orientation with the donor endothelium facing toward the AC. We prefer to use a hand-held slit beam or an intraoperative OCT to confirm the graft orientation. Some surgeons prefer to utilize asymmetric markings along the edge of the trephined graft or an "S" stamp on the DM side of the graft to confirm orientation, while others check for the "Moutsouris sign" using a cannula to identify whether the curl of the graft is directed above or below the cannula.[10,48,49]

Intraoperative Bleeding

We usually make the PI after stripping DM. A potential advantage of making the PI before stripping DM is that the cornea would be less likely to swell further in the event of prolonged intraoperative bleeding. An iridotomy with an Nd:YAG laser can be performed before the day of surgery; however, those can bleed as well. The incidence of intraoperative hyphema secondary to an intraoperative peripheral iridotomy is as high as 41%. We previously reported that intraoperative hyphema is more likely when DMEK is combined with cataract surgery; however, it had no significant effect on graft attachment, endothelial cell loss, or visual acuity.[50] If intraoperative bleeding develops after doing the PI, the intraocular pressure can be raised with irrigation or with an air bubble so the bleeding stops.

Postoperative Complications

Graft Detachment

Graft detachment is the most common complication of DMEK (**Fig. 7**); it can be complete when the entire graft is detached or partial when part of the graft is still attached to the recipient stroma.[51] However, with DMEK, it is prudent to reinject air before there is a total detachment and the graft has curled back up. The mean air injection rate to reattach grafts is 28.8% (range 2.4%–82%), but as the surgeon becomes more experienced in performing DMEK the rate of air injection to treat detachment decreases substantially.[17]

Some precautions can be taken to avoid graft detachment. These include ensuring a correct graft orientation with the endothelium facing the AC, ensuring that the graft is completely unfolded, ensuring correct positioning with no overlapping host-donor DM, maintaining a well-pressurized AC, and minimizing donor damage by avoiding excessive manipulation when preparing the donor, injecting it and unfolding it. In a recent meta-analysis by Marques et al. they reported that use of intraocular sulfur hexafluoride (SF6) 20% instead of air tamponade seemed to be a safe option to reduce the incidence of graft detachment and decrease the need for re-bubbling procedures.[52] However,

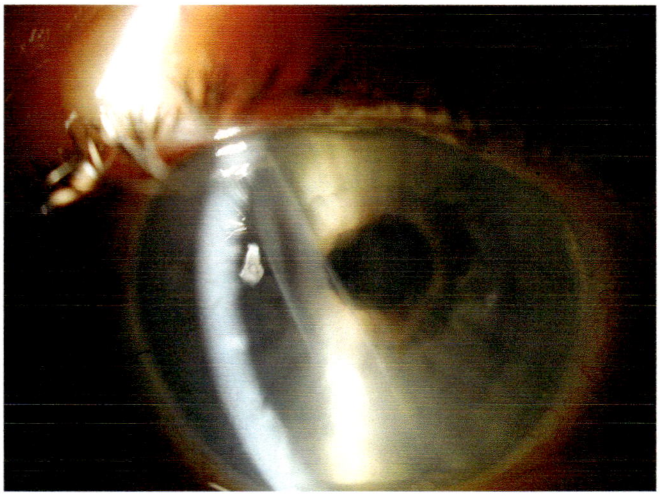

Fig. 7: Slit-lamp image of a total Descemet membrane endothelial keratoplasty graft detachment.

the incidence of posterior synechiae is increased with long-acting gases.

There is no consensus regarding the best timing for re-bubbling. Some surgeons recommend re-bubbling when partial detachments are central or larger than one-third of the DMEK-graft surface.[53] We also re-bubble if we see that the detached areas of the graft are increasing in size or seem to affect vision. Re-bubbling is easier if a residual air bubble is still present because adding more air to the residual bubble helps ensure the new air is not being injected between the graft and the host cornea.

Graft Failure

Early graft failure is the absence of clearance of the cornea despite having a completely attached graft; this implies an initial lack of endothelial function. Persisting nonimproving graft detachment after re-bubbling can also be a sign of graft failure.[54] Early failure of the graft is usually due to surgical trauma, graft detachment, upside down orientation of the graft, etc. The average rate of early DMEK graft failure is 1.9% (range 0–12.5%).[17] Secondary graft failure means that the cornea cleared initially with an attached graft, but decompensated later with or without associated graft rejection or glaucoma filtering surgery. In any case, repeat DMEK should be considered. Prompt replacement of a failed graft provides visual outcomes comparable to primary DMEK,[24] whereas a regraft performed after prolonged corneal edema can have inferior visual outcomes.

Graft Rejection

Graft rejection in DMEK is characterized by AC cell reaction, keratic precipitates (KP), and corneal edema. DMEK has the lowest rejection rate of corneal transplants. The general mean rejection rate has been reported as 1.9% (range 0–5.9%) during follow-up periods ranging from 6 months to 8 years.[17] We previously found that the cumulative incidence of rejection episodes through 1 year with a tapering dose of prednisolone acetate 1%, or with prednisolone acetate for the first month followed by a tapering dose of loteprednol etabonate 0.5% gel or fluorometholone 0.1% were 0%, 0%, and 1.4%, respectively.[19,20] Based on this, we reduce the steroid strength 1–2 months after DMEK.

There is no consensus on when to stop topical corticosteroids, so we conducted a study in which patients could choose whether to stop topical steroids at 1 year after DMEK or continue once daily dosing of a low-strength steroid. The incidence of rejection episodes during the subsequent year was 6% in patients who discontinued topical corticosteroids and 0% in patients who continued low-dose topical corticosteroids.[55] Therefore, we recommend continued once-a-day use of a low strength topical steroid indefinitely. In the event of a graft rejection, immunosuppression with topical corticosteroids can be used to reverse the rejection.

Intraocular Pressure Elevation

Intraocular pressure elevation is the second most common complication after DMEK and occurs in up to one quarter of patients. IOP elevation can occur in association with the gas tamponade or with topical corticosteroid use.

The reported incidence of IOP increase associated with the gas tamponade ranges from 0 to 15%.[17] Strategies for prevention and treatment were discussed in the postoperative management section above.

The risk of steroid-associated IOP elevation can be significantly reduced by reducing the topical corticosteroid strength at 1–2 months after DMEK.[19,20] Patients with a previous glaucoma diagnosis are particularly susceptible to this complication. Steroid-induced IOP elevation can be treated by reducing steroids and/or using glaucoma medications. We prefer to use topical beta-blockers followed by brimonidine and as last resort prostaglandin analogs. Carbonic anhydrase inhibitors should be avoided because they can decrease endothelial cell function.

Other Complications

Other complications include cystoid macular edema, pupillary abnormalities, iris ischemia and pupillary sphincter muscle dysfunction, posterior synechiae formation, subcapsular lens opacities, cataract progression, and IOL calcification.[32,56-60]

OUTCOMES

Visual Outcomes

The principal factors associated with good visual outcomes are graft regularity and thickness. DMEK grafts consist of only isolated DM and endothelium and are thinner and more regular than DSAEK grafts. We previously compared DSAEK and DMEK in fellow eyes of the same patients and found statistically significant better best corrected visual acuity (BCVA) in the DMEK group.[61]

In a recent review of DMEK safety and outcomes conducted by the American Academy of Ophthalmology, the mean BCVA ranged from 20/20 to 20/30 after DMEK during the follow-up period which ranged from 5.3 to 68 months. Seven studies that directly compared visual outcomes of DSEK and DMEK showed better visual recovery after DMEK than after DSEK.[17] Recently Chamberlain et al. conducted a double-masked, randomized controlled trial comparing ultrathin DSAEK with DMEK and found that DMEK delivered better vision than ultrathin DSAEK, which was previously shown in a randomized trial to provide better vision than standard DSAEK[62] (**Table 1**).

Refractive Outcomes

The mean change in the spherical equivalent refraction after DMEK is +0.31 D (range +0.03–+1.2 D) and the mean

Table 1: Studies directly comparing visual outcomes of DSEK and DMEK.

Authors, year	No. of eyes	Follow-up (months)	DMEK BCVA (mean or median)	DSEK BCVA (mean or median)	DMEK BCVA 20/25 or better (%)	DSEK BCVA 20/25 or better (%)
Guerra (Price), 2011[61]	DMEK 13 DSEK 13 (Fellow eye)	12	20/23	20/32	77	23
Rudolph et al. 2012[63]	DMEK 30 DSEK 20	DMEK 6.5 DSEK 22.6	20/29	20/37	–	–
Tourtas et al. 2012[64]	DMEK 38 DSEK 35	6	20/30	20/46	50	6
Hamzaoglu et al. 2015[65]	DMEK 100 DSEK 100	6	20/26	20/32	67	31
Bhandari et al. 2015[66]	DMEK 30 DSEK 30	12	20/30	20/44	–	–
Droutsas et al. 2016[67]	DMEK 25 DSEK 25	12	20/20	20/40	–	–
Heinzelmann et al. 2016[68]	DMEK 450 DSEK 89	42	–	–	53	15
Phillips et al. 2017[69]	DMEK 100 DSEK 100	6	20/24	20/32	55	13
Chamberlain et al. 2019[62]	DMEK 25 UT-DSEK 25	12	20/21	20/28 UT-DSAEK	–	–

(BCVA: best corrected visual acuity; DMEK: Descemet membrane endothelial keratoplasty; DSEK: Descemet stripping endothelial keratoplasty; DSAEK: Descemet stripping automated endothelial keratoplasty)

change in astigmatism is +0.03 D (range: −0.6–+1.11 D).[17] However, there is significant variability between patients, so it is prudent to target −0.75–1.00 D when calculating the IOL power for DMEK combined with cataract surgery to reduce the risk of a hyperopic outcome.[70,71] For patients who desire a toric or multifocal intraocular lens, we prefer doing DMEK first to resolve the corneal edema, and then follow up later with cataract surgery to improve refractive predictability.

Endothelial Cell Density

The greatest endothelial cell loss is in the perioperative period. At 6 months the mean cell loss is 33% (range 25–46%) relative to the baseline donor endothelial cell density reported by the provider eye bank.[17] In an initial sample of 28 eyes, we observed 39% cell loss at 5 years after DMEK, which compared favorably with 5-year cell loss of 53% for DSEK and 70% for PK.[72] More recently, we reported 48% cell loss after 5 years in a larger sample of 289 eyes.[73] The first patient who underwent DMEK by Dr Melles in 2006 had endothelial cell loss at 10 years of 72% in the right eye and 68% in the left eye, with both corneas remaining clear.[74]

Prior glaucoma filtration surgery accelerates endothelial cell loss. Birbal et al. recently reported 71% endothelial cell loss at 12 months in eyes with a glaucoma drainage device.[75]

Graft Survival

We recently reported a cumulative 5-year survival rate of 93% after DMEK which was comparable to that of DSAEK despite the significantly lower risk of rejection episodes with DMEK.[73] These rates are within the ranges reported in previous smaller studies (85–95%).[76,77] Our 5-year survival rates included our first cases when the procedures were still in their infancies and not fully optimized.

CONCLUSION

Descemet membrane endothelial keratoplasty is the surgical technique of choice for the treatment of endothelial dysfunction because of its multiple advantages over DSAEK and PK, including visual and refractive results, but above all safety. Therefore, we prefer to perform DMEK whenever possible including complex cases. However, it is important to know when to choose DSAEK instead of DMEK. Surgeon training through attending courses, practicing in a wet laboratory and watching surgical videos online can be very helpful for achieving favorable results.

REFERENCES

1. Melles GR, Eggink FA, Lander F, Pels E, Rietveld FJ, Beekhuis WH, et al. A surgical technique for posterior lamellar keratoplasty. Cornea. 1998;17(6):618-26.
2. Melles GR, Lander F, Beekhuis WH, Remeijer L, Binder PS. Posterior lamellar keratoplasty for a case of pseudophakic bullous keratopathy. Am J Ophthalmol. 1999;127(3):340-1.
3. Terry MA, Ousley PJ. Deep lamellar endothelial keratoplasty in the first United States patients: Early clinical results. Cornea. 2001;20(3):239-43.
4. Melles GR, Wijdh RH, Nieuwendaal CP. A technique to excise the Descemet's membrane from a recipient cornea (descemetorhexis). Cornea. 2004;23(3):286-8.

5. Price FW Jr, Price MO. Descemet's stripping with endothelial keratoplasty in 50 eyes: A refractive neutral corneal transplant. J Refract Surg. 2005;21(4):339-45.
6. Gorovoy MS. Descemet-stripping automated endothelial keratoplasty. Cornea. 2006;25(8):886-9.
7. Melles GR, Ong TS, Ververs B, van der Wees J. Descemet's membrane endotelial keratoplasty (DMEK). Cornea. 2006;25(8):987-90.
8. Burkhart ZN, Feng MT, Price MO, Price FW. Handheld slit beam techniques to facilitate DMEK and DALK. Cornea. 2013;32(5):722-4.
9. Saad A, Guilbert E, Grise-Dulac A, Sabatier P, Gatinel D. Intra-operative OCT-assisted DMEK: 14 consecutive cases. Cornea. 2015; 34(7):802-7.
10. Veldman BP, Dye PK, Holiman JD, Mayko ZM, Sáles CS, Straiko MD, et al. The S-stamp in Descemet's membrane endothelial keratoplasty safely eliminates upside-down graft implantation. Ophthalmology. 2016;123(1):161-4.
11. Tenkman LR, Price FW, Price MO. Descemet's membrane endothelial keratoplasty donor preparation: navigating challenges and improving efficiency. Cornea. 2014;33(3):319-25.
12. Parekh M, Ruzza A, Salvalaio G, Ferrari S, Camposampiero D, Busin M, et al. Descemet's membrane endothelial keratoplasty tissue preparation from donor corneas using a standardized submerged hydro-separation method. Am J Ophthalmol. 2014;158(2):277-85.e1.
13. Gonzalez A, Price FW Jr, Price MO, Feng MT. Prevention and management of pupil block after Descemet's membrane endothelial keratoplasty. Cornea. 2016;35(11):1391-5.
14. Guell JL, Morral M, Gris O, Elies D, Manero F. Comparison of sulfur hexafluoride 20% versus air tamponade in Descemet's membrane endothelial keratoplasty. Ophthalmology. 2015;122(9):1757-64.
15. Eye Bank Association of America. Eye Banking Statistical Report. 2017. [online] Available from: https://restoresight.org/what-we-do/publications/statistical-report/. [Last accessed August, 2019].
16. Dapena I, Ham L, Melles GR. Endothelial keratoplasty: DSEK/DSAEK or DMEK—the thinner the better? Curr Opin Ophthalmol. 2009;20(4):299-307.
17. Deng SX, Lee WB, Hammersmith KM, Kuo AN, Li JY, Shen JF, et al. Descemet's membrane endothelial keratoplasty: safety and outcomes: A report bye the American Academy of Ophthalmology. Ophthalmology. 2018;125(2):295-310.
18. Anshu A, Price MO, Price FW Jr. Risk of corneal transplant rejection significantly reduced with Descemet's membrane endothelial keratoplasty. Ophthalmology. 2012;119(3):536-40.
19. Price MO, Price FW Jr, Kruse FE, Bachmann BO, Tourtas T. Randomized comparison of topical prednisolone acetate 1% versus fluorometholone 0.1% in the first year after Descemet's membrane endothelial keratoplasty. Cornea. 2014;33(9):880-6.
20. Price MO, Feng MT, Scanameo A, Price FW Jr. Loteprednol etabonate 0.5% gel vs. prednisolone acetate 1% solution after Descemet's membrane endothelial keratoplasty: prospective randomized trial. Cornea. 2015;34(8):853-8.
21. Anshu A, Price MO, Price FW Jr. Descemet's membrane endothelial keratoplasty and hybrid techniques for managing failed penetrating grafts. Cornea. 2013;32(1):1-4.
22. Yoeruek E, Bartz-Schmidt KU. Secondary Descemet's membrane endothelial keratoplasty after failed primary Descemet's membrane endothelial keratoplasty: clinical results. Cornea. 2013;32(11):1414-7.
23. Weller JM, Tourtas T, Kruse FE, Schlötzer-Schrehardt U, Fuchsluger T, Bachmann BO. Descemet's membrane endothelial keratoplasty as treatment for graft failure after Descemet's stripping automated endothelial keratoplasty. Am J Ophthalmol. 2015;159(6):1050-7.e2.
24. Price MO, Feng MT, Mckee Y, Price FW Jr. Repeat Descemet membrane endothelial keratoplasty: secondary grafts with early intervention are comparable with fellow-eye primary grafts. Ophthalmology. 2015;122(8):1639-44.
25. Einan-Lifshitz A, Belkin A, Sorkin N, Mednick Z, Boutin T, Gill I, et al. Descemet's membrane endothelial keratoplasty after penetrating keratoplasty: features for success. Cornea. 2018;37(9):1093-7.
26. Pasari A, Price MO, Feng MT, Price FW Jr. Descemet's membrane endothelial keratoplasty for failed penetrating keratoplasty: visual outcomes and graft survival. Cornea. 2019;38(2):151-6.
27. Pierné K, Panthier C, Courtin R, Mazharian A, Souedan V, Gatinel D, et al. Descemet's membrane endothelial keratoplasty after failed penetrating keratoplasty. Cornea. 2019;38(3):280-4.
28. Price MO, Mehta JS, Jurkunas UV, Price FW Jr. Corneal endothelial dysfunction: Evolving understanding and treatment options. Prog Retin Eye Res. 2021;82:100904.
29. Asi F, Milioti G, Seitz B. Descemet's membrane endothelial keratoplasty for corneal decompensation caused by herpes simplex virus endotheliitis. J Cataract Refract Surg. 2018;44(1):106-8.
30. Hannush SB, Riveroll-Hannush L. Preoperative considerations and decision-making in keratoplasty. In: Mannis MJ, Holland EJ (Eds). Cornea fundamentals, diagnosis and management, 4th edition. New York: Elsevier; 2017. pp. 1256-63.
31. Feng MT, Price FW Jr, Price MO. Complex endothelial keratoplasty. In: Mannis MJ, Holland EJ (Eds). Cornea fundamentals, diagnosis and management, 4th edition. New York: Elsevier; 2017. pp. 1493-500.
32. Burkhart ZN, Feng MT, Price FW Jr, Price MO. One-year outcomes in eyes remaining phakic after Descemet's membrane endothelial keratoplasty. J Cataract Refract Surg. 2014;40(3):430-4.
33. Price FW Jr, Price MO. Will level I evidence trigger a tipping point in endothelial keratoplasty? Ophthalmology. 2019;126(1):27-8.
34. Heinzelmann S, Hüther S, Böhringer D, Eberwein P, Reinhard T, Maier P. Influence of donor characteristics on Descemet's membrane endothelial keratoplasty. Cornea. 2014;33(6):644-8.
35. Schwarz C, Aldrich BT, Burckart KA, Schmidt GA, Zimmerman MB, Reed CR, et al. Descemet's membrane adhesion strength is greater in diabetics with advanced disease compared to healthy donor corneas. Exp Eye Res. 2016;153:152-8.
36. Greiner MA, Rixen JJ, Wagoner MD, Schmidt GA, Stoeger CG, Straiko MD, et al. Diabetes mellitus increases risk of unsuccessful graft preparation in Descemet's membrane endothelial keratoplasty: a multicenter study. Cornea. 2014;33(11):1129-33.
37. Vianna LM, Stoeger CG, Galloway JD, Terry M, Cope L, Belfort R Jr, et al. Risk factors for eye bank preparation failure of Descemet's membrane endothelial keratoplasty tissue. Am J Ophthalmol. 2015;159(5):829-34.e2.
38. Williams RS, Mayko ZM, Friend DJ, Straiko MD, Clay RD, Stoeger CG. Descemet's membrane endothelial keratoplasty (DMEK) tissue preparation: A donor diabetes mellitus categorical risk stratification scale for assessing tissue suitability and reducing tissue loss. Cornea. 2016;35(7):927-31.
39. Price MO, Lisek M, Feng MT, Price FW Jr. Effect of donor and recipient diabetes status on Descemet's membrane endothelial keratoplasty adherence and survival. Cornea. 2017;36(10):1184-8.
40. Feng MF, Burkhart ZN, Price FW Jr, Price MO. Effect of donor preparation-to-use times on Descemet's membrane endothelial keratoplasty outcomes. Cornea. 2013;32(8):1080-2.
41. Birbal RS, Sikder S, Lie JT, Groeneveld-van Beek EA, Oellerich S, Melles GRJ. Donor tissue preparation for Descemet's membrane endothelial keratoplasty: An updated review. Cornea. 2018;37(1):128-35.
42. Giebel AW, Price FW Jr. Descemet's membrane endothelial keratoplasty (DMEK): the bare minimum. In: Price FW, Price MO (Eds). DSEK: All You Need to Know about Endothelial Keratoplasty. Thorofare, NJ: Slack Inc; 2008. pp. 119-46.
43. Price MO, Giebel AW, Fairchild KM, Price FW Jr. Descemet's membrane endothelial keratoplasty: Prospective multicenter study of visual and refractive outcomes and endothelial survival. Ophthalmology. 2009;116(12):2361-8.
44. Veldman PB, Dye PK, Holiman JD, Mayko ZM, Sáles CS, Straiko MD, et al. Stamping an S on DMEK donor tissue to prevent

upside-down grafts: Laboratory validation and detailed preparation technique description. Cornea. 2015;34(9):1175-8.
45. Busin M, Leon P, Scorcia V, Ponzin D. Contact lens-assisted pull-through technique for delivery of tri-folded (endothelium in) DMEK grafts minimizes surgical time and cell loss. Ophthalmology. 2016;123(3):476-83.
46. McKee Y, Price MO, Gunderson L, Price FW Jr. Rapid sequential endothelial keratoplasty with and without combined cataract extraction. J. Cataract Refract. Surg. 2013;39(9):1372-6.
47. Price MO, Jordan CS, Moore G, Price FW Jr. Graft rejection episodes after Descemet stripping with endothelial keratoplasty: Part two: The statistical analysis of probability and risk factors. Br J Ophthalmol. 2009;93(3):391-5.
48. Bachmann BO, Laaser K, Cursiefen C, Kruse FE. A method to confirm correct orientation of Descemet's membrane during Descemet's membrane endothelial keratoplasty. Am J Ophthalmol. 2010;149(6):922-5.e2.
49. Dapena I, Moutsouris K, Droutsas K, Ham L, van Dijk K, Melles GR. Standardized "no-touch" technique for Descemet's membrane endothelial keratoplasty. Arch Ophthalmol. 2011;129(1):88-94.
50. Crews JW, Price MO, Lautert J, Feng MT, Price FW Jr. Intra-operative hyphema in Descemet's membrane endothelial keratoplasty alone or combined with phacoemulsification. J Cataract Refract Surg. 2018;44(2):198-201.
51. Parekh M, Leon P, Ruzza A, Borroni D, Ferrari S, Ponzin D, et al. Graft detachment and re-bubbling rate in Descemet's membrane endothelial keratoplasty. Surv Ophthalmol. 2018;63(2):245-50.
52. Marques RE, Guerra PS, Sousa DC, Ferreira NP, Gonçalves AI, Quintas AM, et al. Sulfur hexafluoride 20% versus air 100% for anterior chamber tamponade in DMEK: a meta-analysis. Cornea. 2018;37(6):691-7.
53. Gerber-Hollbach N, Baydoun L, López EF, Frank LE, Dapena I, Liarakos VS, et al. Clinical outcome of rebubbling for graft detachment after Descemet's membrane endothelial keratoplasty. Cornea. 2017;36(7):771-6.
54. Ćirković A, Schlötzer-Schrehardt U, Weller JM, Kruse FE, Tourtas T. Clinical and ultrastructural characteristics of graft failure in DMEK: 1-year results after repeat DMEK. Cornea. 2015;34(1):11-7.
55. Price MO, Scanameo A, Feng MT, Price FW Jr. Descemet's membrane endotelial keratoplasty: risk of immunologic rejection episodes after discontinuing topical corticosteroids. Ophthalmology. 2016;123(6):1232-6.
56. Santander-García D, Dapena I, Baydoun L, Melles GRJ. DMEK complications: current treatment and recommendations. Expert Rev Ophthalmol. 2018;13(1):33-46.
57. Holtmann C, Spaniol K, Geerling G. Urrets-Zavalia syndrome after Descemet's membrane endothelial keratoplasty. Eur J Ophthalmol. 2015;25(5):e75-7.
58. Arnalich-Montiel F, Pérez-Sarriegui A, Lauzirika G, Porrua L, Hernández-Verdejo JL. Pupillary abnormalities in Descemet's membrane endothelial keratoplasty after nearly full tamponade. Cornea. 2017;36(3):290-4.
59. Musa FU, Cabrerizo J, Quilendrino R, Dapena I, Ham L, Melles GR. Outcomes of phacoemulsification after Descemet's membrane endothelial keratoplasty. J Cataract Refract Surg. 2013;39(6):836-40.
60. Schrittenlocher S, Penier M, Schaub F, Bock F, Cursiefen C, Bachmann B. Intraocular lens calcifications after (triple-) Descemet's membrane endothelial keratoplasty. Am J Ophthalmol. 2017;179:129-36.
61. Guerra FP, Anshu A, Price MO, Price FW. Endothelial keratoplasty: fellow eyes comparison of Descemet's stripping automated endothelial keratoploasty and Descemet's membrane endothelial keratoplasty. Cornea. 2011;30(12):1382-6.
62. Chamberlain W, Lin CC, Austin A, Schubach N, Clover J, McLeod SD, et al. Descemet's endothelial thickness comparison trial: A randomized trial comparing ultrathin Descemet stripping automated endothelial keratoplasty with Descemet's membrane endothelial keratoplasty. Ophthalmology. 2019;126(1):19-26.
63. Rudolph M, Laaser K, Bachmann BO, Cursiefen C, Epstein D, Kruse FE. Corneal higher-order aberrations after Descemet's membrane endothelial keratoplasty. Ophthalmology. 2012;119(3):528-35.
64. Tourtas T, Laaser K, Bachmann BO, Cursiefen C, Kruse FE. Descemet's membrane endothelial keratoplasty versus Descemet's stripping automated endothelial keratoplasty. Am J Ophthalmol. 2012;153(6):1082-90.e2.
65. Hamzaoglu EC, Straiko MD, Mayko ZM, Sáles CS, Terry MA. The first 100 eyes of standardized Descemet's stripping automated endothelial keratoplasty versus standardized Descemet's membrane endothelial keratoplasty. Ophthalmology. 2015;122(11):2193-9.
66. Bhandari V, Reddy JK, Relekar K, Prabhu V. Descemet's stripping automated endothelial keratoplasty versus Descemet's membrane endothelial keratoplasty in the fellow eye for Fuchs endothelial dystrophy: A retrospective study. Biomed Res Int. 2015;2015:750567.
67. Droutsas K, Lazaridis A, Papaconstantinou D, Brouzas D, Moschos MM, Schulze S, et al. Visual outcomes after Descemet's membrane endothelial keratoplasty versus Descemet's stripping automated endothelial keratoplasty-comparison of specific matched pairs. Cornea. 2016;35(6):765-71.
68. Heinzelmann S, Bohringer D, Eberwein P, Reinhard T, Maier P. Outcomes of Descemet's membrane endothelial keratoplasty, Descemet's stripping automated endothelial keratoplasty and penetrating keratoplasty from a single center study. Graefes Arch Clin Exp Ophthalmol. 2016;254(3):515-22.
69. Phillips PM, Phillips LJ, Muthappan V, Maloney CM, Carver CN. Experienced DSAEK surgeon's transition to DMEK: outcomes comparing the last 100 DSAEK surgeries with the first 100 DMEK surgeries exclusively using previously published techniques. Cornea. 2017;36(3):275-9.
70. Schoenberg ED, Price FW Jr, Miller J, McKee Y, Price MO. Refractive outcomes of Descemet's membrane endothelial keratoplasty triple procedures (combined with cataract surgery). J Cataract Refract Surg. 2015;41(6):1182-9.
71. Laaser K, Bachmann BO, Horn FK, Cursiefen C, Kruse FE. Descemet's membrane endothelial keratoplasty combined with phacoemulsification and intraocular lens implantation: advanced triple procedure. Am J Ophthalmol. 2012;154(1):47-55.e2.
72. Feng MT, Price MO, Miller JM, Price FW Jr. Air reinjection and endothelial cell density in Descemet's membrane endothelial keratoplasty: five-year follow-up. J Cataract Refract Surg. 2014;40(7):1116-21.
73. Price DA, Kelley M, Price FW Jr, Price MO. Five-year graft survival of Descemet's Membrane Endothelial Keratoplasty (EK) versus Descemet's stripping EK and the effect of donor sex matching. Ophthalmology. 2018;125(10):1508-14.
74. Baydoun L, Müller T, Lavy I, Parker J, Rodriguez-Calvo-de-Mora M, Liarakos VS, et al. Ten-year clinical outcome of the first patient undergoing Descemet's membrane endothelial keratoplasty. Cornea. 2017;36(3):379-81.
75. Birbal RS, Tong CM, Dapena I, Parker JS, Parker JS, Oellerich S, et al. Clinical outcomes of Descemet's membrane endothelial keratoplasty in eyes with a glaucoma drainage device. Am J Ophthalmol. 2019;199:150-8.
76. Schlögl A, Tourtas T, Kruse FE, Weller JM. Long-term clinical outcome after Descemet's membrane endothelial keratoplasty. Am J Ophthalmol. 2016;169:218-26.
77. Ham L, Dapena I, Liarakos VS, Baydoun L, van Dijk K, Ilyas A, et al. Mid-term results of Descemet's membrane endothelial keratoplasty: 4 to 7 years clinical outcome. Am J Ophthalmol. 2016;171:113-21.

SECTION

5

Specific Techniques in Corneal Transplantation

40 Keratoplasty and Cataract Extraction: Triple Procedure

Mohamed Ibrahime Asif, Namrata Sharma

INTRODUCTION

Triple procedure refers to the combined surgery of keratoplasty, cataract extraction, and intraocular lens (IOL) implantation. Katzin and Meltzer reported combining cataract surgery[1] and penetrating keratoplasty (PK) in 1966 with later addition of IOL implantation in 1976. It is an accepted modality of treatment in patients with visually disabling corneal opacification with associated cataract. The triple procedure not only offers immediate postoperative visual improvement but also precludes the need of another intraocular surgery for cataract in future which might jeopardize the survival of the graft. Apart from full-thickness keratoplasty, lamellar procedures can also be combined with cataract surgery such as Descemet stripping automated endothelial keratoplasty (DSAEK) triple, Descemet membrane endothelial keratoplasty (DMEK) triple or deep anterior lamellar keratoplasty (DALK) triple.

COMBINED VERSUS SINGLE STAGED PROCEDURES

Various studies have shown encouraging results of triple procedure over performing sequential procedures as the graft survival might be jeopardized by subsequent cataract surgery.[2-5]

The advantages of a triple procedure include the need for only one procedure, less expenditure, and hospital stay and the most important is lesser trauma involved to the endothelium of transplanted cornea.[6-8] However, certain disadvantages associated with the triple procedure are IOL power calculations and prolonged surgical time. The difficulty of accurately predicting the IOL power is due to the difficulty in assessing the postoperative keratometric readings. However, if the corneal transplantation is performed first, followed by cataract surgery after keratometric stabilization, the IOL power could be better predicted. The corneal curvature will not be stabilized until all the sutures have been removed. However, Nguyen et al.[9] found that there was no evidence of improved visual or refractive outcome after sequential surgery when compared with the triple procedure. Green et al.[10] showed that the triple procedure carried a similar risk of graft failure or rejection when compared with keratoplasty alone. Therefore, the triple procedure is recommended for quicker visual recovery and less operative procedures.

In a recent study on DSAEK triple, they concluded that a concurrent cataract surgery did not affect the endothelial count whereas, a higher preoperative donor endothelial cell density (ECD) was correlated with higher ECD at 5 years postoperatively.[11]

In cases of DSAEK triple, it is important to remember that the DSAEK graft would induce a hyperopia ranging from 0.75 to 1.5 D.[10,12] Hence, a target refraction of at least 1 D myopia should be aimed at during IOL power calculation. However, DMEK grafts hardly induce any hyperopic shifts.

INDICATIONS

Any visual significant corneal pathology along with cataractous lens could be an indication for triple procedure. In certain scenarios where the visual morbidity associated with cataract is not significant, a triple procedure may still be contemplated, as early cataractous changes may progress following keratoplasty due to intraoperative lens touch, postoperative inflammation, and steroid use.[13] Preoperatively, in most cases, it might be challenging to assess the lenticular opacity in the presence of corneal opacity. Hence, the surgeon has to be prepared for cataract extraction during the surgery and the final decision is usually taken intraoperatively following the removal of the corneal button. In cases where the media is hazy enough to decrease the vision to 20/50 or worse postoperatively, the lens should be removed at the time of keratoplasty. If the nuclear sclerosis grade is more than 2+ (on a scale of 1+ to 4+) and for posterior subcapsular cataract if the grade of the cataract is of 1+ or more, triple procedure should be planned. Various pathologies for which triple procedure are commonly done are discussed here.

Fuchs' Dystrophy

There is a shift from PK to lamellar procedures such as DSAEK and DMEK in Fuchs' dystrophy due to better graft survival.[14] Many patients with Fuchs' dystrophy with no apparent clinical corneal decompensation have an accompanying cataract. Cataract surgery in such patients usually leads to endothelial cell loss below a critical value and the development of bullous keratopathy.

Such cases require specular microscopy, confocal microscopy, and pachymetry in the preoperative evaluation. Van Cleynenbreugel et al.[15] concluded that central corneal thickness (CCT) and backscatter at the basal epithelial valley (EV) are the most important factors in predicting the need for keratoplasty. A cutoff of 1894 scatter units for EV and 630 µm for CCT are considered for combined endothelial keratoplasty with cataract surgery (DSAEK/DMEK triple).

If cataract surgery alone is performed in cases of Fuchs' dystrophy, then intraoperatively viscodispersive ophthalmic viscosurgical device (OVD) such as Viscoat should be used to protect the endothelium. The presence of corneal guttate alone is not an indication for the combined procedure. Multifocal IOL are avoided as DSAEK induces negative asphericity which could degrade visual acuity and reduce contrast sensitivity. In addition, remember the hyperopic refractive shift, hence aim for at least 1–1.5 D myopia while choosing the IOL.

Some authors have advocated that a staged procedure[16] should be done in Fuch, whereas some supported combined procedure.[17,18]

Sykakis et al.[19] concluded that DSAEK triple is associated with increased immediate postoperative complications such as graft dislocation and rebubbling rate, however, the ECD and the final visual outcomes were comparable.

In the Fuchs' endothelial corneal dystrophy (FECD) cases, performing phacoemulsification before DMEK or doing a combined procedure did not seem to affect the rebubbling or survival rate up to 1 year postoperatively.[20]

Das et al.[21] show that the refractive and visual outcome after the PK triple procedure did not differ significantly from that after PK only. Therefore, they recommend the triple procedure in elderly patients with Fuchs' dystrophy and cataract to avoid delayed visual rehabilitation and a second surgical procedure.

Infective Keratitis

In cases of recurrent herpetic keratitis, stromal scarring with associated thinning and vascularization may be present associated with cataract (**Fig. 1**). Cataract when present results from the inflammatory process due to the disease pathology or frequent usage of steroids, particularly in disciform keratitis. In such cases, it is preferable to do a combined procedure of PK along with cataract extraction. It has to be ensured that patients receive prophylactic systemic acyclovir therapy for at least 1 year to reduce the risk of recurrence.[22]

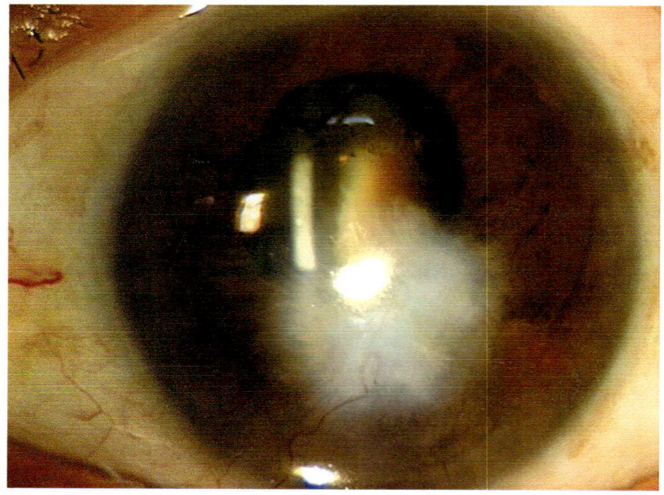

Fig. 1: Slit-lamp examination of healed viral keratitis with adherent leukoma and cataractous lens.

The bacterial keratitis particularly those associated with severe anterior chamber reaction may result in the scarred cornea with cataract. Later in a quiet eye, one can safely do simultaneous cataract extraction and keratoplasty.

Chemical Burns

The chemical burns especially alkali burns due to their potential to penetrate across cornea set up acute uveitis, which could result in cataract. The visual rehabilitation of such patients usually warrants full-thickness keratoplasty with cataract extraction.

Trauma

Penetrating ocular trauma involving cornea may have a clear lens at the time of initial presentation but generally, such cases develop cataract later on and it may be necessary to do combined procedure to remove the cataract. The triple corneal procedure is a useful therapeutic option even in cases of corneolenticular trauma in children where prior repair of the perforating injury has occurred (**Fig. 2**).[23]

Corneal Opacity in Elderly Patients

Some elderly patients with corneal opacities resulting from various diverse causes such as corneal degenerations, dystrophies, etc. present late in life and there may be an associated senile cataract. Such cases need combined triple procedure for optimum visual rehabilitation. Ideally, the surgeon should be prepared to perform a triple procedure if the lens is found to be cataractous intraoperatively while performing PK for cases where preoperative slit-lamp biomicroscopy of the lens could not be performed due to severity of corneal pathology. However, Shimmura et al.[24]

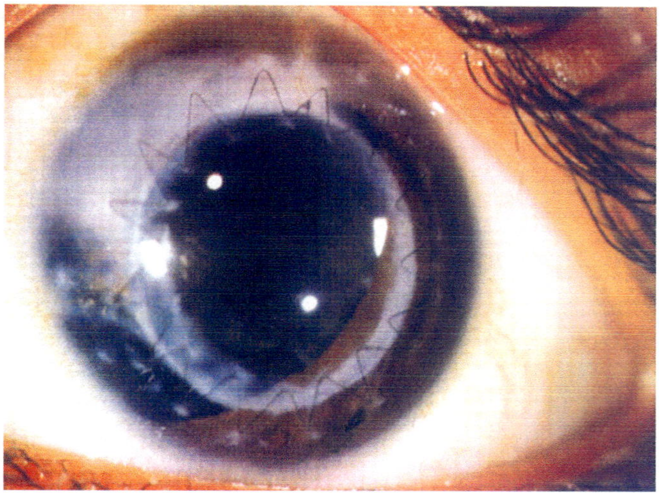

Fig. 2: Triple procedure in a case of corneolenticular injury.

showed that performing secondary cataract surgery after 1 year (second stage) following PK, does not affect the endothelial viability and resulted in lesser refractive error.

PREOPERATIVE EVALUATION

The preoperative evaluation of the patient undergoing triple procedure includes a complete history taking with the ocular examination. The basic investigations, which need to be done before performing the procedure of combined PK with cataract extraction, are similar to those done for PK alone. Special attention should be given to the evaluation of the intraocular pressure assessment and the retinal evaluation. These include ultrasonographic evaluation for the posterior segment, electrophysiological tests [electroretinogram (ERG), visual evoked response (VER)] and macular function tests including the assessment of the potential acuity which can be done by the potential acuity meter or by a laser interferometer. The objectives of the investigations are to evaluate the case thoroughly, to rule out any posterior segment pathology and to assess beforehand the potential visual acuity.

Intraocular Lens Power Calculation

A common problem, a surgeon, faces in the combined procedure is the calculation of the exact IOL power. Axial length determination should be undertaken in both the eyes as a cross-check for accuracy.

Since the involved cornea is scarred and proper keratometry is not possible, hence the various options available with the surgeon are:

- Use keratometry values of the fellow eye
- Use the average normal keratometry of 43.5 D
- The surgeon takes the average postoperative keratometry readings for a series of his/her patients.[25]
- Alternatively, the keratometry value may be selected based on the results of numerous triple procedures with the same trephine and suturing techniques and using personlized constants within the IOL formula could result in improved outcomes. IOL formula per se does not affect the outcome.[26]
- In some cases of Fuchs' dystrophy or bullous keratopathy, it may be possible to do keratometry using handheld noncontact keratometer intraoperatively following epithelial debridement.
- Viestenz et al.[27] proposed correcting multiple regression formula for IOL power prediction may help to improve the postoperative refractive outcome in patients undergoing triple procedures.

Table 1: Intraoperative lens power calculation formula as per axial length.

Axial length (mm)	*Formula*	*Percentage used*
<22	Hoffer Q	8
22.0–24.5	Average of all three	72
24.5–26.0	Holladay	15
>26	Sanders–Retzlaff–Kraff	5

Hoffer technique for intraoperative lens power calculation is based on the axial length and is given in **Table 1**.[6]

A study by Bonfadini et al.[28] found that optimization of the IOL constant rather than using manufacturer IOL constant could improve refractive outcomes after DSAEK triple. Diener et al. found that the corneal power estimation using conventional K for IOL power calculation is invalid in eyes with Fuchs' dystrophy undergoing DMEK.[29] To avoid an overestimation of corneal power and minimize the risk of a postoperative hyperopic shift, conventional K for IOL power calculation should be adjusted. The fictitious preoperative anterior curvature radii ratio and keratometer index may guide further IOL power calculation methods to achieve this. Fritz et al. concluded that hyperopic surprises after triple DMEK particularly occur in corneas that are flatter centrally than the periphery because of edematous changes (oblate posterior profile). Eyes with a positive Q value on Scheimpflug imaging should be considered for additional power at the IOL level.[30]

PREOPERATIVE MANAGEMENT

The preoperative care for patients undergoing the combined triple procedure is similar to those who undergoing any keratoplasty procedure.

The patient may be operated under general or local anesthesia. General anesthesia is preferred in children, mentally challenged, or anxious uncooperative patients, PK triple (open-sky procedure) especially decrease in intraocular pressure and reduction in vitreous volume could help in safe surgery.

A soft eye is considered as essential in performing combined surgery. This can be achieved by a number of methods. Hyperventilation is one of such modalities and can be performed under general anesthesia only. The other methods include applying digital pressure over the globe, use of Honan balloon or Super Pinkey ball. Honan balloon exerts a pressure of 30–35 mm Hg that leads to the reduction of 5–7 mm Hg. The osmotic agents such as intravenous mannitol also reduce intraocular pressure by reducing vitreous volume. Pupillary dilatation is achieved with 10% cyclopentolate and 2.5% phenylephrine, which is given 30, 45 and 60 minutes preoperatively.

SURGICAL TECHNIQUE

Various surgical options for performing the cataract extraction and the transplantation simultaneously include the following:

- Simultaneous extracapsular cataract extraction with corneal transplantation (PK triple)
- Phacoemulsification followed immediately by corneal transplantation (PK triple, DSAEK triple, and DMEK triple)
- Temporary graft for closed system cataract surgery during corneal triple procedures (PK triple)
- Temporary keratoprosthesis to perform cataract extraction with small incision surgery in a closed system followed by corneal transplantation (PK triple)

Simultaneous Extracapsular Cataract Extraction with Corneal Transplantation

Removing cataract through open-sky method after the host cornea has been trephined is the most common and simple technique of triple procedure.

Donor Cornea Trephination

Donor tissue should be trephinated before complete removal of the affected recipient cornea to avoid open globe for a long duration. There are a variety of techniques for donor tissue trephination. This can be done using conventional disposable handheld trephines, suction fixated trephines, endothelial punches or by using a trephine with artificial anterior chamber maintainer. The size of the graft should be greater than the host by 0.25–0.5 mm which allows for some tissue compression effect of the sutures without significant flattening of the central graft curvature.

Recipient Cornea Trephination

Similarly, the recipient cornea trephination can be done using conventional disposable handheld trephines (**Fig. 3A**), suction fixated trephines or by using a trephine with artificial anterior chamber maintainer. With any of the trephine systems, once the anterior chamber is entered, it is imperative to avoid rapid chamber shallowing and inadvertent cutting of the iris or the lens capsule by the blade. The recipient corneal button is excised with the help of the corneoscleral or Vannas scissors (**Fig. 3B**).

Cataract Extraction

There are various methods of cataract extraction following removal of recipient corneal button. Initially, intracapsular cataract extraction (ICCE) with iris fixated or anterior chamber IOL were done. However, the most common method generally employed is the use of open-sky extracapsular cataract extraction with posterior chamber IOL implantation. Open-sky phacoemulsification has also been described.[31]

Capsulotomy and nucleus removal: Performing anterior capsulotomy is more difficult under open-sky method than under a closed system. Staining of the capsule with trypan blue could help in prevention of complications such as capsular tear.[32] After excess viscoelastic and fluid are removed, a capsulotomy is performed. A can-opener, an endocapsular capsulotomy or even a continuous curvilinear capsulorrhexis (CCC) can be undertaken. However, performing a CCC is difficult under open-sky conditions, as there is more tendency for it to extend to periphery.

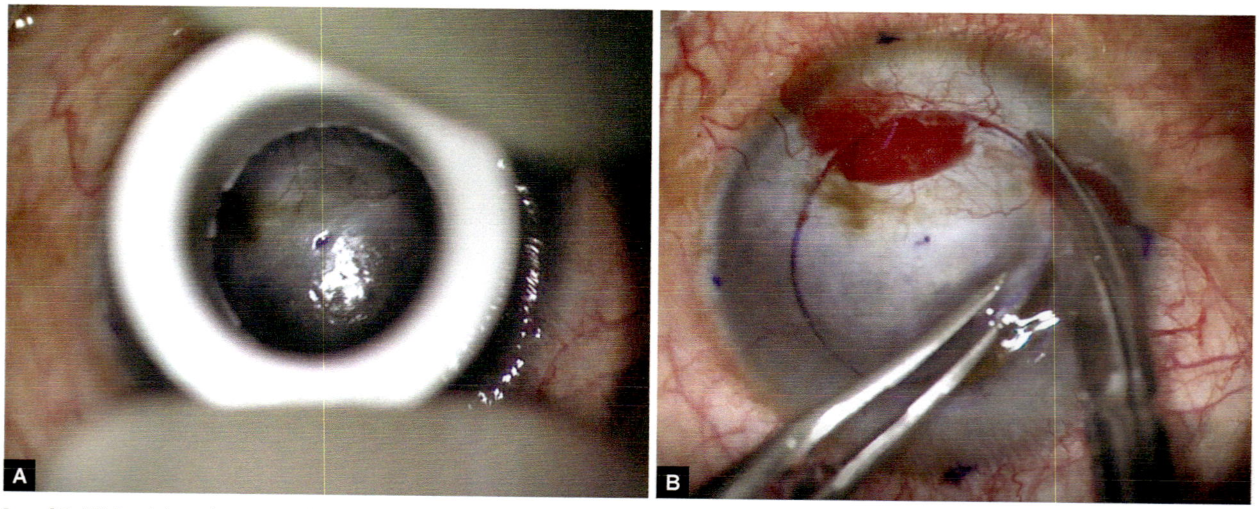

Figs. 3A and B: (A) Partial trephination of the host cornea using a disposable handheld trephine; (B) Cutting the host tissue using curved Vannas scissors.

Following capsulorrhexis, it is imperative to give relaxing incisions in the capsule to facilitate nuclear delivery. Borderie et al. recommend the use of a phaco probe to engage a large nucleus by using phaco power so that the intact nucleus is removed, and the relaxing incisions may not be required.[33]

In some cases, due to positive vitreous pressure, the nucleus of the lens tends to prolapse anteriorly after making the initial nick in the anterior capsule and it causes the rhexis margin to extend to periphery. Under such conditions, Vannas scissors can be used to complete the capsulotomy or the lens can be pushed back with a blunt instrument such as cyclodialysis spatula with one hand and the other hand may be used to complete the capsulotomy.

After completing the capsulotomy, hydrodissection is done and nucleus delivery is facilitated by applying gentle pressure with one instrument at the limbus and counter pressure with the second instrument applied just diagonally opposite to the first point (**Figs. 4A and B**). It is useful to make relaxing incisions in the anterior capsule to facilitate the nucleus delivery.

Irrigation and aspiration of the cortical matter: The cortical material is removed using either the automated irrigating aspirating (I/A) machine or by using a manual aspiration system such as a Simcoe cannula. Less irrigation should be used when undertaking cortical aspiration in open-sky conditions as excess fluid obscures the surgeon's view of the red reflex and creates multiple mirrored images from the fluid surface. The cortical material can be removed by engaging the anterior aspect of the cortex and then peeling out the residual cortex. One may place the irrigation aspiration tip against the posterior cortex and the posterior capsule, pushing it slightly away from the anterior cortex facilitating grasping of the anterior cortex, which will then strip out. Kawamoto K showed that the use of the new soft contact lens significantly reduced the time required for irrigation and aspiration of the lens cortex, the total operative duration and the duration of the open-sky maneuvers.[34]

Sometimes in cases with positive vitreous pressure, posterior lens capsule assumes a convex shape and it becomes difficult to aspirate the cortical matter from the fornices of the capsule. The viscoelastic should be used to counter the vitreous pressure and peripheral cortical matter should be aspirated by gentle posterior pressure on the peripheral posterior lens capsule, while one strips away the cortical matter. It is not mandatory to completely remove cortical matter as there is increased risk for PC tear. Vongthongsri showed that pars plana anterior vitreous tapping is a safe adjunct for triple procedures to prevent positive vitreous pressure and its associated complications.[35]

In some instances of too much positive pressure, we have sutured the graft with 8 sutures and then have aspirated the cortical lens matter through the host-graft junction.

Posterior chamber intraocular lens insertion: After completion of the cortical matter aspiration, viscoelastic is injected to separate the anterior and the posterior lens capsules to facilitate IOL placement in the capsular bag. Care must be taken to ensure that the haptics goes into the capsular bag. This can be ensured by placing the haptic against the posterior capsule cautiously and then gently pushing the IOL inferiorly (**Fig. 5**). After the inferior haptic is in place, the optic of the lens should be introduced through the capsular opening. The second instrument may be used to maintain the pressure on the optic of the IOL, which prevents it from moving. The trailing haptic of the IOL may then be grasped with a McPherson forceps and with a pronation movement of the wrist, the trailing haptic can be introduced into the capsular bag. The lens may then be "dialed" to confirm its position. Core vitrectomy can be done preceding the triple procedure, especially in cases at high-risk for increased posterior chamber pressure which would help in better IOL insertion.[36]

Inadvertent posterior capsule tear: In cases, where the posterior capsular tear occurs, and the tear is small, it may be possible to convert it into a circumscribed continuous tear. In cases, where vitreous presents through the tear,

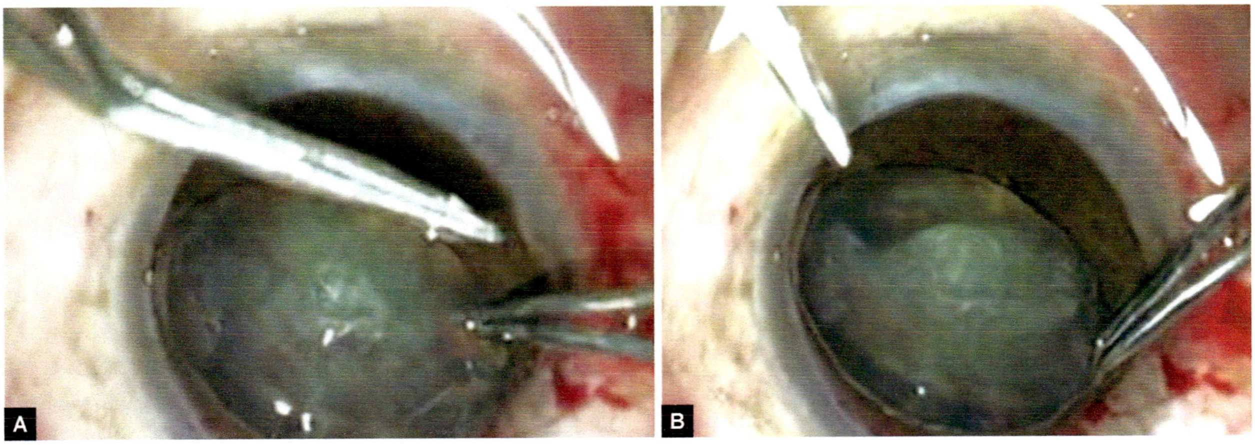

Figs. 4A and B: Open sky extracapsular cataract extraction.

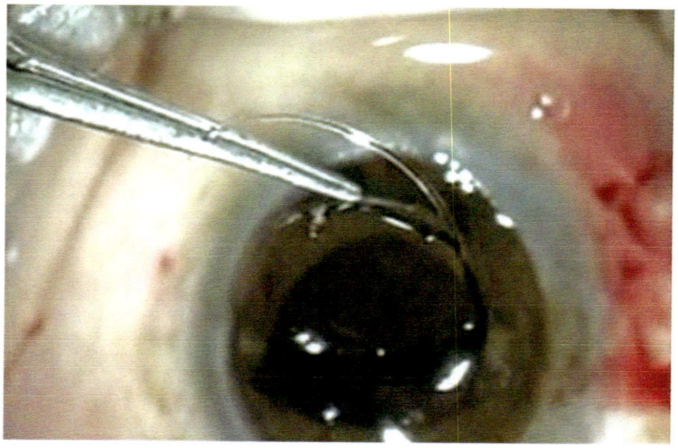

Fig. 5: Open sky intraocular lens implantation.

vitrectomy should be performed, and due care must be taken to preserve as much of posterior capsule as possible. The vitreous must be completely removed from the anterior chamber and no vitreous strand should be left behind. After all the vitreous is removed from the anterior chamber, an IOL is placed in such a way that the haptics lies in the ciliary sulcus in an area where there is more capsular support. In cases, where there is no capsular support, one can put Kelman multiflex anterior chamber IOL or do the scleral fixation of the posterior chamber IOL.

Suturing the Graft

After the IOL is positioned in the bag or the sulcus, intracameral pilocarpine is used to constrict the pupil and to ensure final placement of IOL behind the iris in the bag. Some viscoelastic like Healon (sodium hyaluronate 1%) or Viscoat (3% sodium hyaluronate and 4% chondroitin sulfate) should be put over the exposed surface of iris and IOL to prevent contact between iris and the graft endothelium. The donor corneal tissue is removed from the graft holder and placed over the recipient bed and is secured with four cardinal sutures. The chamber is deepened with viscoelastic or balanced salt solution (BSS) and additional sutures are applied. The suturing technique applied may be interrupted sutures alone, combination interrupted and running sutures, and single or double running sutures.

Adjustment of Suture Tension

Intraoperative adjustment of suture tension may then be done to minimize postkeratoplasty astigmatism. An intraoperative surgical keratometer may be used. Alternatively, in developing countries where the expensive keratometers are not available, the round end of the sterile safety pin may be used. The interrupted or the continuous suture can be relaxed in the steep meridian and tightened in the flat meridian. The oval mire can be converted into a circular configuration, which is the desired endpoint (**Fig. 6**).

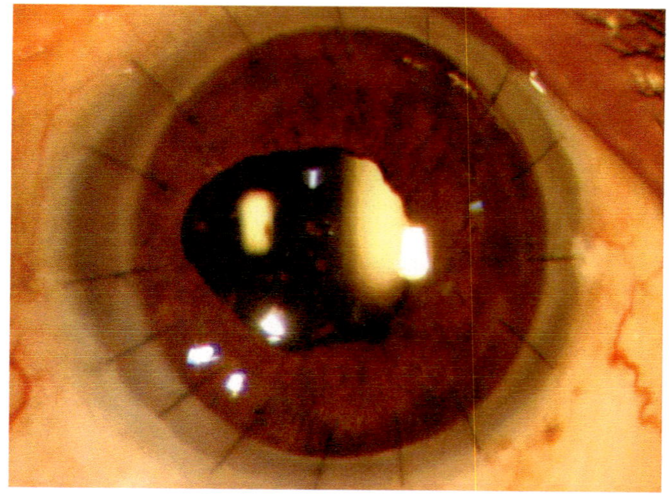

Fig. 6: Postsuturing—look for the configuration of the mires.

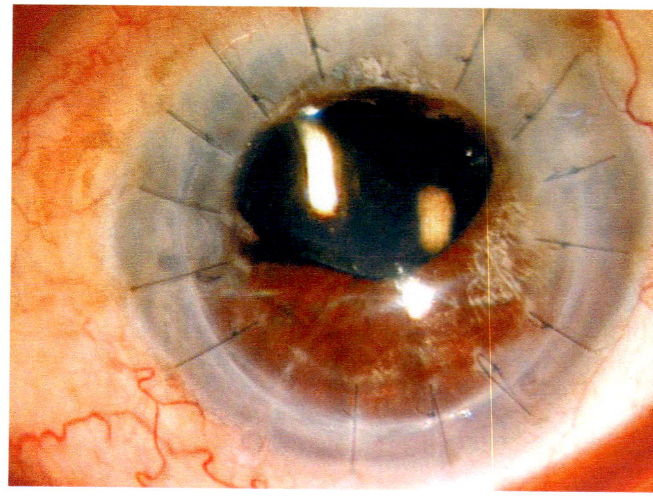

Fig. 7: Post-triple procedure with a clear graft.

Outcomes

Many surgeons have reported the clinical results of triple procedures with generally favorable outcome. The presence of clear grafts (**Fig. 7**) reported in various studies varies from 60 to 100%.[7] The postoperative visual acuity of 20/20 to 20/40 following triple procedure varies in various studies from 33.3[8] to 88%.[3,6,8] A recent study by Javadi et al.[37] found that PK triple is a safe and effective approach to restore vision, however unacceptable postoperative refractive error should be anticipated. Mean refractive error was -2.13 ± 3.02 D which significantly differed from target refraction. At a mean follow-up of 5 years, 89.5% of grafts remained clear.

The various complications following triple procedure include graft rejection (0–11%), graft failure (6–20%), postoperative glaucoma (1.5–19%), posterior capsule opacification (0–6%), cystoid macular edema (0–6%), retinal detachment (0–2%), and endophthalmitis (0–1%). A study done by Jonas[38] showed that the most important factors influencing visual outcome after central penetrating allogeneic keratoplasty combined with IOL surgery are preoperative visual acuity, graft size, and reason for keratoplasty. Other factors such as age, sex, diabetes mellitus, and preoperative refractive error do not substantially influence postoperative visual outcome.

Phacoemulsification Followed Immediately by Corneal Transplantation

This surgery can be undertaken in cases where adequate visualization of the lens is possible through the cornea. Performing phacoemulsification before keratoplasty has certain advantages in the form of controlled procedure, less risk of posterior capsular rupture and choroidal hemorrhage.[39,40] The most difficult time during open-sky method is the removal of cataract and implantation of IOL because of positive vitreous pressure.[38,39] Phacoemulsification may not always be possible as corneas may not be sufficiently clear enough to allow visualization of cataract. Baykara et al.[41] proposed that phacoemulsification, through the recipient bed that is thinned by lamellar dissection, could be safely performed in a short time, under the good view of the lens. Anterior chamber illumination technique using chandelier endoillumination has been found useful in these cases.[42]

Sharma et al. described various modifications in the surgical steps during phacoemulsification.[43] A *scleral tunnel* is preferred over a clear corneal one since the corneal tunnel may interfere with the subsequent keratoplasty procedure. The CCC is quite difficult in these settings due to decreased visibility. Trypan blue dye to stain the anterior capsule is mandatory for capsulorrhexis in these cases. The CCC should be started in the visible and clear area preferably using forceps and it should be continued in a single centripetal motion without leaving the edge underneath the opacity. When visualization of the leading edge is hazy, a blob of dispersive OVD can be placed to increase the magnification for a second, thereby allowing the surgeon to identify the lost edge. The globe can also be manually rotated for better visualization. Nuclear emulsification with primary chop is preferred, whereas in cases of advanced cataract, an eccentric crater followed by chopping can be used.

One can preferably implant a foldable IOL in view of its advantages over the poly(methyl methacrylate) (PMMA) lens. In cases where posterior capsule gets ruptured and vitreous loss occurs, the anterior chamber and wound area is cleaned by doing meticulous vitrectomy and if possible IOL can be implanted in the sulcus. In cases where posterior capsular rent is significant and does not allow either in bag or sulcus IOL, the pupil is constricted after anterior vitrectomy with the use of intracameral pilocarpine and subsequently one can proceed with transplantation surgery as described above. A multiflex Kelman AC IOL may be implanted in these eyes during keratoplasty.

Temporary Graft for Closed System Cataract Surgery during Corneal Triple Procedures

In cases of dense corneal opacities where a closed chamber surgery is not possible, a temporary corneal graft, which is not suitable for PK, may be used to allow phacoemulsification and foldable IOL implantation through a corneal tunnel. The temporary graft is then replaced with a healthy permanent graft following phacoemulsification.[44]

Temporary Keratoprosthesis to Perform Cataract Extraction with Small Incision Surgery in a Closed System Followed by Corneal Transplantation

A temporary keratoprosthesis may be used to perform cataract extraction with small incision surgery in a closed system. This is then followed by corneal transplantation.[45]

Phacoemulsification and Anterior Lamellar Keratoplasty (ALK Triple)

The basic principle involves initial host debulking to improve visibility followed by phacoemulsification, followed by placement and suturing of the graft. Panda et al.[46] found encouraging results with simultaneous DALK and phacoemulsification, with a significant improvement in corrected distance visual acuity (CDVA) to better than 20/60 in all cases. The DALK triple procedure has also been performed successfully in eyes with a bare pre-Descemet layer, which is tougher and more resilient than Descemet membrane and can withstand pressure during phacoemulsification.[47] Microkeratome-assisted superficial anterior lamellar keratoplasty (SALK) has also been combined with phacoemulsification, with good visual outcomes.[48]

Phacoemulsification and Endothelial Keratoplasty (DSAEK/DMEK Triple)

Phacoemulsification can be combined with endothelial keratoplasty in presence of corneal edema and coexisting cataract. Often, these cases are associated with subepithelial haze that can be cleared using simple debridement. Subsequent phacoemulsification followed by endothelial keratoplasty can be performed after any standard technique. Price et al.[49] and Terry et al.[18] reported excellent visual outcomes after the DSAEK triple procedure, with a CDVA of 20/40 or better in 97% of cases and a low-risk for graft dislocation (1.8%). The refractive spherical equivalent at the 1-year follow-up was within ±1.0 D of emmetropia in 73% of cases and within ±2.0 D in 95% of cases.[18] Similar visual outcomes have been reported in other series of endothelial keratoplasty with phacoemulsification,[50-52] with excellent postoperative refractive predictability. The key modification during phacoemulsification with endothelial keratoplasty is that initially, trypan blue-assisted host Descemet membrane removal is performed to improve visibility; this is followed by phacoemulsification. Next, the graft is inserted, which helps to prevent endothelial loss in the graft.

POSTOPERATIVE CARE

The postoperative care is the same as that of any routine keratoplasty patient. One must care for wound integrity, anterior chamber reaction and control of IOP. The postoperative regime should consist of topical corticosteroids such as prednisolone acetate 1–2 hourly/day, topical antibiotic such as 0.5% moxifloxacin four times a day, along with topical preservative-free artificial tears six times/day. Hoerster et al.[53] reported that on intensified topical steroids (hourly) during the first week had significant reduced incidence of cystoid macular edema (CME) compared to five times/day schedule.

Cycloplegics and antiglaucoma medications should be given, wherever indicated.

Posterior capsular opacification occurs with about same frequency as in simple extracapsular cataract extraction and is treated with yttrium aluminum garnet (YAG) laser capsulotomy.

With time, corneal triple surgery has evolved from PK triple to triple-combined with lamellar surgeries. Combining new types of corneal tissue including regenerative medicine, keratoprosthesis, and bioengineered corneas have recently been developed.

REFERENCES

1. Katzin HM, Meltzer JF. Combined surgery for corneal transplantation and cataract extraction. Am J Ophthalmol. 1966;62(3):556-60.
2. Reddy SC, Gupta S, Rao GN. Results of penetrating keratoplasty with cataract extraction and intraocular lens implantation in Fuchs' dystrophy. Indian J Ophthalmol. 1987;35(5-6):161-4.
3. Hunkeler JD, Hyde LL. The triple procedure: combined penetrating keratoplasty, extracapsular cataract extraction and lens implantation. An expanded experience. J Am Intra Ocul Implant Soc. 1983;9(1):20-4.
4. Pineros OE, Cohen EJ, Rapuano CJ, Laibson PR. Triple vs nonsimultaneous procedures in Fuchs' dystrophy and cataract. Arch Ophthalmol. 1996;114(5):525-8.
5. Brady SE, Rapuano CJ, Arentsen JJ, Cohen EJ, Laibson PR. Clinical indications for and procedures associated with penetrating keratoplasty, 1983-1988. Am J Ophthalmol. 1989;108(2):118-22.
6. Hoffer KJ. The Hoffer Q formula: A comparison of theoretic and regression formulas. J Cataract Refract Surg. 1993;19(6):700-12.
7. Taylor DM, Khaliq A. Keratoplasty and intraocular lenses: follow-up study. Ophthalmic Surg. 1977;8(2):49-57.
8. Erb C, Zimmermann-Burg B, Steuhl KP, Weidle EG, Thiel HJ. Retrospective long-term follow-up of the triple procedure (combined keratoplasty and cataract surgery). Folia Med (Plovdiv). 1996;38(2):19-25.
9. Nguyen DQ, Mumford LL, Jones MN, Armitage WJ, Cook SD, Kaye SB, et al. The visual and refractive outcomes of combined and sequential penetrating keratoplasty, cataract extraction, and intraocular lens insertion. Eye (Lond). 2009;23(6):1295-301.
10. Anshu A, Price MO, Tan DT, Price FW Jr. Endothelial keratoplasty: a revolution in evolution. Surv Ophthalmol. 2012;57(3):236-52.
11. Alqudah AA, Bauer AJ, Straiko MD, Sanchez PJ, Terry MA. Descemet stripping automated endothelial keratoplasty: The influence of preoperative endothelial cell density and triple procedures on grafts at 5 years postoperative. Medicine (Baltimore). 2020;99(45):e23139.
12. Dupps WJ, Qian Y, Meisler DM. Multivariate model of refractive shift in Descemet-stripping automated endothelial keratoplasty. J Cataract Refract Surg. 2008;34(4):578-84.
13. Stainer GA, Perl T, Binder PS. Controlled reduction of postkeratoplasty astigmatism. Ophthalmology. 1982;89(6):668-76.
14. Woo JH, Ang M, Htoon HM, Tan D. Descemet's membrane endothelial keratoplasty versus Descemet's stripping automated endothelial keratoplasty and penetrating keratoplasty. Am J Ophthalmol. 2019;207:288-303.
15. van Cleynenbreugel H, Remeijer L, Hillenaar T. Cataract surgery in patients with Fuchs' endothelial corneal dystrophy: when to consider a triple procedure. Ophthalmology. 2014;121(2):445-53.
16. Gorovoy MS. Descemet's-stripping automated endothelial keratoplasty. Cornea. 2006;25(8):886-9.
17. Covert DJ, Koenig SB. New triple procedure: Descemet's stripping and automated endothelial keratoplasty combined with phacoemulsification and intraocular lens implantation. Ophthalmology. 2007;114(7):1272-7.
18. Terry MA, Shamie N, Chen ES, Phillips PM, Shah AK, Hoar KL, et al. Endothelial keratoplasty for Fuchs' dystrophy with cataract: complications and clinical results with the new triple procedure. Ophthalmology. 2009;116(4):631-9.
19. Sykakis E, Lam FC, Georgoudis P, Hamada S, Lake D. Patients with Fuchs endothelial dystrophy and cataract undergoing Descemet's stripping automated endothelial keratoplasty and phacoemulsification with intraocular lens implant: Staged versus combined procedure outcomes. J Ophthalmol. 2015; 2015:172075.
20. Fajardo-Sanchez J, de Benito-Llopis L. Clinical outcomes of Descemet's membrane endothelial keratoplasty in pseudophakic eyes compared with triple-DMEK at 1-year follow-up. Cornea. 2021;40(4):420-4.
21. Das S, Langenbucher A, Jacobi C, Nguyen NX, Kruse FE, Naumann GO, et al. Long-term refractive and visual outcome after penetrating keratoplasty only versus the triple procedure in Fuchs' dystrophy. Graefes Arch Clin Exp Ophthalmol. 2006;244(9):1089-95.
22. Bhatt UK, Abdul Karim MN, Prydal JI, Maharajan SV, Fares U. Oral antivirals for preventing recurrent herpes simplex keratitis in people with corneal grafts. Cochrane Database Syst Rev. 2016;11:CD007824.
23. Vajpayee RB, Angra SK, Honavar SG. Combined keratoplasty, cataract extraction, and intraocular lens implantation after corneolenticular laceration in children. Am J Ophthalmol. 1994;117(4):507-11.
24. Shimmura S, Ohashi Y, Shiroma H, Shimazaki J, Tsubota K. Corneal opacity and cataract: triple procedure versus secondary approach. Cornea. 2003;22(3):234-8.
25. Mattax JB, McCulley JP. The effect of standardized keratoplasty technique on IOL power calculation for the triple procedure. Acta Ophthalmol Suppl. 1989;192:24-9.
26. Flowers CW, McLeod SD, McDonnell PJ, Irvine JA, Smith RE. Evaluation of intraocular lens power calculation formulas in the triple procedure. J Cataract Refract Surg. 1996;22(1):116-22.
27. Viestenz A, Seitz B, Langenbucher A. Intraocular lens power prediction for triple procedures in Fuchs' dystrophy using multiple regression analysis. Acta Ophthalmol Scand. 2005;83(3):312-5.
28. Bonfadini G, Ladas JG, Moreira H, Campos M, Matthaei M, Muñoz B, et al. Optimization of intraocular lens constant improves refractive outcomes in combined endothelial keratoplasty and cataract surgery. Ophthalmology. 2013;120(2):234-9.

29. Diener R, Treder M, Lauermann JL, Eter N, Alnawaiseh M. Assessing the validity of corneal power estimation using conventional keratometry for intraocular lens power calculation in eyes with Fuch's dystrophy undergoing Descemet's membrane endothelial keratoplasty. Graefes Arch Clin Exp Ophthalmol. 2021;259(4):1061-70.
30. Fritz M, Grewing V, Böhringer D, Lapp T, Maier P, Reinhard T, et al. Avoiding hyperopic surprises after Descemet's membrane endothelial keratoplasty in Fuchs dystrophy eyes by assessing corneal shape. Am J Ophthalmol. 2019;197:1-6.
31. Lindquist TD. Open-sky phacoemulsification during corneal transplantation. Ophthalmic Surg. 1994;25(10):734-6.
32. Ozkiriş A, Arslan O, Cicik E, Köylüoglu N, Evereklioglu C. Open-sky capsulorrhexis in triple procedure: with or without trypan blue? Eur J Ophthalmol. 2003;13(9-10):764-9.
33. Borderie VM, Touzeau O, Bourcier T, Carvajal-Gonzalez S, Laroche L. The triple procedure: in the bag placement versus ciliary sulcus placement of the intraocular lens. Br J Ophthalmol. 1999;83(4):458-62.
34. Kawamoto K, Morishige N, Chikama T, Nishida T. Modification of a soft contact lens for use during irrigation and aspiration in the penetrating keratoplasty triple procedure. Arch Ophthalmol. 2006;124(4):550-1.
35. Vongthongsri A, Jakpaiwong W, Preechanon A, Lekhanont K, Chuck RS. Anterior vitreous tapping to manage positive vitreous pressure during triple procedures. Ophthalmology. 2005;112(5):875-8.
36. Shimomura Y, Hosotani H, Kiritoshi A, Watanabe H, Tano Y. Core vitrectomy preceding triple corneal procedure in patients at high risk for increased posterior chamber pressure. Jpn J Ophthalmol. 1997;41(4):251-4.
37. Javadi MA, Feizi S, Moein HR. Simultaneous penetrating keratoplasty and cataract surgery. J Ophthalmic Vis Res. 2013; 8(1):39-46.
38. Jonas JB, Rank RM, Budde WM, Sauder G. Factors influencing visual outcome after penetrating keratoplasty combined with intraocular lens implantation. Eur J Ophthalmol. 2003;13(2):134-8.
39. Caporossi A, Traversi C, Simi C, Tosi GM. Closed-system and open-sky capsulorhexis for combined cataract extraction and corneal transplantation. J Cataract Refract Surg. 2001;27(7): 990-3.
40. Malbran ES, Malbran E, Buonsanti J, Adrogué E. Closed-system phacoemulsification and posterior chamber implant combined with penetrating keratoplasty. Ophthalmic Surg. 1993;24(6):403-6.
41. Baykara M, Ucan G. Modifying the position of cataract incisions in triple procedure. Eur J Ophthalmol. 2008;18(6):891-4.
42. Oshima Y, Shima C, Maeda N, Tano Y. Chandelier retroillumination-assisted torsional oscillation for cataract surgery in patients with severe corneal opacity. J Cataract Refract Surg. 2007;33(12):2018-22.
43. Sharma N, Singhal D, Maharana PK, Dhiman R, Shekhar H, Titiyal JS, et al. Phacoemulsification with coexisting corneal opacities. J Cataract Refract Surg. 2019;45(1):94-100.
44. Nardi M, Giudice V, Marabotti A, Alfieri E, Rizzo S. Temporary graft for closed-system cataract surgery during corneal triple procedures. J Cataract Refract Surg. 2001;27(8):1172-5.
45. Menapace R, Skorpik C, Grasl M. Modified triple procedure using a temporary keratoprosthesis for closed-system, small-incision cataract surgery. J Cataract Refract Surg. 1990;16(2):230-4.
46. Panda A, Sethi HS, Jain M, Nindra Krishna S, Gupta AK. Deep anterior lamellar keratoplasty with phacoemulsification. J Cataract Refract Surg. 2011;37(1):122-6.
47. Zaki AA, Elalfy MS, Said DG, Dua HS. Deep anterior lamellar keratoplasty—triple procedure: A useful clinical application of the pre-Descemet's layer (Dua's layer). Eye (Lond). 2015;29(3):323-6.
48. Agarwal T, Bandivadekar P, Sharma N, Sagar P, Titiyal JS. Sutureless anterior lamellar keratoplasty with phacoemulsification. Cornea. 2015;34(6):615-20.
49. Price FW Jr, Price MO. Combined cataract/DSEK/DMEK: Changing expectations. Asia Pac J Ophthalmol (Phila). 2017; 6(4):388-92.
50. Chaurasia S, Price FW, Gunderson L, Price MO. Descemet's membrane endothelial keratoplasty: Clinical results of single versus triple procedures (combined with cataract surgery). Ophthalmology. 2014;121(2):454-8.
51. Schoenberg ED, Price FW, Miller J, McKee Y, Price MO. Refractive outcomes of Descemet's membrane endothelial keratoplasty triple procedures (combined with cataract surgery). J Cataract Refract Surg. 2015;41(6):1182-9.
52. Yokogawa H, Sanchez PJ, Mayko ZM, Straiko MD, Terry MA. Astigmatism correction with toric intraocular lenses in Descemet's membrane endothelial keratoplasty triple procedures. Cornea. 2017;36(3):269-74.
53. Hoerster R, Stanzel TP, Bachmann BO, Siebelmann S, Felsch M, Cursiefen C. Intensified topical steroids as prophylaxis for macular edema after posterior lamellar keratoplasty combined with cataract surgery. Am J Ophthalmol. 2016;163:174-179.e2.

41

Penetrating Keratoplasty for Aphakic and Pseudophakic Bullous Keratopathy

Sujata Das, Smrutirekha Priyadarshini, Vishal Gupta

INTRODUCTION

Bullous keratopathy is a major complication of cataract surgery. Persistent corneal edema after cataract extraction is the leading indication for penetrating keratoplasty (PKP) in the United States.[1,2] The rate of corneal edema is low due to modern cataract surgical techniques. However, the actual number of afflicted patients is relatively high because a large number of cataract extractions are performed annually. Postoperative corneal edema may occur in the absence or presence of an intraocular lens (IOL) and is accordingly termed aphakic bullous keratopathy (ABK) or pseudophakic bullous keratopathy (PBK) respectively (**Figs. 1A to D**).

Aphakic bullous keratopathy is known to be the leading cause of secondary corneal degeneration for over 100 years[3] although it was described as corneal dystrophy or bullous keratitis in much of the earlier literature.[4] Past rates of ABK

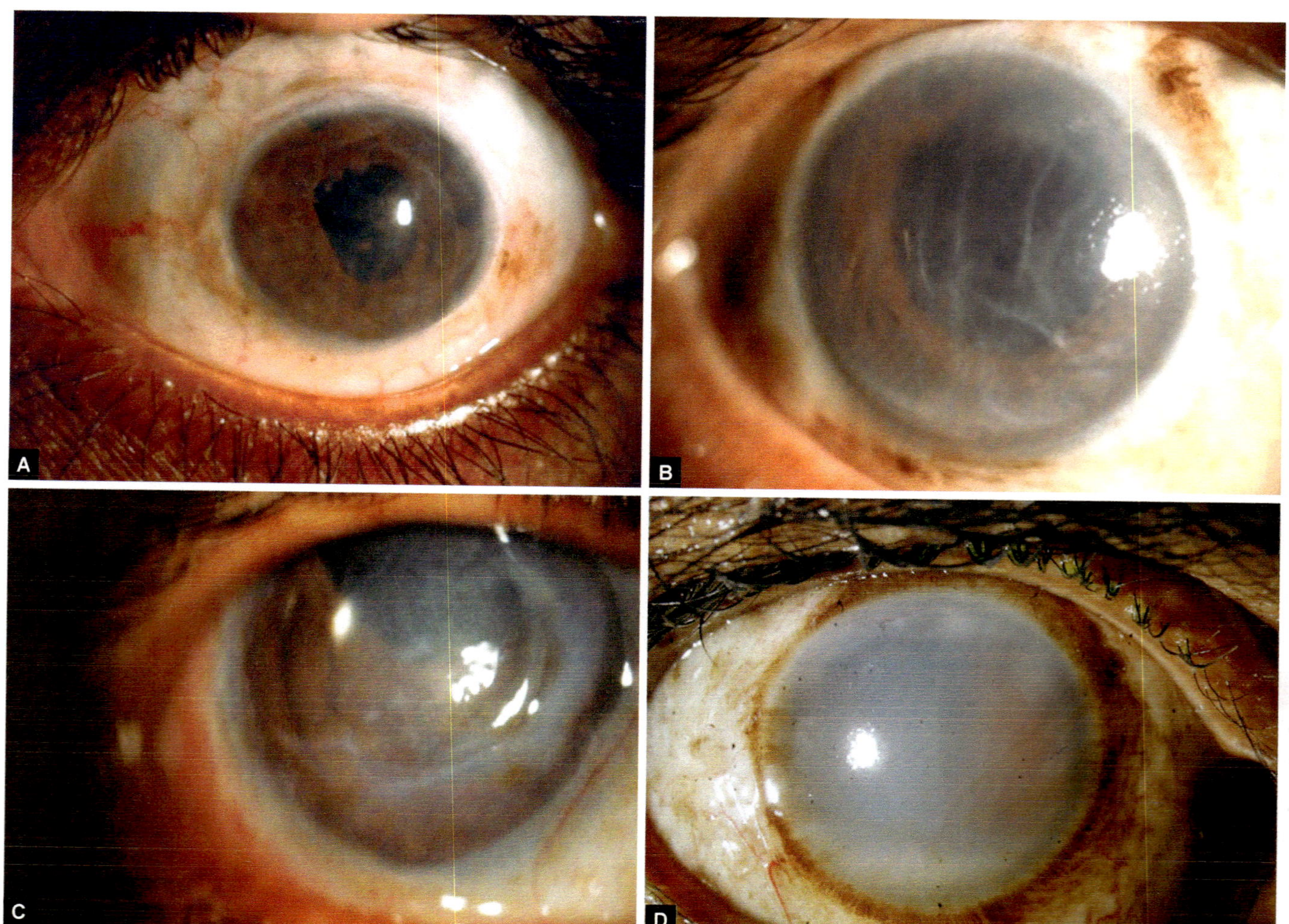

Figs. 1A to D: Pseudophakic bullous keratopathy (A) Early stage; (B) Advanced stage with posterior chamber intraocular lens implant, (C) with anterior chamber intraocular lens implant; (D) Aphakic bullous keratopathy.

are difficult to determine. Comparative series, in the period of early IOL use, has rates of 0–0.8% with intracapsular extraction and no IOL.[5,6] Incidence in eyes with vitreous loss during intracapsular cataract extraction ranged from 0.9 to 11.3% before vitrectomy techniques came into use.[7]

The widespread use of IOLs was followed by a dramatic increase in PBK, especially that associated with early prototypical lens models, beginning with the Ridley lens (1949–1954), early anterior chamber lens (1952–1986), and iris-supported pupillary lenses (1953–1980). These early lenses were characterized by design flaws, manufacturing defects and inadequate quality control.[8,9] The rate of PBK was as high as 50% over 5 years in some of the early European series of the 1950s and in 1960s.[10,11] The incidence of PBK after posterior chamber IOL (PC-IOL) implantation has been reported to be lower than the rate associated with anterior chamber or iris-fixated IOL.[12,13]

In most cases of bullous keratopathy, PKP is the only effective therapy. Survival of a donor cornea in bullous keratopathy has been extensively studied.[14-16] Although the short-term graft survival rate is good, visual improvement is often suboptimal. Corneal transplant surgeons agree on certain goals in the surgical management of patients with pseudophakic and aphakic bullous keratopathy. Because of the optical advantages of IOL over contact lenses or aphakic spectacles, eye should remain pseudophakic after corneal transplant surgery.[17-19] There is consensus that iris plane, closed-loop anterior chamber IOL (AC-IOL), and dislocated IOL be explanted and a careful anterior segment reconstruction including vitrectomy, goniosynechiolysis, and iridoplasty (when indicated) be performed.[20-22] The indications of IOL exchange/removal during PKP are listed in **Box 1**. At present, placement of a flexible open-loop AC-IOL in the angle or suturing of a PC-IOL either to the iris or to the sclera is the method commonly used by most surgeons.

PREOPERATIVE EVALUATION

History

Taking a careful history is a mandatory component. A detailed history of the cause of vision loss is helpful in documenting whether the visual loss is related solely to the corneal disease. The history should also include an assessment of the patient's activities, employment, and the effect of visual loss on these. The most crucial factor here is detailed information of the previous cataract surgery, including techniques used in cataract removal, status of the posterior capsule and zonules, and intraoperative and postoperative complications. The type, power, and configuration of the IOL should be obtained from the records. A history of general medical problems is helpful in planning the pre- and postoperative care and anesthesia.

Box 1: Indications of IOL exchange/removal during PKP.

- An unstable IOL demonstrating dislocation or improper sizing
- Poorly controlled glaucoma
- Recurrent hyphema
- UGH syndrome
- Metal clips or loops on the IOL
- Any closed-loop anterior chamber IOL (AC-IOL)
- Iris-supported IOLs with the optic in front of iris
- Chronic pain attributable to an AC-IOL

(IOL: intraocular lens; PKP: penetrating keratoplasty; UGH: uveitis-glaucoma-hyphema)

Examination of Anterior Segment

Slit-lamp examination is an essential feature of the diagnostic evaluation. Careful attention should be paid to the status of the lids, conjunctiva, and cornea. Measurement of central corneal thickness may document stromal edema when there is mild epithelial edema or Descemet's folding. Serial pachymetry is often helpful in documenting the progression of edema. Specular microscopy of the corneal endothelium may be of some use in the evaluation of eyes with marginal vision and edema. Slit-lamp examination and specular microscopy of the uninvolved eye may provide clue in cases of Fuchs' endothelial corneal dystrophy (FECD).

Documentation of the slit-lamp examination includes variations in corneal thickness, extent and depth of vascularization, and the location of opacities and edema. The status of the anterior chamber, presence of peripheral anterior synechiae (PAS), and position, type, and stability of the IOL, vitreous and capsule are important to observe preoperatively.

A high proportion of eyes with PBK has glaucoma. About 35% of the patients use antiglaucoma medication at the time of keratoplasty.[11] Intraocular pressure should be controlled before keratoplasty is undertaken, if possible, or a combined filtering or valve procedure should be done at the time of corneal grafting.

Evaluation of Intraocular Lens

In the pseudophakic patient who is about to undergo PKP, special attention must be paid to the IOL and its relationship with the surrounding structures. The iris should be examined for synechiae to the IOL, suture to the IOL, erosions and dialysis. Extent and location of PAS should be documented. If the view is inadequate, it can be evaluated by gonioscopy. Gonioscopy not only provides the surgeon with information on the condition of the angle but also on the site of IOL haptics (in case of AC-IOL) and the environment surrounding them. In many eyes with PBK, successful gonioscopy is not possible because of the severity of the corneal edema. High-frequency ultrasound biomicroscopy (UBM) makes it possible to visualize the anterior segment structure at high resolution even in the presence of corneal opacity. It allows the surgeon to predict preoperatively the degree of difficulty that will be encountered in explanting the IOL.[23]

Intraocular Lens Power Calculations

The IOL power calculations are derived from the modified Sanders-Retzlaff-Kraff (SRK) formula that uses the axial length measurements and the keratometry readings. There are various methods by which the keratometry can be assessed.

- The surgeon's average keratometry value can be used, which is the average for all previous postoperative keratometry values, following suture removal.
- Most surgeons use a value of 43.5 or 45.0 D.
- For AC-IOL, horizontal limbal diameter, white-to-white, is measured prior to the attachment to the Flieringa ring. One millimeter is then added to this measurement to determine the size of the new AC-IOL.[17,24] Power of the implanted IOL may be determined from previous surgical records. The new AC-IOL power is achieved by subtracting 1.5 D from the previous AC-IOL, based on the assumption of an average of 1 or 2 D of corneal steepening postoperatively. If the original IOL is of iris plane style, 2.5 D are subtracted.[25]
- For scleral-fixated IOL target of –0.5 D is aimed.[26]

Retinal Evaluation

Preoperative detection of retinal detachment is of particular concern in aphakic and pseudophakic eyes with opaque corneas, particularly when, the original surgery is complicated by vitreous loss or a dislocated nucleus. Indirect ophthalmoscopy must be performed, to the extent possible prior to keratoplasty. B-scan ultrasonography can be performed rapidly as a screening procedure to rule out posterior segment pathology.

Cystoid macular edema (CME) is a major preoperative and postoperative problem in eyes with ABK and PBK.[27] It is a great problem in eyes with iris-supported and AC-IOLs that are inserted after intracapsular cataract extraction. In eyes with older style IOL associated late-onset corneal edema is often associated with late-onset of CME. Although fluorescein angiography usually cannot be performed in eyes with significant corneal edema, fluorescein angioscopy using an indirect ophthalmoscope and a blue filter often allows visualization of late cystoid pulling in the macula. Many patients with CME after PBK experience gradual improvement of their vision as the CME clears over a period of two or more years.[28] Macular function tests (Maddox Rod test, two-point discrimination test, laser interferometry) may be undertaken whenever possible. Visual evoked response (VER) gives much needed information about the retinal and optic pathway integrity.

SURGICAL TECHNIQUE

The challenges in performing keratoplasty in cases of PBK are not only to ensure minimal postoperative astigmatism, but also to evaluate the stability of IOL, and if IOL exchange or removal is contemplated, to facilitate atraumatic removal of the lens from fibrous encashment in delicate uveal tissue, restoration of anterior segment anatomy, and implantation of an IOL which will remain stable and not elicit intraocular inflammation (**Figs. 2A and B**).

The surgery can be performed either under local (peribulbar block) or general anesthesia. In some cases intravenous mannitol (1–2 g/kg body weight) can be administered immediately before the surgery over 20–30 minutes for deturgescence of the vitreous and make the iris diaphragm back.

Aphakic eyes have very low scleral rigidity and are prone to scleral collapse during surgery. Either a single or double Flieringa ring may be fixed to the globe with sutures. Extreme care must be taken in the placement of the scleral support ring because unequal placement of the fixation sutures can cause irregularity in the graft recipient bed and considerable

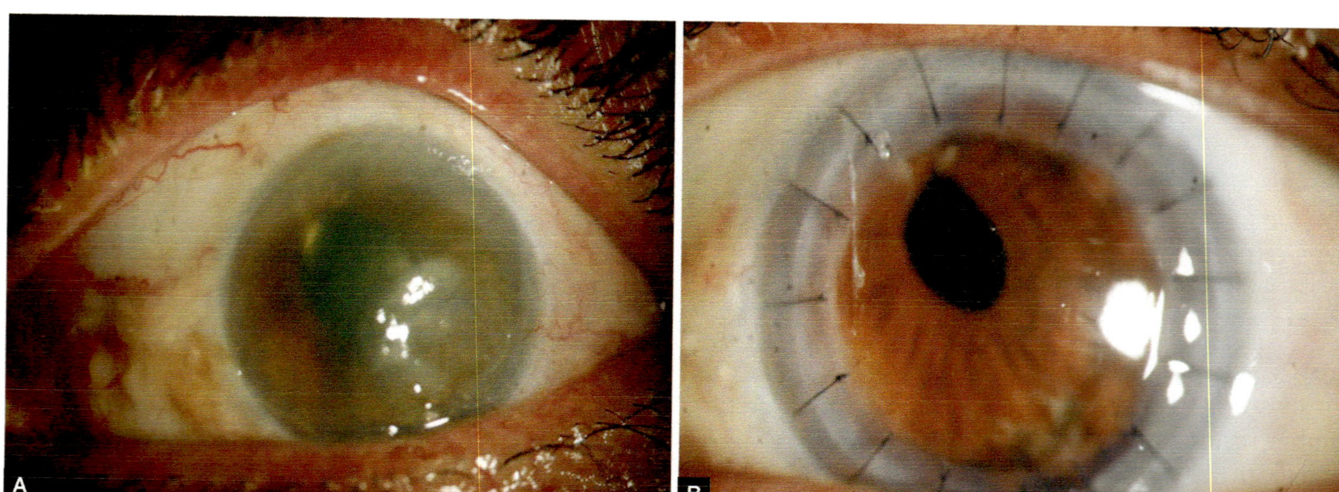

Figs. 2A and B: Pseudophakic bullous keratopathy: (A) Before keratoplasty; (B) After keartoplasty.

graft astigmatism. Because of this problem, many corneal surgeons have discontinued the use of Flieringa ring and instead simply place a bridal suture beneath the superior and inferior rectus muscle.

The recipient cornea should be inspected for any evidence of superficial corneal pannus, corneal neovascularization, or corneal thinning. If corneal pannus is present, it should be scraped off the superficial cornea using a surgical blade. It should be kept completely dry. If the epithelium is edematous and loose, it should be removed with a cellulose sponge or blade at this time as loose epithelium may prohibit achieving adequate suction during trephination. In cases of ABK and PBK, the graft size is relatively large in order to provide the maximum number of healthy endothelial cells. Using a handheld disposable trephine or a Hessburg-Barron vacuum trephine, a partial thickness cut 80–90% deep should be made in the recipient cornea. Corneal tissue is trephined with due care so as not to apply too much pressure on the globe. The trephine should be perpendicular to the corneal surface. Care should be taken to avoid uncontrolled entry into the anterior chamber, especially in eyes with ABK because of the danger of collapse of the globe due to low scleral rigidity. The anterior chamber is slowly entered with a microsharp blade. A 3–4 mm incision is made to allow easy entrance of the corneal scissors, which cuts the rest of the host corneal disk. As the cutting of the cornea is completed, attention should be directed to its endothelial surface where, vitreous attachments and iris adhesions may have to be cut before removal of the corneal tissue. Once the recipient cornea has been removed from the eye, several different approaches may be taken depending on the preoperative and intraoperative finding. These approaches may be differentiated as given here.

Aphakia with Hyaloid Face Intact

If the hyaloid face is intact and away from the cornea, the pupil may be constricted with pilocarpine. A decision to implant an IOL depends on the status of the other eye, physical needs and activities of the patient and the inability to use contact lens. If an IOL is to be inserted into the eye, a small amount of viscoelastic material is first placed over the pupil and on the surface of the iris to help act as a cushion. A flexible open-loop AC-IOL with three-point or quadriflex fixation lens is inserted, if indicated. The donor button is transferred to the recipient bed and sutured in place.

Aphakia with Loose Vitreous in Anterior Chamber

Vitreous manipulation at PKP may be a double-edged sword. Failure to remove vitreous from the anterior chamber results in vitreous incarceration in the wound, contact with the endothelium, and a poor prognosis for graft clarity and macular function. Open-sky automated anterior vitrectomy should be performed in case of loose vitreous in the anterior chamber. This reduces vitreous traction. Some surgeons have also advocated the evacuation of fluid vitreous through the pars plana before entering the anterior chamber depending on the visibility through the overlying edematous cornea. If formed vitreous is encountered in the anterior chamber at the time of removal of the corneal button, care must be taken to cut any adhesion from the posterior surface of the cornea. Once the cornea has been removed, an open-sky vitrectomy is performed. Attempts should be made to free the pupil from vitreous adhesions and to remove any strands of vitreous to the peripheral cornea. Vitrectomy should not be performed if the vitreous face is unbroken and does not protrude anteriorly because this increases the risk of CME and retinal detachment occurring after this procedure.[29]

Pseudophakia with Hyaloid Face Intact

If the hyaloid is unbroken or the posterior capsule is intact, the style of the implant and its effect on the eye primarily determine the surgical approach. Whenever, the IOL has to be explanted, anterior vitrectomy must be performed even if the hyaloid face is undisturbed. Depending on the style of IOL and duration of the surgery, frequently there are strong adhesions to the angle, iris, vitreous, capsular bag, or ciliary sulcus. Explantation of these lenses is extremely difficult and traumatic to the eye structure. Various forms of iris clips and loops must be opened or cut before lysis of iris and vitreous adhesions that surround the implant. The use of blunt and sharp dissection is required for removal of these lenses. Care must be taken to preserve as much of the iris as possible. In some cases, the AC-IOL optic should be cut from the haptic near the optic junction and then carefully rotated free from the dense fibrous tissue in the angle or ciliary sulcus. Anterior vitrectomy should be performed after removal of the lens. IOLs are left in place when they are stable and eye is quiet.

Pseudophakia with Loose Vitreous in Anterior Chamber

In patients with PBK and loose vitreous, the course of action is mainly determined by the type of implant and stability of the lens. In most cases, the removal of IOL and anterior vitrectomy is required. In general, iris plane lenses and closed-loop AC-IOLs are removed.

Gonioplasty

Viscodissection of the angle may be done by injecting viscoelastic. Iris adhesion to the cornea can be reduced by gently stroking it radially toward the pupil with a Sinskey hook or pulling it radially with smooth forceps.[30] If large iridocorneal adhesions are present which are not amenable to separation, iridotomies may be undertaken on either side of the lesion to prevent progression of the angle closure in the postoperative period.

Pupilloplasty

Restoration of the pupil to a central, round configuration by synechiolysis and iridoplasty serves several important functions. These functions include prevention of glaucoma and allograft rejection related to synechia formation, and improvement of the support for an AC-IOL if it has to be used. Pupilloplasty also addresses the postoperative glare seen in large iris defects mostly as a result of a previous eventful course. When suturing the iris with 10-0 polypropylene, it is important to bury the knots in the iris stroma, with short tags at the ends. The sutures are tied tight enough to approximate the iris, but not so tight as to cause buttonholing and cheese wiring of the tissue. If the pupil is eccentric, one can perform sphincterotomies at the pupillary rough where interrupted sutures can be placed starting peripherally along the sphincterotomy defect. Purse string sutures have been used along the pupillary margin to enable the creation of a central and circular pupil.[30] It has been observed that patients with pupilloplasty along with PKP performed for PBK/ABK had a better postoperative visual acuity compared to control group.[31,32]

Intraocular Lens Implantation

Successful vision restoration in eyes with PBK is dependent, to a large extent, on the successful management of the IOL at the time of surgery. The three available options for the management of IOL at the time of keratoplasty are to retain, remove without replacement, or replace the lens. Earlier reports advocated the retention of the original IOL.[33] However, this has not been corroborated by later investigations. The high rate of graft failure associated with retained IOLs prompted the recommendation of routine IOL removal at the time of PKP in these cases.[34] Although this approach produced better graft clarity, it created problems related to binocular vision in patients where the fellow eye was phakic or pseudophakic.[35] This stimulated the introduction of IOL exchange. An algorithm can be used in evaluating IOL exchange (**Flowchart 1**). The various options for replacing the IOL at the time of PKP and IOL exchange include the following:

- Flexible open-loop AC-IOL
- Iris-sutured PC-IOL (IS PC-IOL)
- Posterior chamber IOL in the ciliary sulcus
- Scleral-fixated PC-IOL (SF PC-IOL).[36]

Flexible Open-loop Anterior Chamber Intraocular Lens

Experimental[37] and clinical evidence[38-41] indicates that Kelman-style, one-piece, open-loop polymethylmethacrylate (PMMA) AC-IOL performs more favorably than the closed-loop AC-IOL and is associated with long-term graft survival. Open-loop AC-IOLs can give good postoperative results and functional vision in cases of PBK and ABK.[24] However,

Flowchart 1: Management options for IOL exchange.

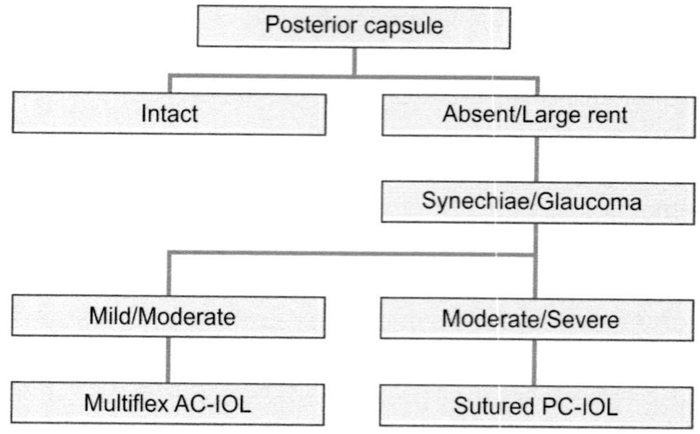

(AC-IOL: anterior chamber intraocular lens; PC-IOL: posterior chamber intraocular lens)

it is contraindicated in cases of intractable glaucoma, PAS greater than 3 clock hours, and insufficient iris tissue.

Advantages
- Technically easy
- Requires less iris manipulation
- Lack of suturing for IOL fixation
- Precludes vitrectomy in many cases
- Less surgical intraoperative time
- Can be used in nearly any eye, even in those with sector iridectomies or inflamed irides.

Disadvantages
- Possibility of progressive endothelial loss
- Potential for development of synechiae and secondary glaucoma.

Technique: After trephination of the recipient, the pupil is constricted with intracameral pilocarpine or acetylcholine hydrochloride as it minimizes the incidence of peripheral iris tuck. Viscoelastic is injected on the anterior surface of the iris and into the peripheral iridocorneal angle. The AC-IOL is then grasped along the edge of the haptic or superior edge of the optic, and inserted using the smallest angle of insertion to minimize the entrapment of the peripheral iris. The other haptic is grasped, flexed, lowered into the keratoplasty opening and then released. The pupil should be monitored to ensure that it is round without any oval distortion; that would indicate the entrapment of peripheral iris. If entrapment of iris is suspected, the involved haptic can be grasped with Kelman-McPherson forceps and gently pulled back from the angle, lifted slightly anteriorly, and reinserted until displacement of the pupil is no longer visualized. Once implanted, the haptic should be drawn toward the optic and elevated with a lens hook to ensure that the foot plates have not captured peripheral iris. Any bleeding is controlled by use of sodium hyaluronate in the angle or compression with a sponge soaked with epinephrine (1:1000). At least one peripheral iridectomy should be done. Care must be taken to avoid placing the foot plates over iridectomies as prolapse through them to the ciliary body may occur.

Most authors have recommended that AC-IOLs should be placed at 90° to the orientation of the explanted IOL, away from goniosynechiae, damaged angle or peripheral iridectomies[40,42] as it could otherwise erode, cause hemorrhage or become a source of persistent inflammation.

Iris-sutured Posterior Chamber Intraocular Lens

Suture-fixating a PC-IOL to the posterior aspect of the iris, through the limbal incision was first reported by Pearce.[43] Several other surgeons[44-46] modified this technique combining it with PKP in aphakic eyes with corneal edema. Graft survival ranged between 93 and 97.7%.

Advantages

- Avoidance of the anterior chamber structure
- Intraocular lens closer to the nodal point of eye.

Disadvantages

- Due to the large area of uveal contact with the IOL, there is increased risk of suture-induced uveitis, iris atrophy, and possible dislocation of the IOL.
- Insufficient iris from previous iridectomies or iris colobomas may not allow iris fixation
- Vitrectomy is required in all cases.
- The iris sutures may also cause an ellipsoid dilation of the pupil.

Technique: Fixation of the optic to the iris is preferred to haptic fixation to ensure better fixation and centration. Either a planar or angled haptic can be used to suture the optic to the iris. A double-armed 10-0 polypropylene (prolene) suture is passed through the positioning holes in a four-hole[47] or two-hole lens.[48] The lens implant is then held over the iris to determine the best position for its placement, avoiding any atrophic areas. The polypropylene suture is then passed through the mid-peripheral iris. The PC-IOL is then slipped behind the iris with each haptic directed into the ciliary sulcus. The sutures are then tied snuggly.[46,49,50] The suture knots are placed between the optic and the iris to reduce the areas of contact.

Posterior Chamber Intraocular Lens in the Ciliary Sulcus

In the past, IOL insertion at the time of PKP for pseudophakic or aphakic bullous keratopathy after intracapsular cataract extraction was limited to an AC-IOL or suturing of PC-IOL to the iris or through the ciliary sulcus. A complicated cataract surgery with AC-IOL placement may leave posterior capsular remnants or a Soemmering's ring. If sufficient amounts of these tissues are available, implantation of the PC-IOL into the ciliary sulcus with posterior support is possible during PKP and IOL exchange.[51]

Advantages

- Technically less demanding
- Less surgical time
- Intraocular lens closer to nodal point
- Least complicated
- Avoids complications of AC-IOLs on the angle of the anterior chamber.

Technique: The residual posterior capsule, the remnants of the anterior capsule and Soemmering's ring should be carefully evaluated by retracting the iris in all four quadrants with an iris retractor or Sinskey hook. Iris repositor, viscodissection, cyclodialysis spatula and/or Vannas scissors can be used to break the posterior synechia. Very little capsular support is required for successful PC-IOL implantation in the sulcus as capsular fibrosis occurs in a few months after the original cataract surgery. The IOLs can be placed with the haptic over the region of greatest capsular support after placing a high viscosity viscoelastic in the capsular remnant.

Scleral-fixated Posterior Chamber Intraocular Lens

This technique involves suturing the haptics into the ciliary sulcus, which then places the IOL in the anatomic position of the lens. This procedure is indicated in cases of preoperative glaucoma or PAS, and insufficient iris.

Advantages

- The posterior location limits endothelial damage
- Lack of iris sutures allows full pupillary dilation.

Disadvantages

- Technically difficult
- More intraoperative manipulation
- Longer surgical time
- Increased risk of vitreous hemorrhage, retinal detachment, suture-wick, endophthalmitis, lens decentration and tilt.[48,52-54]

Technique: Conjunctival peritomies measuring approximate 3 mm in length are created at the 2 and 8 o'clock positions or at the 4 and 10 o'clock positions of the limbus to avoid ciliary blood vessels and the long posterior ciliary nerve at the horizontal meridian. A bipolar cautery may be applied to the episcleral vessels to control any bleeding. Scleral flaps can be constructed to cover the fixation sutures.

The selection of an appropriate PC-IOL is critical to the success of this technique. The recommended PC-IOL includes biconvex, large optic (6.5–7.0 mm) and one-piece all-PMMA construction. The eyelet-to-eyelet diameter is 12–12.5 mm, and the haptics are angled posteriorly to further minimize iris contact. A 10-0 polypropylene suture with double-armed needles is passed through the iris. The surgeon should ensure that both ends of the suture pass the same side of the haptic to avoid any torque effect, which could result in IOL tilt. The transscleral fixation can be approached internally by the ab interno approach or externally by the ab externo procedure.

Ab interno approach: This technique uses two polypropylene sutures on a short-tapered needle. The tip of the needle is held parallel to the iris and gently moved along the posterior surface of the iris until the ciliary sulcus is entered approximately 0.75 mm back from the surgical limbus. Both ends of the double-ended sutures are passed through the ciliary sulcus approximately 3 mm apart. The IOL haptics gently placed into the ciliary sulcus while the fixation sutures are alternatively tightened to avoid further tangling of the sutures and to ensure symmetrical placement of the trans-scleral fixation of PC-IOL (TS-PC-IOL). The IOL is checked for adequate central fixation and tilt by gentle retraction of the pupil. The sutures are then pulled taut and tied themselves. The knots are buried beneath the episclera by gentle rotation of the suture.

Ab externo approach: A straight transcorneal needle with a 10-0 polypropylene suture penetrates the scleral bed parallel to the iris 1.5 mm posterior to the surgical limbus. The needle tip is passed through the ciliary sulcus posterior to the iris and is visualized in the pupillary space. A 28-gauge needle is passed through the sclera 180° from the straight transcorneal needle. The straight needle is threaded into the barrel of the 28-gauge needle and then removed. It is then passed back across the sulcus in the opposite direction parallel to the initial pass but separated by a minimum of 2 mm on the scleral bed.

A recent study by Sewelam et al.[55] reported ultra-biomicroscopic (UBM) evaluation of 20 eyes, who had ab externo approach TS-PC-IOL. They observed 22 haptics (55%) were in the sulcus, 11 (27.5%) were anterior to the sulcus, and 7 (17.5%) were posterior to the sulcus. They recommended use of the endoscopic technique for precise localization of the entry of the needle in the sulcus. Recent studies using fibrin glue-assisted intrascleral fixation of a PC-IOL combined with PKP was found to be a safe and effective method in achieving visual rehabilitation in ABK or PBK with malpositioned IOLs.[36] The IOL fixation was strong enough to sustain the manipulation required for corneal procedures.

Posterior Lamellar Keratoplasty

Although PKP enjoys a high anatomic success rate, visual rehabilitation is often slow due to delayed stromal wound healing, surgically induced astigmatism, suture-related complications, and anisometropia associated with unexpected changes in the postoperative corneal power. In contrast, posterior lamellar corneal surgery allows for selective replacement of diseased host endothelium. Posterior lamellar keratoplasty (PLK) for the management of corneal endothelial disorders was first described in 1998[56-58] and since 2001, the technique has been made popular in the United States as deep lamellar endothelial keratoplasty (DLEK).[59] Instead of a full-thickness transplant, a 7.5-mm diameter posterior lamellar disk is transplanted through a 9-mm sutured scleral incision. In 2000, Melles et al. modified this technique to a sutureless procedure in which a folded 9 mm diameter posterior lamellar disk is transplanted through a self-sealing 5 mm scleral tunnel incision. Despite the excellent postoperative result, visual acuity after DLEK rarely exceeded 20/30 due to presumed optical aberration at the graft-host interface.[60] Unlike DLEK, in Descemet's stripping endothelial keratoplasty (DSEK), the recipient endothelial layer can be removed by stripping of the Descemet's membrane (Descemetorhexis) followed by insertion of a folded donor lamellar donor disk.[61] Price and Price employed mechanical stripping of the diseased host endothelium and replacement with a healthy homograft of the endothelium, Descemet's membrane and a thin layer of the donor's stromal tissue harvested with an automated microkeratome (DSAEK).[62] Melles et al. introduced the technique of Descemet's membrane endothelial keratoplasty (DMEK), where only Descemet's membrane with endothelium without any stroma is being inserted into anterior chamber.[63] DMEK may have several advantages. As in DSEK, the surgical trauma to the recipient's eye is minimized but DMEK also provides a near normal restoration of the grafted cornea.

The main advantages of PLK and its variants are that these techniques induce little postoperative astigmatism, eliminate suture-related complications, and minimize the risk of wound dehiscence. However, from a technical viewpoint, it is challenging to create a dissection plane in a corneoscleral ring that has already been excised.

OUTCOME

The short-term graft survival rate is good (74% at 5 years), however, visual improvement is often poor.[64] The most important positive prognostic factors affecting visual acuity after PKP for bullous keratopathy are well integrated posterior segment, short interval between development of bullous keratopathy and keratoplasty, and simultaneous PC-IOL implantation. The negative prognostic factors affecting visual outcome are the presence of coexisting ocular pathology, presence of AC-IOL, and significantly long gap the development of bullous keratopathy and keratoplasty.[65] Barkana Y et al. have studied that the method of IOL implantation during the cataract surgery is the single most significant predictor of visual acuity after keratoplasty.[66] Better outcome was seen in Bag-fixated or sulcus-fixated posterior chamber IOL than with anterior chamber IOL, scleral-fixated posterior chamber IOL, or aphakia.

CONCLUSION

With the advent of modern surgery and better techniques, PKP is slowly getting replaced by endothelial procedures such as PDEK pre-Descemet's endothelial keratoplasty (PDEK), DSAEK, and DMEK for ABK and PBK. The learning curve may be steeper in the beginning for surgeons, but faster and better outcome has been observed with these newer techniques. However, in cases with very long-standing corneal decompensation and especially with significant scarring involving the visual axis, PKP is still the preferred technique.

REFERENCES

1. Waring GO 3rd. The 50-year epidemic of pseudophakic corneal edema. Arch Ophthalmol. 1989;107:657-9.
2. Lois N, Kowal VO, Cohen EJ, Rapuano CJ, Gault JA, Raber IM, et al. Indications for penetrating keratoplasty and associated procedures, 1989-1995. Cornea. 1997;16:623-9.
3. Hess C. Klinische und experimintelle studie uber die entstehung der streifenformigen hornhauttraubung nach starextraktion. Graefes Arch Clin Experiment Ophthalmol. 1892;38:1.
4. Cogan DG. Experimental production of so-called bullous keratitis. Arch Ophthalmol. 1940;23:918-25.
5. Cataract surgery: interim results and complications of a randomized controlled trial. Oxford Cataract Treatment and Evaluation Team (OCTET). Br J Ophthalmol. 1986;70:402-10.
6. Jaffe NS, Eichenbaum DM, Clayman HM, Light DS. A comparison of 500 Binkhorst implants with 500 routine intracapsular cataract extractions. Am J Ophthalmol. 1978;85:24-7.
7. Vail DJ. After-results of vitreous loss. Am J Ophthalmol. 1965;59:573-86.
8. Apple DJ, Mamalis N, Loftfield K, Googe JM, Novak LC, Kavka-Van Norman D, et al. Complications of intraocular lenses. A historical and histopathological review. Surv Ophthalmol. 1984;29:1-54.
9. Stark WJ, Whitney CE, Chandler JW, Worthen DM. Trends in intraocular lens implantation in the United States. Arch Ophthalmol. 1986;104:1769-70.
10. DeVoe AG. Critical evaluation of current concepts in cataract surgery. The George K. Smelser Lecture. Am J Ophthalmol. 1976;81:715-21.
11. Sugar A. An analysis of corneal endothelial and graft survival in pseudophakic bullous keratopathy. Trans Am Ophthalmol Soc. 1989;87:762-801.
12. Taylor DM, Atlas BF, Romanchuk KG, Stren AL. Pseudophakic bullous keratopathy. Ophthalmology. 1983;90:19-24.
13. Fagadau WR, Maumenee AE, Stark WJ Jr, Datiles M. Posterior chamber intraocular lenses at the Wilmer Institute: a comparative analysis of complication and visual results. Br J Ophthalmol. 1984;68:13-8.
14. Waldock A, Cook SD. Corneal transplantation: how successful are we? Br J Ophthalmol. 2000;84:813-5.
15. Vail A, Gore SM, Bradey BA, Easty DL, Rogers CA. Corneal graft survival and visual outcome. A multicenter Study. Corneal Transplant Follow-up Study Collaborators. Ophthalmology. 1994;101:120-7.
16. Agrawal V, Vagh MM, Sangwan V, Rao GN. Penetrating keratoplasty for pseudophakic bullous keratopathy. Indian J Ophthalmol. 1994;42:75-80.
17. Polack FM. Results of keratoplasty for aphakic or pseudophakic corneal edema with intraocular lens implantation or exchange. Cornea. 1988;7:239-43.
18. Binder PS. Secondary intraocular lens implantation during or after corneal transplantation. Am J Ophthalmol. 1985;99:515-20.
19. Arentsen JJ, Laibson PR. Surgical management of pseudophakic corneal edema: complications and visual results following penetrating keratoplasty. Ophthalmic Surg. 1982;13:371-3.
20. Smith PW, Wong SK, Stark WJ, Gottsch JD, Terry AC, Bonham RD. Complications of semi-flexible closed-loop anterior chamber intraocular lens. Arch Ophthalmol. 1987;105:52-7.
21. Speaker MG, Lugo M, Laibson PR, Rubinfeld RS, Stein RM, Genvert GI, et al. Penetrating keratoplasty for pseudophakic bullous keratopathy. Management of the intraocular lens. Ophthalmology. 1988;95:1260-8.
22. Sugar A, Meyer RF. PKP for PBK—we don't have all the answers. Cornea. 1985-86;4:1-2.
23. Rutnin SS, Pavlin CJ, Slomovic AR, Kwartz J, Rootman DS. Preoperative ultrasound biomicroscopy to assess ease of haptic removal before penetrating keratoplasty combined with lens exchange. J Cataract Refract Surg. 1997;23:239-43.
24. Zaidman GW, Goldman S. A prospective study on the implantation of anterior chamber intraocular lenses during keratoplasty for pseudophakic and aphakic bullous keratopathy. Ophthalmology. 1990;97:757-62.
25. Hunkeler JD. Longer haptic allows for better manipulation. Ophthalmic Surg. 1989;20:599.
26. Hwang AM, Rue KS, Francis BA, Yiu SC. Analysis of Refractive Outcome and Complications of Descemet's Stripping and Automated Endothelial Keratoplasty (DSAEK) with Scleral-fixated Sutured Posterior Chamber Intraocular Lens. Invest Ophthalmol Vis Sci. 2011;52:751.
27. Brightbill FS, Dudley SS. Aphakic bullous keratopathy: preoperative fluorescein angiographic screening for macular edema. Contact Intraocul Lens Med J. 1981;7:144-9.
28. Price FW Jr, Whitson WE. Natural history of cystoid macular edema in pseudophakic bullous keratopathy. J Cataract Refract Surg. 1990;16:163-9.
29. Kramer SG. Cystoid macular edema after aphakic penetrating keratoplasty. Ophthalmology. 1981;88:782-7.
30. Waring GO 3rd. Management of pseudophakic corneal edema with reconstruction of the anterior ocular segment. Arch Ophthalmol. 1987;105:709-15.
31. Arundhati A, Jun BZ, Janardhan P, Tan DT. Iris reconstruction in penetrating keratoplasty-surgical techniques and a case-control study to evaluate effect on graft survival. Am J Ophthalmol. 2008;145:203-9.
32. Arundhati A, Zhou B, Tan DT. Effect of Pupil Reconstruction on Corneal Graft Survival and Visual Outcome—A Case Control Study. Invest Ophthalmol Vis Sci. 2007;48:4673.
33. Speaker MG, Laibson PR, Cohen EJ, Arentsen JJ. Pseudophakic bullous keratopathy. In: Cavanagh HP (Ed). The Cornea: Transactions of the World Congress on the Cornea III. New York: Raven Press; 1988: pp. 319-326.
34. Waring GO 3rd, Welch SN, Cavanagh HD, Wilson LA. Results of penetrating keratoplasty in 123 eyes with pseudophakic or aphakic corneal edema. Ophthalmology. 1983;90:25-33.
35. Alpar JJ. Long-term results of keratoplasty in eyes with intraocular lenses. Ophthalmic Surg. 1986;17:650-4.
36. Sinha R, Shekhar H, Sharma N, Tandon R, Titiyal JS, Vajpayee RB. Intrascleral fibrin glue intraocular lens fixation combined with Descemet-stripping automated endothelial keratoplasty or penetrating keratoplasty. J Cataract Refract Surg. 2012;38:1240-5.
37. Apple DJ, Hansen SO, Richards SC, Ellis GW, Kanka-Van Norman D, Tetz MR, et al. Anterior chamber lenses. Part II: A laboratory study. J Cataract Refract Surg. 1987;13:175-89.
38. Insler MS, Kook MS, Kaufman HE. Penetrating keratoplasty for pseudophakic bullous keratopathy associated with semiflexible, closed-loop anterior chamber intraocular lenses. Am J Ophthalmol. 1989;107:252-6.
39. Lass JH, DeSantis DM, Reinhart WJ, Hossain TS, Hom DL. Clinical and morphometric results of penetrating keratoplasty with one-piece anterior-chamber or suture-fixated posterior-chamber

lenses in the absence of lens capsule. Arch Ophthalmol. 1990;108:1427-31.
40. Hassan TS, Soong HK, Sugar A, Meyer RF. Implantation of Kelman-style, open-loop anterior chamber lenses during keratoplasty for aphakic and pseudophakic bullous keratopathy. A comparison with iris-sutured posterior chamber lenses. Ophthalmology. 1991;98:875-80.
41. Lois N, Cohen EJ, Rapuano CJ, Liabson PR. Long-term graft survival in patients with flexible open-loop anterior-chamber intraocular lenses. Cornea. 1997;16:387-92.
42. Ritterband DC, Seedor JA, Speaker MG. Penetrating keratoplasty for pseudophakic bullous keratopathy. In: Brightbill FS (Ed). Corneal Surgery: Theory, Technique and Tissue, 3rd edition. St. Louis: Mosby, 1999. pp. 292-301.
43. Pearce JL. New lightweight sutured posterior chamber lens implant. Trans Ophthalmol Soc UK. 1976;96:6-10.
44. Waring GO 3rd, Stulting RD, Street D. Penetrating keratoplasty for pseudophakic corneal edema with exchange of intraocular lenses. Arch Ophthalmol. 1987;105:58-62.
45. Hall JR, Muenzler WS. Intraocular lens replacement in pseudophakic bullous keratopathy. Trans Ophthalmol Soc UK. 1985;104:541-5.
46. Soong HK, Meyer RF, Sugar A. Posterior chamber IOL implantation during keratoplasty for aphakic or pseudophakic corneal edema. Cornea. 1987;6:306-12.
47. Drews RC. Posterior chamber lens implantation during keratoplasty without posterior capsule support. Cornea. 1987;6:38-40.
48. Price FW Jr, Whitson WE. Visual results of suture-fixated posterior chamber lenses during penetrating keratoplasty. Ophthalmology. 1989;96:1234-9.
49. Morrison LK, Waltman SR. Management of pseudophakic bullous keratopathy. Ophthalmic Surg. 1989;20:205-10.
50. Soong HK, Meyer RF, Sugar A. Techniques of posterior chamber lens implantation without capsular support during penetrating keratoplasty: a review. Refract Corneal Surg. 1989;5:249-55.
51. Donnenfeld ED, Ingraham HJ, Perry HD, Russell S, Foulks G. Soemmering's ring support for posterior chamber intraocular lens implantation during penetrating keratoplasty. Changing trends in bullous keratopathy. Ophthalmology. 1992;99:1229-33.
52. Rajpal RK, Carney MD, Weinberg RS. Complications of transscleral sutured posterior chamber intraocular lenses. Ophthalmology. 1991;(98 suppl):144.
53. Schecter RJ. Suture-wick endophthalmitis with sutured posterior chamber intraocular lenses. J Cataract Refract Surg. 1990;16:755-6.
54. Heilskov T, Joondeph BC, Olsen KR, Blankenship GW. Late endophthalmitis after transscleral fixation of a posterior chamber intraocular lens. Arch Ophthalmol. 1989;107:1427.
55. Sewelam A, Ismail AM, El Serogy H. Ultrasound biomicroscopy of haptic position after transscleral fixation of posterior chamber intraocular lenses. J Cataract Refract Surg. 2001;27:1418-22.
56. Melles GR, Eggink FA, Lander F, Pels E, Rietveld FJ, Beekhuis WH, et al. A surgical technique for posterior lamellar keratoplasty. Cornea. 1998;17:618-26.
57. Melles GR, Lander F, Beekhuis WH, Remeijer L, Binder PS. Posterior lamellar keratoplasty for a case of pseudophakic bullous keratopathy. Am J Ophthalmol. 1999;127:340-1.
58. Melles GRJ, Lander F, van Dooren BT, Pels E, Beekhuis WH. Preliminary clinical results of posterior lamellar keratoplasty through a sclerocorneal pocket incision. Ophthalmology. 2000;107:1850-7.
59. Terry MA, Ousley PJ. Deep lamellar endothelial keratoplasty in the first United States patients: early clinical results. Cornea. 2001;20:239-43.
60. Terry MA, Ousley PJ. Replacing the endothelium without corneal surface incisions or sutures: the first United States clinical series using the deep lamellar endothelial keratoplasty procedure. Ophthalmology. 2003;110:755-64.
61. Melles GR, Lander F, Rietveld FJ. Transplantation of Descemet's membrane carrying viable endothelium through a small scleral incision. Cornea. 2002;21:415-8.
62. Price FW Jr, Price MO. Descemet's stripping with endothelial keratoplasty in 200 eyes: early challenges and techniques to enhance donor adherence. J Cataract Refract Surg. 2006;32:411-8.
63. Melles GR, Ong TS, Ververs B, van derWees J. Descemet membrane endothelial keratoplasty (DMEK). Cornea. 2006;25:987-90.
64. Williams KA, Muehlberg SM, Lewis RF. The Australian corneal graft registry 1996 report. Adelaide: Mercury Press; 1997. p. 11.
65. Schraepen P, Koppen C, Tassignon M. Visual acuity after penetrating keratoplasty for pseudophakic and aphakic bullous keratopathy. J Cataract Refract Surg. 2003;29:482-6.
66. Barkana Y, Segal O, Krakovski D, Avni I, Zadok D. Prediction of visual outcome after penetrating keratoplasty for pseudophakic corneal edema. Ophthalmology. 2003;110:286-90.

42 Pediatric Corneal Transplants

Gerald W Zaidman

INTRODUCTION

The field of pediatric corneal transplant surgery has reached an exciting stage in its development. Pediatric corneal transplant surgery now includes penetrating keratoplasty, lamellar keratoplasty (LKP), and endothelial keratoplasty (EK). At one time, corneal transplantation in children was considered to have a very high chance of failure and even contraindicated.[1,2] Because of advances in surgical techniques and postoperative care, a clear transplant can now often be obtained in an infant or a child. Therefore, corneal transplant surgery is no longer contraindicated in pediatric patients.[3,4] In fact prompt keratoplasty is the necessary first step in averting irreversible loss of visual function due to amblyopia. The visual results of pediatric corneal transplant surgery, however, are often disappointing. Many unique difficulties encountered in the management of an infant or a child requiring corneal transplantation conspire to make these patients the most challenging for a corneal surgeon. However, appropriate use of these new techniques can lead to successful visual rehabilitation.

PREOPERATIVE ASSESSMENT

Many aspects of an infant or child's preoperative or postoperative care are different from those of an adult undergoing corneal transplantation. The child and the child's parents are usually very anxious when they present for the preoperative evaluation. Also, the difficulty in assessing the visual function of an infant or a young child, the child's inability to cooperate with an eye examination, and the great variability in outcome makes the physician's decision regarding surgery more difficult. A diagnosis is made after an office visit, family history, consultation with a pediatrician and pediatric ophthalmologist to rule out systemic, genetic, and metabolic disorders, and most importantly an examination under anesthesia (EUA).

An EUA is done on all children with congenital corneal opacities and is often indicated for older children depending on their level of cooperation. This is the most accurate way to do a slit-lamp examination, check the intraocular pressure, measure the corneal diameter and perform A-scan and B-scan ultrasonography. At the same time, a refraction, visual evoked response (VER), electroretinography (ERG), optical coherence tomography (OCT), or ultrasound biomicroscopy (UBM) can be done (**Figs. 1 and 2**).

Before surgery, one more factor is considered—the child's social situation. A stable social situation is mandatory. These children require many years of conscientious care; therefore, supportive and motivated parents or caregivers are necessary. In an unstable social environment, surgery is doomed to fail and should not be undertaken. Even in a stable social situation, extensive preoperative counseling is done. Before surgery is scheduled and after the EUA is performed, parents are extensively counseled regarding the risk of surgery. The parents are reminded that they are about to begin a "marathon" of care. Infants are nonverbal and difficult to examine, young children can be extremely uncooperative, and finally in order to increase the chances of graft success all children must be examined very often. The parents are also informed that eyes with more severe anterior segment pathology, such as cataracts or glaucoma have a poorer surgical and visual prognosis. They must understand the difference between surgical success (a clear graft) and visual development. The parents are also informed about amblyopia and its treatment. Finally, the parents are told that the goal is functional, ambulatory (i.e., better than counting fingers) vision and they should not expect perfect vision.

Once surgery is agreed upon, the timing of surgery must be determined. Timing is slightly different in unilateral than bilateral cases because of the higher risk of amblyopia in unilateral cases. The timing of surgery is also influenced by glaucoma. Control of glaucoma is necessary before performing corneal transplant surgery. If the untreated intraocular pressure is within a reasonable range (<30 mm Hg), it can usually be controlled medically. In these patients, therapy is typically begun with latanoprost or other antiprostaglandins, carbonic anhydrase inhibitors, a beta-blocker, or oral acetazolamide. Alpha-agonists are not used because of reports of pulmonary side effects in infants. If

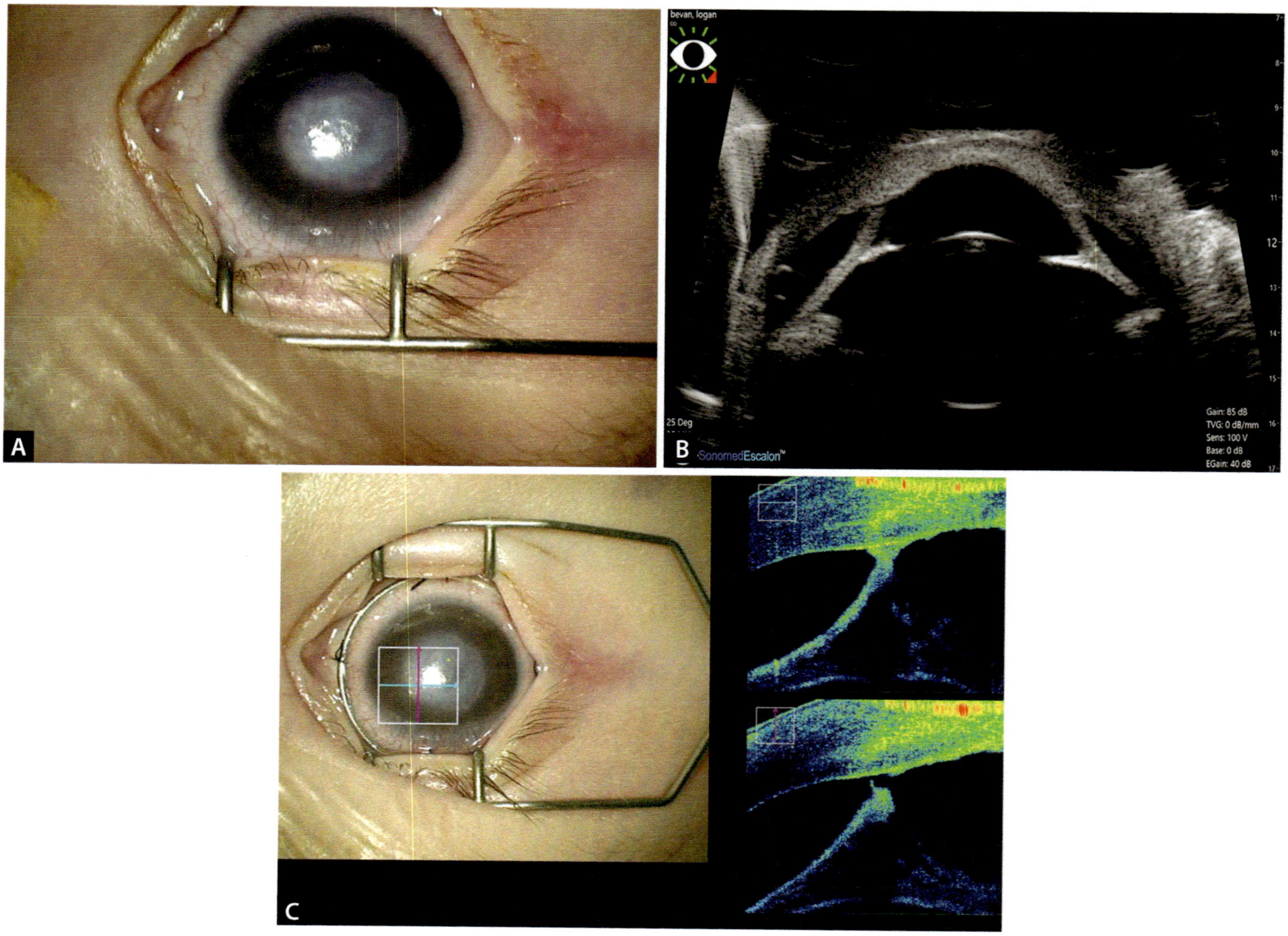

Figs. 1A to C: (A) Preoperative photograph of an infant with congenital central corneal scarring due to Peters' anomaly type I; (B) Preoperative ultrasound biomicroscopy demonstrating synechiae extending from iris to the cornea and a normal non-cataractous lens; (C) Intraoperative optical coherence tomography demonstrating synechiae from iris to the cornea.

medical control is unsuccessful surgery is required. In these cases, a filtering procedure (trabeculectomy) is preferred rather than a valve because of possible irritative effect of the valve on the corneal endothelium or crystalline lens.

INDICATIONS

In North America, the most common cause of a congenital corneal opacity is one of the anterior segment dysgenesis (**Box 1**). This is a group of disorders comprising Peters' anomaly type I and II, sclerocornea, corneal dermoid, and congenital anterior staphyloma. Peters' anomaly is the most common disease in this group. Type I, the milder form, only involves the cornea and the iris. Type II is the more severe form in which the lens is usually adherent to the cornea or is shrunken, dislocated or cataractous. Anterior segment dysgenesis makes up nearly 60% of congenital corneal opacities in North America. The next most common cause is congenital glaucoma, comprising 10–15% of patients. The third group, also consisting of approximately 15% of patients, is the congenital corneal dystrophies. This includes congenital hereditary endothelial dystrophy (CHED), congenital hereditary stromal dystrophy, and posterior polymorphous dystrophy. Finally, trauma, infection, and metabolic congenital disorders make up <10% of the patients.

In young children (generally considered between the ages of 3–6 years), congenital corneal opacities remain the main cause of corneal transplant surgery. In older children (ages 7–14 years), acquired conditions, both traumatic and nontraumatic, are the main reason for transplant surgery. These most frequently include herpes keratitis, bacterial keratitis, trauma, and keratoconus, which have been reported to occur as early as 6 years of age.

TIMING OF SURGERY

Though penetrating keratoplasty remains the predominant form of corneal transplant surgery in children, there are other techniques that are gaining increasing popularity. These consist of selective corneal transplant surgery techniques, such as standard lamellar keratoplasty or deep anterior lamellar keratoplasty (DALK) or EK. Penetrating keratoplasty remains the most common form of corneal

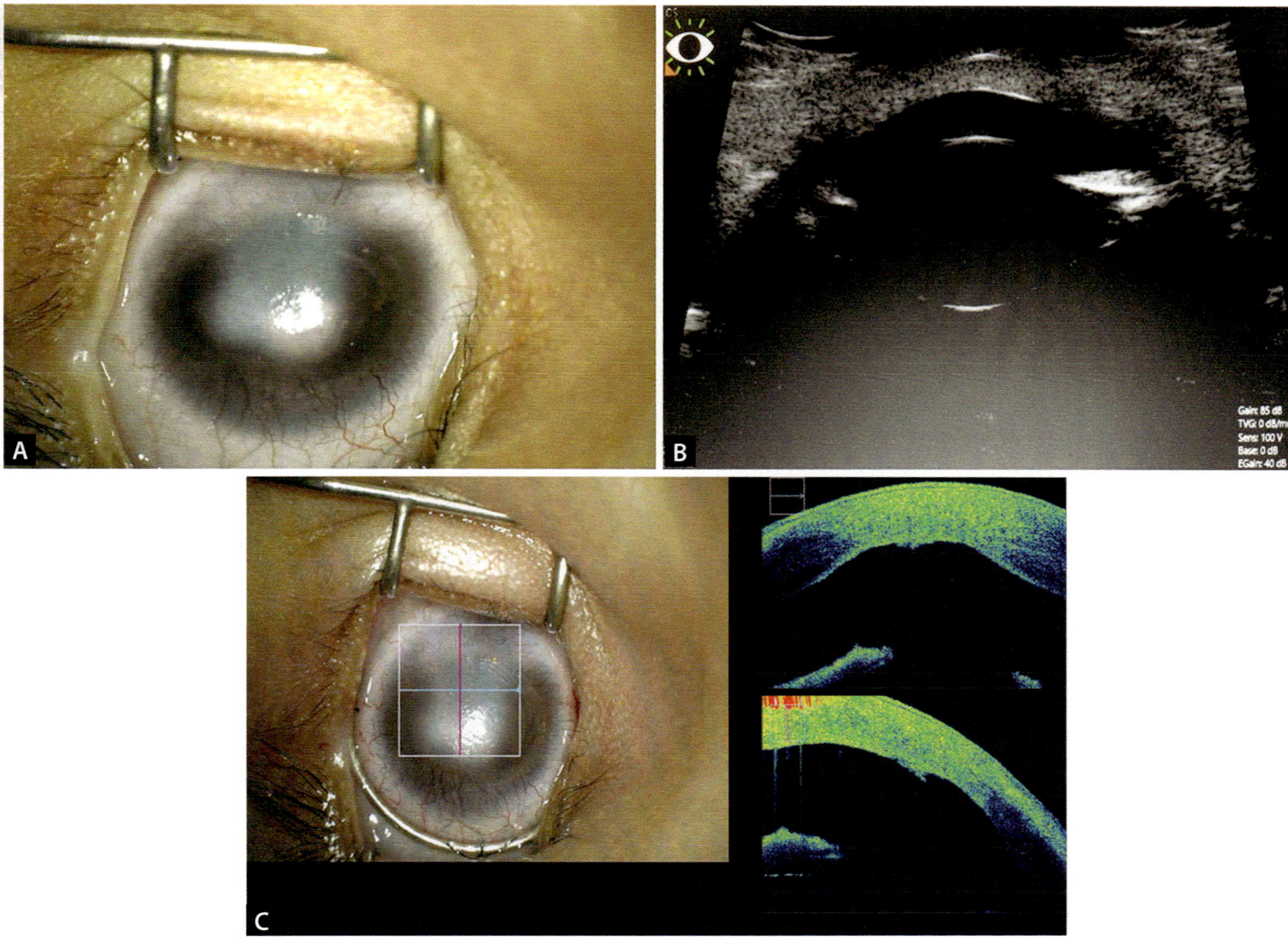

Figs. 2A to C: (A) Preoperative photograph of an infant with congenital central corneal opacity; (B) Preoperative ultrasound biomicroscopy images showing the absence of any synechiae in the anterior chamber; (C) Intraoperative optical coherence tomography of the same infant confirming the absence of any synechiae in the anterior chamber.

Box 1: The indications for pediatric corneal transplant surgery.

Congenital
- Peter's anomaly
- Sclerocornea
- Corneal dermoids
- Congenital glaucoma with corneal edema
- Congenital hereditary endothelial dystrophy
- Posterior polymorphous dystrophy
- Congenital hereditary stromal dystrophy*
- Mucopolysaccharidosis* (can start later in childhood)

Acquired, non-traumatic
- Herpes simplex keratitis
- Keratoconus
- Bacterial keratitis
- Neurotrophic keratitis
- Interstitial keratitis*
- Ophthalmia neonatorum*
- Fungal keratitis*
- Steven-Johnson syndrome*

Acquired, traumatic
- Birth trauma
- Corneal or corneoscleral laceration
- Nonpenetrating injury with scar

*very rare causes of pediatric transplants

transplant surgery in infants and children because of the prevalence of congenital corneal opacities. However, children with CHED can sometimes have an EK done and children with superficial scars may benefit from an LKP.

Because of the small size of the neonatal eye and the significant risk of intraoperative complications, penetrating keratoplasty is not done before the child is 2 months of age. In an ideal situation, the child is first seen in the office at 7–21 days of age. The EUA is scheduled for 3–6 weeks of age. The corneal transplant is done at 8–12 weeks of age. With bilateral opacities, surgery can be delayed slightly, but in general, the first eye is also done between 2 and 3 months of age. In a bilateral case, the more severe eye is not necessarily done first. Because of the risk of amblyopia and the need for the child to develop vision, the less severe eye is often done first. In bilateral cases, the second eye is usually done 2 months after the first. Although this may worsen the amblyopia between the two eyes, at least 4 weeks of postoperative care is required after the first eye to remove stitches, control glaucoma, avoid infection, and validate parenteral compliance. Once these have been accomplished, the second eye is done.

If an EK is done, then an examination under anesthesia is routinely scheduled for 5–7 days postoperatively to confirm adherence of the endothelial graft to the corneal stroma. Also in children having anterior LKP or EK, intraoperative OCT is used during surgery.

SURGICAL TECHNIQUE

Penetrating Keratoplasty

Surgery starts by measuring the corneal diameter and sizing the incision. The donor cornea is generally 0.5 mm larger than the recipient. In cases of sclerocornea, the conjunctiva may have to be recessed to the limbus. A scleral support (Flieringa) ring is sutured to the globe. The donor is removed from its container, excised, and kept in Optisol until needed. A handheld trephine blade is used to make a partial thickness incision into the patient's cornea while stabilizing the globe with the ring. The anterior chamber is very carefully entered with a microsharp (number 75) blade. The surgeon must be sure that a gush of aqueous is seen, indicating that there is a space between the iris and the cornea. Most of these patients have synechiae (often extensive) from the iris to the cornea and a shallow anterior chamber. If available, intraoperative OCT is used throughout the procedure, especially after the initial incision is made. Therefore, if the surgeon is not careful, he can find that he is dissecting above Descemet's membrane or under the iris.

After the anterior chamber is entered, a high-viscosity viscoelastic (usually Viscoat) is injected between the iris and the cornea. It is not necessary to fully reform the anterior chamber at this time. A specially designed cyclodialysis spatula (made by Storz) is used to separate some of the adhesions from the cornea. The spatula is passed through the surgical opening and into the angle and under the central cornea. This viscoelastic and mechanical synechiolysis is a crucial step. It has to be done carefully and with sufficient magnification. After some of the adhesions are separated, Viscoat is again injected and the spatula is reinserted. These two steps are alternated until the surgeon is satisfied that all of the adhesions have been broken. During these maneuvers, bleeding can usually be controlled by viscoelastics, topical epinephrine drops (in a concentration of 1/10,000), gentle pressure or microcautery to the bleeding vessels.

After the synechiolysis, the cornea can be excised. Excision of a cornea from an infant is a very difficult, delicate, and precise maneuver. Because of the inherent instability of the infant eye, the unpredictable variety of anomalies, the tendency for rapid and sudden scleral collapse (even in the presence of a Flieringa ring) and the very high-positive vitreous pressure, surgeons should always "expect the unexpected." These factors can rapidly lead to prolapse of the lens anterior to the iris with extrusion of the lens followed by vitreous loss and more serious complications. This can occur suddenly as the surgeon gently lifts on the patient's cornea or anytime during the synechiolysis. Therefore, the surgeon must be prepared to treat this potentially disastrous complication. There are several maneuvers available. First, the surgeon must be sure that the child is totally paralyzed and hyperventilated. Another dose of mannitol can be given intravenously. In most cases of "average bulging," the surgeon can attempt rapid excision of the diseased cornea and rapid replacement of the donor. This can work, especially in older infants and children and those with minimal anterior segment pathology. In these patients, after removing the cornea, the donor tissue is quickly sutured in place with two 9-0 nylon sutures, one at 12 o'clock and the other at 6 o'clock. A drop of 1% atropine can be used to pull the ciliary body posteriorly at this stage and then two more 9-0 nylon sutures are placed at 3 and 9 o'clock.

However, in most cases, the preferred method of doing the keratoplasty is known as the "Sandwich Technique". The theory behind the sandwich technique is that the surgeon places the donor cornea on top of the host cornea before the host cornea is removed. This controls the positive pressure present in most of these very small eyes. In cases with "gradual severe bulging" of the lens, approximately 270° of the cornea is excised leaving the cornea attached at one quadrant. A layer of viscoelastic is put on top of the patient's cornea. The donor cornea is slid on top of the patient's cornea (on the layer of viscoelastic) and sutured it to the limbal side of the incision with two 9-0 nylon sutures (at 6 and 12 o'clock). Viscoelastic is placed under the host cornea and scissors are slid into the potential space between the host cornea and the iris. The host cornea is then cut and slid out from under the donor cornea.

There are some cases with "rapid and immediate bulging." Almost as soon as you start removing the cornea, the lens and posterior segment begin to bulge forward. In these eyes, each of the four quadrants of the patient's cornea is opened one-by-one and tacked back down with a 7-0 silk suture. After that, some viscoelastic is put on the surface of the cornea and the donor cornea is placed on the top of the viscoelastic. Two 9-0 nylon sutures are passed through the host and donor 180° apart, at 6 and 12 o'clock and tied. Slowly, each 7-0 silk suture is removed. Then the host cornea is slid out from under the donor and two more 9-0 nylon cardinal sutures are placed at 3 and 9 o'clock.

Using these maneuvers, it is possible to prevent lens prolapse in nearly all cases. Once the donor cornea is in position, the eye is closed with multiple interrupted 10-0 sutures (nylon or prolene) removing the 9-0 nylon sutures. The anterior chamber is deepened with either balanced salt solution or viscoelastic. All knots are trimmed and buried, the scleral ring is removed, subconjunctival antibiotics and steroids are given, and the eye is covered with a patch and a shield.

These maneuvers are only worthwhile if the lens is clear and not attached to the cornea. If the lens is cataractous, adherent to the cornea or abnormal in size or location (as in Peters' type II), it is removed. Depending on the extent of positive pressure and the nature of the cataract, a standard extracapsular cataract extraction can be done. Generally, we prefer to keep the posterior capsule intact. If the posterior capsule breaks (or if the lens is small or subluxed or attached to the cornea) then a generous anterior vitrectomy is performed, after lens removal. If cataract surgery is required, heparin, 2,500 units in 500 cc, and epinephrine is added to the I/A bottle of BSS. The heparin is used to decrease fibrin formation. The donor cornea is then sutured in position, the anterior chamber is deepened and the wound closed and the case ended as above. In rare instances, the donor cornea is placed into position and the lens is removed in a "closed-eye" technique. Finally, the new cornea may afford the surgeon the first view of the retina with the indirect ophthalmoscope.

Selective Corneal Transplants—Endothelial Keratoplasty and Deep Anterior Lamellar Keratoplasty

Only a small minority (less than one-sixth) of children are candidates for selective corneal transplants. Endothelial keratoplasty is only used in cases of endothelial dysfunction (such as CHED) or rarely in corneal graft edema. Lamellar keratoplasty can be used in cases of dermoids, anterior corneal scarring (as in HSV) or metabolic disorders (Hurler's syndrome, etc.) (**Figs. 3 and 4**).

In EK, a scleral support ring is typically not used. IV mannitol is given to soften the eye and to prevent intraoperative prolapse of the iris and lens. Additionally, great care is given throughout this procedure to avoid damaging the crystalline lens. During an EK, the first step is to determine the size of the donor and the host, the second step is then to make a peripheral corneal incision. Provisc is injected into the eye, and the corneal endothelium is removed. A peripheral iridectomy is performed and attention is then turned to the donor cornea, which has been typically precut by the eye bank. Usually, an ultrathin donor is used. The donor is harvested in the standard technique and then inserted into the anterior chamber after widening the wound to allow insertion of the endothelial graft. The endothelial graft is irrigated until it unravels and then the anterior chamber is filled with an air bubble to assure adhesion of the graft to the stroma. Typically, an oversize graft is used and then the anterior chamber is filled with a bubble of air. Intraocular drops of Cyclogyl and timolol 0.5% is placed in the eye and the surgeon will wait 60 minutes while the child is under anesthesia to assure that the endothelial graft has become adherent to the stroma. OCT is used intraoperatively to determine the exact position of the graft. At the end of 60 minutes, the procedure is ended and the surgeon will then decide how much air should remain in the eye until the patient is examined the next day.

If one is performing a LKP in cases of anterior stromal scarring from herpes keratitis or in a metabolic disorder such as mucopolysaccharidosis, UBM is performed during the preoperative examination under anesthesia to determine if the posterior cornea is free of disease. If it is, then a typical DALK procedure is performed using a big-bubble technique. The diseased corneal stroma is removed, then after harvesting the corneal donor and removing the endothelium, the corneal donor is sutured in position with interrupted sutures.

CONCOMITANT PROCEDURES

Iris Procedures

Peripheral Iridectomy

This is indicated if there is posterior synechia or persistent intraocular inflammation. This is also performed when lensectomy and vitrectomy are undertaken and is always done in an EK.

Tightening the Iris Diaphragm

In some cases, creating a smaller pupil with 10-0 prolene suture on a noncutting needle will tighten the diaphragm and prevent the formation of synechia.

Pupilloplasty

This may be indicated when the pupil is disfigured.

Concomitant Retinal Surgery

If the eye requires a pars plana vitrectomy for a retinal detachment, use of an intraoperative keratoprosthesis for the retinal surgery allows the retinal surgeon a better view than through a new transplant. After the retinal surgeon completes the retinal procedures, the keratoprosthesis is replaced with a donor cornea.

POSTOPERATIVE CARE

Immediate

After surgery, premature infants and children with systemic diseases should be monitored carefully by the ophthalmologist, pediatrician, and anesthesiologist. All surgeries are done on an outpatient basis, unless the child has some systemic comorbidities that require a one-night stay in the hospital. Generally, this only applies to children that are premature births. Full-term infants and healthy older children are done as outpatients.

Early

In the first few weeks after the surgery, the surgeon's goal is to make certain that the wounds are secure and watertight, monitor and promote re-epithelialization of the graft, monitor and control intraocular pressure, rule out ocular infection, and begin amblyopia therapy. In addition, if the child had an endothelial graft, the surgeon needs to be sure that the donor and cornea are adherent. Also, if the child has had a DALK, one has to make sure that there are no problems with apposition of the donor

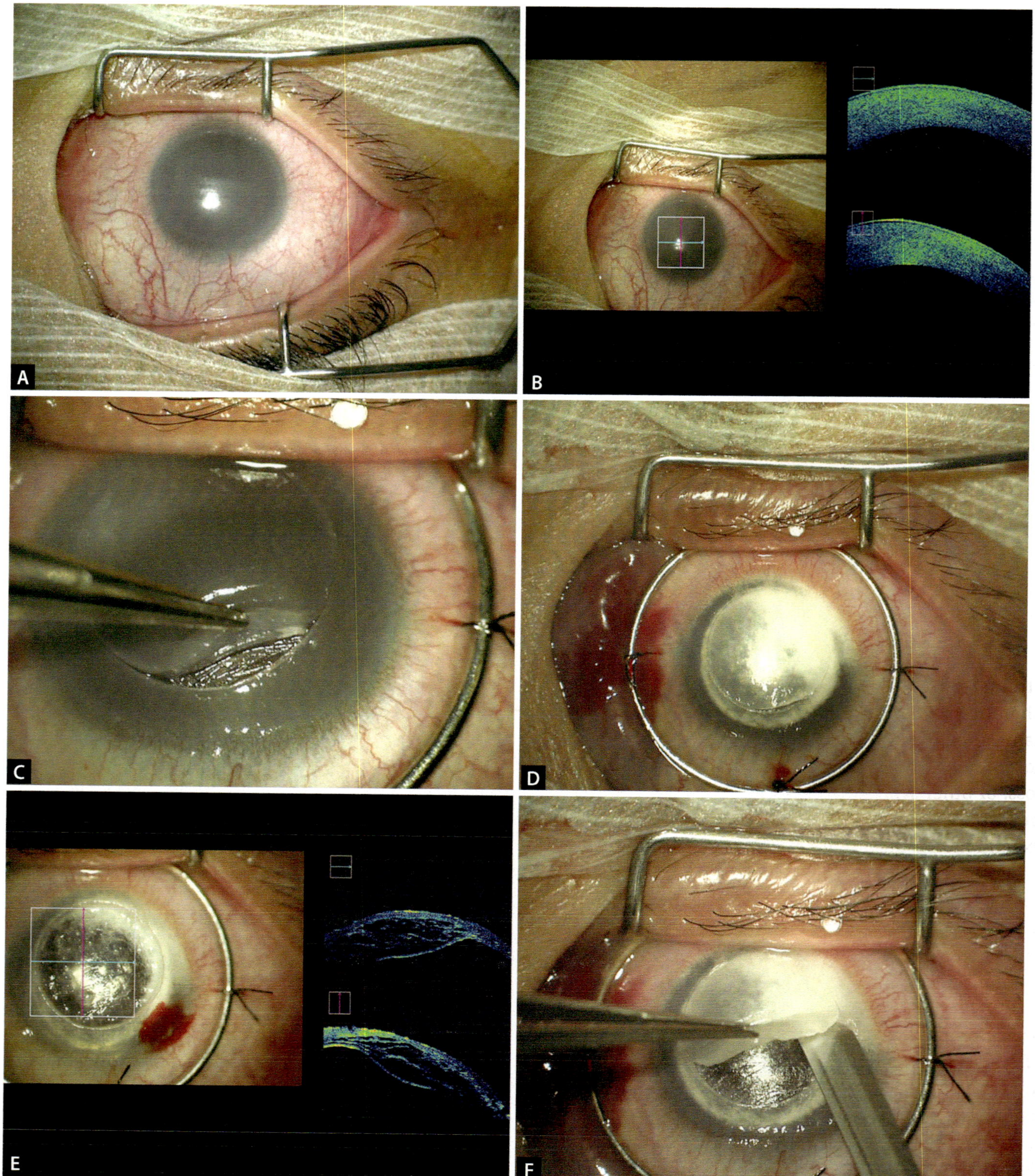

Figs. 3A to F: (A) Preoperative photo of a child with mucopolysaccharidosis Type VII-Sly syndrome; (B) Intraoperative optical coherence tomography (OCT) of the same child prior to undergoing DALK; (C) Intraoperative images showing initial dissection of the cornea, followed by big bubble formation (D) also confirmed on an intraoperative OCT (E). This is followed by anterior keratectomy (F).

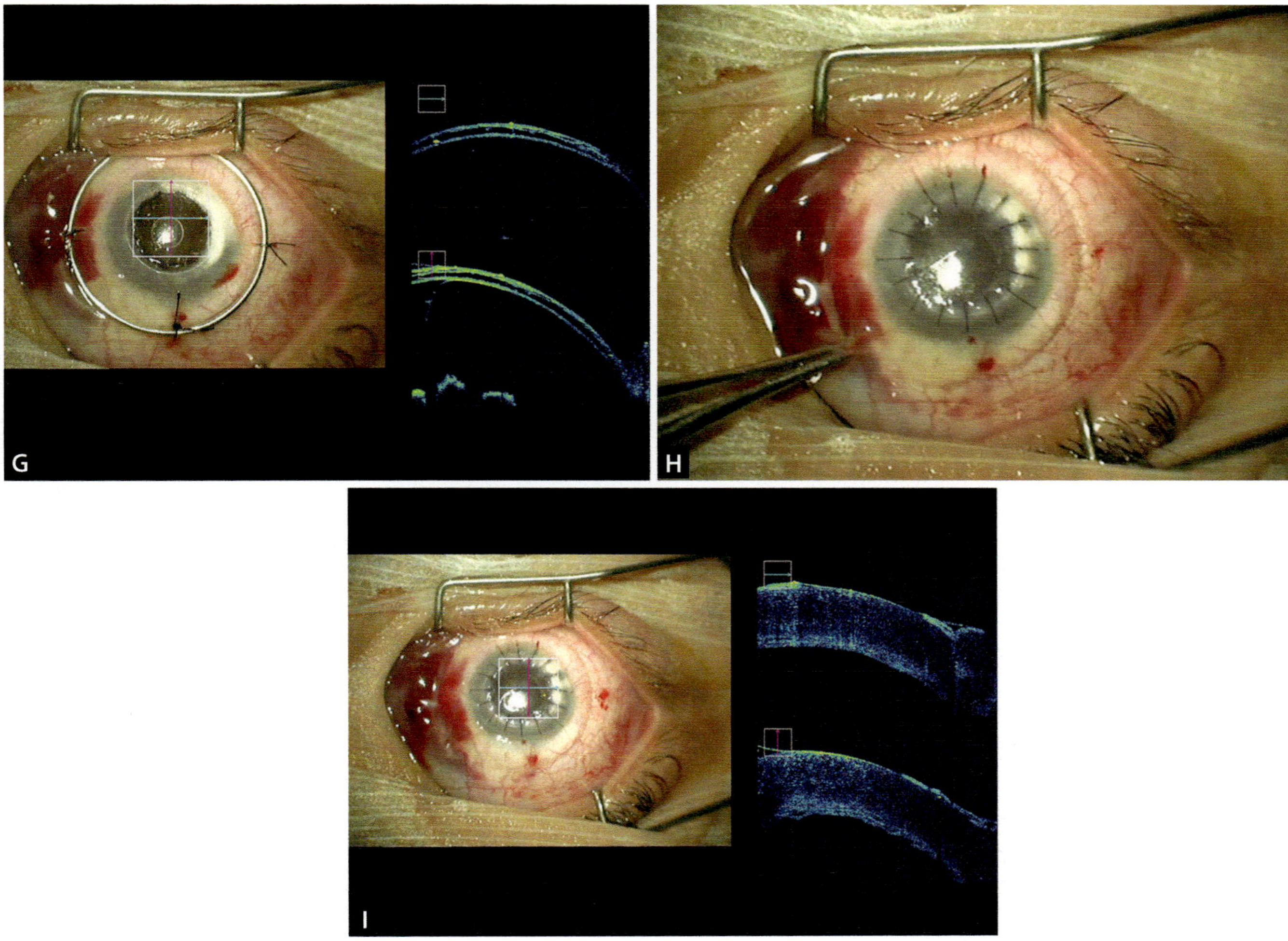

Figs. 3G to I: (G) The depth of which can be assessed on an optical coherence tomography (OCT); (H) Final result after placement of the graft, as visualized under the operating microscope (I) and with an intraoperative OCT attached.

stroma to the host cornea and no secondary anterior chambers. Postoperative complications are usually the same as adults, but infants and young children are unable to communicate as to whether they have pain, visual loss, or other symptoms. Therefore, they require frequent postoperative examinations. The first postoperative examination is the day after surgery.

Postoperatively, the children are treated with prednisolone forte 1% drops eight times a day, a fluoroquinolone antibiotic or another form of antibiotic four times a day, and glaucoma therapy (if needed is continued). No systemic immunosuppressive therapy is used.

In routine penetrating keratoplasties, examinations are done at least 2–3 times a week for the first 3–4 weeks after surgery, then once or twice a week for 4 weeks, once a week for the next month, and then every 2 weeks for 2 months and finally monthly. The monthly examination is continued for 1 year. For children who have had endothelial grafts, the schedule of the postoperative visits is less frequent, but all children who have had an EK have an examination under anesthesia within 5–7 days after surgery to determine if the donor cornea is adherent to the recipient cornea. In penetrating keratoplasty patients, the child will sometimes have an examination under anesthesia performed approximately every 4 weeks. However, depending on the condition of the eye, it can be done as often as every 5–7 days. These EUAs are necessary in order to remove the sutures before they loosen and to check the intraocular pressure. A loose suture in a pediatric graft is a recipe for disaster; loose sutures quickly (sometimes overnight) lead to infection or graft rejection. Therefore, they are removed immediately after they are noticed. The best way to recognize the loose suture is if one sees mucus adherent to the suture—if this is noticed by the ophthalmologist or parents, the child is sedated and the suture removed.

In most young children with an uneventful postoperative course, an average of three EUAs is required usually every 3–4 weeks. For children with endothelial grafts, the number of EUAs is less frequent. After doing the first EUA to ensure adherence to the cornea, the next EUA is done about 8 weeks postoperatively to remove the child's sutures. In children who have had a LKP, EUA is done as often as necessary to remove the sutures.

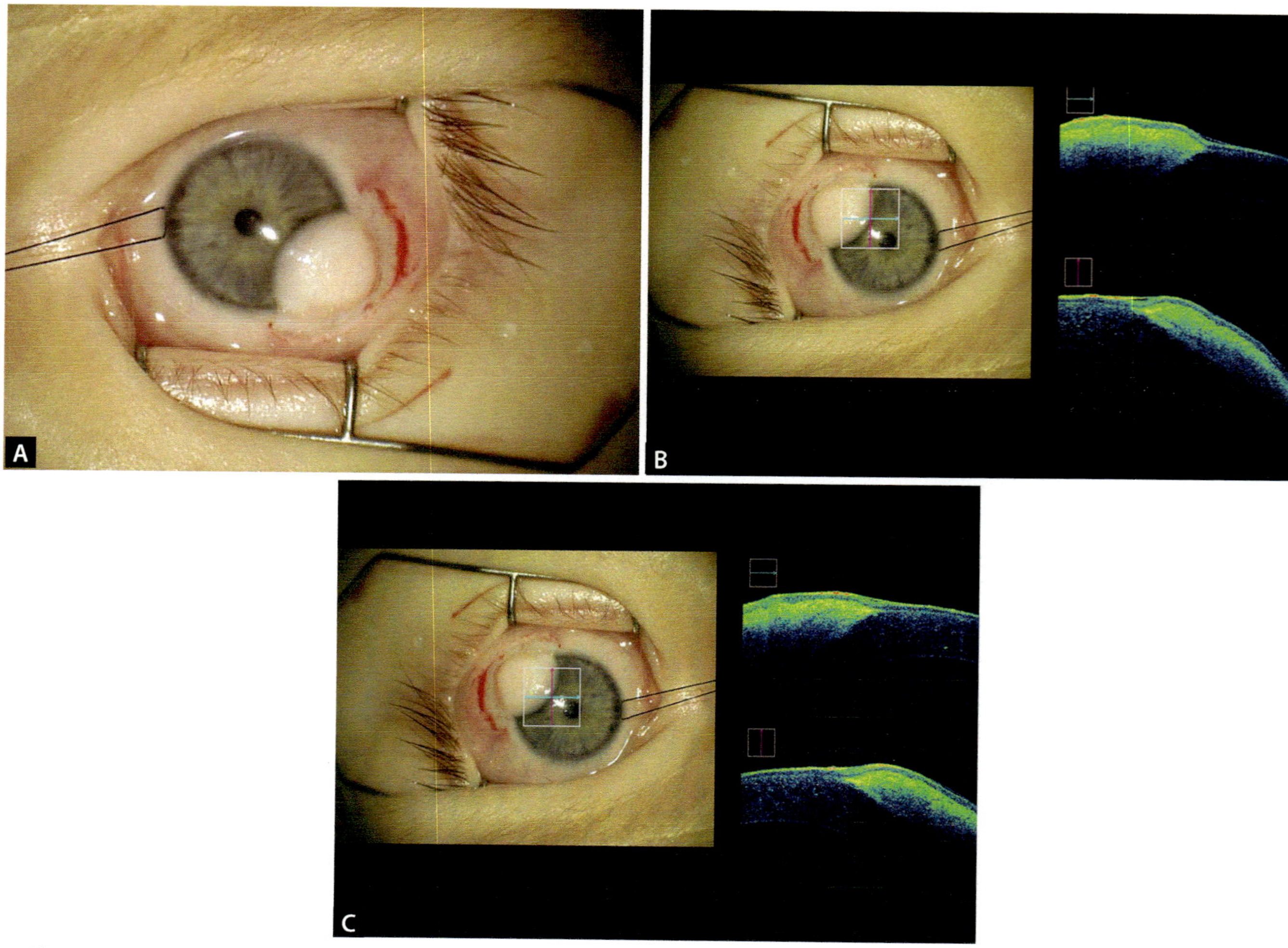

Figs. 4A to C: (A) Preoperative photo of a child with a limbal corneal dermoid; (B and C) Intraoperative photos of the same child using an intraoperative optical coherence tomography.

Steroid drops are tapered very slowly, usually by one drop every 4 weeks, starting at the third month postoperative. Finally, the child is kept on at least once a day steroid drops until 1 year postoperatively and then they are stopped. If the graft begins to reject, the steroid drops are increased until either the graft clears or it fails and oral steroids can be used. If the cornea fails, the drops are rapidly tapered and a regraft is done.

If all goes well with the first eye, the second eye is operated on in 4–8 weeks after the first. During this time, the child is seen by a pediatric ophthalmologist and the management continues indefinitely. As the months pass, the office examinations become less frequent. If the child is too uncooperative for subsequent office visits or if we cannot use either a pneumotonometer, iCare tonometer or Tono-Pen to check the intraocular pressure, then the sedative, such as chloral hydrate (75 mg), is given orally in the office. Once the child falls asleep, the intraocular pressure is checked and a portable slit lamp is used to examine the eye. This process has been made much easier with the developments of the iCare tonometer. The iCare tonometer can be easy to use on even generally uncooperative children and it has avoided sedation in almost every patient.

Finally, the parents are warned that the graft is at risk of rejection whenever the child develops any severe febrile illness or is to be vaccinated. At these times, the steroid drops are increased in frequency for short time. Also, vaccinations are delayed until 1 year after surgery. Then, when it is time to vaccinate, the steroid drops are increased to four times a day for 4 days before and 4 days after the vaccination.

ALTERNATIVES TO KERATOPLASTY

Some children with congenital corneal opacities can be treated without a penetrating keratoplasty. These alternative operations consist of an optical iridectomy, rotating keratoplasty or lamellar keratoplasty. The first two can be used when the child has a peripheral opacity that just impinges on the visual axis. Surgically enlarging the pupil (in an optical iridectomy) or moving the scar out of the way (rotating keratoplasty) can enable the child to see around the opacity. In some children, especially those with corneal dermoids or scars secondary to infectious keratitis, the corneal opacity is not full thickness. In these cases, we first remove the opacity with a lamellar dissection; if a relatively clear posterior cornea remains then a lamellar graft is placed on top of the patient's residual cornea. The main problem with any of these procedures is that they can result in significant astigmatism. Also, interface haze may be present after a lamellar graft. However, each procedure avoids a full-thickness keratoplasty eliminating the risk of an endothelial graft rejection. Also the postoperative regimen is less demanding than a full-thickness graft.

OPTICAL CORRECTION AND AMBLYOPIA THERAPY

Without effective optical correction and amblyopia therapy, a pediatric penetrating keratoplasty will be useless. The younger the patient, the deeper the amblyopia, especially if the eye has a structural and refractive abnormality that limits vision. However, amblyopia is more easily reversed in younger patients if it is treated promptly and appropriately.

Correction of the refractive error is a vital part of amblyopia therapy. At about the second to third postoperative week, the epithelium has usually healed and the graft has cleared sufficiently to perform cycloplegic retinoscopy. Retinoscopy may be difficult and the refraction will change as the wound heals and sutures are removed; but a correction of a moderate or large refractive error could be prescribed at this time. The refraction should be repeated periodically until a few months after all the sutures have been removed. Thereafter, refraction should be repeated as needed. Refraction of an aphakic eye can be confirmed if the axial length is known. The following formula is an approximation for an aphakic eye and assumes a keratometry measurement of 45 D and a vertex distance of 10 mm.

$$\text{Distance Spectacle Power} = 63.7 - (2.28 \times \text{Axial length in mm}).$$

The results from this formula can be modified by keratometry measurements. For an aphakic eye, an infant is generally prescribed a near correction that is approximately +2.50 D sphere over the distance correction. Eventually the aphakic child should be put in a bifocal, with the top of the segment at the inferior border of the pupil. Contact lenses are also useful in visual rehabilitation of pediatric keratoplasty patients especially in monocular aphakes. Silicone lenses offer the highest oxygen permeability of all lenses and are often well-tolerated in aphakic patients with normal corneas.

If the contralateral eye is normal, occlusion therapy should be started as soon as the graft is partially clear and after correction of any refractive error. Optimally, this should not be later than 3–4 postoperative weeks. Occlusion during the first 6 months of life usually is limited to one-fourth to three-fourths of infant's waking hours. If the child is older than 6 months, full time occlusion therapy should be started. The vision in both eyes is monitored carefully to check for improvement of the amblyopic eye or worsening of the normal eye.

Suture Removal

Typically all sutures can be removed safely according to the following schedule. During the first year of life, sutures are removed by 5–6 weeks after surgery, in 1-year-old by 2–3 months postoperative; in 2 and 3 years old at 3–4 postoperative months, and in 4–8 years old by 5–6 months postoperatively. Children older than that require removal of all sutures before 1 year after surgery.

RESULTS

In our experience, if this peri- and postoperative regimen is followed children can have good surgical results. Graft clarity is obtained in 70–75% of the young children with acquired corneal opacities (infections, trauma, etc.).[5-9] In the milder form of Peters' anomaly, Peters' anomaly type I, and in congenital corneal dystrophies, graft clarity is possible in 80–90% of children. The remainder of the children, even if they have a translucent graft, have better visual potential than if they had their original opaque cornea.[10-14] We recently reviewed our experience with children with Peters, anomaly type I.[15] We followed our children for >3 years after their original transplants and noted that nearly 90% had clear grafts; additionally, 54% of the children had obtained vision ≥20/100.

Children with sclerocornea, Peters' anomaly type II or severe glaucoma do less well.[5-8] However, also in these children the visual potential is usually better with a cloudy keratoplasty than their original opaque cornea.

Finally one must continually remind the parents that visual acuity is dependent both on the status of the graft and on aggressive amblyopia therapy. The child must continue to see a pediatric ophthalmologist throughout the postoperative period (and beyond) in order to develop and maintain the best possible vision.

REFERENCES

1. Dana MR, Schaumberg DA, Moyes AL, Gomes JA. Corneal transplantation in children with Peter's anomaly and mesenchymal dysgenesis. Arch Ophthalmol. 1977;104:1580-6.
2. Developmental anomalies of size and shape. In: Cornea. Krachmer, et al. (Eds). St. Louis, Mosby, Chapter. 1977;76:871-84.
3. Zaidman GW, Juechter K. Peters' anomaly associated with protruding corneal pseudostaphyloma. Cornea. 1998;17:163-8.
4. Fruech BE, Brown SI. Transplantation of congenitally opaque corneas. Br J Ophthalmol. 1997;8:1064-9.

5. Dana MR, Moyes AL, Gomes JA, Rosheim KM, Schaumberg DA, Laibson PR, et al. The indications for and outcome in pediatric keratoplasty. A Multicenter Study. Ophthalmology. 1995;102:1129-38.
6. Dana MR, Schaumberg DA, Moyes AL, Gomes JA, Laibson PR, Holland EJ, et al. Outcome of penetrating keratoplasty after ocular trauma in children. Arch Ophthalmol. 1995;113:1503-7.
7. Gollamudi SR, Traboulsi EI, Chamon W, Stark WJ, Maumenee IH. Visual outcome after surgery for Peters' anomaly. Ophthalmic Genet. 1994;15:31-5.
8. Parmley VC, Stonecipher KG, Rowsey JJ. Peter's anomaly: a review of 26 penetrating keratoplasties in infants. Ophthalmic Surgery. 1993;24:31-5.
9. Cameron JA. Good visual result following early penetrating keratoplasty for Peter's anomaly. J Ped Ophthal Strabismus. 1993;30:109-12.
10. Heon E, Barsoum-Homsy M, Cevrette L, Jacob JL, Milot J, Palemeno R, et al. Peters' anomaly. The spectrum of associated ocular and systemic malformations. Ophthal Ped Genetics. 1992;13:137-43.
11. Tucker SM, Enzenauer RW, Levin AV, Morin JD, Hellmann J. Corneal diameter, axial length and intraocular pressure in premature infants. Ophthalmology. 1992;99:1296-300.
12. Cowden JW. Penetrating keratoplasty in infants and children. Ophthalmology. 1990;97:324-9.
13. Brown SI, Salamon SM. Wound healing of grafts in congenitally opaque infant corneas. Am J Ophthalmol. 1983;95:641-4.
14. Rahman W, Anwar S. An unusual case of keratoconus. JAPOS. 2006;43:373-5.
15. Zaidman, GW. Lamellar Keratoplasty for Anterior Corneal Scarring in Infants and Young Children. In Surgical Techniques in Anterior and Posterior Lamellar Corneal Surgery. John, T (Ed). Jaypee Brothers, New Delhi, India, 2005.

43 Therapeutic Keratoplasty

Eric Donnenfeld, Nandyala Sushma, Ritu Nagpal

INTRODUCTION

Therapeutic keratoplasty is a surgical procedure, the main purpose of which is (1) to restore the structural integrity of the eye (tectonic keratoplasty) or (2) to resolve an infectious/inflammatory keratitis which is refractory to conventional medical therapy. Often, therapeutic keratoplasty is performed when both of these indications are present, such as in the treatment of a corneal ulcer that has been unresponsive to antibiotics, and has perforated. Therapeutic keratoplasties are generally emergent or urgent procedures in which the survival of the globe is in jeopardy. Thus, unlike optical penetrating keratoplasty, in which visual restoration is the primary goal, acute visual rehabilitation remains of secondary importance in therapeutic keratoplasty. Visual rehabilitation if necessary can always be accomplished at a later date under more controlled circumstances.

INDICATIONS FOR THERAPEUTIC KERATOPLASTY

Despite recent advances in the medical management of infectious keratitis, there remains a subgroup of bacteria, fungi, ameba, parasites, and viruses that does not respond to antimicrobial therapy.[1-7] Therapeutic keratoplasty is indicated when, inflammatory or infectious corneal disease is progressing despite maximal medical therapy, and the integrity of the globe is compromised. Medical therapy should be continued or altered, if necessary, until there is no reasonable expectation that the infection or inflammation can be controlled or until there is a significant risk of corneal perforation or scleral extension. Corneal perforation dramatically increases the risk of endophthalmitis and reduces the survival of the keratoplasty, while infectious scleritis should be avoided due to the severe morbidity of this disease.[8-11] Noninvasive surgical treatment, such as conjunctival flaps and tarsorrhaphies, can be attempted if indicated.

A therapeutic keratoplasty offers a surgical debridement of an infectious process. The goal of therapeutic keratoplasty is to completely remove the infectious inoculum or to decrease the organisms in the cornea to a level at which exogenous anti-infective/anti-inflammatory agents and the patient's endogenous host defense mechanisms can be effective.[12] Robin et al.[13] reviewed 497 penetrating keratoplasty buttons and noted that penetrating keratoplasty was performed for active ulcerative keratitis in 7% of these patients and for viral keratitis in 6% of patients.[13] Killingsworth et al.[12] reviewed 80 consecutive therapeutic keratoplasties performed in Florida, over a 9-year period. Twenty-six therapeutic keratoplasties were performed for bacterial infections, 15 for fungal infections, 11 for active herpetic keratitis, 4 for persistent epithelial defects following herpes simplex keratitis, 12 for dry eyes, 10 for nonherpetic persistent epithelial defects, and 2 for *Acanthamoeba* keratitis. Similarly, a review in India of 100 cases by Sony et al.[14] demonstrated that most therapeutic keratoplasties were performed for bacterial keratitis refractory to maximal medical therapy, while fewer cases were for fungal keratitis unresponsive to maximal medical management. A recent series from Singapore showed that the most common infectious organisms requiring a therapeutic keratoplasty were, *Pseudomonas aeruginosa* (58.7%) and *Fusarium* species (32.3%).[15] Eighty patients received a penetrating keratoplasty and 12 underwent a lamellar keratoplasty. Mean transplant diameter was 9.5 mm. One-year therapeutic survival for bacterial and fungal keratitis was 76.6 and 72.4%, respectfully.

When an acute ulceration threatens perforation, the patient should be receiving systemic as well as topical therapy to reduce the likelihood of intraocular involvement. Subconjunctival antibiotics do not appear to offer a significant advantage over aggressive topical therapy.[16,17] Once, an acute infectious corneal perforation has occurred, topical antimicrobials should be continued, but the physician and patient should be aware of the risk of intraocular toxicity.[18-20] An attempt to seal the perforation with cyanoacrylate adhesives can be considered.[21-23] After the integrity of the anterior chamber has been re-established, topical antimicrobial treatment can be reinstituted safely without the risk of intraocular toxicity. Closing the perforation with cyanoacrylate restores the integrity of the anterior chamber, opens the angle and prevents the formation of synechial angle closure glaucoma. Sealing the perforation with cyanoacrylate may often be de management, but if the perforation does progress to require therapeutic keratoplasty, the patient will have been temporized with additional antimicrobials and hopefully the ulceration will have been sterilized. When cyanoacrylate is applied, the patient must be monitored closely because bacterial infections have been shown to progress beneath the cyanoacrylate glue.[24]

When perforations or descemetoceles are treated with therapeutic keratoplasties, outcomes are generally satisfactory. Jonas et al. examined a series of 60 cases of keratoplasty for these indications, and found that 90% achieved some improvement in preoperative visual acuity. Ten patients (17%) required repeat keratoplasties for recurrent corneal ulcers.[25] In a series of 20 patients who experienced a corneal perforation graft transparency rate was 67% in 15 eyes that underwent central penetrating keratoplasty and 85% of eyes had improved visual acuity following their therapeutic keratoplasty.[26]

Therapeutic Keratoplasty for Bacterial Keratitis

Certain bacteria, notably *Pseudomonas aeruginosa*,[27] can infect the cornea and progress to corneal perforation over 24–48 hours. These bacteria may produce collagenase, which results in rapid corneal thinning. Most bacterial infections, when, managed expediently, respond to therapy, but due to delay in patients seeking or obtaining medical treatment, the infections may rapidly progress to corneal perforation. (**Fig. 1**).[27,28] Bacterial keratitis has been treated with both lamellar and penetrating keratoplasty in an attempt to reduce the infectious organism count in the cornea when medical treatment has not been successful. Lamellar and penetrating grafts have also been used to prevent and/or treat perforation. Malik and Singh[3] managed 36 *Pseudomonas* ulcers with lamellar and penetrating grafts. All eight of the lamellar grafts became reinfected and one eye was enucleated. Only four of the 28 penetrating therapeutic grafts became reinfected (**Figs. 2 and 3**). The authors concluded that penetrating grafts are more efficient in treating active infection than lamellar grafts. Hill[1] in 1986 presented 23 patients with deep, indolent ulceration and/or descemetocele that were treated with therapeutic keratoplasty. Early surgery did not jeopardize the outcome of the keratoplasty. The period of morbidity was shorter, and more rapid visual rehabilitation occurred with early keratoplasty, possibly secondary to the fact that corneal neovascularization was prevented by earlier surgical management. Removal of the infected cornea may necessitate a larger than customary keratoplasty in order to debride the infected tissue. Cowden et al.[29] presented 14 penetrating keratoplasty patients using 9.5 mm or larger diameter grafts (**Figs. 4A and B**). Five of these patients had bacterial keratitis. They concluded that larger diameter penetrating keratoplasties can salvage an eye

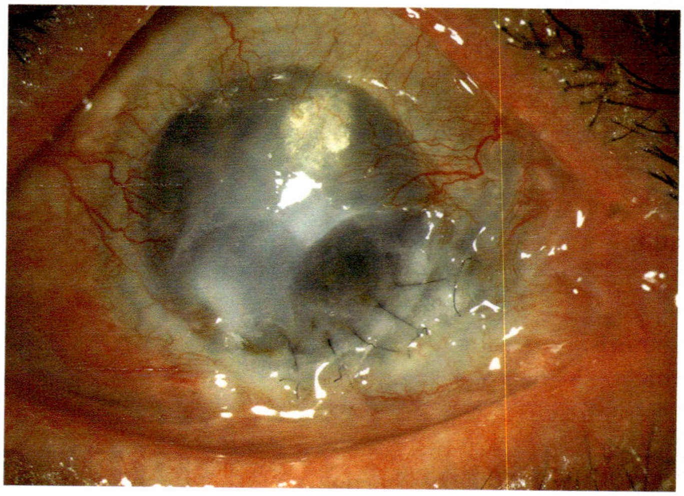

Fig. 2: Diffuse illumination slit-lamp photograph of a patient with Pseudomonas keratitis over a full thickness graft causing melt, uveal show and loosening of sutures.

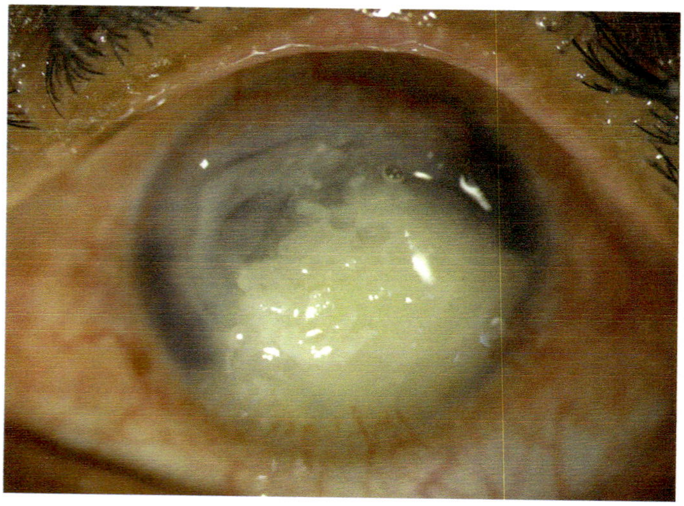

Fig. 1: Diffuse illumination slit-lamp photograph of a patient with Pseudomonas keratitis causing central stromal thinning and melting.

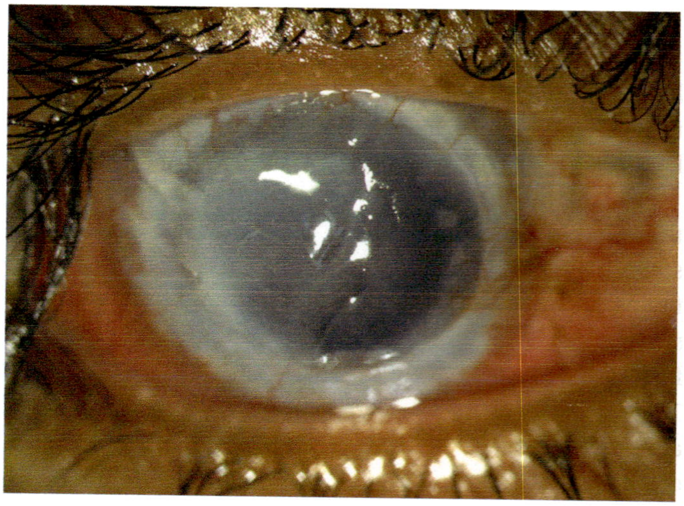

Fig. 3: Diffuse illumination slit-lamp photograph of a patient with Pseudomonas keratitis over a full thickness graft, causing diffuse stromal haze and melt.

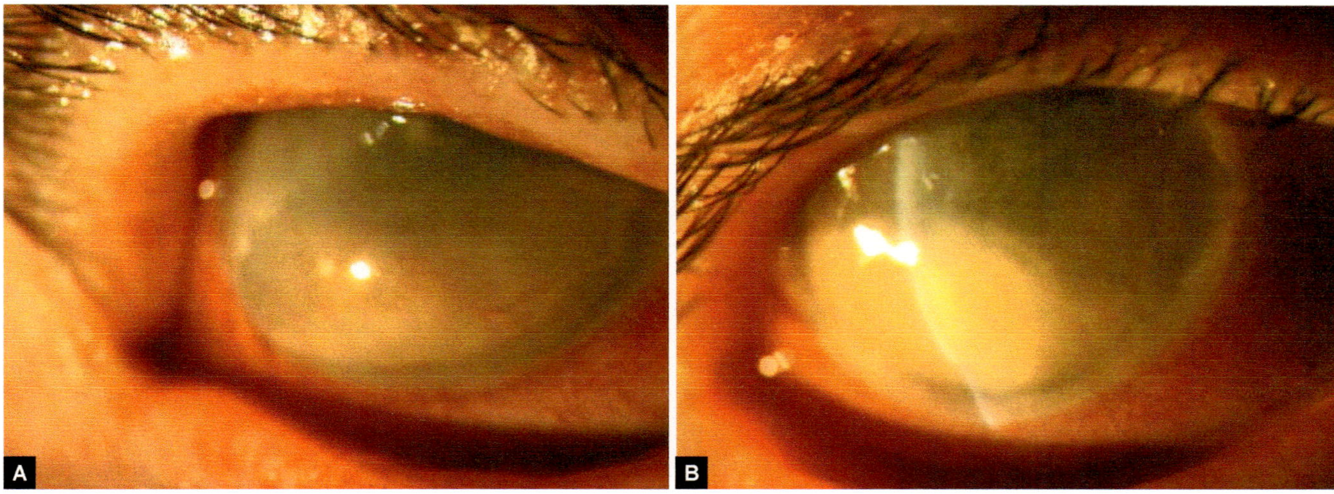

Figs. 4A and B: (A) This 82-year-old female developed microbial keratitis in the setting of pseudophakic bullous keratopathy with epithelial bullae; (B) Cultures grew *Moraxella* spp. sensitive to the antimicrobials used, but the ulcer persisted with minimal improvement after 4 weeks. The patient underwent successful penetrating keratoplasty with an improvement of preoperative visual acuity.

that may have otherwise been lost, with reasonable visual rehabilitation. Although visual prognosis is best when the surgery is performed in a sterilized, minimally inflamed eye, perforation or threatened perforation with uncontrolled progression of the disease and/or a necrotic stroma all mandate early intervention. Lam and Cooper[30] presented 13 patients treated with therapeutic keratoplasty for bacterial suppurative keratitis with satisfactory long-term optical results.

A separate subgroup of bacterial keratitis, which may require therapeutic keratoplasty, is bacterial infections that are unresponsive to conventional medical therapy. These infections are generally opportunistic and indolent, but continue to progress despite aggressive treatment. This subgroup includes crystalline keratopathy (most commonly due to alpha-hemolytic *Streptococcus*),[12,31,32] but can be seen with a variety of bacteria as well as *Candida* and *Mycobacterium fortuitum*.[2,12] These infections are most commonly seen following corneal surgery, and will relentlessly progress until a therapeutic keratoplasty is performed. Although >50% of cases of infectious crystalline keratopathy fail to respond to medical management, as there is minimal inflammation in this disorder, therapeutic keratoplasty is generally successful.[32]

Koçluk et al.[33] evaluated and compared the efficacy of therapeutic keratoplasty performed in the early and late stages of disease. A total of 13 patients were operated in the early stage of keratitis and 12 were operated in the later stages of the disease. The cohort consisted of bacterial, fungal as well as mixed keratitis (bacterial and fungal) cases. 100% of grafts in the group that underwent keratoplasty at an early stage of disease, remained clear while in the other group, only 83% grafts could retain clarity. Postoperative complications were significantly higher in the latter group. Low complication rate in the former group was attributed to less number of cases with preoperative evidence of limbal or scleral extension. Another recent study by Gümüş G et al.,[34] a total of 59 patients undergoing therapeutic keratoplasty were analyzed. 12 patients developed reinfection, of which 10 required rekeratoplasty. Mean time interval between diagnosis of reinfection and rekeratoplasty was 12 days. The success rate of rekeratoplasty was found to be significantly better when the recurrence of keratitis was dealt early on. Also, a significant relationship was noted between functional success and the absence of postoperative complications.

Therapeutic Keratoplasty for Fungal Keratitis

The introduction of topical antifungal agents has reduced the need for therapeutic penetrating keratoplasty for fungal keratitis and has also improved the prognosis and visual outcome of patients with medically uncontrolled fungal ulcers. Forster and Rebell[4] emphasized the importance of intensive antifungal treatment prior to therapeutic keratoplasty to help stabilize the cornea and improve the prognosis. They reviewed 61 eyes with corneal fungal infections, of which 13 were considered treatment failures. Nine of the 13 patients with treatment failure underwent therapeutic keratoplasty. Five of these nine patients achieved a visual acuity of 20/70 or better. In all nine patients who underwent penetrating keratoplasty, the fungal disease process was halted by the therapeutic keratoplasty.[4] Polack et al.[35] had reviewed 30 patients with keratomycosis. Of the 22 treated surgically, penetrating keratoplasty was far superior to lamellar keratoplasty. Pathological examination revealed that fungal filaments appeared to penetrate Descemet's membrane, causing a high recurrence rate in lamellar keratoplasty grafts. Forster[36] observed that 17 of 29 corneas infected by fungi remained culture-positive at the time of keratoplasty, and 26 of the eyes had viable hyphal elements on pathology (**Fig. 5**).[36] Killingsworth et al.[12] obtained a 100% cure rate in 15 fungal ulcers treated with therapeutic keratoplasty (**Figs. 6A and B**).[12] Postoperatively, fungal infection may infiltrate the grafted tissue.[37-39]

Xie et al.[40] studied 108 eyes with fungal keratitis in which therapeutic keratoplasty was performed. Eighty percent of eyes remained clear during follow-up with no recurrence of infection and visual acuity ranging from 20/100 to 20/20. A later study by Xie et al.[41] investigated the effectiveness of lamellar keratoplasty in treating fungal keratitis. They achieved therapeutically beneficial results in 93% of eyes (51 of 55 operations performed) with a resulting visual acuity ranging from 20/63 to 20/20.[41] In four cases there was a recurrence of the fungal infection within 2 weeks, which was cured by a therapeutic keratoplasty. The authors point out that corneal tissue used in lamellar keratoplasty may be obtained more readily than healthy tissue used in penetrating keratoplasty, and that lamellar keratoplasty is a viable option for treating fungal keratitis.[41]

The mainstay for treatment after therapeutic keratoplasty has been corticosteroids to prevent allograft rejection and control postoperative inflammation. However, in the management of mycotic keratitis, corticosteroids have been discouraged because of the risks of exacerbating an existing infection or introducing a superinfection.[42] In a prospective, nonrandomized interventional case series of three patients, topical cyclosporine A (tCSA) 0.5% has been shown to be a safe and useful adjunct in the treatment of therapeutic keratoplasties for fungal keratitis to avoid or reduce the use of corticosteroids.[43] Furthermore, compared to corticosteroids, tCSA has been shown in vitro to have a statistically significant suppressive effect on fungal growth.[44,45] The most common fungal organisms isolated preceding and during therapeutic keratoplasty include *Fusarium*, *Aspergillus*, and *Candida*.[4,15,46]

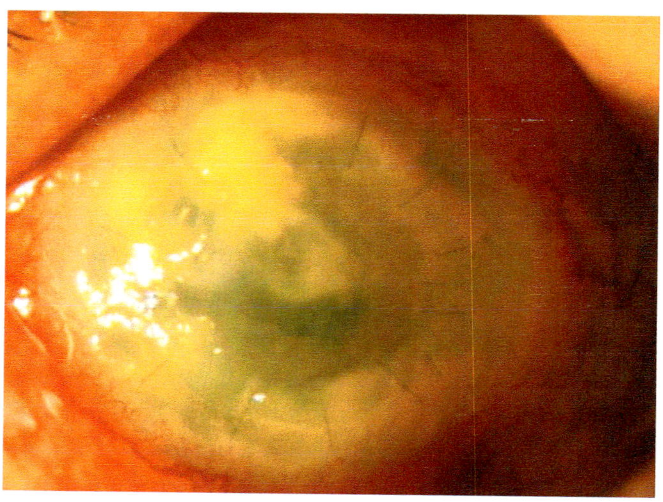

Fig. 5: Recurrence of *Candida albicans* in a corneal graft

In a large retrospective observational study performed in southern part of India, 198 eyes of fungal keratitis which underwent therapeutic penetrating keratoplasty were evaluated.[47] *Aspergillus flavus* was the most common fungal species identified in the culture plates smeared using corneal scrapings. Size of the corneal infiltrate was found to be a risk factor, significantly associated with graft survival. Timely surgical intervention should be considered in eyes not responding appropriately to medical therapy. A similar study from a tertiary eye care center of North India proved that early intervention before the keratitis progresses to cause corneal perforation or involves the adjacent structures is associated with a better postoperative outcome.[48]

There are several factors that influence the success of a therapeutic graft performed in eyes with fungal keratitis. Graft diameter is one such important factor. Although the recurrence rate of infection is similar with small and large diameter grafts, the chances of complications such as glaucoma and graft rejection are significantly higher in eyes receiving large diameter grafts (8 mm or more).[49]

Therapeutic keratoplasty in eyes with bacterial keratitis usually has a better prognosis than fungal keratitis. Sharma et al. however, reported no significant

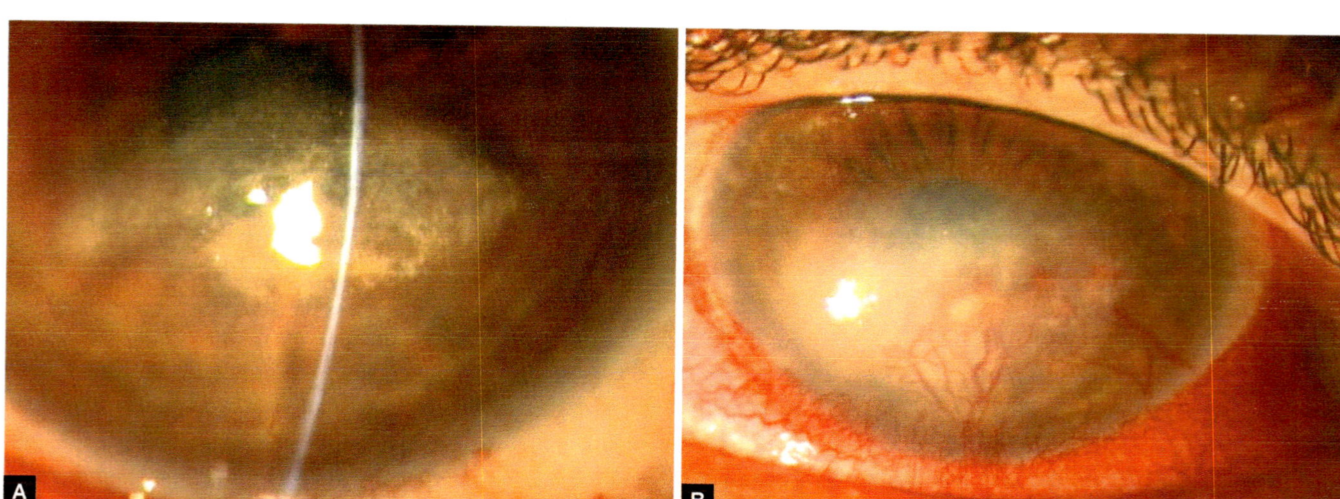

Figs. 6A and B: (A) An inactive scar from herpes simplex interstitial keratitis, with cholesterol deposits within the stroma; (B) Active herpetic stromal disease with prominent vascularization and significant inflammation.

difference in outcomes of surgery between bacterial and fungal keratitis cases. The authors attributed their findings to the practice of anterior chamber wash using intracameral antifungal drugs at the end of the surgical procedure and performing keratoplasty at an early stages to improve the overall outcome. This study also revealed that keratitis attributed to pathogens mixed etiology has poorer therapeutic keratoplasty outcomes than pure bacterial or fungal ulcer.[48]

Therapeutic Keratoplasty for *Interface Infectious Keratitis*

Interface keratitis is a rare but vision threatening complication, which can be develop after any form of lamellar keratoplasty. The virtual space between the graft and the host corneal tissue is the site of the origin of infection. Although these tend to remain localized for a long time with slow spread, but have a potential to cause serious complications such as endophthalmitis and sequential severe visual loss.

The entity is not very common, so the literature is not very replete with the outcome studies. Fungal pathogens, most commonly the *Candida* species have been implicated as the most common pathogens implicated in the causation of interface keratitis in most studies. In most instances, the source of infection has been documented to be a donor-host transmission.[50-52]

Sharma et al. reported growth of coagulase-negative *Staphylococcus* in one of the two cases, developing microbial keratitis following Descemet stripping automated endothelial keratoplasty (DSAEK).[53]

Nahum Y et al. in another study of 10 eyes, which developed interface keratitis following DSAEK, *Staphylococcus* species was identified in three cases.[54]

Medical therapy is usually the first line of treatment, but is ineffective alone in majority of cases due to the sequestered nature of infection. Targeted drug therapy in the form of injection of drugs directly at the graft-host interface has been tried with variable results and complications in the form of graft dislocation, dissemination of infection, and interface scarring. The largest systematic review included 62 cases of interface keratitis, occurring after a lamellar keratoplasty.[50] 39 out of 62 patients required therapeutic graft due to nonresponse to medical therapy alone.

Donor graft removal helps to lessen the microbial load besides providing adequate sample for microbiological evaluation, serving to guide the postoperative management. Additional use of intracameral and intravitreal antifungal injections helps to reduce the risk of dissemination of infection.[51,52] Early intervention is the key to successful outcome in these cases. Excisional keratoplasty with complete removal of the infected tissue is advocated as early as possible to minimize the risk of endophthalmitis. Obtaining donor rim cultures is another important part of the management algorithm to help isolate the infectious agent. Nahum et al. described the results of early excisional penetrating keratoplasty combined with intracameral injection, at the end of surgery. No study patient developed endophthalmitis, with retainment of good visual acuity and graft clarity in most patients.[54]

Therapeutic Keratoplasty for *Acanthamoeba* Keratitis

The respective roles of medical and surgical intervention in *Acanthamoeba* keratitis are controversial. Some patients diagnosed early have been successfully treated with medication alone.[55,56] Early penetrating keratoplasty has been advocated to remove the bulk of infection and reduce the risk of intractable scleral contamination.[57] In a report by Ficker et al.,[58] graft survival for *Acanthamoeba* keratitis was poor with >50% incidence of recurrence in the graft. Cullen et al.,[59] in a seven patient experience, concluded that early diagnosis helped with successful medical treatment, but penetrating keratoplasty continues to have a central role in the management of cases that are advanced or unresponsive to medical therapy. Cryotherapy of the host cornea has also been suggested in conjunction with penetrating keratoplasty for cases unresponsive to medical treatment.[60] In a series of 32 patients, the most common complication of therapeutic keratoplasty for *Acanthamoeba* keratitis was glaucoma with over half of these patients developing graft failure and mydriatic, fixed pupils.[61] The acute management of these active cases is to sterilize the infection as rapidly as possible and to delay surgical management until the patient receives adequate antiamebic therapy.[62] Adequate control of infection by using antiamebic drugs and control of glaucoma help to improve the overall prognosis of graft.[63]

Robaei D et al.[64] evaluated the outcomes of keratoplasty; either therapeutic or optical (anterior lamellar), performed in 50 eyes with *Acanthamoeba* keratitis. Visual outcomes were significantly better in patients belonging to the optical keratoplasty group compared to those who underwent therapeutic keratoplasty. Therapeutic keratoplasty was associated with 13-fold increased risk of poor visual outcome compared to optical keratoplasty. Similar findings of favorable visual outcomes and graft survival following optical keratoplasty were also observed by Kitzmann A et al.[65]

Studies analyzing the correlation between clinical presentation and the ultimate prognosis have shown the need for surgical treatment to be significantly associated with factors such as delayed diagnosis (>30 day interval between the onset of symptoms and establishment of diagnosis), poor presenting visual acuity (<20/200), large infiltrate size (>3 mm), presence of corneal perforation, and corneal neovascularization.[66]

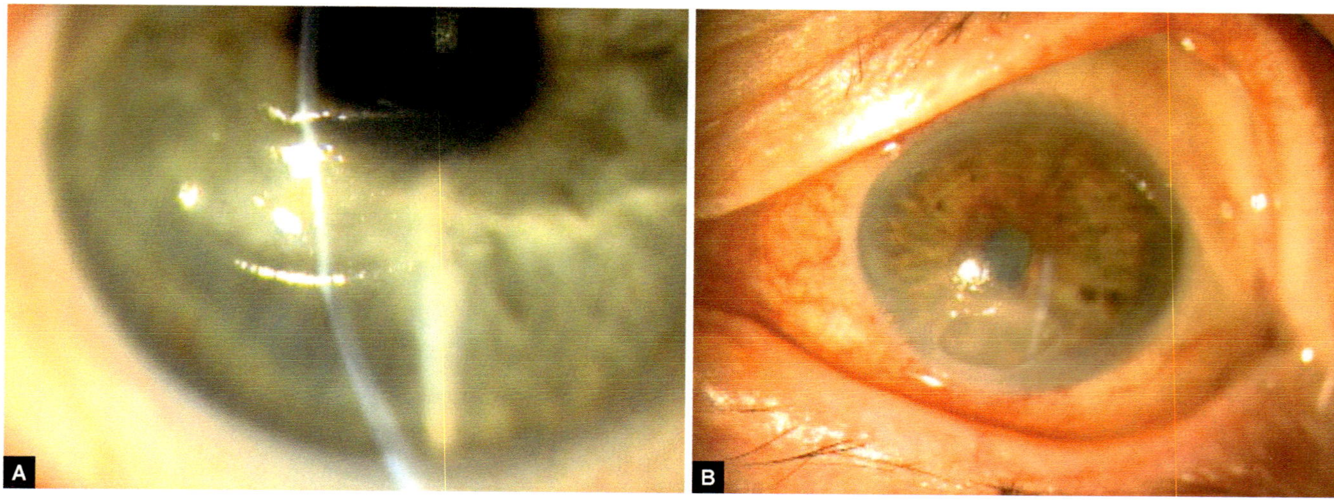

Figs. 7A and B: (A) A chronic, stable neurotrophic ulcer; (B) Microbial keratitis occurring in the setting of a neurotrophic ulcer. Cultures grew *Moraxella* spp.

Therapeutic Keratoplasty for Herpetic Keratitis

Herpes simplex viral disease of the cornea often requires surgical intervention. Most commonly, this is done for significant corneal scarring and is performed under quiescent, controlled circumstances. Adjunctive medical management has made possible successful penetrating keratoplasty in the active stromal stage of herpes simplex keratitis. Therapeutic keratoplasty can be employed for significant ulceration and/or perforation, or to remove viral antigenic material responsible for repeated immune inflammatory episodes. Success of the keratoplasty depends, as noted by Langston et al.,[67] on the degree of inflammation, presence of neovascularization, use of sutures, and high doses of topical steroids in the immediate postoperative period.

Adjunctive use of oral acyclovir has been shown to improve prognosis as well (**Figs. 7A and B**).[68,69] Topical antiviral prophylaxis during the immediate postoperative period and during allograft rejection episodes while topical corticosteroids are used may prevent recurrent herpetic disease.[70] Ficker et al.[71] found that the combination of prophylactic antivirals and corticosteroids increased the success rate in inflamed eyes undergoing therapeutic keratoplasty for herpes simplex keratitis to a rate comparable to that of quiescent eyes. The use of interrupted sutures, prompt removal of loose sutures, and the previously noted antivirals and topical steroid treatment combination reduced the recurrence of herpes simplex virus to 15%. Killingsworth et al.[12] divided 15 patients who required therapeutic penetrating keratoplasty for herpes simplex keratitis into two groups. The first group included patients with severe stromal keratitis who did not respond to medical treatment and patients who progressed to perforation. The second group consisted of patients who developed corneal perforation secondary to persistent epithelial defects with little or no active stromal inflammation. Only four of the 11 patients in the first group achieved clear grafts, while all four patients in the second group were successful.

The prognosis for therapeutic keratoplasty in herpes zoster keratitis is generally worse than for herpes simplex keratitis. Patients with herpetic corneal disease commonly have neurotrophic corneas. However, the anesthesia tends to be more severe for herpes zoster than for herpes simplex. One of the most important prognostic variables for herpes zoster therapeutic keratoplasty is the level of corneal sensation. Therapeutic keratoplasty in patients with herpes zoster keratitis perforations often requires adjunctive therapy, such as conjunctival flaps or tarsorrhaphies. Careful management of external and corneal disease can improve the outcomes in therapeutic keratoplasty for varicella-zoster keratitis. Tanure et al.[72] published results from a series of 15 keratoplasties performed for varicella-zoster keratopathy from 1989 through 1998 (12 with zoster and 3 with varicella), and found that 87% of grafts remained clear at an average follow-up of 50 months. To reduce complications from neurotrophic keratopathy, four eyes received lateral tarsorrhaphies in conjunction with the keratoplasties, and frequent lubrication was prescribed.

Therapeutic Keratoplasty for Persistent Epithelial Defects and Sterile Melts

An additional subgroup, which may require therapeutic keratoplasty, is severe external disease resulting in a persistent epithelial defect that progresses to stromal loss. Killingsworth et al.[12] found that 26 of 80 patients (33%) in their series had therapeutic keratoplasty for a persistent epithelial defect. This subgroup may often be secondarily infected. The underlying disease process may be extremely varied, but all have in common the inability to maintain a normal ocular surface and tear film. This category can be divided into three subclasses: (1) neurotrophic disease, (2) exposure keratitis, and (3) dry eye.

Neurotrophic corneal perforation may be due to systemic disease, trigeminal nerve dysfunction, or localized to the eye. Systemic diseases include Riley-Day[73] syndrome (familial dysautonomia) and Wilson's disease (hepatolenticular degeneration).[74] Trigeminal nerve dysfunction produces corneal tissue damage by a poorly understood mechanism. The pathogenesis may be related to neurologically controlled mediators of the epithelium.[75] Trigeminal dysfunction may occur in 15–18% of patients following trigeminal ganglionectomies or inadvertent surgical trauma.[76] Additional nonsurgical causes of trigeminal dysfunction include cerebrovascular accidents, multiple sclerosis, tumors, and aneurysms. The most common cause of neurotrophic corneal disease is the herpes virus family.[77] Neurotrophic keratitis following herpes zoster ophthalmicus may be particularly debilitating.[78] Corneal anesthesia leading to perforation has been described following *Acanthamoeba* keratitis,[48,79-81] anesthetic abuse,[82] and penetrating keratoplasty.[83,84] Corneal perforation may be particularly devastating, as the patient is often unaware of the severity of the disease process because of the lack of pain.

Exposure keratitis may predispose to corneal perforation and the need for a therapeutic keratoplasty. In exposure keratitis, the common finding is breakdown of the epithelium and the loss of corneal integrity. Exposure keratitis can occur due to a variety of lid abnormalities, including facial nerve paralysis,[85] Parkinson's disease, entropion, ectropion, lid notching, and lid imbrication syndrome.[86] The combination of fifth and seventh nerve dysfunction can be particularly dangerous.[87]

Severe dry eye may also predispose to corneal perforation and therapeutic keratoplasty.[88] The dry eye may affect the mucin, aqueous, or lipid component in the tear film, or any combination of the above.[89] Severe dry eye may be associated with systemic conditions,[90] such as collagen vascular disease, ocular cicatricial pemphigoid,[91] rosacea, Riley-Day syndrome,[74] or Stevens-Johnson syndrome.[92,93] Localized causes of severe dry eye include radiation[94] and chemical injuries.[95] When a therapeutic keratoplasty is required and the patient has neurotrophic disease, exposure keratitis, or severe dry eye, attention must be paid to the underlying condition.

PRESURGICAL EVALUATION

Antimicrobial Therapy

Before therapeutic keratoplasty for infectious keratitis, the patient should be treated with topical and systemic therapy directed towards the offending microbe. This treatment applies to bacterial, fungal, herpetic, and parasitic infections. Regardless of the infectious etiology, we always recommend topical antibiotic therapy to prevent bacterial superinfection. In sterile corneal necrosis with corneal perforation, the preoperative antibiotic prophylaxis should be broad spectrum and nontoxic to help promote re-epithelialization. In addition, we prefer an antibiotic that penetrates well into the cornea, aqueous, and vitreous to achieve levels above the minimal inhibitory concentration (MIC)[100] of most pathogenic bacteria.[98] We currently use a topical fourth-generation fluoroquinolone in conjunction with a systemic fluoroquinolone. After the patient is hospitalized, we often place the patient on intravenous vancomycin and tobramycin.

Donor Material

Exclusion criteria for therapeutic keratoplasties are similar to those for optical penetrating keratoplasties. Most eye banks will respond to an emergent request, and either find a local donor or bring in a donor cornea from another eye bank. Under emergent circumstances, the donor cornea may not be of the same quality as it is for an optical penetrating keratoplasty. Older donor corneas, that have decreased endothelial cell counts, or have been in storage media too long to be used for optical penetrating keratoplasty, can be ideal for a therapeutic keratoplasty. When, fresh tissue is not available, cryopreserved, glycerine-preserved corneal tissue, or even sclera, can be acceptable.[99-101] The surgeon should have a reasonable expectation of the size of keratoplasty prior to entering the operating room. In many operating rooms, small trephines <7.0 mm and trephines larger than 8.5 mm may not be readily available. It is the surgeon's responsibility to make certain these devices are available if there is any expectation that they are going to be needed. When the therapeutic keratoplasty is to be small, and off the visual axis, the donor cornea quality is not as important as when the visual axis is involved. Central therapeutic keratoplasties often become optical penetrating keratoplasties, and the availability of good donor tissue in these cases is even more important.

SURGICAL TECHNIQUE

At the time of therapeutic keratoplasty, the size of the graft should be carefully determined by placing the appropriate trephine over the cornea and creating an indentation in the epithelium. The goal of surgery is to excise all necrotic or infected tissue during the trephination. If possible, a 1-mm rim of healthy corneal tissue should also be removed to leave a stable, noninfected recipient bed. We routinely suture a Flieringa ring in place to provide scleral support. Once, the size of the recipient bed has been determined, the donor cornea can be trephined and is usually 0.25–0.5 mm larger than the host trephine. The donor trephination is the same as for optical penetrating keratoplasty.

During trephination of the recipient bed, care should be taken not to place pressure on the globe, which could lead to extrusion of the intraocular contents or an expulsive choroidal hemorrhage. Avoidance of pressure is particularly important in therapeutic keratoplasty for corneal perforation. A self-retaining lid speculum or lid sutures are very helpful to prevent pressure on the globe. The host trephination in a therapeutic keratoplasty for a corneal perforation can be difficult due to loss of scleral rigidity with decreased intraocular pressure. Femtosecond laser trephination for lamellar or therapeutic keratoplasty may offer the advantage of reduced pressure on the globe while stabilizing the corneal perforation.[102,103] Femtosecond laser trephinations may also be customized to fit the corneal perforation. When cyanoacrylate adhesive has not successfully sealed a corneal perforation prior to therapeutic keratoplasty, it can often be attempted during the operation. A limbal incision or peripheral corneal stab incision can be made to sweep iris with a cyclodialysis spatula from the perforation under viscoelastic protection. When there is vitreous in the perforation, an anterior vitrectomy can often be performed through the limbal incision. When there is significant chamber shallowing with vitreous pressure a pars plana vitrectomy can be invaluable to deepen the anterior chamber and prevent expulsion of the crystalline lens. If cyanoacrylate adhesive can be applied preoperatively or intraoperatively, the anterior chamber can be reformed with viscoelastic, and the host trephination can be performed under a more controlled environment.

The corneal trephination should be centered over the infection or perforation to leave the maximal, noninfected tissue between the ulceration and the recipient bed. The one exception is the case of a small perforation or infection in which decentering the therapeutic keratoplasty would provide a better optical result. Occasionally, the therapeutic transplantation is located near the limbus. This possibility occurs most frequently with limbal wound infections after cataract surgery, infections after pterygium surgery with adjunctive mitomycin or irradiation, and peripheral inflammatory disorders such as Mooren's ulceration. Small therapeutic grafts can be performed in a normal fashion with a corneal trephine straddling the limbus. Jonas et al. performed a series of 60 therapeutic keratoplasties for patients with perforated or pre-descemetal corneal ulcers, and found that sclerokeratoplasties were necessary in eight patients with paralimbal ulcers.[25] With larger, eccentric therapeutic keratoplasties, however, a round trephine will not adequately excise the affected tissue. In these severe cases, a freehand graft is often required. The therapeutic patch graft can be excised with a corneal trephine and then approximated into the corneal defect by serially excising tissue from the donor cornea, until it fits into the appropriate corneal scleral defect. Trephining a cornea in an eye with a flat anterior chamber or markedly decreased intraocular pressure can be challenging. Care should be taken to avoid pressure on the eye if a perforation is present. We recommend using an extremely sharp trephine and applying a minimal amount of pressure to the globe. Suction trephines, such as a Hessburg–Barron trephine,[104] can be advantageous. We have had success with a motorized trephine.

Rarely, an undiagnosed infectious keratitis patient will be brought to the operating room for a therapeutic keratoplasty. In a review by Cohen et al.,[105] two cases of *Acanthamoeba* keratitis were found on retrospective pathologic evaluation. At the time of keratoplasty, suppurative areas of the specimen should be aggressively cultured on multiple media. In addition to chocolate agar, blood agar, Sabouraud's, and thioglycolate, we frequently culture specimens on Löwenstein–Jensen, brain-heart infusion, and blood agar with an *Escherichia coli* overlay, as indicated by the clinical findings. In undiagnosed infectious keratitis, we also perform multiple scrapings and send a portion of the specimen for frozen-section pathological evaluation. Establishing the diagnosis in the operating room allows us to alter intraoperative therapy, including the use of intravitreal antimicrobial injections, if we are suspicious of a concomitant endophthalmitis. Establishing a diagnosis also allows the surgeon to modify the subconjunctival injections, soak a collagen shield in an appropriate medication, and initiate directed postoperative therapy.

Lamellar keratoplasty should generally be avoided for therapeutic grafts in active infections, as there is an increased risk of the infection spreading into the deeper tissue, particularly in cases of fungal ulcerative keratitis.[35] Fungi appear to have a tropism for Descemet's membrane. When the deeper cornea is viable, however, we recommend an 80% depth trephination with approximately 1 mm of beveling of the incision to create a deep lip of tissue, which provides support for the therapeutic keratoplasty and decreases the risk of postoperative wound leaks. Suturing technique in any inflamed or infectious keratitis should almost always be interrupted. The sutures should be approximately 75% corneal depth and should not be full thickness, as this increases the risk for a conduit of infectious organisms from the cornea into the anterior chamber. The interrupted sutures should be placed radially and farther into the recipient bed than for a noninflamed optical penetrating keratoplasty. We use an increased number of sutures, but try to maintain only moderate suture tension. The goal of the longer interrupted sutures with moderate tension is to avoid "cheese-wiring" of the sutures through a potentially necrotic host-bed. The interrupted sutures also allow early suture removal for excessive sectoral inflammation, vascularization, or recurrent infection.

At the time of keratoplasty, we recommend performing the minimum intraocular surgery necessary. When possible, the crystalline lens should be left in place, as it provides a barrier against vitreous seeding and infectious endophthalmitis.[96] The anterior chamber should be irrigated aggressively with balanced salt solution and the iris should be inspected for infectious foci. Any iris lesions should be excised and cultured. When infection of the vitreous is suspected, particularly in aphakic eyes, the vitreous should be thoroughly cultured. When the organism is known, intravitreal injections of an appropriate antimicrobial are indicated. When the organism is in question, broad-spectrum intravitreal injections are indicated. We currently use intravitreal vancomycin (1 mg in 0.1 mL) and ceftazidime (2.5 mg in 0.1 mL) for suspected bacterial endophthalmitis.

At the time of surgery, any predisposing factors that have contributed to the need for a therapeutic keratoplasty should be addressed. As previously mentioned, many patients who require a therapeutic keratoplasty have underlying external disease that has been a significant part of their disease process. After a therapeutic keratoplasty, the donor cornea will be more anesthetic than preoperatively, and the tear film will be significantly altered. Failure to address the predisposing external disease problem, in conjunction with the changes induced by the surgery, often leads to severe postoperative complications, including persistent epithelial defects, sterile corneal melts, infectious keratitis, wound leaks, and corneal neovascularization. All lid abnormalities should be corrected. Patients with mild dry eyes should have punctal occlusion. Patients with moderate to severe dry eye should undergo tarsorrhaphy. Patients with severe dry eyes or anesthetic corneas, in which postoperative wound healing is jeopardized, should either have large tarsorrhaphies or should be offered a conjunctival flap at the time of therapeutic keratoplasty. A conjunctival flap is often a definitive procedure, which is further indicated if the eye has limited visual prognosis. A conjunctival flap is never indicated if there is active infection or perforation.

Patients who have undergone previous penetrating keratoplasty may develop recurrence of the original disease or have a neurotrophic cornea that leads to corneal melting. In these cases, an anterior lamellar keratoplasty (ALK) can be considered. Ang M et al. reported eight consecutive cases of ALK following penetrating keratoplasty.[106] Three of these cases were therapeutic and two were tectonic. All patients had an improvement in visual acuity although one patient required a repeat ALK for recurrence of the infectious process.

POSTOPERATIVE MANAGEMENT OF THERAPEUTIC PENETRATING KERATOPLASTIES

The postoperative management of a therapeutic keratoplasty is often as challenging as the operation. Several basic principles should be followed:

- *Eradicate all remnants of infection and prevent reinfection*: The therapeutic keratoplasty often provides a surgical excision of an infection. When there is a reasonable doubt, however, anti-infectious therapy should be maintained until the corneal epithelium has healed. Duration of treatment depends on the severity of the infection and the causative organism. In general, the more opportunistic infections, such as *Acanthamoeba* and fungi, are the most resistant to therapy and require the longest postoperative antimicrobial treatment to prevent reinfection. This treatment may be as prolonged as several months.
- *Promote re-epithelialization of the cornea and wound healing*: Avoid prolonged overtreatment of the cornea with toxic medications, such as fortified antibiotics, amphotericin B, and antivirals. Systemic acyclovir appears to offer the efficacy of topical antivirals without the risk of keratitis medicamentosa. We routinely maintain patients with a therapeutic keratoplasty for herpes simplex keratitis on acyclovir 400 mg twice daily or valacyclovir 500 mg once a day for 6 months after surgery.[69] When treating epitheliopathy in therapeutic keratoplasties postoperatively, nonpreserved tears and lubricants are often useful. When these agents are ineffective, a cyanoacrylate temporary tarsorrhaphy can often resolve a persistent epithelial defect.[107] Milder medications should be substituted for toxic antibiotics when indicated.
- *Control inflammation with corticosteroids*: The use of topical corticosteroids following a therapeutic keratoplasty for an infectious organism is controversial. Most bacterial corneal infections are responsive to antibiotics. Therefore, the concomitant use of corticosteroids is justified in an inflamed eye. In a therapeutic keratoplasty for herpetic keratitis, the corticosteroids can be given without significant risk, as long as the patient is managed with topical or oral antiviral therapy. There is controversy regarding the use of corticosteroids after therapeutic keratoplasty involving infections that do not respond readily to treatment, such as fungal or *Acanthamoeba* corneal ulceration. When there is any sign of active fungal or *Acanthamoeba infection* following a therapeutic keratoplasty, corticosteroids should be avoided.[20,108] When the eye has been treated extensively and a wide surgical debridement has been performed, however, corticosteroids are indicated and can be used safely.[12,109] For severe inflammation, the use of systemic corticosteroids should be considered.
- *Intraocular pressure control*: Postoperatively, the patient's intraocular pressure should be followed carefully. Glaucoma is seen in approximately 50% of optical penetrating keratoplasties. Following therapeutic keratoplasty, the patient may develop anterior synechiae, iritis, and trabeculitis, which may further contribute to an elevated intraocular pressure. The pupil should be dilated with cyclopentolate 1% to reduce ciliary spasm, prevent pupillary block, and decrease peripheral anterior synechiae. Prevention of glaucomatous visual field loss following therapeutic keratoplasty often requires aggressive medical and surgical management.[97]

VISUAL PROGNOSIS FOR THERAPEUTIC KERATOPLASTY

The final visual prognosis for therapeutic keratoplasties depends on multiple variables. The infecting organism and its susceptibility to treatment are extremely important. Therapeutic keratoplasty for bacterial keratitis has a much better prognosis than for *Acanthamoeba* or fungal infections. Killingsworth et al.[12] reported clear therapeutic grafts in 73% of bacterial corneal ulcers, 60% of fungal corneal ulcers, 50% of *Acanthamoeba* corneal ulcers, and 36% of herpes ulcerations with inflammation. Underlying corneal pathology also affects postoperative visual rehabilitation. Ocular surface disease, such as dry eye and neurotrophic disease, significantly decreases the viability of the donor cornea. In severe ocular surface disease, the visual prognosis is extremely poor and the keratoplasty is generally performed for tectonic rather than visual purposes.

The severity of ocular inflammation at the time of surgery has direct impact on graft survival. Active inflammation increases the risk of anterior synechiae, glaucoma, corneal neovascularization, and graft rejection. Although eradication of the corneal infection is paramount, inflammation control is also important. Superimposing the trauma of a penetrating keratoplasty on an underlying inflammatory condition can result in increased inflammation in the donor cornea.[31,56] This inflammation can progress to donor cornea melting, vascularization, and allograft rejection. When a therapeutic keratoplasty is semiemergent and the infection is controlled, a short pulse of topical corticosteroids prior to surgery may improve visual outcome. Corneal neovascularization also decreases the success of therapeutic keratoplasty. The more extensive the stromal vascularization, the more likely graft rejection will occur.

Finally, the size of the therapeutic keratoplasty is important in graft survival. Keratoplasties of >9.5 mm diameter appear to have a significantly decreased chance of long-term viability.[12,30] Larger transplants that are closer to the limbus can increase the risk of allograft rejection and peripheral anterior synechiae with glaucoma. These larger keratoplasties often provide tectonic support for smaller optical penetrating keratoplasties, which can be performed later.

Therapeutic keratoplasty is generally an emergent, high-risk procedure that challenges the surgical and medical skills of the corneal surgeon. It requires meticulous attention to detail and careful postoperative monitoring. Nevertheless, advances in microsurgical technique, antimicrobial therapy, and control of inflammation have resulted in an improved prognosis for therapeutic keratoplasty.

REFERENCES

1. Hill JC. Use of penetrating keratoplasty in acute bacterial keratitis. Br J Ophthalmol. 1986;70:502-6.
2. Dugel PU, Holland GN, Brown HH, Pettit TH, Hofbauer JD, Simons KB, et al. Mycobacterium fortuitum keratitis. Am J Ophthalmol. 1988;105:661-9.
3. Malik SR, Singh G. Therapeutic keratoplasty in Pseudomonas pyocyanea corneal ulcers. Br J Ophthalmol. 1971;55:326-30.
4. Forster RK, Rebell G. Therapeutic surgery in failures of medical treatment for fungal keratitis. Br J Ophthalmol. 1975;59:366-71.
5. Grimmett MR, Holland EJ, Krachmer JH. Therapeutic keratoplasty after radial keratotomy. Am J Ophthalmol. 1994;118:108-9.
6. Polack FM, Kaufman HE. Penetrating keratoplasty in herpetic keratitis. Am J Ophthalmol. 1970;73:908-12.
7. Foster CS, Duncan J. Penetrating keratoplasty for herpes simplex keratitis. Am J Ophthalmol. 1981;92:336-43.
8. Eiferman RA. Cryotherapy of Pseudomonas keratitis and scleritis. Arch Ophthalmol. 1979;97:1637-9.
9. Reynolds MG, Alfonso E. Treatment of infectious scleritis and keratoscleritis. Am J Ophthalmol. 1991;112:543-7.
10. Jackson WB. Infections of the sclera. In: Tabbera RK, Hyndiuk RA (Eds). Infections of the Eye. Boston: Little Brown; 1986. pp. 477-86.
11. Alfonso E, Kenyon KR, Ormerod LD, Stevens R, Wagoner MD, Albert DM. Pseudomonas corneoscleritis. Am J Ophthalmol. 1987;103:90-8.
12. Killingsworth DW, Stern GA, Driebe WT, Knapp A, Dragon DM. Results of therapeutic penetrating keratoplasty. Ophthalmology. 1993;100:534-41.
13. Robin JB, Gindi JJ, Koh K, Schanzlin DJ, Rao NA, York KK, et al. An update of the indications for penetrating keratoplasty. 1979 through 1983. Arch Ophthalmol. 1986;104:87-9.
14. Sony P, Sharma N, Vajpayee RB, Ray M. Therapeutic keratoplasty for infectious keratitis. A review of the literature. CLAO J. 2002;28:111-8.
15. Ti SE, Scott JA, Janardhanan P, Tan DT. Therapeutic keratoplasty for advanced suppurative keratitis. Am J Ophthalmol. 2007;143(5):755-62.
16. Davis SD, Sarff LD, Hyndiuk RA. Comparison of therapeutic routes in experimental Pseudomonas keratitis. Am J Ophthalmol. 1975;87:710-6.
17. Baum J, Barza M. Topical vs subconjunctival treatment of bacterial corneal ulcers. Ophthalmology. 1983;90:162-8.
18. Hirst LW, Smiddy WR, Stork WJ. Corneal perforations. Ophthalmology. 1982;89:630-5.
19. Foster CS, Lass JH, Moran-Wallace K, Giovanoni R. Ocular toxicity of topical antifungal agents. Arch Ophthalmol. 1981;99:1081-4.
20. Driebe WT Jr, Stern GA, Epstein RJ, Visvesvara GS, Adi M, Komadina T. Acanthamoeba keratitis: potential role for topical clotrimazole in combination chemotherapy. Arch Ophthalmol. 1988;106:1196-201.
21. Partnoy SL, Insler MS, Kaufman HE. Surgical management of corneal ulceration and perforation. Surv Ophthalmol. 1989;34:47-58.
22. Eiferman RA, Snyder JW. Cyanoacrylate glue. Arch Ophthalmol. 1984;102:192-4.
23. Leahey A, Gottsch JD, Stark WJ. Clinical experience with N-butyl cyanoacrylate (Nexacryl) tissue adhesive. Ophthalmology. 1993;100:173-80.
24. Cavanaugh TB, Gottsch JD. Infectious keratitis and cyanoacrylate adhesive. Am J Ophthalmol. 1991;111:466-72.
25. Jonas JB, Rank RM, Budde WM. Tectonic sclerokeratoplasty and tectonic penetrating keratoplasty as treatment for perforated or pre-descemetal corneal ulcers. Am J Ophthalmol. 2001;132:14-8.
26. Hanada K, Igarashi S, Muramatsu O, Yoshida A. Therapeutic keratoplasty for corneal perforation: Clinical results and complications. Cornea. 2008;27:156-60.
27. Hyndiuk RA. Experimental Pseudomonas keratitis. Trans Am Ophthalmol Soc. 1981;79:540-624.
28. Ogawa GSH, Hyndiuk RA. Ulcerative keratitis. In: Smolin G, Thoft RA (Eds). The Cornea. Boston: Little Brown; 1994. pp. 125-67.

29. Cowden JW, Copeland RA, Schneider MS. Larger diameter therapeutic penetrating keratoplasties. Refract Corneal Surg. 1989;5:244-8.
30. Lam GC, Cooper RL. "Hot" corneal grafts—a long-term study. Aust N Z J Ophthalmol. 1989;17:395-8.
31. Stern GA. Infectious crystalline keratopathy. Int Ophthalmol Clin. 1993;33:1-7.
32. Sharma N, Vajpayee RB, Pushker N, Vajpayee M. Infectious crystalline keratopathy. CLAO J. 2000;26:40-43.
33. Koçluk Y, Sukgen EA. Results of therapeutic penetrating keratoplasty for bacterial and fungal keratitis. Int Ophthalmol. 2017;37(5):1085-93.
34. Gümüş G, Kırgız A, Yıldırım Y, Kandemir Beşek N, Genç S, Kepez Yıldız B, et al. Prognostic Factors Affecting Graft Survival in Patients Undergoing Penetrating Keratoplasty for Infectious Keratitis. Turk J Ophthalmol. 2020;50(6):324-31.
35. Polack FM, Kaufman HE, Newmark G. Keratomycosis. Medical and surgical treatment. Arch Ophthalmol. 1971;85:410-6.
36. Forster RK. The role of excisional keratoplasty in microbial keratitis. In: Cavanagh HD (Ed). The Cornea. Transactions of the World Congress on the Cornea. III. New York: Raven; 1988. pp. 529-33.
37. Gomes JA. Positive donor rim culture in penetrating keratoplasty. Cornea. 1995;14:457-62.
38. Kloess PM, Stulting RD, Waring GO 3rd, Wilson LA. Bacterial and fungal endophthalmitis after penetrating keratoplasty. Am J Ophthalmol. 1993;115:309-16.
39. Sutphin JE, Pfaller MA, Hollis RJ, Wagoner MD. Donor-to-host transmission of Candida albicans after corneal transplantation. Am J Ophthalmol. 2002;134:120-1.
40. Xie L, Dong X, Shi W. Treatment of fungal keratitis by penetrating keratoplasty. Br J Ophthalmol. 2001;85:1070-4.
41. Xie L, Shi W, Liu Z, Li S. Lamellar keratoplasty for the treatment of fungal keratitis. Cornea. 2002;21:33-7.
42. Baratz KH, Hattenhauer MG. Indiscriminate use of corticosteroid-containing eye drops. Mayo Clin Proc. 1999;74:362-6.
43. Perry HD, Doshi SJ, Donnenfeld ED, Bai GS. Topical cyclosporin A in the management of therapeutic keratoplasty for mycotic keratitis. Cornea. 2002;21:161-3.
44. Wong TY, Au Eong KG, Chan WK, Tseng PS. Fusarium keratitis following the use of topical antibiotic-corticosteroid therapy in traumatized eyes. Ann Acad Med Singapore. 1996;25:862-5.
45. Bell NP, Karp CL, Alfonso EC. Effects of methylprednisolone and cyclosporine A on fungal growth in vitro. Cornea. 1999;18:306-13.
46. Sanders N. Penetrating keratoplasty in treatment of fungal keratitis. Am J Ophthalmol. 1970;24-30.
47. Mundra J, Dhakal R, Mohamed A, Jha G, Joseph J, Chaurasia S, et al. Outcomes of therapeutic penetrating keratoplasty in 198 eyes with fungal keratitis. Indian J Ophthalmol. 2019;67(10):1599-605.
48. Sharma N, Jain M, Sehra SV, Maharana P, Agarwal T, Satpathy G, et al. Outcomes of therapeutic penetrating keratoplasty from a tertiary eye care centre in northern India. Cornea. 2014;33(2):114-8.
49. Li C, Zhao GQ, Che CY, Lin J, Li N, Jia WY, et al. (2012). Effect of corneal graft diameter on therapeutic penetrating keratoplasty for fungal keratitis. Int J Ophthalmol. 2012;5(6):698-703.
50. Gao Y, Li C, Bu P, Zhang L, Bouchard CS. Infectious interface keratitis (IIK) following lamellar keratoplasty: A literature review. Ocul Surf. 2019;17(4);635-43.
51. McElnea E, Power B, Murphy C. Interface Fungal Keratitis after Descemet Stripping Automated Endothelial Keratoplasty: A Review of the Literature with a Focus on Outcomes. Cornea. 2018;37(9):1204-11.
52. Fontana L, Moramarco A, Mandarà E, Russello G, Iovieno A. Interface infectious keratitis after anterior and posterior lamellar keratoplasty. Clinical features and treatment strategies. A review. Br J Ophthalmol. 2019;103(3):307-14.
53. Sharma N, Agarwal PC, Kumar CS, Mannan R, Titiyal JS. (2011). Microbial keratitis after descemet stripping automated endothelial keratoplasty. Eye Contact Lens. 2011;37(5):320-2.
54. Nahum Y, Russo C, Madi S, Busin M. (2014). Interface infection after descemet stripping automated endothelial keratoplasty: outcomes of therapeutic keratoplasty. Cornea. 2014;33(9):893-8.
55. Holland GN, Donzis PB. Rapid resolution of early Acanthamoeba after epithelial debridement. Am J Ophthalmol. 1987;104:87-9.
56. Bacon AS, Frazer DG, Dart JK. A review of 72 cases of Acanthamoeba keratitis, 1984–1992. Eye. 1993;7:719-25.
57. Hirst LW, Green WR, Merz W, Kaufmann C, Visvesvara GS, Jensen A, et al. Management of Acanthamoeba keratitis. A case report and review of the literature. Ophthalmology. 1984;91:1105-11.
58. Ficker LA, Kirkness C, Wright P. Prognosis for keratoplasty in Acanthamoeba keratitis. Ophthalmology. 1993;100:105-10.
59. Cullen EJ, Parlato CJ, Arentsen JJ, Genvert GI, Eagle RC Jr, Wieland MR, et al. Medical and surgical treatment of Acanthamoeba keratitis. Am J Ophthalmol. 1987;103:615-25.
60. Binder PS. Cryotherapy for medically unresponsive Acanthamoeba keratitis. Cornea. 1989;8:106-14.
61. Kashiwabuchi RT, de Freitas D, Alvarenga LS, Vieira L. Corneal graft survival after therapeutic keratoplasty for Acanthamoeba keratitis. Acta Ophthalmol. 2008;86:666-9.
62. Lindquist TD. Treatment of Acanthamoeba keratitis. Cornea. 1998;17:11-6.
63. Awwad ST, Parmar DN, Heilman M, Bowman RW, McCulley JP, Cavanagh HD. Results of penetrating keratoplasty for visual rehabilitation after Acanthamoeba keratitis. Am J Ophthalmol. 2005;140(6):1080-4.
64. Robaei D, Carnt N, Minassian DC, Dart JK. Therapeutic and optical keratoplasty in the management of Acanthamoeba keratitis: risk factors, outcomes, and summary of the literature. Ophthalmology. 2015;122(1):17-24.
65. Kitzmann AS, Goins KM, Sutphin JE, Wagoner MD. Keratoplasty for treatment of Acanthamoeba keratitis. Ophthalmology. 2009;116(5):864-9.
66. Bouheraoua N, Gaujoux T, Goldschmidt P, Chaumeil C, Laroche L, Borderie VM. Prognostic factors associated with the need for surgical treatments in acanthamoeba keratitis. Cornea. 2013;32(2):130-6.
67. Langston R, Pavan-Langston D, Dohlman CH. Penetrating keratoplasty for herpetic keratitis. Trans Am Acad Ophthalmol Otolaryngol. 1975;79:577.
68. Barney NP, Foster CS. A prospective randomized trial of oral acyclovir after penetrating keratoplasty for herpes simplex keratitis. Cornea. 1994;13:232-6.
69. Akova YA, Onat M, Duman S. Efficacy of low-dose and long-term oral acyclovir therapy after penetrating keratoplasty for herpes simplex keratitis. Ocul Immunol Inflamm. 1999;7:51-60.
70. Cobo LM, Coster DJ, Rice NS, Jones BR. Prognosis and management of corneal transplantation for herpetic keratitis. Arch Ophthalmol. 1980;98:1755-9.
71. Ficker LA, Kirkness CM, Rice NS, Steele AD. Changing management and improved prognosis for corneal grafting and herpes simplex keratitis. Ophthalmology. 1989;96:1587-96.
72. Tanure MA, Cohen EJ, Grewal S, Rapuano CJ, Laibson PR. Penetrating keratoplasty for varicella-zoster virus keratopathy. Cornea. 2000;19:135-9.
73. Liebman SD. Ocular manifestations of Riley-Day syndrome; familial dysautonomic dysfunction. AMA Arch Ophthalmol. 1956;56:719-25.
74. Wilson SAK. Progressive lenticular degeneration: a familial nervous disease associated with cirrhosis of the liver. Brain. 1912;34:295-507.

75. Alper MG. The anesthetic eye: an investigation of changes in the anterior ocular segment of the monkey caused by interrupting the trigeminal nerve of various levels along its course. Trans Am Ophthalmol Soc. 1975;73:323-65.
76. Sweet WH, Wepsic JG. Controlled thermocoagulation of trigeminal ganglion and rootlets for differential destruction of pain fibers. 1. Trigeminal neuralgia. J Neurosurg. 1974;40:143-56.
77. Gundersen T. Herpes corneae: with special reference to its treatment with strong solution of iodine. Arch Ophthalmol. 1936;12:225-49.
78. Straus SE. Clinical and biological differences between recurrent herpes simplex virus and varicella-zoster virus infections. JAMA. 1989;262:3455-8.
79. Auran JD, Starr MD, Jakobiec FA. Acanthamoeba keratitis. A review of the literature. Cornea. 1987;6:2-26.
80. Perry HD, Donnenfeld ED, Foulks GN, Moadel K, Kanellopoulos AJ. Decreased corneal sensation as an initial feature of Acanthamoeba keratitis. Ophthalmology. 1995;102:1565-8.
81. Wilhelmus KR. Acanthamoeba keratitis. In: Smolin G, Thoft RA (Eds). The Cornea. Boston: Little Brown; 1994. pp. 262-6.
82. Zagelbaum BM, Donnenfeld ED, Perry HD, Buxton J, Buxton D, Hersh PS. Corneal ulcer caused by combined intravenous and anesthetic abuse of cocaine. Am J Ophthalmol. 1993;116:241-2.
83. Rexed B, Rexed V. Degeneration and regeneration of corneal nerves. Br J Ophthalmol. 1951;35:38-49.
84. Mathers WD, Jester JV, Lemp MA. Return of human corneal sensitivity after penetrating keratoplasty. Arch Ophthalmol. 1988;106:210-1.
85. Foster CS. Corneal manifestations of neurologic disease. In: Smolin G, Thoft RA (Eds). The Cornea. Boston: Little Brown; 1994. pp. 488-9.
86. Donnenfeld ED, Perry HD, Schrier A, Zagelbaum B, Rodgers R. Lid imbrication syndrome. Diagnosis with rose bengal staining. Ophthalmology. 1994;101:763-6.
87. Donzis PB, Mondino BS. Management of non-infectious corneal ulcers. Surv Ophthalmol. 1987;32:94-110.
88. Pster RR, Murphy GG. Corneal ulceration and perforation associated with Sjögren's syndrome. Arch Ophthalmol. 1980;98:89-94.
89. Jones DB. Prospects in the management of tear-deficiency states. Trans Sect Ophthalmol Am Acad Ophthalmol Otolaryngol. 1977;83:693-70.
90. Ralph RA. Conjunctival goblet cell density in normal subjects and in dry eye syndromes. Invest Ophthalmol. 1975;14:299-302.
91. Ormerod LD, Fong LP, Foster CS. Corneal infection in mucosal scarring disorder and Sjögren's syndrome. Am J Ophthalmol. 1988;105:512-8.
92. Howard GM. The Stevens-Johnson syndrome. Ocular prognosis and treatment. Am J Ophthalmol. 1963;55:893-900.
93. Potz A. Ocular involvement in erythema multiforme. Arch Ophthalmol. 1950;43:244-56.
94. Donnenfeld ED, Ingraham HJ, Abramson DH. Effects of ionizing radiation on the conjunctiva, cornea and lens. In: Sagerman RH, Alberti WE (Eds). Radiotherapy of Intraocular and Orbital tumors(Medical Radiology/Radiation Oncology). Germany: Springer-Verlag; 1993. pp. 261-70.
95. Pster RR. The effect of chemical injury on the ocular surface. Ophthalmology. 1983;90:601-9.
96. Speaker MG, Menikoff JA. Prophylaxis of endophthalmitis with topical povidone iodine. Ophthalmology. 1991;98:1769-75.
97. Foulks GN. Glaucoma associated with penetrating keratoplasty. Ophthalmology. 1987;94:871-4.
98. Donnenfeld ED, Schrier A, Perry HD, Aulicino T, Gombert ME, Snyder R. Penetration of topically applied ciprofloxacin, norfloxacin, and ofloxacin into the aqueous humor. Ophthalmology. 1994;101:902-5.
99. Capella JA, Kaufman, HE, Robbins JE. Preservation of viable corneal tissue. Arch Ophthalmol. 1965;74:669-73.
100. Eastcott HH, Gross AG, Leigh AG, North DP. Preservation of corneal grafts by freezing. Lancet. 1954;266:237-9.
101. Mueller FO, Casey TA, Trevor-Roper PD. Use of deep frozen human cornea in full thickness grafts. Br Med J. 1964;2:473.
102. Yoo SH, Kymionis GD, Koreishi A, Ide T, Goldman D, Karp CL, et al. Femtosecond laser-assisted sutureless anterior lamellar keratoplasty. Ophthalmology. 2008;115:1303-7, 1307.e1.
103. Farid M, Kim M, Steinert RF. Results of penetrating keratoplasty performed with a femtosecond laser zigzag incision initial report. Ophthalmology. 2007;114:2208-12.
104. Hessburg PC, Barron M. A disposable corneal trephine. Ophthalmic Surg. 1980;11:730-3.
105. Cohen EJ, Buchanan HN, Laughrea PA, Adams CP, Galentine PG, Visvesvara GS, et al. Diagnosis and management of Acanthamoeba keratitis. Am J Ophthalmol. 1985;100:389-95.
106. Ang M, Mehta JS, Arundhati A, Tan DT. Anterior lamellar keratoplasty over penetrating keratoplasty for optical, therapeutic, and tectonic indications: A case series. Am J Ophthalmol. 2009; 147:697-702.e2.
107. Donnenfeld ED, Perry HD, Nelson DB. Cyanoacrylate temporary tarsorrhaphy in the management of corneal epithelial defects. Ophthalmic Surg. 1991;22:591-3.
108. Moore MB, McCulley JP. Acanthamoeba keratitis associated with contact lenses. Six consecutive cases of successful management. Br J Ophthalmol. 1989;73:271-5.
109. Stern GA, Buttrosski H. Use of corticosteroids in combination with antimicrobial drugs in the treatment of infectious corneal disease. Ophthalmology 1991;98:847-53.

44 Shaped Penetrating Keratoplasty

Priyadarshini K, Bhavana Sharma, Namrata Sharma, Rasik B Vajpayee

INTRODUCTION

Since the evolution of penetrating keratoplasty, there has been an emphasis on optimizing the graft-host junction to improve the anatomical as well as the functional outcomes. Shaped keratoplasty techniques use circular or noncircular grafts with complex graft-host junction morphology, in order to enhance their tensile strength. The advantages of performing shaped grafts over regular grafts are as follows:[1-6]

- Increased wound strength
- Accelerated wound healing
- Early suture removal and visual rehabilitation
- Improved refractive outcomes
- Reduced rates of graft rejection

Obtaining grafts with complex wound designs while maintaining the integrity of graft-host junction can be challenging. Any minor decentration or vertical tilt during manual trephination at the time of donor preparation can lead to suboptimal visual outcomes caused by astigmatism.[7,8] Non-contact laser assisted trephination has helped to overcome the drawbacks of manual trephination. Following are the advantages of laser-assisted trephination over conventional manual trephination.

- Accurate construction of surgical wounds[7,9]
- Reduced risk of horizontal torsion[10]
- Expanded range of graft designs with complex wound architecture without compromising the congruency of graft-host junction.

Various patterns of shaped penetrating keratoplasty based on the configuration of graft-host junction have been described below.

TOP-HAT KERATOPLASTY

First described by Busin et al. in 2003, it consists of a small anterior stromal button with a large posterior stromal endothelial disk, which is separated by a stepped lamellar incision.[11] This gives an appearance of a "top-hat" (TH), and hence the nomenclature (**Fig. 1A**).

Indications

Endothelial diseases such as Fuchs' endothelial corneal dystrophy and bullous keratopathy in association with stromal scarring.

Donor Preparation

A partial thickness trephination is done from the epithelial surface, following which a lamellar dissection from the trephined edge to the limbus is performed. A trephine of larger diameter is then used to perform a full thickness trephination from the endothelial surface.

Recipient Bed Preparation

This is done using femtosecond laser for greater precision and reduction of surgical time.

Surgical Modification

A half-TH modification has been described by Kaiserman et al., wherein the same size trephine, which is used for the preparation of anterior corneal button is also used for the full-thickness trephination of host cornea.[12] This brings the lamellar wings of the graft in contact with the posterior surface of the host cornea. The visual outcomes using both techniques have been found to be comparable.[12] However, it might have the advantage of obtaining a better graft-host junction apposition.

Advantages

- Increased mechanical stability, due to stepped pattern of the graft edge
- Early suture removal at 3–7 months promoting faster visual rehabilitation and lesser suture-related complications[1]
- Reduced rates of graft rejection.[1]

Disadvantages

Descemet membrane folds and postoperative wound leak due to graft-host junction mismatch can occur, which can be addressed using femtolaser-assisted technique.[12]

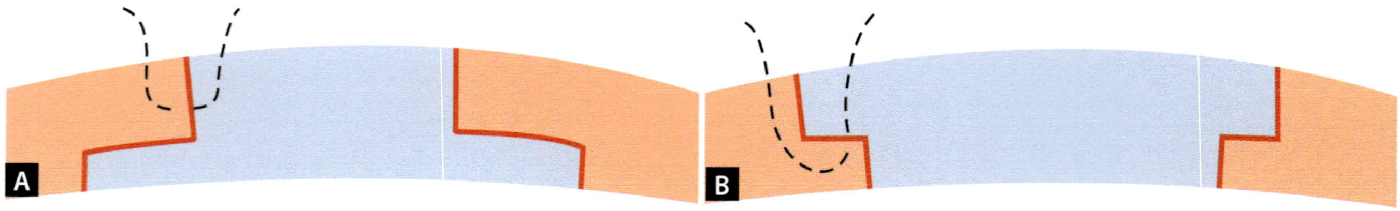

Figs. 1A and B: (A) Schematic diagram of a top-hat keratoplasty; (B) Schematic diagram of a mushroom keratoplasty.

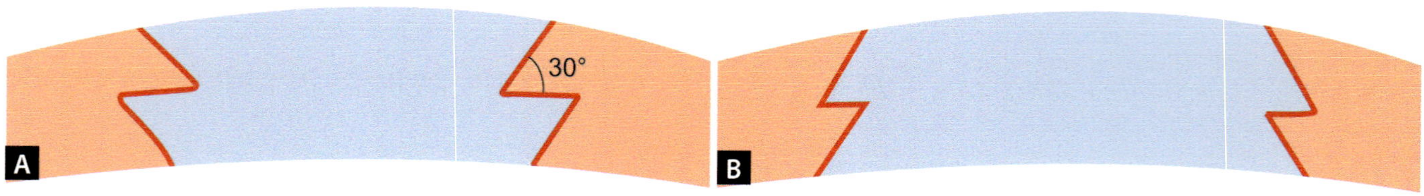

Figs. 2A and B: (A) A schematic representation of zigzag keratoplasty; (B) A schematic representation of Christmas tree keratoplasty.

MUSHROOM KERATOPLASTY

Described by Franceschetti et al. in 1951, this type of corneal graft has a large anterior stromal disk (lesser postoperative astigmatism) with a small posterior stalk (reduced risk of graft rejection).[13] It is a graft with inverse configuration compared that of a TH-keratoplasty (**Fig. 1B**).

Indications

Deep stromal corneal opacities, keratoconus with hydrops, postinfectious keratitis sequelae or chemical burns in which deep anterior lamellar keratoplasty (DALK) can be challenging.

Donor Preparation

A partial thickness trephination followed by centripetal lamellar dissection of 2 mm is made. The full thickness button is then removed by dissecting through the posterior stroma and endothelial layers.

The graft can also be made using microkeratome wherein the anterior and posterior lamellae are punched with a 9 and 5 mm trephine, respectively. Both are then secured at the recipient bed and the anterior graft is sutured.

Recipient Bed Preparation

It is prepared in a manner, similar to that of the donor tissue.[14] Femtosecond and excimer lasers can also be used for the preparation of recipient bed.[15,16]

Advantages

- Reduced rates of postoperative astigmatism (2.8 D vs. 3.9 D—M-PK vs. PK)[4]
- Reduced rates of graft rejection (7.7% vs. 9.1%—M-PK vs. PK)[4]
- Reduced endothelial cell loss (32.1% vs. 38.7%—M-PK vs. PK)[4]

Disadvantages[13,14,16]

- Posterior button detachment
- Microcystic edema overlying the lamellar interface
- Protrusion of anterior lamella between sutures

ZIGZAG KERATOPLASTY

In this type of keratoplasty, the corneal graft has a multi-level, stepped edge and a corresponding shaped recipient bed, so that the graft-host junction is interlocked together, achieving higher wound stability due to a larger surface area of graft-host interface[17] (**Fig. 2A**).

Indications

Corneal ectatic disorders, corneal scarring, bullous keratopathy, Fuchs' endothelial corneal dystrophy.

Donor Preparation

Femtosecond laser is used for donor preparation. Using femtosecond laser, multiple angular incisions are made at 30° angle, with intervening horizontal steps.

Recipient Bed Preparation

Femtosecond laser is used for host preparation as well by making angular incisions complementing with that of donor button incisions.

A modification of this technique has been reported experimentally which has an inverted zigzag configuration, termed as Christmas tree keratoplasty[18] (**Fig. 2B**).

Advantages

- Better visual acuity in comparison to penetrating keratoplasty[19]
- Faster visual recovery

- Reduced postoperative astigmatism[19]
- Reduced suture tension required in wound apposition.[20]

Disadvantage

Requirement of femtosecond laser, leading to higher cost of the procedure.

TUCK-IN PENETRATING KERATOPLASTY

Described by Vajpayee et al. in 2005, the donor button contains a full thickness graft centrally with a peripheral flange consisting of deep stroma and endothelium, which is tucked intrastromally in the recipient bed.[6] This gives the combined advantage of a penetrating keratoplasty with the wound strength of a lamellar procedure (**Fig. 3**).

Indication

Keratoglobus with concurrent endothelial dysfunction.

Donor Preparation

A partial thickness trephination is performed which is followed by a peripheral lamellar dissection, excising the peripheral superficial corneal tissue. A full thickness trephination is then performed the endothelial side using a large size trephine to the graft.

Recipient Bed Preparation

Partial thickness trephination is followed by creation of an intrastromal pocket extending up to the limbus. The central host button is then excised. Following this, the donor is placed on the recipient bed and the peripheral flange is tucked into the stromal pocket. The donor is then sutured to the host using full thickness corneal sutures.

Advantages

- Faster healing due to wound configuration
- Early suture removal and reduced suture-related complications

Disadvantage

Full thickness corneal suture can act as conduit for infection into the anterior chamber. However, it has not been reported yet in the literature.

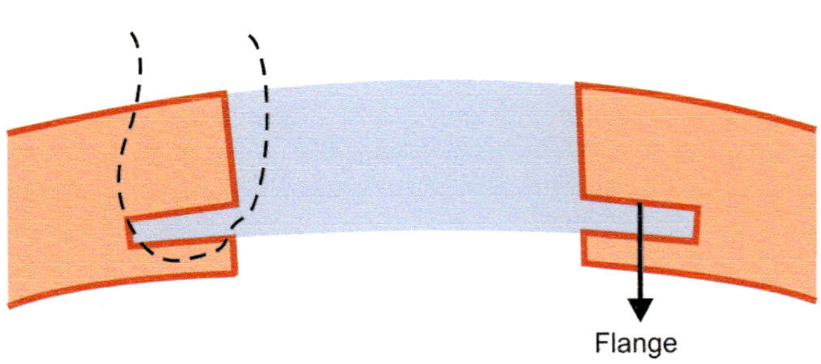

Fig. 3: A schematic representation of tuck-in penetrating keratoplasty.

OTHER CONFIGURATIONS OF GRAFT-HOST JUNCTION

Dovetail Keratoplasty

In this technique described by Lee et al., femtosecond laser is used to create an initial vertical side cut followed by a lamellar cut and an oblique posterior side cut in the host cornea, with a complementary configuration in the donor.[21] Thus, it gives the graft-host junction a tongue and groove configuration providing greater graft stability (**Fig. 4A**).

Anvil-profiled Grafts

Femtosecond laser is used to cut the anterior face of the graft at 135° after which a ring lamellar incision is made, which is then completed by cutting the posterior face at 90° (**Fig. 4B**).[22]

TECHNIQUES OF NONCIRCULAR CORNEAL TRANSPLANTATION

The techniques described above have a circular graft with different configurations at the graft-host junction. However, in certain circumstances, there is a prerequisite for noncircular grafts. These are diseases involving the peripheral cornea, such as, Terrien's marginal degeneration, pellucid marginal degeneration, and peripheral ulcerative keratitis. This is done to avoid using large diameter grafts in these conditions, which can result in increased risk of graft rejection. The various techniques of performing noncircular penetrating keratoplasty are as follows.

Plastic Drape Template Technique

This is indicated in cases of peripheral inflammatory corneal ulceration or perforation to preserve the healthy tissue. A plastic drape material is used to make a template of the area to be resected in the host. This is used to resect the desired host tissue and then the donor tissue accordingly using freehand technique.[23]

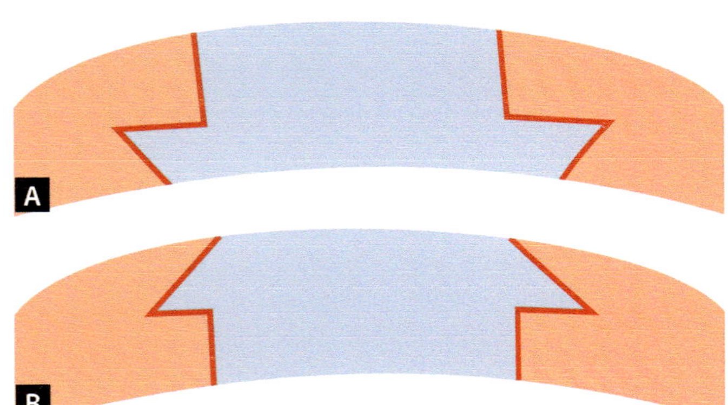

Figs. 4A and B: (A) A schematic representation of dovetail keratoplasty; (B) A schematic representation of anvil-profiled keratoplasty.

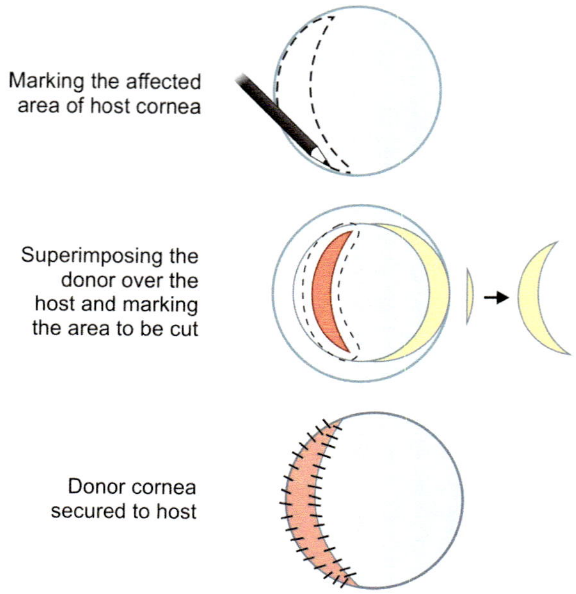

Fig. 5: A schematic diagram representing the copy and fix technique of noncircular grafts.

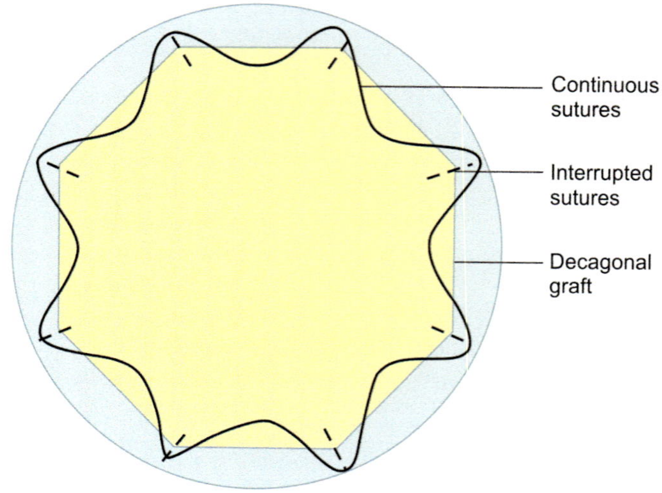

Fig. 6: A schematic diagram of decagonal keratoplasty with combined use of interrupted and continuous sutures.

Copy and Fix Technique

Described by Samarawickrama et al., it allows precise preparation of freehand-horseshoe tectonic grafts. The extent of corneal involvement is marked. The donor is then superimposed over the host bed and the defect is then outlined in the donor cornea, which is then cut freehand (**Fig. 5**).[24]

Print and Prick Keratoplasty

Similar to the copy and fix technique, a 26-G needle is used to mark an outline of the host tissue defect on a superimposed plastic sheet before cutting it. The sheet is used as a template to prepare the donor cornea.[25]

Decagonal Keratoplasty

Reported by Proust et al., it was done in cases of Fuchs' endothelial corneal dystrophy, bullous keratopathy, corneal amyloidosis, and keratoconus.[26] Femtosecond laser is used to create a decagonal-shaped incision in the host as well as the donor cornea. The short-term visual and refractive results of the procedure are encouraging. However, it lacks long-term data and hence, is not widely performed (**Fig. 6**).

CONCLUSION

The advent of shaped penetrating keratoplasty procedures opens up a wide range of treatment options for various corneal diseases, tailored to the needs of the patient. Though these procedures carry the advantage of better visual outcomes with faster visual rehabilitation and increased wound strength, the techniques require surgical expertise and hence a longer learning curve. The need for femtosecond laser for better precision limits the use of certain techniques in all clinical settings, due to its cost and equipment constraints. Comparative studies between various techniques show a lot of heterogeneity, the superiority of one technique over the others is not clearly documented. With further research, a more comprehensive data about these techniques might be available in the future to recommend these procedures with better affirmation.

REFERENCES

1. Bahar I, Kaiserman I, Srinivasan S, Berger Y, McAllum P, Slomovic A, et al. Manual top hat wound configuration for penetrating keratoplasty. Cornea. 2008;27:521-6.
2. Fung SSM, Aiello F, Maurino V. Outcomes of femtosecond laser-assisted mushroom configuration keratoplasty in advanced keratoconus. Eye. 2016;30:553-61.
3. Kaushal S, Jhanji V, Sharma N, Tandon R, Titiyal JS, Vajpayee RB. "Tuck in" lamellar keratoplasty (TILK) for corneal ectasias involving corneal periphery. Br J Ophthalmol. 2008;92:286-90.
4. Levinger E, Trivizki O, Levinger S, Kremer I. Outcome of "mushroom" pattern femtosecond laser-assisted keratoplasty versus conventional penetrating keratoplasty in patients with keratoconus. Cornea. 2014;33:481-5.
5. Maier P, Böhringer D, Birnbaum F, Reinhard T. Improved wound stability of top-hat profiled femtosecond laser-assisted penetrating keratoplasty in vitro. Cornea. 2012;31:963-6.
6. Vajpayee RB, Sharma N, Bhartiya P, Agarwal T, Tandon R, Titiyal JS. Central penetrating keratoplasty with peripheral intrastromal tuck. Cornea. 2005;24:947-50.
7. Seitz B, Langenbucher A, Naumann GO. [Perspectives of excimer laser-assisted keratoplasty]. Ophthalmologe. 2011;108:817-24.
8. Krumeich J, Binder PS, Knulle A. The theoretical effect of trephine tilt on postkeratoplasty astigmatism. CLAO J. 1988;14:213-9.
9. Seitz B, Langenbucher A, Kus MM, Küchle M, Naumann GO. Nonmechanical corneal trephination with the excimer laser improves outcome after penetrating keratoplasty. Ophthalmology. 1999;106:1156-64; discussion 1165.
10. Behrens A, Seitz B, Küchle M, Langenbucher A, Kus MM, Rummelt C, et al. "Orientation teeth" in non-mechanical laser corneal trephination for penetrating keratoplasty: 2.94 microm Er:YAG v 193 nm ArF excimer laser. Br J Ophthalmol. 1999;83:1008-12.
11. Busin M. A new lamellar wound configuration for penetrating keratoplasty surgery. Arch Ophthalmol. 2003;121:260-5.

12. Kaiserman I, Bahar I, Slomovic AR, Rootman DS. Half top hat wound configuration for penetrating keratoplasty: 1-year results. Br J Ophthalmol. 2009;93:1629-33.
13. Franceschetti A. [Combined lamellar and perforant keratoplasty (mushroom graft)]. Bull Schweiz Akad Med Wiss. 1951;7:134-45.
14. Roberts RW. The mushroom graft. Trans Am Acad Ophthalmol Otolaryngol. 1961;65:913-8.
15. Elkamshoushy A, Gonnah R, Madi S, Beltz J. Single-piece femtosecond-assisted mushroom keratoplasty in children. J AAPOS. 2019;23:28.e1-28.e5.
16. Della Valle V, Bonci P. Excimer laser mushroom penetrating keratoplasty: new technique. Eur J Ophthalmol. 2014;24:186-90.
17. Shehadeh Mashor R, Bahar I, Rootman DB, Kumar NL, Singal N, Slomovic AR, et al. Zig zag versus top hat configuration in intraLase-enabled penetrating keratoplasty. Br J Ophthalmol. 2014;98:756-9.
18. Bahar I, Kaiserman I, Srinivasan S, Ya-Ping J, Slomovic AR, Rootman DS. Comparison of three different techniques of corneal transplantation for keratoconus. Am J Ophthalmol. 2008;146:905-12.e1.
19. Farid M, Steinert RF, Gaster RN, Chamberlain W, Lin A. Comparison of penetrating keratoplasty performed with a femtosecond laser zig-zag incision versus conventional blade trephination. Ophthalmology. 2009;116:1638-43.
20. Shumway CL, Aggarwal S, Farid M, Muniz-Castro H, Jarstad A, Garg S, et al. Penetrating keratoplasty using the femtosecond laser: a comparison of postoperative visual acuity and astigmatism by suture pattern. Cornea. 2018;37:1490-6.
21. Lee J, Winokur J, Hallak J, Azar DT. Femtosecond dovetail penetrating keratoplasty: surgical technique and case report. Br J Ophthalmol. 2009;93:861-3.
22. Menabuoni L, Canovetti A, Rossi F, Malandrini A. The 'anvil' profile in femtosecond laser-assisted penetrating keratoplasty. Acta Ophthalmol. 2013;91:e494-5.
23. Bessant DA, Dart JK. Lamellar keratoplasty in the management of inflammatory corneal ulceration and perforation. Eye (Lond). 1994;8 (Pt 1):22-8.
24. Samarawickrama C, Goh R, Vajpayee RB. "Copy and fix": a new technique of harvesting freehand and horseshoe tectonic grafts. Cornea. 2015;34:1519-22.
25. Parmar GS, Ghodke B, Bose S, Meena AK. Stenciling-based "prick and print" technique for harvesting shaped corneal grafts for management of peripheral corneal perforations. Cornea. 2019;38:105-9.
26. Proust H, Baeteman C, Matonti F, Conrath J, Ridings B, Hoffart L. Femtosecond laser-assisted decagonal penetrating keratoplasty. Am J Ophthalmol. 2011;151:29-34.

45

Noncircular Corneal Transplantation

Rashmi Deshmukh, Louis J Stevenson, Rasik B Vajpayee

INTRODUCTION

Surgical management of peripheral corneal pathologies poses several challenges. Peripheral corneal melting and perforation is not uncommon in conditions such as Mooren's ulcer, pellucid marginal degeneration (PMD), Terrien's marginal degeneration (TMD), and peripheral ulcerative keratitis (PUK). Tectonic or therapeutic corneal grafting in these situations would require a very large or eccentric circular graft. This results in unnecessary excision of healthy, unaffected corneal tissue. Moreover, these grafts are also more prone to rejection,[1] and if eccentric, can produce severe astigmatism or require sutures in the visual axis.[2]

Noncircular corneal transplantation techniques have been developed to manage peripheral corneal melting and perforations by creating corneal grafts of corresponding shape and size. These procedures have the advantage of resecting just the affected part of the cornea, and leaving behind the central and largely unaffected cornea. Failure or rejection of such grafts is less likely to affect the patient's visual acuity (VA) as well.

PERIPHERAL CORNEAL DISORDERS

Mooren's Ulcer

Mooren's ulcer is a chronic, severe, painful, peripheral ulceration of the cornea that tends to progress circumferentially and centrally. Scleritis is characteristically absent and there is no association with systemic diseases.[3] Patients usually present with a red, painful eye, intense photophobia and watering. Corneal ulceration typically begins peripherally in the interpalpebral area and then progresses circumferentially and centrally. There is a characteristic undermining of the central ulcerated area giving the edge of the ulcer an "overhanging" appearance.[4]

Wood and Kaufman classified Mooren's ulcer into two types, based on clinical presentation and prognosis:[5]

- *Type I*: Benign type is usually unilateral. It is seen in older patients and they have mild to moderate symptoms. This type of ulcer responds well to treatment.
- *Type II*: Seen in younger individuals and is bilateral. The symptoms are more severe and it responds poorly to treatment. This type is considered as the malignant type of ulcer.

Clinically, Mooren's ulcer is graded by the severity of corneal disease:[4]

- *Grade I*: Corneal thinning in one or more quadrants. Subdivided into: (a) mild: thinning of up to 25% of the corneal circumference; (b) moderate: thinning of 25–50% of the corneal circumference; and (c) severe: thinning of >50% of the corneal circumference.
- *Grade II*: Impending corneal perforation.
- *Grade III*: Perforation >2 mm in size.

The rate of perforation following Mooren's ulcer has been reported to be ranging from 7 to 36%.[6-8] Perforations in these cases are typically peripheral and irregular, with the central cornea unaffected.

Initial management includes topical or systemic immunosuppressive agents such as steroids, cyclosporin, and tacrolimus. Additional interventions such as conjunctival resection might be needed to halt the stromal melt. Despite these efforts, corneal perforation can occur necessitating lamellar or penetrating keratoplasty.[9]

Terrien's Marginal Degeneration

Terrien's marginal degeneration is a slowly progressive, peripheral corneal ectatic disease, which initially affects the superior or superonasal cornea and progresses circumferentially.[10,11] It is more commonly seen above the age of 40 years and affects men more commonly than women.[11] Although the disease is bilateral, presentation could be asymmetric.[11] Patients usually remain asymptomatic until corneal thinning causes corneal astigmatism and subsequent decrease in vision.[12,13]

Clinically, TMD progresses through five stages:[14]

- *Stage I*: Peripheral corneal opacification resembling gerontoxon, associated with vascularization.
- *Stage II*: Corneal thinning commences marked by an indentation parallel to the limbus.

- *Stage III*: Progressive corneal thinning and beginning of corneal ectasia. This stage is limited to the peripheral cornea and may continue for years. Complications such as corneal perforations and iris prolapse may occur.
- *Stage IV*: Ectasia progresses centrally similar to keratoconus.
- *Stage V*: Central cornea becomes opacified. This stage is rarely seen as patients present earlier due to advanced ectasia or perforation.

Terrien's marginal degeneration is known to progress very slowly;[13] however, around 1.68 D of astigmatism has been reported within 3 years of diagnosis.[15] As corneal thinning begins superiorly, astigmatism is typically against-the-rule.[12] Early stages of disease may be associated with atypical pterygia or pseudopterygia appearing at locations other than the usual 3 and 9 o'clock.[16] A steeply sloped leading edge is seen with a relatively gentle slope on the posterior lip. There is an uninvolved area of cornea between the limbus and the area of stromal thinning. Lipid deposition and vascularization often accompanies stromal thinning.[17] Around 11–15% cases are known to perforate with most perforations located in the superior cornea[13,15] and minimum accompanying symptoms.[12]

The cause of TMD remains unknown. It is thought to be a degenerative process due to a lack of inflammatory signs, bilaterality, and slow progression. However, TMD has been associated with several systemic and ocular inflammatory diseases including rheumatoid arthritis,[18] erythema elevatum diutinum,[19] vernal keratoconjunctivitis,[20] posterior polymorphous corneal dystrophy,[21] lattice corneal dystrophy,[22] and deep episcleritis.[13]

Terrien's marginal degeneration has been classified into two types: (1) inflammatory and (2) quiescent,[23] younger patients being more often affected by the inflammatory subtype.[24,25] Clinical signs of inflammation, stromal infiltration, and cellularity are seen[10] in addition to activated keratocytes on confocal microscopy.[17]

Patients having visual symptoms alone can be managed conservatively with spectacles/contact lenses to correct astigmatism. Surgical management in the form of corneal lamellar keratoplasties, amniotic membrane transplantation, and conjunctival flaps may be needed in severe corneal thinning.[12] Small perforations may be amenable to treatment with corneal glue while tectonic patch grafts are needed for larger perforations.[26]

Peripheral Ulcerative Keratitis

Peripheral ulcerative keratitis is characterized by progressive, crescent-shaped, stromal degradation, and thinning, accompanied by an epithelial defect within 2 mm of the limbus. Involvement of adjacent conjunctiva, episclera and sclera may predispose to rapid stromal melt and corneal perforation.[27,28] The juxtalimbal cornea is particularly susceptible to immune-mediated ulcerative keratitis. This could be due to the proximity to the vascular and lymphatic arcades of the limbus[29] allowing deposition of immune complexes, and activation of the complement system mobilizing inflammatory cells into the area.[30] These inflammatory cells release collagenases leading to stromal thinning and melt.[31]

Approximately 50% of cases are associated with collagen vascular disease, rheumatoid arthritis being the most common.[32,33] Wegener's granulomatosis, relapsing polychondritis, systemic lupus erythematosus (SLE), polyarteritis nodosa and Churg-Strauss syndrome are the other common autoimmune associations.[33] Association with infections is not uncommon. Ocular and systemic infection secondary to *Streptococcus* and *Staphylococcus* species, spirochetes (*Treponema pallidum*), acanthamoeba, mycobacteria, fungi, and viruses such as hepatitis C, herpes simplex and herpes zoster have been found to be associated with PUK.[34]

Around 22–47% of the cases might get perforated, depending on the severity, with around 3% of patients with severe disease presenting with impending corneal perforation.[35] Management involves immunosuppressive drugs therapy including glucocorticoids, alkylating agents such as cyclophosphamide or alternative agents such as methotrexate, azathioprine, and mycophenolate mofetil. Conjunctival resection may help reduce localized inflammation adjacent to the cornea and arrest ongoing melt. Small or impending perforations necessitate corneal gluing or keratoplasty procedures depending on the size of the perforation.[32,36]

Pellucid Marginal Degeneration

Pellucid marginal degeneration is a noninflammatory corneal ectasia characterized by peripheral corneal thinning and protrusion of the cornea above the area of maximal thinning. There is a band of unaffected cornea of 1–2 mm from the limbus.[37] The inferior cornea is characteristically affected, however, a variant affecting the superior cornea exists.[38] Patients usually present between second and fifth decade of life and males are more commonly affected.[39,40]

Clinically, patients present with an against-the-rule astigmatism causing gradual progressive decrease in vision.[37] Rarely, patients may develop hydrops or corneal perforation causing acute pain and sudden loss of vision.[41-43] Examination shows a 1–2 mm wide, clear band of corneal thinning, with a protruding cornea superior to the thinned out area,[39,44] and a characteristic "crab-claw" pattern on corneal topography.[45]

Most cases are managed by contact lenses alone, although nearly 10–15% cases require surgical intervention.[46] Lamellar crescentic resection,[47] corneal wedge resection,[48] and tuck-in lamellar keratoplasty[49] have all been described in the management of advanced cases. Corneal perforations are managed with tissue adhesives and bandage contact lenses, however, eccentric keratoplasties may be performed in case where conservative management fails.[50]

SURGICAL TECHNIQUES

Eyes suffering from the peripheral corneal thinning and perforations might require tectonic grafts to maintain ocular integrity. Various surgical techniques have been described to achieve noncircular host dissection and harvest matched donor corneal grafts to manage peripheral corneal pathology.

Plastic Drape Template for Shaped Grafts

Bessant and Dart described this technique in 1994, for harvesting unusually shaped grafts for tectonic keratoplasty.[51] The area to be excised is first marked on the recipient cornea and a surgical drape is used to create a matching with the marked area. A superficial incision made along the marked outline on the recipient cornea. This incision is then progressed to the desired depth using a stepped diamond knife. The drape template is used to harvest a donor graft of a similar shape to match the excised area on the host cornea. This technique is effective at providing tectonic support and maintaining globe integrity, although two cases out of the 10 reported by the authors, had a disease recurrence necessitating repeat procedure. Visual outcomes are impaired due to surface irregularity and lipid deposition postoperatively.

Crescentic Lamellar Keratoplasty

Crescentic lamellar keratoplasty was first described by Schanzlin et al. in the management of PMD.[52] A crescent-shaped area is marked to involve the area of thinning. Two trephines of different sizes are used to create a crescent-shaped recipient bed and excise the marked tissue. A donor graft is then fashioned, using corneoscleral scissors, to match the shape of the resected area and the graft sutured in place using 10-0 nylon sutures. Lamellar keratoplasties restore corneal thickness and provide tectonic support and address visually significant astigmatism in cases of peripheral thinning and ectasias.[47,52]

Crescentic Tuck-in Lamellar Keratoplasty

Arora et al. described a modification of above technique and called it crescentic tuck-in lamellar keratoplasty. First, a layer-by-layer lamellar dissection is performed in the area of peripheral thinning followed by creating a subscleral, 2 mm wide groove adjacent to the dissected area. A corresponding peripheral flange is created on the donor tissue by dissecting stromal tissue obliquely, which is then tucked into the subscleral groove. This technique not only provides tectonic support, but also avoids damage to the limbus. In addition, the placement of tight sutures in vertical meridian, helps in dramatic reduction of the astigmatism as well.[53]

Intrastromal Crescentic Lamellar Keratoplasty

This technique involves creating an intrastromal pocket in the host cornea and inserting crescentic-shaped donor tissue into it.[54] The diseased area is delineated using a dermographic pen. A 200-mm diamond knife is used to create a 2-mm long, partial thickness radial incision. An intrastromal pocket is created at a depth of approximately 50% of the corneal thickness. Corneal epithelium and endothelium is removed from the donor cornea which is then cut to match the shape of the host bed. The crescent-shaped donor corneal stroma is then inserted into the intrastromal recipient pocket and the radial incision is sutured. In the initial report, postoperative astigmatism was reduced from 5.5–4.4 D up to 3 months postoperatively, after which, refraction stabilized.

This technique preserves the limbus and avoids corneal vascularization. It also reduces the risk of endothelial graft rejection and the use of a single corneal suture helps to decrease postoperative astigmatism. The authors also suggest that as the thickness of the inferior cornea is increased, further management of astigmatism is possible using laser ablative procedures.[54]

Sclerocorneal Intrastromal Lamellar Keratoplasty

Sclerocorneal intrastromal lamellar keratoplasty (SILK) is a modification of the intrastromal crescentic lamellar keratoplasty and has been described in the management of PMD.[55] The conjunctiva is reflected, a scleral tunnel created and an intrastromal corneal pocket dissected to the edge of the ectatic tissue. The donor cornea is dissected using a 300-mm microkeratome and the epithelium and endothelium removed before being cut to match the area of recipient corneal thinning. The stromal tissue is then inserted into the intrastromal pocket and the conjunctival flap sutured. In addition to the advantages offered by intrastromal lamella keratoplasty, this technique avoids corneal sutures and therefore has favorable astigmatic outcomes.[55]

Compressive C-shaped Lamellar Keratoplasty

Compressive C-shaped lamellar keratoplasty has been described in the management of advanced PMD and small peripheral corneal perforations.[43,56] Crescentic-shaped donor lamellar tissue is intentionally undersized and tightly sutured in place, creating a compressive effect.

Corneal trephines are used to mark the inner and outer circumference of the ectatic corneal tissue; the desired C-shape completed using a dermatological trephine (**Fig. 1**). A freehand, vertical, partial-thickness incision is then performed using a diamond knife. The donor cornea is then similarly marked and a graft, undersized by 0.25–0.5 mm, obtained and sutured in place.[57] Good postoperative VA and astigmatic results have been reported with this technique. Peripheral vascularization is not typically an issue, however a long-term drift toward against-the-rule astigmatism can occur.[57]

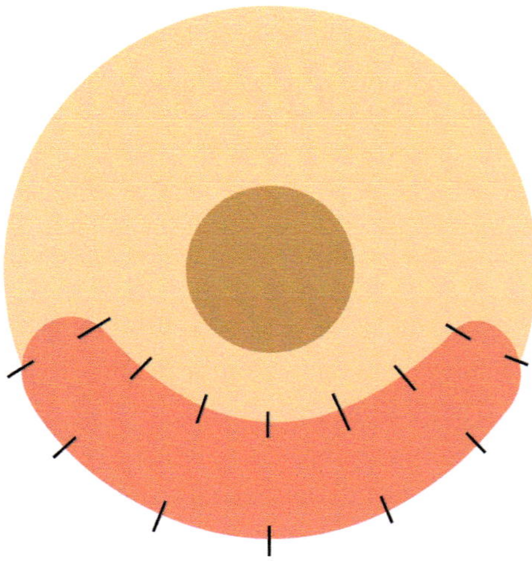

Fig. 1: C-shaped donor corneal lamellar tissue sutured on the recipient bed.

Copy and Fix Technique (Figs. 2A to D)

This technique allows full-thickness or lamellar grafts to be constructed freehand and is therefore useful in creating complex graft patterns for tectonic peripheral keratoplasty.[58] The host cornea is marked and a full-thickness or lamellar freehand incision is performed using a diamond knife followed by corneal scissors or lamellar dissector (**Fig. 2A**). The host corneoscleral tissue is then used as a stencil to trace an outline onto the donor tissue under direct visualization (**Fig. 2B**). Viscoelastic is placed between the donor and the recipient tissue to protect the endothelium. The donor tissue is then mounted on an artificial anterior chamber and a full-thickness or lamellar graft obtained before being sutured in the recipient bed (**Fig. 2C**). The graft can be equally or slightly oversized.

This technique allows the tissues to be precisely matched regardless of location of the pathology (central vs. limbal) or graft type used (lamellar, penetrating, and tuck-in procedures). Additionally, there is minimal requirement for specialized equipment.

This technique was initially described in the management of a corneal perforation secondary to microbial keratitis, and

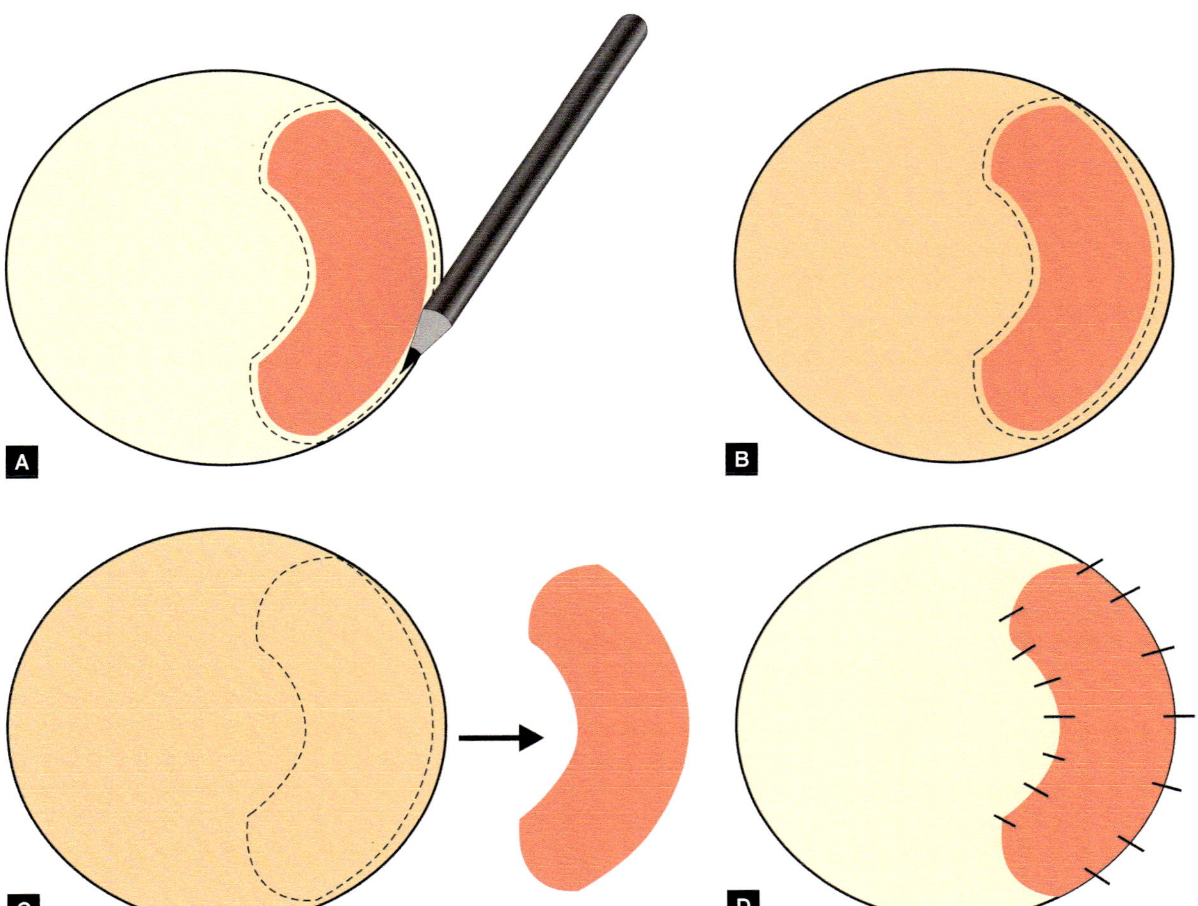

Figs. 2A to D: (A) Diseased area identified and marked on the host cornea using marker pen; (B) Donor corneoscleral rim is placed on the host cornea and the area to be grafted is traced onto the donor tissue with a marker pen; (C) Marked donor tissue is mounted on artificial anterior chamber and graft is harvested; (D) Donor tissue is secured to the recipient bed using interrupted 10-0 nylon sutures.

a patient with bilateral TMD. In the case of the perforation, preservation of healthy corneal, limbal, and scleral tissue was achieved; however, a recurrence of infection in the graft occurred at 3 months. The patient with TMD achieved an improvement in VA from 20/200 to 20/80 with a superior and inferior graft in one eye, with 4.4 D of residual astigmatism. In the fellow eye, the VA improved from 20/400 to 20/60 at 6 months with a superior graft.

Stencilling using the "Prick and Print" Technique

This technique uses a stencil created from a plastic sheet to create a graft.[59] The diseased cornea is first outlined with a marking pen (**Fig. 3A**). A transparent plastic sheet is then placed on the host cornea and the perimeter of the diseased tissue traced using a 26-G needle (**Fig. 3B**) before a 15-degree lancet tip is use to create linear, interrupted slits outside the needle pricks (**Fig. 3C**). The donor corneoscleral tissue is then mounted on an artificial anterior chamber and an imprint created on the graft using the stencil and a marking pen (**Fig. 3D**) before the graft is excised (**Fig. 3E**). The plastic sheet should be thin (approximately 20 µm) so that it conforms to the shape of the cornea. Despite this, an excavated lesion in the extreme periphery may be challenging, as the stencil may not conform adequately. The advantages of this technique include the lack of direct contact between the donor tissue and recipient bed and its applicability to scleral tissue if needed.

Ring-shaped Lamellar Keratoplasty

This technique has been use to manage advanced peripheral corneal thinning secondary to TMD, where tectonic keratoplasty is required.[60] The area of diseased cornea is marked using trephines and the graft is sized such that the inner edge has a margin 0.5-mm smaller than the area of thinning, while the outer edge has a margin of 1.5 mm larger. This results in the recipient bed being 2 mm larger than the graft. A diamond knife is then used to deepen the groove to 80% of the corneal thickness at the inner edge and 30% of the scleral thickness at the outer edge. A ring-shaped outline is achieved and lamellar dissection of the recipient bed is performed. This removes all stromal fibers and exposes Descemet's membrane (**Fig. 4**).

Intraoperative optical coherence tomography (OCT) is used to avoid perforation during dissection of the thinned cornea. A donor graft is obtained from the corresponding area of the corneal button, ensuring a normal postoperative contour. The inner edge of the donor graft is cut to the same size as the recipient bed. In contrast, the outer edge of the donor tissue is cut using a trephine undersized by 0.5 mm.

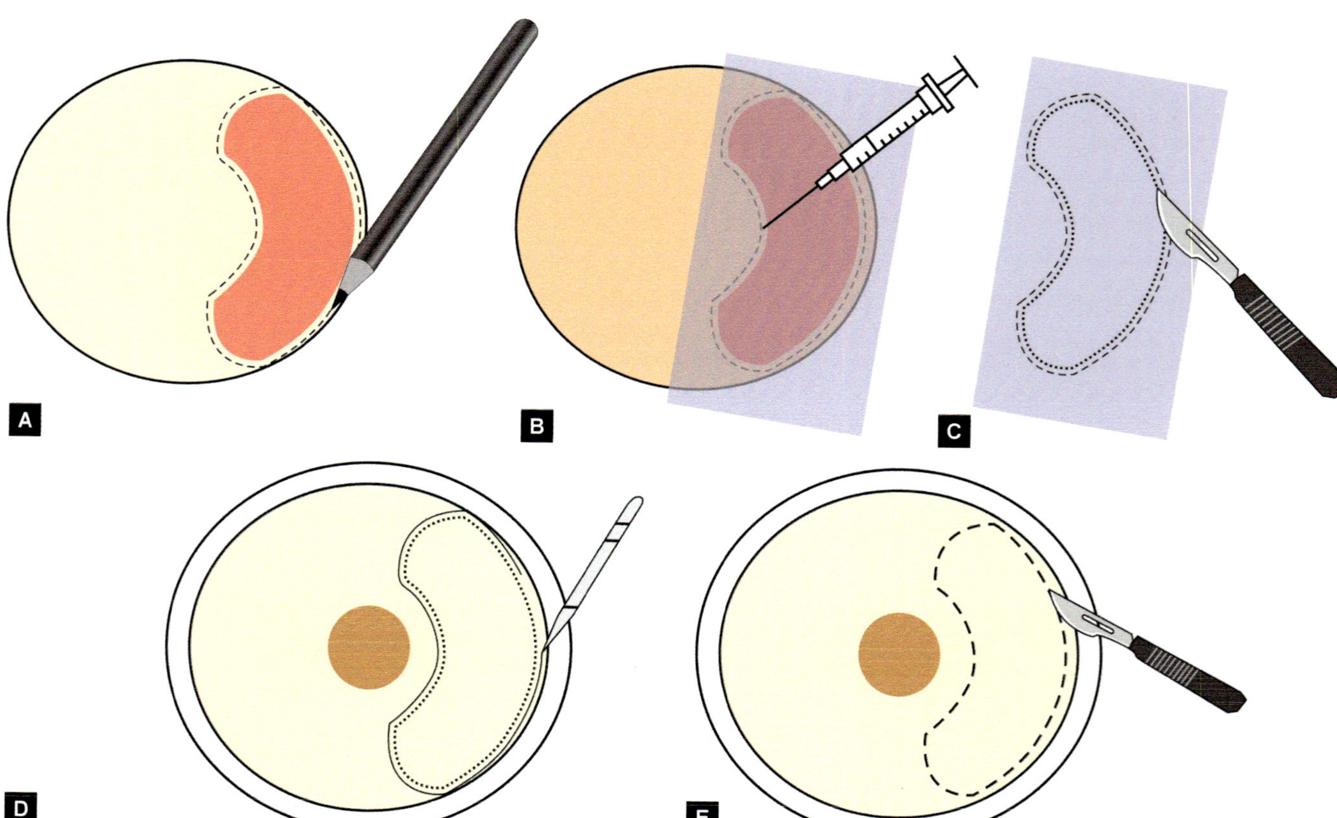

Figs. 3A to E: (A) Host cornea is marked using marker pen; (B) A transparent plastic sheet is placed on host cornea and the shape is traced on the sheet using a 26-G needle to make a "stencil"; (C) Linear, interrupted slits are created just outside the needle pricks using 15-degree blade; (D) Stencil is placed on the donor cornea and marker pen used to create an imprint of the desired shape onto the donor tissue; (E) Donor corneal tissue excised.

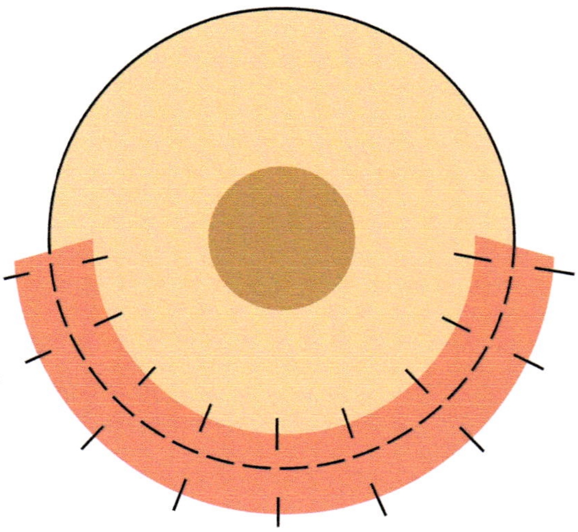

Fig. 4: Ring-shaped area is dissected from the host cornea to bare the Descemet's membrane and donor tissue harvested from the same area in the corneaoscleral rim is sutured to the recipient bed.

Once the graft is cut, Descemet's membrane is stripped. The ring-shaped graft is then fixed in position using interrupted sutures and the tension adjusted using a Placido-disk reflex to minimize astigmatism (*see* **Fig. 4**). The deliberate undersizing of the graft helps achieve a compressive effect and reduce astigmatism, while the ring-shaped graft is anatomically stable.

In their series, Wang et al. treated 25 eyes with a mean operative best corrected visual acuity (BCVA) and astigmatism of 6/36 and 13.39 D, respectively. At 2 years, all grafts were stable with clear graft-host interfaces and there was no disease recurrence. The mean postoperative BCVA and astigmatism were 6/9 and 4.37 D, respectively, with the mean BCVA being 6/9.

FUTURE DIRECTIONS

Noncircular grafts are useful in managing peripheral corneal lesions. The various methods described above allow for full-thickness or lamellar grafting as required. Although these methods achieve excellent tectonic stability, improved astigmatic outcomes are needed.

Femtosecond laser achieves reproducible, precise corneal incisions, and has been used to create a wide range of complex circular grafts including "top-hat", "mushroom" and "zigzag" wound designs. Such grafts have been demonstrated to have satisfactory postoperative results with minimal astigmatism and may be improve noncircular graft outcomes.[61,62]

Radiofrequency technology is also being explored for its potential to create precise, nontraumatic, and traction-less incisions. The Fugo blade creates corneal incisions using a plasma blade, that combines radiochemical and radiomechanical interactions to ablate tissue.[63] Further evaluation of this technology may allow it to enter clinical use in the future.

CONCLUSION

To summarize, peripheral corneal lesions are increasingly being managed using noncircular grafts, instead of conventional large circular penetrating keratoplasties. Various methods have been described and this field is still evolving in an effort to improve clinical outcomes. Developments in this field may see the use of femtosecond laser or Fugo blade technology to further optimize these procedures, in particular, reduce astigmatism, improve the precision of graft-donor wound construction, and further minimize damage to the healthy corneal tissue.

REFERENCES

1. Boisjoly HM, Bernard PM, Dubé I, Laughrea PA, Bazin R, Bernier J. Effect of factors unrelated to tissue matching on corneal transplant endothelial rejection. Am J Ophthalmol. 1989;107(6):647-54.
2. van Rij G, Cornell FM, Waring GO, Wilson LA, Beekhuis WH. Postoperative astigmatism after central vs eccentric penetrating keratoplasties. Am J Ophthalmol. 1985;99(3):317-20.
3. Sangwan VS, Zafirakis P, Foster CS. Mooren's ulcer: Current concepts in management. Indian J Ophthalmol. 1997;45(1):7-17.
4. Alhassan MB, Rabiu M, Agbabiaka IO. Interventions for Mooren's ulcer. Cochrane Database Syst Rev. 2014;(1):CD006131.
5. Wood TO, Kaufman HE. Mooren's ulcer. Am J Ophthalmol. 1971;71(1 Pt 2):417-22.
6. Chen J, Xie H, Wang Z, Yang B, Liu Z, Chen L, et al. Mooren's ulcer in China: A study of clinical characteristics and treatment. Br J Ophthalmol. 2000;84(11):1244-9.
7. Kietzman B. Mooren's ulcer in Nigeria. Am J Ophthalmol. 1968;65(5):679-85.
8. Yang L, Xiao J, Wang J, Zhang H. Clinical characteristics and risk factors of recurrent Mooren's Ulcer. J Ophthalmol. 2017;2017:8978527.
9. Li S, Deng Y, Du C, Huang H, Zhong J, Chen L, et al. Rapid deterioration of Mooren's ulcers after conjunctival flap: A review of 2 cases. BMC Ophthalmol. 2017;17(1):93.
10. Pouliquen Y, Dhermy P, Renard G, Goichot-Bonnat L, Foster G, Savoldelli M. Terrien's disease: Clinical and ultrastructural studies, five case reports. Eye (Lond). 1989;3(Pt 6):791-802.
11. Beauchamp GR. Terrien's marginal corneal degeneration. J Pediatr Ophthalmol Strabismus. 1982;19(2):97-9.
12. Richards WW. Marginal degeneration of the cornea with perforation. Arch Ophthalmol. 1963;70:610-5.
13. Austin P, Brown SI. Inflammatory Terrien's marginal corneal disease. Am J Ophthalmol. 1981;92(2):189-92.
14. Süveges J, Léval G, Alberth B. Pathology of Terrien's disease. Histochemical and electron microscopic study. Am J Ophthalmol. 1972;74(6):1191-200.
15. Chan AT, Ulate R, Goldich Y, Rootman DS, Chan CC. Terrien marginal degeneration: Clinical characteristics and outcomes. Am J Ophthalmol. 2015;160(5):867-72.e1.
16. Goldman KN, Kaufman HE. Atypical pterygium. A clinical feature of Terrien's marginal degeneration. Arch Ophthalmol. 1978;96(6):1027-9.
17. Ceresara G, Migliavacca L, Orzalesi N, Rossetti L. In vivo confocal microscopy in Terrien marginal corneal degeneration: A case report. Cornea. 2011;30(7):820-4.
18. Zarei-Ghanavati S, Javadi MA, Yazdani S. Bilateral Terrien's marginal degeneration and posterior polymorphous dystrophy in a patient with rheumatoid arthritis. J Ophthalmic Vis Res. 2012;7(1):60-3.
19. Shimazaki J, Yang HY, Shimmura S, Tsubota K. Terrien's marginal degeneration associated with erythema elevatum diutinum. Cornea. 1998;17(3):342-4.

20. Kremer I. Terrien's marginal degeneration associated with vernal conjunctivitis. Am J Ophthalmol. 1991;111(4):517-8.
21. Wagoner MD, Teichmann KD. Terrien's marginal degeneration associated with posterior polymorphous dystrophy. Cornea. 1999;18(5):612-5.
22. Zhang Y, Jia H. Terrien's marginal degeneration accompanied by latticed stromal opacities. Optom Vis Sci. 2014;91(5):e110-6.
23. Iwamoto T, DeVoe A, Farris RL. Electron microscopy in cases of marginal degeneration of the cornea. Invest Ophthalmol. 1972;11(4):241-57.
24. Chung J, Jin KH, Kang J, Kim TG. Spontaneous corneal perforation in Terrien's marginal degeneration in childhood: A case report. Medicine (Baltimore). 2017;96(49):e9095.
25. Srinivasan S, Murphy CC, Fisher AC, Freeman LB, Kaye SB. Terrien marginal degeneration presenting with spontaneous corneal perforation. Cornea. 2006;25(8):977-80.
26. Fernandes M, Vira D. Patch graft for corneal perforation following trivial trauma in bilateral Terrien's marginal degeneration. Middle East Afr J Ophthalmol. 2015;22(2):255-7.
27. Galor A, Thorne JE. Scleritis and peripheral ulcerative keratitis. Rheum Dis Clin North Am. 2007;33(4):835-54, vii.
28. Mondino BJ. Inflammatory diseases of the peripheral cornea. Ophthalmology. 1988;95(4):463-72.
29. Freeman RD. Oxygen consumption by the component layers of the cornea. J Physiol. 1972;225(1):15-32.
30. Allansmith MR, McClellan BH. Immunoglobulins in the human cornea. Am J Ophthalmol. 1975;80(1):123-32.
31. Gregory JK, Foster CS. Peripheral ulcerative keratitis in the collagen vascular diseases. Int Ophthalmol Clin. 1996;36(1):21-30.
32. Tauber J, Sainz de la Maza M, Hoang-Xuan T, Foster CS. An analysis of therapeutic decision making regarding immunosuppressive chemotherapy for peripheral ulcerative keratitis. Cornea. 1990; 9(1):66-73.
33. Sainz de la Maza M, Foster CS, Jabbur NS, Baltatzis S. Ocular characteristics and disease associations in scleritis-associated peripheral keratopathy. Arch Ophthalmol. 2002;120(1):15-9.
34. Dana MR, Qian Y, Hamrah P. Twenty-five-year panorama of corneal immunology: emerging concepts in the immunopathogenesis of microbial keratitis, peripheral ulcerative keratitis, and corneal transplant rejection. Cornea. 2000;19(5):625-43.
35. Sharma N, Sinha G, Shekhar H, Titiyal JS, Agarwal T, Chawla B, et al. Demographic profile, clinical features and outcome of peripheral ulcerative keratitis: a prospective study. Br J Ophthalmol. 2015;99(11):1503-8.
36. Messmer EM, Foster CS. Vasculitic peripheral ulcerative keratitis. Surv Ophthalmol. 1999;43(5):379-96.
37. Krachmer JH. Pellucid marginal corneal degeneration. Arch Ophthalmol. 1978;96(7):1217-21.
38. Bower KS, Dhaliwal DK, Barnhorst DA, Warnicke J. Pellucid marginal degeneration with superior corneal thinning. Cornea. 1997;16(4):483-5.
39. Krachmer JH, Feder RS, Belin MW. Keratoconus and related noninflammatory corneal thinning disorders. Surv Ophthalmol. 1984;28(4):293-322.
40. Sridhar MS, Mahesh S, Bansal AK, Nutheti R, Rao GN. Pellucid marginal corneal degeneration. Ophthalmology. 2004;111(6):1102-7.
41. Carter JB, Jones DB, Wilhelmus KR. Acute hydrops in pellucid marginal corneal degeneration. Am J Ophthalmol. 1989;107(2):167-70.
42. Akpek EK, Altan-Yaycioglu R, Gottsch JD, Stark WJ. Spontaneous corneal perforation in a patient with unusual unilateral pellucid marginal degeneration. J Cataract Refract Surg. 2001;27(10):1698-700.
43. Lucarelli MJ, Gendelman DS, Talamo JH. Hydrops and spontaneous perforation in pellucid marginal corneal degeneration. Cornea. 1997;16(2):232-4.
44. Robin JB, Schanzlin DJ, Verity SM, Barron BA, Arffa RC, Suarez E, et al. Peripheral corneal disorders. Surv Ophthalmol. 1986;31(1):1-36.
45. Karabatsas CH, Cook SD. Topographic analysis in pellucid marginal corneal degeneration and keratoglobus. Eye Lond Engl. 1996;10(Pt 4):451-5.
46. Tzelikis PF, Cohen EJ, Rapuano CJ, Hammersmith KM, Laibson PR. Management of pellucid marginal corneal degeneration. Cornea. 2005;24(5):555-60.
47. Javadi MA, Karimian F, Hosseinzadeh A, Noroozizadeh HM, Sa'eedifar MR, Rabie HM. Lamellar crescentic resection for pellucid marginal corneal degeneration. J Refract Surg. 2004;20(2):162-5.
48. MacLean H, Robinson LP, Wechsler AW. Long-term results of corneal wedge excision for pellucid marginal degeneration. Eye (Lond). 1997;11(Pt 5):613-7.
49. Kaushal S, Jhanji V, Sharma N, Tandon R, Titiyal JS, Vajpayee RB. "Tuck In" lamellar keratoplasty (TILK) for corneal ectasias involving corneal periphery. Br J Ophthalmol. 2008;92(2):286-90.
50. Lee WB, O'Halloran HS, Grossniklaus HE. Pellucid marginal degeneration and bilateral corneal perforation: case report and review of the literature. Eye Contact Lens. 2008;34(4):229-33.
51. Bessant DA, Dart JK. Lamellar keratoplasty in the management of inflammatory corneal ulceration and perforation. Eye (Lond). 1994;8(Pt 1):22-8.
52. Schanzlin DJ, Sarno EM, Robin JB. Crescentic lamellar keratoplasty for pellucid marginal degeneration. Am J Ophthalmol. 1983;96(2):253-4.
53. Arora R, Manudhane A, Jain P, Goyal JL. Crescentic tuck in lamellar keratoplasty-A novel technique in a case of advanced pellucid marginal corneal degeneration. Eye Contact Lens. 2018;44 Suppl 1:S345-7.
54. Jabbarvand M, Hashemian H, Khodaparast M, Hassanpour N, Mohebbi M. Intrastromal lamellar keratoplasty in patients with pellucid marginal degeneration. J Cataract Refract Surg. 2015;41(1):2-8.
55. Guindolet D, Petrovic A, Doan S, Cochereau I, Gabison EE. Sclerocorneal intrastromal lamellar keratoplasty for pellucid marginal degeneration. Cornea. 2016;35(6):900-3.
56. Symes RJ, Catt CJ, Sangiampornpanit T, Males JJ. Corneal perforation associated with pellucid marginal degeneration and treatment with crescentic lamellar keratoplasty: two case reports. Cornea. 2007;26(5):625-8.
57. Cheng CL, Theng JTS, Tan DTH. Compressive C-shaped lamellar keratoplasty: a surgical alternative for the management of severe astigmatism from peripheral corneal degeneration. Ophthalmology. 2005;112(3):425-30.
58. Samarawickrama C, Goh R, Vajpayee RB. "Copy and Fix": A new technique of harvesting freehand and horseshoe tectonic grafts. Cornea. 2015;34(11):1519-22.
59. Parmar GS, Ghodke B, Bose S, Meena AK. Stenciling-Based "Prick and Print" Technique for harvesting shaped corneal grafts for management of peripheral corneal perforations. Cornea. 2019;38(1):105-9.
60. Wang T, Shi W, Ding G, Li S, Liu M, Gao H. Ring-shaped corneoscleral lamellar keratoplasty guided by high-definition optical coherence tomography and Scheimpflug imaging for severe Terrien's marginal corneal degeneration. Graefes Arch Clin Exp Ophthalmol. 2012;250(12):1795-801.
61. Asota I, Farid M, Garg S, Steinert RF. Femtosecond laser-enabled keratoplasty. Int Ophthalmol Clin. 2013;53(2):103-14.
62. Ibrahim T, Goernert P, Rocha G. Femto-second laser (FSL) techniques and consistency in corneal surgery: Experimental study. Can J Ophthalmol. 2018;53(4):324-9.
63. Peponis V, Rosenberg P, Reddy SV, Herz JB, Kaufman HE. The use of the Fugo Blade in corneal surgery: a preliminary animal study. Cornea. 2006;25(2):206-8.

46

Crescentic Tuck in Lamellar Keratoplasty

Ritu Arora, Shipra Sarda

INTRODUCTION

Pellucid marginal corneal degeneration (PMCD) is a bilateral, peripheral, corneal, ectatic disorder, characterized by a band of corneal thinning in the inferior cornea (**Figs. 1A to C**). This term pellucid was reported by Schlaeppi.[1] PMCD is considered as a variant of keratoconus[2] and both of them can be present simultaneously (**Figs. 2A and B**). The corneal protrusion takes place above the thinned area. Patients may remain asymptomatic or may present with progressive visual deterioration due to high and irregular astigmatism. Most patients are initially managed with spectacles or contact lenses. In advanced cases contact lenses are ineffective.

Conventional penetrating keratoplasty in these ectatic disorders is challenging with lower chances of gaining good optical results.[3] In cases of PMCD, a large eccentric graft is required for penetrating keratoplasty to obtain a clear central visual axis. Early graft vascularization and early suture erosion is common in these large eccentric graft due to close proximity to inferior limbus.

Wedge resection[4] along with relaxing incisions has been described to reduce astigmatism in PMCD. The procedure involves removal of a wedge of affected corneal tissue and reapposing normal cornea in order to restore normal contour. The results have been unpredictable with large amount of undercorrections or overcorrections.

Crescentic lamellar resection[5] is performed by placing a crescent-shaped incision up to mid-stroma and deeper dissection carried out up to Descemet's membrane followed by suturing of superior and inferior normal cornea. In crescentic lamellar resection, abnormal tissue is removed in contrast to penetrating keratoplasty where full thickness cornea is removed thereby reducing chances of graft rejection. Although associated with lesser chances of rejection, it has short-lived effect and is associated with peripheral vascularization. The combined technique of peripheral crescentic lamellar keratoplasty with central penetrating keratoplasty[6] gave encouraging results (**Fig. 3**). Lamellar keratoplasty restores normal thickness to the inferior cornea and provides tectonic support for good edge-to-edge apposition at the time of penetrating keratoplasty, thus reducing chances of postkeratoplasty astigmatism (**Fig. 4**). The combined procedure usually done in one sitting, hence same donor cornea can be used thus reducing antigenic load. Combined procedure has an added advantage of early visual rehabilitation and the drift toward against-the-rule astigmatism is almost negligible postoperatively. Risk of full-thickness corneal graft rejection always exists.

A C-shaped compression keratoplasty[7] causes flattening of ectatic area and corrects astigmatism as a result of deliberate undersizing of donor tissue and tight suturing. There exists the risk of thinning of the cornea adjacent to the peripheral graft because of constant pulling of undersized graft.

Tuck in lamellar keratoplasty (TILK) is an excellent technique to manage extremely ectatic peripheral and central corneal disorders, i.e., advanced pellucid marginal corneal degeneration and keratoglobus as it provides strength and support by increasing corneal thickness of the ectatic area (**Figs. 5A and B**).[8] Varied surgical procedures have been described for tectonic purpose and eventual improvement in functional vision in patients with advanced PMCD.

In TILK, the central part is full thickness graft with a thin peripheral flange, tucked into a pocket created intrastromally in host's peripheral cornea. The advantages being reduced risk of graft rejection, minimal damage to limbus. A possible limitation of TILK is interface haze over a few years.[8] A modification done in form of C in TILK has been found to be beneficial.[9]

SURGICAL TECHNIQUE FOR C-SHAPED TUCK IN LAMELLAR KERATOPLASTY

The surgery is performed under peribulbar/general anesthesia. Intraoperatively ultrasonic pachymetry is done to mark the zone of peripheral thin cornea (**Fig. 6A**). Horizontal ends of the arc are outlined with 3-mm trephine

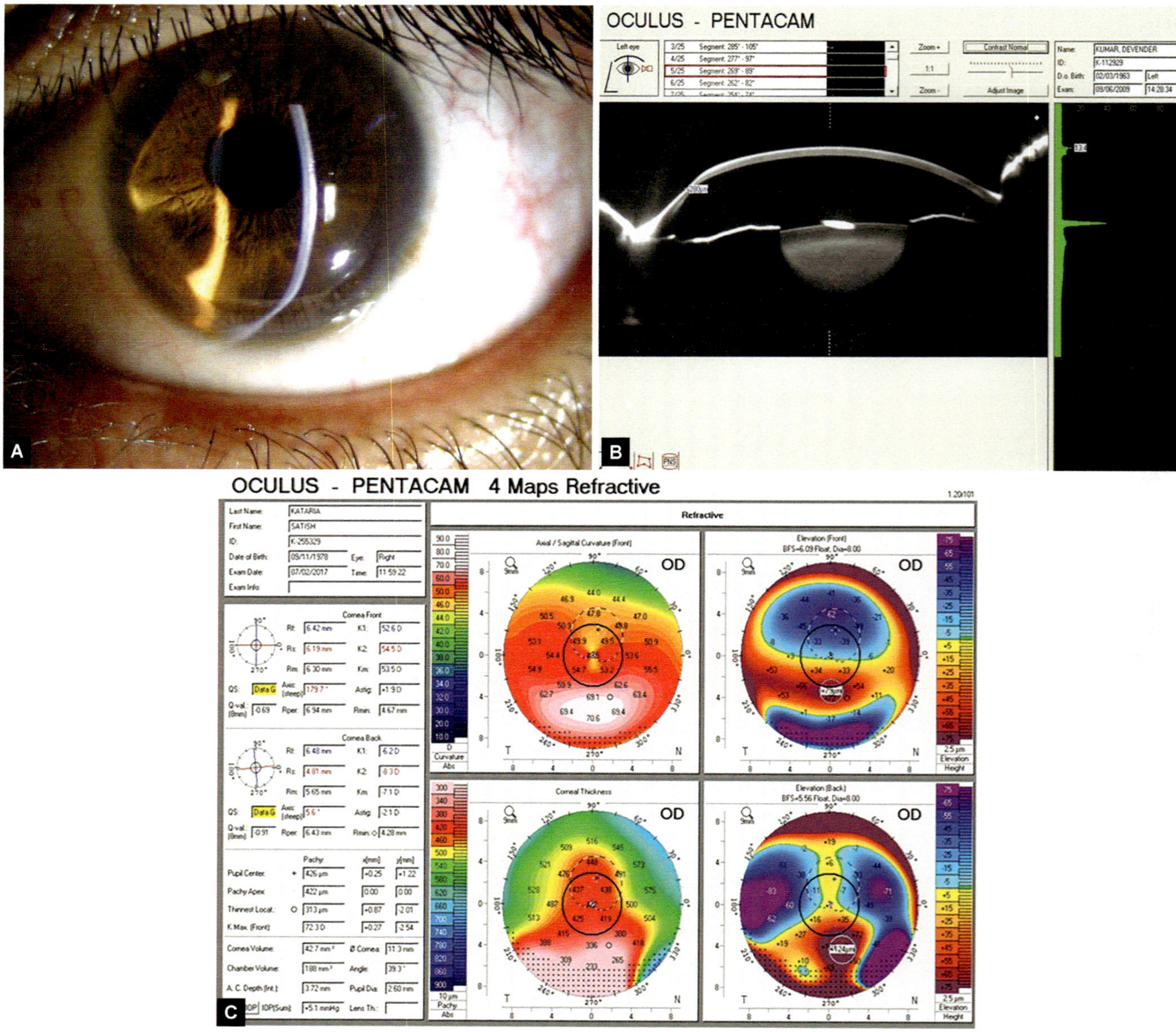

Figs. 1A to C: Advanced pellucid marginal degeneration. (A) Slit-lamp image showing inferior corneal thinning with ecstatic area above it; (B) Scheimpflug image of pellucid marginal corneal degeneration mapping severe peripheral corneal thinning; (C) Pentacam showing typical crab claw appearance with against-the-rule astigmatism.

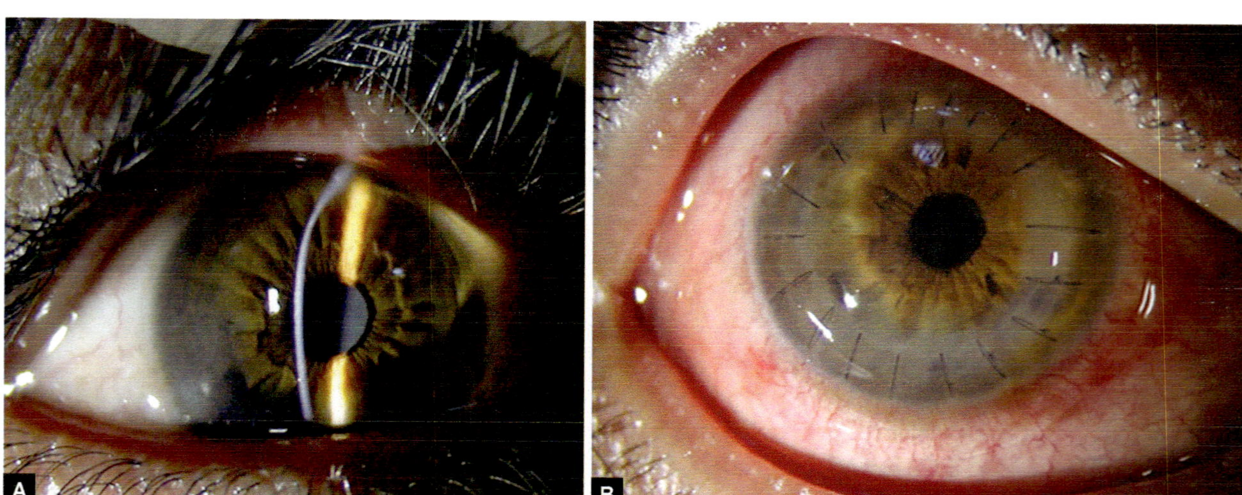

Figs. 2A and B: Superior pellucid marginal corneal degeneration (PMCD) with keratoconus. (A) Slit-lamp image showing superior PMCD with keratoconus; (B) Postoperative image of deep lamellar keratoplasty in the same patient of PMCD with keratoconus.

each (**Fig. 6B**). In PMCD, there is a band of peripheral corneal thinning. Outer and inner circumferences of peripheral corneal thinning are marked with corresponding trephines (usually 11 and 7/7.5 mm). The horizontal ends of the arc are marked to get well-defined rounded edges merging into the normal host cornea. Manual corneal dissection is done layer-by-layer using crescent blade (**Figs. 6C to E**). Peripheral limboscleral dissection is performed for 2 mm in the subscleral zone (**Fig. 6F**).

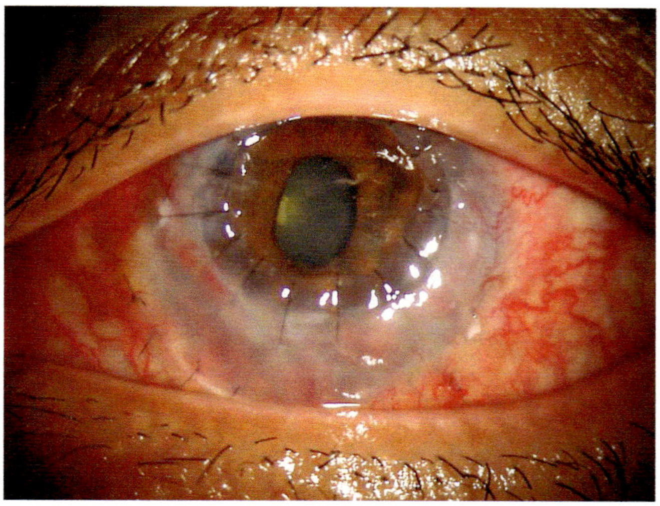

Fig. 3: Postoperative image of combined technique of peripheral crescentic lamellar keratoplasty with central penetrating keratoplasty.

Donor corneal endothelium is stripped manually and a crescent-shaped graft (**Fig. 6G**) is trephined using the same trephines as for the recipient bed. A peripheral flange of 1 mm width is created toward the outer circumference in the donor cornea (**Fig. 6H**). This is performed by removing stromal tissue in an oblique fashion (**Fig. 7**). The donor cornea is sutured by interrupted sutures using 10-0 nylon on the corneal side. The peripheral flange is tucked in under the scleral groove, and 10-0 nylon suture bites are taken full thickness from donor cornea to overlying sclera (**Fig. 6I**). This modified C-shaped TILK has shown early visual rehabilitation and optimum long-term survival (**Figs. 8A and B**). Postoperatively anterior segment optical coherence tomography (ASOCT) can be done to monitor graft-host apposition, tuck in of donor graft and residual host corneal thickness left (**Fig. 8C**).

SUMMARY

Tuck in lamellar keratoplasty has been described for ectatic corneal disorders involving central and peripheral cornea. It provides tectonic support by improving corneal thickness of the diseased area, prevents dissection and damage of limbus, and reduces the risk of allograft rejection. Modification of the TILK in a C shape with peripheral subscleral tuck in and tight suturing induced compressive effect and resultant flattening of the cornea

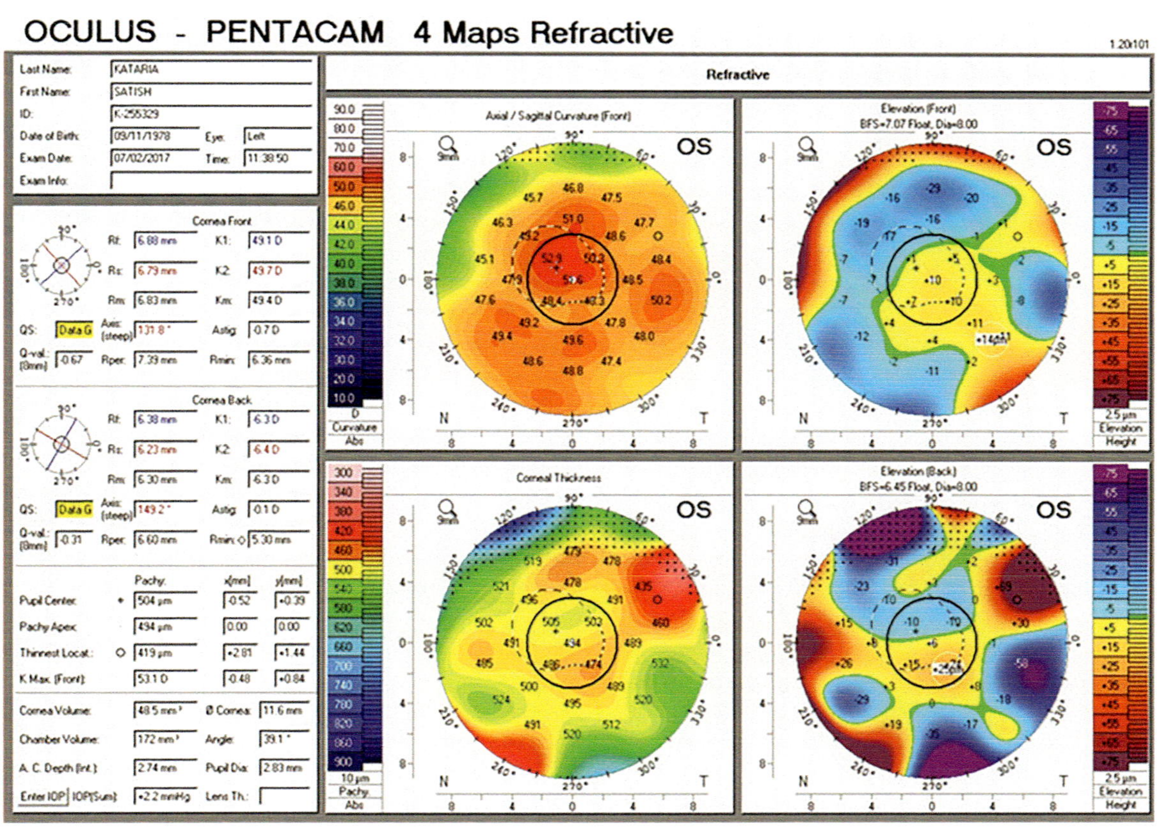

Fig. 4: Pentacam in case of postoperative lamellar keratoplasty in case of advanced pellucid marginal corneal degeneration (PMCD) with reduced astigmatism and steepening.

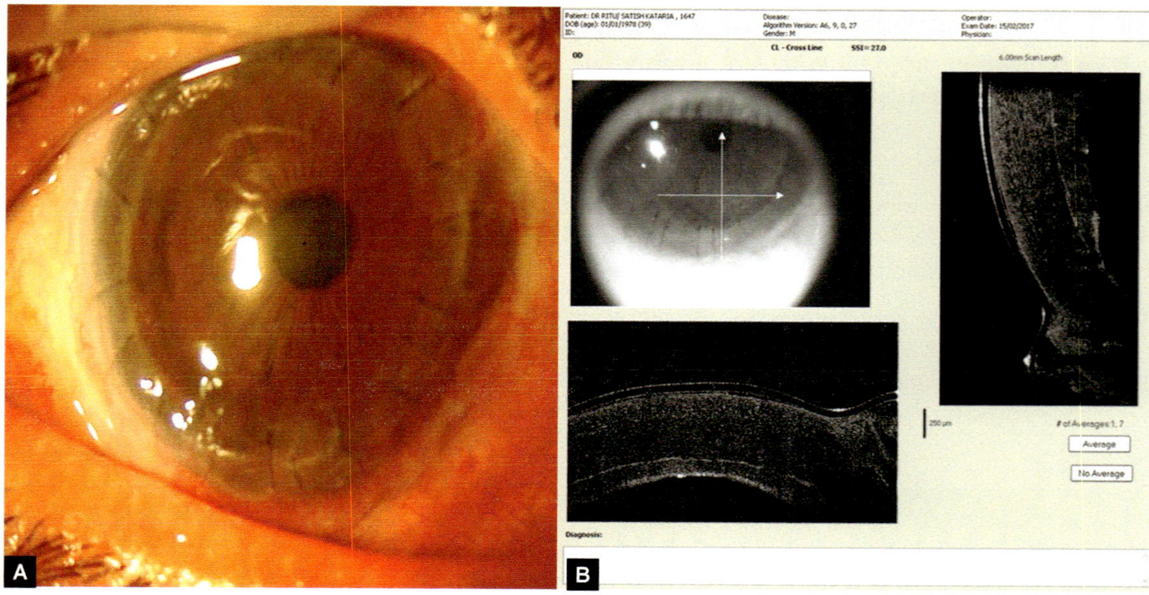

Figs. 5A and B: Tuck in lamellar keratoplasty done in a patient with pellucid marginal corneal degeneration (PMCD). (A) Slit-lamp image; (B) Anterior segment optical coherence tomography (ASOCT) image of graft tucked in pocket created intrastromally.

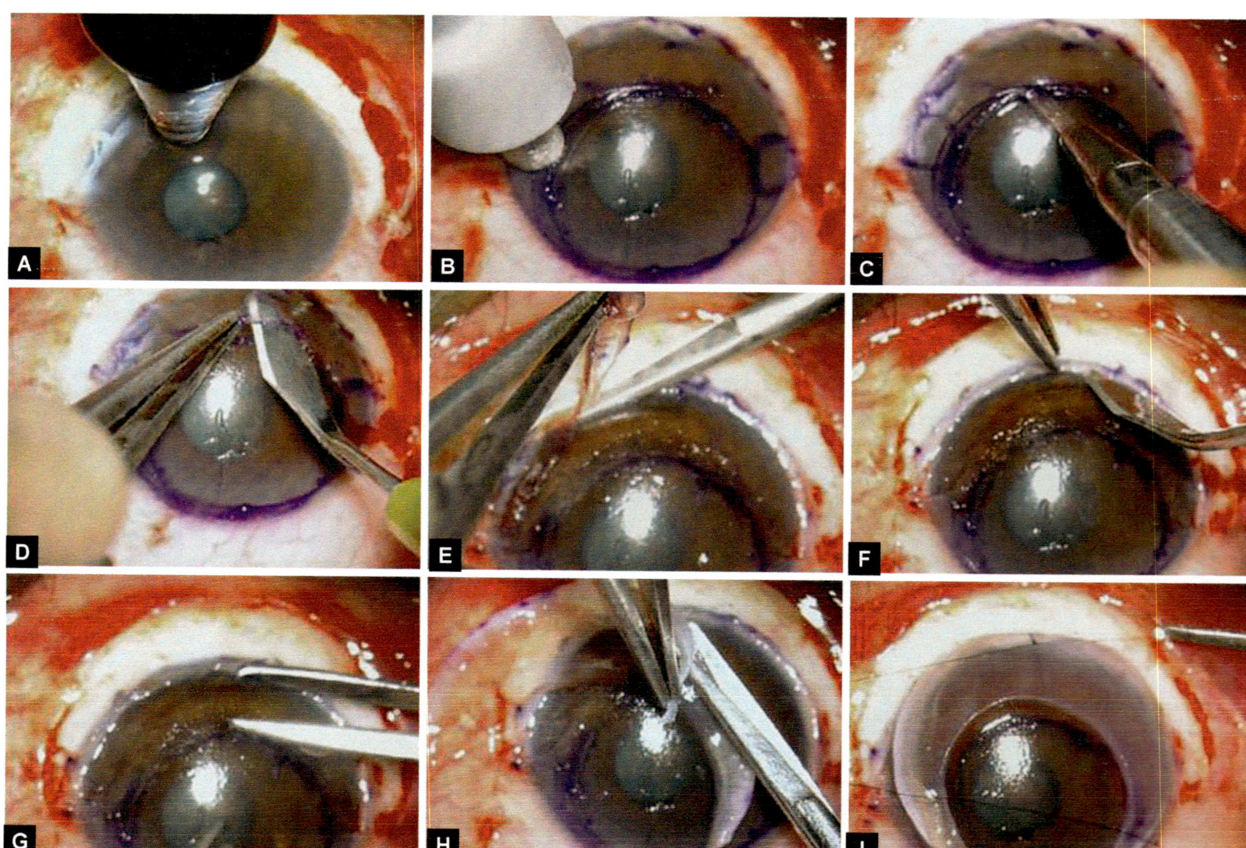

Figs. 6A to I: Surgical technique of preparation host bed and donor lenticule in crescentic tuck in lamellar keratoplasty. (A) Intraoperative pachymetry done. Area of maximum thinning noted; (B) 4 o'clock and 8 o'clock area marked with 3-mm corneal trephine; (C) Corneal marking deepened using diamond knife and peripheral groove dissected; (D) Manual lamellar corneal dissection done; (E) Superficial lamellar crescentic tissue dissected; (F) Sclerolimbal dissection done. Host bed prepared for tuck in; (G) Defect of host bed measured; (H) A 3.5-mm wide, crescent-shaped, donor lamellar tissue harvested and peripheral flange created; (I) Donor cornea sutured to host bed with 10-0 nylon using interrupted sutures and peripheral flange tucked in.

perpendicular to the circumference, that is, horizontal meridian. Crescentic TILK offers refractive advantage with tectonic support without posing any threat to the central cornea.

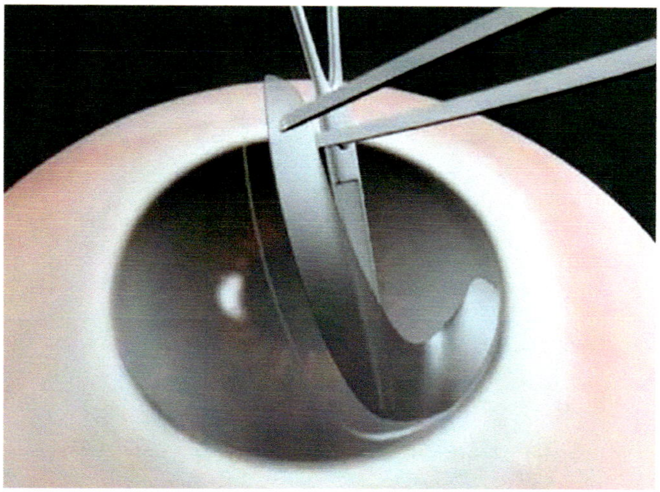

Fig. 7: Schematic representation of preparation of donor lenticule. A peripheral flange of 1-mm width was created in the crescentic donor lenticule by removing stromal tissue in an oblique fashion.

REFERENCES

1. Schlaeppi V. La dystophiemarginaleinferieurepellucide de la cornee. Mod Prabl Ophthalmol. 1995;1:672-7.
2. Kayazawa F, Nishimura K, Kodama Y, Tsuji T, Itoi M. Keratoconus with pellucid marginal corneal degeneration. Arch Ophthalmol. 1984;102:895-6.
3. Kaushal S, Jhanji V, Sharma N, Tandon R, Titiyal JS, Vajpayee RB. "Tuck In" Lamellar Keratoplasty (TILK) for corneal ectasias involving corneal periphery. Br J Ophthalmol. 2008;92:286-90.
4. Dubroff S. Pellucid marginal corneal degeneration: Report on corrective surgery. J Cataract Refract Surg. 1989;15:89-93.
5. Cameron JA. Results of lamellar crescentic resection for pellucid marginal corneal degeneration. Am J Ophthalmol. 1992;113:296-302.
6. Rasheed K, Rabinowitz YS. Surgical treatment of advanced pellucid marginal degeneration. Ophthalmology, 2000;107:1836-40
7. Cheng CL, Theng JT, Tan DT. Compressive C-shaped lamellar keratoplasty: A surgical alternative for the management of severe astigmatism from peripheral corneal degeneration. Ophthalmology. 2005;112:425-30.
8. Vajapyee RB, Bhartiya P, Sharma N. Central lamellar keratoplasty with peripheral intralamellar tuck: A new technique for keratoglobus. Cornea. 2002;21:657-60.
9. Arora R, Manudhane A, Jain P, Goyal JL. Crescentic tuck in lamellar keratoplasty—A novel technique in a case of advanced pellucid marginal corneal degeneration. Eye Contact Lens. 2018;44 Suppl 1:S345-S347.

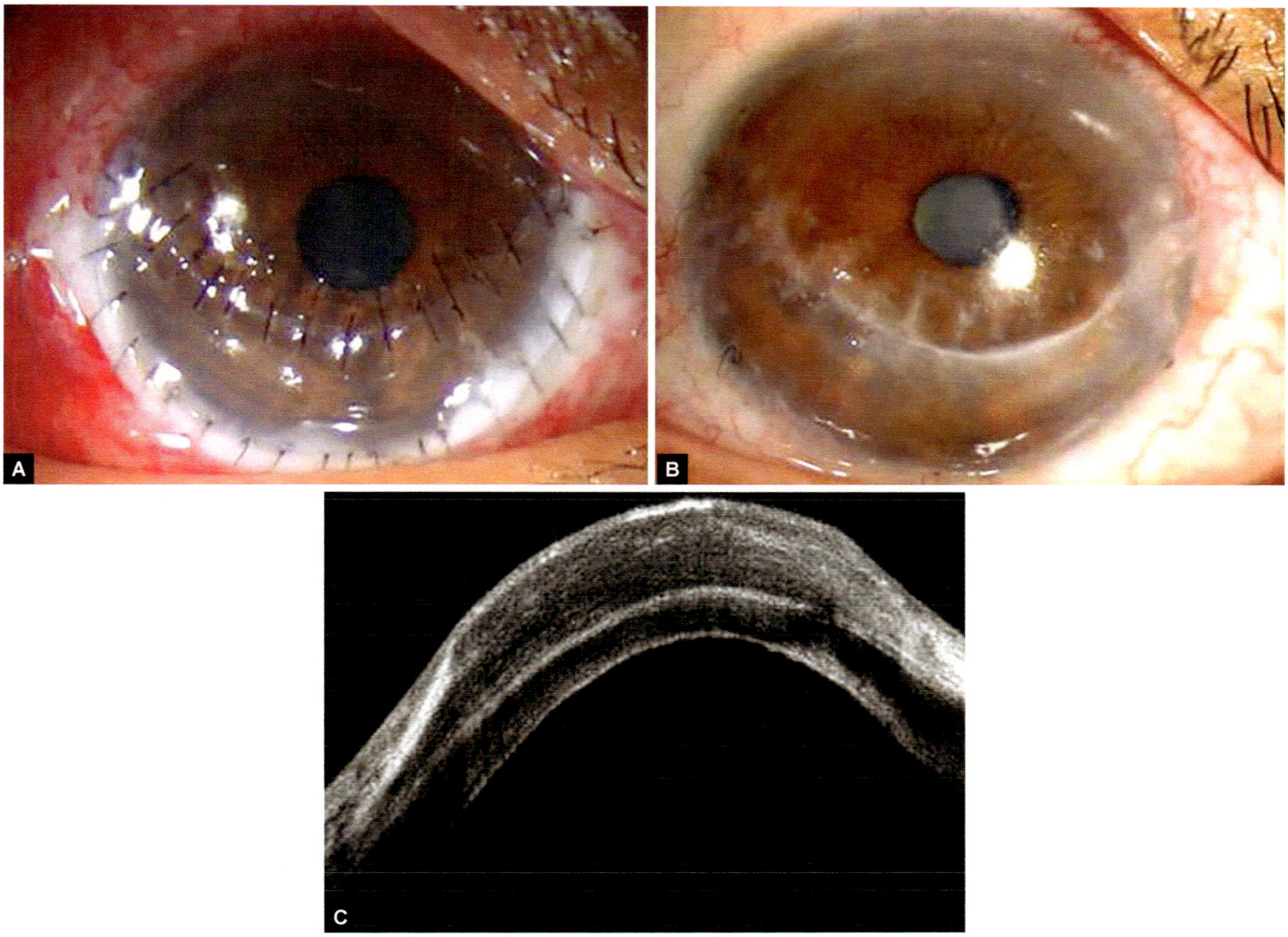

Figs. 8A to C: Crescentic (C-shaped) tuck in lamellar keratoplasty (TILK). (A) Postoperative day 1; (B) Postoperative 6 months; (C) Anterior segment optical coherence tomography (ASOCT) image showing a well-integrated donor lamellar graft with an epithelium continuous with the recipient's central cornea.

47

Hemi-automated Lamellar Keratoplasty

Hassan Mansoor, Jodhbir S Mehta

INTRODUCTION

Over the last two decades, corneal transplantation has undergone a gradual transition, from conventional penetrating keratoplasty (PK) to the replacement of only the diseased layers of the cornea. Technological advancements in eye banking, innovative surgical techniques, and availability of laser platforms have allowed a paradigm shift in corneal grafting. These have all contributed to improved anatomical and visual outcomes after corneal transplantation.[1,2] Targeted lamellar transplantation has also enabled better utilization of donor corneal tissue. Furthermore, it also circumvents problems associated with the scarcity of donor corneas, especially in the developing world.[1-3]

Anterior lamellar keratoplasty (ALK) has emerged as a surgical option for the management of anterior stromal pathologies and superficial corneal scars.[1-6] The keratometric and visual outcomes of ALK have been shown to be comparable to PK.[4-6] However, ALK is an extraocular procedure, and hence, as compared to PK, there is a reduced risk of expulsive hemorrhage and endophthalmitis. The globe is also tectonically stronger postoperatively.[7,8] Unlike PK, ALK has the added advantage of retaining the healthy host endothelium that eliminates the risk of endothelial rejection.[1,2]

The advent of microkeratome technology has enabled clinicians to prepare donor corneal tissue and the recipient bed in a precise manner.[7,9,10] Automated lamellar therapeutic keratoplasty (ALTK) combines the use of an artificial anterior chamber (AAC) maintainer, with a microkeratome, of a changeable head thickness, for the lamellar dissection of the donor. The surgeon prepares the recipient corneal bed with the help of a microkeratome.[2] In brief, the surgeon relies on preoperative anterior segment optical coherence tomography (AS-OCT) to plan the depth of the lamellar cut in the recipient cornea. The AAC maintainer of the ALTK system is used to harvest the donor corneal tissue from a corneoscleral button.[11,12] The diameter of the lamellar cut in the donor tissue is matched with the diameter of the lamellar cut in the recipient bed, using appropriate applanation lenses and adjustment rings. The donor corneal flap is then sutured on the recipient bed using 10-0 monofilament nylon sutures.[11]

Automated lamellar therapeutic keratoplasty is typically used to treat corneal pathology affecting the anterior 200–300 microns of the cornea.[11-13] It is easier and more convenient for the corneal surgeon to use the ALTK system for preparing the donor and recipient cornea.[11] There is also minimal risk of inadvertently perforating the donor or recipient corneal tissue, during automated lamellar therapeutic keratoplasty.[11-13]

Automated lamellar therapeutic keratoplasty has been used in patients with corneal scarring, secondary to nonviral microbial keratitis, herpetic eye disease, localized trauma due to a corneal foreign body or an alkali burn, epithelial and stromal dystrophies, and corneal degenerations.[11-15] ALTK has been advocated as a better alternative to PK in the treatment of post-photorefractive keratectomy (PRK) corneal thinning and scarring.[16] The microkeratome cut, in ALTK, facilitates a smooth graft-host interface that leads to improved visual outcomes, reproducibility, and curtails surgical time compared to performing a deep anterior lamellar keratoplasty (DALK).[1,7,8]

Alternatively, topography-guided photorefractive keratectomy (TG-PRK) can serve as a treatment modality in selected cases of corneal scarring.[17] TG-PRK reduces irregular astigmatism and can decrease the density of corneal scars.[17] The surgical planning of TG-PRK in irregular corneas (such as those with corneal scars, keratoconus, postkeratoplasty astigmatism and refractive surgery complications) relies on corneal topography images, which are analyzed by proprietary algorithms to generate an ablation profile, thereby reducing the surface irregularities.[17,18] The commercially available laser ablation platforms licensed with TG-PRK include Allegretto Wave Eye-Q Excimer laser platform (Alcon Laboratories Inc., Ft Worth, Texas, USA), CRS-Master (Carl Zeiss Meditec, Jena, Germany), Nidek Advanced Vision Excimer (NAVEX, Nidek, Gamagori, Japan), Corneal Interactive Programmed

Topographic Ablation (CIPTAmax, iVis Technology, Taranto, Italy) and the Pulsar Z1 platform (CV Laser Pty Ltd., Perth, Australia).[17]

Any corneal topographic change will lead to an accompanying shift in refraction, hence, TG-PRK may cause a refractive surprise that is unpredictable and could compromise the postoperative visual outcomes.[17,18] Therefore, a stepwise approach is advisable, in which the corneal surface is regularized first, followed by refractive error correction.[17] However, the need for two laser ablation procedures to achieve desired visual outcomes may increase the overall treatment duration and cost.[17] It is also challenging to acquire corneal topography images for optimal TG-PRK planning in highly irregular corneas, which could further affect the predictability and efficacy of the procedure. To address the limitations mentioned above, some surgeons have developed different nomograms and techniques [topographic neutralization technique (TNT)] to improve outcomes.[19]

The clinical cases that might benefit from TG-PRK are cases that have a scar depth of less than 200 microns with an acceptable residual stromal bed that allows correction for any refractive shift post-TG-PRK.[17] However, if the corneal thickness does not allow adequate laser ablation for dense or deep corneal scars, ALTK may be a better treatment option.

Nonetheless, ALTK has some constraints that limit its use to superficial corneal stromal pathologies with relatively regular corneal topographies.[2,20] Microkeratomes applanate the corneal surface before lamellar dissections and therefore tend to replicate corneal surface irregularities in the recipient corneal bed.[7,21] The depth of the lamellar cut and symmetry in the thickness of the dissected lamellar flap depends on the transition speed of microkeratome.[12] Therefore, inter-surgeon and intra-surgeon variability, in the transition speed of the microkeratome, can affect the precision of the harvested lamellar flap. Deeper stromal lesions are also more challenging due to the selection of available microkeratome heads, and the larger standard deviation of deeper cuts, which makes them less accurate.[22] Hence, there is a chance that the resulting graft-host interface may be irregular and compromise visual outcomes postoperatively.[1,7] In addition, the side-cuts produced by the microkeratome are also meniscus-shaped and not vertical, which can further hamper optimal alignment of the graft-host junction.[1] There can also be donor-host diameter mismatch, due to variations of different suction pressure between donor and recipient lamellar cuts.[1,2] Furthermore, the use of microkeratomes for lamellar dissection in eccentrically steep and thin corneas has an inherent risk of incomplete recipient flaps and buttonhole formation.[2,20,23]

A modified ALTK technique has been introduced to bypass some of the limitations of conventional ALTK. In brief, the procedure is completed in two-stages, 4–6 weeks apart, and it differs from the original technique as it couples conventional ALTK with a Hanna trephination, to enable precise control of diameter and depth during lamellar dissection.[14] A femtosecond laser (FSL) may also achieve this.[14] The vertical side-cuts attained with modified ALTK technique and FSL, promote optimal alignment of the graft-host junction.[14]

An alternative technique, the "hemi-automated lamellar keratoplasty" (HALK) was described in 2011.[20] HALK is a hybrid technique. It combines the advantages of a sharp manual lamellar dissection of the recipient bed, respecting the intended anatomical surgical plane, with the automated preparation of donor corneal tissue, using conventional ALTK technique and microkeratome.[20,24] HALK provides a smooth graft-host interface in anterior corneal scars with topographical irregularities where ALTK is contraindicated.[20,24]

INDICATIONS

The technique is especially useful for localized corneal scars, which arise due to infectious keratitis, corneal dystrophies, corneal degenerations, and nonpenetrating ocular trauma, as these scars are often associated with corneal thinning and surface irregularities.[24] It has been reported that a stromal scar secondary to contact lens-associated infectious keratitis (10/35, 29%) was the most common indication for HALK, which was followed by scars of unknown origin (9/35, 26%), and scars related to corneal dystrophies (5/35, 14%), respectively.[24]

Infectious Keratitis

The corneal scars that follow the acute resolution of infectious keratitis may involve the visual axis and adversely affect the visual potential of the patient. Therefore, it becomes inevitable to remove these corneal scars for visual rehabilitation in patients who have no significant visual improvement with the use of contact lenses or show intolerance to their use.[25] Moreover, the scars often have a stromal involvement with topographical irregularities (**Figs. 1A to H**).[24]

Corneal Dystrophies

Hemi-automated lamellar keratoplasty is a suitable treatment option for anterior/midstromal dystrophies. These corneal dystrophies can cause recurrent corneal erosions, foreign body sensation, ocular discomfort, and visual loss.[26] Moreover, the disease recurrence following conventional keratoplasty in corneal dystrophies remains a challenge, which may affect the visual prognosis and may require a re-operation.[26,27] HALK is a useful surgical technique to treat anterior/midstromal dystrophies (*see* **Figs. 1A to H**), as the donor corneal button can be exchanged with a new donor in the event of recurrence, with minimal risk of intraoperative complications.[24]

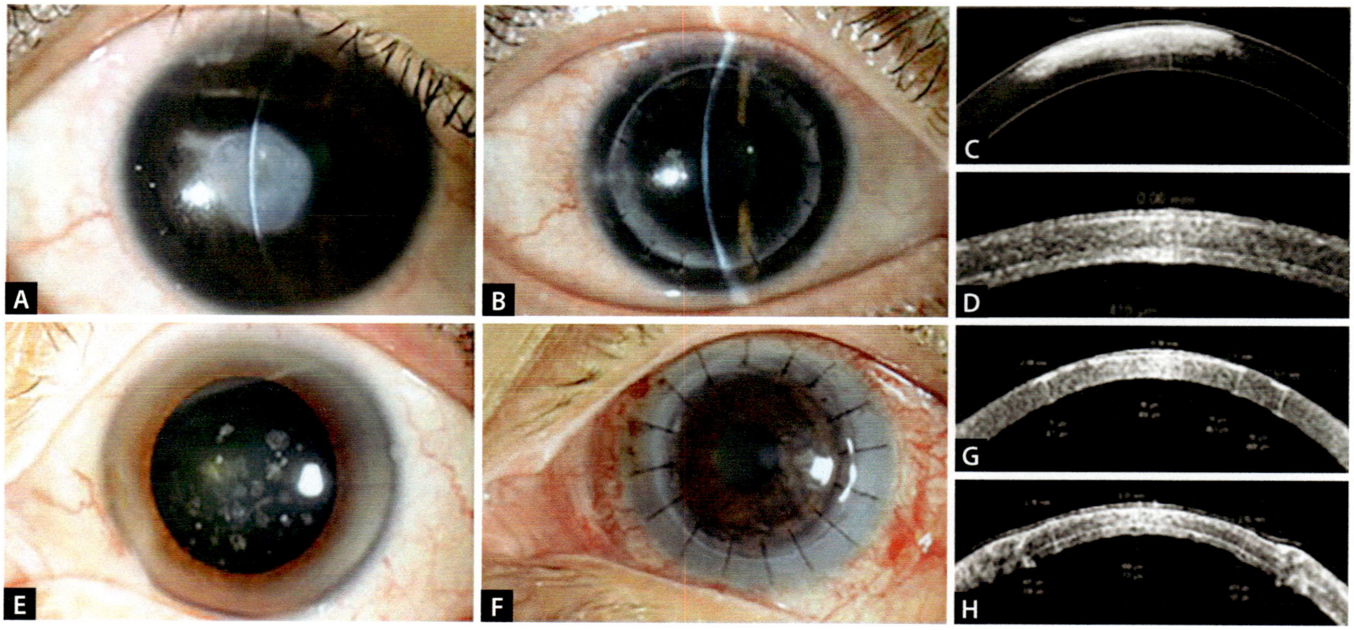

Figs. 1A to H: Preoperative slit-lamp (A and E) and optical coherence tomography (OCT) (C and G) pictures, showing contact lens-associated infectious keratitis scar and granular dystrophy, respectively, treated with hemi-automated lamellar keratoplasty, as well as postoperative slit-lamp (B and F) and OCT (D and H) pictures.

Corneal Degenerations

Salzmann's nodular degeneration (SND) and spheroidal degeneration are slowly progressive corneal pathologies that affect the corneal epithelium, Bowman's membrane, and anterior corneal stroma.[28,29] They are caused by the deposition of hyaline plaques or immunoglobulins/albumins in the superficial corneal layers, respectively.[28,29] Superficial keratectomy has been used as a useful tool to treat diffuse opacities and scars that involve the superficial corneal layers only.[28,29] However, lesions associated with involvement of the anterior stroma, can be treated by performing HALK.[24]

Herpes Simplex Virus Keratitis Scars

Keratoplasty in patients with herpes simplex virus (HSV) keratitis is primarily for the removal of corneal scarring to restore visual acuity. It is advisable to have an inflammation-free interval of at least 6 months, before considering corneal grafting.[30] HALK may be used to treat superficial corneal scars with surface irregularities following herpetic keratitis.[24]

It is necessary to use antiviral prophylaxis in the postoperative period (at least 1 year or longer).[31] Both acyclovir (400 mg twice daily) and valacyclovir (500 mg once or twice daily) are equally effective in preventing the recurrence of HSV keratitis after corneal transplantation.[32]

Post-refractive Surgery Complications

Post-PRK haze and rarely, post-infection corneal scars that may occur after PRK and LASIK (laser-assisted in-situ keratomileusis) can lead to suboptimal best-corrected vision.[33] HALK can be considered to remove the haze or scarred corneal tissue, in the anterior or midstroma region, and replace it with an optically clear donor cornea button.[24]

Other Corneal Scars

Hemi-automated lamellar keratoplasty may also be used to treat congenital linear corneal scars and deep traumatic scars as they are localized in nature and often associated with corneal thinning and surface irregularities.[24]

Contraindications

Hemi-automated lamellar keratoplasty is not advisable for patients with active infection and inflammation, advanced keratoconus, patients with grossly irregular topographies, scarring involving the posterior one-fourth of the corneal stroma and patients with tears/folds in the Descemet's membrane (DM). It has been shown that HALK did not improve the best spectacle-corrected visual acuity increased (BSCVA) beyond 20/160 in a patient with advanced keratoconus due to folds in the DM that resolved with a DALK at a later stage and improved the BSCVA to 20/32.[24] HALK is also contraindicated in any case of corneal endothelial dysfunction.

Preoperative Consideration

The preoperative assessment of HALK follows the same guidelines as any other keratoplasty procedure. Uncorrected visual acuity (UCVA) and BSCVA assessment, and slit-lamp/fundus examination, the preoperative evaluation should also include rigid gas-permeable (RGP) contact lens fitting trial, contrast sensitivity, corneal front- and back-scatter estimation, potential acuity meter measurement (PAM), as well as ultrasound pachymetry (USP) and AS-OCT imaging. The ocular surface disease can compromise the long-term corneal graft survival.[34] Therefore, it needs to be managed preoperatively.

A precise analysis of the scar-depth in the host is essential in the surgical planning of HALK; otherwise, there is an increased risk of incomplete removal of the scar tissue and/or perforation. This assessment, commonly is performed by AS-OCT, can often be very challenging due to the artifacts and optical shadowing caused by the stromal pathology.[24] Imaging enhancement software may aid in sharper scar delineation.[35] HALK can be performed under the peribulbar or general anesthesia (GA).

The eligibility criterion of the donor cornea for HALK is less strict than PK, since HALK replaces the anterior 200–300 microns of the corneal stroma and preserves the host's endothelium. Therefore, HALK can potentially use tissue that would otherwise be discarded, such as corneas with clear stroma and low endothelial cell counts.[24] Also, eye banks may provide precut donor corneal tissue, based on the assessment of thickness and depth of the corneal scar in the recipient.

HEMI-AUTOMATED LAMELLAR KERATOPLASTY PROCEDURE

The surgical technique of HALK involves manual lamellar dissection of the recipient corneal bed, coupled with an automated and microkeratome-assisted preparation of the donor corneal tissue. Broadly, the technique can be divided into the following three steps:

1. The host's trephination and manual lamellar dissection.
2. The preparation of the donor (OT/Eye Bank).
3. The suturing of the donor on the host's stromal bed.

The Host's Trephination and Manual Lamellar Dissection

The recipient bed is usually prepared before the corneal donor cap is harvested. At times, the precut corneal donor button can be provided by the eye bank. Optical coherence tomography (OCT) can be used both preoperatively and intraoperatively to determine the depth of the corneal scar accurately. The recipient's central corneal thickness (CCT) is confirmed again intraoperatively using a USP (CorneoGage Plus, Sonogage, Cleveland, Ohio, USA). It is advisable to take a minimum of three readings by the USP to avoid inconsistencies in the assessment of irregular corneal surfaces. A vacuum trephine is then used to trephine the recipient corneal tissue partially. The depth of the partial trephination should be 20–50 microns deeper than the depth of the stromal pathology. However, the diameter of the partial trephination should correspond to the planned diameter of the lamellar dissection that was assessed preoperatively. The recipient's trephination diameter in HALK usually ranges from 7.5 to 8.75 mm.[24]

The vacuum trephines used on the recipient cornea are commercially available in different diameters. The Moria's single-use vacuum trephine (Moria, Antony, France) provides an adjustable preset depth setting and straight-walled cuts without parallax errors. [Diameters available: 6.00 mm, from 6.50 to 9.00 mm (0.25 mm increments), 9.50 mm and 10.00 mm]. The use of Hanna Vacuum Trephine System (Moria, Antony, France) allows adjustment within 50 microns in the depth of trephination. In addition, the Hessburg-Barron Vacuum Trephine (Katena Products Inc., Denville, NJ; Diameters available: 6.00–9.00 mm) and the Coronet Recipient Vacuum Trephine (Coronet™ Technology, UK; Diameters available: 6.50–9.50 mm) are other available options. However, it has been reported that the Hanna Vacuum Trephine System (Moria, Antony, France) has greater accuracy in depth and angle of trephination than the Hessburg-Barron Vacuum Trephine (Katena Products Inc., Denville, NJ) when evaluated using light microscopy, AS-OCT and elliptical curve fitting models.[36]

The partial trephination of the host cornea serves as a guide for the manual lamellar dissection. After partial trephination, a standard 2.25-mm crescent blade (BD Visitec, Oxford, UK) is used in a sweeping movement, for the sharp lamellar dissection, in the predetermined anatomical surgical plane, which facilitates complete removal of the anterior stromal pathology.[20,24] If needed, a second or third lamellar dissection can be performed at deeper planes to ensure complete removal of the abnormal scar tissue. The crescent blade dissects the corneal tissue anteriorly and on the sides, whereas, it is blunt inferiorly (**Fig. 2A**). However, if the crescent blade is not kept flat during lamellar dissection, there is an increased risk of creating an alternative dissection plane and penetrating into the anterior chamber.

The dissected corneal lamellae are excised at the trephination margin, using Anwar corneal scissors (Duckworth and Kent, Hertfordshire, UK) (**Fig. 2B**). A USP or an intraoperative OCT can be used to calculate the thickness of the residual stromal bed. Unlike microkeratome-assisted preparation of the recipient bed in ALTK, the sharp manual lamellar dissection in HALK does not replicate the topographical irregularities in the plane of the lamellar cut, which facilitates an optimal graft-host interface.

The Preparation of the Donor Cap (OT/Eye Bank)

The donor corneal button preparation in HALK combines the use of an AAC maintainer, with a microkeratome, of a changeable head thickness, for tailoring the lamellar dissection to the desired depth. The donor cap can either be prepared by the surgeon in the operation theater or provided by the eye bank as a precut tissue, which shortens the surgery time considerably.

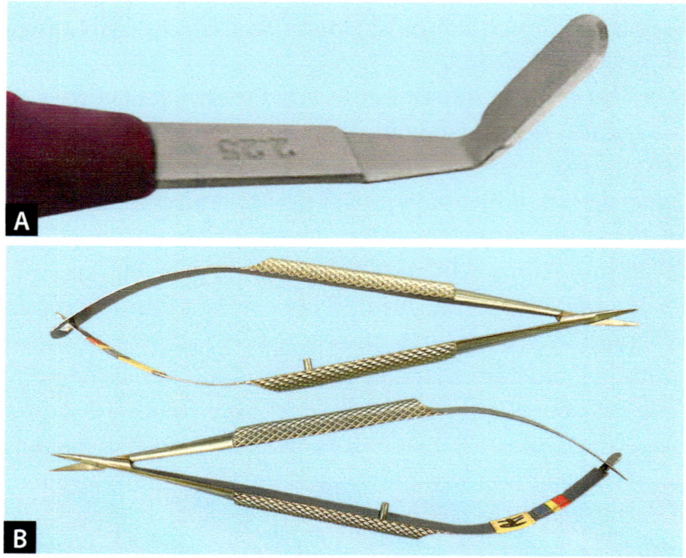

Figs. 2A and B: (A) Standard 2.25-mm crescent blade (BD Visitec, Oxford, UK); (B) Anwar corneal scissors (Duckworth and Kent, Hertfordshire, UK).

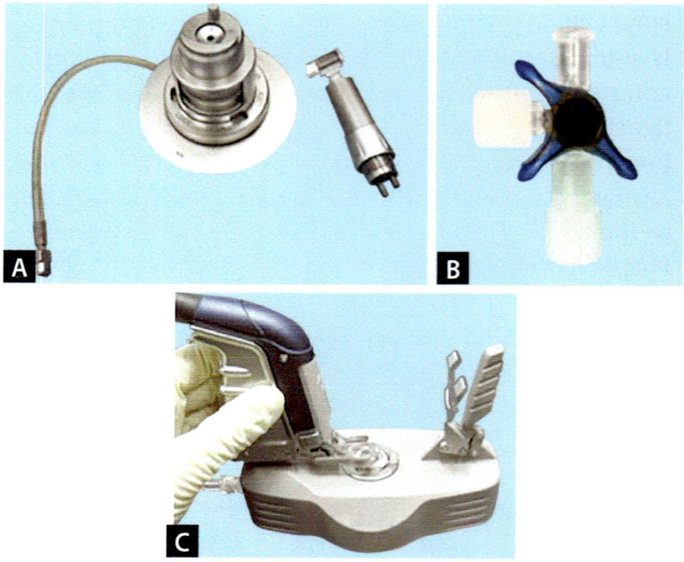

Figs. 3A to C: (A) The artificial anterior chamber (AAC) and microkeratome of Moria ALTK system (Moria SA, Antony, France Inc.); (B) Two-way valve; (C) Amadeus II AAC system (SIS, Ziemer Ophthalmic, Port, Switzerland).

Artificial Anterior Chambers

There are two types of AACs. The "reusable AACs" can be used repeatedly after sterilization, and include the Moria (manual, Moria SA, Antony, France Inc.), the Moria ALTK system (Moria SA, Antony, France Inc.), Amadeus II AAC (SIS, Ziemer Ophthalmic, Port, Switzerland), Med-Logics ML7 Microkeratome System (Med-Logics, Inc.) and the Bausch and Lomb (B&L manual) AAC. Whereas, the Barron AAC (Katena Inc., Denville, NJ, USA) is a type of "disposable AAC", which mounts the donor corneal button and maintains an adequate intra-chamber pressure, during the lamellar dissection or full-thickness trephination.[37]

Moria ALTK System (Moria SA, Antony, France Inc.)

The Moria ALTK system (Moria SA, Antony, France Inc.) is a stainless steel device that is designed to be used with a microkeratome.[37,38] The microkeratome cut of the Moria ALTK system (Moria SA, Antony, France Inc.) has been shown to create the smoothest graft-host interface, in a comparative analysis, with the horizon microkeratome and the FSL (Intralase FS60).[37,38] The Moria ALTK system (Moria SA, Antony, France Inc.) uses an Evolution 3 console (Moria, Inc.) that is compatible with all the available microkeratomes manufactured by the Moria (CB, M2 and LSK units).[37,38]

The AAC of the Moria's ALTK system (Moria SA, Antony, France Inc.) has a central post for placing the donor corneoscleral button with the endothelial side down (**Fig. 3A**). The AAC is also connected to an infusion reservoir through a two-way valve (**Fig. 3B**). The corneoscleral donor is then centred on the central post, and stabilized with the graft-tightening ring, keeping the infusion on, to avoid air bubbles. The encasing cylindrical unit is put in place and rotated clockwise to hold the donor cornea in position.[24,37]

During the donor preparation, it is important for the donor corneoscleral tissue to have a 360° scleral skirt, of at least 3.6 mm, to avoid tissue slippage and loss of intra-chamber pressure.[37,39] Also, it is advisable to maintain a pressure of 60–80 mm Hg or higher in the AAC during the preparation of the donor corneal lenticule.[24,37] This can be achieved either by raising the height of the infusion bottle to at least 1.50 m above the AAC, by applying an inflatable pressure cuff around the infusion reservoir[11,12,24] or using the recently introduced automated pressure machine (Moria SA, Antony, France Inc.). The Barraquer tonometer can confirm the pressure in the AAC.[11,12,24]

The corneal epithelium should be removed to avoid errors in the calculation of corneal thickness. The USP is then used to measure the total thickness of the donor cornea.[24] The depth of the recipient dissection determines the targeted thickness of the donor corneal cap, which can be achieved using a suitable microkeratome head (130–400 microns).[37] As discussed before, the depth of the lamellar cut and the symmetry in the thickness of the donor corneal button is dependent on the transition speed of microkeratome and the pressure inside the AAC during the procedure.[12] The microkeratome cut should be carried out with a smooth and continuous movement, at a constant speed, to avoid interface ridges and provide an optimal graft-host interface.

Amadeus II AAC System (SIS, Ziemer Ophthalmic, Port, Switzerland)

The Amadeus II AAC System (SIS, Ziemer Ophthalmic, Port, Switzerland) enables the surgeon or the technician to have both hands free during the dissection of the donor cap (**Fig. 3C**). The donor cornea is placed on the AAC body that is connected to an infusion reservoir through a three-way stopcock. The forward movement of the microkeratome is automated, and the speed of the microkeratome pass is adjustable that ensures a consistent cutting speed. Moreover, the shape of the AAC guides the mounted microkeratome into the correct position over the center of the donor cornea. A wide range of cutting depths (200–450 microns) is available with the Amadeus II AAC System (SIS, Ziemer Ophthalmic, Port, Switzerland).

Horizon Microkeratome System (Refractive Technologies, Cleveland, OH)

The Horizon Microkeratome System (Refractive Technologies, Cleveland, OH) uses a disposable microkeratome, which dissects the donor cornea that is mounted on a plastic AAC filled with pressurized air. The Horizon Microkeratome System (Refractive Technologies, Cleveland, OH) provides a smooth donor-host interface; however, it has some limitations. Unlike other AACs that are filled with fluid, the AAC of the Horizon Microkeratome System (Refractive Technologies, Cleveland, OH) requires a specially calibrated USP to measure the thickness of the donor cornea. Besides, the calibrated USP cannot measure the stromal bed thickness accurately if it is below 300 microns.[38] Therefore, it becomes difficult to calculate the thickness of the residual stromal bed after the microkeratome cut.[38]

Med-Logics ML7 Microkeratome System (Med-Logics, Inc.)

The Med-Logics ML7 Microkeratome System (Med-Logics, Inc.) uses an AAC that fixates the donor corneoscleral button easily. It also has a digital gauge to monitor the pressure in the AAC in real time. Moreover, the ML7 microkeratome has an automated advancement that is assisted by a motor and at an adjustable speed. This avoids the inter-surgeon and intra-surgeon variability in the transition speed of the microkeratome during the lamellar dissection.

In HALK, the recipient dissection can range between 150 and 250 microns.[24] Therefore, it is advisable to use a 350 μm microkeratome head to achieve a postoperative central corneal thickness of 550–600 μm.[24] The donor anterior lamella is removed from the head of the microkeratome, once it is dissected. The thickness of the donor corneal anterior lamella is calculated, by subtracting the thickness of the residual stromal bed from the initially measured total thickness of the donor cornea, using the USP.

Thereafter, the diameter of the donor corneal button has to be matched with the recipient bed for precise donor-host tissue apposition. The donor cap is placed on a punch block and trephined with a Hanna trephine (Moria Inc., Antony, France) or any other preferred trephine of the surgeon. The diameter of the trephines used on the recipient and the donor corneas are always the same. The trephine ensures accurate diameter sizing of both the recipient and donor, and also provides vertical side-cuts that promote optimal graft-host alignment.[24]

The Suturing of the Donor Cap on the Host's Stromal Bed

Once the donor lamella is prepared, the graft-host interface is rinsed with a balanced salt solution to remove any debris present. The donor corneal button can then be sutured onto the recipient bed using 10-0 nylon (Ethicon, Johnson and Johnson, New Brunswick, NJ, USA) interrupted sutures or any other preferred suturing technique of the surgeon. If available, an intraoperative keratoscope can be used to adjust the sutures for controlling postoperative astigmatism.[24]

An alternative is, sutureless ALK, using a microkeratome and fibrin glue, which can be considered as a treatment option for corneal opacities that are more superficial.[40] If the donor cap is placed on the recipient bed without suturing, it is essential to dry the edges of the graft-host junction with a sponge to promote graft-host adherence.[14]

Upon completion of the surgical procedure, subconjunctival injections of 14 mg/mL gentamicin (Schering AG, Berlin-Wedding, Germany), 50 mg/mL cefazolin (GlaxoSmithKline, Durham, NC, USA), and dexamethasone 0.1% (Merck and Co., Rahway, NJ, USA) are administered. A bandage contact lens (BCL) is also placed and kept for at least 5–7 days, or until the epithelium is healed completely. It is advisable to prescribe topical prednisolone acetate 1%, every qds for 1 month, to patients who undergo HALK. A topical antibiotic (levofloxacin 0.5%) can also be prescribed for a short duration. Besides, the topical steroid regime should be tapered over 4 months to avoid steroid-induced complications (glaucoma and cataract).[24]

COMPLICATIONS

Intraoperative Complications

Multiple Intralamellar Dissection Planes

Manual lamellar dissection of the recipient bed can be a challenging procedure due to the inherent limitation of judging the depth of dissection accurately. Multiple intralamellar dissection planes in the host cornea can lead to an irregular donor-host interface with compromised visual outcomes postoperatively. Moreover, shallower dissection planes than intended require multiple dissections with an increased risk of interface ridges and irregularities.

On the contrary, a deeper dissection plane has an added risk of perforating the recipient cornea. Therefore, it is important to maintain a uniplanar lamellar dissection by staying in the predetermined surgical plane.[24]

Challenges in Harvesting the Donor Cap

It is vital that surgeons have the expertise and training before using the different commercially available ALTK systems to dissect the donor cap. The head of the microkeratome must always be checked before the procedure to ensure that it corresponds to the target thickness.

In case of compression during the microkeratome pass, the resected donor lenticule may often be thicker than the planned cut.[41] It is essential to keep this in mind to avoid inaccuracies in the thickness of the donor lenticules and to mitigate the risk of perforation during deeper resections. It is also advisable to avoid the reuse of microkeratome blades as it can erroneously harvest donor caps that are too thin and have an inherent risk of buttonhole formation.

Early Postoperative Complications

Descemet's Membrane Wrinkles

The thickness of the donor cap in HALK can be altered predictably.[24] However, if the donor corneal lamella is too thick, it will compress the posterior residual stromal bed and lead to DM wrinkling, thus, adversely influencing the postoperative visual results.[24] The interface wrinkling can regress with time, but if it does not, the transplanted donor cap has to be exchanged with thinner tissue.[24] In a recent study, two patients (n = 2, 2/35) developed wrinkles in the DM or the graft-host interface following HALK, owing to thick donor lamellae, and required graft replacement with thinner donor caps.[24]

Postkeratoplasty Atopic Keratoscleritis

Postkeratoplasty atopic keratoscleritis (PKAS) is a rare phenomenon, which is associated with loose sutures, and causes acute inflammation of the ocular surface. The PKAS can occur during the early postoperative period after HALK and can lead to melting of the graft.[42] It should be treated with the removal of the loose sutures coupled with intensive topical and systemic immunosuppression.[42]

Interface Infections

Interface infections have been reported after lamellar keratoplasty.[43] The most common pathogens associated with interface infections are Candida, gram-positive bacteria, gram-negative bacteria, and herpes simplex.[43] During the procedure, the microorganisms can be sequestered in the graft-host interface. Hence, these microorganisms may resist topical antifungal/antibacterial therapy and should be followed up rigorously.[43] Since it is relatively easy to remove the donor cap in HALK, therefore, it is advisable to lift the donor button and irrigate the graft-host interface with an antifungal/antibacterial solution. Besides, in the event of therapeutic failure, the existing donor corneal button can be exchanged with new donor tissue.[24]

Epithelial Ingrowth

Corneal epithelial ingrowth after HALK is the presence of ectopic corneal epithelial cells in the graft-host interface.[44] Epithelial ingrowth can happen in HALK but has not been reported in the literature to date. It may cause troublesome glare, photophobia, foreign body sensation, decreased visual acuity, astigmatism, and keratolysis.[44] The treatment involves complete mechanical removal of the corneal epithelium from the posterior surface of the donor cap and the recipient stromal bed. Additionally, alcohol, mitomycin C, neodymium:yttrium aluminum garnet laser and fibrin glue can be used for recurrent or refractory cases.[45] Thereafter, the same or a freshly prepared donor button can be sutured or placed on the host's stromal bed.

Suture-related Problems

Suture-related factors can cause graft infections that often effect graft survival.[40] Besides, sterile suture infiltrates, suture-related corneal ulceration, suture loosening (secondary to corneal deturgescence, after suture-tract infections or biodegradation of the suture material)[46] with subsequent wound dehiscence, involve a cascade of events that can complicate the postoperative course of HALK. Periodic monitoring and prompt intervention can prevent suture-related complications in HALK.[46]

Dellen

A corneal dellen is a localized saucer-like excavation that may arise due to an irregular graft-host junction after HALK. The corneal dellen can interfere with the normal tear film distribution by causing a localized break in its oily layer, thus, causing stromal dehydration, thinning, tissue loss, scarring, and astigmatism. The treatment includes rehydration with artificial lubricants and addressing the contributory cause of corneal dellen.[47]

Late Postoperative Complications

Steroid-induced Glaucoma

Steroids can raise the intraocular pressure (IOP) by altering the extracellular matrix around the trabecular meshwork and increasing the outflow resistance.[48] The transient or persistent rise in IOP is detrimental to the health of the optic nerve, with more pronounced effects in the children and adults, who have preexisting glaucomatous optic neuropathy.[48] Steroid-induced ocular hypertension has been reported in patients who underwent HALK.[24] However, rapid tapering of the steroids and instillation of IOP lowering drugs proved effective in controlling steroid-induced glaucoma.[24]

Graft Rejection

Graft rejection after ALK has been reported in the literature.[49] The stroma is the most common site of graft rejection in ALK.[49] However, stromal rejections are less aggressive and more amenable to treatment than the corneal endothelial rejections that can be seen in penetrating and endothelial keratoplasties. Steroids (topical, oral, and subconjunctival routes) and immunosuppressive agents can be used to prevent and treat corneal graft rejections.[49]

Graft Failure

Graft failure is defined as a cornea that was cloudy on the first postoperative day and did not clear within 8 weeks (primary or early donor graft failure, depending upon whether the donor-graft failure occurred in the absence or presence of operative complications, respectively) or a cornea that initially cleared and subsequently became cloudy for 3 months (late donor graft failure).[50] In HALK, graft failure can be due to residual scarring in the recipient's stromal bed, wrinkles in the DM or infectious keratitis.[24] Following graft failure, the scarred/opaque donor cap can be replaced by secondary procedure.

Recurrence of Corneal Degenerations and Dystrophies

The recurrence of corneal degenerations and corneal dystrophies after corneal grafting is well known.[51] Likewise, after HALK, recurrence of lattice dystrophy in the peripheral graft-host margin has been noted (**Fig. 4**).[24]

Recurrence of Herpes Simplex Virus Keratitis

It has been suggested that trauma to corneal nerves during corneal transplantation can lead to reactivation of HSV at the site of its latency.[52] During the process, HSV is released from the nerve endings in the cornea. Recurrence of HSV keratitis with subepithelial corneal infiltrates after HALK has been reported.[24] A combination therapy comprising of topical acyclovir ointment and steroids is required.[24] The recurrence of HSV keratitis following HALK can also lead to graft failure.[24]

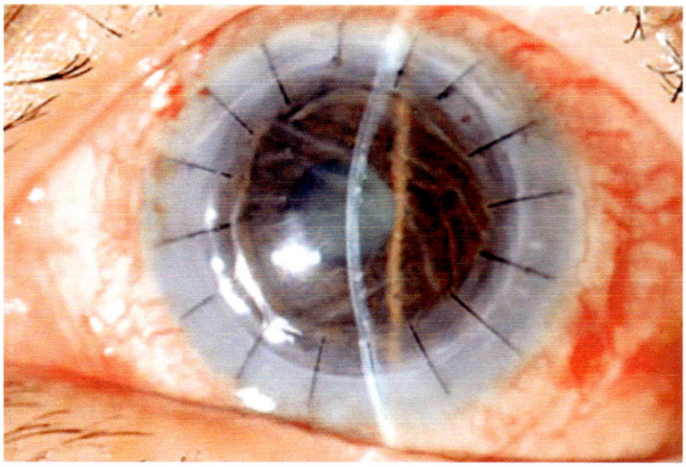

Fig. 4: Postoperative slit-lamp picture of a patient with recurrence of lattice dystrophy after hemi-automated lamellar keratoplasty.

Postoperative Astigmatism

Astigmatism is a significant challenge that is associated with sutured-keratoplasty.[40] Postoperative astigmatism in HALK patients can lead to decreased visual acuity, image distortion, aniseikonia, and diplopia. Varying suture techniques with intraoperative adjustments, better trephination, and use of femtosecond technology may reduce the occurrence of postoperative astigmatism.[53] Moreover, spectacles, rigid gas-permeable contact lenses, corneal topography-guided suture adjustment and/or removal, relaxing incisions, PRK, and LASIK are options to manage postoperative astigmatism in HALK patients.

OUTCOMES OF HEMI-AUTOMATED LAMELLAR KERATOPLASTY

In HALK, it is imperative to do a smooth manual lamellar dissection and ensure complete removal of the anterior stromal pathology, without replicating the surface irregularities in the interface. Recently, Fuest et al. have shown the long-term outcomes of HALK by following the patients for a mean period of 61.4 ± 29.2 months.[24]

Visual Acuity

Hemi-automated lamellar keratoplasty has been shown to improve the postoperative visual acuity significantly.[24] UCVA improved from 0.91 ± 0.31 to 0.58 ± 0.35 logMAR ($p < 0.001$), whereas BSCVA from 0.66 ± 0.30 to 0.21 ± 0.20 logMAR ($p < 0.001$) at the last follow-up. The postoperative BSCVA in HALK patients was 0.28 logMAR at 1-year follow-up.[24] It was better than BSCVA seen after the ALTK, which was reported by Acar et al. (0.34 ± 0.15 logMAR)[54] and Vajpayee et al.[11] (0.33 ± 0.30 logMAR at 6 months). Both the groups used a microkeratome for the preparation of donor and the recipient corneal caps to treat different anterior stromal pathologies with surface irregularities. The inferior outcomes of BSCVA, in the studies conducted by Acar and Vajpayee, could be attributed to the aforementioned limitations of the microkeratomes with surface irregularities.

Stromal Remodeling

Interestingly, BSCVA continued to improve throughout the follow-up period in HALK patients. It was attributed to the stromal remodeling of the graft-host interface by the corneal keratocytes. The higher corneal keratocyte density in the anterior stroma leads to faster and more extensive stromal remodeling in HALK.[55] However, a denser keratocyte population has also been associated with an increased risk of interface scarring.[55] However, in HALK, the latter is minimized because the sharp manual lamellar dissection of the host cornea ensures optimal graft-host interface.

Astigmatism and Spherical Equivalent

In HALK patients, the overall postoperative change in astigmatism and spherical equivalent (SE) at the last follow-up visit was statistically insignificant ($p = 0.2$ and $p = 0.8$, respectively).[24] The mean postoperative refractive cylinder (3.14 ± 1.86 D)[24] following HALK was comparable to the postoperative cylindrical values seen after ALTK (2.33 ± 0.98 D to 4.50 ± 1.05 D)[54] and FSL-assisted ALK (–3.74 ± 2.62 D).[56] The mean postoperative SE (–2.21 D) seen in HALK patients[24] was also comparable to the mean SE reported after ALTK (–1.5 D and –3.45 ± 0.77 D).[54]

Central Corneal Thickness

The reported mean donor-cap thickness for HALK, harvested with a 350 μm microkeratome head, was of 349.4 ± 51.3 μm, whereas, the mean recipient's residual stromal bed thickness was of 194.2 ± 34.8 μm.[24] Therefore, the central corneal thickness (CCT) increased from 490 to 560 μm ($p = 0.004$) postoperatively.[24] Targeting a thicker postoperative CCT may have its advantages. A thicker stroma provides the surgeon with an opportunity to perform a planned refractive surgery procedure, at a future date, in the likely event of a residual/unexpected postoperative refractive error.

Endothelial Cell Loss

The surgical plane in HALK is usually away from the DM. Therefore, the surgery-induced endothelial cells loss in HALK is negligible ($p = 0.4$).[24]

Graft Survival

The graft survival in primary HALK cases and patients with prior keratoplasty is very encouraging.[24] In Fuest's study, the Kaplan-Meier estimated survival for all HALK cases was 90.6 months (95% confidence interval 82.6–98.5). Furthermore, the survival probability was 96% at 12 months and 92% at 3, 5, and 7 years follow-up postoperatively.[24] None of the HALK cases underwent a rejection episode during the follow-up period.

Femtosecond Laser-assisted HALK: A Futuristic Perspective

The technological advancements in FSL platforms, development of new nomograms, and a better understanding of laser-tissue interaction have made FSL-assisted lamellar dissection a possibility. FSL-assisted ALTK has shown a BSCVA of 0.20 logMAR (12 months follow-up),[56] which is comparable to 0.28 logMAR (12 months follow-up), seen in HALK patients.[24] Nonetheless, some of the available FSL platforms use a flat applanation cones, which can reproduce the surface irregularities in the graft-host interface and affect the postoperative visual outcomes. In addition, the high cost and the limited availability of the FSL platforms have restricted their widespread use worldwide. Besides, the laser beam can undergo scattering and has limited penetration, as it passes through significant corneal opacities, which may further limit the use of FSL platforms.[24]

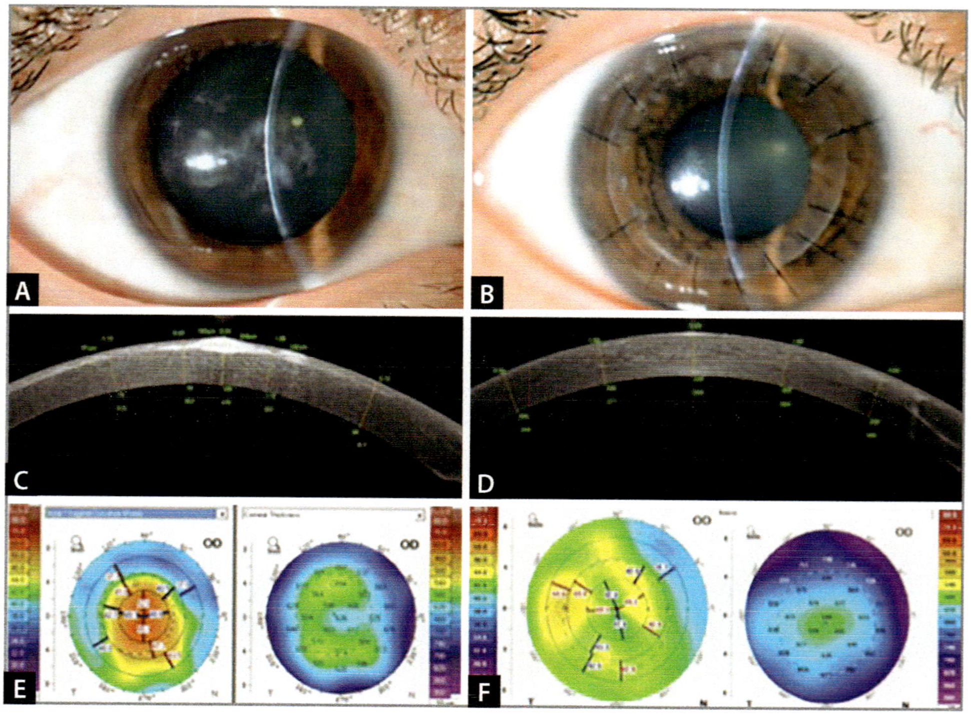

Figs. 5A to F: Preoperative slit-lamp (A) and optical coherence tomography (OCT) (C) pictures, showing refractive surgery-associated anterior stromal scar, suitable for femtosecond laser (FSL)-assisted hemi-automated lamellar keratoplasty (HALK) treatment, as well as postoperative slit-lamp (B) and OCT (D) pictures. The corneal topographic measurements before (E) and 8 months after FSL-assisted HALK (F) show improvement in astigmatism.

Despite the limitations, FSL-assisted ALK is gaining popularity because of its precision in corneal dissection at a customizable depth, thereby enabling surgeons to reach a dissection plane just inferior to the stromal pathology.[57] The highly reproducible dimensions of the cuts at the graft-host margin and the adjustable orientation of the vertical side-cuts that is achieved with FSL technology, also enhance the precision in ALK.[58] Moreover, FSL technology allows a donor-lenticule harvest of uniform thickness.[58] In addition, curtailed surgical time, decreased risk of microkeratome-related complications (e.g., button-hole, cap tears) are other potential advantages of FSL-assisted ALK.[57,58] Considering the benefits of FSL technology, FSL-assisted HALK has been used in our clinical setting to treat corneal scars (secondary to post-PRK haze and interstitial keratitis) with topographical irregularities that obscured the visual axis as shown in **Figures 5A to F**. Postoperatively, BSCVA increased by two Snellen lines in both the cases, whereas, the astigmatism decreased from 4.7 to 1.6 D and from 4.1 to 1.0 D, respectively at the last follow-up.

In conclusion, HALK is a hybrid surgical technique that combines manual recipient and automated-microkeratome donor dissection. HALK is useful for the treatment of corneal scars, corneal degenerations, corneal dystrophies, and post-PRK haze that involve the anterior or middle stroma and have associated topographical irregularities. Besides, HALK retains the host's endothelium and is superior to PK regarding repeatability, tectonic strength, and intraoperative complications.[24] HALK is also surgically less demanding than DALK with a reduced risk of conversion to PK.[24] However, HALK is not recommended for patients with active infection or inflammation, posterior stromal pathologies, Descemet membrane's scarring/folds, and endothelial dysfunction.

Funding sources: The authors did not receive any specific grants from funding agencies in the public, commercial, or not-for-profit sectors.

REFERENCES

1. Jhanji V, Mehta JS, Sharma N, Sharma B, Vajpayee RB. Targeted corneal transplantation. Curr Opin Ophthalmol. 2012;23(4):324-9.
2. Tan DT, Mehta JS. Future directions in lamellar corneal transplantation. Cornea. 2007;26(9 Suppl 1):S21-8.
3. Tan DT, Anshu A, Mehta JS. Paradigm shifts in corneal transplantation. Ann Acad Med Singapore. 2009;38(4):332-8.
4. Noble BA, Agrawal A, Collins C, Saldana M, Brogden PR, Zuberbuhler B. Deep anterior lamellar keratoplasty (DALK): Visual outcome and complications for a heterogeneous group of corneal pathologies. Cornea. 2007;26(1):59-64.
5. Watson SL, Tuft SJ, Dart JK. Patterns of rejection after deep lamellar keratoplasty. Ophthalmology. 2006;113(4):556-60.
6. Watson SL, Ramsay A, Dart JK, Bunce C, Craig E. Comparison of deep lamellar keratoplasty and penetrating keratoplasty in patients with keratoconus. Ophthalmology. 2004;111(9):1676-82.
7. Wiley LA, Joseph MA, Pemberton JD. Microkeratome-assisted anterior lamellar keratoplasty. Arch Ophthalmol. 2008;126(3):404-8.
8. Jiménez-Alfaro I, Pérez-Santonja JJ, Gómez Tellería G, Bueno Palacín JL, Puy P. Therapeutic lamellar keratoplasty with an automated microkeratome. J Cataract Refract Surg. 2001;27(8):1161-5.
9. Hafezi F, Mrochen M, Fankhouser F 2nd, Seiler T. Anterior lamellar keratoplasty with a microkeratome: a method for managing complications after refractive surgery. J Refract Surg. 2003;19:52-7.
10. Alio JL, Shah S, Barraquer C, Bilgihan K, Anwar M, Melles GR. New techniques in lamellar keratoplasty. Curr Opin Ophthalmol. 2002;13(4):224-9.
11. Vajpayee RB, Vasudendra N, Titiyal JS, Tandon R, Sharma N, Sinha R. Automated lamellar therapeutic keratoplasty (ALTK) in the treatment of anterior to mid-stromal corneal pathologies. Acta Ophthalmol Scand. 2006;84(6):771-3.
12. Bhogal MS, Allan BD. Graft profile and thickness as a function of cut transition speed in Descemet-stripping automated endothelial keratoplasty. J Cataract Refract Surg. 2012;38(4):690-5.
13. Guber I, Bergin C, Othenin-Girard P, Munier F, Majo F. 12-year outcomes of microkeratome-assisted anterior lamellar therapeutic keratoplasty (ALTK) for disorders of the anterior part of the corneal stroma - a comparative review of adult and children. Klin Monbl Augenheilkd. 2018;235(4):404-8.
14. Fogla R, Knyazer B. Microkeratome-assisted two-stage technique of superficial anterior lamellar keratoplasty for Reis-Bücklers corneal dystrophy. Cornea. 2014;33(10):1118-22.
15. Wiley LA, Joseph MA, Springs CL. Tectonic lamellar keratoplasty utilising a microkeratome and an artificial anterior chamber system. Cornea. 2002;21(7):661-3.
16. Tan DT, Ang LP. Automated lamellar therapeutic keratoplasty for post-PRK corneal scarring and thinning. Am J Ophthalmol. 2004;138(6):1067-9.
17. Sorkin N, Einan-Lifshitz A, Boutin T, Showail M, Borovik A, Chan CC, et al. Topography-guided photorefractive keratectomy in the treatment of corneal scarring. J Refract Surg. 2017;33(9):639-44.
18. Holland S, Lin DT, Tan JC. Topography-guided laser refractive surgery. Curr Opin Ophthalmol. 2013;24(4):302-9.
19. Wallerstein A, Caron-Cantin M, Gauvin M, Adiguzel E, Cohen M. Primary topography-guided LASIK: refractive, visual, and subjective quality of vision outcomes for astigmatism ≥2.00 diopters. J Refract Surg. 2019;35(2):78-86.
20. Yuen LH, Mehta JS, Shilbayeh R, Lim L, Tan DT. Hemi-automated lamellar keratoplasty (HALK). Br J Ophthalmol. 2011;95(11):1513-8.
21. Li EY, Mohamed S, Leung CK, Rao SK, Cheng AC, Cheung CY, et al. Agreement among 3 methods to measure corneal thickness: ultrasound pachymetry, Orbscan II and Visante anterior segment optical coherence tomography. Ophthalmology. 2007;114(10):1842-7.
22. Tan DT, Ang LP. Modified automated lamellar therapeutic keratoplasty for keratoconus: a new technique. Cornea. 2006;25(10):1217-9.
23. Jackson DW, Wang L, Koch DD. Accuracy and precision of the amadeus microkeratome in producing LASIK flaps. Cornea. 2003;22(6):504-7.
24. Fuest M, Liu YC, Arundhati A, Li L, Tan D, Mehta JS. et al. Long-term outcomes of hemi-automated lamellar keratoplasty. Clin Exp Ophthalmol. 2018;46(9):1017-27.
25. Zimmerman AB, Nixon AD, Rueff EM. Contact lens associated microbial keratitis: practical considerations for the optometrist. Clin Optom (Auckl). 2016;8:1-12.
26. Bourges JL. Corneal dystrophies. J Fr Ophtalmol. 2017;40(6):e177-92.

27. Aggarwal S, Peck T, Golen J, Sharma B, Vajpayee RB. Macular corneal dystrophy: A review. Surv Ophthalmol. 2018;63(5):609-17.
28. Maharana PK, Sharma N, Das S, Karcioglu ZA. Salzmann's nodular degeneration. Ocul Surf. 2016;14(1):20-30.
29. Farjo QA, Sugar A. Corneal degenerations. In: Yanoff M, Duker JS (Eds). Ophthalmology, 3rd edition. St. Louis: Mosby/Elsevier; 2009. pp. 318-23.
30. Ficker LA, Kirkness CM, Rice NS, Steele AD. Longterm prognosis for corneal grafting in herpes simplex keratitis. Eye (Lond). 1988; 2(Pt 4):400-8.
31. Larkin DF. Corneal transplantation for herpes simplex keratitis. Br J Ophthalmol. 1998;82(2):107-8.
32. Goldblum D, Bachmann C, Tappeiner C, Garweg J, Frueh BE. Comparison of oral antiviral therapy with valacyclovir or acyclovir after penetrating keratoplasty for herpetic keratitis. Br J Ophthalmol. 2008;92(9):1201-5.
33. Rao SK, Fogla R, Seethalakshmi G, Padmanabhan P. Excimer laser phototherapeutic keratectomy: indications, results and its role in the Indian scenario. Indian J Ophthalmol. 1999;47(3):167-72.
34. Ho YJ, Wu CH, Chen HC, Hsiao CS, Hsueh YJ, Ma DH. Surgical outcome of deep anterior lamellar keratoplasty with air-assisted manual dissection for corneas with previous inflammation or fibrosis. Taiwan J Ophthalmol. 2017;7(4):191-8.
35. Girard MJ, Ang M, Chung CW, Farook M, Strouthidis N, Mehta JS, et al. Enhancement of corneal visibility in optical coherence tomography images using corneal adaptive compensation. Transl Vis Sci Technol. 2015;4(3):3.
36. Moshirfar M, Calvo CM, Kinard KI, Williams LB, Sikder S, Neuffer MC. Comparison of Hanna and Hessburg-Barron trephine and punch systems using histological, anterior segment optical coherence tomography, and elliptical curve fitting models. Clin Ophthalmol. 2011; 5:1121-5.
37. Brightbill FS, McDonnell PJ, McGhee CN, Farjo AA, Serdarevic ON. Corneal Surgery: Theory, Technique and Tissue, 4th edition. Mosby/Elsevier; 2009. pp. 1-912.
38. Mootha VV, Heck E, Verity SM, Petroll WM, Lakshman N, Muftuoglu O, et al. Comparative study of descemet stripping automated endothelial keratoplasty donor preparation by Moria CBm microkeratome, horizon microkeratome, and Intralase FS60. Cornea. 2011;30(3):320-4.
39. John T, Selvadurai D, Ruszkowski E, et al. Evaluation of three artificial anterior chamber using donor human corneoscleral explants. Presented at the annual meeting of The Cornea Society and Eye Bank Association of America, Federal Scientific Session Meeting. New Orleans, LA: The Cornea Society and Eye Bank Association of America; 2004.
40. Agarwal T, Bandivadekar P, Sharma N, Sagar P, Titiyal JS. Sutureless anterior lamellar keratoplasty with phacoemulsification. Cornea. 2015;34(6):615-20.
41. Jones YJ, Goins KM, Sutphin JE, Mullins R, Skeie JM. Comparison of the femtosecond laser (IntraLase) versus manual microkeratome (Moria ALTK) in dissection of the donor in endothelial keratoplasty: initial study in eye bank eyes. Cornea. 2008;27(1):88-93.
42. Lyons CJ, Dart JK, Aclimandos WA, Lightman S, Buckley RJ. Sclerokeratitis after keratoplasty in atopy. Ophthalmology. 1990;97(6):729-33.
43. Lyall DA, Srinivasan S, Roberts F. A case of interface keratitis following anterior lamellar keratoplasty. Surv Ophthalmol. 2012;57(6):551-7.
44. Nicolas M, Abouzeid H, Deprez M, Hafezi F, Munier FL, Varga Z, et al. Epithelial ingrowth cells after LASIK/ALTK (automated lamellar therapeutic keratoplasty): are they corneal epithelial stem cells? Br J Ophthalmol. 2012;96(7):1043-6.
45. Ting DS, Srinivasan S, Danjoux JP. Epithelial ingrowth following laser in situ keratomileusis (LASIK): prevalence, risk factors, management and visual outcomes. BMJ Open Ophthalmol. 2018;3(1):e000133.
46. Christo CG, van Rooij J, Geerards AJ, Remeijer L, Beekhuis WH. Suture-related complications following keratoplasty: a 5-year retrospective study. Cornea. 2001;20(8):816-9.
47. Accorinti M, Gilardi M, Giubilei M, De Geronimo D, Iannetti L. Corneal and scleral dellen after an uneventful pterygium surgery and a febrile episode. Case Rep Ophthalmol. 2014;5(1):111-5.
48. Nuyen B, Weinreb RN, Robbins SL. Steroid-induced glaucoma in the pediatric population. J AAPOS. 2017;21(1):1-6.
49. Borderie VM, Guilbert E, Touzeau O, Laroche L. Graft rejection and graft failure after anterior lamellar versus penetrating keratoplasty. Am J Ophthalmol. 2011;151(6):1024-9.e1.
50. Terry MA, Aldave AJ, Szczotka-Flynn LB, Liang W, Ayala AR, Maguire MG, et al. Cornea Preservation Time Study Group. Donor, recipient, and operative factors associated with graft success in the cornea preservation time study. Ophthalmology. 2018;125(11):1700-9.
51. Marcon AS, Cohen EJ, Rapuano CJ, Laibson PR. Recurrence of corneal stromal dystrophies after penetrating keratoplasty. Cornea. 2003;22(1):19-21.
52. Nicholls SM, Shimeld C, Easty DL, Hill TJ. Recurrent herpes simplex after corneal transplantation in rats. Invest Ophthalmol Vis Sci. 1996;37(2):425-35.
53. Bahar I, Levinger E, Kaiserman I, Sansanayudh W, Rootman DS. IntraLase-enabled astigmatic keratotomy for postkeratoplasty astigmatism. Am J Ophthalmol. 2008;146(6):897-904.e1.
54. Acar BT, Arslan OS, Buttanri IB, Sevim MŞ, Acar S. Comparing deep anterior lamellar keratoplasty and automated lamellar therapeutic keratoplasty in patients with keratoconus. Jpn J Ophthalmol. 2011;55(4):327-32.
55. Patel S, McLaren J, Hodge D, Bourne W. Normal human keratocyte density and corneal thickness measurement by using confocal microscopy in vivo. Invest Ophthalmol Vis Sci. 2001;42(2):333-9.
56. Mosca L, Fasciani R, Tamburelli C, Buzzonetti L, Guccione L, Mandarà E, et al. Femtosecond laser-assisted lamellar keratoplasty: early results. Cornea. 2008;27(6):668-72.
57. Yoo SH, Kymionis GD, Koreishi A, Ide T, Goldman D, Karp CL, et al. Femtosecond laser-assisted sutureless anterior lamellar keratoplasty. Ophthalmology. 2008;115(8):1303-7.e1
58. Shetty R, Nagaraja H, Veluri H, Shivanna Y, Kugar T, Nujits R, et al. Sutureless femtosecond anterior lamellar keratoplasty: a 1-year follow-up study. Indian J Ophthalmol. 2014;62(9):923-6.

48

Compressive C-shaped Lamellar Keratoplasty

Namrata Sharma, Prakhyat Roop, Ritu Nagpal

INTRODUCTION

The management of advanced peripheral corneal ectasias has always been challenging for the corneal surgeons. Peripheral corneal ectasias such as the pellucid marginal degeneration (PMD) and the Terrien's marginal degeneration (TMD) cause eccentric thinning with high irregular astigmatism, in their advanced stages.[1-4] Rehabilitation of any eye with irregular astigmatism involves regularizing the corneal surface so as to minimize the astigmatism, or at the very least, make it resolvable in two orthogonal axes. In the early stages of disease, visual rehabilitation can be achieved using rigid gas permeable lenses[1] and scleral contact lenses. Advanced stages, however, cannot be dealt with contact lenses only and therefore need surgical intervention for regularization of the anterior corneal surface. While, the standard keratoplasty techniques; lamellar or full are the straightforward answers while dealing with corneal ectasias involving the central cornea only, eyes with peripheral corneal ectasias are much more complex.

Since PMD presents with thinning and ectasia involving the perilimbal inferior cornea,[1] carrying out a full-thickness keratoplasty entails using either a very large graft to include the limbus or using a relatively small size graft which is placed eccentrically.[5] In either situation, complications such as distorted anterior chamber angle anatomy with peripheral anterior synechiae formation, uncontrolled intraocular pressure causing glaucoma and the increased risk of graft rejection,[6] are inevitable. Over the years, different surgical techniques have been tried and tested in order to avoid these problems and to limit the unjustified removal of healthy corneal tissue. The initial techniques of thermokeratoplasty[6] and epikeratophakia, both gave dismal outcomes and therefore are now out of favor. Resection techniques, either lamellar or full-thickness wedge resection although involve removal of the ectatic tissue only, suffer from disadvantages of unpredicted postoperative refraction with progressive loss of the desired effect over a period of time.[5,7] Crescentic lamellar keratoplasty, described by Schanzlin et al.,[8] involves free-hand dissection of both donor and host tissues, followed by placement of a similar sized graft. Compressive C-shaped lamellar keratoplasty is another surgical technique, described by Cheng et al. for addressing advanced peripheral ectasias. The technique involves lamellar dissection of the pathologically thinned out stromal tissue, followed by placement of an undersized donor tissue. The dissected area is replaced using a donor tissue which is narrow in width, compared to the area of original dissection. Graft-host junction apposition is obtained by drawing the edges of the recipient bed closer toward a narrow width graft and placement of tight compressive sutures. The inward drawing of the host edges in order to approximate with a narrow-sized donor tissue creates a strong compressive effect which causes flattening of the anterior corneal surface. Using a narrower graft helps in maintaining the compressive effect, even after the sutures are removed (**Figs. 1A to H**).

SURGICAL TECHNIQUE

The surgical procedure is carried out under general anesthesia.

Host preparation: Preparation of host begins by peritomy, performed adjacent to the area of corneal ectasia. The conjunctiva adjacent to the area of corneal ectasia is incised and retracted away, in order to completely reveal the extent of corneal thinning. The inner and outer dimensions of the thinned out area are then identified and marked using handheld trephines of various diameters. The ends of the inner and outer limits of the marked area are joined using a dermatological trephine of appropriate size, so as to have a C-shaped strip demarcating the area to be dissected. Using a diamond knife, a partial thickness vertical incision is made to create a vertical edge which is used to carry out lamellar dissection along the marked area of corneal ectasia.

Donor preparation: The donor lamellar graft is prepared by a technique described by Wong et al.,[9] wherein the corneoscleral button is firmly sutured over a draped glass orbital implant. Suturing of donor tissue ensures adequate stability in order to dissect out a lamellar graft which exactly matches the area of defect in shape as well

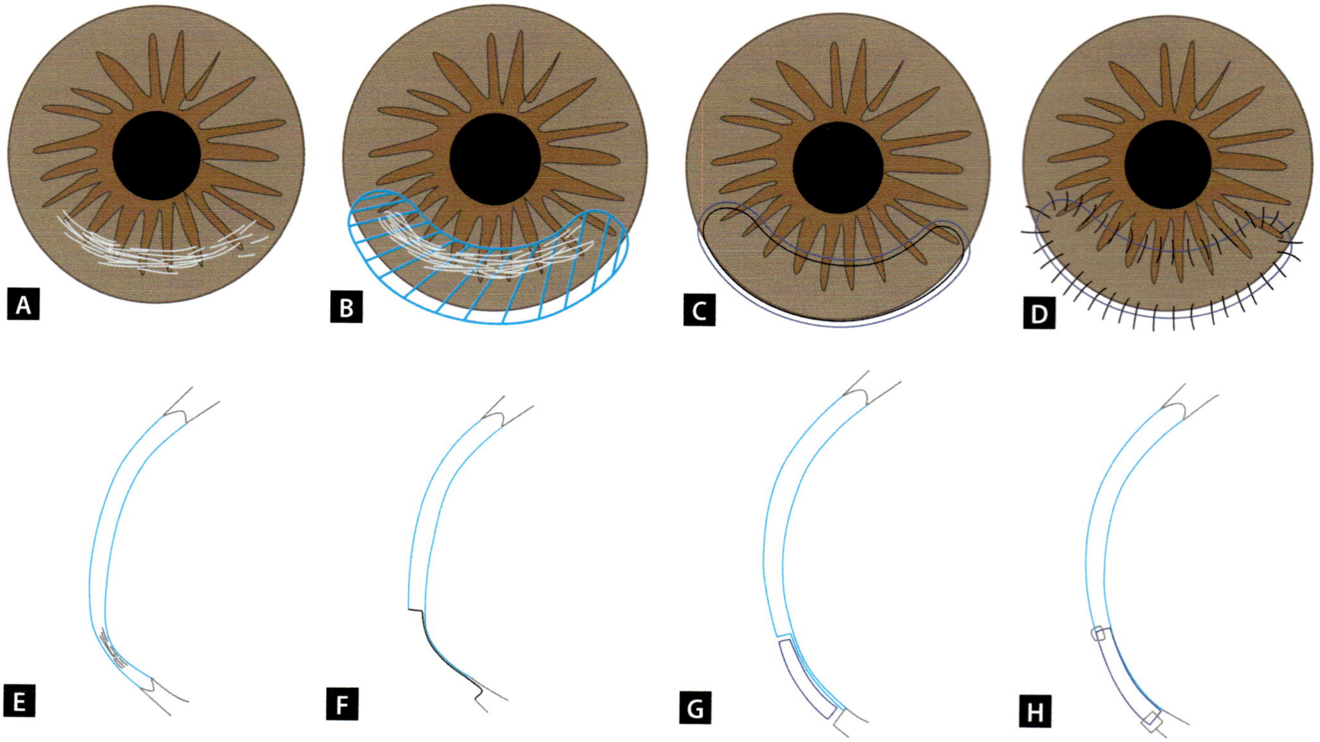

Figs. 1A to H: Schematic diagram showing various steps of compressive C-shaped keratoplasty. A and E depict the area of inferior corneal ectasia, adjacent to limbus in diffuse and slit view respectively. B and F show the C-shaped area to be dissected out in diffuse and slit view respectively. C shows a C-shaped graft, narrower in width as compared to the host bed, placed over it. The edges of the graft do not correspond with the superior and inferior dimensions of the dissected area. G shows the undersized graft placed over the host bed in slit view. D and H show the narrower graft well-secured over the host bed with interrupted sutures in diffuse and slit view respectively.

as in size. Using similar size trephines as used to mark the host bed, a lamellar graft is fashioned out. Width of the graft is however kept 0.25–0.5 mm lesser than the width of the area marked over the host bed. The graft is secured over the host bed using a combination of 10/0 and 9/0 nylon interrupted sutures. Use of 9/0 nylon sutures help to provide the necessary strength to keep the junction apposed, since a small-sized graft is used. Compression sutures are placed under direct keratoscopic guidance so as to ensure overcorrection of astigmatism by approximately 50%, in the required axis.

OUTCOMES OF COMPRESSIVE KERATOPLASTY

In a retrospective case series by Cheng et al.,[10] four eyes of three patients with either pellucid or Terrien's marginal corneal degeneration were treated with compressive C-shaped lamellar keratoplasty. 100% eyes were able to achieve visual acuity of 20/40 or better with stable astigmatism ranging from 0 to –2.75 D within 6 months, following the surgical procedure. None of the eyes experienced complications such as recurrence of the original corneal pathology or peripheral corneal vascularization till 6 months follow-up.

Progression of cataract requiring surgical intervention was seen in three out of four eyes. Cataract surgery with intraocular lens implantation was performed with good visual outcomes and no graft-related complications were seen in the immediate postoperative period. In two eyes, however, a recurrence of original corneal pathology was observed requiring astigmatic keratotomy and compression sutures, following which a stable refraction was maintained till 40 months of follow-up. None of the eye experienced any episode of graft rejection at any point of time.

CONCLUSION

Overall, the surgical technique of compressive C-shaped lamellar keratoplasty helps to achieve good postoperative visual results due to regularization of the anterior corneal surface and reduction in astigmatism. Success of the procedure requires careful dissection of corneal stroma, especially in areas of extreme ectasia, in order to avoid inadvertent corneal perforation. Postoperative complications such as recurrence of the original corneal pathology are amenable to treatment by a second stage refractive procedure without compromising the integrity of the graft.

REFERENCES

1. Krachmer JH. Pellucid marginal degeneration. Arch Ophthalmol. 1978;96:1217-21.
2. Karabatsas CH, Cook SD. Topographic analysis in pellucid marginal corneal degeneration and keratoglobus. Eye. 1996;10:451-5.

3. Rao SK, Fogla R, Padmanabhan P, Sitalakshmi G. Corneal topography in atypical pellucid marginal degeneration. Cornea. 1999;18:265-72.
4. Bower KS, Dhaliwal DK, Barnhorst DA, Warnicke J. Pellucid marginal degeneration with superior corneal thinning. Cornea. 1997;16:483-5.
5. Dubroff S. Pellucid marginal corneal degeneration: report on corrective surgery. J Cataract Refract Surg. 1989;15:89-93.
6. Varley GA, Macsai MS, Krachmer JH. The results of penetrating keratoplasty for pellucid marginal corneal degeneration. Am J Ophthalmol. 1990;110:149-52.
7. Cameron JA. Results of lamellar crescentic resection for pellucid marginal corneal degeneration. Am J Ophthalmol. 1992;113:296-302.
8. Schanzlin DJ, Sarno EM, Robin JB. Crescentic lamellar keratoplasty for pellucid marginal degeneration [letter]. Am J Ophthalmol. 1983;96:253-4.
9. Wong DW, Chan WK, Tan DT. Harvesting a lamellar graft from a corneoscleral button: a new technique. Am J Ophthalmol. 1997;123:688-9.
10. Cheng CL, Theng JTS, Tan DTH. Compressive C-shaped lamellar keratoplasty. Ophthalmology. 2005;112(3):425-30.

49 Femtosecond Laser-assisted Keratoplasty

Nir Sorkin, David S Rootman

FEMTOSECOND LASER IN CORNEAL SURGERY

Femtosecond laser technology was developed by Dr Kurtz at the University of Michigan in the early 1990s,[1] and rapidly became an integral part of ophthalmic surgery. Femtosecond lasers emit infrared pulses of short duration (10^{-15} s) at a wavelength of 1053 nm, that cause photodisruption of the tissue with minimum collateral damage.[2] The laser vaporizes the tissue, producing plasma, shock wave, cavitation, and gas (CO_2 and H_2O) bubbles. By aligning multiple adjacent bubbles close to each other, the laser creates an incision plane with tissue separation. Using computer guidance, the laser is able to perform extremely precise bladeless incisions within translucent ocular tissue, producing various patterns and depths. Some of the commercially available femtosecond laser platforms today capable of making corneal incisions, include: Intralase (Johnson and Jonson vision, Jacksonville, Florida, USA), Femtec (20/10 PerfectVision; GmbH, Heidelberg, Germany), Femto LDV (Ziemer Ophthalmic Systems AG, Port, Switzerland), Victus (Bausch and Lomb, Rochester, New York, USA), VisuMax (Carl Zeiss Meditec AG, Jena, Germany), and Wavelight (Alcon, Fort Worth, Texas, USA).

In the field of corneal surgery, femtosecond lasers have been commonly used to fashion uniform thickness cuts in laser in situ keratomileusis (LASIK) flaps, small incision lenticule extraction (SMILE) surgery, intracorneal ring segment channels, astigmatic keratotomy incisions, intrastromal pockets for presbyopic corneal inlays, and surgical incisions for intraocular surgery. Since approximately 2005, femtosecond lasers have also been incorporated into corneal transplantation procedures, including penetrating keratoplasty (PKP), deep anterior lamellar keratoplasty (DALK), Descemet membrane endothelial keratoplasty (DMEK), Descemet stripping automated endothelial keratoplasty (DSAEK), and anterior lamellar keratoplasty (ALK).[3-11] The precision of femtosecond incisions has the potential to provide better surgical alignment which can reduce early astigmatism, increase wound strength, and enable faster wound healing. It can also potentially reduce graft-host slippage which causes late astigmatism.

FEMTOSECOND PENETRATING KERATOPLASTY

First described in human patients in 2007 by both Holzer et al.[3] and Buratto et al.,[4] femtosecond laser-assisted PKP involves trephination of both donor and recipient tissues using a femtosecond laser. While manual trephines can only perform straight vertical side cuts, the femtosecond laser is able to perform a variety of complex trephination patterns. These include "top-hat" (the posterior corneal diameter is larger than the anterior corneal diameter), "mushroom" (the anterior corneal diameter is larger than the posterior corneal diameter), "zigzag", and "Christmas tree" configurations (**Fig. 1A to E**).

Wound Strength

The femtosecond laser is able to perform identical incisions in both the donor and recipient tissue, thus enabling excellent alignment of the two (**Fig. 2**). The first advantage of customized side-cut patterns is increased mechanical strength of the graft-host junction with higher resistance to separation forces induced by intraocular pressure (IOP). Ex vivo models have shown that top-hat and mushroom configurations

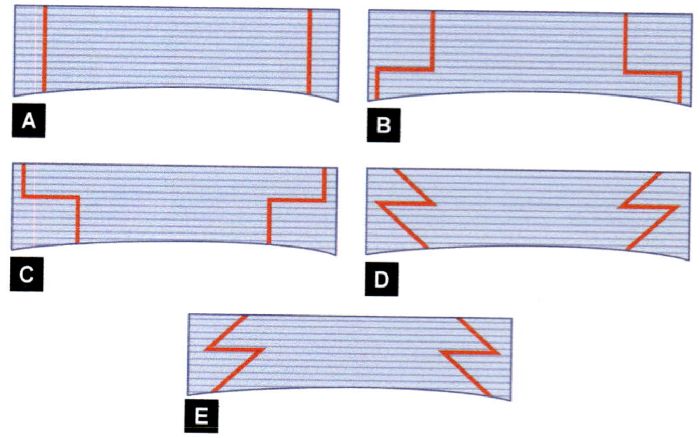

Figs. 1A to E: Customized trephination patterns with femtosecond laser-enabled keratoplasty. (A) Standard straight and vertical manual cut; (B) "Top-hat"; (C) "Mushroom"; (D) "Zigzag"; (E) "Christmas tree".
Courtesy: Reproduced from Asota I, Farid M, Garg S, Steinert RF. Femtosecond laser-enabled keratoplasty. Int Ophthalmol Clin. 2013;53:103-14.

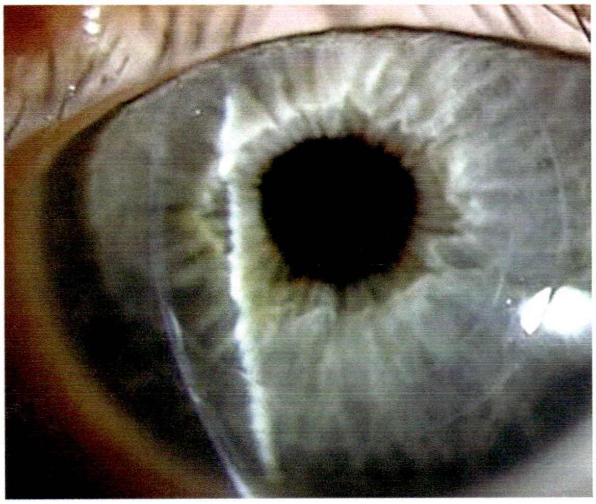

Fig. 2: Postoperative slit-lamp photograph showing a mushroom configuration femtosecond penetrating keratoplasty. The larger circle represents the larger anterior part of the graft and the smaller circle represents the smaller posterior part of the graft.

withstand higher levels of IOP compared with straight vertical cuts performed by manual rephines.[12] In addition, it has been shown that the strength of zigzag and Christmas tree patterns is lower than that of top-hat and mushroom patterns, and that in fact, zigzag and Christmas tree patterns do not provide a significant increase in strength compared with manual trephination.[12,13] While unsutured wounds may not be much stronger, the wounds do clinically heal more securely and in our experience with repeat femto-keratoplasty, the wounds can be difficult to separate. Despite the increased mechanical strength of custom side-cut patterns, they are not sufficient to hold the corneal structure on their own, and femtosecond incised corneas still require suturing in a manner similar to standard PKP. In our institutions, we employ either 16 interrupted sutures or 8 interrupted and one running suture (as with our standard PKPs).

Surgical Technique

Preoperative and postoperative management of femtosecond PKP is largely identical to standard PKP, with the exception of earlier commencement of suture removal. Preoperative and postoperative management of standard PKP is described in detail elsewhere in this book. We here in focus on surgical technique of femtosecond PKP done with the Intralase iFS femtosecond platform (Johnson and Jonson Vision, Jacksonville, Florida, USA):

- The choice between the commonly described configurations can be guided by the clinical situation. In corneas with peripheral thinning (such as in ectasia or peripheral scarring), choosing a mushroom configuration may add peripheral mechanical strength. In corneas with endothelial pathology, choosing a top-hat configuration will increase the surface area of transplanted endothelium.
- The patient is placed supine under an operating microscope.
- The host corneal diameter is measured ("white-to-white"), and trephination diameter is set at approximately 3 mm less than the measured horizontal "white-to-white".
- Corneal thickness is measured at 8 points at the planned trephination perimeter using an ultrasound pachymeter. Corneal thickness measurements can also be obtained using either corneal tomography or anterior segment optical coherence tomography (AS-OCT), yet we recommend to confirm pachymetry measurements intraoperatively using an ultrasound pachymeter.
- Peripheral corneal markings are done using a surgical marking pen, to enable easy centration of the femtosecond laser's docking apparatus. We do not recommend central marking on the donor as it may cause delay in healing and some haze. Also, in keratoconic corneas, the central mark may be shifted due to the extra surface area of a steep cone.
- Recipient femtosecond laser parameters are programmed according to the set trephination diameter and side-cut pattern (we use either a top-hat or mushroom configuration).
- When programming the laser, four parameters need to be input (**Fig. 3A**):
  1. *Anterior side cut*: Diameter of anterior side cut, and anterior and posterior depth of the cut, resulting in a vertical circular incision.
  2. *Horizontal ring-lamellar cut*: Depth of horizontal ring-lamellar cut (usually 300 μm), inner and outer diameters of ring-lamellar cut
  3. *Posterior side cut*: Diameter of posterior side cut and anterior and posterior depth of posterior side cut. Depth of the posterior side cut is set to penetrate on the donor only, we do not penetrate on the recipient and make the posterior side cut on the recipient about 100 μm less than thinnest measurement in that zone.
  4. *Suture alignment markings*: Eight superficial radial marking lines that can guide precise suture placement. Additionally, incision angles can also be specified (in top-hat and mushroom configuration we use 90° angulation—vertical and horizontal cuts only).
- Vertical cuts overlap 0.1 mm horizontally and 30 μm vertically with the horizontal lamellar cut at a 90° angulation to the corneal surface to ensure completely cut intersecting wound edges.
- The only differences in set parameters between the recipient and the donor tissues are: (A) The outer diameter of the donor may be oversized by 0.1–0.2 mm or same sized compared to the recipient, (B) An uncut gap of 50 μm is left between the posterior side cut and lamellar cut in the recipient's cornea only, in order to avoid corneal perforation during the laser cut, and keep the globe closed until the patient is transferred safely to the

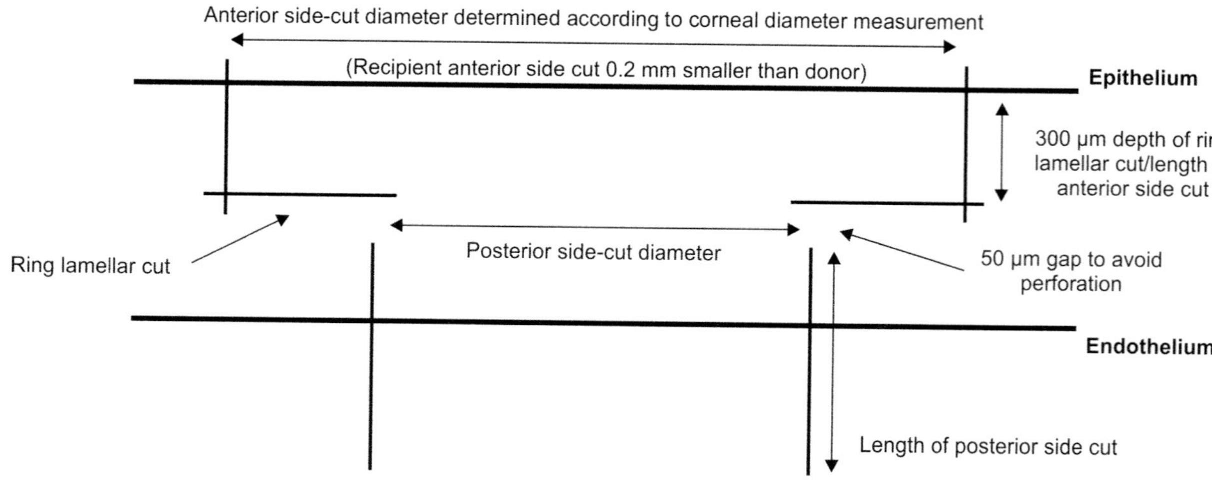

Fig. 3A: Side view of recipient femtosecond penetrating keratoplasty incision profile (mushroom configuration).

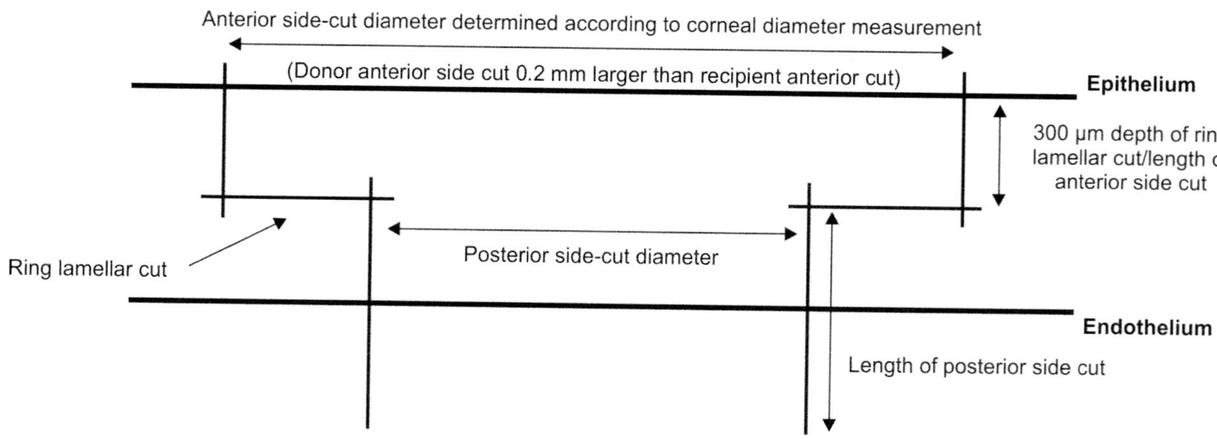

Fig. 3B: Side view of donor femtosecond penetrating keratoplasty incision profile (mushroom configuration).

operating room (*see* **Fig. 3A**). A second option to avoid perforation instead of leaving a gap between the posterior side cut and lamellar cut is to keep the posterior side cut shallower than penetration on the recipient. In our opinion, this option is more secure and has become our preferred method. This gap is bluntly dissected during surgery using a Sinskey hook, to achieve a continuous full-thickness incision and removal of the recipient's corneal button.

- The laser apparatus is docked on the eye, centered on the peripheral corneal marking, and femtosecond recipient incisions are performed (**Video 1**).
- The donor cornea is removed from the storage solution, mounted on an artificial anterior chamber and brought under the femtosecond laser (**Video 2**).
- Laser settings are changed to the donor parameters (outer diameter 0.1–0.2 mm larger than the recipient and no uncut 50 μm gap), the laser is docked and activated to create donor incisions (**Fig. 3B**).
- In the operating room, the recipient donor button is removed after blunt dissection of the uncut gap using a reverse Sinskey hook.
- The donor button is positioned and sutured using 10-0 nylon sutures with care to match to position of the alignment marks (**Video 3**).

Wound Healing and Outcomes

The excellent alignment of femtosecond incisions, as well as their custom configurations which increase the contact area between the graft and the host, both contribute to improved wound healing. Publications in the literature demonstrate that femtosecond PKP provides more rapid wound healing which enables earlier suture removal and visual rehabilitation with reduced astigmatism magnitudes, when compared with standard PKP. The majority of these differences, however, become nonsignificant beyond the first few postoperative months, signifying that once sutures are removed, there is not much clinical difference between femtosecond and standard PKP in terms of astigmatism.[14-17] Surgeons should also be aware that in cloudy corneas, the femtosecond laser may not be able to penetrate the opacity, and an incomplete cut may form. Future prospective, randomized, comparative trials can help us understand better the potential advantages of femtosecond PKP.

FEMTOSECOND DEEP ANTERIOR LAMELLAR KERATOPLASTY

Initially described by Farid et al.[5] and Price et al.[6] in 2009, femtosecond DALK involves partial thickness trephination of the recipient stroma, as well as full thickness trephination of the donor tissue, using a femtosecond laser. This is followed by baring of recipient Descemet membrane using standard big-bubble or manual techniques. Ideally, the femtosecond laser would perform a deep lamellar incision just above Descemet membrane, facilitating complete removal of host stroma, thus obviating the need to perform dissection of Descemet's using big-bubble or manual techniques. However, current femtosecond technology is still unable to perform such a precise deep incision, parallel to the posterior surface in a safe manner due to several limitations:

- Current femtosecond technology is unguided in real time. The depth of femtosecond ablation is set according to pachymetry measurements taken prior to activation of the laser, and the laser cannot be adjusted according to immediate thickness changes along the incision path. Femtosecond incisions performed close to Descemet's without penetrating it would need to be guided by real-time 3D mapping of the posterior corneal surface. Liu et al.[18] recently described outcomes of OCT-guided femtosecond DALK, where the Femto LDV laser used OCT guidance to create a precise stromal big-bubble cannulation channel reaching a depth that was 50 µm away from Descemet membrane. They reported successful creation of a big-bubble in all 14 eyes of the series. While OCT did not guide the femtosecond laser directly in Liu et al.'s study, it may have improved DALK success rate, showing the potential of OCT-guided femtosecond DALK.
- Deep femtosecond incisions that are close to Descemet's, may damage endothelial cells.[13]
- Deep stromal femtosecond incisions (such as those performed close to Descemet) have been shown to be more irregular than superficial incisions. This affects clarity and regularity of the DALK interface and reduces visual outcomes.[19,20]
- Since the femtosecond laser applanates the cornea, any irregularities present on the corneal surface would transfer onto the incised stromal surface. Therefore, in irregular corneas, deep stromal incisions will produce an irregular DALK interface.

For these reasons, current femtosecond DALK includes vertical incisions (with a midstromal ring lamellar incision to create a mushroom or top-hat configuration), but does not include deep lamellar incision close to Descemet membrane. Nonetheless, the femtosecond laser performs vertical incisions with precise depth which may facilitate big-bubble or manual dissection. Additionally, with a mushroom configuration, there is less surface area needed for the deep lamellar dissection.

Surgical Technique

Femtosecond DALK technique is largely similar to the femtosecond PKP technique described earlier in this chapter. The differences are:

- The posterior side-cut incisions in the recipient do not penetrate the anterior chamber, but terminate in the deep stroma. The depth where the posterior side-cut incisions terminate is set at 100 µm above the thinnest measured pachymetry (**Fig. 4**).
- An additional deep horizontal lamellar incision can be performed to enable easy debulking of host stroma instead of dissecting stroma manually. However, this incision is not at full stromal depth for the reasons mentioned earlier. Baring of Descemet membrane is still performed using big-bubble or manual techniques.
- In areas of focal thinning that are not discovered by preoperative or intraoperative pachymetry, the posterior side-cut incision might penetrate the anterior chamber, producing a full-thickness perforation which may necessitate conversion to PKP.
- Donor tissue is prepared in a manner similar to femtosecond PKP (*see* **Fig. 3B and Video 2**), with the difference of Descemet membrane being stripped off the donor (manually as in standard DALK—**Video 4**).

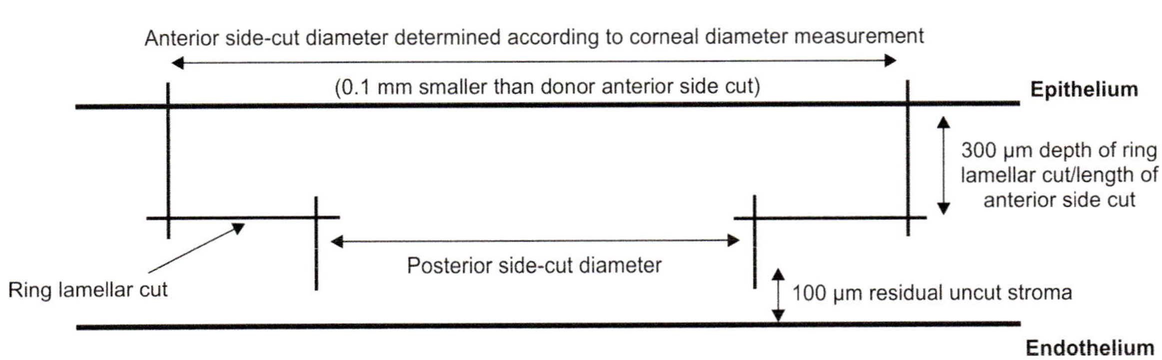

Fig. 4: Side view of recipient femtosecond deep anterior lamellar keratoplasty incision profile (mushroom configuration).

Wound Healing and Outcomes

The previously-mentioned characteristics of femtosecond PKP wound profile and wound healing, also apply to femtosecond DALK. Data in the literature is conflicting regarding outcome differences between femtosecond DALK and standard DALK. While some studies suggest that femtosecond DALK produces better visual acuity and lower astigmatism,[21] others found no outcome differences between femtosecond and standard DALK, but for reduced residual myopia.[22-24] Other studies showed superiority of femtosecond DALK in early suture removal and visual recovery together with reduced astigmatism, all of which were evident during the first few postoperative months, and became insignificant thereafter (a trend similar to published data on femtosecond PKP).[24-26] Similar to femtosecond PKP, future prospective comparative studies evaluating the efficacy and cost-effectiveness of femtosecond DALK, could help establish its role in the field of corneal transplantation. We are involved in such study at our institution.

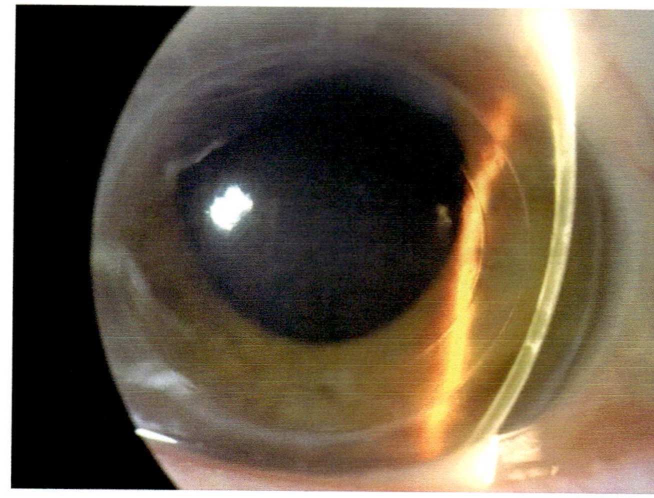

Fig. 5: Postoperative slit-lamp photograph of a patient with a femtosecond Descemet membrane endothelial keratoplasty (DMEK) graft performed under a failed penetrating keratoplasty (PKP). The larger circle represents the PKP graft edge, and the smaller circle represents the femtosecond descemetorhexis, and DMEK graft diameters which were same-sized in this case. PKP functionality and clarity were restored following femtosecond DMEK.

FEMTOSECOND DESCEMET MEMBRANE ENDOTHELIAL KERATOPLASTY

In DMEK surgery, the recipient's Descemet membrane is peeled manually (descemetorhexis), to allow adherence of the donor DMEK tissue to the recipient's stroma. Complete removal of the recipient's Descemet membrane at the transplant site is important, since remnant tags, and islands of Descemet's tissue may lead to graft detachment—the most common DMEK postoperative complication. In femtosecond DMEK, the femtosecond laser outlines the descemetorhexis.[7] Recent literature shows good early and longer-term outcomes of femtosecond DMEK in Fuchs' dystrophy patients. Specifically, femtosecond DMEK was found to have reduced detachment and rebubble (reinjection of air into the anterior chamber to treat a detached graft) rates, as well as reduced rates of endothelial cell loss, compared with standard DMEK.[27,28] The proposed mechanism for reduced detachment rates in femtosecond DMEK is the lack of remnant Descemet membrane tags and islands which can interfere with donor tissue adherence, as well as perhaps mild postoperative inflammation induced by the laser, which may promote tissue adherence. The proposed cause for reduced cell-loss rates in femtosecond DMEK is the more precise removal of recipient Descemet membrane that matches the donor trephination cut (usually, manual descemetorhexis may have a jagged profile with excess removal of peripheral endothelial cells) and leaves less denuded areas that need to be repopulated by endothelial cells. Also, given the low detachment rate in femtosecond DMEK, the descemetorhexis and graft can be same-sized, which further reduces the bare area which lacks endothelium.

In recent years, secondary PKP graft failure from late endothelial decompensation can be managed with endothelial keratoplasty to replenish the endothelial layer and restore graft function and clarity (**Fig. 5**). This obviated the need to replace the entire PKP graft. DMEK performed in this setting is associated with high rates of postoperative graft detachment.[29,30] Recent literature shows that femtosecond DMEK performed under a failed PKP graft, has reduced postoperative detachment rates,[31] much lower when compared with standard DMEK performed in a similar setting.[32]

Surgical Technique

Femtosecond descemetorhexis diameter is usually the same as DMEK graft diameter (or 0.1 mm larger). In cases of DMEK performed under a failed PKP, descemetorhexis diameter is at least 0.25 mm smaller than the PKP graft to avoid the graft-host interface. Corneal thickness is measured using an ultrasound pachymeter at 8 points along the circumference of the planned descemetorhexis incision. The femtosecond laser is docked and creates a vertical ring cut at a depth that extends from 100 μm above the thinnest measured corneal thickness to 100 μm below the thickest measured corneal thickness (**Fig. 6 and Video 5**). Descemet membrane is then dissected using a reverse Sinskey hook. It is not recommended to start dissection from the location of the femtosecond incision itself since the femtosecond incision extends into the stroma and it may be difficult to achieve an initial Descemet's flap due to the stromal resistance to peel at the point of the stromal incision. Instead, dissection should start slightly more central. Once a Descemet's flap has been lifted, dissection can continue normally or using forceps after

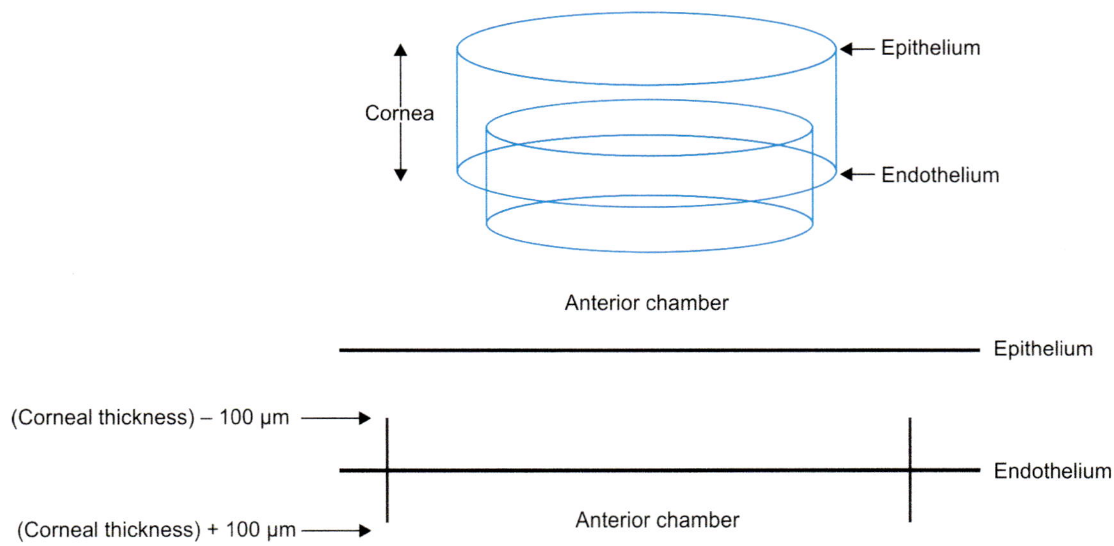

Fig. 6: Schematic overview of femtosecond Descemet membrane endothelial keratoplasty (DMEK): The laser creates a round vertical ring cut at a depth that extends from 100 µm above the thinnest measured corneal thickness to 100 µm below the thickest measured corneal thickness. *Courtesy*: Reproduced from Einan-Lifshitz A, Sorkin N, Boutin T, Showail M, Borovik A, Alobthani M, et al. Comparison of femtosecond laser-enabled descemetorhexis and manual descemetorhexis in Descemet membrane endothelial keratoplasty. Cornea. 2017;36:767-70.

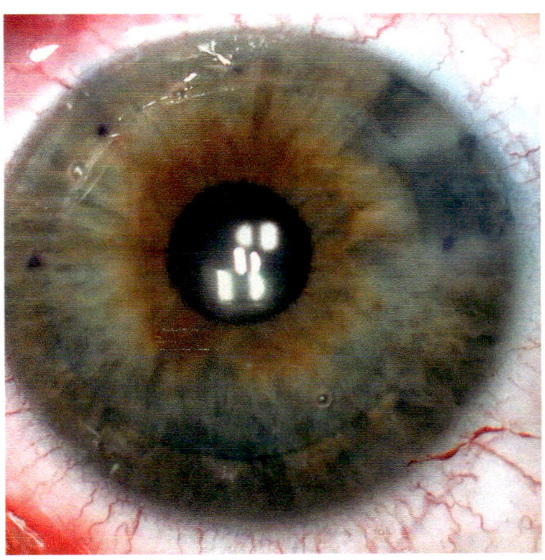

Fig. 7: Intraoperative photograph of femtosecond Descemet membrane endothelial keratoplasty following stripping of Descemet and trypan blue staining to confirm complete removal of Descemet membrane. The photograph demonstrates the perfect femtosecond descemetorhexis circle with no remnant Descemet islands or tags.

staining with a blue dye (**Fig. 7, and Video 6**). The rest of the DMEK procedure is performed in a manner identical to standard DMEK.

FEMTOSECOND DESCEMET STRIPPING AUTOMATED ENDOTHELIAL KERATOPLASTY

The femtosecond laser can be used for preparation of posterior donor disks for DSAEK. Ex vivo studies have shown that the femtosecond laser can produce thin DSAEK grafts with good endothelial cell counts.[33] Despite some clinical studies showing good outcomes of DSAEK performed using femtosecond graft preparation,[8] other comparative studies have shown femtosecond DSAEK to have reduced visual acuity outcomes compared with microkeratome DSAEK.[34] This is likely due to the fact that deep femtosecond incisions tend to be more irregular, thus producing a more irregular graft interface compared with that of a microkeratome.[34] A prospective study comparing ultra-thin DSAEK to femtosecond DSAEK was suspended due to significantly reduced clinical outcomes in the femtosecond DSAEK group, including visual acuity, graft dislocation rates, and interface haze rates.[35]

FEMTOSECOND ANTERIOR LAMELLAR KERATOPLASTY

Corneal pathologies involving the anterior cornea can be managed by ALK. These include epithelial and stromal dystrophies, traumatic scarring, postkeratitis scarring, and recalcitrant stromal haze. ALK can be performed manually, semi-mechanized with an automated microkeratome or with an excimer laser.[9] However, these technologies can result in irregular stromal interface between the donor and recipient lamellae that could bring out stromal haze, irregular astigmatism, and loss of visual acuity. The femtosecond laser can produce precise incisions with perfect alignment of donor and host tissue, as well as creation of highly regular incision surfaces in the anterior layers of the cornea. This makes the femtosecond laser ideal for ALK incisions. Femtosecond ALK has been shown to have good outcomes in treatment of anterior corneal pathologies.[9-11] Most studies describe ALK in depths of up to 250 µm and beyond that, many surgeons will opt to perform DALK. The femtosecond ALK graft can be sutured, but femtosecond ALK can also be sutureless, owing to the square side-cut femtosecond incision profile (as opposed to a thin edge with a microkeratome incision) and perfect alignment, which reduce the risk of graft dislocation.[36,37] It should be noted, as mentioned earlier, that since the femtosecond laser applanates the cornea and produces a cut which is parallel to the anterior surface, any irregularities present on the corneal surface will transfer onto the incised stromal surface. Therefore, in corneas with significant surface irregularity, the use of femtosecond ALK should be avoided as it will be unlikely to produce a good outcome without a rigid contact lens. The scar may be removed, but irregular astigmatism will persist.

CONCLUSION

Femtosecond laser technology is an effective tool in corneal transplant surgery, providing precise cuts with stronger and quicker-healing wounds. In anterior lamellar transplantation, it produces precise recipient-donor matching which is unmatched by manual surgery. In posterior lamellar transplantation, it creates perfectly circular Descemet incisions which improve DMEK outcomes. Its advantages over standard keratoplasty and its cost-effectiveness may become more obvious with further study and advances in delivery technology.

REFERENCES

1. Soong HK, Malta JB. Femtosecond lasers in ophthalmology. Am J Ophthalmol. 2009;147:189-197.e2.
2. Stern D, Schoenlein RW, Puliafito CA, Dobi ET, Birngruber R, Fujimoto JG. Corneal ablation by nanosecond, picosecond, and femtosecond lasers at 532 and 625 nm. Arch Ophthalmol. 1989;107:587-92.
3. Holzer MP, Rabsilber TM, Auffarth GU. Penetrating keratoplasty using femtosecond laser. Am J Ophthalmol. 2007;143:524-6.
4. Buratto L, Böhm E. The use of the femtosecond laser in penetrating keratoplasty. Am J Ophthalmol. 2007;143(5):737-42.
5. Farid M, Steinert RF. Deep anterior lamellar keratoplasty performed with the femtosecond laser zigzag incision for the treatment of stromal corneal pathology and ectatic disease. J Cataract Refract Surg. 2009;35:809-13.
6. Price FW Jr, Price MO, Grandin JC, Kwon R. Deep anterior lamellar keratoplasty with femtosecond-laser zigzag incisions. J Cataract Refract Surg. 2009;35:804-8.
7. Pilger D, von Sonnleithner C, Bertelmann E, Joussen AM, Torun N. Femtosecond laser-assisted descemetorhexis: A novel technique in Descemet membrane Endothelial Keratoplasty. Cornea. 2016;35:1274-8.
8. Feng Y, Qu HQ, Ren J, Prahs P, Hong J. Corneal endothelial cell loss in femtosecond laser-assisted Descemet's stripping automated endothelial keratoplasty: A 12-month follow-up study. Chin Med J (Engl). 2017;130:2927-32.
9. Lu Y, Yang L, Ge Y, Chen X, Huang Z. Femtosecond laser-assisted anterior lamellar keratoplasty for the treatment of stromal corneal pathology. BMC Ophthalmol. 2015;15:15.
10. Shousha MA, Yoo SH, Kymionis GD, Ide T, Feuer W, Karp CL, et al. Long-term results of femtosecond laser-assisted sutureless anterior lamellar keratoplasty. Ophthalmology. 2011;118:315-23.
11. Almousa R, Samaras KE, Khan S, Lake DB, Daya SM. Femtosecond laser-assisted lamellar keratoplasty (FSLK) for anterior corneal stromal diseases. Int Ophthalmol. 2014;34:49-58.
12. Bahar I, Kaiserman I, McAllum P, Rootman D. Femtosecond laser-assisted penetrating keratoplasty: Stability evaluation of different wound configurations. Cornea. 2008;27:209-11.
13. Kopani KR, Page MA, Holiman J, Parodi A, Iliakis B, Chamberlain W. Femtosecond laser-assisted keratoplasty: Full and partial-thickness cut wound strength and endothelial cell loss across a variety of wound patterns. Br J Ophthalmol. 2014;98:894-9.
14. Bahar I, Kaiserman I, Lange AP, Levinger E, Sansanayudh W, Singal N, et al. Femtosecond laser versus manual dissection for top hat penetrating keratoplasty. Br J Ophthalmol. 2009;93:73-8.
15. Farid M, Steinert RF, Gaster RN, Chamberlain W, Lin A. Comparison of penetrating keratoplasty performed with a femtosecond laser zig-zag incision versus conventional blade trephination. Ophthalmology. 2009;116:1638-43.
16. Chamberlain WD, Rush SW, Mathers WD, Cabezas M, Fraunfelder FW. Comparison of femtosecond laser-assisted keratoplasty versus conventional penetrating keratoplasty. Ophthalmology. 2011;118:486-91.
17. Gaster RN, Dumitrascu O, Rabinowitz YS. Penetrating keratoplasty using femtosecond laser-enabled keratoplasty with zig-zag incisions versus a mechanical trephine in patients with keratoconus. Br J Ophthalmol. 2012;96:1195-9.
18. Liu YC, Wittwer VV, Yusoff NZM, Lwin CN, Seah XY, Mehta JS, et al. Intraoperative optical coherence tomography-guided femtosecond laser-assisted deep anterior lamellar keratoplasty. Cornea. 2019;38:648-53.
19. Zhang C, Liu L, Tang M, Li Y, Chamberlain W, Huang D. Laboratory evaluation of femtosecond laser lamellar cuts in gamma-irradiated corneas. Cornea. 2015;34:1499-503.
20. Phillips PM, Phillips LJ, Saad HA, Terry MA, Stolz DB, Stoeger C, et al. "Ultrathin" DSAEK tissue prepared with a low-pulse energy, high-frequency femtosecond laser. Cornea. 2013;32:81-6.
21. Li S, Wang T, Bian J, Wang F, Han S, Shi W. Precisely controlled side cut in femtosecond laser-assisted deep lamellar keratoplasty for advanced keratoconus. Cornea. 2016;35:1289-94.
22. Blériot A, Martin E, Lebranchu P, Zimmerman K, Libeau L, Weber M, et al. Comparison of 12-month anatomic and functional results between Z6 femtosecond laser-assisted and manual trephination in deep anterior lamellar keratoplasty for advanced keratoconus. J Fr Ophtalmol. 2017;40:e193-e200.
23. Salouti R, Zamani M, Ghoreyshi M, Dapena I, Melles GRJ, Nowroozzadeh MH. Comparison between manual trephination versus femtosecond laser-assisted deep anterior lamellar keratoplasty for keratoconus. Br J Ophthalmol. 2019:103(12):1716-23.
24. Alio JL, Abdelghany AA, Barraquer R, Hammouda LM, Sabry AM. Femtosecond laser assisted deep anterior lamellar keratoplasty outcomes and healing patterns compared to manual technique. Biomed Res Int. 2015;2015:397891.
25. Shehadeh-Mashor R, Chan CC, Bahar I, Lichtinger A, Yeung SN, Rootman DS. Comparison between femtosecond laser mushroom configuration and manual trephine straight-edge configuration deep anterior lamellar keratoplasty. Br J Ophthalmol. 2014;98:35-9.
26. Shehadeh-Mashor R, Chan C, Yeung SN, Lichtinger A, Amiran M, Rootman DS. Long-term outcomes of femtosecond laser-assisted mushroom configuration deep anterior lamellar keratoplasty. Cornea. 2013;32:390-5.
27. Einan-Lifshitz A, Sorkin N, Boutin T, Showail M, Borovik A, Alobthani M, et al. Comparison of femtosecond laser-enabled descemetorhexis and manual descemetorhexis in Descemet membrane endothelial keratoplasty. Cornea. 2017;36:767-70.
28. Sorkin N, Mednick Z, Einan-Lifshitz A, Trinh T, Santaella G, Telli A, et al. Three-year outcome comparison between femtosecond laser-assisted and manual Descemet membrane endothelial keratoplasty. Cornea. 2019;38(7):812-6.
29. Einan-Lifshitz A, Belkin A, Sorkin N, Mednick Z, Boutin T, Gill I, et al. Descemet membrane endothelial keratoplasty after penetrating keratoplasty: features for success. Cornea. 2018;37:1093-7.

30. Pasari A, Price MO, Feng MT, Price FW Jr. Descemet membrane endothelial keratoplasty for failed penetrating keratoplasty: visual outcomes and graft survival. Cornea. 2019;38:151-6.
31. Sorkin N, Trinh T, Einan-Lifshitz A, Mednick Z, Santaella G, Telli A, et al. Outcomes of femtosecond laser-assisted Descemet membrane endothelial keratoplasty for failed penetrating keratoplasty. Can J Ophthalmol. 2019:54(6):741-5.
32. Sorkin N, Mimouni M, Santaella G, Trinh T, Cohen E, Einan-Lifshitz A, et al. Comparison of Manual and Femtosecond Laser-Assisted Descemet Membrane Endothelial Keratoplasty for Failed Penetrating Keratoplasty. Am J Ophthalmol. 2020;214:1-8.
33. Liu YC, Teo EP, Adnan KB, Yam GH, Peh GS, Tan DT, et al. Endothelial approach ultrathin corneal grafts prepared by femtosecond laser for descemet stripping endothelial keratoplasty. Invest Ophthalmol Vis Sci. 2014;55:8393-401.
34. Vetter JM, Butsch C, Faust M, Schmidtmann I, Hoffmann EM, Sekundo W, et al. Irregularity of the posterior corneal surface after curved interface femtosecond laser-assisted versus microkeratome-assisted descemet stripping automated endothelial keratoplasty. Cornea. 2013;32:118-24.
35. Ivarsen A, Hjortdal J. Clinical outcome of Descemet's stripping endothelial keratoplasty with femtosecond laser-prepared grafts. Acta Ophthalmol. 2018;96:e655-e656.
36. Jabbarvand M, Hashemian H, Khodaparast M, Ghadimi H, Khalilipour E. Femtosecond laser-assisted sutureless anterior lamellar keratoplasty for superficial corneal opacities. J Cataract Refract Surg. 2014;40:1805-12.
37. Shetty R, Nagaraja H, Veluri H, Shivanna Y, Kugar T, Nujits R, et al. Sutureless femtosecond anterior lamellar keratoplasty: a 1-year follow-up study. Indian J Ophthalmol. 2014;62:923-6.

50 Femtosecond Laser-assisted Deep Lamellar Endothelial Keratoplasty

Jorge L Alió del Barrio, Verónica Vargas, Bruce D Allan

INTRODUCTION

Descemet's stripping automated endothelial keratoplasty (DSAEK) and Descemet's membrane endothelial keratoplasty (DMEK) have become the gold standard treatment for corneal endothelial diseases.[1,2] In DMEK, the recipient dysfunctional Descemet membrane (DM) and endothelial layers are excised and replaced by a healthy DM-endothelium from a donor cornea (same for DSAEK, but with the exception that the donor lenticule also contains a thin layer of stroma), restoring corneal transparency by a resolution of the preexisting corneal edema.

Posterior lamellar keratoplasty (PLK) was originally described by Melles in 1998.[3] The surgery was later modified by Terry in 2001 and was termed deep lamellar endothelial keratoplasty (DLEK).[4-6] In DLEK, the failed endothelium, DM and a thin lamella of posterior corneal stroma were replaced by a healthy disk of donor corneal tissue which was positioned in the reciprocal host dissection. Manual host lamellar dissection in DLEK was time-consuming and the posterior side cut in particular was technically challenging. Despite femtosecond laser-assisted tissue preparation was utilized by a number of investigators to simplify corneal tissue dissection,[7,8] DLEK was largely abandoned in favor of Descemet's stripping techniques which do not require host stromal dissection (DSEK, DSAEK, and DMEK), and it is now a largely forgotten endothelial keratoplasty (EK) modality.

Descemet's membrane endothelial keratoplasty and other modalities of EK are not able to restore the transparency if well-established stromal scars are already present, being penetrating keratoplasty (PK) the elective procedure for such cases. However, if corneal opacity is limited exclusively to the posterior cornea, the removal of the deeper stromal layers together with the DM and endothelium would still allow to perform an EK instead of a PK, avoiding all well-known drawback of latest (long visual rehabilitation, suture-related complications, significant residual ametropia, risk of rejection, and glaucoma).[9] On this regard, a few recent publications of our group pointed out the importance of recovering DLEK as a successful alternative treatment option for such uncommon cases, suggesting a modified DLEK technique that integrates the recent advances in femtosecond laser technology and donor corneal tissue preparation to significantly simplify the technique.[10,11] This simplified form of DLEK [femtosecond laser-assisted deep lamellar endothelial keratoplasty (Femto-DLEK)] combined with conventional DSAEK or DMEK donor preparation and insertion techniques demonstrated to be safe and effective for the treatment of corneal endothelial diseases associated with posterior stromal opacities.[10,11]

INDICATIONS

Main indications of Femto-DLEK are those visually impairing pathologies involving exclusively the deeper posterior corneal stroma and DM, with or without endothelial failure and corneal edema (**Fig. 1**). It is critical to have a healthy epithelium and anterior/mid stroma for the correct success of this technique.

Alternative indications are:

- Endothelial failure or retained deep scarring after deep anterior lamellar keratoplasty (DALK) (**Figs. 2A and B**).
- Revision of a failed DSAEK in cases of pseudophakic bullous keratopathy with an anterior chamber intraocular lens (AC-IOL). If a pseudophakic AC-IOL is properly placed within the AC, Femto-DLEK allows to enhance the AC depth and so increases the distance between the IOL and the new donor tissue, thereby reducing the risk of repeat failure due to endothelial touch (**Fig. 3C**).

PREOPERATIVE CONSIDERATIONS

Before surgery, the extension and depth of the deep corneal opacity should be well identified and measured with an anterior segment optical coherence tomography (AS-OCT) (*see* **Fig. 1**).

Surgical Technique

Once established the extension and depth of the posterior opacification, an overlying manual lamellar dissection plane

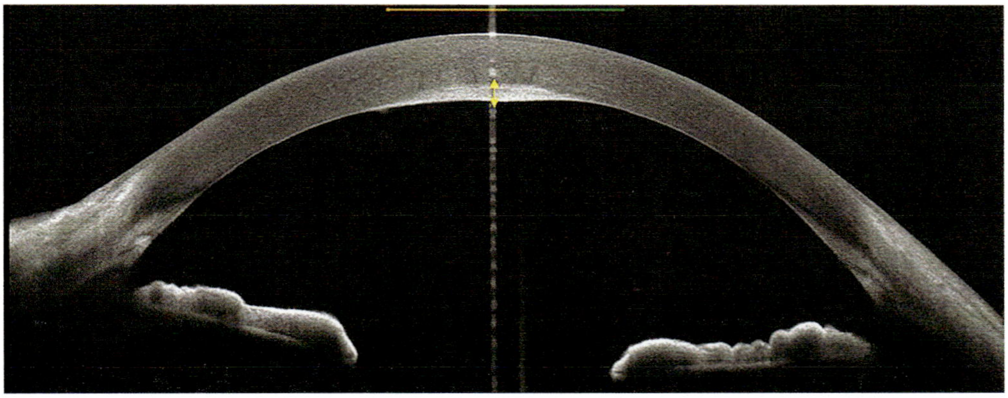

Fig. 1: Anterior segment optical coherence tomography (AS-OCT) image of a pseudophakic bullous keratopathy associated with a severe deep stromal scar without involving other corneal layers. We can measure the precise depth of the scar (yellow arrows).

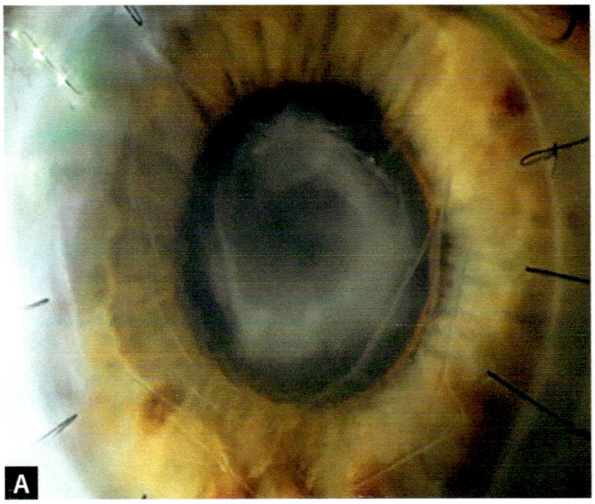

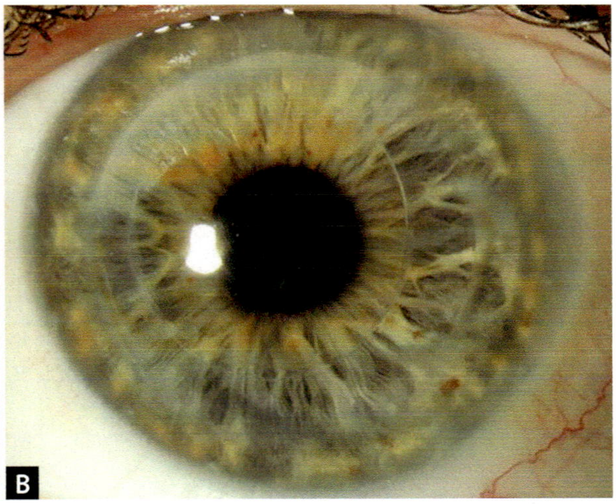

Figs. 2A and B: Femtosecond laser-assisted deep lamellar endothelial keratoplasty (Femto-DLEK) (B) for retained deep stromal opacity after deep anterior lamellar keratoplasty (DALK) (A).

is created 1 week prior to the EK surgery at approximately 75–85% depth through a 5.0-mm superior scleral incision, using a combination of blunt dissection with the Morlet lamellar dissector (Duckworth and Kent, England) and sharp dissection with a Crescent knife (Alcon), always assisted by an AC air fill. Accuracy of the manually dissected pocket location should be confirmed with AS-OCT prior to the EK surgery (**Fig. 4**).

Then, under local anesthesia with sedation, the IntraLase iFS femtosecond laser (AMO Inc, Irvine, Calif) is used to create an intersecting posterior side cut of 7.0–8.5 mm of diameter (depths should be determined by AS-OCT depending on the exact depth of the lamellar dissected plane; femtosecond laser energy settings as previously described).[10] Subsequently, the dissected posterior recipient disk is removed from the AC through a 3.2-mm limbal incision placed temporally (**Fig. 5**). A 7.0–8.5-mm DSAEK or DMEK graft is then inserted into the AC and attached to the recipient stroma using a standard DSAEK or DMEK technique (following each surgeon's preference) (**Figs. 3A and B**).

In cases of failure or scarring of the recipient bed after DALK, the posterior side cut is performed in isolation as the deep lamellar dissection is already performed from the original lamellar surgery.

POSTOPERATIVE MANAGEMENT

Postoperative care and patient positioning do not differ to the one used for a standard DSAEK or DMEK surgery.

COMPLICATIONS

Probably, the most critical step in Femto-DLEK is the manual dissection of the lamellar plane just over the deep stromal opacification (*see* **Fig. 4**). It is not a technically demanding step and its performance do not differ to the one used for manual DALK as described previously by Melles.[12] However, an unsatisfactory dissection plane, either because of a too superficial plane or an incorrect one that leaves part of the opacity on the anterior cornea in relation with the dissection, will force us to abort this technique and to convert into a PK. If available, intraoperative corneal OCT imaging systems could highly simplify this step by allowing and easy "in live" assessment of the correct dissection depth. Alternatively, the femtosecond laser can be used in single pass mode for the recipient posterior corneal lamellar dissection by creating a posterior intrastromal lamellar cut of 7.5–9.0 mm in diameter at 400–450 μm depth (depending on the preoperative corneal pachymetry as measured by AS-OCT). However, we recommend to perform manually this posterior lamellar plane 1 week in advance (and only perform a Femto posterior side cut at the moment of the EK surgery) as tissue bridges become a problem if it is performed with femtosecond laser. Moreover, the posterior side cut negates the anchoring counter traction required for easy lamellar dissection, so these tissue bridges usually have to be divided using sharp dissection and counter traction with vitrectomy forceps, what involves a challenging maneuver that may compromise to host interface smoothness. The reason for this is due to the fact that deep stromal femtosecond laser dissections leave a relatively rougher and more irregular interface compared with the more superficial ones, probably in relation with the scattering of the energy and the anatomical differences between the anterior and the less compacted posterior stromal collagen fibers.[13-15]

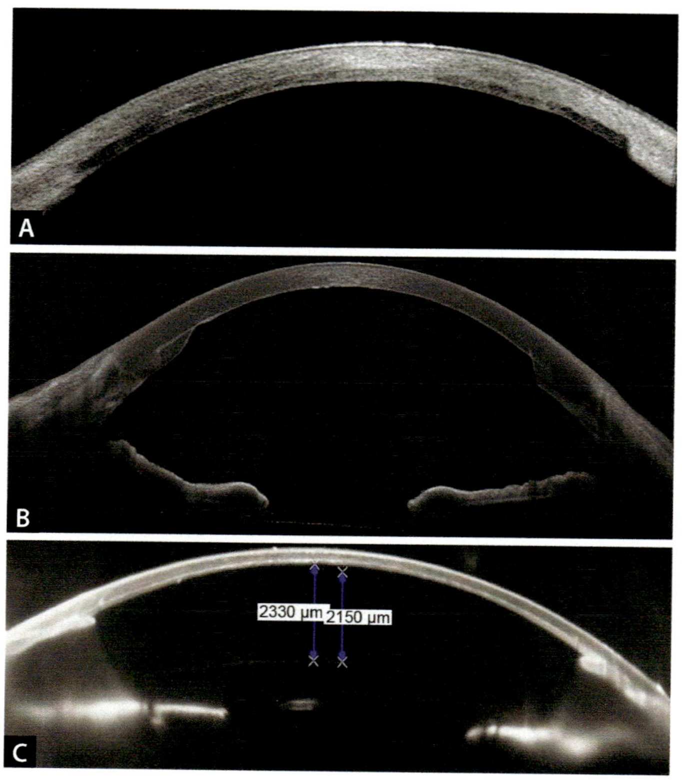

Figs. 3A to C: (A) Anterior segment optical coherence tomography (AS-OCT) image of femtosecond laser-assisted deep lamellar Descemet's stripping automated endothelial keratoplasty (Femto DL-DSAEK). Observe how the DSAEK lenticule fills the space left after the recipient's posterior cornea removal; (B) AS-OCT image of femtosecond laser-assisted deep lamellar Descemet membrane endothelial keratoplasty (Femto DL-DMEK). Observe how the DMEK lenticule does not fill the space left after the recipient's posterior cornea removal, remaining a step in between the central and peripheral posterior corneal surfaces; (C) Scheimpflug image of a Femto-DL-DSAEK after previous failed DSAEK providing enhanced clearance between the donor endothelium and the anterior chamber lens in a case of pseudophakic bullous keratopathy.

In Femto-DLEK, after removing the recipient diseased lamellae of posterior cornea, there will remain a step in between the central and peripheral posterior corneal surfaces, space that will be filled with the endothelial donor tissue (*see* **Figs. 3A and B**). Because of this, a correct centration of the DSAEK or DMEK graft into the recipient bed becomes more important than for a standard EK case, as graft decentration may increase the risk for graft detachment due to the fact of having the EK graft covering the posterior surface step.

OUTCOMES

Existing published evidence (n = 8; six cases associated with a DSAEK graft and two associated with a DMEK graft) do not allow to determine the Femto-DLEK specific rate of other postoperative complications such as rejection, primary failure or graft detachment, but probably they do not differ from those already published for standard DSAEK or DMEK cases as far as the EK graft is well centered within the posterior recipient bed. In our series, only two eyes required re-bubbling of the graft for partial detachment 1 week after surgery, and no cases of graft rejection, primary or secondary failure or glaucoma have been observed with more than 1 year follow-up in all cases. Regarding efficacy, all published eyes have reached a spectacle corrected distance vision of 6/9 or better except two cases (in relation with ocular copathology).

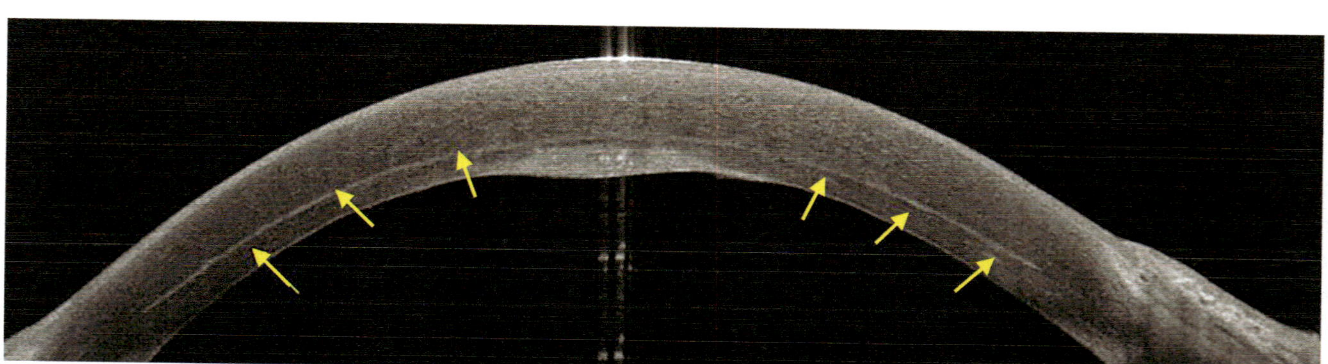
Fig. 4: Anterior segment optical coherence tomography (AS-OCT) image in which the manually dissected pocket location is confirmed (yellow arrows).

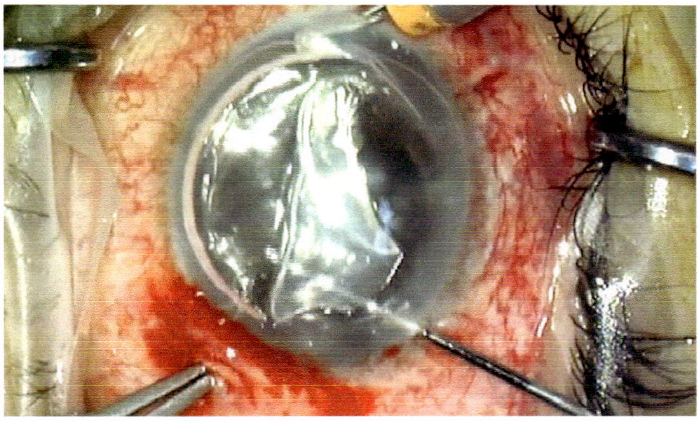

Fig. 5: With a reverse Sinskey hook, the diseased endothelium-Descemet membrane—posterior stroma complex is stripped out from the cornea through a 3.2-mm limbal incision.

The addition of a DMEK graft after Femto-DLEK [femtosecond laser-assisted deep lamellar Descemet membrane endothelial keratoplasty (Femto DL-DMEK)] may enhance the outcomes by adding the advantages of DMEK over DSAEK (better visual potential, lower rejection rate, and faster visual rehabilitation), although a larger sample is still necessary to confirm this statement (*see* **Fig. 3B**).[11,16]

It is still uncertain the potential refractive impact of removing a thick lamella of posterior stroma, mainly when a DMEK donor grafts is used as it does not supply additional donor stromal tissue (as it happens with DSAEK lenticules) (*see* **Figs. 3A and B**), and further studies will have to explore this. However, considering published evidence and excluding those cases of Femto-DLEK after DALK, no significant impact on the refractive sphere or cylinder has been observed: mean spherical equivalent of +2.85 D and mean refractive cylinder of -0.8 D (n = 4).[10,11]

CONCLUSION

Deep lamellar endothelial keratoplasty was abandoned due to the fact of being a technically demanding and challenging surgical technique, but the addition of femtosecond laser has facilitated the most critical step, the posterior side cut in host dissection. Femto DL-DMEK (*see* **Fig. 3B**) or Femto DL-DSAEK (*see* **Fig. 3A**) are the successful and alternative treatment option for the treatment of posterior corneal diseases. As far as the anterior and mid stroma are not affected, opacifications of the posterior cornea with or without endothelial dysfunction can benefit from EK advantages through a Femto-DLEK procedure, avoiding all well-known drawback of PK.[9] The question of whether to exchange AC IOLs for suture fixated posterior chamber IOLs in cases of pseudophakic bullous keratopathy is unresolved. The goal of exchange for a scleral or iris fixated posterior chamber IOL (where the existing AC IOL is stable) is to reduce the risk of optic/endothelial touch. Potential complications of AC IOL exchange include intraoperative hemorrhage, iris trauma, cyclodialysis, pupil distortion, chronic cystoid macular edema, and late failure of fixation with posterior IOL dislocation.[17,18] Femto-DLEK (and mainly DL-DMEK) allows to deepen the AC and theoretically reduce the risk for graft secondary failure (*see* **Fig. 3C**).

Conflict of interest: None of the authors have any conflict of interest to disclose.

REFERENCES

1. Gorovoy MS. Descemet-stripping automated endothelial keratoplasty. Cornea. 2006;25:886-9.
2. Melles GR, Ong TS, Ververs B, van der Wees J. Descemet membrane endothelial keratoplasty (DMEK). Cornea. 2006;25:987-90.
3. Melles GR, Eggink FA, Lander F, Pels E, Rietveld FJ, Beekhuis WH, et al. A surgical technique for posterior lamellar keratoplasty. Cornea. 1998;17:618-26.
4. Terry MA, Ousley PJ. Endothelial replacement without surface corneal incisions or sutures: Topography of the deep lamellar endothelial keratoplasty procedure. Cornea. 2001;20:14-8.
5. Terry MA. Deep lamellar endothelial keratoplasty (DLEK): Pursuing the ideal goals of endothelial replacement. Eye (Lond). 2003;17:982-8.
6. Terry MA, Ousley PJ. Deep lamellar endothelial keratoplasty: Visual acuity, astigmatism, and endothelial survival in a large prospective series. Ophthalmology. 2005;112:1541-8.
7. Terry MA, Ousley PJ, Will B. A practical femtosecond laser procedure for DLEK endothelial transplantation: Cadaver eye histology and topography. Cornea. 2005;24:453-9.
8. Lee DH, Chung TY, Chung ES, Azar DT. Case report: Femtosecond laser-assisted small incision deep lamellar endothelial keratoplasty. Korean J Ophthalmol. 2008;22:43-8.
9. Maier AK, Gundlach E, Gonnermann J, Klamann MK, Eulufi C, Bertelmann E, et al. Fellow eye comparison of descemet membrane endothelial keratoplasty and penetrating keratoplasty. Cornea. 2013;32:1344-8.
10. Alió del Barrio JL, Ziaei M, Bhogal M, Allan BD. Femtosecond laser-assisted deep lamellar endothelial keratoplasty: A new approach to a forgotten technique. Cornea. 2015;34:1369-74.
11. Alió Del Barrio JL, Vargas V. Femtosecond laser-assisted deep lamellar descemet membrane endothelial keratoplasty for the treatment of endothelial dysfunction associated with posterior stromal scarring. Cornea. 2019;38(3):388-91.
12. Melles GR, Lander F, Rietveld FJ, Remeijer L, Beekhuis WH, Binder PS. A new surgical technique for deep stromal, anterior lamellar keratoplasty. Br J Ophthalmol. 1999;83(3):327-33.
13. Rousseau A, Bensalem A, Garnier V, Savoldelli M, Saragoussi JJ, Renard G, et al. Interface quality of endothelial keratoplasty buttons obtained with optomised femtosecond laser settings. Br J Ophthalmol. 2012;96:122-7.
14. Vetter JM, Butsch C, Faust M, Schmidtmann I, Hoffmann EM, Sekundo W, et al. Irregularity of the posterior corneal surface after curved interface femtosecond laser-assisted versus microkeratome-assisted Descemet stripping automated endothelial keratoplasty. Cornea. 2013;32:118-24.
15. Phillips PM, Phillips LJ, Saad HA, Terry MA, Stolz DB, Stoeger C, et al. "Ultrathin" DSAEK tissue prepared with a low-pulse energy, high-frequency femtosecond laser. Cornea. 2013;32:81-6.
16. Goldich Y, Showail M, Avni-Zauberman N, Perez M, Ulate R, Elbaz U, et al. Contralateral eye comparison of Descemet membrane endothelial keratoplasty and Descemet stripping automated endothelial keratoplasty. Am J Opthalmol. 2015;159:155-9.
17. Hayashi K, Hirata A, Hayashi H. Possible predisposing factors for in-the-bag and out-of-the-bag intraocular lens dislocation and outcomes of intraocular lens exchange surgery. Ophthalmology. 2007;114:969-75.
18. Gonnermann J, Klamann MK, Maier AK, Rjasanow J, Joussen AM, Bertelmann E, et al. Visual outcome and complications after posterior iris-claw aphakic intraocular lens implantation. J Cataract Refract Surg. 2012;38:2139-43.

51 Bowman's Layer Transplantation

Bhavana Sharma, Harsha Saxena, Rasik B Vajpayee

INTRODUCTION

Keratoconus (KC) is an ectatic disorder of eye, which results in progressive thinning of cornea leading to visual and structural abnormalities. Surgical management of KC has undergone a paradigm shift over last decade with advent of newer treatment modalities, which have evolved from full thickness penetrating keratoplasty (PK) to component corneal transplantation techniques. Recently, the technique of Bowman's layer transplantation (BLT) through a midstromal implant of an isolated Bowman's layer graft has been introduced by van Dijk K et al. for management of KC.[1-6] This procedure has shown to be beneficial in reducing the ectasia in advanced KC by flattening the corneal curvature with minimal intraoperative and postoperative complications. The donor BLT into the midstroma functions to strengthen the corneal structure in addition to flattening the anterior corneal surface. Bowman's layer transplantation has also been evaluated in management of persistent subepithelial haze after excimer laser surface procedure with good outcomes.[7]

Flowchart 1: Indications of Bowman's layer transplantation.

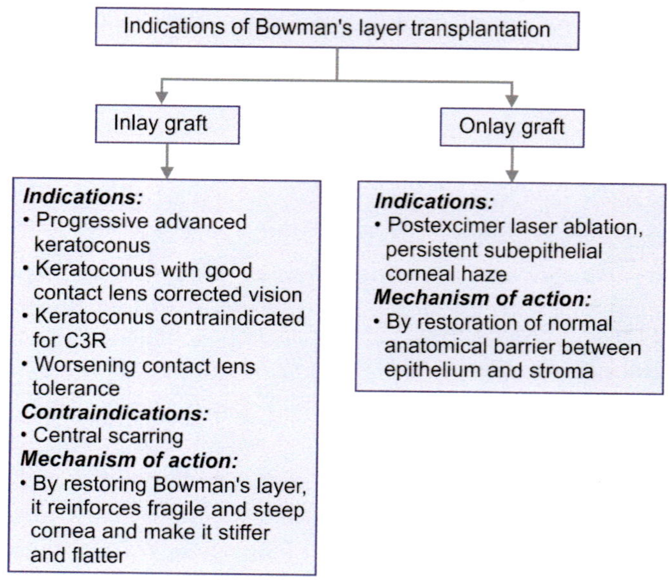

INDICATIONS OF BOWMAN'S LAYER TRANSPLANTATION

Isolated donor BLT has been utilized mainly in two surgical procedures: as an (1) inlay graft into the midstroma of cornea for treatment of KC; and (2) onlay graft for the treatment of persistent subepithelial haze after excimer laser surface ablation (**Flowchart 1**). The patients who can be benefited with BLT are those with progressive and advanced KC, who are not eligible for collagen crosslinking and have increasingly worsening contact lens tolerance. Patients with associated central scarring due to healed hydrops are potentially not suitable for the procedure.

Keratoconus

Bowman's layer transplantation has been considered to be safer then PK and deep anterior lamellar keratoplasty (DALK) with regards to postoperative ectasia and graft rejection. BLT in a keratoconic eye reinforces the thin and structurally fragile ecstatic cornea making it flatter and stronger.[4-6] Further it is hypothesized to arrest the progression of KC and serves to achieve stability of vision. The flatter corneal surface, so achieved helps in preserving, and in some cases restoring, contact lens tolerance, which serves to postpone or avoid surgical alternatives of DALK/PK.[1,3]

Postexcimer Laser Corneal Haze

Subepithelial corneal haze is one of the important complications of excimer laser surface ablation and can sometimes be associated with loss of best-corrected vision. Patients with persistent dense subepithelial haze after photorefractive keratectomy (PRK) have been reported to be benefitted with isolated BLT. The technique involves superficial dissection of scar followed by isolated BLT.[7] The hypothesized cause of subepithelial haze in such a case is the loss of barrier between epithelium and stroma, which in turn leads to abnormal wound-healing response.[8] Bowman's graft functions to restore the requisite anatomical barrier between the epithelium and the underlying stroma.

SURGICAL TECHNIQUES OF BOWMAN'S LAYER TRANSPLANTATION

Preparation of Bowman's Layer Lenticule

The donor tissue is harvested manually by peeling the Bowman's layer (BL) from the anterior stroma of donor cornea. It can be harvested from either whole donor globes mounted on a holder—Technique I, or corneoscleral rims mounted on an artificial chamber—Technique II (**Flowchart 2**).[1,9] Successful harvesting of BL is comparable between the whole globes and the corneoscleral rims [69.4% (25/36) and 72.2% (26/36) for techniques I and II, respectively].[9]

Bowman's membrane can be harvested from donor whole globes, which may not be suitable for keratoplasty either PK or lamellar keratoplasty. When prepared from corneoscleral rims, multiple tissue layers can be harvested from one donor cornea. The anterior part can be used for BL graft preparation and the posterior layers can be used for Descemet's membrane endothelial keratoplasty.[1,9,10]

An ideal BL graft has a thin layer of stromal tissue on its under-surface. A thick BL with substantial stromal tissue attached to BL would not roll making the subsequent surgery difficult. Also presence of an extra-stromal tissue attached to BL can compromise the visual quality after transplantation due to haze at the graft-recipient interface. Tearing of the BL during tissue preparation and a thick graft can be encountered in event of inappropriate dissection.

Femtosecond laser is now being investigated for harvesting the donor BL.[11,12] Though it has been reported to create a thick graft, however has a relatively smooth posterior cut edge as compared to isolated BL with irregular nests of dispersed stroma.[11,12]

Bowman's Layer Transplantation Procedure

Implantation of BL graft is done in the midstroma of recipient cornea. The procedure originally described by Van Dijk et al., involves creation of a midstromal pocket at 50% depth in the recipient cornea over complete circumference from limbus to limbus. The precise dissection can be ensured with air-endothelial reflex visualized over the edge of dissection. Subsequently, the harvested BL graft is stained with trypan blue stain and is transplanted in the stromal pocket with the help of a glide (**Flowchart 3**).

OUTCOMES

Short-term follow-up outcomes have demonstrated that isolated BLT can reduce and stabilize corneal ectasia in eyes with progressive and advanced KC.[1-5] Corneal densitometry and higher-order aberrations (HOAs) after BLT have been studied by Luceri et al.[13] They reported that HOAs like spherical aberration, decreased for both anterior and posterior corneal surfaces, however with an increase in corneal back scattering.

The results in post-PRK haze have been encouraging in early follow-up, showing an improvement in contact lens-corrected visual acuity of 20/18 within 2 months.[2] Although the surgical technique and lamellar dissection currently

Flowchart 2: Preparation of Bowman's layer lenticule.

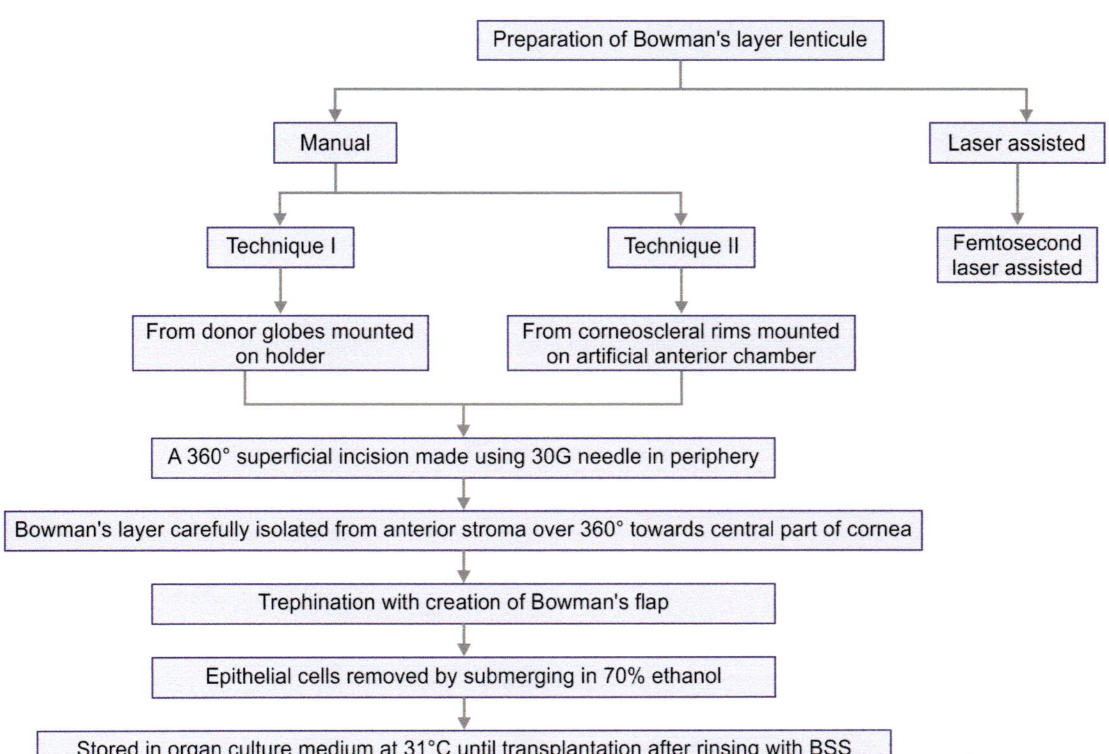

Flowchart 3: Bowman's layer transplantation procedure.

Step 1: Local anesthesia
Retrobulbar block with digital ocular massage and application of Honan's balloon to soften the eye

↓

Step 2: Corneoscleral tunnel
Superior conjunctival peritomy and a 5 mm corneoscleral tunnel is fashioned with a crescent blade, around 1.5 mm outside the limbus

↓

Step 3: Paracentesis
Paracentesis and the anterior chamber filled with air

↓

Step 4: Midstromal pocket
Using DALK dissection spatulas, midstromal pocket is made 360°, in a controlled fashion with constant monitoring of depth, from limbus to limbus, by the air endothelial reflex method

↓

Step 5: Placement of graft using glide
A glide is placed into the mouth of tunnel, the graft after staining with trypan blue dye, placed on top of the glide and pushed inside, unfolded using a bent cannula

↓

Step 6: Tamponade
With graft fully unfolded, eye is pressurized by filling the anterior chamber with balanced salt solution

require a potentially steep-learning curve, femtosecond laser assistance may render this technique easily reproducible, precise, and consistent.

Advantages of BLT can be summarized as:

- Absence of surface incisions and sutures cause minimal changes on ocular surface and keeping the ocular surface intact. BLT can thus be carried out on patients with comorbid ocular surface abnormality.
- BL tissue being acellular and therefore would be unlikely to incite an immune reaction and subsequent rejection.
- BLT carries lower risk for glaucoma than other procedures being a minimally invasive technique.
- Donor tissue from which BL lenticule has been harvested can be used for endothelial keratoplasties at a later date.
- BL is an acellular elastic layer hence offers considerable resistance to inadvertent tears during preparation.

Disadvantages associated with the procedure are:

- *DM perforation*: Similar to other lamellar surgical options like DALK, BLT may also result in inadvertent DM perforation particularly in thin and steep corneas. However if perforation occurs, surgery can be converted to full thickness procedure.
- BLT is a complex surgical procedure requiring expertise with a steep learning curve.
- BLT offers only a modest improvement without a significant functional/anatomical rehabilitation.

CONCLUSION

Bowman's layer transplantation, though in its infancy has proved to be a good alternative in terms of structural outcome. Though associated with only a modest visual improvement, reduction and stabilization of corneal ectasia can still be achieved to prevent further progression. However, long-term results are still awaited from other centers, especially with respect to flattening of posterior corneal surface. The technique being a fairly new one necessitates more evidence, to be recommended as a routine surgical modality.

REFERENCES

1. Van Dijk K, Parker J, Tong CM, Ham L, Lie JT, Groeneveld-van Beek EA, et al. Midstromal isolated Bowman's layer graft for reduction of advanced keratoconus: A technique to postpone penetrating or deep anterior lamellar keratoplasty. JAMA Ophthalmol. 2014;132(4):495-501.
2. Dragnea DC, Birbal RS, Ham L, Dapena I, Oellerich S, van Dijk K, et al. Bowman's layer transplantation in the treatment of keratoconus. Eye Vision. 2018;5:24.
3. van Dijk K, Parker JS, Baydoun L, Ilyas A, Dapena I, Groeneveld-van Beek EA, et al. Bowman's layer transplantation: 5-year results. Graefes Arch Clin Exp Ophthalmol. 2018;256(6):1151-8.
4. Tong CM, van Dijk K, Melles GRJ. Update on Bowman's layer transplantation. Curr Opin Ophthalmol. 2019;30(4):249-55.
5. Parker J, van Dijk K, Cooper E, Melles GRJ. Bowman's layer transplantation for advanced keratoconus. Catar Refract Surg Today Eur. 2017:30-3.
6. Sharma B, Dubey A, Prakash G, Vajpayee RB. Bowman's layer transplantation: Evidence to date. Clin Ophthalmol. 2018;12:433-7.
7. Lie J, Droutsas K, Ham L, Dapena I, Ververs B, Otten H, et al. Isolated Bowman's layer transplantation to manage persistent subepithelial haze after excimer laser surface ablation. J Cataract Refract Surg. 2010;36(6):1036-41.
8. Lagali N, Germundsson J, Fagerholm P. The role of Bowman's layer in corneal regeneration after phototherapeutic keratectomy: A prospective study using in vivo confocal microscopy. Invest Ophthalmol Vis Sci. 2009;50(9):4192-8.
9. Groeneveld-van Beek EA, Parker J, Lie JT, Ham L, van Dijk K, van der Wees J, et al. Donor tissue preparation for Bowman's layer transplantation. Cornea. 2016;35(12):1499-502.
10. Parker JS, van Dijk K, Melles GR. Treatment options for advanced keratoconus: A review. Surv Ophthalmol. 2015;60(5):459-80.
11. Parker JS, Huls F, Cooper E, Graves P, Groeneveld-van Beek EA, Lie J, et al. Technical feasibility of isolated Bowman's layer graft preparation by femtosecond laser: a pilot study. Eur J Ophthalmol. 2017;27(6):675-7.
12. García de Oteyza G, Dibildox LAG, Vázquez-Romo KA, Vázquez AT, Alquisiras JHD, Martínez-Báez BE, et al. Bowman's layer transplantation using a femtosecond laser. 2019;45(3):261-6.
13. Luceri S, Parker J, Dapena I, Baydoun L, Oellerich S, van Dijk K, et al. Corneal densitometry and higher order aberrations after Bowman's layer transplantation: 1-year results. Cornea. 2016; 35(7):959-66.

52

Tectonic Patch Grafts

Nikhil S Gokhale

INTRODUCTION

Patch graft is a tectonic graft, which may be used to restore the integrity of the globe with minimal intraocular surgical manipulation in an inflamed eye. This technique is performed in corneal lesions that are too large to be treated with tissue adhesives, but small enough to preclude the conventionally sized penetrating keratoplasty. Though a patch graft is usually preferred in peripheral corneal lesions (**Figs. 1 and 2**), the central lesions may also be repaired with the patch grafts (**Figs. 3A and B**). Depending on the thickness of the patch grafts, they can be either full thickness or lamellar. Though technically difficult, lamellar patch is effective in reinforcing a thin, necrotic stroma with or without descemetocele. A full thickness patch graft is an easier alternative. Full thickness tectonic patch grafts are particularly useful in eyes with uveal prolapse, where additional structural support is required (**Figs. 4A and B**).

In an acutely inflamed eye such as corneal perforation or melting, it may be safer to perform a lamellar patch graft than a more invasive penetrating graft. The lamellar patch graft serves as an interim procedure to stabilize the eye in such cases, so that the vision restoring penetrating keratoplasty may be performed at a later date, when the eye becomes quiet. Tectonic patch grafts, lamellar or full thickness are useful in the treatment of severe corneal melts, as they not only provide structural support, but also help in the interim period until systemic immunosuppressive medications halt the collagenolytic break down of the cornea (**Figs. 5A and B**).[1]

INDICATIONS

Inflammatory diseases of the cornea result in collagenolytic destruction of the stroma leading to corneal melting and loss of vision. The use of a tectonic patch graft in these conditions aids in providing structural support to the cornea, thus stabilizing the globe.[2,3] The excision and removal of the involved necrotic areas eliminates the devitalized tissue, which is a source of collagenolytic enzyme collagenase[4-7] and the presence of the patch graft provides tectonic support

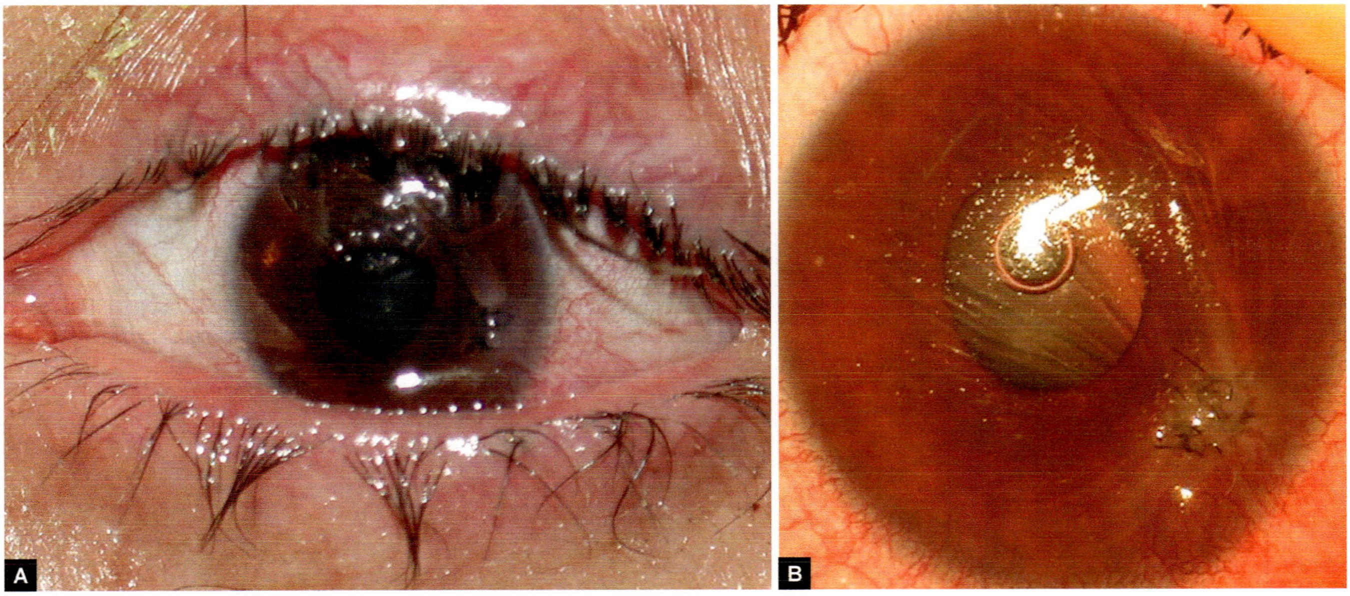

Figs. 1A and B: An 18-year-old girl with rosacea and perforated corneal melt where primary suturing was unsuccessfully attempted elsewhere.

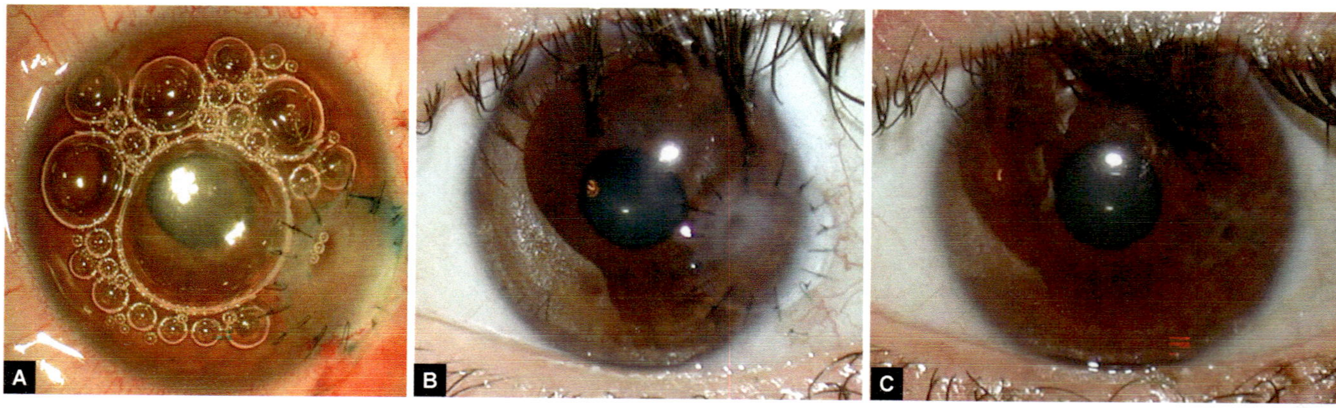

Figs. 2A to C: Intraoperative picture of the same patient showing the perforation site following a lamellar patch graft. 1 year and 5 years postoperative pictures.

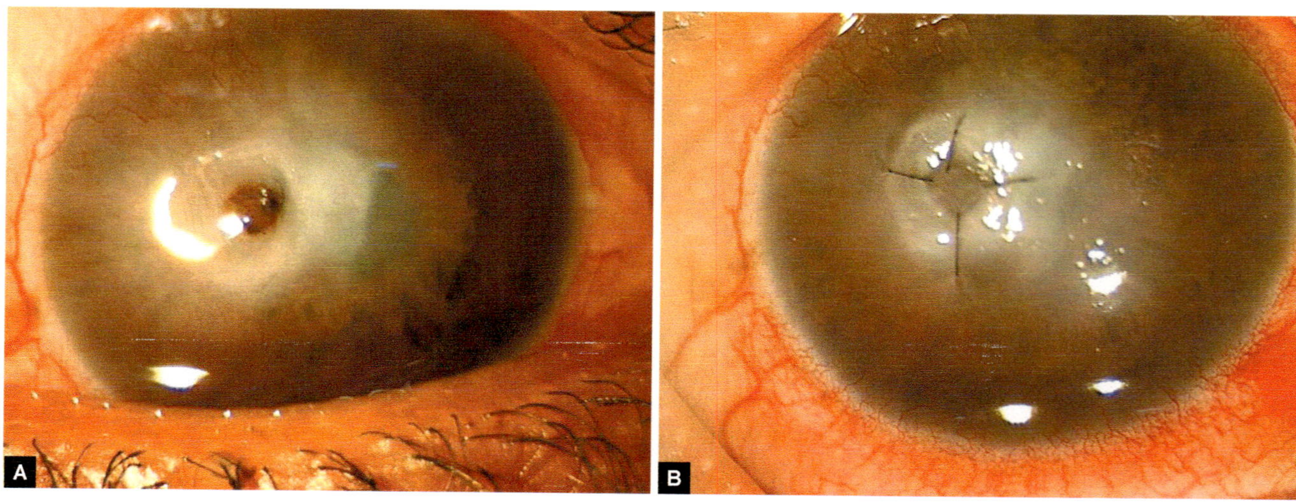

Figs. 3A and B: Central perforation repaired with a patch graft.

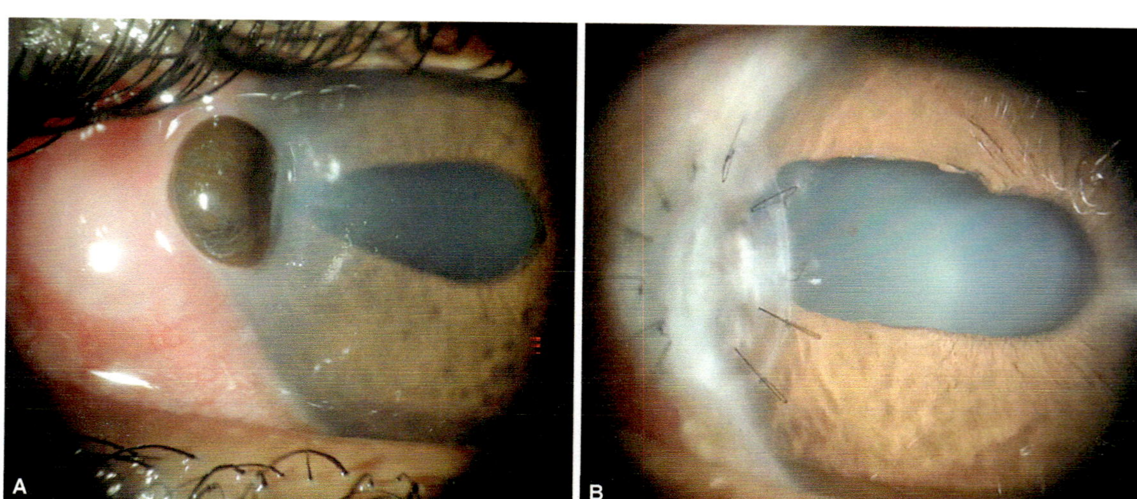

Figs. 4A and B: Perforation with iris prolapse following severe untreated phlyctenular inflammation. Patch graft with iris abscission.

to the globe. The underlying causes of the melt need to be carefully identified and appropriate measures need to be taken to treat them, otherwise the melts can recur in the graft or elsewhere on the cornea.

Reconstructive lamellar patch graft is also indicated in corneal ectasia, descemetocele, and following corneal dermoid excision (**Figs. 6A to C**).[1] In nonseeing eyes with corneal fistulas a tectonic patch graft can be done to prevent late endophthalmitis due to retrograde spread of infection. Similarly, in nonseeing eyes with melts or perforation not amenable to glue application, a patch graft is a good option (**Fig. 7**).

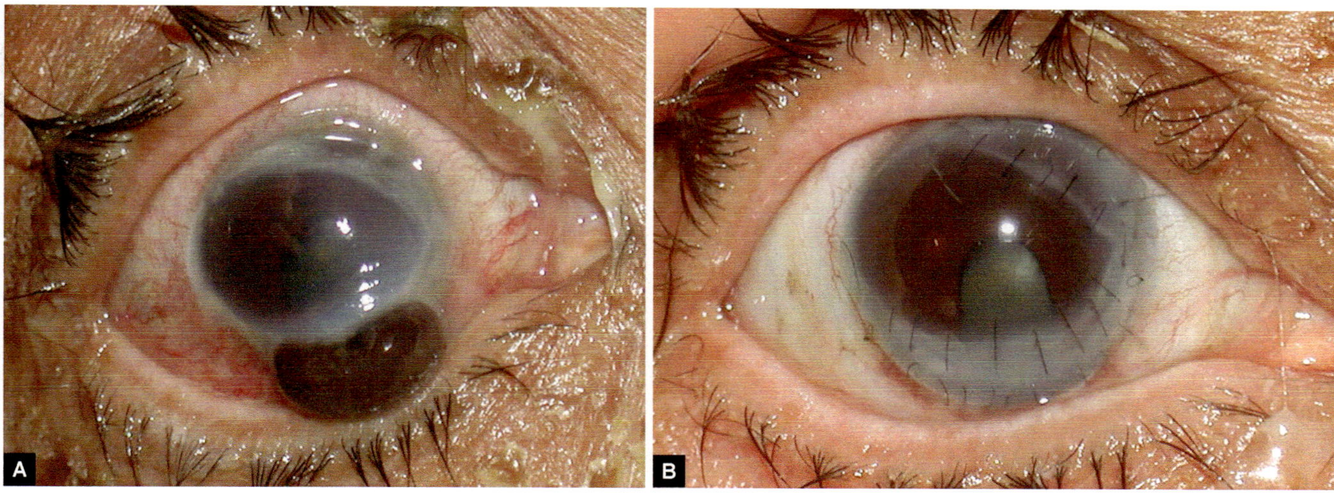

Figs. 5A and B: Tectonic grafts in perforated peripheral ulcerative keratitis.

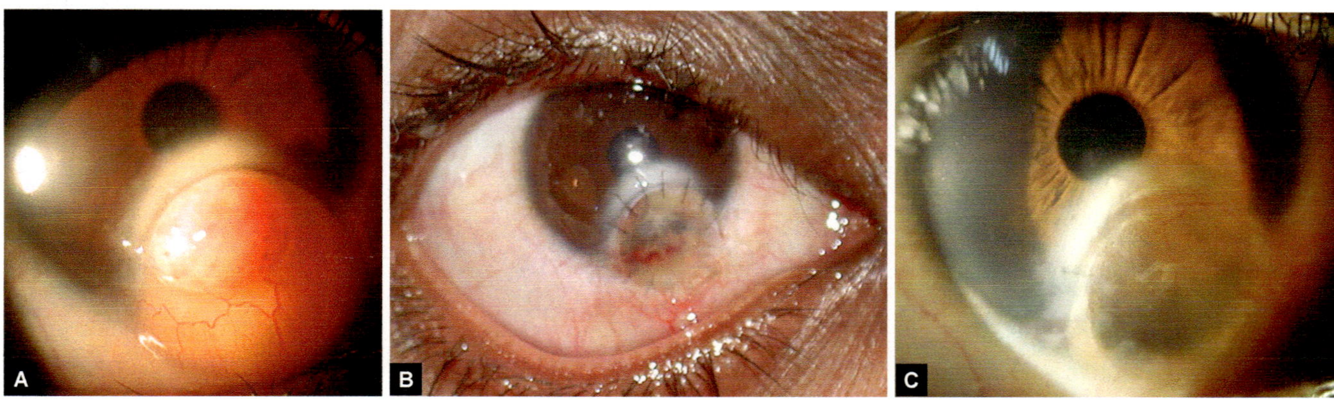

Figs. 6A to C: Patch graft following dermoid excision.

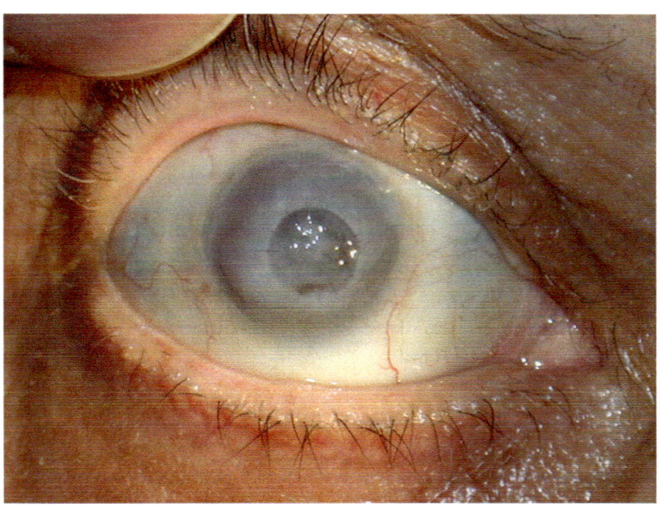

Fig. 7: Patch graft in a nonseeing eye.

Scleral patch grafts are used in eyes with severe scleral thinning or melting as in scleromalacia perforans or after pterygium excision (**Box 1**).

ADVANTAGES OVER TISSUE ADHESIVES

Tissue adhesives are not useful in eyes with corneal perforations larger than 2 mm. In a central corneal melt or perforation the tissue adhesives produce opaque tissue reaction and obscure the visual axis. Tissue adhesives promote corneal vascularization tend to attract new blood vessels in the cornea. Although these new blood vessels may aid in halting the melting process and hasten healing, the risk of immune rejection in a subsequent full thickness graft is enhanced.[1] The healing period following tissue adhesive application is often 2–3 months and delays the recovery process. For perforations with sloping edges glue is usually successful however for punched out melts with vertical

Box 1: Indications of tectonic patch graft.

Corneal patch graft
- Corneal perforation not amenable to closure with tissue adhesives or bandage contact lens (BCL)
- Descemetocele with impending corneal perforation
- Corneal perforation larger than 2 mm but smaller than 5 mm
- Chronic nonhealing corneal ulceration
- Traumatic irreparable corneal tissue loss
- Corneal fistulas
- Corneal ectasia
- Postcorneal dermoid excision

Scleral patch graft
- Scleromalacia perforans
- Following pterygium excision

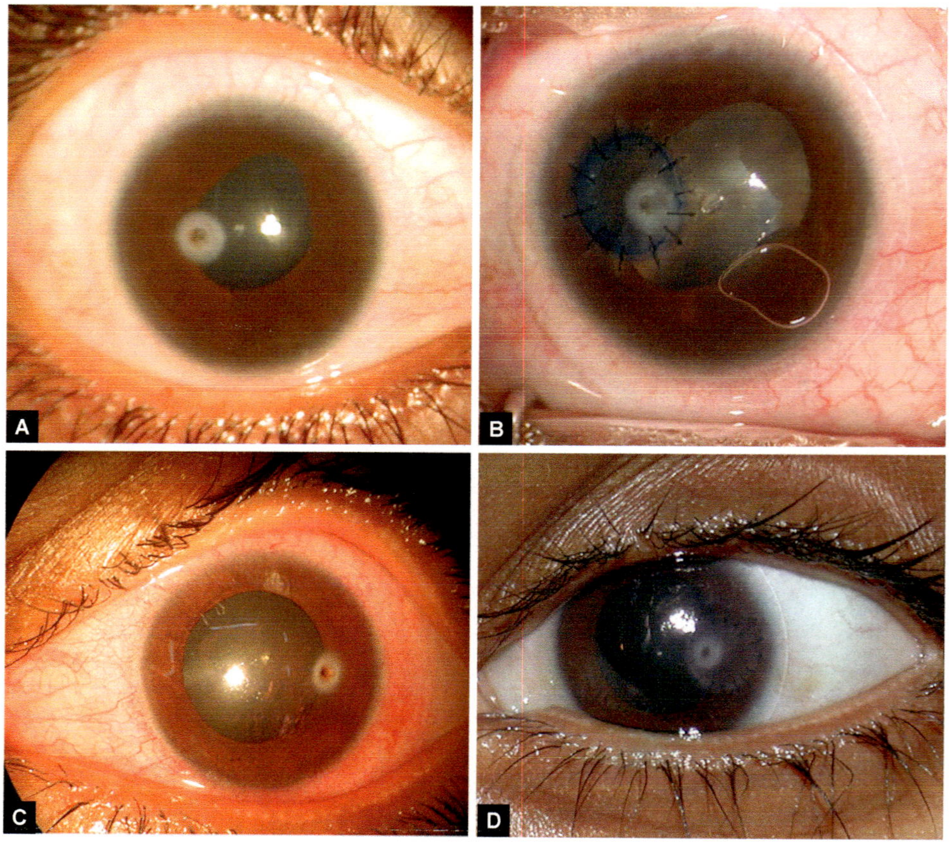

Figs. 8A to D: Lamellar patch grafts to close two cases of post foreign body removal perforations.

walls or in fistulous tracks, it may often fail. Also the scarring and vascularization may cause loss of vision. As seen in **Figures 8A to D** a lamellar patch graft was done for a corneal perforation following removal of a deep foreign body. This allowed a quick closure of the perforation and good recovery of visual acuity. Well-placed superficial lamellar inlay grafts can result in minimal astigmatism and much better visual results than a glue application.

Tectonic patch grafts on the other hand, provide better structural support and early stabilization of the globe in addition to the removal of necrotic stroma, which is a source of collagenase. The visual axis remains clear particularly, if care has been taken to avoid the graft-host junction or suture placement in the center of the cornea. Large penetrating grafts carry a high-risk of long-term failures, which can be obviated if a lamellar patch graft can achieve the same result of providing tectonic support and not affecting vision.

SURGICAL TECHNIQUE

The various types of patch grafts can be lamellar patch grafts, full thickness patch grafts, and sclera patch grafts. Algorithms have been described on the choice of patch grafts depending on the size and severity of lesion.[8-13]

Lamellar Patch Graft

Preoperative preparation for patch graft is similar to that of penetrating keratoplasty. Small sized trephines from 4–6.5 mm are required additionally. Surgery is performed under local or general anesthesia. The eyelids are separated with a Barraquer lid speculum. Conjunctival peritomy or scleral dissection is occasionally required in peripheral corneal lesions. The anterior chamber is formed with a viscoelastic substance or air injected through a self-sealing paracentesis site. The dimensions of the perforation are measured. The host cut should encompass the entire involved area of the cornea and at least 1 mm clear area around the circumference of the perforation. The boundaries of the lamellar bed are marked with a handheld disposable, sharp, obturator-guided trephine blade up to the desired depth. Alternatively, a Hanna vacuum trephine may be set at a depth of 0.45 mm and the recipient cornea is trephined which is centered at the perforation site. The devitalized necrotic tissue is removed from the recipient bed. Lamellar dissection is then facilitated by further inflation of the anterior chamber with viscoelastics or air.

The lamellar dissection of the recipient bed is done by means of a Tooke's knife, or a crescent knife. The dissection is begun peripherally at the trephine wound circumferentially proceeding centrally toward the lesion. Preparation of a smooth recipient bed is necessary to ensure proper apposition of the graft.

The lamellar donor patch is prepared from the donor cornea after fixing it in a King's clamp or on an artificial anterior chamber. The donor button should be of the same size or 0.25 mm larger than that of the recipient size. A complementary partial thickness lamellar graft is then fashioned from the donor cornea. The donor graft is now secured in place over the recipient bed with interrupted 10-0 nylon sutures. Suture bites through the central visual axis should either be avoided or should be intentionally placed shorter.

Full Thickness Patch Graft

The surgical technique is almost similar to that of penetrating keratoplasty. Preoperative mannitol may be required to soften the eye. After trephination, the anterior chamber is entered with a sharp blade. Viscoelastic is injected into the anterior chamber in order to push back the iris. The host cornea is removed with a curved corneal scissors, holding it vertically to avoid beveling. Any adherent iris tissue must be separated gently and meticulously.

A full thickness donor graft oversized by 0.5 mm is prepared and secured in place with interrupted 10-0 nylon sutures. Sutures are buried and anterior chamber is formed with balanced salt solutions and the wound is checked for any leakage.

Scleral Patch Graft

A scleral patch graft is occasionally indicated in cases of localized scleral necrosis caused by scleromalacia or following scleral thinning following recurrent pterygium surgery[14] (**Figs. 9 and 10**). Initially conjunctival peritomy is done in the affected area. The scleral bed is prepared by removing the entire necrotic tissue and delineating a healthy scleral margin. A trephine mark, which includes the necrotic area, may help in the scleral dissection. At least 1 mm healthy scleral area must be included inside the trephine. Scleral incision may be deepened with a blade and dissection is performed manually. A full thickness same sized scleral graft is trephined from a donor globe and the graft is secured in place with 10-0 nylon sutures. The graft is preferably covered, at least partially, with conjunctiva.

Sangwan et al. recommend that scleral grafting with overlying conjunctival or amniotic membrane graft is an effective and simple measure for preserving globe integrity both structurally and functionally.[15]

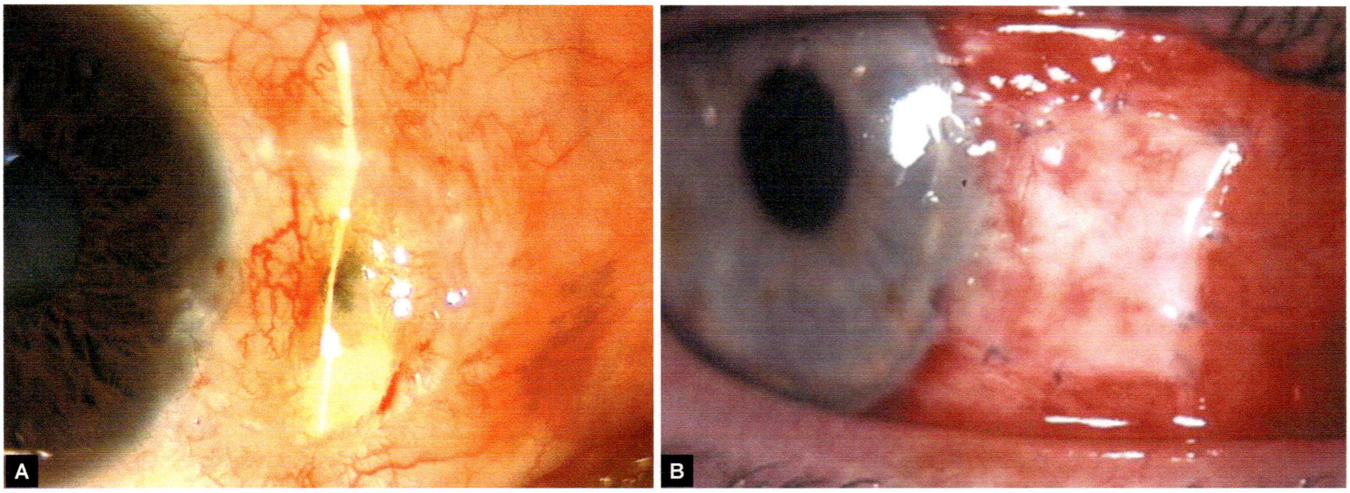

Figs. 9A and B: Scleral melting following pterygium surgery and post-scleral graft.

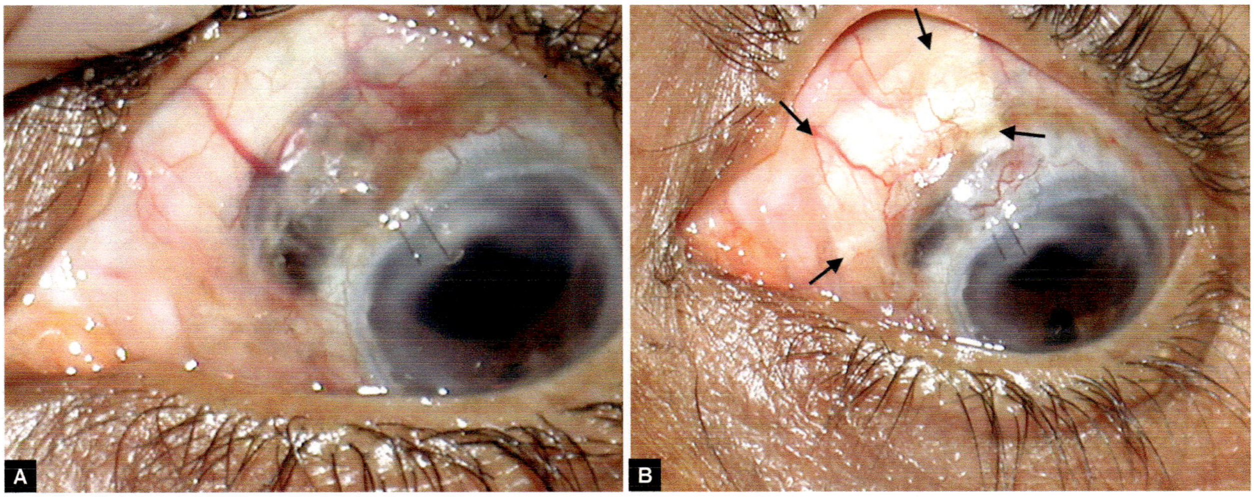

Figs. 10A and B: Scleral patch graft to repair a postinflammatory staphyloma.

REFERENCES

1. Soong HK, Farzo AA, Katz D, Meyer RF, Sugar A. Lamellar corneal patch grafts in the management of corneal melting. Cornea. 2000;19:126-34.
2. Raziman MB, Sainz de la Maza M, Foster CS. Tectonic patch graft in peripheral ulcerative keratitis. Cornea. 1991;10:312-16.
3. Taylor DM, Stern AL. Reconstructive keratoplasty in the management of conditions leading to corneal destruction. Ophthalmology. 1980;87:892-904.
4. Kenyon KR. Corneal perforations: discussion. Ophthalmology. 1982;89:634-5.
5. Eiferman RA, Snyder JW. Antibacterial effect of cyanoacrylate glue. Arch Ophthalmol. 1983;101:955-60.
6. Kenyon KR, Berman MB, Hanninen LA. Tissue adhesive prevents ulceration and inhibits inflammation of the thermal burned rabbit cornea. Invest Ophthalmol Vis Sci. 1979;18:96.
7. Kenyon KR. Decision-making in the therapy of external eye disease: non-infected corneal ulcers. Ophthalmology. 1982;89:44- 51.
8. Vanathi M, Sharma N, Titiyal JS, Tandon R, Vajpayee RB. Tectonic grafts for corneal thinning and perforations. Cornea. 2002;21:792-7.
9. Orlin SE, Sulewski ME. Spontaneous corneal perforation in pellucid marginal degeneration. CLAO J. 1998;24:186-7.
10. Lam DS, Wah C, Lai JS. Short-term results of using corneoscleral patch graft for the Ahmed glaucoma valve implant surgery. Yan Ke Xue Bao. 1997;13:109-12.
11. Seino Jy, Anderson SF. Mooren's Ulcer. Optom Vis Sci. 1998;75:783-90.
12. Rumelt S, Rehany U. A donor corneal patch graft for an incompetent scleral flap following trabeculectomy. Ophthalmic Surg Lasers. 1996;27:878-80.
13. Vrabec MP, Jordan JJ. A surgical technique for the treatment of central corneal perforations. J Refract corneal Surg. 1994;10:365-7.
14. Nguyen OD, Foster CS. Scleral patch graft in the management of necrotizing scleritis. Int Ophthalmol Clin. 1999;39:109-31.
15. Sangwan VS, Jain V, Gupta P. Structural and functional outcome of scleral patch graft. Eye. 2007;21:930-5.

53 Autokeratoplasty

Tushar Agarwal, Sohini Mandal, Namrata Sharma, Rasik B Vajpayee

INTRODUCTION

Penetrating or lamellar keratoplasty using donor corneal tissue is the standard approach for managing corneal scars. However, this option is not always feasible as there is a shortage of optical grade corneas in many parts of the world. This scarcity forces corneal surgeons to look at alternatives of allograft corneal tissue in order to visually rehabilitate patients with corneal opacification. Autokeratoplasty is a type of surgery which uses patients' own cornea for visual rehabilitation.[1] This is especially applicable to patients who are at a high risk for corneal graft rejection.

TYPES OF AUTOKERATOPLASTY

Autokeratoplasty can be of two types:

1. *Contralateral autokeratoplasty*: This procedure is carried out in patients who have one eye affected by a corneal pathology and the fellow eye is blind due to posterior segment or optic nerve pathology but has a normal cornea.[1] In such a case, corneas of the two eyes are surgically so as to provide a clear cornea to the eye with a potential for vision.
2. *Rotational autokeratoplasty*: This procedure is carried out in patients with partial corneal opacification, the cornea of the patient is surgically rotated, so as to move the corneal opacity away from the pupillary axis.[2-5]

CONTRALATERAL AUTOKERATOPLASTY

Case Selection

Contralateral autokeratoplasty is considered in any patient whose one eye is affected by a corneal pathology and the other by a blinding posterior segment pathology.

Examination and Investigations

For sake of clarity, we term the eye with the diseased cornea as the host eye and the contralateral eye from which the clear cornea is to be harvested as the donor eye.

Donor Eye

Important features to be looked for in eye being considered as a potential donor are:

- Absence of light perception
- The cornea is clear and of normal size and shape. The cornea should be free from any synechiae. Examination by specular reflection should be done to rule out any endothelial abnormalities like guttae.
- Intraocular pressure (IOP) should be assessed. Any long-standing glaucoma can cause damage to the endothelial cells. Important investigations are:
  - *Specular count*: Endothelial cell count of 1,000 cells/mm^3 should be the cut off for considering an eye's suitability for corneal harvesting.
  - *Videokeratography*: Videokeratography using a slit-scan based machine like Orbscan is should be performed to rule out any ectatic disorders of the cornea.
  - *Visual evoked response*: This is done to document the absence of any visual potential.

Host Eye

Baseline investigations should be done as in any case being taken up for penetrating keratoplasty. Points to be noted specifically in relation to contralateral autokeratoplasty are:

- Corneal thickness should be assessed using ultrasonic pachymetry. The cornea should not be extraordinarily thin at any point. This would make its apposition with the donor eye difficult.
- Iris and lens status has to be examined carefully. If the lens is cataractous then cataract surgery is also planned along with autokeratoplasty. If the eye is pseudophakic, the intraocular lens (IOL) position and stability should be assessed if visible. If corneal opacity precludes a proper clinical evaluation, then ultrasound biomicroscopy can be done to determine the IOL position. If the posterior chamber IOL is found to be displaced anteriorly or there is an anterior chamber IOL then IOL explanation can be planned.

The goals of examination and investigations are:

- To ensure that the donor eye's cornea is suitable for harvesting.
- Plan in advance the anterior segment surgical steps other than keratoplasty in the host eye.

Surgical Technique

The surgery should be undertaken in general anesthesia as bilateral keratoplasty is a time taking procedure. It is advisable to administer intravenous mannitol in a dose of 1–1.5 g/kg, 45 minutes before surgery to reduce the vitreous pressure.

Both eyes of the patient are cleaned and draped. Two separate instrument trolleys are prepared, one for each eye. The operating room floor is organized to ensure that the surgeon can switch between the two eyes anytime during the surgical procedure. To understand the surgery better, surgical procedure is divided into discrete surgical steps. The aim of these steps is to ensure that the host eye is left open sky for a minimum possible period of time to reduce the risk of expulsive hemorrhage in the seeing eye.

Step One (Host Eye)

A 7–8 mm trephine is used to remove a central button from the host cornea. After completely dissecting the host button, it is set aside carefully in a graft holder. It is important to remember at this stage that this cornea is to be used to close the donor eye and so, it is handled carefully.

If any anterior segment reconstruction or anterior vitrectomy is required, it is performed at this time. Once the anterior segment surgical procedures are completed, the diseased corneal button is temporarily sutured back to the host with the help of four cardinal sutures. The anterior chamber is formed with viscoelastic containing 0.9% sodium hyaluronate.

Step Two (Donor Eye)

The donor cornea is trephined using a vacuum trephine which is 0.25 mm larger than that used for trephination of the host cornea. One should make sure that the donor cornea is cut with minimal manipulation of the tissue. Once the cut is completed, the donor cornea is carefully set aside on a graft holder with the endothelial side up and covered with a viscoelastic. The donor eye is covered with a wet swab.

Step Three (Host Eye)

The cardinal sutures are cut and the diseased cornea is removed from the host. It is placed on a graft holder with the endothelial side up and covered with a viscoelastic. The donor cornea which has been prepared in step two is placed on the host and tied with four cardinal sutures to the host bed.

Step Four (Donor Eye)

The diseased cornea is sutured to the donor eye with four cardinal sutures.

Step Five (Host Eye)

Suturing of the donor cornea to the host bed is completed with sixteen 10-0 monofilament nylon sutures. Wound is checked for any leaks and is supplemented with sutures if required.

Step Six (Donor Eye)

The diseased cornea is securely sutured to the donor site. This may require a larger number and tighter than normal sutures as the corneal button is 0.25 mm undersized. Again, the wound is checked for any leaks and supplemented with sutures as required.

Postoperative Management

Topical broad-spectrum antibiotics, corticosteroids, and preservative-free lubricants are prescribed for both eyes. Intraocular pressure is carefully monitored for both eyes separately.

Outcomes

Contralateral autokeratoplasty may have similar or better long-term anatomical survival rates than low-risk corneal allografts. Barraquer et al.[6] found an anatomical survival rate of 74 and 63% at 5 and 10 years of follow-up, respectively, while the study by Sanjuán et al. reported 79 and 72% success rates at the same follow up time points. Autokeratoplasty is an effective alternative for cases at high risk for developing corticosteroid induced complications. Furthermore, it would completely eliminate the risk of graft rejection. Although, progression of preexisting glaucoma stays as the most important risk factor for long-term corneal decompensation and loss of visual function.[7] Matsuda and Manabe described endothelial cell loss of up to 55% in the first 2 years after autokeratoplasty with minimal cell loss subsequently.[8] In a study by Sanjuán et al., 52% patients achieved anatomical and functional success at the end of the follow-up and functional failures always preceded anatomical failures.

ROTATIONAL AUTOKERATOPLASTY

The principle of rotational autokeratoplasty is to surgically rotate a patient's cornea that is affected by a localized corneal opacity, so that the opacified part of the cornea is moved away from the pupil.

Case Selection

Selecting cases suitable for this type of surgery and planning the trephine size and its placement are the important decisive factors.

Mathematical Method

Bourne et al. described a mathematical model for deciding the suitability of a patient for this type of surgery and the trephine size to be used.[3]

To determine the suitability two measurements are taken. First the diameter of the largest circle of the clear cornea is measured. Second, the shortest distance from the edge of the circle to the geometric center of the cornea is assessed. This is considered positive if the opacity involved the center of the cornea and negative if the opacity is within the largest area of the clear cornea.

The required trephine size is obtained with the following equation:

1.5 × diameter of the largest clear circle + shortest distance from the circle to the corneal center

Computer Simulation

The cases can also be selected and the surgery planned on the basis of preoperative computer simulation and digital imaging.[9]

A central photo of the cornea is captured using a digital photo slit lamp (**Fig. 1A**). This image is imported into a commercially available image editing software like Photoshop. Using the circle drawings tool, a circle approximating the pupil is drawn over the cornea (**Fig. 1B**). This is done on a new, transparent layer created on the original image. Then switching back to the original layer, a circle is drawn on the cornea to simulate corneal trephination (*see* **Fig. 1B**). The corneal area within this circle is rotated on the image to simulate rotational autokeratoplasty (**Fig. 1C**). This step is repeated a number of times using varying sizes and position of the larger circle, which simulates the corneal trephine, to include maximum clear cornea in the pupillary axis. The position of the rotated cornea that provides the maximum clearing of the pupil is chosen as the final intended position of the cornea (*see* **Fig. 1C**). The size of the larger circle (trephine) and its distance from the limbus is measured. The layers of the image can be fused at this stage and printout be taken for reference during the surgery.

Surgical Technique

The surgery is performed under peribulbar anesthesia. The size and site of trephination is preplanned. The reference points from the limbus are marked on the cornea and it is trephined. The cornea is freed from any attachments to the host rim. Cataract surgery is performed if required (**Fig. 1D**). The cornea is placed in the rotated position as per the preoperative simulation (*see* **Fig. 1D**). It is sutured to the eye in this position with interrupted 10-0 monofilament nylon sutures. Special care is required while suturing the opaque parts as they are likely to be of uneven thickness. Extra sutures can be placed to properly approximate the graft host junction. The wound is checked for leaks at the end of surgery.

Femtosecond Laser-assisted Ipsilateral Rotational Lamellar Autokeratoplasty

Several studies have reported the efficacy of femtosecond laser-assisted anterior lamellar keratoplasty (ALK) for corneal scars that do not involve the posterior 250 μm of stroma.[10-15] Ipsilateral rotational penetrating autokeratoplasty has been described previously in the literature but has not found widespread use. Indeed, few patients are suitable for this procedure.[16,17] Corneal lenticules created with the femtosecond laser present a more planar architecture. Moreover, the femtosecond laser provides greater precision in the lenticule diameter and thickness. Although the femtosecond laser can enhance the precision of an eccentric cut, it might also introduce some interface complications compared to penetrating or deep anterior lamellar procedures. Cassagne et al. described the surgical technique and reported the outcomes of two patients treated

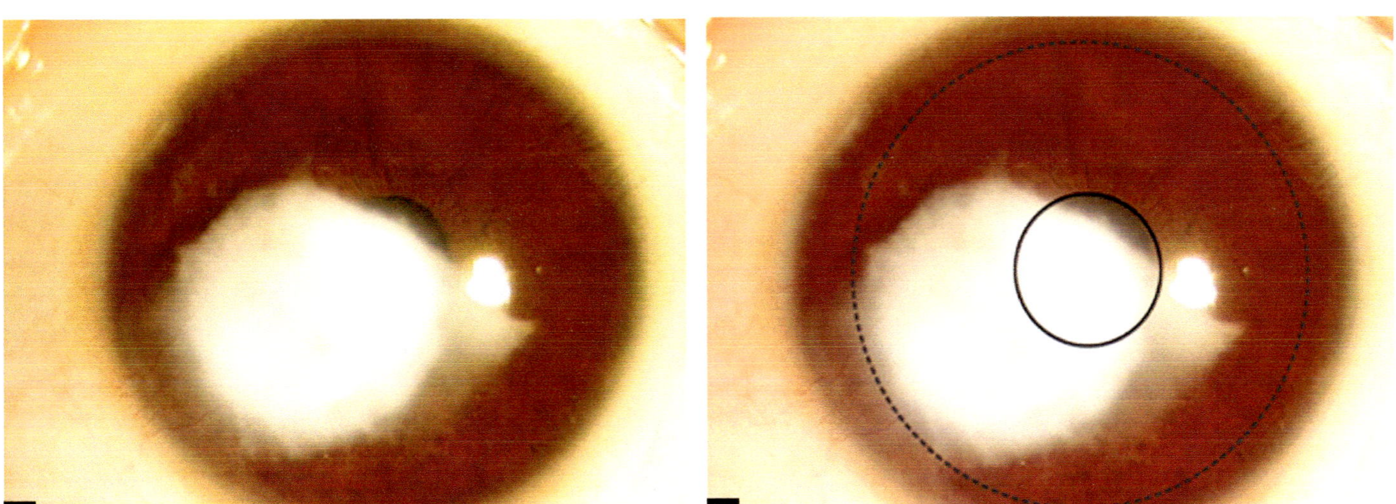

Figs. 1A and B: (A) Central photo of cornea is captured using digital photo slit lamp which is then imported in commercially available imaging editing software; (B) A circle is drawn on cornea to simulate corneal trephination and another circle is drawn to simulate the pupil.

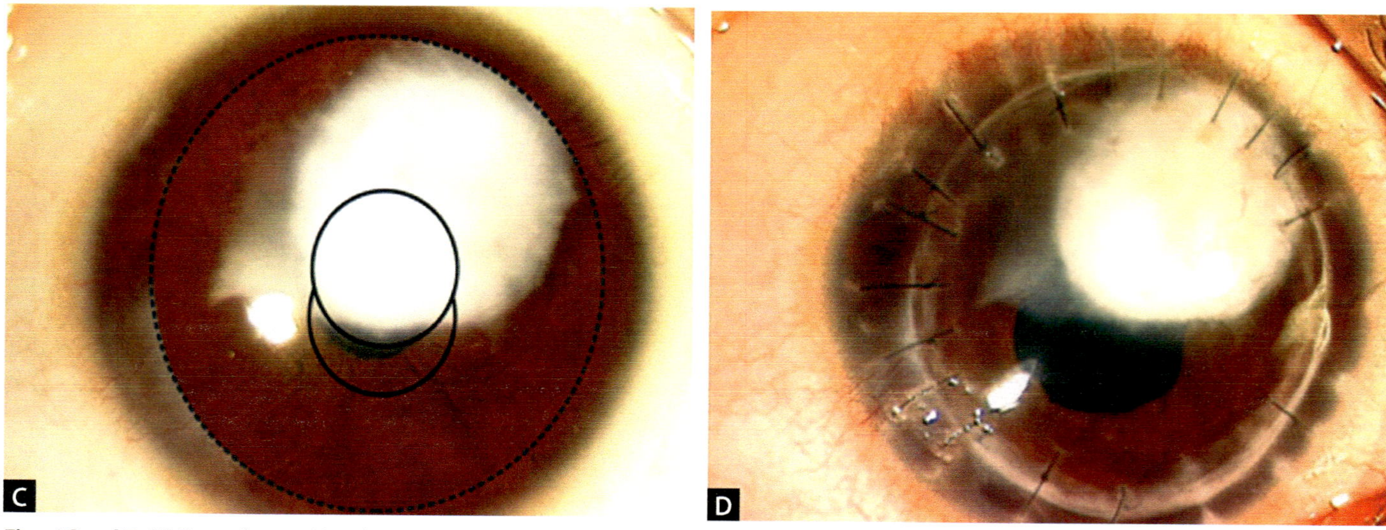

Figs. 1C and D: (C) Corneal area within the circle is rotated to simulate rotational autokeratoplasty; (D) Cataract surgery, pupilloplasty and rotational corneal transplantation are done as guided by computer simulation.

for central corneal scars. The corneal scar depth was mapped using preoperative optical coherence tomography. An eccentric lamellar lenticule was cut with a femtosecond laser and rotated to decenter the corneal opacity and clear the pupillary area. The surgical plan was set after simulating lenticule rotation with a digital corneal image and computer software. The corneal scar was decentered inferiorly, out of the pupillary area, resulting in improved postoperative visual acuity.

Postoperative Management

Postoperatively the patient are prescribed topical broad-spectrum antibiotics, topical steroids and preservative-free lubricants. Steroids can be tapered off after 4 weeks.

Outcomes and Complications

- *Astigmatism*: The study by Jonas et al.[18] is the only one to have compared visual outcomes with that of a control group of penetrating allografts, and found significantly higher astigmatism in nine patients receiving autografts. Potential reasons for increased astigmatism are eccentric trephination, disparity of corneal thickness between the peripheral clear cornea and the central scarred cornea, and the close proximity of one edge of trephination to the pupillary zone.[18]
- *Visual acuity*: From the four studies in which the results of individual cases are reported[2,4,5,19] 48% of patients were 6/12 or better, although it is not clear whether this was unaided or with contact lenses.
- *Transplant survival and endothelial cell loss*: Long-term results are unknown, but Bertelmann et al.[20] showed that the mean endothelial cell loss was 15% in rotational autografts compared with 40% in homografts at 1 year, such that the survival of autografts can be expected to compare well with the failure rates of 20% after 10 years due to the continued attrition of endothelial cells and the high rate of transplant rejection in penetrating corneal homografts.[21,22]

Advantages

The biggest advantage of autokeratoplasty is that the patient is totally free from the risk of graft rejection. This is a major benefit for patients who are at a high risk of graft rejection including those with previous failed grafts and vascularized corneas. Since no external donor is required, there is no waiting period associated. The surgery can be scheduled at the convenience of both the patient and the surgeon. There is no risk of transmission of donor related infections as is a possibility with allografts. Also, there is a decreased requirement for postoperative steroids. This is especially helpful in patients who are steroid responders. Finally, there are no risks associated with the use of corneal preservative media.

Disadvantages

There are a few disadvantages for the patient. Since the opacity is not removed completely and merely shifted from one eye to the other in contralateral keratoplasty, it might not be cosmetically welcoming for all patients.

Contralateral autokeratoplasty is a bilateral simultaneous procedure, requiring general anesthesia which adds an element of additional risk. These are higher chances of astigmatism with rotational autokeratoplasty as tighter sutures are required for securing a same sized graft. Also, the corneal thickness of the central and peripheral part of the cornea that are being apposed are dissimilar.

Patient Counseling

The treating physician should speak in detail with the patient regarding the procedure. Patient should be explained about the relative advantages and disadvantages of the procedure. It is important for the patient to have an understanding of the procedure and have realistic expectations regarding the outcomes. He should be aware that the opacity is going to persist, although it may be covered by the eyelids in a rotational graft. Also the visual outcome is expected to be suboptimal.

An informed consent highlighting these points should be obtained from the patient.

CONCLUSION

Autokeratoplasty is a good alternative to corneal allograft transplantation for high risk cases. It provides the benefits of zero risk of graft rejection and donor-transmitted infections, faster recovery, and reduced dependence on steroids, and other immunosuppressives. Along with these advantages, they provide the benefit of elimination of dependence on the availability of donor corneal tissue. There are some pitfalls such as moderate visual recovery, persistence of corneal opacity, and bilateral surgery in cases of contralateral autokeratoplasty. In properly selected cases, the risk benefit ratio may be skewed in favour of patients.

REFERENCES

1. Price FW Jr, Hanna Si. Bilateral penetrating autokeratoplasty. J Refract Surg. 1995;11:494-6.
2. McDonnell PJ, Falcon MG. Rotational autokeratoplasty. Eye. 1989;3:576-80.
3. Bourne WM, Brubaker RF. A method for ipsilateral rotational autokeratoplasty. Ophthalmology. 1978;85:1312-6.
4. Verma N, Melengas S, Garap JA. Ipsilateral rotational autokeratoplasty for the management of corneal opacities. Aust N Z J Ophthalmol. 1999;27:21-5.
5. Murthy S, Bansal AK, Sridhar MS, Rao GN. Ipsilateral rotational autokeratoplasty: an alternative to penetrating keratoplasty in nonprogressive central corneal scars. Cornea. 2001;20:455-7.
6. Barraquer RI, Pareja-Aricò L, Gómez-Benlloch A, Michael R. Risk factors for graft failure after penetrating keratoplasty. Medicine (Baltimore). 2019;98(17):e15274.
7. Sanjuán P, Julio G, Bolaños J, Álvarez de Toledo J, García de Oteyza G, Temprano J, et al. Long-term anatomical and functional outcomes after autokeratoplasty. Br J Ophthalmol. 2021;105(8):1063-8.
8. Matsuda M, Manabe R. The corneal endothelium following autokeratoplasty. A case report. Acta Ophthalmol. 1988;66:54-7.
9. Bower KS, Mines MJ, Stutzman RD. Digital imaging to assist preoperative planning for ipsilateral rotational autokeratoplasty. J Telemed Telecare. 2006;12:374-6.
10. Yoo SH, Kymionis GD, Koreishi A, Ide T, Goldman D, Karp CL, et al. Femtosecond laser-assisted sutureless anterior lamellar keratoplasty. Ophthalmology. 2008;115:1303-7.
11. Shousha MA, Yoo SH, Kymionis GD, Ide T, Feuer W, Karp CL, et al. Long-term results of femtosecond laser-assisted sutureless anterior lamellar keratoplasty. Ophthalmology. 2011;118: 315-23.
12. Bonfadini G, Moreira H, Jun AS, Campos M, Kim EC, Arana E, et al. Modified femtosecond laser-assisted sutureless anterior lamellar keratoplasty. Cornea. 2013;32:533-7.
13. Almousa R, Samaras KE, Khan S, Lake DB, Daya SM. Femtosecond laser-assisted lamellar keratoplasty (FSLK) for anterior corneal stromal diseases. Int Ophthalmol. 2014;34:49-58.
14. Jabbarvand M, Hashemian H, Khodaparast M, Ghadimi H, Khalilipour E. Femtosecond laser-assisted sutureless anterior lamellar keratoplasty for superficial corneal opacities. J Cataract Refract Surg. 2014;40:1805-12.
15. Kymionis GD, Mikropoulos DG, Portaliou DM, Boboridis KG, Voudouragkaki IC, Dragoumis ND, et al. New perspectives on lamellar keratoplasty. Adv Ther. 2014;31:494-511.
16. Agarwal T, Sharma N, Jhanji V, Vajpayee RB. Computer simulation-assisted rotational autokeratoplasty with pupillary enlargement for management of cases with partial corneal opacification. Br J Ophthalmol. 2010;94:24-5.
17. Ramappa M, Pehere NK, Murthy SI, Chaurasia S, Rao HL, Sangwan VS. Rotational autokeratoplasty in pediatric patients for nonprogressive paracentral corneal scars. Ophthalmology. 2012;119:2458-62.
18. Jonas JB, Rank RM, Budde WM. Autologous ipsilateral rotating penetrating keratoplasty. Am J Ophthalmol. 2001;131:427-30.
19. Groden LR, Arentsen JJ. Ipsilateral rotating autokeratoplasty. Ann Ophthalmol. 1983;15:899-901.
20. Bertelmann E, Hartmann C, Scherer M, Rieck P. Outcome of rotational keratoplasty: comparison of endothelial cell loss in autografts vs allografts. Arch Ophthalmol. 2004;122:1437-40.
21. Armitage WJ, Dick AD, Bourne WM. Predicting endothelial cell loss and long-term corneal graft survival. Invest Ophthalmol Vis Sci. 2003;44:3326-31.
22. Ing JJ, Ing HH, Nelson LR, Hodge DO, Bourne WM. Tenyear postoperative results of penetrating keratoplasty. Ophthalmology. 1998;105:1855-65.

54

Autorotational Keratoplasty

Namrata Sharma, Sohini Mandal, Nandyala Sushma, Rasik B Vajpayee

INTRODUCTION

Penetrating or lamellar keratoplasty using corneal allografts is the standard approach for the management of visually significant corneal opacities. However, this option may not always be feasible, due to scarcity of optical grade corneas resulting in a long waiting period for the affected patients. This paucity has forced corneal surgeons to look at alternatives to the use of allografts for visual rehabilitation of patients with corneal opacification. Although, these techniques are not practiced routinely, their appropriate utilization helps the surgeons to offer an interim modality of treatment for these patients with the added benefits of using an autograft such as the absence of rejection and complication of long term corticosteroid use. Autokeratoplasty is a procedure that uses patients' own cornea for the purpose of visual restoration.[1] Although, visual outcomes may not be comparable to that of a conventional keratoplasty; it would at least reduce the dependency on the availability of an optical grade donor cornea. Autokeratoplasty offers several advantages such as absence of immunologic rejection, and a simpler postoperative care. Autokeratoplasty does have its disadvantages, that include stringent criteria for patient selection and a high rate of postoperative astigmatism, anterior synechiae formation, and glaucoma.

TYPES OF AUTOKERATOPLASTY

Autokeratoplasty can be of two types:

1. *Bilateral/contralateral autokeratoplasty*: Contralateral autokeratoplasty is considered when one eye has blindness attributed to a posterior segment pathology and the other eye has visual impairment due to corneal opacification. It is not very common to find such a combination. The procedure involves replacing the cornea of an eye with good visual potential from the cornea obtained from the contralateral eye with retinal pathology.
2. *Ipsilateral rotational autokeratoplasty (IRA)*: This surgical procedure can be attempted in eyes with partial corneal opacification where the diseased cornea of the patient is surgically rotated by eccentric trephination, so as to move the corneal opacity away from the pupillary axis.[2] The first account of an IRA was reported in the year 1914.[3] Subsequently, since the 1960s, various authors have described numerous surgical techniques such as rectangular,[4] triangular[5] and "Figure 8" grafts[6] in order to reduce the incision size. Nonetheless, these procedures have been seldom practiced. This might be due to the requirement of modified instrumentation in cases of "Figure 8" grafts and difficult wound apposition with rectangular grafts (**Fig. 1**). As a result of which, eccentric trephination got substituted by other techniques in subsequent decades.[7]

INDICATIONS

Ipsilateral rotational autokeratoplasty is known to be associated with poor visual gain due to high amount of corneal astigmatism in the postoperative period compared to a conventional partial or full-thickness keratoplasty.[8] However, appropriate patient selection might be able to cut back on these problems. Following principles have been suggested for the same:

1. Type of Opacity

Nonprogressive corneal scars (resulting from blunt and penetrating corneal trauma, infectious keratitis, congenital opacities, and chemical injuries)[2,9,10] and progressive cases of idiopathic or postherpetic (zoster and simplex) lipid keratopathy are some of the ideal cases to be considered.[11]

2. Size of Opacity

At least 4 mm[2,11] or 5 mm[10,12] of peripheral clear cornea should be present even though one study has suggested a minimum of 3 mm.[9] It is necessary to obtain a clear entrance pupil of 3 mm, free of suture track scars. The ideal clear pupillary area is probably 5 mm to minimize glare,[7] but this can only be achieved with opacification that involves <50% of the mean corneal diameter. This is because an additional 1.5 mm of clear cornea is needed to allow for a suture bite

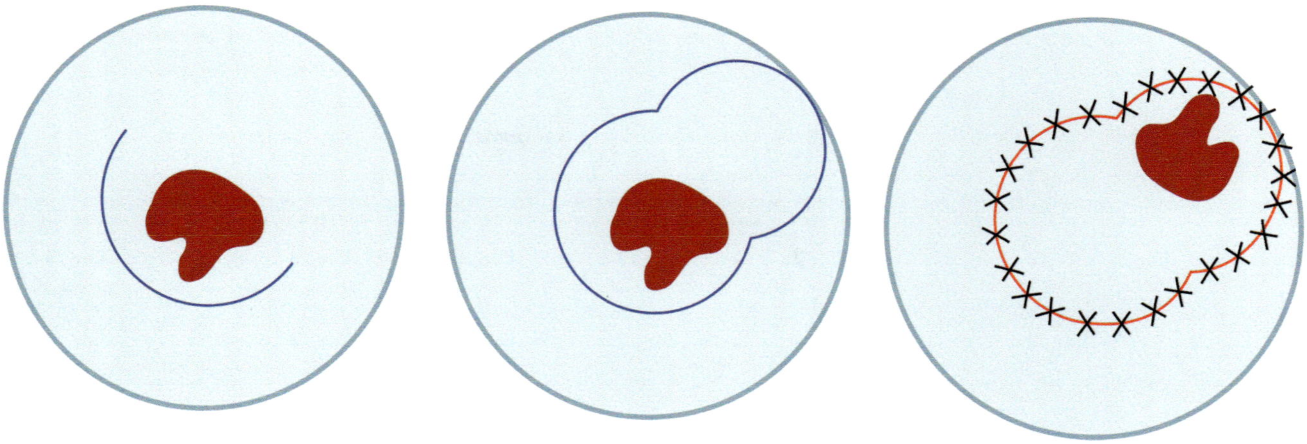

Fig. 1: Schematic representation of the technique of "Figure 8" ipsilateral rotational autokeratoplasty.

length of 0.75 mm, and scars of such small size may not require surgery.

3. Endothelial Cell Count

The technique may not work in cases with endothelial cell counts <1,000 mm^2. The reliance is often placed on the quality of specular reflex and the presence of normal pachymetry in the peripheral clear cornea.

4. Patients with High Risk of Rejection

Corneal leucomatous opacities with deep vascularization[11] and corneal transplants in the pediatric age group may be considered for autokeratoplasty because of their higher risk of rejection with the standard allograft transplantation.[10]

5. Reduced Availability of Donor Material

This technique is particularly beneficial in countries where donor corneal tissue is scarce and expensive, or donation is outlawed.[9]

SURGICAL TECHNIQUE

On the lines of principle, the procedure is indistinguishable from a conventional corneal transplant. The host cornea is eccentrically trephined and rotated, in a way so as to move the scarred corneal away from the visual axis. Any added anterior segment surgeries such as synechiolysis, pupilloplasty, and cataract surgery with or without lens implantation may be performed in the same sitting.[8-10] Continuous suturing might lead to early suture loosening and therefore, interrupted sutures are recommended, especially those that are in close proximity to the sclera. The outcome of surgery is predominantly determined by the size and position of the trephination and the relative site of the rotated scar. Various methods and mathematical deductions have been described in the literature to help predict the practicability of the surgical technique to attain optimal visual outcomes (**Fig. 2**).

Determining the Size and Location of Trephination

The surgical technique chosen is entirely based on the surgeon's decision.[9,10,13] A few approaches have been elaborated to aid in decision-making process and these have been described below.

SURGICAL GUIDELINES

The study by Verma et al. mentions that a minimum of 3 mm of clear peripheral cornea and trephine size of 6–7 mm are acceptable to achieve an optically clear zone. However, clear corneal edge placement at the corneal geometric center is a major limitation associated with this technique.[9] The other study by McDonnell et al. recommends:[2]

- Patient selection with at least 4 mm of clear peripheral corneal zone and trephine size to be 8–9 mm.
- Eccentric trephination such that the edge of the graft lies in close proximity to the limbus.
- Central edge of the graft should be sutured at least 3 mm away from the visual axis.
- If feasible, the scar should be rotated under the upper lid to be cosmetically acceptable.

Few simple intraoperative calculations have been formulated by Rao and Lam et al.[14] that can help in determining the size and ideal centration of the autograft.

MATHEMATICAL FORMULATIONS

Table 1 lists the most commonly used formulae for calculating the trephine size.

The method devised by Bourne and Brubaker as shown in **Table 1** is the most frequently mentioned one in literature.[7,10,11,15] They reported a simple geometric system to define the maximum extent of clear postoperative central cornea and size of the trephine, in which the trephine is placed at the limbus. This method serves as a reliable guide for the exact site of trephination, when pupil cannot be identified due to the dense nature of corneal opacity. Harris[16] advocated marking the center of the pupil, instead of

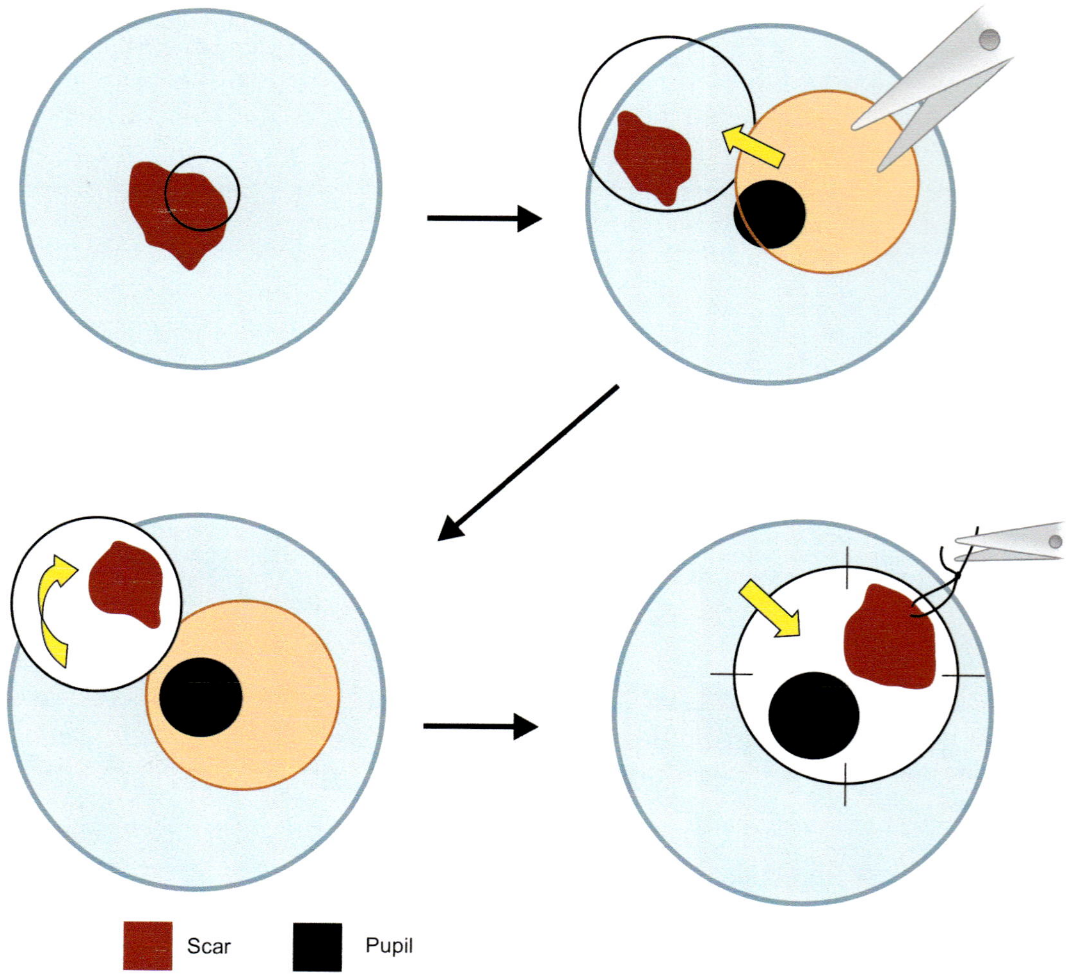

Fig. 2: Procedure of an ipsilateral rotational autograft. The central corneal opacity is moved from the visual axis by making an eccentric trephination, rotating the scar to a position near the limbus, and resuturing the cornea into its new orientation.

Table 1: Commonly used formulae for calculating the trephine size.

Authors	*Mathematical formula*	*Measurements*
Bourne et al.[7]	Dt = 1.5 × Dcl + e^a	• The diameter of the largest disk of optically clear cornea • The shortest distance between the geometric center of the cornea to the junction of the opacity and the circle of clear cornea
Jonas et al.[8]	Dt = 0.75 × Dcd – 0.5 × e	• Overall corneal diameter in the axis of the greatest maximum extent of scarring • The shortest distance between the geometric center of the cornea to the junction of the opacity and the circle of clear cornea

(Dcd: overall corneal diameter in the axis of the largest diameter of clear cornea; Dcl: diameter of the largest area of clear cornea; Dt: size of trephine; e: The shortest distance between the geometric center of the cornea to the junction of the opacity and the circle of clear cornea. e^a is positive if the scar is at the center of the cornea and negative if the corneal center is in the largest circle of clear cornea)

the geometric center of the cornea in order to maximize the visual outcome. A third formula has also been designed to estimate the degree of rotation of a linear corneal scar so as to transpose it away from the pupil.[17] However, this formula by Harris makes presumptions that are questionable. It has limited applications, and no longer in use.[16]

DIGITAL IMAGE MANIPULATION

An earlier study reported the use of a computer software assisted digitized two-dimensional corneal image to optimize the center and diameter of trephination.[12] Thereafter, several papers have described the use of Photoshop 5.0, Adobe which is extensively accessible digital image guidance software for planning the size, site, and optimal graft rotation required to achieve perfect centration. Miscalculations may often lead to an unsightly residual opacity or a wound extending too far peripherally closer to the limbus.[18] Agarwal et al.[19] have also described a similar method of computer simulation-assisted rotational autokeratoplasty, in which five cases with partial corneal opacification were selected and a central photograph of the eye was taken using the Haag–Streit slit lamp (Photo Slit lamp 900 P-BQ; Haag-Streit AG, Koeniz, Switzerland) which was then imported into a commercially available image-editing software (Adobe Photoshop, version 5.0). A circle approximating the pupil was drawn on a new transparent layer created on the original image of the eye using a drawing tool. Subsequently, a circle was drawn on the original photograph of the cornea to simulate corneal trephination. The corneal part within this circle was rotated on the image as per convenience to simulate IRA. This step was repeated using various sizes and position of the larger circle, which simulated the corneal trephine, to include the maximum area of clear cornea within the pupillary axis. At this point, an enlargement in the pupillary area was planned in order to provide an adequately sized optical window. Hence, the traced-out pupil was enlarged to simulate the new pupil.

OUTCOMES

The results of 16 patients who had undergone IRA have been presented out of which 13 patients gained significant visual improvement, and eight patients achieved an acuity of ≥6/12 with no significant preoperative or postoperative complications.[2] In the past two decades, there have been only a handful of reports regarding rotational autokeratoplasty. Gundersen and Calnan,[20] Stocker,[21] Bourne and Brubaker,[7] and Casey and Mayer[22] all report rotational grafting in individual or small numbers of cases. There are only two papers that have reported a case series who have undergone IRA: Naumann, Volcker, and Gackle D[23] who reported 14 cases, and Groden and Arentsen[13] who reported 10 cases. The baseline characteristics of all these patients were alike. Most of them belonged to a younger age group and the corneal opacity was usually due to trauma and there was frequently other anterior segment injury that needed surgical intervention. Both series stressed on the fact that there were no serious intraoperative or postoperative complications. The visual results were moderately decent: in Naumann's series[23] 11 of the 14 cases had detailed follow-up and eight of these had significant visual improvement although the refraction details were missing. Groden and Arentsen[13] reported visual improvement in eight out of 10 cases and the refraction details in five patients were described as comparable to routine penetrating keratoplasty. The findings in the series of 16 patients that was presented by McDonnell et al. are similar to those previously reported (**Table 2**).[2]

ADVANTAGES

There are a series of important advantages to autokeratoplasty, the most important of them being complete elimination of the possibility of graft rejection. The postoperative course of treatment is usually much smoother with mild to moderate anterior segment inflammation restricted to the early postoperative period only because of which the postoperative steroid is required for initial month. Healing accordingly proceeds rapidly thus prompting for an earlier suture removal in these cases. Moreover, the risk of steroid-induced glaucoma and cataract formation will be minimal. Furthermore, vascularization of the graft does not seem to occur. Other advantages are that the surgery can be performed as an elective procedure according to the patient and surgeon convenience as there is no dependency on the eye bank for suitable donor corneal tissue, and there is complete absence of risk of transmission of infection such as human immunodeficiency virus or hepatitis.

FEMTOSECOND LASER-ASSISTED IPSILATERAL ROTATIONAL LAMELLAR AUTOKERATOPLASTY

Theoretically, femtosecond laser-assisted ipsilateral rotational lamellar autokeratoplasty combines the advantages of both anterior lamellar keratoplasty (ALK) and autokeratoplasty. The success of femtosecond laser ALK is the result of accurate cuts of the donor lenticule and recipient cornea, which enables close apposition of the donor and recipient tissues. The donor lenticule was set to 0.1 mm larger in diameter and 10–20% thicker than the recipient lenticule, to compensate for donor tissue swelling.[24,25] A sutureless approach for IRA may be preferable and is being considered in the future for astigmatism purposes. The femtosecond laser provides the precision to produce anterior lamellar and trephination cuts at the desired depth, diameter, and localization according to the preset treatment plan for each individual. A planar-shaped corneal lenticule after a femtosecond cut might also allow for better tissue apposition and avoid differences in the thicknesses of the central and peripheral cornea, which have been observed with penetrating autokeratoplasty and are accountable for most of the postoperative astigmatism. Although the femtosecond laser can enhance the precision of the cut, it might also introduce some interface problems such as interface haze or fibrosis as has previously been reported after femtosecond laser-assisted ALK.[26-28] However, incomplete removal of the hazy cornea is a known complication after femtosecond laser-assisted procedure.[29] The residual scar tissue can be the result of miscalculation of the scar depth or the inability to remove the entire involved hazy corneal tissue because the aim is to leave a 250-mm residual stromal bed.

COMPLICATIONS

Astigmatism

Jonas et al.[8] evaluated and compared the visual outcomes following IRA and in control group comprising full-thickness allografts. The authors found a significantly higher amount of astigmatism in eyes wherein IRA was performed. Factors attributed to a higher amount of astigmatism included the

Table 2: Brief summary of the outcomes of various studies on ipsilateral rotational autokeratoplasty.

Author/Year	N	Age range (years)	Indications	Visual outcome	Mean/median astigmatism [(Range (D)]	Complications	Mean follow-up (months)	Number of additional surgeries performed	Endothelial cell loss
McDonnell et al./ 1989[2]	16	3–63	Trauma (n = 14), Trachoma (n = 2)	8 patients attained vision ≥6/12	2 (0–4)	None	27 (2–83)	N = 15	
Jonas et al./2001[8]	9	2–48	Post-traumatic corneal lacerations	100% had visual improvement	6 (5.5–10)	None	31.27 ± 21.54	None	-
Verma et al./1999[9]	17	5–42	Not mentioned	Postoperative visual acuity ranged between 5/60 and 6/9. 8 patients had visual acuity ≥6/12				N = 6	-
Murthy et al./2001[10]	27	0.25–60	Trauma (N = 12), healed keratitis (N = 8), chemical injury (N = 4), congenital etiology (N = 2), unknown cause (N = 1)	13 patients attained visual acuity ≥20/80 with 7 reaching up to ≥20/40	4.25 (1–9)	3 patients had graft failure, one of which was attributed to glaucoma	12	N = 12	-
Sah et al./1997[11]	4	13–53	Lipid keratopathy	Postoperative visual acuity ranged from 20/200 to 20/25 with 100% eyes experiencing visual improvement	4 (2.5–4.5)	Suture track vascularization (N = 1), progressive cataract (N = 1)	11–24	None	-
Groden et al./ 1983[13]	10	3–77	Trauma (N = 7), Interstitial keratitis (N = 2), post pterygium surgery (N = 1)	9 out of 10 patients experienced visual improvement with visual acuity ranging from 6/15 to 6/9	5 (1–9)	0		4/10	-
Bertelmann et al./ 2004[15]	7	20–85	Trauma (N = 4), healed keratitis (N = 3)	Mean vision improved by 3.5 lines (range 20/200–20/25)	4.75 ± 1.5	Corneal decompensation (N = 1), retinal detachment (N = 1)	39	3	15%

eccentric nature of trephination, discrepancy in corneal thickness between the peripheral clear cornea and the scarred central cornea, and the proximity of one edge of trephination to the central cornea.

Graft Survival and Endothelial Cell Loss

Bertelmann et al.,[15] in their study, found a cell loss rate of 15% following IRA at 1-year follow-up. The autograft survival is expected to compare well with a failure rate of 20% after 10 years. This is attributed to the ongoing reduction in the endothelial cell density and higher risk of allograft rejection following penetrating keratoplasty.[30,31] However, there is a paucity of long-term studies in the literature.

CONCLUSION

Ipsilateral rotational autokeratoplasty results in higher astigmatism, compared to a full-thickness keratoplasty resulting in suboptimal-corrected distance visual acuity. The risk of allograft rejection remains higher in cases of pediatric keratoplasty and in eyes with a vascularized cornea episodes. In these scenarios, IRA seems to have an upper hand compared to a penetrating allograft.

Various benefits of IRA have been enlisted here:

- The host endothelium is kept intact, thereby preventing the likelihood of an endothelial rejection.
- The constancy of the endothelial cell population in autografts which is expected to end up in graft failure after 2–3 decades.[30]
- Reduced frequency of postoperative corticosteroid use, and thus the associated complications such as glaucoma, cataract, and infection.[32-34]

One of the major limitations of IRA is limited visual outcome. This might overshadow the potential short-term advantages of a penetrating allograft. In this background, a trial of autograft should be given when there is expected visual gain, particularly in cases, where the other eye is healthy and patients for whom some potential vision improvement is satisfactory. Unfortunately, because of stringent prerequisites, only a few patients become suitable for this procedure. Only patients with uninvolved peripheral cornea of at least 4–5 mm are suitable. Patients with only 2–3 mm uninvolved peripheral cornea may get comparably minimal vision improvement. Yet this would be limited by the prospect of inadequate centration of the clear cornea with the line of sight.[35] The failure rate may increase in corneas with extensive corneal opacification, because of the endothelial cell loss resulting from the primary trauma and further loss as a result of ancillary anterior segment procedures in the primary sitting. The precise assessment of endothelial cell morphology and density is highly impossible preoperatively owing to poor visualization of endothelium through the scarred cornea and difficulty in assessing the peripheral endothelial cell counts in the remaining clear cornea.

REFERENCES

1. Price FW Jr, Hanna Si. Bilateral penetrating autokeratoplasty. J Refract Surg. 1995;11:494-6.
2. McDonnell PJ, Falcon MG. Rotational autokeratoplasty. Eye (Lond). 1989;3:576-80.
3. Kraupa E. Transposition durch Lappendrehung eine neue Methode der Keratoplastik. Zbl Augenh. 1914;38:132-3.
4. Mortada A. Rectangular autogenous lamellar keratoplasty. Br J Ophthalmol. 1963;47:232-6.
5. Forster AE. A review of keratoplastic surgery and some experiments in keratoplasty. Am J Ophthalmol. 1923;6:366-75.
6. Wilson RS. 'Figure 8' ipsilateral autokeratoplasty. A modification using standard corneal trephines. Arch Ophthalmol. 1976;94:121-2.
7. Bourne WM, Brubaker RF. A method for ipsilateral rotational autokeratoplasty. Ophthalmology. 1978;85:1312-6.
8. Jonas JB, Rank RM, Budde WM. Autologous ipsilateral rotating penetrating keratoplasty. Am J Ophthalmol. 2001;131:427-30.
9. Verma N, Melengas S, Garap JA. Ipsilateral rotational autokeratoplasty for the management of corneal opacities. Aust N Z J Ophthalmol. 1999;27:21-5.
10. Murthy S, Bansal AK, Sridhar MS, Rao GN. Ipsilateral rotational autokeratoplasty: an alternative to penetrating keratoplasty in nonprogressive central corneal scars. Cornea. 2001;20:455-7.
11. Sah WJ, Myoung YW, Hahn TW, Kim JH. Rotational autokeratoplasty in advanced lipid keratopathy. Ophthalmic Surg Lasers. 1997;28:1020-4.
12. Karpouzas I, Pouliquen YJ. Computerized method for rotational autokeratoplasty. Cornea. 1991;10(5):369-71.
13. Groden LR, Arentsen JJ. Ipsilateral rotating autokeratoplasty. Ann Ophthalmol. 1983;15:899-901.
14. Rao SK, Lam DS. Calculating graft size and position in rotational corneal autografting: a simplified approach. Indian J Ophthalmol. 2008;56:228-30.
15. Bertelmann E, Hartmann C, Scherer M, Rieck P. Outcome of rotational keratoplasty: comparison of endothelial cell loss in autografts vs allografts. Arch Ophthalmol. 2004;122:1437-40.
16. Harris DJ Jr. Centration of clear zone over the pupil is the best strategy for rotational autografts. Arch Ophthalmol. 2007;125:992-3.
17. Afshari NA, Duncan SM, Tanhehco TY, Azar DT. Optimal size and location for corneal rotational autografts: a simplified mathematical model. Arch Ophthalmol. 2006;124:410-3.
18. Bower KS, Mines MJ, Stutzman RD. Digital imaging to assist preoperative planning for ipsilateral rotational autokeratoplasty. J Telemed Telecare. 2006;12(7):374-6.
19. Agarwal T, Sharma N, Jhanji V, Vajpayee RB. Computer simulation-assisted rotational autokeratoplasty with pupillary enlargement for management of cases with partial corneal opacification. Br J Ophthalmol. 2010;94(1):24-5.
20. Gundersen T, Calnan AF. Corneal autografts, ipsilateral and contralateral. Arch Ophthalmol. 1965;73:164-8.
21. Stocker FW. Rotating autokeratoplasty. South Med J. 1969;62:1183-4.
22. Casey TA, Mayer DJ. Corneal Grafting, Principles and Practice. London: WB Saunders; 1984.
23. Naumann GOH, Volcker HE, Gackle D. Ipsilaterale Rotations-Autokeratoplastik. Klin Mbl Augenheilk. 1977;170:488-93.
24. Yoo SH, Kymionis GD, Koreishi A, Ide T, Goldman D, Karp CL, et al. Femtosecond laser-assisted sutureless anterior lamellar keratoplasty. Ophthalmology. 2008;115:1303-7.
25. Shousha MA, Yoo SH, Kymionis GD, Ide T, Feuer W, Karp CL, et al. Long-term results of femtosecond laser-assisted sutureless anterior lamellar keratoplasty. Ophthalmology. 2011;118:315-23.

26. Almousa R, Samaras KE, Khan S, Lake DB, Daya SM. Femtosecond laser-assisted lamellar keratoplasty (FSLK) for anterior corneal stromal diseases. Int Ophthalmol. 2014;34:49-58.
27. Jabbarvand M, Hashemian H, Khodaparast M, Ghadimi H, Khalilipour E. Femtosecond laser-assisted sutureless anterior lamellar keratoplasty for superficial corneal opacities. J Cataract Refract Surg. 2014;40:1805-12.
28. Kymionis GD, Mikropoulos DG, Portaliou DM, Boboridis KG, Voudouragkaki IC, Dragoumis ND, et al. New perspectives on lamellar keratoplasty. Adv Ther. 2014;31:494-511.
29. Cassagne M, Soler V, Malecaze F, Fournié P. Femtosecond laser-assisted ipsilateral rotational lamellar autokeratoplasty. 2018;37(4):532-6.
30. Armitage WJ, Dick AD, Bourne WM. Predicting endothelial cell loss and long-term corneal graft survival. Invest Ophthalmol Vis Sci. 2003;44:3326-31.
31. Ing JJ, Ing HH, Nelson LR, Hodge DO, Bourne WM. Tenyear postoperative results of penetrating keratoplasty. Ophthalmology. 1998;105:1855-65.
32. Donshik PC, Cavanaugh HD, Boruchoff SA, Dohlman CH. Posterior subcapsular cataracts induced by topical corticosteroids following keratoplasty for keratoconus. Ann Ophthalmol. 1981;13:29-32.
33. Greenlee EC, Kwon YH. Graft failure: III. Glaucoma escalation after penetrating keratoplasty. Int Ophthalmol. 2008;28:191-207.
34. Sharif KW, Casey TA. Penetrating keratoplasty for keratoconus: complications and long-term success. Br J Ophthalmol. 1991;75:142-6.
35. Uozato H, Guyton DL. Centering corneal surgical procedures. Am J Ophthalmol. 1987;103:264-75.

55

Limbal Stem Cell Transplantation

Swapna S Shanbhag, Anahita Kate, Sayan Basu

SEVERE OCULAR SURFACE DISEASE AND LIMBAL STEM CELLS

Severe ocular surface disease (OSD) following chemical burns or Stevens-Johnson syndrome (SJS) is a rare but severe form of corneal blindness. It is characterized by loss of corneal transparency due to conjunctival overgrowth on the corneal surface along with vascularization (**Figs. 1A to D**). Initially surgeons believed that corneal transplantation alone could restore vision in eyes with severe OSD. In fact, the first successful corneal transplantation, by the Austrian surgeon Eduard Zirm in 1905, was in the left eye of a farmer with bilateral chronic lime burns.[1,2] However, with experience surgeons realized that almost all corneal grafts performed for ocular burns failed within the first year due to epithelial healing problems.[3] In the late 1970s and early 1980s, Richard Thoft showed that conjunctival transplantation as opposed to corneal transplantation was effective in stabilizing the corneal surface and moderately improving the visual function in eyes with chemical burns.[4] However, he later credited this to the peripheral cornea, giving rise to the x-y-z hypothesis of epithelial migration and differentiation.[5] Soon in 1986, Sun and associates actually demonstrated the presence of stem cells in the basal layers of the limbus which were slow-cycling, did not express cytological markers for either the conjunctiva or the cornea and were capable of proliferation in-vitro.[6] This discovery led to a paradigm shift

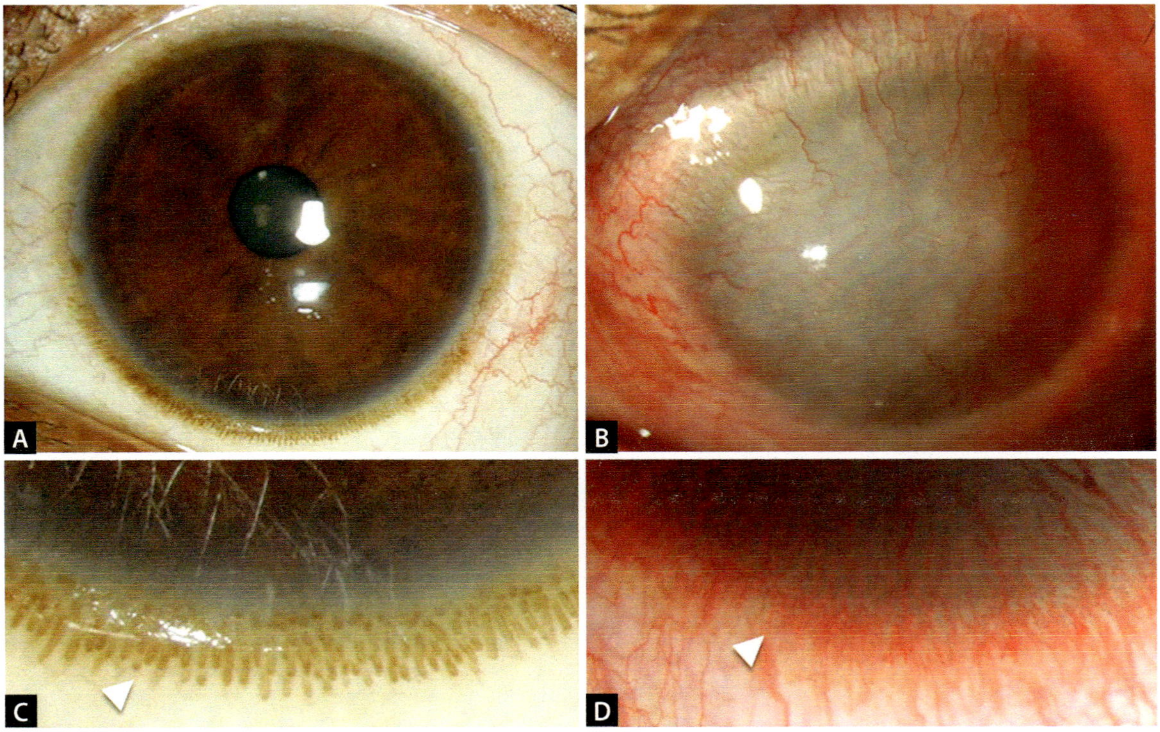

Figs. 1A to D: *Clinical features of limbal stem cell deficiency (LSCD).* Clinical photographs showing the appearance of a normal ocular surface (A) and that of a disease ocular surface due to total LSCD (B). While the normal cornea is transparent, the diseased cornea with LSCD is covered by hazy conjunctival epithelium with scarring and vascularization. The bottom row shows the normal appearance of the palisades of Vogt on the left (white arrowhead, C) and the distortion of the palisades in LSCD (white arrowhead, D). The limbal epithelial stem cells are located in the basal layers of the palisades and the absence of clinically identifiable palisades is the hallmark of LSCD.

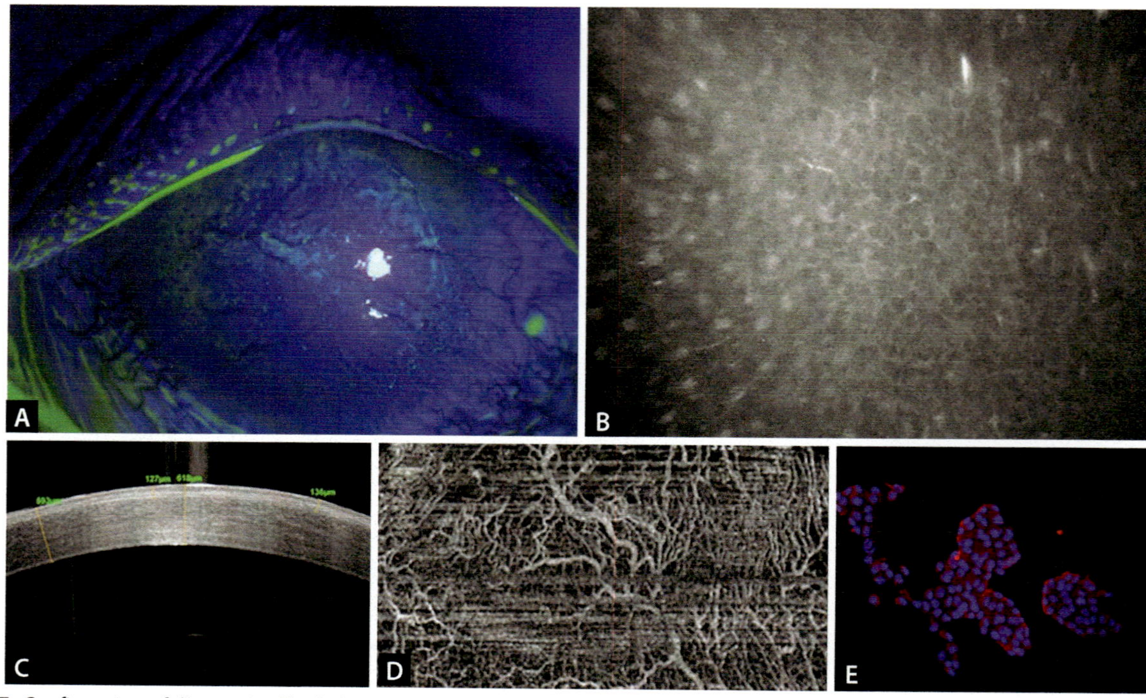

Figs. 2A to E: *Confirmation of diagnosis of limbal stem cell deficiency (LSCD).* The clinical diagnosis of LSCD can be confirmed by presence of diffuse fluorescein staining of the corneal surface (A), decreased basal cell density or nerve fiber density on confocal microscopy (B), presence of thick (>50 μ) and bright (hyperreflective) abnormal epithelium on anterior segment optical coherence tomography (ASOCT) (C), distortion of the normal vascular pattern of the limbus on ASOCT-angiography (D) and detection of conjunctival cytokeratin (CK19) on corneal impression cytology (E).

in the understanding of the pathophysiology of severe OSD suggesting that limbal stem cell deficiency (LSCD) was the reason behind this pathology (**Figs. 2A to E**).[7]

LIMBAL STEM CELL TRANSPLANTATION

The obvious implication of this new knowledge was whether LSCD could be treated by performing limbal transplantation?[7] Following successful preclinical animal trials,[8] Kenyon and Tseng in 1989 provided the first proof-of-concept of limbal stem cell transplantation (LSCT) for patients of unilateral acute and chronic chemical burns.[9] This technique of LSCT, which is now termed conjunctival-limbal autograft (CLAu), involved removing as much as six clock hours of donor limbal tissue from healthy donor eyes and transplanting them to the affected eye.[9] Although this technique was extremely effective,[10-16] other groups who tried to replicate the results reported rare incidents of iatrogenic LSCD in the donor eyes.[17-20] In 1997, Pellegrini and associates solved this problem by developing a technique of culturing the limbal cells ex-vivo in a laboratory to form a transplantable sheet of epithelium from less than one clock hour of donor limbal tissue.[21] Following this, several large clinical trials have established the safety and efficacy of autologous cultivated limbal epithelial transplantation (CLET) for the treatment of unilateral LSCD.[22-45] However, CLET is prohibitively expensive and needs a clinical grade laboratory, which is available only in select centers around the world.[10] Other issues include the risk of disease transmission due to use of xenogeneic laboratory reagents.[46] To address these problems of accessibility and affordability, Sangwan et al., in 2012, described an innovative approach called simple limbal epithelial transplantation (SLET). In SLET, a one-clock-hour of limbal tissue is obtained from the donor eye, divided into multiple pieces and secured over the donor eye over a human amniotic membrane (hAM) graft.[47] This is akin to in-vivo cultivation, as the cornea re-epithelizes using the natural environment of the ocular surface instead of laboratory reagents in a petridish. Several large studies have subsequently established the long-term safety and efficacy of SLET in the treatment of severe OSD and LSCD, particularly in chemical burns.[48-51]

Indications of LSCT

Limbal transplantation, irrespective of the technique used, is indicated in conditions that cause irreversible damage to the limbal stem cells. The clinical diagnosis of LSCD is based on the signs of vascularization in the superficial corneal, diffuse staining of the corneal surface which may or may not be associated with persistent epithelial defects, conjunctivalization of the cornea and no discernible palisades of Vogt. This can be confirmed by diagnostic tests like confocal microscopy, impression cytology, and anterior segment optical coherence tomography.[52,53]

The different causes of LSCD are as follows:

A. Inflammation and trauma
  1. Chemical burns (alkali or acid burns)
  2. Thermal burns
  3. Iatrogenic LSCD (due to multiple surgeries at the limbus)

4. Radiation
5. Contact lens wear

B. Immunological
1. Stevens-Johnson syndrome (SJS)
2. Mucous membrane pemphigoid (MMP)
3. Vernal keratoconjunctivitis (VKC)
4. Graft-versus-host disease (GVHD)
5. Keratoconjunctivitis Sicca (Primary and secondary Sjogren's syndrome)

C. Idiopathic

D. Hereditary
1. Congenital aniridia
2. Epidermolysis bullosa
3. Xeroderma pigmentosum
4. Multiple endocrine deficiency
5. Ectodermal dysplasia (**Figs. 3A to D**)

The most common indication for LSCT is LSCD due to chemical burns, which is mostly unilateral.[54] Unilateral LSCD can be treated with autologous LSCT, where the donor tissue is usually obtained from the healthy contralateral eye or sometimes even the unaffected area of the same eye. Autologous LSCT has the benefit of not needing any systemic or long-term immunosuppression. Bilateral LSCD is also most commonly due to chemical burns and immunological conditions like SJS, MMP, VKC, and GVHD.[54] Idiopathic and hereditary causes of LSCD are extremely rare. Bilateral LSCD requires allogeneic LSCT from a living or cadaveric donor and long-term and perhaps life-long systemic immunosuppression. The allogeneic counterparts of CLAu are termed conjunctival-limbal allografting (CLAL) or kerato-limbal allografting (KLAl), depending on whether the source is living or cadaveric, respectively.[55-60]

SURGICAL TECHNIQUE OF LSCT

A. Preoperative considerations

i. *Diseased eye:*

- The ideal case for LSCT is an uninflamed eye with a wet ocular surface without any adnexal pathologies with a clear/translucent underlying stroma.
- Adnexal pathologies may be common in cases of chemical/thermal burns, SJS/TEN, OCP and these should be identified and addressed before undertaking LSCT.
- In eyes with severe symblepharon, the symblepharon should be addressed before or during LSCT with a conjunctival autograft (in unilateral LSCD) or mucous membrane graft (in bilateral cases).
- In eyes with an opaque stroma, LSCT may help in achieving an avascular epithelized surface, but a penetrating keratoplasty (PK) or a lamellar keratoplasty (LK) may be required for achieving functional success in terms of vision.

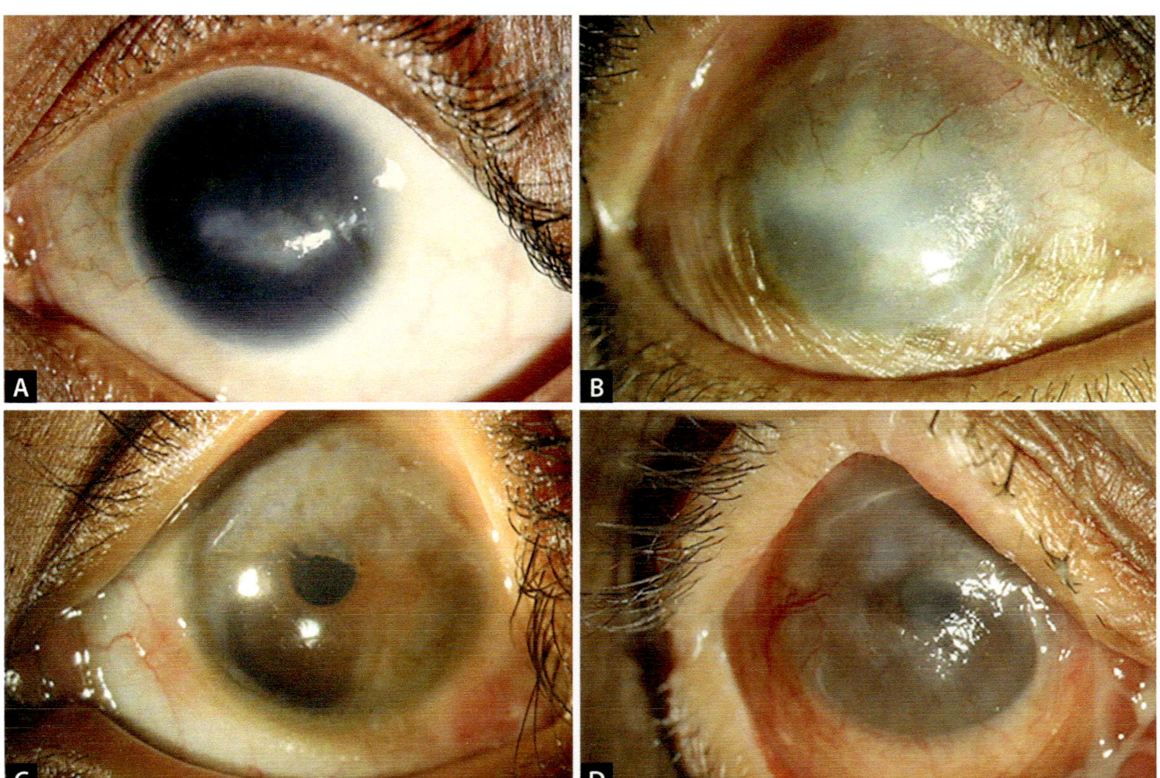

Figs. 3A to D: *Causes of limbal stem cell deficiency (LSCD).* Other than ocular burns LSCD can occur due to congenital causes like aniridia (A) or immunological diseases like mucous membrane pemphigoid (B), allergic conjunctivitis (C) and Stevens-Johnson syndrome (D).

ii. *Donor eye*: The donor eye in a case of autologous LSCT or live-related allogeneic LSCT should have a wet ocular surface and should not have any history of trauma, inflammation or surgery. The superior limbal area is the favored site to harvest the limbal tissue. For cadaveric LSCT, the donor age should be ≤50 years, and the corneoscleral button should be used within 48 hours of harvesting. It should have clearly discernible palisades with an intact epithelium in order to ascertain that the proliferative potential of the donor sample similar to that of live tissue.[61,62]

iii. *Contraindications for LSCT*:
  1. Dry eye disease (repeated Schirmer's score at 5 minutes of ≤10 mm of wetting).
  2. Disorganized anterior segment (adherent leucoma or anterior staphyloma).
  3. Presence of uncorrected eyelid pathologies such as ectropion, entropion, and trichiasis.
  4. Lagophthalmos, eye-lid retraction or excessive exposure.

B. *Harvesting of the limbal graft*: The fundamental difference between the techniques is that in CLAu the limbal lenticules are obtained along with adjacent conjunctival and clear-corneal tissue while in CLET and SLET, the donor tissue includes only the limbus without any adjacent conjunctiva or cornea. The other major difference is the size of the donor tissue: in CLAu, usually 2 donor lenticules of 2–3 clock-hours each are obtained from the superior and inferior limbus while in CLET and SLET, a 2–4 mm (1-clock-hour) biopsy is harvested from the superior limbus alone.

C. *Cell expansion*: This additional step is only relevant for CLET. The limbal biopsy is transferred to a clinical grade laboratory facility. Under good manufacturing practice (GMP) conditions the cells are cultivated on a suitable substrate until a confluent epithelial sheet is obtained in 10–14 days. Different groups have reported various methods of cell culture (suspension/explant) using myriad reagents (fetal bovine serum/human serum) and growth factors.[63,64] It is unclear if one cultivation technique is better in any way than others.

D. *Transplantation*: While in CLAu/CLAL/KLAL and SLET the donor-tissue is directly transplanted onto the affected/recipient eye, in CLET this is done as a separate second-stage procedure.

  i. *Preparation of the recipient eye*: First, the conjunctivalized pannus covering the cornea is separated from the cornea by performing a peritomy all around about 2–3 mm from the corneal margin. The bleeding points can be cauterised with the help of bipolar wet field cautery. The pannus is dissected, first circumferentially around the limbus and then centripetally using both sharp and blunt dissection. A tenotomy scissors is used to recess the surrounding conjunctiva. An amniotic membrane is then placed with its basement membrane side up and secured with fibrin glue over the recipient cornea and tucked under the conjunctival edge in all quadrants. Using a blunt spatula, all the folds of the membrane are smoothened out over the corneal surface.

  ii. *CLAu*: The donor grafts are transferred to the prepared bed and sutured to corneal and scleral beds with 10-0 nylon sutures to the superior and inferior limbal areas. The cornea may then be covered with a large diameter bandage contact lens (BCL).

  iii. *CLET*: The cultivated limbal epithelial cells are expanded ex-vivo and placed over a hAM. Using fibrin glue, the membrane is secured over the host corneal bed. At the end of surgery, the lids are closed for the next 2–3 days to prevent displacement of the transplanted tissue.

  iv. *SLET*: The limbal tissue, which was previously stored in BSS, is then retrieved and divided into smaller (6–10) pieces using Vannas scissors.[65] These pieces are positioned with their epithelial side up, concentrically in the corneal mid-periphery over the amniotic membrane. Each implant is then coated with fibrin glue to ensure its adherence to the underlying membrane. The polymerization of the glue takes around a minute following which a BCL is placed. A suture tarsorrhaphy is performed in very young children and retained for 1–2 weeks to avoid the dislocation of the BCL or the implants in the immediate postoperative period. This tarsorrhaphy can be released after 1–2 weeks (**Figs 4 A to J**).

POSTOPERATIVE MANAGEMENT AFTER LSCT

The postoperative topical steroid regimen for both the donor and host eyes are similar. The steroid drops are started at 6 times/day for a week, which is then continued over six weeks in a weekly tapering fashion. Topical antibiotics are started 4 times/day in both eyes and continued until complete corneal epithelization has occurred. At the first week postoperative visit, the cornea is stained with fluorescein and checked for epithelial defects after removing the BCL. If the epithelial healing is incomplete, then the bandage lens is placed again. The same process is repeated for the donor eye until the biopsy site is completely epithelialized. For autografts, topical steroids are generally not required after 6 weeks and lubricants can be used if required, but patients are often off of medications completely. In case a temporary suture tarsorrhaphy is performed, a topical steroid-antibiotic ointment is prescribed in the immediate postoperative period, until the tarsorrhaphy is removed.

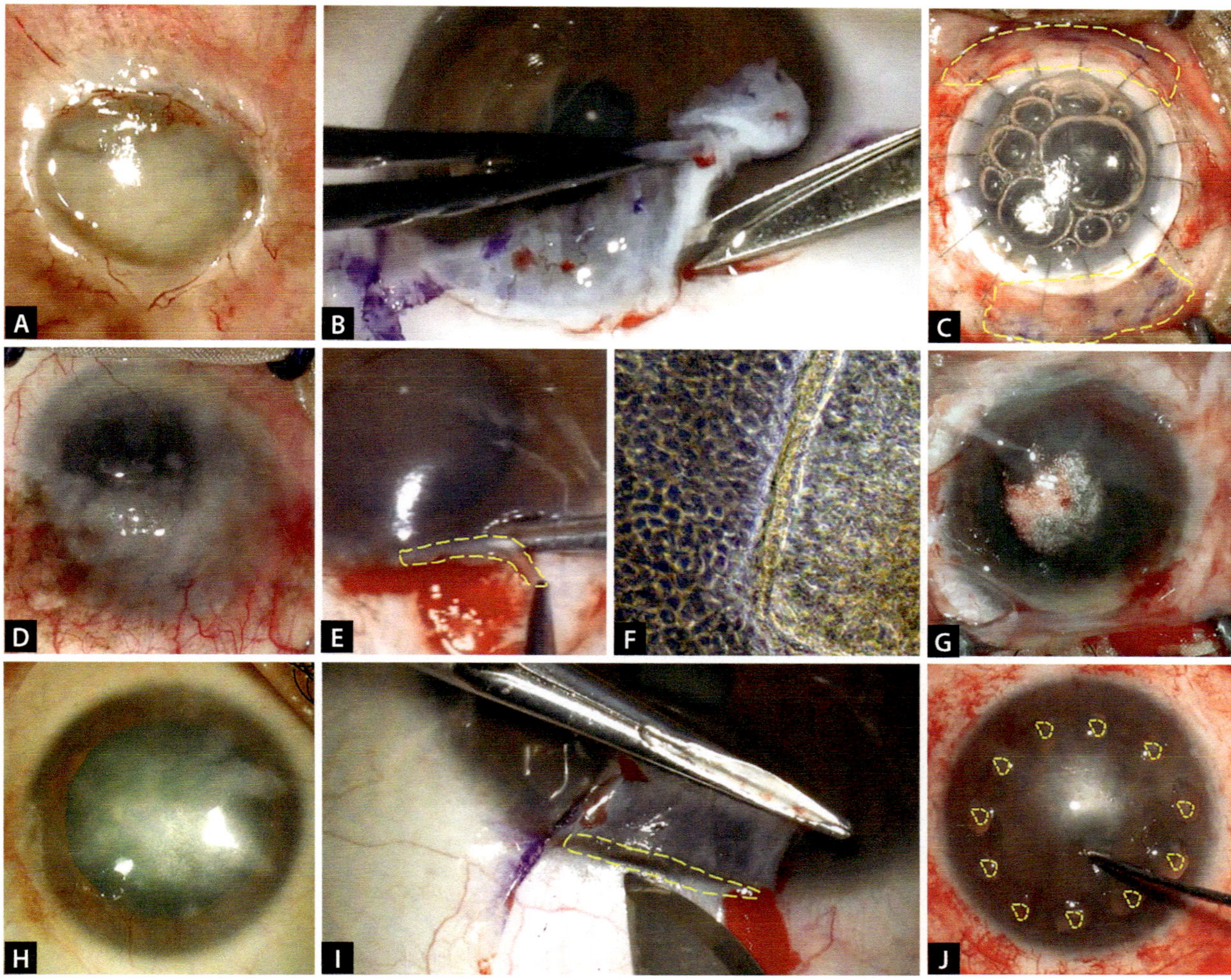

Figs. 4A to J: *Surgical technique of limbal stem cell transplantation (LSCT).* Each row describes the different surgical approaches of LSCT. The top row describes conjunctival-limbal grafting in patient with severe chemical burn-induced limbal stem cell deficiency (LSCD) (A). Two-three clock-hour long conjunctival limbal biopsies are harvested from the healthy fellow eye (B) and transplanted in the anatomical position superiorly and inferiorly (yellow-dotted lines) after replacing the scarred cornea with a penetrating keratoplasty (C). The middle row describes ex-vivo cultivated limbal epithelial transplantation for a patient with chronic ocular allergy induced LSCD (D). A one-clock hour long limbal biopsy is obtained from a living-related donor (E) and cultured on a human amniotic membrane scaffold in the laboratory, where epithelial cells grow out as a sheet from the limbal tissue (F); this sheet of epithelium is then transplanted on to the affected eye (G). The bottom-row describes simple limbal epithelial transplantation for a case of unilateral chemical burn (H), where a one-clock-hour long limbal biopsy is obtained from the healthy fellow eye (I) and transplanted directly onto the affected eye over a hAM graft after dividing it into smaller pieces (J).

Systemic immunosuppression is required in cases of allogeneic LSCT done for bilateral LSCD. Often a combination of multiple agents is used with oral corticosteroids and the latter is slowly tapered off while the patient is maintained on steroid-sparing immunosuppressive agents.[66]

COMPLICATIONS AND THEIR MANAGEMENT

Recipient Eye

a. *Early complications*:
    1. Postoperative loss of limbal transplants: This can be prevented by avoiding the use of excessive glue. The loss of the transplants results in the failure of the surgical procedure.
    2. Postoperative loss of hAM with limbal transplants: This can be prevented by securing the hAM in the correct orientation with the basement membrane facing upwards and ensuring that an adequate amount of fibrin glue is placed to secure the hAM. This usually leads to surgical failure.
    3. Hemorrhage under the hAM: This is normal and self-limiting and may not adversely affect the outcome of the surgery.

b. *Late complications*:
    1. Focal recurrence of LSCD in the first 6 months after surgery: The rate of recurrence is around 20–30% for all types of LSCT.[67] This may be non-progressive and should be observed initially. If this is progressive, a conjunctival autograft may be performed. The incidence of recurrence of LSCD is more when a concurrent symblepharon is not corrected intraoperatively.
    2. Failure of corneal epithelialization: This could lead to a multitude of problems such as persistent epithelial

defect, sterile keratitis, microbial keratitis, corneal melt, or perforation.

3. Recurrence of corneal vascularization
4. Eyes where an allogeneic procedure has been carried out are at a higher risk for developing steroid-induced glaucoma.[68]

Donor Eye

The donor eye may be at a risk of developing iatrogenic nonprogressive focal LSCD at the site of the limbal biopsy.

OUTCOMES

The outcomes of autologous CLET for unilateral LSCD are summarized in **Table 1**.[21-23,26,28,29,31-34,36-45] The clinical outcomes of CLAu for eyes with unilateral LSCD are shown in **Table 2**.[9-18,20,49] The clinical outcomes of CLAL/KLAL for patients with bilateral LSCD are mentioned in **Table 3**.[55-60] The clinical outcomes of allogeneic CLET for bilateral LSCD are mentioned in **Table 4**.[25,32,33,38,39,43,45,69-74] The clinical outcomes of SLET for unilateral LSCD are summarized in **Table 5**.[47-51,75-79] There are unfortunately no randomized controlled trials that compare one technique of LSCT to another. It is also difficult to compare different techniques of allografting because of the variances in postoperative systemic immunosuppressive regimens. A recent systematic review that compared the different techniques of autologous LSCT found that CLAu and SLET had significantly better outcomes than CLET, in patients with unilateral LSCD which were mostly due to ocular

Table 1: Techniques and outcomes of autologous CLET for unilateral LSCD.

Author	*Year*	*Culture technique*	*Substrate*	*Culture time*	*Eyes*	*Clinical success (%)*	*2-line visual gain (%)*	*Follow-up (years)*	
								Mean	*Range*
Feeder-free and xeno-free cell cultures									
Sangwan et al.[23]	2011	Explant	hAM	10–14	200		60.5	3	1–7.6
Kolli et al.[28]	2010	Explant	hAM	12–14	8	100	63	1.6	1–2.5
Di Girolamo et al.[29]	2009	Explant	CL	10	2	100	50	0.9	0.7–1.1
Feeder-free but not xeno-free cell cultures									
Baradaran-Rafii et al.[31]	2010	Explant	hAM	14	8	88	63	2.8	0.5–4
Pauklin et al.[32]	2010	Explant	hAM	14	30	77	73	2.4	0.8–6
Shortt et al.[39]	2008	Suspension	hAM	14–21	3	78	22	0.8	0.5–1.1
Shimakazi et al.[33]	2007	Explant	hAM	14.6	16	50	37.5	2.5	0.5–7.1
Nakamura et al.[43]	2006	Explant	hAM	15–16	2	100	67	1.2	0.5– 1.6
Sangwan et al.[34]	2006	Explant	hAM	11–15	88	73	37	1.5	0.3– 3.3
Sangwan et al.[26]	2003	Explant	hAM	10–14	2	100	50	1	1
Grueterich et al.[40]	2002	Explant	hAM	21	1	100	100	3.1	3.1
Tsai et al.[36]	2000	Explant	hAM	14–21	3	100	50	2	0.3–10
Neither feeder-free nor xeno-free cell cultures									
Fasolo et al.[82]	2017	Suspension	Fibrin	N/A	59	42	N/A	6	1–13
Ganger et al.[83]	2015	Explant	hAM	N/A	54	72	23	1.8	0.3–3.3
Zakaria et al.[84]	2014	Explant	hAM	14	12	58	17	1.6	0.3–3.6
Sejpal et al.[85]	2013	Explant	hAM	10–14	107	46.7	54.2	3.4	1–9.3
Prabhaswat et al.[86]	2012	Suspension	hAM	14–21	12	75	58.3	2.3	0.5–3.9
Di lorio et al.[41]	2010	Suspension	Fibrin	N/A	166	80	N/A	N/A	N/A
Rama et al.[22]	2010	Suspension	Fibrin	14–16	107	68	54	2.9	1–10
Kawashima et al.[42]	2007	Explant	hAM	N/A	2	100	67	2.7	1.7–3.7
Nakamura et al.[37]	2004	Explant	hAM	23	1	100	100	1.6	1.6
Rama et al.[44]	2001	Suspension	Fibrin	14–16	18	74	33	1.5	1–2.2
Schwab et al.[38]	2000	Suspension	hAM	21–28	10	60	36	1.1	0.5–1.6
Schwab et al.[45]	1999	Suspension	hAM	28–35	17	76	16	0.9	0.2–2
Pellegrini et al.[21]	1997	Suspension	3T3s	16–19	2	100	50	N/A	N/A

(hAM: human amniotic membrane; CL: contact lens; N/A: not available; CLET: cultivated limbal epithelial transplant; LSCD: limbal stem cell deficiency)

Modified from Shukla et al.[67]

Table 2: Clinical outcomes of conjunctival limbal autografting for eyes with unilateral limbal stem cell deficiency.

Author	Year	Eyes	Clinical success (%)	2-line vision gain (%)	Follow-up (months)
Moreria et al.[87]	2015	15	33	N/A	1.5
Barreiro et al.[88]	2014	23	87	79	1.7
Burcu et al.[89]	2013	69	69	69	7.6
Baradar an-Rafii et al.[90]	2012	88	88	N/A	1.4
Miri et al.[20]	2011	25	N/A	N/A	41
Miri et al.[10]	2010	12	100	81.3	46
Santos et al.[11]	2005	10	80	61	33
Ozdemir et al.[12]	2004	15	87	80	13.9
Dua et al.[13]	2000	6	100	83	18.8
Rao et al.[14]	1999	16	94	82	19.3
Basti et al.[17]	1999	3	100	100	N/A
Frucht-Pery et al.[15]	1998	9	100	100	N/A
Tan et al.[18]	1996	9	77	77	27.1
Morgan et al.[16]	1996	6	83	83	12.6
Kenyon et al.[9]	1989	26	77	65	18

(N/A: not available; LSCD: limbal stem cell deficiency)
Modified from Shukla et at.[67]

Table 3: Clinical outcomes of conjunctival limbal allografts (CLAL)/ keratolimbal allograft (KLAL) for patients with bilateral limbal stem cell deficiency.

	Holland et al.[55]	Tsubota et al.[60]	Ilari and Daya[56]	Solomon et al.[57]	Maruyama-Hosoi et al.[58]	Shi et al.[59]	Cheung et al.[91]
Year published	1996	1999	2002	2002	2006	2008	2020
No. of eyes	25	43	23	39	85	23	224/63#
Mean follow-up (months)	26.4	38.8	60	34	46.6	32	86.4
Stable ocular surface (%)	72	51	27.3	23.7	65.9	56.5	64.7/82.5
Improved VA (%)	66	60	82.6	44.6	N/A	43.5	69.6/81.1
Complications Epithelial/Lenticule rejection (%)	40	N/A	39.4	N/A	13.1	48	43.3./30.2
PED (%)	40	60	24.2	35.9	34.1	9	N/A
Glaucoma (%)	N/A	30	26.1	25.6	33.1	0	N/A
Infection (%)	N/A	N/A	13	7.7	8.3	N/A	N/A
Melting/perforation (%)	N/A	N/A	13	N/A	4.1	N/A	N/A

KLAL was performed in 224 eyes and 63 eyes underwent CLAL
(N/A: not available; PED: persistent epithelial defect; VA: visual acuity)

Table 4: A comparison of the methods and outcomes of allogeneic CLET for bilateral LSCD.

Author (year)	Donor source (n)	Culture technique	Feeder cell	Serum	Air-lifting	Xenofree	Success (n/N) (%)	Follow-up, months (range)
Basu et al. (2011)[69]	LR (28)	Explant	No	AuS	No	Yes	71.4	58 (12–114)
Pauklin et al. (2010)[32]	LR (4), Cadaveric (10)	Explant	No	AuS	No	No	50	28.5 (9–72)
Meller et al. (2009)[70]	HLA matched donor (1)	Explant	No	AuS	No	No	100	31
Shortt et al. (2008)[39]	Cadaveric (7)	Suspension	No	F-BS	No	No	100	9.9 (6–13)

(Contd...)

(Contd.)

Author (year)	Donor source (n)	Culture technique	Feeder cell	Serum	Air-lifting	Xenofree	Success (n/N) (%)	Follow-up, months (range)
Ang et al. (2007)[25]	Cadaveric (3)	Suspension	Yes	F-BS	Yes	No	100	48
Shimazaki et al. (2007)[33]	LR (8), Cadaveric (12)	Suspension	Yes	F-BS	Yes	No	50	29 (6–85)
		Explant	No	AuS	Yes			
Nakamura et al. (2006)[43]	Cadaveric (7)	Suspension	Yes	AuS	Yes	No	100	14.4 (6–20)
Daya et al. (2005)[77]	LR (1), Cadaveric (9)	Suspension	Yes	F-BS	No	No	70	28 (12–50)
Sangwan et al. (2005)[72]	LR (4)	Explant	No	F-BS	No	No	100	15.3 (7–24)
Nakamura et al. (2003)[73]	Cadaveric (3)	Explant	Yes	F-BS	Yes	No	100	13 (12–14)
Koizumi et al. (2001)[74]	Cadaveric (13)	Explant	Yes	F-BS	Yes	No	100	11.2 (9–13)
Schwab et al. (2000)[38]	LR (4)	Suspension	Yes	F-BS	Yes	No	100	11.5 (6–19)
Schwab et al. (1999)[45]	LR (2)	Suspension	Yes	F-BS	No	No	50	13 (16–19)

(LSCD: limbal stem cell deficiency; LRL: live-related; CD: cadaveric; AuS: autologous serum; F-BS: fetal bovine serum)

Table 5: Outcomes of SLET for the management of ocular surface disorders.

Most common indication (number of eyes)[‡]	Author	Year	Number of eyes	Success rate in percentage (Number of eyes)	Percentage of eyes with 2-line improvement in BCVA (Number of eyes)	Eyes which underwent keratoplasty*	Mean follow-up in years (range)
Chemical burn (5)	Sangwan et al.[47]	2012	6	100 (6/6)	100 (6/6)	None	0.8 (0.6–1)
Chemical burn (2)	Amescua et al.[75]	2014	4	100 (4/4)	N/A	None	0.6 (0.5–0.75)
Simultaneously after primary pterygium excision (9)	Hernadez-Bogantes et al.[76]	2015	9	100 (9/9)	N/A	N/A	0.67
Chemical burn (125)	Basu et al.[48]	2016	125	76 (95/125)	75 (94/125)	8 (10/125)	1.5 (1–4)
Chemical burn (62)	Vazirani et al.[49]	2016	68	84 (57/68)	65 (44/68)	7 (5/68)	1 (0.5–4.9)
Chemical burn (4)	Quieroz et al.[77]	2016	4	50 (2/4)	24 (1/4)	None	0.5
Chemical burn (26)	Gupta et al.[50]	2018	30	70 (21/30)	50 (15/30)	10 (3/30)	1.1 (0.5–3.4)
Simultaneously after OSSN excision (8)	Kaliki et al.[78]	2017	8	100 (8/8)	N/A	N/A	1
Simultaneously after recurrent pterygium excision (4)	Mednick et al.[79]	2018	4	100 (4/4)	N/A	N/A	1.2 (0.7–2.5)
Chemical burn–eyes with previous failed CLET (30)	Basu et al.[51]	2018	30	80 (24/30)	N/A	13 (4/30)	2.3 (0.8–3.8)
Chemical burn (7)	Prabhasawat et al.[92]	2021	28	82 (23/28)	N/A	25 (7/28)	2.4 (1.4–3.3)
Chemical burn (9)	Wang et al.[93]	2021	13	77 (10/13)	60 (6/10)	15 (2/13)	0.5 (0.2–1.6)

*Simultaneous/subsequent lamellar/penetrating keratoplasty

[‡]In previous unsuccessful CLET

(OSSN: ocular surface squamous neoplasia; N/A: not available)

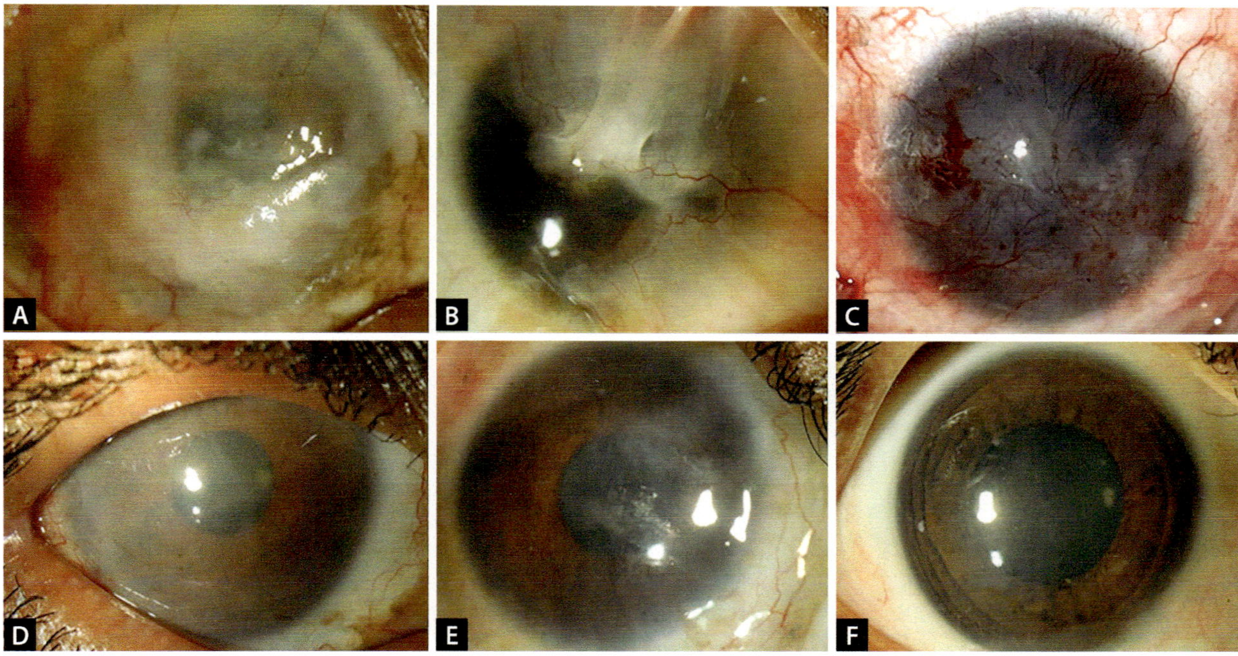

Figs. 5A to F: *Clinical outcomes of limbal stem cell transplantation.* The top row shows preoperative images of cases with limbal stem cell deficiency (A to C). The bottom row shows the corresponding 1-year postoperative outcomes with cultivated limbal epithelial transplantation (D), conjunctival limbal autografting (E) and simple limbal epithelial transplantation (F). All cases show significant improvement in corneal clarity and regression of vascularization and conjunctivalization.

burns. The average success rates for CLAu and SLET in restoring an avascular, epithelized and stable corneal surface were 81% and 78%, respectively, while it was 61.4% for CLET. Similarly, a two-line improvement in vision was seen in 74.4% and 68.6% cases of CLAu and SLET, respectively, while it was 53% in CLET (**Figs. 5A to F**).[80] Another systematic review revealed the anatomical success rates between the different types of LSCT to be similar, but the functional outcomes were better with SLET and KLAL.[81]

COMBINING LSCT AND CORNEAL TRANSPLANTATION

In eyes with LSCD and corneal scarring the visual benefit of PK without prior limbal transplantation is short-lived as the transplanted allogeneic epithelium has limited proliferative potential and the resultant ocular surface instability invariably leads to graft failure.[3] Conversely, successful restoration of the ocular surface by limbal transplantation without replacing the scarred cornea does not always improve vision.[94,95] Although the two procedures can be performed simultaneously or sequentially, a two-stage approach is known to prolong corneal allograft survival in eyes undergoing allogeneic limbal transplantation.[55,56,60,66] In comprehensive reviews of cultivated allogeneic or autologous limbal epithelial transplantation for unilateral or bilateral LSCD by Shortt et al.[63] and Baylis et al.[64] it was shown that 27.5% required one or more keratoplasties in order to visually rehabilitate the patients. Basu et al.,[27] Sangwan et al.,[34] and Di Iorio et al.[41] reported the corneal allograft survival rates of 58–90%.[5,7,12] Basu et al. also showed that corneal allograft survival after a two-stage limbal and corneal transplantation (80%) was superior compared to that reported in eyes with corneal transplantation alone (33.3–46.2%)[3,94] or in eyes which were at high-risk for graft failure (32–67%).[95-97] The increased incidence of both corneal and limbal graft failure in eyes with a single-stage surgery can possibly be attributed to the additive inflammatory effect induced by combining an extraocular and an intraocular procedure. In cases where an anterior LK can be performed instead of a PK, the outcomes are likely to be better as the immunological risk of endothelial rejection is absent.

CONCLUSION

While the basic concept of LSCT has remained unchanged since stem cells were discovered at the limbus over 3 decades ago, not only have three different surgical approaches evolved with time, but they also continue to be practiced concurrently. Although the long-term outcomes of the different LSCT techniques are well known, there is no unanimity on whether one technique is better than the others. At present this choice is based on the surgeon's preference, training, familiarity, and the practice pattern of local peers, rather than evidence. However, it is abundantly clear from the reported outcomes that LSCT works, irrespective of the technique used. This efficacy of an average success rate of around 77%[63,64] needs to be placed in context of the fact that before the advent of LSCT, the prognosis for patients with LSCD was abysmally poor.[3,94] Corneal grafts were performed in desperation and inevitably failed and severe ocular surface disease was considered as one of the causes of incurable corneal blindness. It is worthwhile to take a step back and appreciate the fact that the field of ocular surface has advanced leaps and bounds, and it has indeed come a long way since then.

The innovative technique of SLET has many obvious advantages over CLET or CLAu/CLAL/KLAL, chiefly the need for minimal donor tissue and the avoidance of ex-vivo laboratory cultivation.[65] As a result, there is also a significant decrease in the cost incurred while performing SLET when compared to CLET.[98] This has resulted in SLET becoming increasingly popular in recent years. However, that does not mean in any way that the other techniques will have no relevance in the future. The different techniques of LSCT can be considered analogous to different techniques of treating corneal endothelial diseases. While most surgeons may now prefer isolated endothelial keratoplasty in the form of Descemet membrane endothelial keratoplasty, there would still be more complex cases that would require a Descemet stripping endothelial keratoplasty or even a PK. Extending the same line of thinking for LSCT, while the most straightforward cases of LSCD would be amenable to SLET, the complex cases with extensive limbal and conjunctival damage would still need conjunctival-limbal grafting. Also, in cases of LSCD due to genetic diseases, ex-vivo cultivation with gene editing may be a better approach than others. At present it appears that individual surgeons can continue to practice their preferred technique without needing to upgrade or transition to a different approach.

ACKNOWLEDGMENTS

The authors would like to acknowledge the contributions of Dr Shobhit Varma (MBBS, DNB) and Dr Abhinav Reddy (PhD) who were working as ophthalmology resident and graduate student, respectively at the time of writing of this manuscript, for their help with acquiring the images used in **Figure 2**.

REFERENCES

1. Zirm EK. Eine erfolgreiche totale Keratoplastik (A successful total keratoplasty). 1906. Refract Corneal Surg. 1989;5(4):258-61.
2. Armitage WJ, Tullo AB, Larkin DF. The first successful full-thickness corneal transplant: a commentary on Eduard Zirm's landmark paper of 1906. Br J Ophthalmol. 2006;90(10):1222-3.
3. Brown SI, Bloomfield SE, Pearce DB. A follow-up report on transplantation of the alkali-burned cornea. Am J Ophthalmol. 1974;77(4):538-42.
4. Thoft RA. Conjunctival transplantation as an alternative to keratoplasty. Ophthalmology. 1979;86(6):1084-92.
5. Thoft RA, Friend J. The X, Y, Z hypothesis of corneal epithelial maintenance. Invest Ophthalmol Vis Sci. 1983;24(10):1442-3.
6. Schermer A, Galvin S, Sun TT. Differentiation-related expression of a major 64K corneal keratin in vivo and in culture suggests limbal location of corneal epithelial stem cells. J Cell Biol. 1986;103(1):49-62.
7. Cotsarelis G, Cheng SZ, Dong G, Sun TT, Lavker RM. Existence of slow-cycling limbal epithelial basal cells that can be preferentially stimulated to proliferate: implications on epithelial stem cells. Cell. 1989;57(2):201-9.
8. Tsai RJ, Sun TT, Tseng SC. Comparison of limbal and conjunctival autograft transplantation in corneal surface reconstruction in rabbits. Ophthalmology. 1990;97(4):446-55.
9. Kenyon KR, Tseng SC. Limbal autograft transplantation for ocular surface disorders. Ophthalmology. 1989;96(5):709-22.
10. Miri A, Al-Deiri B, Dua HS. Long-term outcomes of autolimbal and allolimbal transplants. Ophthalmology. 2010;117(6):1207-13.
11. Santos MS, Gomes JA, Hofling-Lima AL, Rizzo LV, Romano AC, Belfort R Jr. Survival analysis of conjunctival limbal grafts and amniotic membrane transplantation in eyes with total limbal stem cell deficiency. Am J Ophthalmol. 2005;140(2):223-30.
12. Ozdemir O, Tekeli O, Ornek K, Arslanpençe A, Yalçindağ NF. Limbal autograft and allograft transplantations in patients with corneal burns. Eye (Lond). 2004;18(3):241-8.
13. Dua HS, Azuara-Blanco A. Autologous limbal transplantation in patients with unilateral corneal stem cell deficiency. Br J Ophthalmol. 2000;84(3):273-8.
14. Rao SK, Rajagopal R, Sitalakshmi G, Padmanabhan P. Limbal autografting: comparison of results in the acute and chronic phases of ocular surface burns. Cornea. 1999;18(2):164-71.
15. Frucht-Pery J, Siganos CS, Solomon A, Scheman L, Brautbar C, Zauberman H. Limbal cell autograft transplantation for severe ocular surface disorders. Graefes Arch Clin Exp Ophthalmol. 1998;236(8):582-7.
16. Morgan S, Murray A. Limbal autotransplantation in the acute and chronic phases of severe chemical injuries. Eye (Lond). 1996;10(Pt 3):349-54.
17. Basti S, Mathur U. Unusual intermediate-term outcome in three cases of limbal autograft transplantation. Ophthalmology. 1999;106(5):958-63.
18. Tan DT, Ficker LA, Buckley RJ. Limbal transplantation. Ophthalmology. 1996;103(1):29-36.
19. Jenkins C, Tuft S, Liu C, Buckley R. Limbal transplantation in the management of chronic contact-lens-associated epitheliopathy. Eye (Lond). 1993;7(Pt 5):629-33.
20. Miri A, Said DG, Dua HS. Donor site complications in autolimbal and living-related allolimbal transplantation. Ophthalmology. 2011;118(7):1265-71.
21. Pellegrini G, Traverso CE, Franzi AT, Zingirian M, Cancedda R, De Luca M. Long-term restoration of damaged corneal surfaces with autologous cultivated corneal epithelium. Lancet. 1997;349(9057):990-3.
22. Rama P, Matuska S, Paganoni G, Spinelli A, De Luca M, Pellegrini G. Limbal stem-cell therapy and long-term corneal regeneration. N Engl J Med. 2010;363(2):147-55.
23. Sangwan VS, Basu S, Vemuganti GK, Sejpal K, Subramaniam SV, Bandyopadhyay S, et al. Clinical outcomes of xeno-free autologous cultivated limbal epithelial transplantation: a 10-year study. Br J Ophthalmol. 2011;95(11):1525-9.
24. Basu S, Ali H, Sangwan VS. Clinical outcomes of repeat autologous cultivated limbal epithelial transplantation for ocular surface burns. Am J Ophthalmol. 2012;153(4):643-50.e1-2.
25. Ang LP, Sotozono C, Koizumi N, Suzuki T, Inatomi T, Kinoshita S. A comparison between cultivated and conventional limbal stem cell transplantation for Stevens-Johnson syndrome. Am J Ophthalmol. 2007;143(1):178-80.
26. Sangwan VS, Vemuganti GK, Iftekhar G, Bansal AK, Rao GN. Use of autologous cultured limbal and conjunctival epithelium in a patient with severe bilateral ocular surface disease induced by acid injury: a case report of unique application. Cornea. 2003;22(5):478-81.

27. Basu S, Mohamed A, Chaurasia S, Sejpal K, Vemuganti GK, Sangwan VS. Clinical outcomes of penetrating keratoplasty after autologous cultivated limbal epithelial transplantation for ocular surface burns. Am J Ophthalmol. 2011;152(6):917-24.e1.
28. Kolli S, Ahmad S, Lako M, Figueiredo F. Successful clinical implementation of corneal epithelial stem cell therapy for treatment of unilateral limbal stem cell deficiency. Stem Cells. 2010;28(3):597-610.
29. Di Girolamo N, Bosch M, Zamora K, Coroneo MT, Wakefield D, Watson SL. A contact lens-based technique for expansion and transplantation of autologous epithelial progenitors for ocular surface reconstruction. Transplantation. 2009;87(10):1571-8.
30. Zakaria N, Koppen C, Van Tendeloo V, Berneman Z, Hopkinson A, Tassignon MJ. Standardized limbal epithelial stem cell graft generation and transplantation. Tissue Eng Part C Methods. 2010;16(5):921-7.
31. Baradaran-Rafii A, Ebrahimi M, Kanavi MR, Taghi-Abadi E, Aghdami N, Eslani M, et al. Midterm outcomes of autologous cultivated limbal stem cell transplantation with or without penetrating keratoplasty. Cornea. 2010;29(5):502-9.
32. Pauklin M, Fuchsluger TA, Westekemper H, Steuhl KP, Meller D. Midterm results of cultivated autologous and allogeneic limbal epithelial transplantation in limbal stem cell deficiency. Dev Ophthalmol. 2010;45:57-70.
33. Shimazaki J, Higa K, Morito F, Dogru M, Kawakita T, Satake Y, et al. Factors influencing outcomes in cultivated limbal epithelial transplantation for chronic cicatricial ocular surface disorders. Am J Ophthalmol. 2007;143(6):945-53.
34. Sangwan VS, Matalia HP, Vemuganti GK, Fatima A, Ifthekar G, Singh S, et al. Clinical outcome of autologous cultivated limbal epithelium transplantation. Indian J Ophthalmol. 2006;54(1):29-34.
35. Sangwan VS, Vemuganti GK, Singh S, Balasubramanian D. Successful reconstruction of damaged ocular outer surface in humans using limbal and conjunctival stem cell culture methods. Biosci Rep. 2003;23(4):169-74.
36. Tsai RJ, Li LM, Chen JK. Reconstruction of damaged corneas by transplantation of autologous limbal epithelial cells. N Engl J Med. 2000;343(2):86-93.
37. Nakamura T, Inatomi T, Sotozono C, Koizumi N, Kinoshita S. Successful primary culture and autologous transplantation of corneal limbal epithelial cells from minimal biopsy for unilateral severe ocular surface disease. Acta Ophthalmol Scand. 2004;82(4):468-71.
38. Schwab IR, Reyes M, Isseroff RR. Successful transplantation of bioengineered tissue replacements in patients with ocular surface disease. Cornea. 2000;19(4):421-6.
39. Shortt AJ, Secker GA, Rajan MS, Meligonis G, Dart JK, Tuft SJ, et al. Ex vivo expansion and transplantation of limbal epithelial stem cells. Ophthalmology. 2008;115(11):1989-97.
40. Grueterich M, Espana EM, Touhami A, Ti SE, Tseng SC. Phenotypic study of a case with successful transplantation of ex vivo expanded human limbal epithelium for unilateral total limbal stem cell deficiency. Ophthalmology. 2002;109(8):1547-52.
41. Di Iorio E, Ferrari S, Fasolo A, Böhm E, Ponzin D, Barbaro V. Techniques for culture and assessment of limbal stem cell grafts. Ocul Surf. 2010;8(3):146-53.
42. Kawashima M, Kawakita T, Satake Y, Higa K, Shimazaki J. Phenotypic study after cultivated limbal epithelial transplantation for limbal stem cell deficiency. Arch Ophthalmol. 2007;125(10):1337-44.
43. Nakamura T, Inatomi T, Sotozono C, Ang LP, Koizumi N, Yokoi N, et al. Transplantation of autologous serum-derived cultivated corneal epithelial equivalents for the treatment of severe ocular surface disease. Ophthalmology. 2006;113(10):1765-72.
44. Rama P, Bonini S, Lambiase A, Golisano O, Paterna P, De Luca M, et al. Autologous fibrin-cultured limbal stem cells permanently restore the corneal surface of patients with total limbal stem cell deficiency. Transplantation. 2001;72(9):1478-85.
45. Schwab IR. Cultured corneal epithelia for ocular surface disease. Trans Am Ophthalmol Soc. 1999;97:891-986.
46. Schwab IR, Johnson NT, Harkin DG. Inherent risks associated with manufacture of bioengineered ocular surface tissue. Arch Ophthalmol. 2006;124(12):1734-40.
47. Sangwan VS, Basu S, MacNeil S, Balasubramanian D. Simple limbal epithelial transplantation (SLET): a novel surgical technique for the treatment of unilateral limbal stem cell deficiency. Br J Ophthalmol. 2012;96(7):931-4.
48. Basu S, Sureka SP, Shanbhag SS, Kethiri AR, Singh V, Sangwan VS. Simple limbal epithelial transplantation: long-term clinical outcomes in 125 cases of unilateral chronic ocular surface burns. Ophthalmology. 2016;123(5):1000-10.
49. Vazirani J, Ali MH, Sharma N, , Gupta N, Mittal V, Atallah M, et al. Autologous simple limbal epithelial transplantation for unilateral limbal stem cell deficiency: multicenter results. Br J Ophthalmol. 2016;100(10):1416-20.
50. Gupta N, Joshi J, Farooqui JH, Mathur U. Results of simple limbal epithelial transplantation in unilateral ocular surface burn. Indian J Ophthalmol. 2018;66(1):45-52.
51. Basu S, Mohan S, Bhalekar S, Singh V, Sangwan V. Simple limbal epithelial transplantation (SLET) in failed cultivated limbal epithelial transplantation (CLET) for unilateral chronic ocular burns. Br J Ophthalmol. 2018;102(12):1640-5.
52. Le Q, Xu J, Deng SX. The diagnosis of limbal stem cell deficiency. Ocul Surf. 2018;16(1):58-69.
53. Deng SX, Borderie V, Chan CC, Dana R, Figueiredo FC, Gomes JAP, et al. Global consensus on the definition, classification, diagnosis and staging of limbal stem cell deficiency. Cornea. 2019;38(3):364.
54. Vazirani J, Nair D, Shanbhag S, Wurity S, Ranjan A, Sangwan V. Limbal Stem Cell Deficiency-Demography and Underlying Causes. Am J Ophthalmol. 2018;188:99-103.
55. Holland EJ. Epithelial transplantation for the management of severe ocular surface disease. Trans Am Ophthalmol Soc. 1996;94:677-743.
56. Ilari L, Daya SM. Long-term outcomes of keratolimbal allograft for the treatment of severe ocular surface disorders. Ophthalmology. 2002;109(7):1278-84.
57. Solomon A, Ellies P, Anderson DF, Touhami A, Grueterich M, Espana EM, et al. Long-term outcome of keratolimbal allograft with or without penetrating keratoplasty for total limbal stem cell deficiency. Ophthalmology. 2002;109(6):1159-66.
58. Maruyama-Hosoi F, Shimazaki J, Shimmura S, Tsubota K. Changes observed in keratolimbal allograft. Cornea. 2006;25(4):377-82.
59. Shi W, Gao H, Wang T, Xie L. Combined penetrating keratoplasty and keratolimbal allograft transplantation in comparison with corneoscleral transplantation in the treatment of severe eye burns. Clin Exp Ophthalmol. 2008;36(6):501-7.
60. Tsubota K, Satake Y, Kaido M, Shinozaki N, Shimmura S, Bissen-Miyajima H, et al. Treatment of severe ocular-surface disorders with corneal epithelial stem-cell transplantation. N Engl J Med. 1999;340(22):1697-703.
61. Vemuganti GK, Kashyap S, Sangwan VS, Singh S. Ex-vivo potential of cadaveric and fresh limbal tissues to regenerate cultured epithelium. Indian J Ophthalmol. 2004;52(2):113-20.
62. Kethiri AR, Basu S, Shukla S, Sangwan VS, Singh V. Optimizing the role of limbal explant size and source in determining the outcomes of limbal transplantation: An in vitro study. PloS One. 2017;12(9):e0185623.
63. Shortt AJ, Secker GA, Notara MD, Limb GA, Khaw PT, Tuft SJ, et al. Transplantation of ex vivo cultured limbal epithelial stem cells: a review of techniques and clinical results. Surv Ophthalmol. 2007;52(5):483-502.
64. Baylis O, Figueiredo F, Henein C, Lako M, Ahmad S. 13 years of cultured limbal epithelial cell therapy: a review of the outcomes. J Cell Biochem. 2011;112(4):993-1002.

65. Shanbhag SS, Patel CN, Goyal R, Donthineni PR, Singh V, Basu S. Simple limbal epithelial transplantation (SLET): Review of indications, surgical technique, mechanism, outcomes, limitations, and impact. Indian J Ophthalmol. 2019;67(8):1265.
66. Deng SX, Kruse F, Gomes JAP, Chan CC, Daya S, Dana R. Global consensus on the management of limbal stem cell deficiency. Cornea. 2020;39(10):1291-1302.
67. Shukla S, Shanbhag SS, Tavakkoli F, Varma S, Singh V, Basu S. Limbal epithelial and mesenchymal stem cell therapy for corneal regeneration. Curr Eye Res. 2020;45(3):265-77.
68. Le Q, Chauhan T, Yung M, Tseng C-H, Deng SX. Outcomes of limbal stem cell transplant: a meta-analysis. JAMA Ophthalmol. 2020;138(6):660-70.
69. Basu S, Fernandez MM, Das S, Gaddipati S, Vemuganti GK, et al. Clinical outcomes of xeno-free allogeneic cultivated limbal epithelial transplantation for bilateral limbal stem cell deficiency. Br J Ophthalmol. 2012;96(12):1504-9.
70. Meller D, Fuchsluger T, Pauklin M, Steuhl KP. Ocular surface reconstruction in graft-versus-host disease with HLA-identical living-related allogeneic cultivated limbal epithelium after hematopoietic stem cell transplantation from the same donor. Cornea. 2009;28(2):233-6.
71. Daya SM, Watson A, Sharpe JR, Giledi O, Rowe A, Martin R, et al. Outcomes and DNA analysis of ex vivo expanded stem cell allograft for ocular surface reconstruction. Ophthalmology. 2005;112(3):470-7.
72. Sangwan VS, Murthy SI, Vemuganti GK, Bansal AK, Gangopadhyay N, Rao GN. Cultivated corneal epithelial transplantation for severe ocular surface disease in vernal keratoconjunctivitis. Cornea. 2005;24(4):426-30.
73. Nakamura T, Koizumi N, Tsuzuki M, Inoki K, Sano Y, Sotozono C, et al. Successful regrafting of cultivated corneal epithelium using AMniotic membrane as a carrier in severe ocular surface disease. Cornea. 2003;22(1):70-1.
74. Koizumi N, Inatomi T, Suzuki T, Sotozono C, Kinoshita S. Cultivated corneal epithelial stem cell transplantation in ocular surface disorders. Ophthalmology. 2001;108(9):1569-74.
75. Amescua G, Atallah M, Nikpoor N, Galor A, Perez VL. Modified simple limbal epithelial transplantation using cryopreserved amniotic membrane for unilateral limbal stem cell deficiency. Am J Ophthalmol. 2014;158(3):469-75.e2.
76. Hernández-Bogantes E, Amescua G, Navas A, Garfias Y, Ramirez-Miranda A, Lichtinger A, et al. Minor ipsilateral simple limbal epithelial transplantation (mini-SLET) for pterygium treatment. Br J Ophthalmol. 2015;99(12):1598-600.
77. Queiroz AG, Barbosa MM, Santos MS, Barreiro TP, Gomes JÁ. Assessment of surgical outcomes of limbal transplantation using simple limbal epithelial transplantation technique in patients with total unilateral limbal deficiency. Arq Bras Oftalmol. 2016;79(2):116-8.
78. Kaliki S, Mohammad FA, Tahiliani P, Sangwan VS. Concomitant simple limbal epithelial transplantation after surgical excision of ocular surface squamous neoplasia. Am J Ophthalmol. 2017;174:68-75.
79. Mednick Z, Boutin T, Einan-Lifshitz A, Sorkin N, Slomovic A. Simple limbal epithelial transplantation for recurrent pterygium: A case series. Am J Ophthalmol Case Rep. 2018;12:5-8.
80. Shanbhag SS, Nikpoor N, Rao Donthineni P, Singh V, Chodosh J, Basu S. Autologous limbal stem cell transplantation: a systematic review of clinical outcomes with different surgical techniques. British Journal of Ophthalmology. 2020;104(2):247-53.
81. Ganger A, Singh A, Kalaivani M, Gupta N, Vanathi M, Mohanty S, et al. Outcomes of surgical interventions for the treatment of limbal stem cell deficiency. Indian J Med Res. 2021;154(1):51-61.
82. Fasolo A, Pedrotti E, Passilongo M, Marchini G, Monterosso C, Zampini R, et al. Safety outcomes and long-term effectiveness of ex vivo autologous cultured limbal epithelial transplantation for limbal stem cell deficiency. Br J Ophthalmol. 2017;101(5):640-9.
83. Ganger A, Vanathi M, Mohanty S, Tandon R. Long-term outcomes of cultivated limbal epithelial transplantation: Evaluation and comparison of results in children and adults. Biomed Res Int. 2015;2015:480983.
84. Zakaria N, Possemiers T, Dhubhghaill SN, Leysen I, Rozema J, Koppen C, et al. Results of a phase I/II clinical trial: Standardized, non-xenogenic, cultivated limbal stem cell transplantation. J Transl Med. 2014;12(1):1-13.
85. Sejpal K, Ali MH, Maddileti S, Basu S, Ramappa M, Kekunnaya R. Cultivated limbal epithelial transplantation in children with ocular surface burns. JAMA Ophthalmol. 2013;131(6):731-6.
86. Prabhasawat P, Ekpo P, Uiprasertkul M, Chotikavanich S, Tesavibul N. Efficacy of cultivated corneal epithelial stem cells for ocular surface reconstruction. Clinical Ophthalmology (Auckland, NZ). 2012;6:1483.
87. Moreira PB, Magalhães RS, Pereira NC, Oliveira LA, Sousa LB. Limbal transplantation at a tertiary hospital in Brazil: a retrospective study. Arq Bras Oftalmol. 2015;78(4):207-11.
88. Barreiro TP, Santos MS, Vieira AC, de Nadai Barros J, Hazarbassanov RM, Gomes JÁ. Comparative study of conjunctival limbal transplantation not associated with the use of amniotic membrane transplantation for treatment of total limbal deficiency secondary to chemical injury. Cornea. 2014;33(7):716-20.
89. Burcu A, Yalniz-Akkaya Z, Ozdemir MF, Erdem E, Onat MM, Ornek F. Surgical rehabilitation following ocular chemical injury. Cutan Ocul Toxicol. 2014;33(1):42-8.
90. Baradaran-Rafii A, Eslani M, Jamali H, Karimian F, Tailor UA, Djalilian AR. Postoperative complications of conjunctival limbal autograft surgery. Cornea. 2012;31(8):893-9.
91. Cheung AY, Eslani M, Kurji KH, Wright E, Sarnicola E, Govil A, et al. Long-term outcomes of living-related conjunctival limbal allograft compared with keratolimbal allograft in patients with limbal stem cell deficiency. Cornea. 2020;39(8):980-5.
92. Prabhasawat P, Chirapapaisan C, Ngowyutagon P, Ekpo P, Tangpagasit W, Lekhanont K, et al. Efficacy and outcome of simple limbal epithelial transplantation for limbal stem cell deficiency verified by epithelial phenotypes integrated with clinical evaluation. Ocul Surf. 2021;22:27-37.
93. Wang Y, Hu X, Yang K, Zhang Y, Deng S, Wang Z, et al. Clinical outcomes of modified simple limbal epithelial transplantation for limbal stem cell deficiency in Chinese population: A retrospective case series. Stem Cell Res Ther. 2021;12(1):259.
94. Maguire MG, Stark WJ, Gottsch JD, Stulting RD, Sugar A, Fink NE, et al. Risk factors for corneal graft failure and rejection in the collaborative corneal transplantation studies. Ophthalmology. 1994;101(9):1536-47.
95. Hill JC. Systemic cyclosporine in high-risk keratoplasty: long-term results. Eye (Lond). 1995;9(Pt 4):422-8.
96. Poon AC, Forbes JE, Dart JK, Subramaniam S, Bunce C, Madison P, et al. Systemic cyclosporin A in high risk penetrating keratoplasties: a case-control study. Br J Ophthalmol. 2001;85(12):1464-9.
97. Rumelt S, Bersudsky V, Blum-Hareuveni T, Rehany U. Systemic cyclosporin A in high failure risk, repeated corneal transplantation. Br J Ophthalmol. 2002;86(9):988-92.
98. Thokala P, Singh A, Singh VK, Rathi VM, Basu S, Singh V, et al. Economic, clinical and social impact of simple limbal epithelial transplantation for limbal stem cell deficiency. Br J Ophthalmol. 2021:bjophthalmol-2020-318642.

56 Large-diameter Anterior Lamellar Keratoplasty

Sohini Mandal, Namrata Sharma, Rasik B Vajpayee

INTRODUCTION

Deep anterior lamellar keratoplasty (DALK) has undeniable benefits over full-thickness keratoplasty in terms of endothelial graft rejection and open-sky related difficulties, and the same has been proven through various studies in the recent decades.[1-8] However, several corneal surgeons are hesitant enough to master this procedure, primarily because of the steep learning curve associated with successful pneumatic dissection. Various other explanations behind this might be that the refractive and visual outcomes following DALK are reportedly similar to those of penetrating keratoplasty (PK). Large-diameter grafts may be used instead to improve postoperative refractive outcomes as they have been reported to be associated with more regular astigmatism.[9]

To our existing knowledge, PK grafts with size >8 mm are invariably accompanied with a higher chance of endothelial rejection. So, as an alternative, large diameter lamellar grafts can be used, due to the lack of possibility of endothelial graft rejection. Stromal and epithelial rejections are usually self-limiting and can be managed efficaciously with medical management alone in majority of the cases. However, large-diameter DALK (L-DALK) is not extensively conducted as a procedure of choice, because up to one-fourth of cases undergoing DALK as a primary procedure carry a risk of intraoperative conversion to PK.

INDICATIONS

Large-diameter lamellar grafts have been classically described in literature for the following indications:

- Keratoconus[10-12]
- Ocular surface disease with limbal stem cell deficiency[13]
- Severe ocular burns[14]

SURGICAL PROCEDURE

Recipient Preparation

Anesthesia and akinesia can be achieved by means of general anesthesia preferably or by a peribulbar[11] or retrobulbar block.[12] A trial of pneumatic dissection is given by a cannula that is advanced centripetally following a partial thickness trephination at a depth at least 100 µm less than the thinnest pachymetry and measuring 8.25–9 mm in diameter. Alternatively, a 30-gauge needle, bent at an angle of 60° at 5 mm from the tip, connected to a 5 mL air-filled syringe can be introduced in a deeper plane in the supradescemetic area and air is injected to create a cleavage plane between the posterior corneal stroma and the Descemet's membrane (DM).[15] A Hessburg–Barron suction trephine (Katena, Denville, New Jersey, USA)[12] is preset to a depth depending on the thinnest corneal pachymetry to reduce the chances of perforation.[12] Regardless of a successful pneumatic dissection, debulking should be routinely performed, in all cases in order to debulk the anterior stroma. A viscocohesive material is placed on top of the bubble and entered with a 15 no. blade. The blunted tip of the Vannas scissor is then introduced into the supradescemetic space, and the opening is widened so as to permit the introduction of corneoscleral scissors to remove the remaining deep stromal layer. Layer-by-layer manual dissection is performed if pneumatic dissection is unsuccessful.

Donor Preparation

A Barron donor punch or a disposable handheld trephine is used to cut the donor cornea and the DM is stripped from the posterior stroma using a wet cellulose sponge after staining it with trypan blue dye 0.06%. Alternatively, the donor cornea can be mounted on an artificial anterior chamber of the automated lamellar therapeutic keratoplasty (ALTK) system (Moria, Antony, France) and automated dissection is completed by means of a microkeratome. The anterior lamella is trephined to the desired diameter and sutured to the recipient bed using interrupted or continuous 10-0 monofilament nylon sutures. At the end of the surgery, balanced salt solution is injected into the anterior chamber through a side port. Gentamicin sulfate 0.3% and dexamethasone is injected subconjunctivally at the end of the procedure. From first postoperative day, patient is started on following medications—0.1% dexamethasone phosphate and 0.3% tobramycin sulfate.

LIMITATIONS OF THE PROCEDURE

The rate of conversion of L-DALK to PK remains substantially high during the initial phase of a surgeon's learning curve due to inadvertent iatrogenic perforation of DM. Thus, a full-thickness optical grade larger graft would be mandatory to address this kind of complication. This would definitely upsurge the risk for immunologic endothelial rejection.[16]

To add to the list of limitations, pneumatic dissection usually remains limited to the central 7.5–8.0 mm of cornea. Hence dissection needs to carry out manually in the peripheral part, thus posing an added task to the surgeon that would further higher the odds of DM perforation, needing conversion to full-thickness keratoplasty.

Addressing the Limitations

To address these shortcomings, Busin et al. have adapted the technique of L-DALK by familiarizing the notion that the anterior lamellar graft size can be larger (9 mm) as compared to that of the central corneal stromal clearance. A 9-mm lamellar graft was transplanted in all eyes in their series, with a central clear optical zone of 6 mm in the recipient bed.[11] Central 6 mm optical zone of the recipient cornea is measured and marked with a handheld trephine after debulking of the anterior stroma by approximately 80%. Therefore, the ultimate corneal architecture would include a peripheral corneal rim of 1.5 mm because of the overlap of the donor lamella and the residual deep stroma of the recipient, as well as a 6.0 mm central optical zone (**Figs. 1A and B**).

Intraoperative conversion to mushroom-shaped penetrating keratoplasty (MK): Two-piece microkeratome-assisted mushroom-shaped PK has been a recent addition to the armamentarium of novel techniques for cases with either insufficient clearance of the optical zone of a full-thickness opacity or an inadvertent intraoperative macroperforation of the DM.[17] After performing anterior keratectomy in the central 9 mm, the central 6 mm optical zone is excised further, leaving a 1.5 mm posterior corneal crown of approximately 100–150 μm thickness. Using the ALTK system (Moria SA, Antony, France), the donor cornea is dissected into anterior and posterior lamellae by using a 350 μm microkeratome head and the anterior and posterior lamellae are punched to the corresponding diameters of 9 and 6 mm, respectively. The donor stem of the mushroom (endothelium and deep stroma) is placed into the central pit of the recipient bed of 6 mm without sutures and the anterior lamella is placed on top and sutured into position with double continuous running sutures (**Fig. 2**).[10]

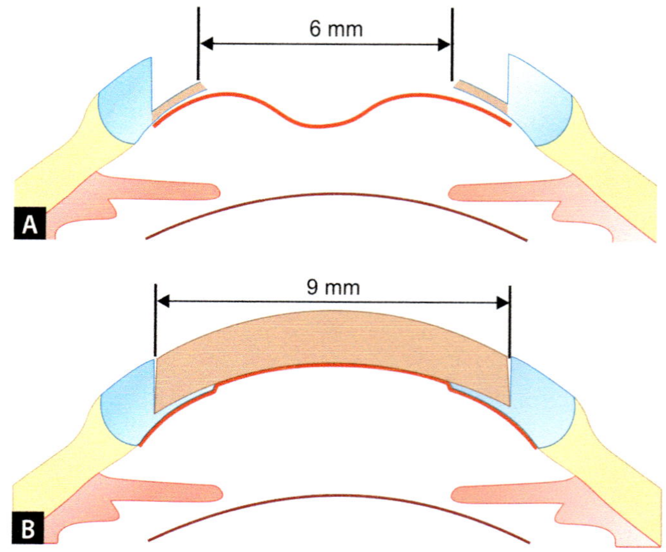

Figs. 1A and B: Schematic representation of modified deep anterior lamellar keratoplasty (DALK).[11] (A) Exposure of a central predescemetic area bounded by a peripheral rim of 1.5 mm deep stroma; (B) Ultimate corneal architecture reveals apposition of the anterior donor lamellae with the predescemetic part of the recipient bed in the central 6 mm area.

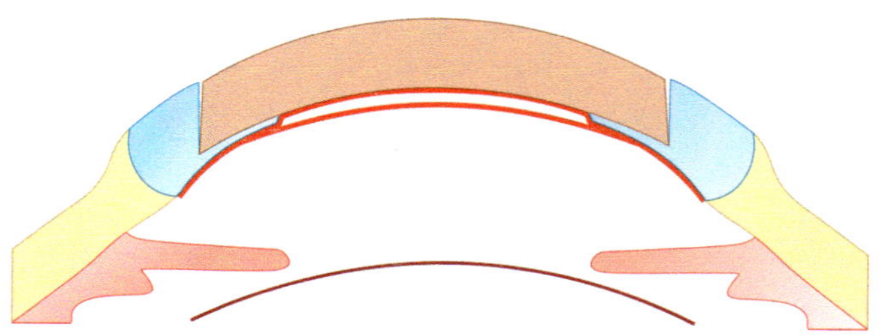

Fig. 2: Schematic diagram of two-piece microkeratome-assisted mushroom-shaped penetrating keratoplasty (MK) illustrating the donor stem of the mushroom (endothelium and deep stroma) (in red) is placed into the central pit of the recipient bed of 6 mm without sutures and the anterior lamella is placed on top (in orange) and sutured into position with double continuous running sutures.

OUTCOMES FOLLOWING LARGE-DIAMETER DEEP ANTERIOR LAMELLAR KERATOPLASTY IN KERATOCONUS

Visual outcomes: Few authors have reported that best spectacle-corrected visual acuity (BSCVA) following successful pneumatic dissection is significantly better than manual layer-by-layer dissection.[3,6,18-20] This finding is quite similar to what has been reported in literature.[7,21-23] On the contrary, Busin et al. in their study were unable to report any such significant difference following suture removal which perhaps could have been accredited to the different residual stromal thickness left behind by various surgeons. In a study by Borderie et al.,[3] the mean residual stromal thickness in the manual dissection cohort ranged from 87 to 150 μm, whereas the study by Busin et al. was unable to detect any residual stroma after complete suture removal both on slit lamp as well as by ASOCT.

Refractive outcomes: As reported in a small study, large-diameter lamellar grafts may provide improved refractive outcomes than that of a standard graft size.[12] The average refractive astigmatism at the last follow-up visit noted in the series by Busin et al. was three-diopter (3D) approximately,[11] similar to what has been reported in literature.[9,12] In contrary to other articles in literature, postoperative astigmatism was reported as high as 8–9 D and even more.[22,24] Huang et al. observed a tendency towards lower myopia in the L-DALK group compared to the standard DALK group.[12] However, the difference in myopic refractive outcomes between the two treatment groups might be attributed to different graft diameters as there was complete absence of residual stroma on the recipient bed. In this study, corneal buttons of 8.50 mm size were designated as large grafts, whereas corneal buttons of 8.0 mm size were designated as standard grafts. The L-DALK group had less manifest astigmatism than the S-DALK group (absolute value 3.8 ± 1.2 D vs. 4.5 ± 1.7 D at 24 months postoperatively). It might appear that large grafts not only lead to less postoperative astigmatism but also change the nature of the astigmatism. It is predicted that corneal grafts ranging from 8.75 to 10.0 mm in diameter might result in more satisfactory correction of corneal ectasia, and even induce the reversal of astigmatism, than grafts of standard diameter. The MK group had statistically higher refractive astigmatism but achieved the same best-corrected visual acuity (BCVA).[10]

Conversion to PK: Large-diameter PK always comes with a drawback of higher chance of immunologic graft rejection due to proximity to the limbal vasculature.[25-27] The study by Myerscough et al. described the 5-year follow-up outcomes of 416 L-DALK cases for keratoconus, with 16.4% of cases needing conversion to a two-piece MK. The cases that needed conversion to MK showed no significant variability in postoperative BCVA, yet showed significantly higher refractive astigmatism even after 18 months to 5 years of suture removal. In literature, however L-DALK (8.5–9 mm) has been proven to show better refractive outcomes when compared to smaller grafts. More than half of the cases that required conversion were scheduled for a layer-by-layer lamellar dissection, which is a known independent risk factor for conversion from DALK to PK. Other risk factors include occurrence of a type 2 bubble, manual layer-by-layer dissection, presence of corneal scarring (healed hydrops), and the relative inexperience of the surgeon.[10]

Endothelial cell loss: Only a single study had compared the rate of endothelial cell loss between the two groups comprising L-DALK and MK. Significant endothelial cell loss at 2 years was also seen following MK (DALK—17.70% vs. MK—46.24%).[10]

Large-diameter Lamellar Keratoplasty in Ocular Surface Diseases with Limbal Insufficiency

Automated large-diameter lamellar keratoplasty offers a safe and fruitful substitute to limbal transplantation for limbal deficiency with corneal opacity. This allows the surgery to be performed as a single-stage procedure using a single donor that would further lower the chances of graft rejection. To add to the list of advantages, optimum refractive outcomes are expected postoperatively due to the higher interface quality and lack of corneal sutures. The final refractive corneal surface achieved is more uniform. Due to lack of corneal sutures the recovery is faster. The main drawback pertaining to this surgery is the requirement for a specific technology, which is not always available or affordable.

SURGICAL TECHNIQUE

In cases of ocular surface diseases with limbal stem cell deficiency, large-diameter lamellar keratoplasty is performed by utilizing a novel head and ring of the ALTK® (Moria®, France) microkeratome system under general or peribulbar anesthesia according to surgeon's preference. With this new technique, lamellar grafts of 13–14 mm in diameter and thickness of 100–150 μm can be obtained including the limbal area with retained stem cells.[28] To ensure smooth passage of the microkeratome, prior perilimbal conjunctival dissection has to be completed as a prerequisite. The recipient stromal bed is trephined (8–10 mm) using a 130–150 μm head of the ALTK system® (Moria®, France), or a larger head up to 250 or 350 μm when there is presence of deeper stromal opacification. The graft edge is tucked underneath the scleral bed and sutured to the host bed with eight interrupted radial 10-0 nylon sutures. Peritomy is closed and secured to the episclera with 8-0 Vicryl sutures. When opacification involves the posterior stroma as well, the recipient bed is punched with a 7.5–8 mm trephine to include the deeper layers. The deep donor button is subsequently sutured to the recipient bed with nylon sutures and the large-diameter anterior lamellar graft is sutured on top.

Vajpayee et al. evaluated the efficacy of large-diameter lamellar keratoplasty in nine cases of severe ocular alkali burns (grade 3 or 4) exhibiting corneal vascularization, conjunctivalization, and chronic inflammation. There was a significant improvement in vision in six eyes postoperatively. None of the eye showed any evidence of recurrence of corneal vascularization or rejection over a mean follow-up of 7.4 ± 3.2 months.[14]

REFERENCES

1. Chen G, Tzekov R, Li W, Jiang F, Mao S, Tong Y. Deep anterior lamellar keratoplasty versus penetrating keratoplasty: a meta-analysis of randomized controlled trials. Cornea. 2016;35:169-74.
2. Reinhart WJ, Musch DC, Jacobs DS, Lee WB, Kaufman SC, Shtein RM. Deep anterior lamellar keratoplasty as an alternative to penetrating keratoplasty: a report by the American Academy of Ophthalmology. Ophthalmology. 2011;118:209-18.
3. Borderie VM, Sandali O, Bullet J, Gaujoux T, Touzeau O, Laroche L. Long-term results of deep anterior lamellar versus penetrating keratoplasty. Ophthalmology. 2012;119:249-55.

4. Keane M, Coster D, Ziaei M, Williams K. Deep anterior lamellar keratoplasty versus penetrating keratoplasty for treating keratoconus. Cochrane Database Syst Rev. 2014;(7):CD009700.
5. Sutphin JE, Goins KM, Wagoner MD. Deep anterior lamellar keratoplasty: when should it replace penetrating keratoplasty? Am J Ophthalmol. 2009;148:629-31.
6. Han DC, Mehta JS, Por YM, Htoon HM, Tan DT. Comparison of outcomes of lamellar keratoplasty and penetrating keratoplasty in keratoconus. Am J Ophthalmol. 2009;148:744-51.e1.
7. Kubaloglu A, Sari ES, Unal M. Long-term results of deep anterior lamellar keratoplasty for the treatment of keratoconus. Am J Ophthalmol. 2011;151:760-7.
8. Fogla R, Padmanabham P. Results of deep lamellar keratoplasty using the big-bubble technique in patients with keratoconus. Am J Ophthalmol. 2006;141:254-9.
9. Seitz B, Langenbucher A, Küchle M, Naumann GO. Impact of graft diameter on corneal power and the regularity of postkeratoplasty astigmatism before and after suture removal. Ophthalmology. 2003;110:2162-7.
10. Myerscough J, Roberts H, Yu AC, Elkadim M, Bovone C, Busin M. Five-year outcomes of converted mushroom keratoplasty from intended deep anterior lamellar keratoplasty (DALK) mandate 9-mm diameter DALK as the optimal approach to keratoconus. Am J Ophthalmol. 2020;220:9-18.
11. Busin M, Leon P, Nahum Y, Scorcia V. Large (9 mm) deep anterior lamellar keratoplasty with clearance of a 6-mm optical zone optimizes outcomes of keratoconus surgery. Ophthalmology. 2017;124(7):1072-80.
12. Huang T, Hu Y, Gui M, Zhang H, Wang Y, Hou C. Large-diameter deep anterior lamellar keratoplasty for keratoconus: visual and refractive outcomes. Br J Ophthalmol. 2015;99(9):1196-200.
13. Mendicute J, Bidaguren A, Martínez-Soroa I, Gibelalde A. Automatized large diameter lamellar keratoplasty and stem cell transplantation for the treatment of ocular surface diseases with limbal insufficiency. Eur J Ophthalmol. 2008;18(4):641-4.
14. Vajpayee RB, Thomas S, Sharma N, Dada T, Tabin GC. Large-diameter lamellar keratoplasty in severe ocular alkali burns: A technique of stem cell transplantation. Ophthalmology. 2000;107(9):1765-8.
15. Busin M, Scorcia V, Leon P, Nahum Y. Outcomes of air injection within 2 mm inside a deep trephination for deep anterior lamellar keratoplasty in eyes with keratoconus. Am J Ophthalmol. 2016;164:6-13.
16. Skeens HM, Holland EJ. Large-diameter penetrating keratoplasty: indications and outcomes. Cornea. 2010;29:296-301.
17. Busin M, Madi S, Scorcia V, Santorum P, Nahum Y. A two-piece microkeratome-assisted mushroom keratoplasty improves the outcomes and survival of grafts performed in eyes with diseased stroma and healthy endothelium (An American Ophthalmological Society Thesis). Trans Am Ophthalmol Soc. 2015;113:T1.
18. Fontana L, Parente G, Tassinari G. Clinical outcomes after deep anterior lamellar keratoplasty using the big-bubble technique in patients with keratoconus. Am J Ophthalmol. 2007;143:117-24.
19. Anwar M, Teichmann KD. Big-bubble technique to bare Descemet's membrane in anterior lamellar keratoplasty. J Cataract Refract Surg. 2002;28:398-403.
20. Tan DT, Anshu A, Parthasarathy A, Htoon HM. Visual acuity outcomes after deep anterior lamellar keratoplasty: a case-control study. Br J Ophthalmol. 2010;94:1295-99.
21. Feizi S, Javadi MA, Jamali H, Mirbabaee F. Deep anterior lamellar keratoplasty in patients with keratoconus: big-bubble technique. Cornea. 2010;29:177-82.
22. Sarnicola V, Toro P, Gentile D, Hannush SB. Descemetic DALK and predescemetic DALK: outcomes in 236 cases of keratoconus. Cornea. 2010;29:53-9.
23. Knutsson KA, Rama P, Paganoni G. Modified big-bubble technique compared to manual dissection deep anterior lamellar keratoplasty in the treatment of keratoconus. Acta Ophthalmol. 2015;93:431-8.
24. Riss S, Heindl LM, Bachmann BO, Kruse FE, Cursiefen C. Pentacam-based big bubble deep anterior lamellar keratoplasty in patients with keratoconus. Cornea. 2012;31:627-32.
25. The collaborative corneal transplantation studies (CCTS). Effectiveness of histocompatibility matching in high-risk corneal transplantation. The Collaborative Corneal Transplantation Studies Research Group. Arch Ophthalmol. 1992;110:1392-403.
26. Cowden J, Copeland R, Schneider M. Large diameter therapeutic penetrating keratoplasties. J Refract Corneal Surg. 1989;5:244-8.
27. Tuberville AW, Foster CS, Wood TO. The effect of donor cornea epithelium removal on the incidence of allograft rejection reactions. Ophthalmology. 1983;90:1351-6.
28. Behrens A, Shah SB, Li L, Côté MA, Liaw LL, Sweet PM, et al. Evaluation of a microkeratome-based limbal harvester device for limbal stem cell transplantation. Cornea. 2002;21:51-5.

57

Femtosecond Laser-assisted Tuck-in Penetrating Keratoplasty

Jorge L Alió del Barrio, Olena Al-Shymali, Jorge L Alió

INTRODUCTION

Keratoglobus (KTG) is a rare noninflammatory corneoscleral ectasia.[1] It is a bilateral disorder characterized by generalized corneal thinning especially peripherally[2] that results in the globular protrusion of the cornea. Previously, it was thought-out equivalent to congenital glaucoma and megalocornea, until it was described by Verrey as an individual clinical entity in 1947.[3] Afterward, this was backed by Cavara in 1950.[4]

Although the exact etiology of the KTG remains unknown, it has been described in both acquired and congenital forms.[1] The former has been associated with vernal keratoconjunctivitis and chronic marginal blepharitis due to frequent eye rubbing, dysthyroid eye disease and idiopathic orbital inflammation.[5,6] Congenital KTG has been linked to Leber's congenital amaurosis, blue sclera syndrome, osteogenesis imperfecta, and connective tissue disorders such as Ehlers-Danlos syndrome, type IV in particular, Marfan syndrome and Rubinstein-Taybi syndrome.[1,7-9]

The extreme corneal thinning and protrusion in patients with KTG lead to visual deterioration due to the extreme myopia, irregular astigmatism, and scarring.[10] The condition can be complicated by acute hydrops causing pain[11] or by corneal perforations occurring spontaneously or following minimal trauma.[1,12]

Since KTG is a rare ectasia, diverse algorithms were proposed but no agreement on a standard method was reached. Using conservative methods such as spectacles or contact lenses in correcting myopia and astigmatism are not always possible especially in children and sometimes are not effective with a corneal perforation risk owing to trauma. Surgical approach consists of various lamellar keratoplasty and epikeratoplasty techniques that provide structural support to these extremely weakened corneas. However, in patients where hydrops or endothelial damage are present, a two-step procedure with a second central corneal penetrating graft will be necessary which means two corneoscleral buttons per eye are required.[2,10] Although conventional penetrating keratoplasty (PKP) is the gold standard procedure for many corneal diseases, it is impracticable in KTG because of the peripheral thinning. Therefore, large limbus to limbus grafts are used which may cause limbal stem cells and angle structure disruptions as well as increase the risk of neovascularization and graft rejection.[1,13]

Recently our team proposed a one-step technique for KTG cases with endothelial damage, femtosecond laser-assisted tuck-in PKP, where both extreme peripheral thinning and corneal endothelial damage exists.[14] On account of the thinning disorders in KTG, the aim of our technique is to insure tectonic support and optimal thickness to the extremely subtle peripheral cornea, in addition to replace the damaged central part of the cornea.

INDICATIONS

Femtosecond laser-assisted tuck-in PKP is indicated in patients with KTG that have both peripheral corneal thinning and endothelial damage due to hydrops or Descemet membrane tears. In this way, we enhance the thickness of the peripheral recipient stroma and simultaneously exchange the central damaged part of the KTG cornea by a full-thickness penetrating corneal graft.

SURGICAL TECHNIQUE

Preoperative Considerations

An explicit examination of the cornea in a KTG patient should be done under the slit lamp. Moreover, a detailed pachymetric map must be made, especially of the corneal periphery. For this technique, we advise a minimum thickness of 300 μm peripherally in order to have a higher chance of succeeding during this technically demanding surgery. If no Descemet membrane tears and endothelial damage are present, then may be the surgeon should opt to a conventional lamellar keratoplasty or a tuck-in lamellar keratoplasy technique.[2,15,16] However, when in addition to the peripheral thinning we have a damaged Descemet membrane or endothelium, we have two options: the two-step procedure[10] of a lamellar epikeratoplasty followed by a central corneal penetrating graft which takes longer time and needs two corneoscleral buttons per eye, or we go for our described femtosecond laser-assisted tuck-in PKP,[14] a one-step surgery that requires only one corneoscleral button per eye.

Technique

Donor Cornea Preparation

In an artificial anterior chamber (AC) assisted by the iFS femtosecond laser (AMO Inc., Irvine, CA), an anterior side cut of 8.5 mm in diameter and 310 μm deep is performed, continued by a 300 μm deep ring lamellar cut up to 9.5 mm of diameter (8.4–9.5 mm). Then, following the ring lamellar dissection plane through the anterior side cut, a crescent blade is used to complete the lamellar dissection until the limbal area. Once this maneuver is finished, a final full-thickness trephination with an 11 mm trephine from the endothelial side is done. Eventually, a donor button that is 11 mm in total diameter with an 8.5 mm central full-thickness area and a 1.25 mm partial thickness circumferential peripheral edge is obtained (**Fig. 1A**).

Recipient Cornea Preparation

Once the preparation of the donor cornea is finished, the recipient cornea is prepared using the same pattern with the femtosecond laser, performing an anterior side cut of 8.5 mm in diameter at 160 μm depth, and a ring lamellar cut depth of 150 μm with 9.5 mm in diameter (recipient side cut depth should be estimated as half of the mean preoperative peripheral recipient corneal thickness). In a similar way as done in the donor cornea, a crescent blade is used to complete the peripheral lamellar dissection following the previously dissected ring lamellar plane, creating a lamellar pocket. The dissection is aimed to the most corneal periphery by reaching the limbus. After the injection of viscoelastic into the AC through a paracentesis, the AC is entered using a 15-degree sharp blade following the contour of the 8.5 mm diameter anterior side cut. Further, the central recipient cornea is excised with the assistance of Vannas scissors. Subsequently, a recipient peripheral stromal pocket made of an anterior and posterior portion is obtained (**Fig. 1B**).

Donor-recipient Apposition

The donor cornea is then sutured using 10/0 nylon interrupted sutures. The thread is passed through the donor 8.5 mm full-thickness button in a partial thickness manner (up to the level where the peripheral rim starts) and the anterior portion of the recipient stromal pocket as close as it could be to the limbus (**Fig. 1C**). In a similar fashion, all 16 sutures are placed on the whole cornea. Then, in order to make sure that the peripheral donor edge remains within the peripheral recipient stromal pocket, this peripheral donor edge is unfolded and tucked in the stromal recipient pocket with the assistance of a blunt spatula (**Fig. 1D**).

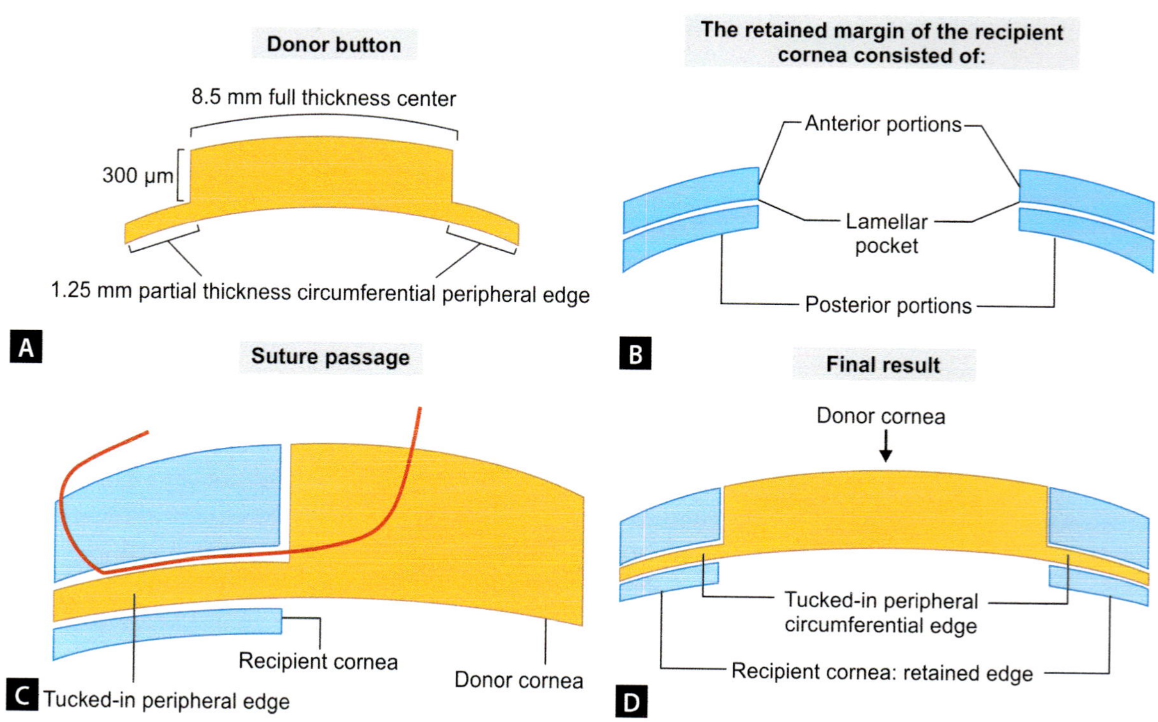

Figs. 1A to D: Femtosecond laser-assisted tuck-in penetrating keratoplasty (PKP) surgical diagram: (A) final appearance of the donor cornea; (B) final appearance of the peripheral recipient stromal pocket; (C) the thread passes through the central 8.5 mm portion of the donor cornea with partial-thickness bite and the anterior portion of the recipient's stromal pocket; and (D) the peripheral circumferential donor rim remains tucked into the recipient's stromal pocket, enhancing the peripheral corneal thickness.

Postoperative Management

Postoperative care do not differ to the one used for a standard PKP surgery: topical antibiotic four times a day for 1 week and topical steroids every 2 hours for 1 week and four times a day thereafter.

COMPLICATIONS

The experience with this technique is still limited, and the only postoperative complications that we have observed were an Urrets-Zavalia syndrome due to retained viscoelastic, and a suture-related infectious keratitis. However, intra- and postoperative potential complications with this Femto tuck-in PKP technique should be equivalent to those described for standard PKP. Especially important for this technique is the fact of performing an adequate preoperative plan for the femtosecond laser dissection planes (diameters and depths) in relation with the peripheral preoperative pachymetry in order to avoid too superficial or too deep surgical planes with subsequent risk of anterior or posterior perforation.

Probably, the most challenging step is the manual expansion of the lamellar plane with the crescent blade on the recipient cornea along the creation of the lamellar recipient pocket. In this step, it is critical to keep the correct depth, but as we are working inside a thin peripheral cornea, inadvertent tears of the anterior lip of the cornea may occur, what will require extra suturing to reconstruct the tear and ensure the correct positioning of the donor cornea.

OUTCOMES

As already discussed, published evidence with this technique is still short and it is limited to a publication of our group describing the outcome obtained from both eyes of the same KG patient (**Figs. 2A to C**).[14] This patient experienced a great bilateral visual improvement (corrected distance vision of 20/50 in both eyes), with residual refractive cylinder of 5 diopters. Corneal topography showed high but regular astigmatism, and the anterior segment OCT is an adequate restoration of the peripheral corneal thickness (**Figs. 3A and B**).

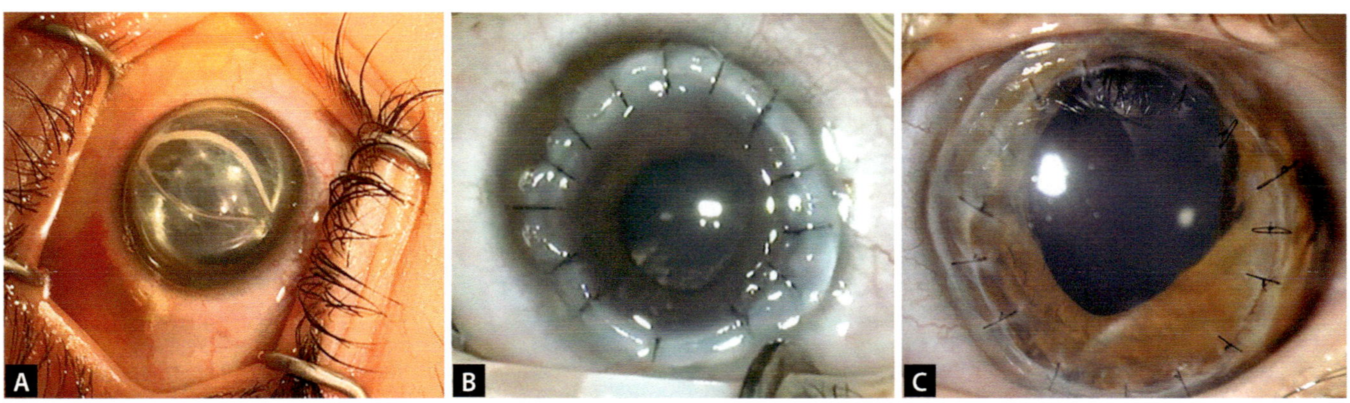

Figs. 2A to C: Preoperative external anterior segment photograph after intracameral air injection of a patient with keratoglobus and chronic hydrops in relation with a severe tear of the corneal endothelium (A); intraoperative photograph immediately after completing the tuck-in penetrating keratoplasty (PKP) (B); and Slit-lamp postoperative anterior segment picture 6 months after the transplant (C). Observe the complete transparency recovery and the peripheral partial thickness donor rim tucked into the host cornea.

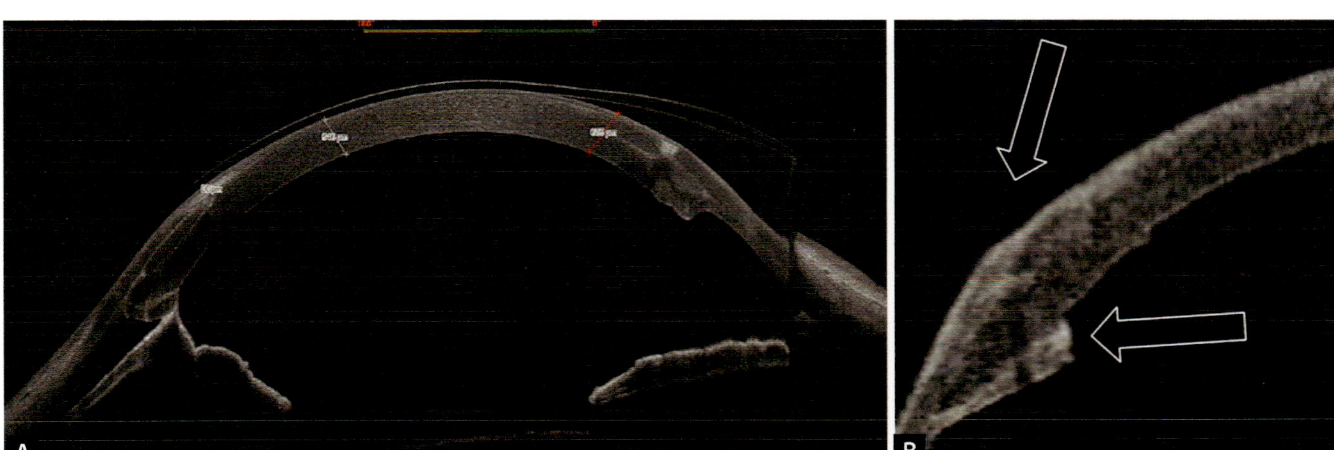

Figs. 3A and B: Anterior segment optical coherence tomography (OCT) (A and B). The peripheral donor partial thickness rim is tucked into the host stromal pocket (B, thick arrows). In those areas not covered by the peripheral donor rim the thickness remains low (A).

CONCLUSION

When severe KTG associates with previous corneal hydrops and severe endothelial damage, routine PKP with an almost limbus to limbus diameter graft associates with a poor visual outcome due to a high-risk of rejection and secondary glaucoma.[13] Such cases were previously managed with a tuck-in or epikeratoplasty lamellar technique to first reinforce the peripheral corneal thickness, followed by a PKP several months later for the visual rehabilitation.[10] However, this approach requires two surgical procedures and the use of two donor corneas. On the other hand, femtosecond laser-assisted tuck-in PKP offers an alternative option to rehabilitate these patients but with a single surgical procedure and only one donor cornea.

Tuck-in PKP in KTG eyes with previous corneal hydrops combines the advantages of PKP (the central full-thickness graft rehabilitates the stroma and the endothelium) and tuck-in lamellar techniques (the peripheral partial thickness rim tucked into the host intrastromal pocket integrates perfectly and provides tectonic support to the recipient tissue). Simultaneously, damage to the recipient's limbal stem cells is avoided as the limbal region is not manipulated. The addition of the femtosecond laser to assist the host and donor cornea partial thickness trephinations is not essential, but it reduces the risk of a full-thickness cut that may happen with manual suction trephines in these extremely thin corneas, and it is more accurate than a free-hand manual technique with surgical blades. Also, the short ring lamellar cut assists the depth of the peripheral dissection that is performed up to the limbal area.

Conflict of interest: None of the authors have any conflict of interest to disclose.

REFERENCES

1. Wallang B, Das S. Keratoglobus. Eye. 2013;27:1004-12.
2. Javadi MA, Kanavi MR, Ahmadi M, Yazdani S. Outcomes of epikeratoplasty for advanced keratoglobus. Cornea. 2007;26:154-7.
3. Verrey F. Keratoglobe aigu. Ophthalmologica. 1947;114:284-8.
4. Cavara V. Keratoglobus and keratoconus. A contribution to the nosological interpretation of keratoglobus. Br J Ophthalmol. 1950;34(10):621-6.
5. Cameron J, Al-Rajhi A, Badr I. Corneal ectasia in vernal keratoconjunctivitis. Ophthalmology. 1989;96:1615-23.
6. Jacobs D, Green W, Maumenee A. Acquired keratoglobus. Am J Ophthalmol. 1974;77:393-9.
7. Koenekoop R. An overview of Leber congenital amaurosis: a model to understand human retinal development. Surv Ophthalmol. 2004;49:379-98.
8. Cameron J. Corneal abnormalities in Ehlers-Danlos syndrome type VI. Cornea. 1993;12:54-9.
9. Nelson M, Talbot J. Keratoglobus in Rubinstein Taybi syndrome. Br J Ophthalmol. 1989;73:385-7.
10. Jones DH, Kirkness CM. A new surgical technique for keratoglobus-tectonic lamellar keratoplasty followed by secondary penetrating keratoplasty. Cornea. 2001;20:885-7.
11. Grewal S, Laibson P, Cohen E, Rapuano C. Acute hydrops in the corneal ectasias: associated factors and outcomes. Trans Am Ophthalmol Soc. 1999;97:187-98.
12. Baillif S, Garweg J, Grange J, Burillon C, Kodjikian L. Keratoglobus: review of the literature. J Fr Ophthalmol. 2005;28:1145-9.
13. Cowden J, Copeland R, Schneider M. Large diameter therapeutic penetrating keratoplasties. Refract Corneal Surg. 1989;5:244-8.
14. Alió Del Barrio J, Al-Shymali O, Alió J. Femtosecond laser-assisted tuck-in penetrating keratoplasty for advanced keratoglobus with endothelial damage. Cornea. 2017;36(9):1145-9.
15. Kaushal S, Jhanji V, Sharma N, Tandon R, Titiyal JS, Vajpayee RB. "Tuck In" Lamellar Keratoplasty (TILK) for corneal ectasias involving corneal periphery. Br J Ophthalmol. 2008;92:286-90.
16. Vajpayee RB, Bhartiya P, Sharma N. Central lamellar keratoplasty with peripheral intralamellar tuck: a new surgical technique for keratoglobus. Cornea. 2002;21:657-60.

58 Microscope-integrated Intraoperative Optical Coherence Tomography-guided Keratoplasty

Namrata Sharma, Priyadarshini K, Pranita Sahay, Rahul Kumar Bafna, Ritu Nagpal

INTRODUCTION

Microscope-integrated optical coherence tomography (MI-OCT) is a recent introduction in the field of ophthalmology that has helped to optimize outcomes, and thus revolutionized the surgical management of numerous anterior and posterior segment disorders.[1,2] This instrument is equipped with a feedback mechanism, hence providing vivid cross-sectional anatomic information of the screened area during surgery without any disruption in the flow of surgery. There are various MI-OCT systems, such as The RESCAN 700 (Carl Zeiss Meditec, Germany), ZEISS OPMI LUMERA 700 (Carl Zeiss Meditec, Inc., Oberkochen, Germany), and the Leica Proveo 8 (Leica Microsystems, Wetzlar, Germany) that are widely used to aid in various ophthalmic surgeries. The techniques of various keratoplasties have been continuously evolving with time and the advent of MI-OCT has further helped to optimize the outcomes of these procedures. The heads-up display provided by the MI-OCT system has added value in decision making and tackling various difficult circumstances intraoperatively in keratoplasties. The impact of MI-OCT on various types of keratoplasties has been discussed here.

PENETRATING KERATOPLASTY

Penetrating keratoplasty is usually performed in full-thickness corneal opacities, which hamper visualization of the anterior chamber anatomy, bringing in hurdles to prior surgical planning. The visualization of iris incarceration and iridocorneal adhesions can help in better manipulation of the uveal tissue and decrease iris trauma intraoperatively. Thus, a better host dissection and release of pre-existing iridocorneal adhesions with minimal trauma to the iris are possible with the aid of MI-OCT in patients with full-thickness corneal opacities. This has been possible with the help of MI-OCT systems. It can also show the various levels of corneoiridic adhesions in a raster pattern intraoperatively to enhance better manipulation and dissection of the adherent uveal tissue (**Figs. 1A to C**).

In a case report by Eguchi et al., it was observed that intraoperative iris incarceration at the graft-host interface during suturing was noted with the aid of MI-OCT, which is difficult to appreciate in a conventional microscope.[3] This could be corrected with the additional manipulation of repositing the iris to the original position using a spatula or irrigation needle in the exact site of adhesion. In conventional microscopes, the visualization of these adhesions is difficult in the peripheral cloudy cornea and blind manipulations can induce further iris incarceration or iridocorneal adhesions and can also cause damage to the endothelial layer. The much-feared complication of penetrating keratoplasty, which is secondary glaucoma, can be avoided by intraoperatively detecting these iridocorneal adhesions and managing them. This also paves way for better graft survival in these patients.

Even in follow-up sequential interventions, such as synechiolysis postpenetrating keratoplasty, MI-OCT helps in better visualization during surgical manipulation. Petrovic et al. have described a case in which synechiolysis postpenetrating keratoplasty was better performed using the aid of MI-OCT.[4] Though it is not required in all cases of keratoplasty with the development of peripheral anterior synechiae, some surgeons advocate it to prevent the onset of secondary glaucoma and reduce the risk of graft failure.

DEEP ANTERIOR LAMELLAR KERATOPLASTY

According to the American Academy of Ophthalmology, deep anterior lamellar keratoplasty (DALK) is the gold standard of management in advanced corneal ectasias and stromal dystrophies. While eliminating the risk of endothelial rejection, it provides visual results similar to penetrating keratoplasty in these conditions.[5,6] Various techniques have been described in DALK. However, Anwar's big bubble technique is widely popular to optimize stromal dissection, wherein the success rate of obtaining a large bubble is at the rate of 66–90%.[7,8] The advent of MI-OCT has optimized various steps of DALK dissection, thus reducing conversion rates to penetrating keratoplasty.[9]

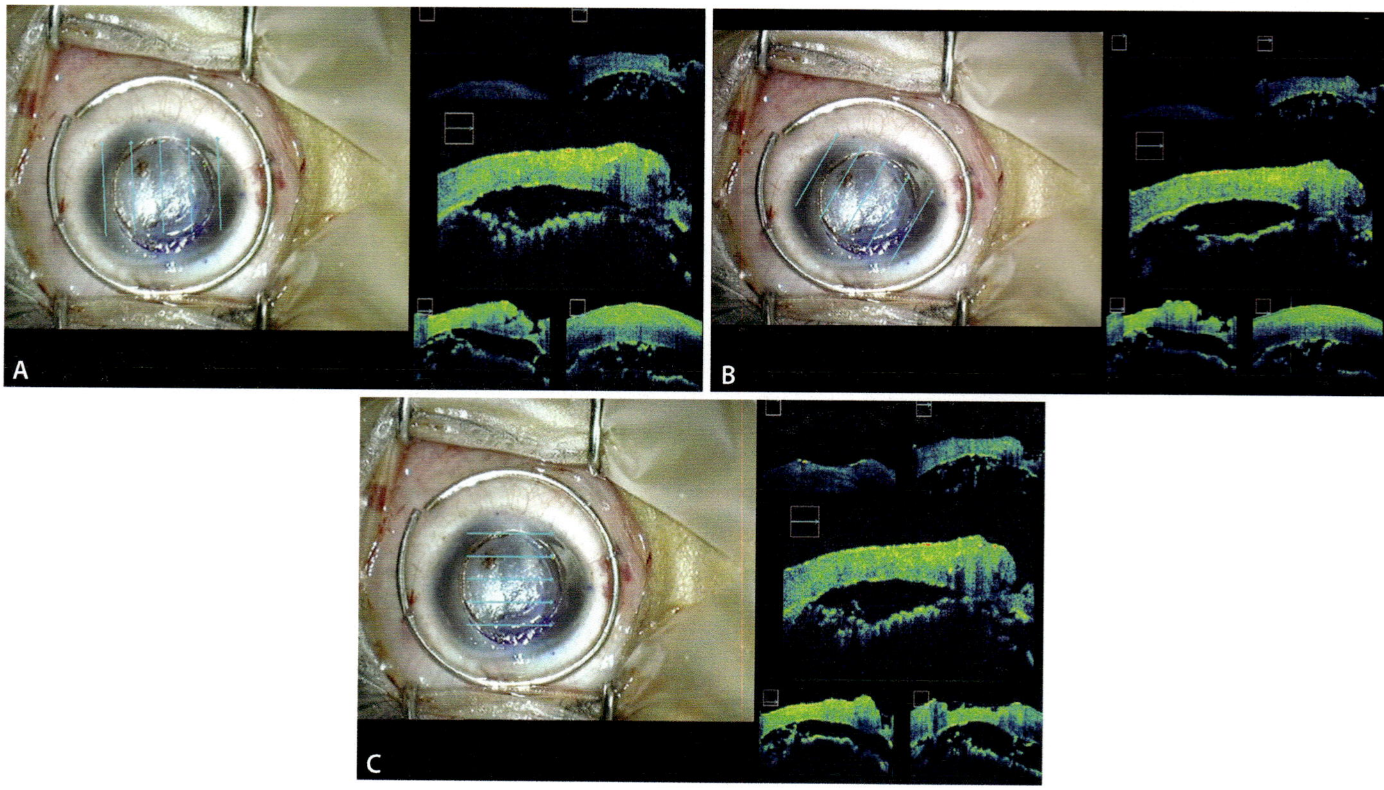

Figs. 1A to C: MI-OCT images showing the iridocorneal adhesions after partial dissection during penetrating keratoplasty in various orientations in a raster pattern.

The first documentation of the use of MI-OCT during DALK surgery was published by Geering et al. in 2005.[10] It was, however, noted that, though all steps in the surgery could be done better with MI-OCT assistance, the shadowing of metallic instruments was an apparent constraint while using this technology.

Beginning with trephination depth, MI-OCT can assist the surgeon in every step of decision-making during DALK. Steven et al. have described the stepwise monitoring using MI-OCT during DALK.[11] Very low or extremely deep trephination depth can thus be identified before proceeding to the next step. The depth of needle insertion can be accurately identified before proceeding with the big bubble technique (**Fig. 2A**). According to a study done by Scorcia et al., it was found that the depth of air injection affected the success rate of big bubble formation. Thus, the plane of air injection can be modified with the assistance of MI-OCT for better success of big bubble formation and avoiding microperforations.[12] A subgroup of patients of the PIONEER study was analyzed by Au et al. in which it was understood that the depth of trephination assessment using MI-OCT in a decision to manually deepen the dissection by 40% before proceeding to big bubble injection.[13] Santorum et al. further reaffirmed the utility of this technology he used MI-OCT-guided trephination and obtained 75% success in big bubble formation.[14]

Diffuse stromal opacification of posterior stroma can occur while attempting a big bubble injection, in which the MI-OCT can help in identifying if the big bubble has formed beneath this area of stromal opacity. In case of incomplete bubble formation, the precise area where a nick can safely be made without damaging the underlying Descemet membrane (DM) can be identified using this technology. MI-OCT can also guide in identifying the dissection plane of the gap between the posterior stroma and the DM, guiding the surgeon in further completion of dissection (**Fig. 2B**). MI-OCT identifies any bumps in the underlying DM and prevents microperforations during dissection. It also helps the surgeon attempt a big bubble again after an initial failed attempt. The residual depth of the corneal bed can also be assessed using MI-OCT to understand the endpoint of dissection (**Fig. 2C**). Graft placement onto the recipient bed and suturing depth can also be monitored to prevent accidental microperforation of DM. At the end of the surgery, the interface can be assessed to ensure complete graft attachment. Any residual interface fluid noted on MI-OCT can be removed by gentle massage on the corneal surface or anterior chamber air injection. This lowers the chances of a double anterior chamber formation postoperatively, reducing the need for additional procedures such as intracameral gas/air injection.

In situations, where the primary surgery is complicated by microperforations, surgeons tend to still proceed with the completion of DALK. Such instances may result in a postoperative Descemet membrane detachment (DMD), which is a known complication of DALK. MI-OCT has also

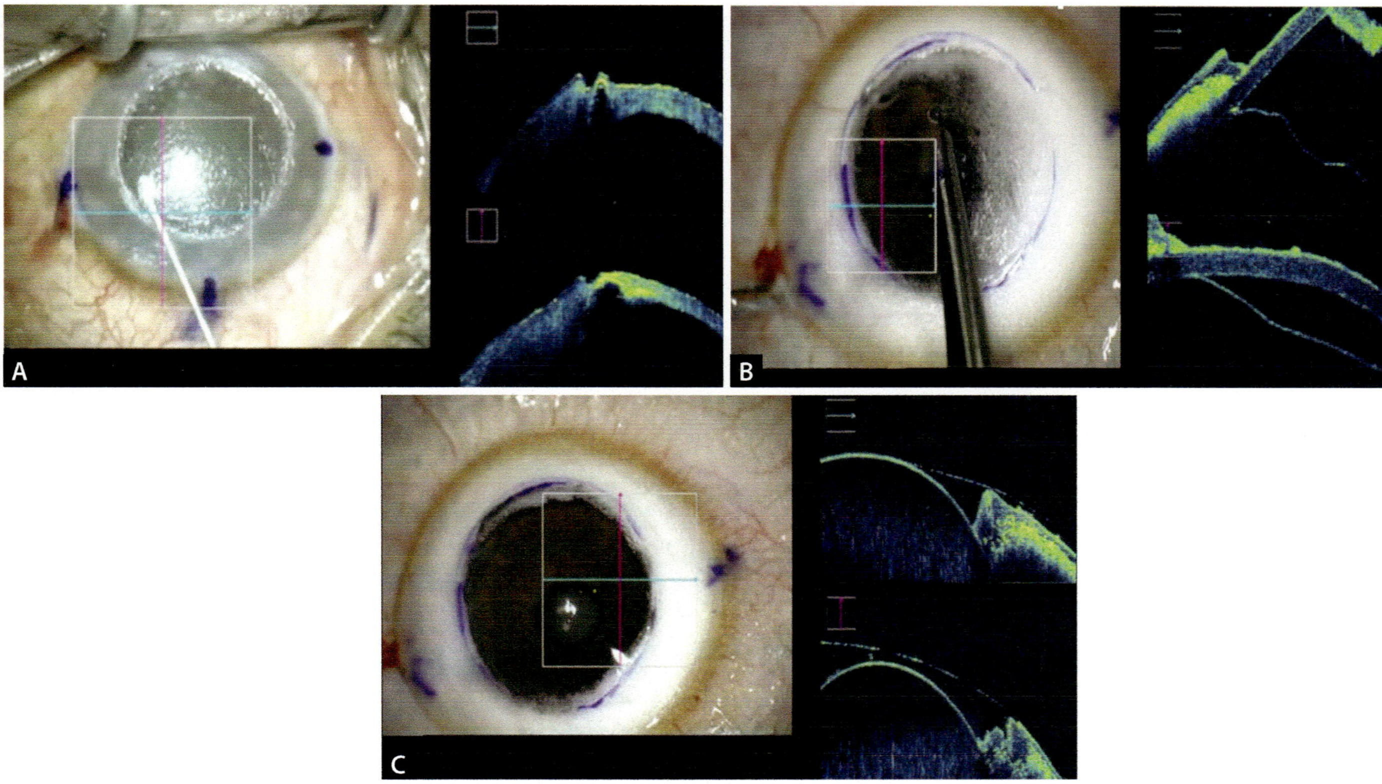

Figs. 2A to C: (A) Depth of needle in the cornea assessed with the aid of MI-OCT after trephination and partial lamellar dissection; (B) MI-OCT-guided visualization of the gap between the posterior stroma and Descemet membrane during dissection in DALK; (C) MI-OCT-guided visualization of the residual stromal bed with bare DM seen after dissection of posterior stroma in DALK.

successfully been used in aiding gas injection and ensuring the attachment of DM in such cases. MI-OCT-assisted gas injection, along with its use of it in choosing the area of venting incision for better apposition of DM has also been described by Sharma et al.[15]

Liu et al. obtained 100% success in type I big-bubble formation using the femtosecond laser (FSL) MI-OCT-guided DALK technique, which was initially done in the preclinical phase in porcine eyes followed by a clinical phase in human eyes.[16] In another study, higher accuracy of intrastromal tunnel depths was obtained in MI-OCT-assisted FSL-DALK over Scheimpflug imaging-assisted FSL-DALK.[17]

ENDOTHELIAL KERATOPLASTY

With the gradual shift toward lamellar surgeries, endothelial keratoplasties have gained popularity for circumventing the risks of open-sky penetrating keratoplasties in cases of endothelial dystrophies and pseudophakic and aphakic corneal edema. From scoring the DM till the end of surgery to ensure graft apposition MI-OCT aids in completely guiding the surgeon during endothelial keratoplasty. In highly edematous thick corneas, MI-OCT can aid in complete DM removal of the host, by allowing the surgeon to identify remnant DM tags intraoperatively. It can aid in locating extremely thin endothelial lenticules and identifying any rolls or folds in them. Toward the end of the surgery, a good graft-host apposition can be visualized in MI-OCT, and any interface fluid remaining can be removed using various techniques such as corneal massage, internal air tamponade, or venting incisions for better graft apposition. Thus, it plays a vital role and has evolved along with the evolution of endothelial keratoplasties, enhancing the results of the procedure.

Descemet's Stripping Anterior Lamellar Keratoplasty

The donor preparation is an important part of Descemet's stripping anterior lamellar keratoplasty (DSAEK), wherein MI-OCT plays a vital role. The initial donor cornea thickness is measured using MI-OCT, and then a suitable microkeratome blade is chosen accordingly, usually in the range of 350–450 μm. The residual corneal thickness can again be measured using MI-OCT. With the advent of MI-OCT, the double-pass microkeratome technique can be used, in which the first pass is made n residual corneal thickness measure and the second pass is titrated to obtain a very thin DSAEK lenticule.[18] Though, even with the single-pass technique, MI-OCT aids in a good selection of microkeratome blades.

The areas of peripheral anterior synechiae can be visualized in MI-OCT and incisions planned accordingly before proceeding with the surgery on the host cornea. The next challenge occurs during the DM scoring, especially in cases of congenital hereditary endothelial dystrophy

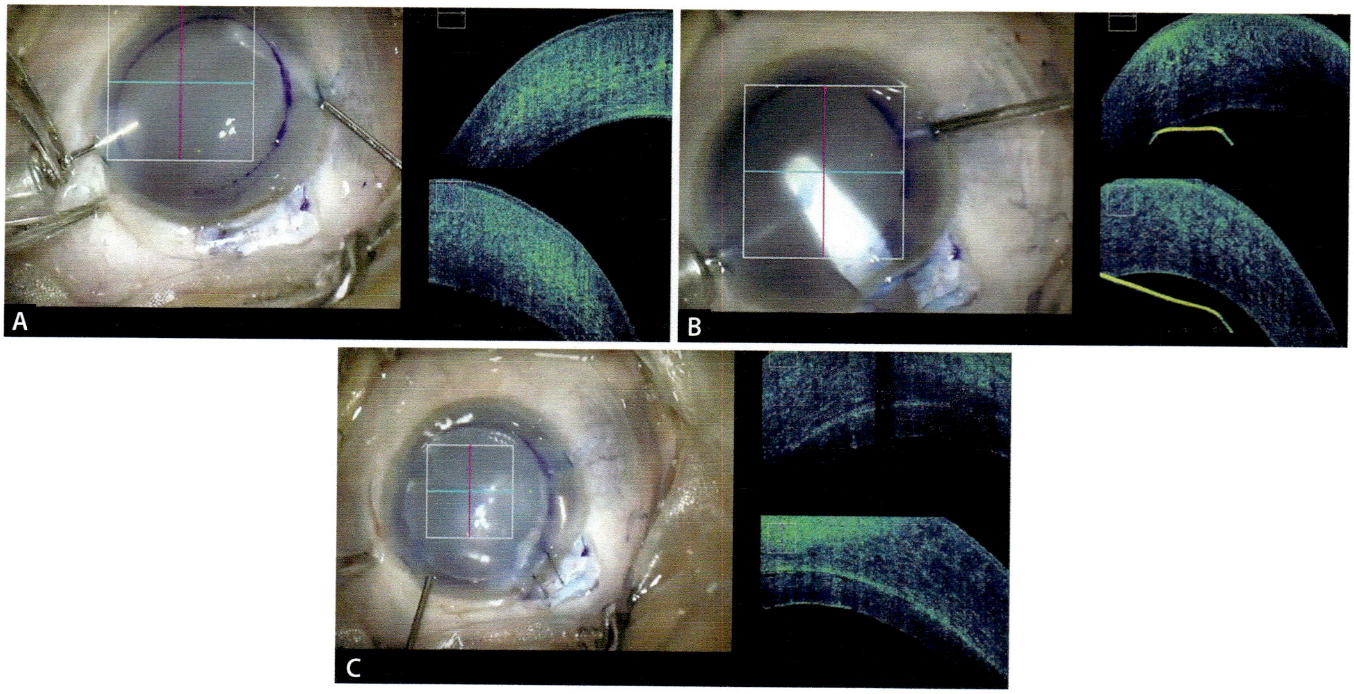

Figs. 3A to C: (A) MI-OCT-guided Descemet membrane scoring during DSAEK in a case of congenital hereditary endothelial dystrophy (CHED); (B) MI-OCT-guided removal of remnant DM tags using a crescent blade during DSAEK in the same patient; (C) MI-OCT-guided assessment of graft host interface showing a well-attached DSAEK lenticule at the end of surgery.

(CHED) and advanced cases of Pseudophakic bullous keratopathy, in which the visibility is very poor. In these cases, MI-OCT was found to aid the surgeon in better visualizing any remnant DM tags and removing them completely (**Figs. 3A and B**).[19,20]

The graft attachment is the crucial step in DSAEK, which limits the success of the procedure. MI-OCT serves as an important aid in ensuring continued visibility of the graft from the time of injection till complete attachment is ensured. There have been various studies that have affirmed the use of MI-OCT in ensuring graft attachment and apposition (**Fig. 3C**). MI-OCT can aid in visualizing the graft in hazy, thick corneas, recognizing any folds or rolls in it, understanding the presence of interface fluid, and performing additional maneuvers to remove it. The PIONEER study highlighted that 48% of eyes enrolled in the study underwent changes in surgical strategy based on graft apposition and persisting interface fluid noted in MI-OCT.[2] In the DISCOVER study, MI-OCT was again found to have altered surgical decision making regarding graft apposition in 41% of the cases: 19% revealed interface fluid wherein the surgeon thought the graft was well apposed, whereas 47% showed well-apposed graft-host interface wherein the surgeon was not sure about the graft apposition thus reducing unnecessary prolongation of surgical time.[1] Titiyal et al. used MI-OCT for finding the optimum time and maneuvers required to reduce surgical timing in DSAEK.[21] It was found that simultaneous positive intracameral pressure and external corneal massage helped in the attachment of the donor lenticule in 1–3 minutes.

Descemet Membrane Endothelial Keratoplasty

Though Descemet membrane endothelial keratoplasty (DMEK) results in faster visual rehabilitation with a better visual outcome and reduced risk of graft rejection, there are several challenges in the surgical technique such as graft preparation, unfolding of the DMEK graft in the anterior chamber, and difficulty in visualizing the DMEK roll in hazy cornea and postoperative risk of detachment.[22-29] These challenges have limited the use of this technique to cases having relatively clear cornea and normal anterior segment anatomy. Unlike most of the published series in DMEK, the majority of cases in developing nations present at a delayed stage of corneal endothelial decompensation, thus making them either unsuitable or surgically challenging for endothelial keratoplasty.[30]

Microscope-integrated optical coherence tomography helps in improvising visibility and hence improving decision making in the various surgical steps of DMEK. During the Descemet scoring of the host cornea, MI-OCT can aid in identifying areas of remnant DM or tags of DM, as during DSAEK. Therefore, complete removal of the residual DM tags can be ensured (**Figs. 4A and B**). This is a critical step for postoperative graft attachment in a thin DM roll. It was found in a study by Sharma et al. that DM tags otherwise unidentified were identified in 92% of the eyes with the aid of MI-OCT in cases of pseudophakic bullous keratopathy.[31] Unnecessary attempts of DM scraping, which can result in postoperative stromal haze can also be avoided by identifying areas of missing DM with the guidance of MI-OCT. During

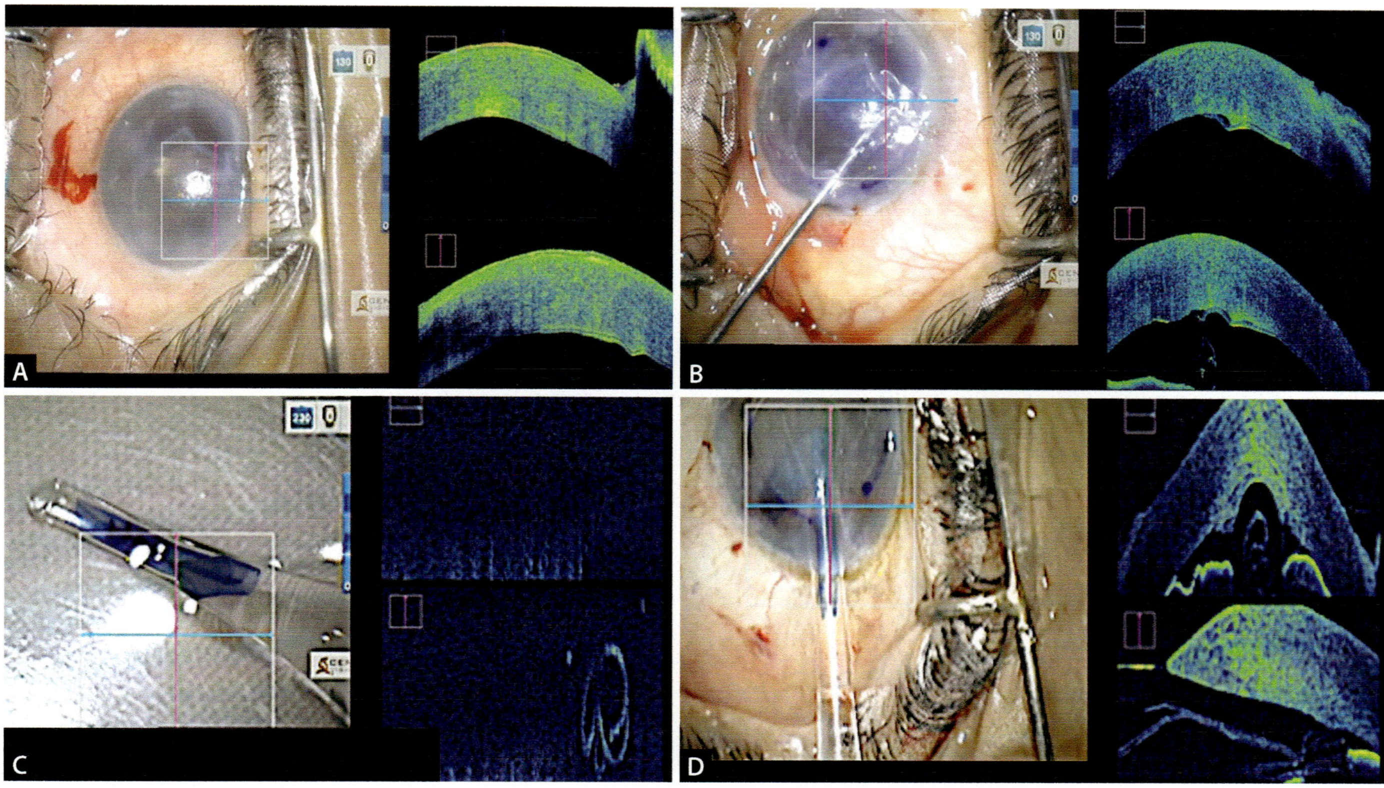

Figs. 4A to D: (A) MI-OCT assisted visualization of the adherent Descemet membrane (DM); (B) MI-OCT assisted DM scoring; (C) Image showing DMEK roll orientation in the Descemet membrane endothelial keratoplasty (DMEK) injector with the orientation of DM facing downward; (D) Unscrolling of graft in the anterior chamber with DM oriented to the right.

injection of the DMEK roll into the anterior chamber, the MI-OCT can assist the surgeon in identifying the orientation of the DM roll in the injector so that the orientation of the injector can be changed to allow injection of the DM roll in the proper orientation (**Figs. 4C and D**). Also, the orientation of the DM roll in the anterior chamber can be assessed with its help before the injection of air. This is especially useful in cases with increased corneal haze wherein the exact orientation of the "S" mark on the donor tissue is difficult to identify intraoperatively (**Figs. 5A to D**). Peripheral DM folds in the graft and their orientation can be precisely assessed with this equipment and it can help in the unfolding of donor tissue as well. This reduces the surgical time as well as inadvertent damage to the graft with repeated attempts to unfold it. It was found that MI-OCT-guided DMEK resulted in the safe completion of this procedure with 72% of the grafts attached on day 3, 16% requiring bubbling, and 100% of grafts attached on 6-month follow-up even in eyes with poor visibility in which DMEK would not have been possible in a conventional microscope.[31]

Microscope-integrated optical coherence tomography was found to decrease the operating time of DMEK as well at various steps of the procedure. Saad et al. noted that the graft unfolding time was found to be 6.1 minutes, which is much faster than 8.9 minutes for a surgeon without this technology.[32] This is in agreement with the DISCOVER study which also noted a graft unfolding time of 6 minutes 15 seconds with the aid of this technology which was identifiable in all cases.[33] With the MI-OCT-guided technique for identifying the tissue orientation, the graft unscrolling time was found to be lesser than the "S" stamp technique.[33,34] MI-OCT also reduced the over-pressurizing time from around 12 minutes to <2 minutes, thus decreasing the chances of elevation of intraocular pressures and damage to the retinal nerve fiber layer.[35] It was also found to alter surgical decision making in 42% of the cases concerning the presence of interface fluid, thus reducing unnecessary prolongation of surgery in well-attached grafts.[35]

PEDIATRIC KERATOPLASTY

Keratoplasty in the pediatric population is an extremely challenging procedure due to various intraoperative morphologic and functional aspects, such as less surgical space due to small globe size, anteriorly displaced iris lens diaphragm, positive vitreous pressure, and decreased rigidity of cornea and sclera. Postoperative complications such as severe inflammatory reaction, secondary glaucoma, graft rejection, repeated examinations under anesthesia, repeat surgical interventions, and suboptimal visual gain are much more common than in adults.[36,37]

Microscope-integrated optical coherence tomography helps to obtain high-resolution images preoperatively, which can aid in the surgical planning in pediatric patients. Siebelman et al. in their study, concluded that screening

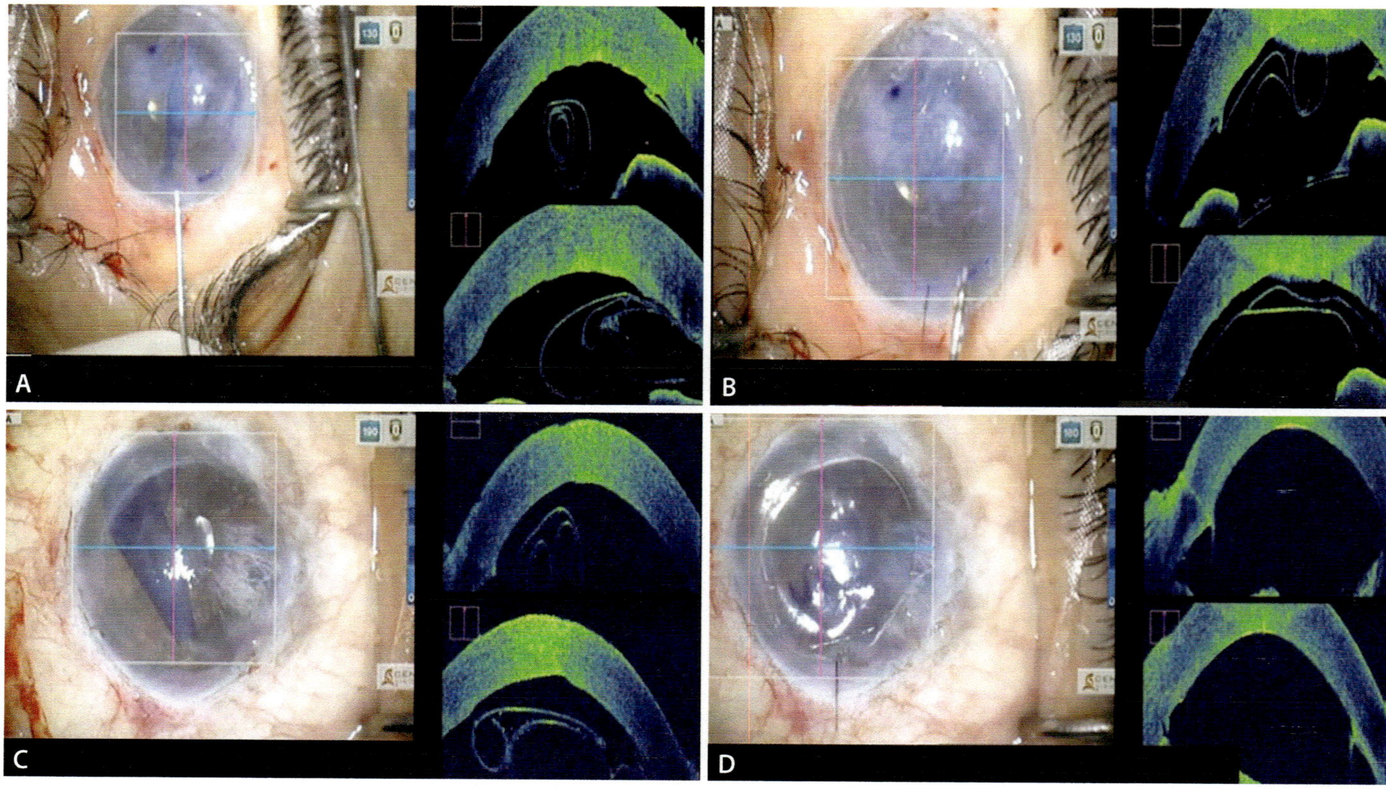

Figs. 5A to D: MI-OCT showing various orientations of the DM roll in the anterior chamber: (A) Tight scroll in the anterior chamber; (B) Double scroll with DM up and endothelium down, which is the right orientation; (C) Double scroll with DM down and endothelium up, which is the inverted orientation; (D) Well attached DM graft at the end of surgery.

pediatric corneal opacities with MI-OCT facilitates minimally invasive operative approaches such as lamellar keratoplasty by allowing dynamic visualization of those anterior segment details that would otherwise be missed by routine surgical microscopic examination.[38] Both MI-OCT and ultrasound biomicroscope (UBM) were indeed found to be superior to the conventional ophthalmic microscope in detecting various anterior segment abnormalities preoperatively in children. However, a fully integrated MI-OCT was found to have a better ability than UBM in detecting retrocorneal membranes, details of iris adhesions, peripheral anterior synechiae, and AC depth, in lieu of its higher resolution and magnification (**Figs. 6A and B**).[39] The knowledge about these details helps in better dissection, avoiding trauma and thus, reducing chances of increased inflammation, rise in intraocular pressure, and graft failure. This technology also aids in the visualization of the posterior capsule and ciliary sulcus rim for intraocular lens placement. Thus, simultaneous interventions such as cataract extraction, synechiolysis, and pupilloplasty can also be planned accordingly, avoiding the need for subsequent procedures and repeated exposure to anesthesia. The adequacy of graft-host apposition and the depth of suture can also be assessed using MI-OCT, which is very vital in cases of pediatric penetrating keratoplasties.

Tibrewal et al. demonstrated more efficient completion of lamellar procedures in a series of 12 children with the aid of MI-OCT.[40] The use of this technology helps to prevent inadvertent perforations during trephination and stromal dissection, thus reducing conversion rates to penetrating keratoplasty during anterior lamellar procedures.[39] This is very important regarding the pediatric population, considering the longer lifespan, and higher graft failure rates in younger eyes. It also helps in better interface assessment, which is again important to prevent rebubbling and gas injection procedures in these patients and reduce the need for repeated anesthesia. In DSAEK, the visualization of remnant DM tags was augmented with this device and helped in precise DM scoring in these patients with CHED as documented in a study done by Asif et al.[19] This helps in avoiding unnecessary manipulation and blind sweeping of angle with instruments, thus reducing inflammation and enhancing the graft-host interface alignment. Sharma et al. documented that the use of MI-OCT had impacted surgical decision-making in 33% of pediatric eyes operated with DSAEK, thus optimizing surgical time with an average unscrolling time of 5:56 ± 2:42 minutes for complete graft-host adherence.[39] The optimization of surgical timing in pediatric cases plays an important role in avoiding unnecessary prolongation of anesthesia.

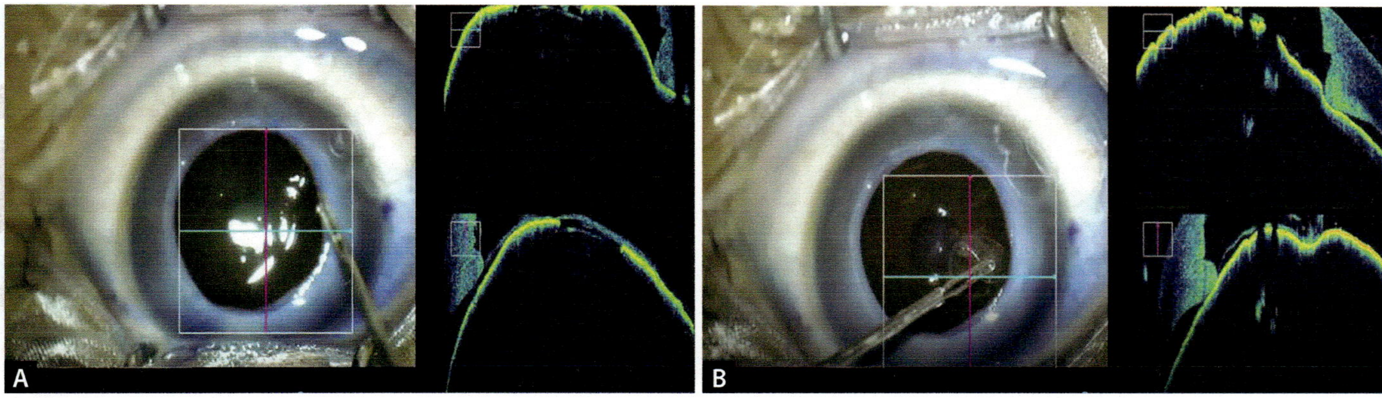

Figs. 6A and B: (A) MI-OCT-guided visualization of retrocorneal membrane posthost dissection in a pediatric eye undergoing penetrating keratoplasty; (B) MI-OCT-guided peeling of the retrocorneal membrane in the same eye.

CONCLUSION

It is understood from various studies that MI-OCT has added value in optimizing the surgical decision making, and intraoperative time and has made life easier for corneal transplant surgeons. It has proven to be useful in performing various steps in penetrating and lamellar keratoplasties. It also plays an important role in performing keratoplasties in pediatric eyes which are difficult to assess and plan preoperatively. However, the major limitation is the cost and availability of this technology. The shadowing seen while using metallic instruments is another drawback, which can be circumvented by the use of plastic cannulas and so on in the future. Further evidence-based randomized controlled trials are required to establish its definitive superiority over conventional microscopes in the management of corneal pathologies with keratoplasties.

REFERENCES

1. Ehlers JP, Modi YS, Pecan MD, Goshe J, Dupps WJ, Rachitskaya A, et al. Feasibility and usefulness of microscope-integrated Intraoperative OCT during ophthalmic surgery (DISCOVER) Study: 3-year results. Am Acad Ophthalmol. 2018;125(7):1014-27.
2. Ehlers JP, Dupps WJ, Kaiser PK, Goshe J, Singh RP, Petkovsek D, et al. The Prospective Intraoperative and Perioperative Ophthalmic ImagiNg with Optical CoherEncE TomogRaphy (PIONEER) Study: 2-year results. Am J Ophthalmol. 2014;158 (5): 999-1007.
3. Eguchi H, Kusaka S, Arimura-Koike E, Tachibana K, Tsujioka D, Fukuda M, et al. Intraoperative optical coherence tomography (RESCAN® 700) for detecting iris incarceration and iridocorneal adhesion during keratoplasty. Int Ophthalmol. 2017;37(3):761-5.
4. Petrovic A, Gianniou C, Hashemi K, Kymionis G. Intraoperative anterior optical coherence tomography-guided synechiolysis in a post-penetrating keratoplasty patient with peripheral corneal opacification. Ther Clin Risk Manag. 2018;14:1387-90.
5. Han DC, Mehta JS, Por YM, Htoon HM, Tan DT. Comparison of outcomes of lamellar keratoplasty and penetrating keratoplasty in keratoconus. Am J Ophthalmol. 2009;148:744-51.
6. Riss S, Heindl LM, Bachmann BO, Kruse FE, Cursiefen C. Pentacam-based big bubble deep anterior lamellar keratoplasty in patients with keratoconus. Cornea. 2012;31:627-32.
7. Anwar M, Teichmann KD. Big-bubble technique to bare Descemet's membrane in anterior lamellar keratoplasty. J Cataract Refract Surg. 2002;28:398-403.
8. Huang T, Zhang XY, Wang Y, Zhang H, Hu AD, Gao N. Outcomes of deep anterior lamellar keratoplasty using the big-bubble technique in various corneal diseases. Am J Ophthalmol. 2012;154:282-9.
9. Siebelmann S, Steven P, Cursiefen C. Intraoperative optical coherence tomography in deep anterior lamellar keratoplasty. Klin Monbl Augenheilkd. 2016;233:717-21.
10. Geerling G, Muller M, Winter C, Hoerauf H, Oelckers S, Laqua H, et al. Intraoperative 2-dimensional optical coherence tomography as a new tool for anterior segment surgery. Arch Ophthalmol Chic. 2005;123:253-7.
11. Steven P, Le Blanc C, Lankenau E, Krug M, Oelckers S, Heindl LM, et al. Optimising deep anterior lamellar keratoplasty (DALK) using intraoperative online optical coherence tomography (iOCT). Br J Ophthalmol. 2014;98:900-4.
12. Scorcia V, Busin M, Lucisano A, Beltz J, Carta A, Scorcia G. Anterior segment optical coherence tomography-guided big-bubble technique. Ophthalmology. 2013;120:471-6.
13. Au J, Goshe J, Dupps WJ Jr, Srivastava SK, Ehlers JP. Intraoperative optical coherence tomography for enhanced depth visualization in deep anterior lamellar keratoplasty from the PIONEER study. Cornea. 2015;34:1039-43.
14. Santorum P, Yu AC, Bertelli E, Busin M. Microscope-Integrated Intraoperative optical coherence tomography-guided big-bubble deep anterior lamellar keratoplasty. Cornea. 2022;41:125-9.
15. Sharma N, Aron N, Kakkar P, Titiyal JS. Continuous intraoperative OCT guided management of post-deep anterior lamellar keratoplasty Descemet's membrane detachment. Saudi J Ophthalmol. 2016;30:133-6.
16. Liu YC, Wittwer VVN, Yusoff NZM, Lwin CN, Seah XY, Mehta JS, et al. Intraoperative optical coherence tomography guided femtosecond laser-assisted deep anterior lamellar keratoplasty. Cornea. 2019;38:648-53.
17. Buzzonetti L, Laborante A, Petrocelli G. Standardized big-bubble technique in deep anterior lamellar keratoplasty assisted by the femtosecond laser. J Cataract Refract Surg. 2010;36:1631-6.
18. Hsu M, Hereth WL, Moshirfar M. Double-pass microkeratome technique for ultra-thin graft preparation in Descemet's stripping automated endothelial keratoplasty. Clin Ophthalmol. 2012;6:425-32.
19. Asif MI, Bafna RK, Sharma N, Kaginalkar A, Sinha R, Agarwal T, et al. Microscope integrated optical coherence tomography guided Descemet stripping automated endothelial keratoplasty in congenital hereditary endothelial dystrophy. Clin Ophthalmol. 2021;15:3173-81.

20. Pasricha ND, Shieh C, Carrasco-Zevallos OM, Keller B, Izatt JA, Toth CA, et al. Real-time microscope-integrated OCT to improve visualization in DSAEK for advanced bullous keratopathy. Cornea. 2015;34(12):1606.
21. Titiyal JS, Kaur M, Falera R, Jose CP, Sharma N. Evaluation of time to donor lenticule apposition using intraoperative optical coherence tomography in Descemet stripping automated endothelial keratoplasty. Cornea. 2016;35:477-81.
22. Singh A, Zarei-Ghanavati M, Avadhanam V, Liu C. Systematic review and meta-analysis of clinical outcomes of Descemet membrane endothelial keratoplasty versus Descemet stripping endothelial keratoplasty/Descemet stripping automated endothelial keratoplasty. Cornea. 2017;36(11):1437-43.
23. Melles GRJ, Ong TS, Ververs B, van der Wees J. Descemet membrane endothelial keratoplasty (DMEK). Cornea. 2006;25(8):987-90.
24. Maharana PK, Sahay P, Titiyal JS, Sharma N. Sinsky hook assisted roll preparation (SHARP): A modified technique for Descemet membrane endothelial keratoplasty donor preparation. Saudi J Ophthalmol. 2019;33(1):28-33.
25. Terry MA, Straiko MD, Veldman PB, Talajic JC, VanZyl C, Sales CS, et al. Standardized DMEK technique: Reducing complications using prestripped tissue, novel glass injector, and sulfur hexafluoride (SF6) gas. Cornea. 2015;34(8):845-52.
26. Siebelmann S, Gehlsen U, Le Blanc C, Stanzel TP, Cursiefen C, Steven P. Detection of graft detachments immediately following Descemet membrane endothelial keratoplasty (DMEK) comparing time-domain and spectral-domain OCT. Graefes Arch Clin Exp Ophthalmol. 2016;254(12):2431-7.
27. Gorovoy MS. DMEK Complications. Cornea. 2014;33(1):101-4.
28. Muraine M, He Z, Toubeau D, Guedry J, Thuret G, Lefevre S, et al. Validation of a novel device to easy the preparation of endothelial graft for DMEK. Acta Ophthalmologica. 2014;92. doi:10.1111/j.1755-3768.2014.4771.x.
29. Yu CQ, Ta CN, Terry MA, Lin CC. Successful DMEK after intraoperative graft inversion. Cornea. 2015;34(1):97-8.
30. Sharma N, Sachdev R, Pandey RM, Titiyal JS, Sinha R, Tandon R, et al. Study of factors for unsuitability of DSAEK in cases of corneal decompensation following cataract surgery. Int Ophthalmol. 2012;32(4):313-9.
31. Sharma N, Sahay P, Maharana PK, Kumar P, Ahsan S, Titiyal JS. Microscope integrated intraoperative optical coherence tomography-guided DMEK in corneas with poor visualization. Clin Ophthalmol. 2020;14:643-51.
32. Saad A, Guilbert E, Grise-Dulac A, Sabatier P, Gatinel D. Intraoperative OCT-assisted DMEK: 14 consecutive cases. Cornea. 2015;34:802-7.
33. Cost B, Goshe JM, Srivastava S, Ehlers JP. Intraoperative optical coherence tomography-assisted Descemet membrane endothelial keratoplasty in the DISCOVER study. Am J Ophthalmol. 2015;160:430-37.
34. Sáles CS, Terry MA, Veldman PB, Mayko ZM, Straiko MD. Relationship between tissue unscrolling time and endothelial cell loss. Cornea. 2016;35:471-6.
35. Muijzer MB, Soeters N, Godefrooij DA, van Luijk CM, Wisse RPL. Intraoperative optical coherence tomography-assisted Descemet membrane endothelial keratoplasty: Toward more efficient, safer surgery. Cornea. 2020;39:674-9.
36. Vanathi M, Panda A, Vengayil S, Chaudhuri Z, Dada T. Pediatric keratoplasty. Surv Ophthalmol. 2009;54(2):245-71.
37. Stulting RD, Sumers KD, Cavanagh HD, Waring GO 3rd, Gammon JA. Penetrating keratoplasty in children. 281 Ophthalmology. 1984;91:1222-30.
38. Siebelmann S, Hermann M, Dietlein T, Bachmann B, Steven P, Cursiefen C. Intraoperative optical coherence tomography in children with anterior segment anomalies. Ophthalmology. 2015;122(12):2582-4.
39. Sharma N, Priyadarshini K, Agarwal R, Bafna RK, Nagpal R, Sinha R, et al. Role of microscope-intraoperative optical coherence tomography in pediatric keratoplasty: A comparative study. Am J Ophthalmol. 2021; 221:190-8.
40. Tibrewal S, Troia A, Espandar L, Nischal K. Use of integrated intraoperative optical coherence tomography in pediatric cornea surgery. Journal of American Association for Pediatric Ophthalmology and Strabismus. 2018;22(4):50-1.

59

Amniotic Membrane Transplantation

Ahmad Kheirkhah, Sean Tighe, Olivia Mead, Scheffer CG Tseng

INTRODUCTION

Human amniotic membrane (AM), the innermost layer of the placental membrane, is 20–150 µm thick and consists of a simple epithelium, a thick basement membrane, and an avascular stroma rich in hyaluronic acid. While the tough, semi-transparent nature of AM renders it valuable as a graft for ocular surface reconstruction, it is the unique, inherent biological action of AM that has spawned increasing interest in its use for ophthalmic indications over the past decade.

Historically, AM has been used predominantly as a surgical "dressing" over different parts of body, including the eye. De Rötth[1] was the first to describe the use of *fresh* placental membranes in 1940, using both amnion and chorion for the management of conjunctival defects. Several years later, Sorsby et al.[2,3] used chemically processed "dry" AM as a temporary patch for the treatment of acute ocular burns. Thereafter, the use of AM disappeared from medical literature for several decades, until Kim and Tseng[4] reintroduced the use of cryopreserved AM for ophthalmic uses in 1995. Since then, transplantation of cryopreserved AM has been widely accepted in ophthalmology and is well recognized as a standard of care (CPT Codes 65778, 65779 and 65780), which is supported by several hundred peer-reviewed publications. AM has been shown to promote epithelial healing and reduce inflammation, scarring and emerging angiogenesis on the ocular surface (for reviews see[5,6]). The heavy chain 1-hyaluronic acid/pentraxin 3 (HC-HA/PTX3) matrix is the major active tissue component responsible for the multifactorial therapeutic actions of cryopreserved AM, as summarized in a recent review.[5] Although AM has been used in various ocular surface surgeries, this chapter will summarize only the applications for corneal indications.

TWO MODES OF CLINICAL USES

The corneal indications for amniotic membrane transplantation (AMT) can be categorized according to whether cryopreserved AM is used as an *inlay graft* or an *overlay patch.*

When used as an *inlay graft*, AM helps fill in corneal stromal defects and restore the structural integrity of the corneal stroma. Because of the remarkable aforementioned biological actions of cryopreserved AM, the resultant corneal stroma often regains clarity. Therefore, AMT better preserves the aesthetic appearance of the ocular surface when compared to tarsorrhaphy or conjunctival flap. If corneal transplantation is required, AM helps promote surgical success by reducing inflammation. Because the cryopreserved AM graft does not include *live* allogeneic cells, the risk of allograft rejection observed with lamellar corneal transplantation is mitigated; thus, patients are not required to take any topical or systemic immunosuppressive or anti-inflammatory medications after healing. If additional surgeries are needed to improve vision, excimer laser ablation, such as phototherapeutic keratectomy (PTK), can be used, as scarring is minimized. AM as an inlay graft can be secured with sutures or fibrin glue. However, the surgical time is significantly reduced when sutures are not used, thus allowing the surgery to be performed under topical anesthesia and facilitating the ease of postoperative care and patient recovery. Corneal indications for AMT as an *inlay graft* are listed in **Box 1**.

When AM is used as an *overlay patch (biological patch),* its aim is to reduce either acute or chronic ocular surface inflammation caused by various diseases and insults and promote epithelial healing with minimal or no scarring. Corneal indications for AMT as an *overlay patch* are mentioned in **Box 2**. AM can be sutured as a biological

Box 1: Corneal indications for inlay amniotic membrane graft.

- Persistent corneal epithelial defects and stromal defects
- Descemetocele or perforation
- Infectious keratitis with stromal defect
- Painful bullous keratopathy
- Band keratopathy
- Following superficial keratectomy (such as to remove scar before phototherapeutic keratectomy is contemplated)
- Limbal stem cell deficiency

patch to cover the cornea at the site of interest, however, many of these indications can now be managed using PROKERA® (see next), which is a sutureless and self-retained cryopreserved AM (**Figs. 1A to C**). Because PROKERA can be placed in the office or at the bedside, it further enhances the ease of patient care, avoids suture-induced inflammation, and reduces medical costs associated with surgery.

Box 2: Corneal indications for overlay amniotic membrane.

- Persistent or recurrent epithelial defect
- Corneal ulcer
- Recurrent corneal erosions
- Acute chemical/thermal burns
- Band keratopathy post-debridement
- Filamentary keratitis
- Neurotrophic keratitis
- Nodular corneal degeneration post-debridement
- Corneal sequelae from dry eye disease
- Acute Stevens-Johnson syndrome/toxic epidermal necrolysis
- Infectious keratitis with stromal defect
- After high-risk corneal grafts (to reduce complications)
- After excision of corneal lesions/pterygium/tumors
- After excimer laser ablation (PRK/PTK) (to prevent haze)
- Corneal dystrophies (epithelial, lattice, macular, etc.)
- Plastic indications as conformer (to prevent lid/lash mechanical insult to the cornea)
- Limbal stem cell deficiency
- Corneal buffering during plaque radiation therapy
- Implantation of keratoprosthesis

(PRK/PTK: photorefractive keratectomy/phototherapeutic keratectomy)

AMNIOTIC MEMBRANE AS AN INLAY GRAFT

Persistent Epithelial Defects with Different Depths

Corneal ulcers are a serious and urgent clinical problem that can be complicated by microbial infection and threaten patient's vision. Corneal ulcers can be caused by various insults, e.g., exogenously from chemical burns, infection, radiation, or surgeries, while endogenous causes include aging, diabetes mellitus, viral (herpes) infection, and autoimmune disorders, with the common denominator being neurotrophic keratopathy (reviewed by Solomon et al.[7]). When the ulceration persists despite exhausting conservative treatment options, conventional surgical treatment with lamellar or full-thickness corneal transplantation (patch graft), tarsorrhaphy, or conjunctival flap is warranted. AMT in these cases offers the following advantages: avoidance of potential allograft rejection and

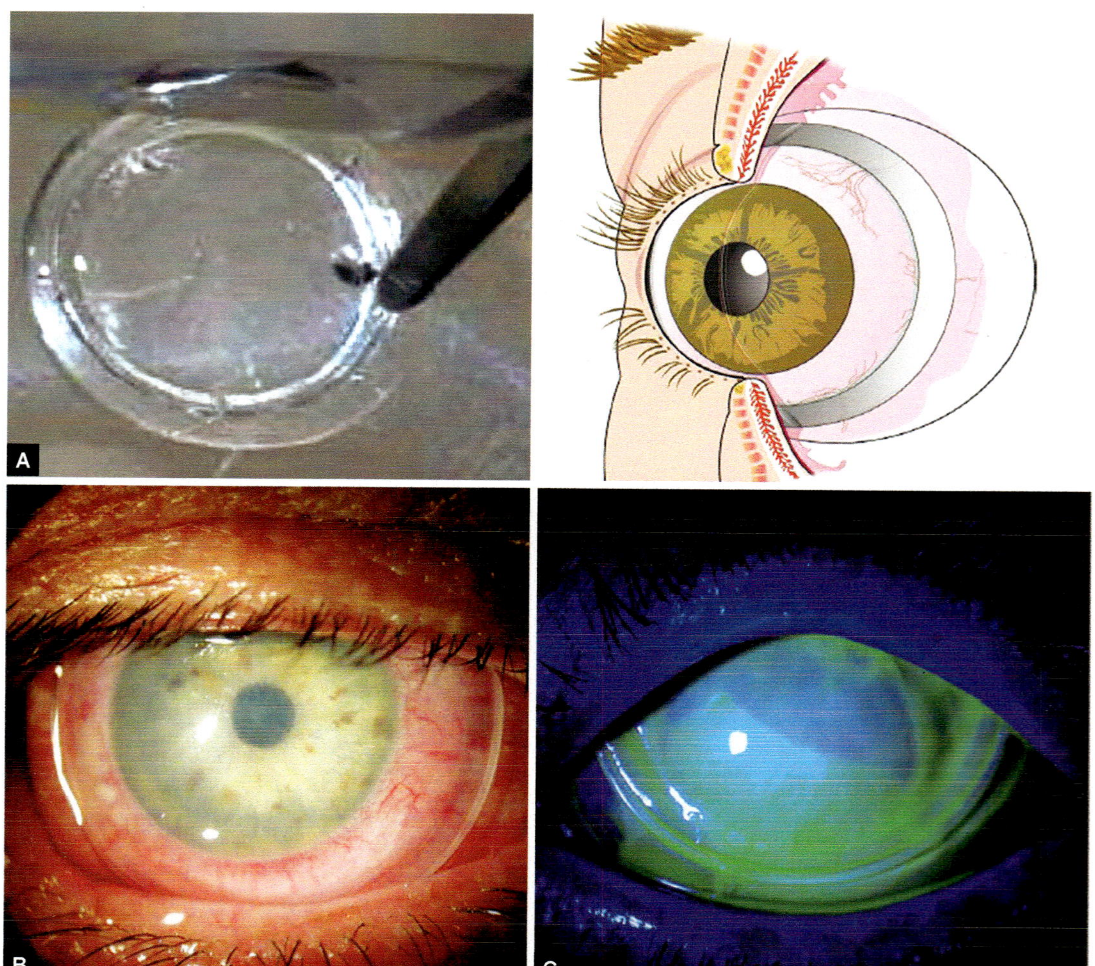

Figs. 1A to C: *Sutureless amniotic membrane transplantation with PROKERA.* PROKERA classic is a dual ring system that fastens a sheet of semi-transparent cryopreserved AM (A). The slit-lamp photograph (B and C) depict its appearance when inserted in the eye. While inserted, the status of epithelialization can be monitored by fluorescein staining without removing PROKERA.

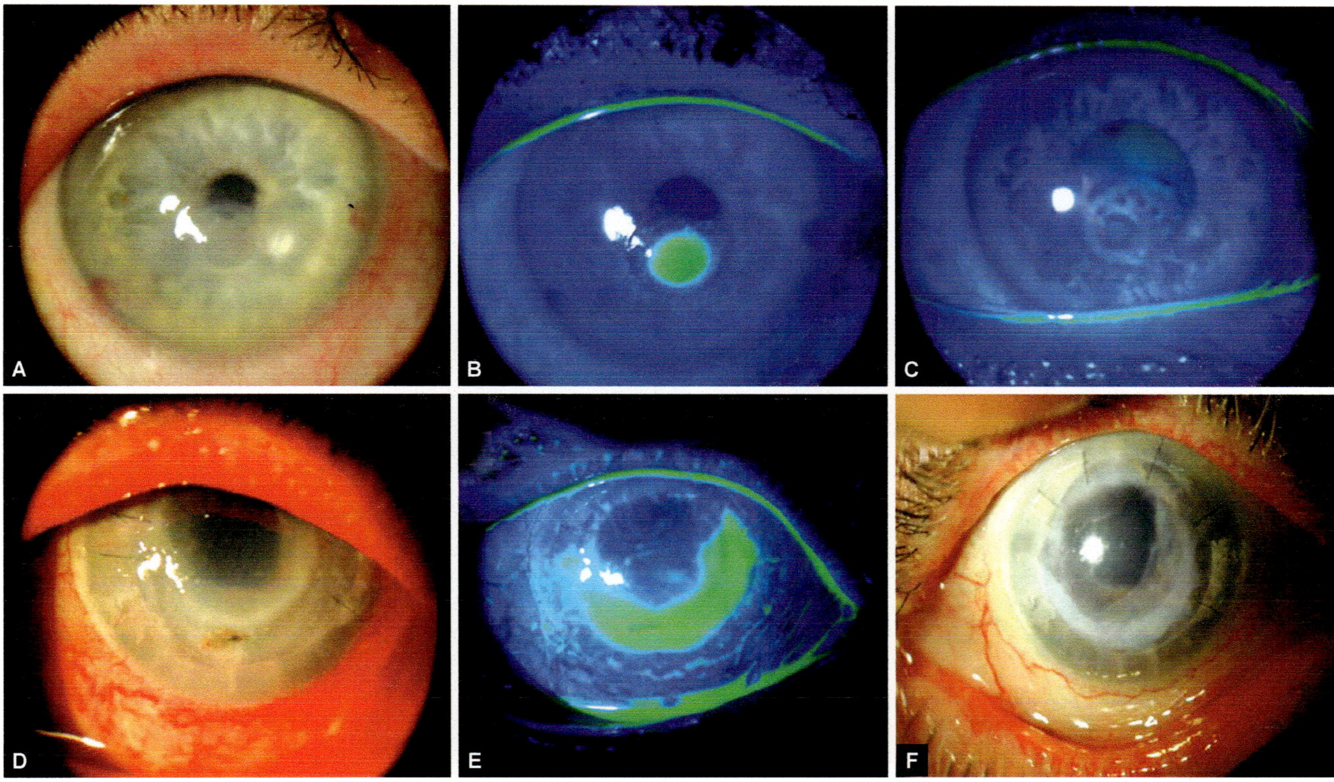

Figs. 2A to F: *Transplantation of amniotic membrane for persistent epithelial defects.* This eye developed superficial persistent corneal epithelial defect associated with corneal stromal neovascularization at 3- and 8-o'clock positions (A). Fluorescein staining showed a circumscribed defect (B). Overlay patch with AMT using PROKERA resulted in complete healing of the corneal surface with resolution of peripheral corneal neovascularization (C). This eye showed persistent epithelial defect associated with stromal ulceration at the donor-recipient junction (D and E). A temporary overlay AM using PROKERA was used together with an inlay graft to provide additional protection while ensuring epithelialization. Favorable outcomes ensued, with complete healing of the defect and resolution of inflammation (F).

postoperative astigmatism of tectonic corneal grafts, ease and convenience of use, feasibility in the event of corneal tissue shortage, and preservation of aesthetic appearance. Even if corneal transplantation is necessary, AMT reduces postoperative inflammation and promotes surgical success. When the corneal ulcer is superficial (e.g., limited to the epithelium), AMT as an overlay patch is generally sufficient in healing the ocular surface (**Figs. 2A to C**). However, when epithelial defects are accompanied by stromal ulceration, a temporary overlay AM is used together with an inlay graft to provide additional protection while promoting epithelialization (**Figs. 2D to F**).[8,9] When used as an inlay graft, a single layer or multiple layers of AM can be used.

A number of studies have shown that AMT has an average success rate of ~79% (range: 67–91%), and rapid healing is usually completed in 1–4 weeks.[8,10–22] In many cases, healing at the ulcer site is accompanied with a reduction in ocular inflammation and improvement in visual acuity. Variable success rates may be attributed to different underlying etiologies and concomitant or subsequent treatments in managing neurotrophic keratopathy. For example, AM rapidly dissolves (within 1 week) if there is severe exposure and dryness caused by neurotrophic keratopathy. The corneal surface breakdown is likely to recur if severe neurotrophic keratopathy is left untreated. Therefore, it is advised to perform punctal occlusion before AMT or temporary tarsorrhaphy at the time of AMT and add extended high DK contact lens or permanent tarsorrhaphy after healing with AMT. It should be noted that AMT alone is not sufficient to heal corneal epithelial defects caused by total limbal stem cell deficiency but can significantly reduce the amount of limbal stem cells needed for transplantation from the fellow eye.

Sterile Corneal Stromal Thinning, Descemetocele, and Perforation

For deeper stromal ulcers down to descemetocele, multiple layers of AM can be used to restore corneal thickness.[8,11,15,17,18,23,24] When there is frank perforation up to 3 mm in diameter, AMT may be used to seal the ulcer[17] with or without additional tissue adhesive[18,23] (**Figs. 3A and B**). Prabhasawat et al.[25] used multiple layers of AMT for corneal epithelial defects with stromal thinning (13 eyes) and corneal perforations up to 1 mm (5 eyes), achieving success rates of 84.6% and 80% in these two groups, respectively. Similarly, Solomon et al.[8] found 28 of 34 eyes (82.3%) with descemetoceles or corneal perforations less than 0.5 mm attained successful outcomes following 3–4 layers of AMT. Rodriguez-Ares et al.[17] used two layers of AM for perforations smaller than 0.5 mm (n = 6) and 3–4 layers for perforations

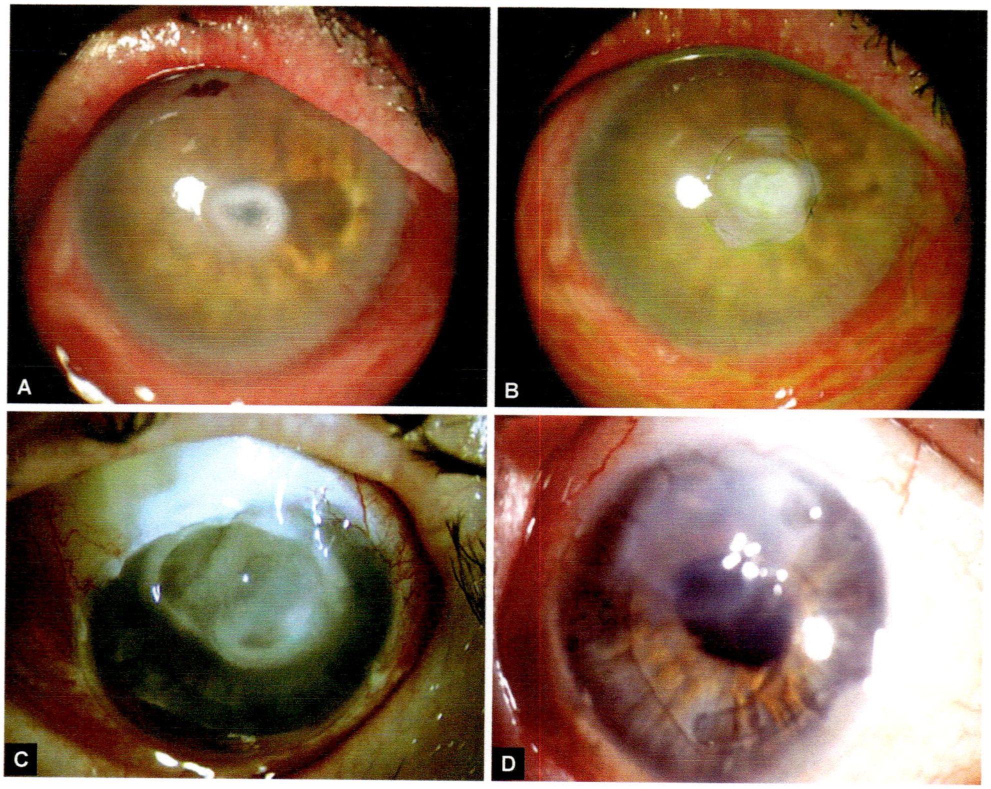

Figs. 3A to D: *Transplantation of amniotic membrane for descemetocele and infectious keratitis.* This eye had sterile corneal ulceration with descemetocele due to severe dry eye in Stevens-Johnson syndrome (A). Multiple layers of AM were laid in the ulcer bed, and a larger piece of AM was then placed over the ulcer and the healthy surface with the stromal side down and secured with a running 10-0 nylon suture onto the surrounding healthy tissue. This resulted in restoration of the normal corneal thickness (B). This eye developed descemetocele after glaucoma drainage implantation and pseudomonas infection (C). Multi-layer AMT restored corneal thickness and resulted in improved vision and a non-inflamed, healed surface without corneal transplantation (D).

>0.5 mm (n = 9) and observed success in 73% (11/15) of eyes. Three of the four failed cases (75%) involved perforations >3 mm in diameter; of the five eyes with perforations >1.5 mm in diameter, only two (40%) were successfully treated. Hick et al.[18] performed single-layer AMT with fibrin glue in 14 eyes with corneal perforation up to 3 mm in diameter, with 93% of perforations successfully sealed. Collectively, multiple layers of AM as an inlay graft, along with a larger AM overlay patch can be used for cases with stromal loss. Multilayered AMT is also reported to seal long-term corneal fistula, not amenable to tissue adhesives[26] (**Figs. 3A to D**).

Infectious Keratitis

Corneal ulcers with bacterial, fungal, or viral causes have been successfully managed with AMT with proper infection control (**Figs. 3C and D**). Chen et al.[27] performed AMT in six eyes with *Pseudomonas* keratitis associated with prominent stromal melting and extensive stromal loss. The lesion became sterile in five cases, with decreased inflammation and rapid re-epithelialization within 9.4 ± 2.1 days. After controlling the infection with proper antimicrobial treatment, Kim et al.[28] performed AMT in 21 eyes with infectious corneal ulcers caused by *Staphylococcus* species (n = 4), *Pseudomonas* species (n = 5), *Acanthamoeba* species (n = 3), fungi (n = 2), and herpes virus (n = 7). Prior to transplantation, the AM was soaked in anti-infective agents. Postoperatively, the corneal surface successfully healed in all cases without recurrence of microbial infection. Ma et al.[24] performed AMT in seven eyes with infectious corneal ulcers complicated with scleral melting (n = 4) or corneal perforation (n = 3) after appropriate treatment with topical and systemic antibiotics. Etiologies included *Pseudomonas* (n = 4), fungi (n = 2), and atypical *Mycobacterium* (n = 1). Following AMT, decreased melting and inflammation was observed at the lesion site and complete epithelialization was attained in 15.7 ± 8.7 days. No recurrent infection was encountered.

Chen et al.[29] performed AMT in 23 eyes with persistent corneal ulcers and perforations secondary to fungal infection during the active phase (positive culture) in 16 patients and during the inactive phase (negative fungal culture) in seven patients. A single-layer of AM was used in 17 patients, and a double-layer was used in six patients with corneal perforation and anterior chamber collapse. After AMT, complete epithelialization was observed in 12 patients (75%) in the active group and in all seven patients (100%) in the inactive group. Treatment failure requiring tectonic penetrating keratoplasty was observed in four patients (25%)

in the active group, with persistent fungal keratitis noted in two eyes. They concluded that AMT is effective in promoting epithelialization and preventing corneal perforations in acute fungal keratitis.

Experimental studies have shown that AMT results in rapid closure of epithelial defects and profound regression of corneal inflammation and neovascularization in eyes with necrotizing keratitis secondary to herpes simplex virus (HSV).[30,31] Heiligenhaus et al.[32] used AMT for the management of seven eyes with acute ulcerative and necrotizing herpes simplex and zoster stromal keratitis; improvement of stromal inflammation was noted after 16.4 ± 2.5 days, epithelialization occurred in 17 ± 2.7 days. In another study, Shi et al.[33] reported the use of multilayer AMT combined with antiviral and corticosteroid medications for the treatment of HSV necrotizing stromal keratitis. Corneal ulcers healed within 1–3 weeks postoperatively, and corneal stromal edema dissipated within 1 month.

Despite potential concerns that AM may prevent penetration of antimicrobial agents when treating infectious corneal ulcers, AM has been found to be permeable to drugs, acting as a reservoir that slowly releases antibiotics following impregnation.[34-37] In a study by Mencucci et al.[34] AM fragments soaked in netilmicin inhibited bacterial growth, with antibiotic uptake occurring rapidly in a dose-dependent manner. The drug was released from the membrane, and the antibacterial effect was present in the elution media at least 3 days after treatment. They concluded that AM can absorb this antibiotic and may be used in the future as a slow-releasing membrane to deliver antibiotics as reported for collagen shields and other medical prosthetic devices.

Symptomatic Bullous Keratopathy

Bullous keratopathy is caused by damage to the corneal endothelium due to a dystrophy (Fuch's endothelial dystrophy), surgical trauma, intractable glaucoma, or corneal graft failure. Eyes with recurrent erosions, poor visual potential, and inadequate pain relief often undergo surgical treatment with cauterization, anterior stromal puncture, excimer laser photoablation, or conjunctival flap. AMT has been shown to alleviate pain, with an overall success rate of more than 85%.[38-44] The AM-covered corneal surface heals in 3 weeks with reduced inflammation, with more than 90% of eyes exhibiting no recurrent breakdown of the ocular surface (**Figs. 4A and B**).

Espana et al.[41] performed AMT after epithelial debridement in 18 eyes with symptomatic bullous keratopathy. During a mean follow-up of 25.1 months, pain relief was obtained in 88% of patients. Complete corneal epithelial healing was attained in all except one eye (94.4%). Chansanti et al.[44] noted postoperative pain relief in 14 of 17 eyes (82.4%) with bullous keratopathy after AMT and complete corneal epithelial healing in 15 eyes (88.2%) during a mean follow-up of 14.1 months. Sonmez et al.[42] performed anterior stromal micropuncture and AMT in five eyes with painful bullous keratopathy. All eyes showed an intact, smooth corneal epithelial surface 1 month after the procedure without recurrence of bullae formation during an average follow-up period of 21 months.

Band Keratopathy

Band keratopathy is a chronic, degenerative condition characterized by the deposition of calcium salts in the subepithelial corneal stroma. Causes are either systemic or local, occurring in various corneal diseases marked by chronic inflammation. Conventional treatment includes superficial keratectomy to remove calcified deposits and corneal stromal tissue, which is often supplemented with EDTA chemical chelation to facilitate more complete removal of the calcium deposits. AMT following conventional treatment has been shown to alleviate pain in more than 90% of cases, restore a smooth, stable corneal epithelium, and improve vision in 27–44% of eyes (**Figs. 4C and D**).[45-49] In one case report by Esquenazi et al.,[49] a 91-year-old man with recurrent band and bullous keratopathy underwent surgical debridement followed by placement of AM with fibrin glue for recurrent, painful epithelial defects due to recurrent erosions. Wound healing was completed in 10 days, and a stable, transparent ocular surface was restored postoperatively without pain and recurrence for up to 9 months.

Partial Limbal Stem Cell Deficiency

The corneal epithelial stem cells are located exclusively at the limbus.[50] Destructive loss of the limbal epithelial stem cells and/or dysfunction of the limbal stroma results in limbal stem cell deficiency (LSCD), which is characterized by conjunctivalization over the corneal surface, vascularization, destruction of the basement membrane, chronic inflammation, and corneal scarring.[51] LSCD can be caused by a number of corneal conditions and diseases such as chemical and thermal burns, Stevens-Johnson syndrome, mucous membrane pemphigoid, severe microbial infections, radiation keratopathy, aniridia, etc. Conventional corneal transplantation invariably fails, as inflammation can cause graft rejection with no stem cells transplanted. In cases with *total* LSCD, transplantation of autologous or allogeneic limbal epithelial stem cells is required.[52,53] In eyes with *partial* LSCD, AMT alone can successfully reconstruct human corneas.[45-48,54-58] The idea of using AMT in such capacity was first demonstrated in a rabbit model of LSCD,[4,59] which suggested that AM aids in the expansion of residual limbal stem cells, thus avoiding the need for limbal stem cell transplantation (**Figs. 4E and F**). This also explains why AMT can be used to restore the donor eye undergoing removal of the normal limbus and the recipient eyes receiving conjunctival limbal autograft for

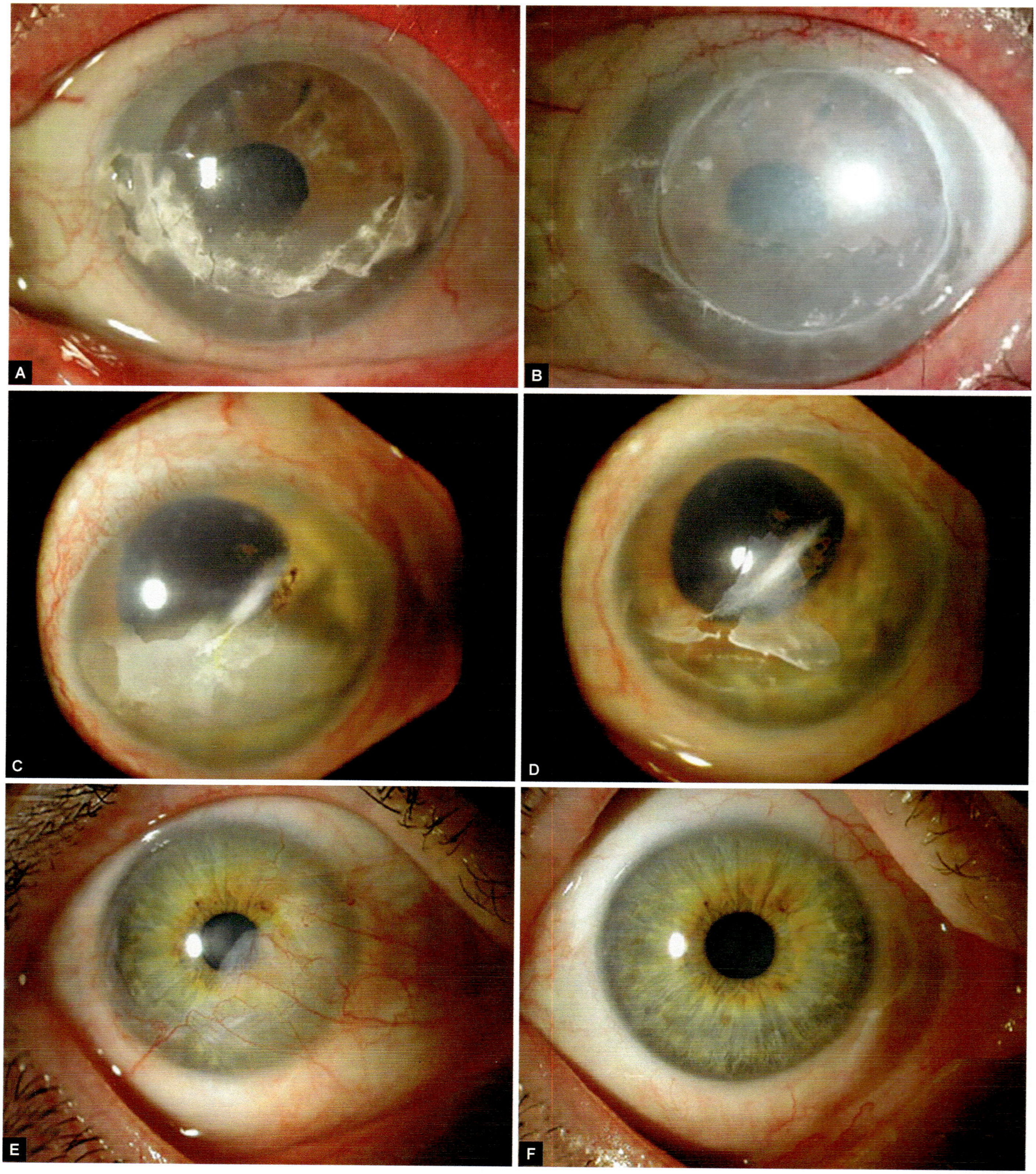

Figs. 4A to F: *Transplantation of amniotic membrane (AM) as an inlay graft to restore corneal integrity.* In this eye with combined band keratopathy and bullous keratopathy (A), the loose and calcified epithelium is removed by superficial keratectomy using a #64 blade. A superficial trephination is followed by a lamellar pocket created 360° toward the limbus by a crescent blade, and AM is inserted into this pocket and secured with a running 10-0 nylon suture, resulting in a non-inflamed, healed and stable corneal surface (B). In this eye, band keratopathy caused erosion and pain (C). Superficial keratectomy removed calcium deposits, and a layer of AM is secured on the denuded surface with fibrin glue. This sutureless AMT results in a smooth and stable corneal surface with less scarring (D). In this eye, there is partial limbal stem cell deficiency in the inferior cornea (E); after removal of pannus, AMT aids in the expansion of residual stem cells to attain a smooth corneal surface without necessitating stem cell transplantation (F).

unilateral *total* limbal stem cell deficiency.[60] The addition of AMT has reduced the necessary size of conjunctival limbal autograft for unilateral total LSCD to 60°.[61] Simple limbal epithelial transplantation (SLET) has been introduced more recently for unilateral partial or total LSCD, which involves fixing small pieces of a limbal graft on a single AM graft with fibrin glue or sandwiching them between two AM grafts.[62,63] The use of AM in SLET has successfully reduced the size of limbal stem cell removal from the fellow eye down to ~1 clock hour. Moreover, for bilateral *total* LSCD, AMT has been used in conjunction with keratolimbal allograft to facilitate re-epithelialization of the cornea.[55,64]

Ex Vivo Expansion of Epithelial Stem Cells

In 1997, Pellegrini et al.[65] used tissue culture techniques to cultivate epithelial cell sheets from a small limbus biopsy obtained from the healthy eyes of two patients with unilateral severe alkali burn injuries. The epithelial sheets were transplanted onto the damaged fellow-eyes, and the regenerated corneal epithelial autograft remained stable over a 2-year period. This *ex vivo* expansion technique of limbal tissue has obvious advantages in cases where there is limited availability of limbal tissue in a diseased donor eye and poses less potential risk to a healthy donor eye. There is also no risk of allograft rejection and no need for systemic immunosuppression.

Using AM as a substrate offers several favorable advantages over Pellegrini's original method, as AM assists with *ex vivo* expansion of limbal epithelial cells by providing:

- A natural, thick supporting substrate.
- Easier transfer of tissue graft from the laboratory to the operating room and onto the patient's eye.
- Unique biological actions of the AM on surrounding tissue.

The validity of this method has now been proven in culture systems,[66-68] laboratory animals,[69,70] and human patients.[71-73] The various techniques of ex vivo expansion including the steps of epithelial isolation, the expansion medium, the use of airlifting, and the use of additional feeder layers has been recently reviewed.[74] However, now that we understand the importance of limbal niche cells in supporting limbal epithelial cell function, it is important to re-examine these variables to ensure a surrogate niche has been restored and maintained to preserve cell function throughout expansion.[54]

AMNIOTIC MEMBRANE AS AN OVERLAY PATCH

The main indication of using AM as an *overlay patch* is to suppress ocular surface inflammation caused by various diseases and insults and ultimately promote epithelial healing with minimal or no scarring. As shown in **Box 2**, clinical indications include severe ocular surface inflammation and epithelial erosion caused by acute chemical and thermal burns[75-83] (**Figs. 5A to C**) and the acute stage of Stevens-Johnson syndrome (SJS)/toxic epidermal necrolysis (TEN)[84-86] (**Figs. 6A to C**). Conventional therapies for these diseases have limited success. In contrast, early intervention with AMT (e.g., within the first week) not only reduces inflammation and facilitates epithelial wound healing, but also prevents the late cicatricial complications that may cause corneal blindness, motility restriction in the conjunctiva, mechanical micro-trauma (by misdirected lashes and keratinization), and dryness in the lids and fornix.[85] As previously mentioned, AM as an overlay patch can be used without sutures through PROKERA to facilitate early intervention. Additional details about PROKERA and the different types will be discussed in the Procedural section next. Besides the aforementioned biological effects, PROKERA can be used as a symblepharon ring that reduces conjunctival inflammation/swelling following reconstruction of the orbit/socket, lids, or fornix.

In addition, cryopreserved AM can also be used as an *overlay patch* to treat chronic recalcitrant inflammation with or without persistent epithelial defect caused by several

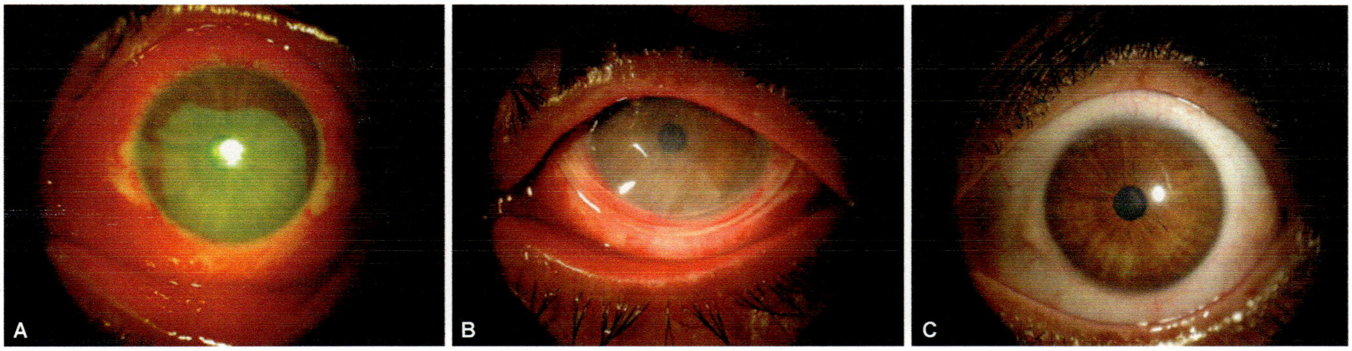

Figs. 5A to C: *Amniotic membrane transplantation (AMT) as an overlay patch for acute chemical burn.* Chemical injury with acid resulted in severe conjunctival inflammation and large corneal-limbal epithelial defect in this eye (A). AMT using PROKERA was done at 1 day after the burn (B). Complete epithelialization of the cornea with resolution of conjunctival inflammation was obviously observed 2 weeks after AMT (C).

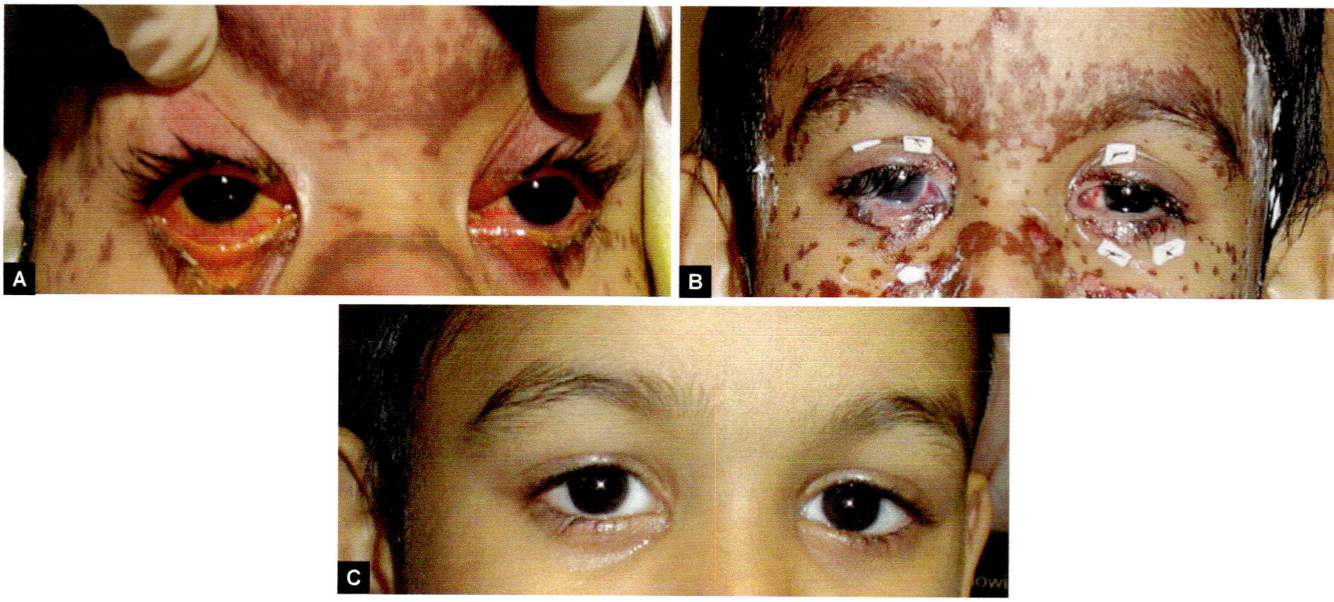

Figs. 6A to C: *Amniotic membrane transplantation (AMT) as an overlay patch for acute Stevens-Johnson syndrome.* This patient with acute manifestations of Stevens-Johnson syndrome had severe conjunctival inflammation with corneal epithelial defect in both eyes (A). AMT was used as an overlay patch to cover the entire ocular surface of both eyes within the first week of presentation (B). The ocular surface was completely restored with a 20/20 vision in both eyes (C).

ocular surface diseases including neurotrophic keratitis caused by herpes zoster virus or herpes simplex virus[30,87] and vernal keratoconjunctivitis.[88] When epithelial defects are accompanied with stromal ulceration, an overlay AM patch can be used together with an inlay graft to provide additional protection while ensuring epithelialization.[8] AM has been shown to promote healing and reduce inflammation in high-risk eyes receiving penetrating or lamellar keratoplasties,[87] reduce corneal haze induced by excimer laser ablation,[89-93] and improve implantation of keratoprosthesis.[94,95] Additionally, cryopreserved AM has been used as an overlay patch for bullous keratopathy, partial LSCD, epithelial basement membrane dystrophy, recurrent corneal erosions, graft versus host disease, and moderate-to-severe dry eye disease with corneal manifestations.

PROCUREMENT, PROCESSING, AND PRESERVATION OF AMNIOTIC MEMBRANE

To date, various procurement and processing methods have been developed for AM. In general, AM is procured from donors undergoing cesarian section with live, healthy babies after obtaining full informed consent. The mothers are generally screened at delivery for infectious, malignant, neurological and autoimmune diseases and other exposures or social habits to determine the suitability for human transplantation. The suitability of the donation is determined by reviewing medical records, physical examinations, and history of possible transmissible diseases. Mothers are also serologically tested at the time of delivery and must be non-reactive for HIV, Hepatitis B and C, West Nile Virus, HTLV 1 and 2, and syphilis using FDA licensed, approved, or cleared test kits.

The placenta is generally cleaned under aseptic conditions with Balanced Salt Solution, and the AM is separated from the chorion using blunt dissection. AM can be preserved using various methods including cryopreservation and dehydration. Cryopreservation refers to the storage and transportation of tissue at low temperatures with cryoprotectants, which devitalize the living cells but retains the natural structural and biological characteristics relevant to this tissue.[96,97] In contrast, dehydration commonly refers to subjecting the tissue to high temperatures to remove the moisture therein.[96]

PROCEDURAL TECHNIQUE

Amniotic membrane transplantation is conventionally performed using sutures when used as either an overlay or inlay. In this section, we will focus on the sutureless approach, which provides the following advantages: Shorter surgical time, feasibility of doing surgery under topical anesthesia, ease of postoperative care, and lack of suture-related complications, thus facilitating patient care and reducing overall medical costs.[98-100]

As an Inlay Graft

Amniotic membrane transplantation is performed using standard surgical instruments and microsurgical equipment. In the United States, AmnioGraft® (Bio-Tissue, Miami, FL) is the only cryopreserved AM recognized by the US Food and Drug Administration (FDA) with anti-inflammatory, anti-scarring, and anti-angiogenic properties for ocular surface reconstruction. Because the cryopreservation method of AmnioGraft® kills allogeneic amniotic cells,[97] the need for

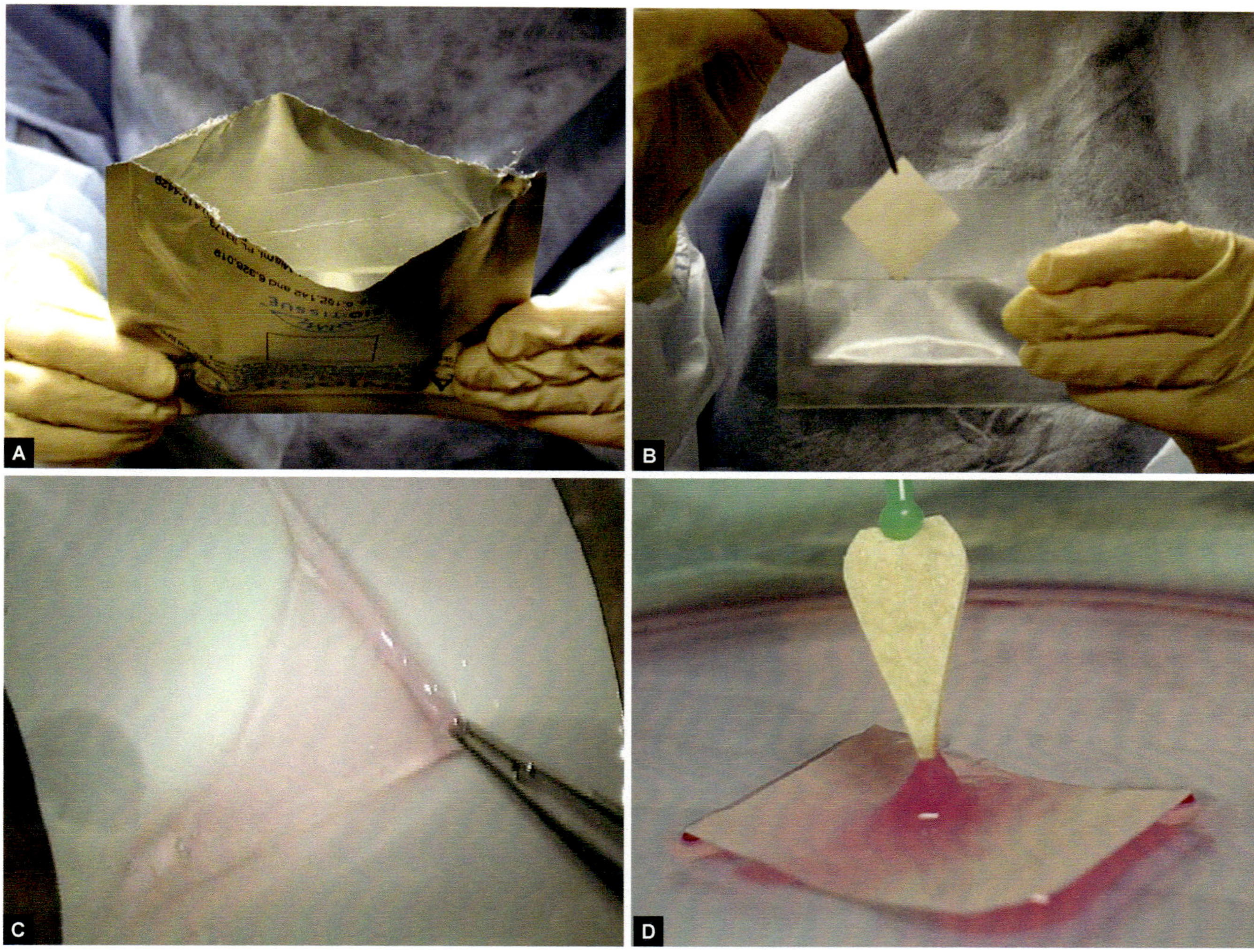

Figs. 7A to D: *Handling of cryopreserved amniotic membrane.* AmnioGraft® obtained from Bio-Tissue is stored in a foil package in a frozen state. After thawing at room temperature, the AM is aseptically retrieved from the inner clear plastic pouch, which is attached to one side of nitrocellulose paper (A and B). Once the AM has been transferred to the operating field, it can be easily peeled off the paper using two forceps to grab the corners while the nurse peels the paper away (C). In general, AmnioGraft® is placed with the stromal side on the recipient bed; the stromal side can be discerned using the tip of a dry surgical sponge. The stromal side, but not epithelial side, sticks to the sponge (D).

immunosuppression is eliminated while maintaining the integrity of its extracellular matrix.

AmnioGraft® comes in various sizes and can be selected based on the indication. AmnioGraft® is distributed in a foil package in a frozen state. After thawing at room temperature, it can be retrieved aseptically from the inner clear plastic pouch, and the membrane is attached to one side of nitrocellulose paper (**Figs. 7A to D**). Once transferred to the operating field, the membrane can be easily peeled off from the paper using two forceps to grab the two corners while the nurse peels the paper away. The tissue is immediately ready for transplantation after removing it from the carrier paper without the need for rehydration. In general, AmnioGraft® is placed with the stromal side on the recipient bed. The stromal side can be discerned by touching it with the tip of a dry surgical sponge such as MicroSponge™ or Weck-cel®; the stromal side, but not epithelial side, sticks to the sponge (*see* **Figs. 7A to D**).

Following Superficial Keratectomy

Topical anesthesia using 0.5% proparacaine hydrochloride, 0.5% tetracaine hydrochloride, or 2% xylocaine jelly (AstraZeneca, Wimington, DE) is adequate if AMT is performed without sutures using fibrin glue (e.g., Tisseel®, Artiss, EVICEL®) to secure AmnioGraft® to the corneal surface.

AmnioGraft® (1.5 × 1.0 cm or 2.0 × 1.5 cm size) can be used as a single layer to cover the defect produced by superficial keratectomy (**Fig. 8A**). For large defects, the AM is placed over the cornea with the stromal side down (**Fig. 8B**). Half of the membrane is folded over the other half, exposing the stromal surface (**Fig. 8C**). Thrombin solution is applied over the corneal surface (**Fig. 8D**), and fibrinogen solution is applied on the stromal surface of the membrane (**Fig. 8E**). This half of the membrane is flipped back using two forceps (**Fig. 8F**), and a muscle hook is used to stretch the membrane over the cornea (**Fig. 8G**). The same procedure is done for the other half of the membrane, and excess membrane is trimmed off (**Fig. 8H**). For

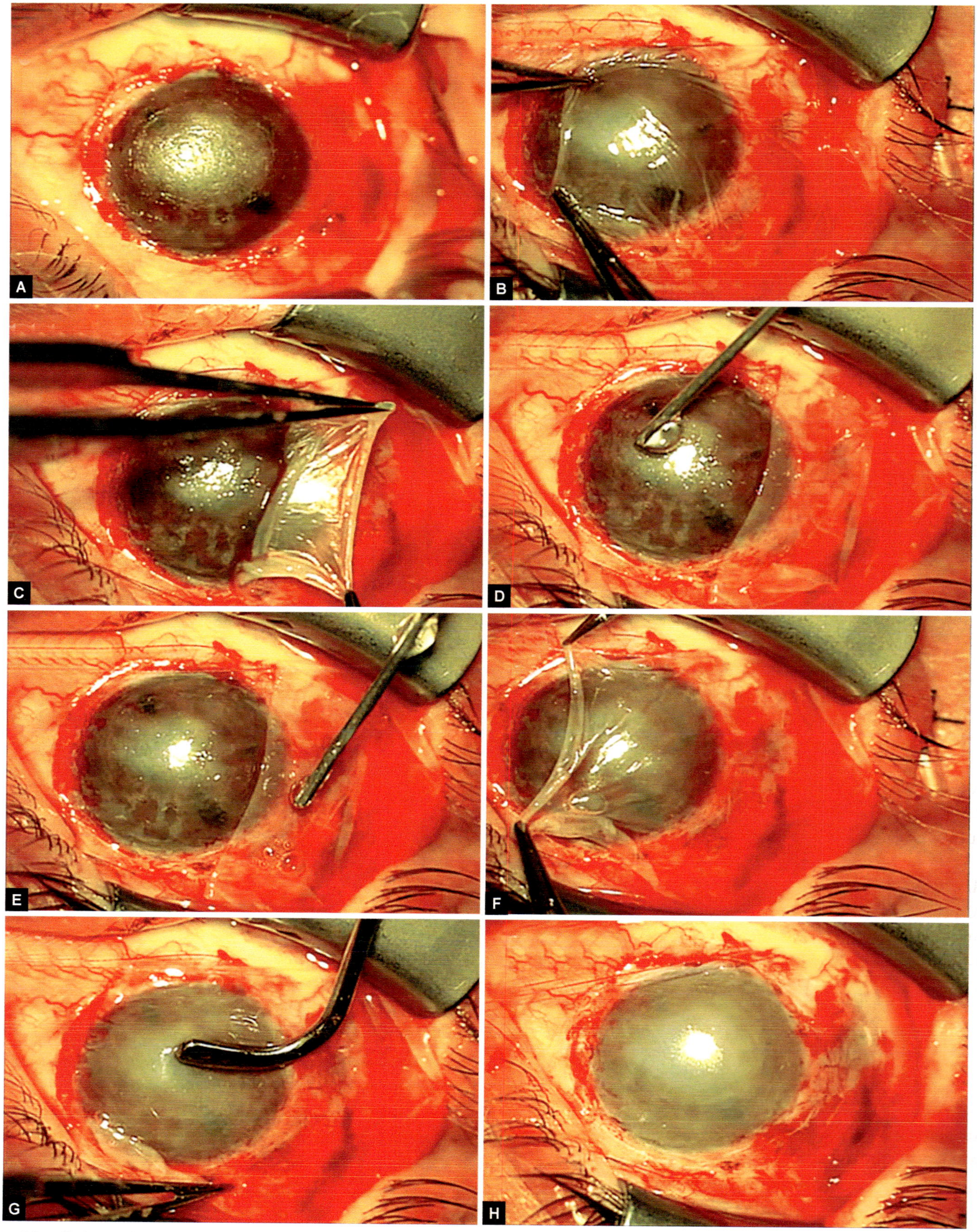

Figs. 8A to H: *Surgical steps of sutureless transplantation of cryopreserved amniotic membrane as an inlay graft to cover the corneal surface with Fibrin glue following superficial keratectomy.* After performing superficial keratectomy (A), AmnioGraft® is laid on the cornea with the stromal side facing down (B). Then, AM is flipped so that the stromal side is facing up (C). The thrombin solution is applied on the corneal surface (D) and the fibrinogen solution on the stromal side of the membrane (E). AmnioGraft® is then flipped back (F), and a muscle hook is used to flatten and attach the membrane onto the corneal surface (G). Excess amniotic membrane is trimmed off (H).

small defects, AmnioGraft® is trimmed to the size of the defect. The membrane is placed outside of the defect with stromal side up. After applying thrombin to the corneal surface and fibrinogen on the stromal side of the AM, the AM is placed over the defect stromal side down, and a muscle hook is used to stretch the membrane over the cornea.

For Corneal Ulcers

A single layer of AmnioGraft® (2.5 × 2.0 cm or 2.0 × 1.5 cm size) can be used for corneal ulcers or multiple layers can be used to fill in the stromal defect depending on the depth of the ulcer. The orientation of the bottom layers does not matter and can be secured using fibrin glue, while the top AM layer, which is intended to promote epithelialization, is placed with the stromal side down and secured tightly to the corneal surface with either interrupted or running 10-0 nylon sutures.

For Bullous and Band Keratopathy

To ensure that epithelialization will take place on top of the membrane, and not underneath, a lamellar pocket can be prepared with a crescent blade to enable insertion of the membrane. After removal of band keratopathy and bullous epithelium, a very superficial trephination is performed on the corneal surface. Afterwards, a 2 mm wide lamellar pocket is created in 360° of the cornea. AM is secured over the corneal surface and into the pocket using fibrin glue.

For Partial Limbal Stem Cell Deficiency

After removal of fibrovascular tissue from the corneal surface, AMT is performed similar to the procedure mentioned for superficial keratectomy.

About sutures: If fibrin glue is not used, the cryopreserved AM can be secured with several interrupted or running 10-0 nylon sutures on peri-limbal bulbar conjunctiva and with 8-0 Vicryl sutures in a mattress fashion, parallel to the fornix, with solid episcleral bites to seal the fornix border.

As an Overlay Patch

To Cover the Entire Ocular Surface

To cover both corneal and conjunctival surfaces, especially for acute chemical/thermal burns or acute SJS/TEN, two large pieces of AmnioGraft® (3.5 × 3.5 cm size) are needed. These grafts are secured to the skin surface of the upper lid margin with suture in an interrupted or running manner and then tugged into the upper fornix with a muscle hook and secured there by passing a double-armed 4-0 black silk or 6-0 polypropylene in a mattress fashion to the skin surface with a bolster (**Fig. 9**) (see Meller et al.[76]). The remaining AM is spread to cover the upper bulbar conjunctiva and part of the upper corneal surface. The other piece is secured to the lower lid and the lower fornix in a similar fashion; it is overlapped with the first AmnioGraft® on the corneal surface and secured with a 10-0 nylon suture in the same manner as described above. If there is an exposure concern due to large scleral exposure or infrequent blinking as a result of a neurotrophic state, temporary tarsorrhaphy can be utilized to minimize the lid fissure.

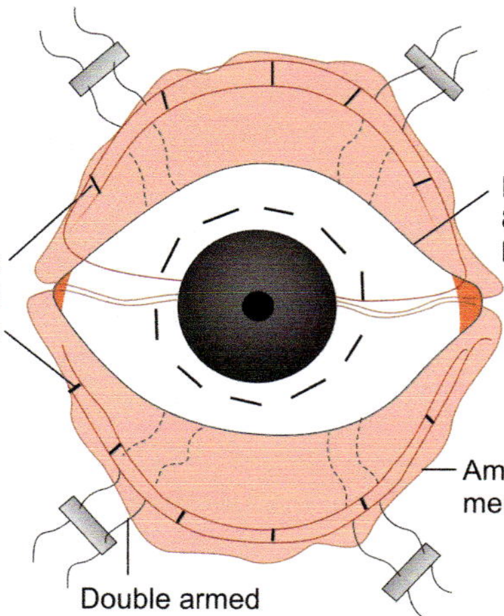

Fig. 9: *Amniotic membrane as an overlay patch to cover the entire ocular surface.* To cover both corneal and conjunctival surfaces, two large pieces of AmnioGraft® (3.5 × 3.5 cm size) are needed. One of these membranes is secured to the skin of the upper lid margin by a 10-0 nylon suture in an interrupted or running manner. It is then tugged into the upper fornix with a muscle hook and secured there by passing a double-armed 4-0 black silk in a mattress fashion to the skin surface with a bolster. The remaining AM is spread over the upper bulbar conjunctiva and part of the upper corneal surface. The other piece is secured to the lower lid and the lower fornix in a similar fashion, overlapped with the first AmnioGraft® on the corneal surface, and secured by a 10-0 nylon suture placed in the same manner as described above.

Shanbhag et al.[101,102] have described a combination of a custom made symblepharon ring to secure AM over the entire ocular surface and cyanoacrylate glue to secure AM to the eyelid margins in cases of acute SJS/TEN. It is a quick and painless bedside technique that can be performed under intravenous sedation and with topical anesthesia. The distance between the superior and the inferior fornix rims is calculated to determine the diameter of the symblepharon ring, which is made of intravenous (IV) tubing (Ultra Small Bore Extension Sets, Reference Number MX453HL, Smiths Medical, Dublin, OH). One end of the IV tubing is cut with an oblique beveled edge which is threaded into the straight edge. Instead of gluing the AM to the eyelid margin, one may use 4-0 black silk or 6-0 polypropylene mattress sutures and bolsters.

To Cover Only the Corneal Surface

AmnioGraft® (2.5 × 2.0 cm size) is secured using a 10-0 nylon suture 2–3 mm from the limbus in a purse-string running fashion for a total of 8–10 episcleral bites, covering the corneal surface as a biological bandage.

PROKERA

PROKERA is a self-retaining biologic corneal bandage comprised of a cryopreserved AM fastened to a dual polycarbonate ring system, allowing the membrane to act as a biological bandage when in contact with the cornea. PROKERA obtained clearance as a Class II Medical Device on December 12, 2003 in the USA and is a Class IV medical device regulated by Health Canada. The PROKERA family comprises four device models: PROKERA, PROKERA Plus, PROKERA Slim, and PROKERA Clear. The PROKERA Plus model has two AM layers, providing double thickness. Both PROKERA Slim and PROKERA Clear have smaller thickness rings (less plastic). PROKERA Clear has central aperture clearance.

With availability of this device, AMT as an overlay patch can be done at the bedside or at the office without any need for operation room facilities. Placement of PROKERA is described within the Current Procedural Terminology (CPT) procedure code 65778, "Placement of membrane on the ocular surface; without sutures" and is considered to be a covered service, subject to medical necessity criteria by Medicare, Medicaid, and nearly all commercial health insurance plans. While individual plan coverage policies vary, the most commonly covered uses include the following: neurotrophic keratitis;[103] corneal ulcers and melts;[103-105] after corneal transplantation;[106] bullous keratopathy; partial limbal stem cell deficiency;[61,107] acute SJS with primary corneal involvement;[108-114] recurrent corneal erosions;[115,116] persistent corneal epithelial defects; [103] severe dry eye (DEWS 3 or 4) with ocular surface damage and inflammation;[103] and acute ocular chemical/thermal burn.[103,117-120]

For PROKERA insertion, first allow the PROKERA to sit at controlled room temperature (20–25°C) in its original, unopened packaging for at least 5 minutes to allow the AM to thaw. Next, peel open the lid, and handle the tray using aseptic techniques. Discard the storage media contained within the tray. Thoroughly rinse the PROKERA device while inside the tray with sterile saline solution to remove the storage media. Remove the center retainer piece from the tray to access the PROKERA device. For insertion into the eye, topical anesthetic eye drops are instilled, and a lid speculum is used to open the eye. Conversely, the physician can use their hands to hold the upper eyelid. Then, PROKERA is inserted into the upper superior fornix while the patient is looking downward, and then it is tucked under the lower lid. The PROKERA device should be checked to ensure it is properly centered over the cornea. If not properly centered, the physician should move the device or perform a tape-tarsorrhaphy over the lid creases to limit movement of the device over the cornea.

Postoperative Care

Postoperative care varies depending on the clinical setting in which AMT is performed. On the first postoperative day, medications can be prescribed such as prednisolone acetate 1% tapered over 6–8 weeks and broad-spectrum antibiotics for the first 1–2 weeks until the epithelium heals. There is no need for any systemic immunosuppressants. During the postoperative course, corneal epithelialization can be assessed using fluorescein staining[121] (*see* **Fig. 1C**), and intraocular pressure can be monitored without removing PROKERA or AmnioGraft® using Tonopen.[122] When used as an overlay, the AM does reduce light transmission, causing blurry vision. For patients with additional nocturnal exposure (e.g., lagophthalmos), pressure patching is recommended, especially for sunken globes. A rigid eye shield should be used for floppy eye lids prior to sleeping.

Upon complete healing in 1–2 weeks times, PROKERA can be easily removed from the ocular surface with forceps under a slit-lamp microscope. Severe ocular inflammation or dryness can result in early dissolution of the AM; causes that are often overlooked include floppy eyelid syndrome and sunken globes. For the former, delayed tear clearance should be ruled out especially if excessive discharge was present prior to PROKERA use and additional inflammation can be mitigated with additional non-preserved steroids. If the AM is dissolved (due to dryness or inflammation) or cloudy (due to attracting inflammatory cells), the PROKERA should be removed and a new one inserted if medically necessary. For eyes with severe neurotrophic keratopathy or incomplete blinking, a small permanent tarsorrhaphy may be necessary.

Complications and Limitations

When using AM as an inlay graft, the healing process is also dependent on the surrounding host tissue, as the cryopreserved AM does not contain live cells and requires migration of host epithelial cells. Therefore, if the surrounding tissue is intrinsically abnormal, e.g., severe squamous metaplasia with frank keratinization, healing of the AM-covered area may not be normal unless AMT is performed with adjunctive measures such as conjunctival autograft. Furthermore, if there is total LSCD, AMT along with transplanted stem cells is needed. Premature AM degradation or displacement may warrant repeated transplant or adjunctive treatment such as tarsorrhaphy as mentioned above. The degree of ocular dryness and exposure are limiting factors that should be addressed. Lastly, as with the use of any human tissue, the possibility of infectious agent transmission cannot be completely eliminated, although screening and microbial testing are performed as mentioned in the section PROCUREMENT, PROCESSING AND PRESERVATION.[123] Overall, AM can be used to promote epithelial healing and reduce inflammation, scarring, and unwanted angiogenesis on the ocular surface. AM can be used either as an inlay or overlay Patch for many indications such as such as keratitis, band keratopathy, burns, keratoconjunctivitis, ulcers, basement membrane dystrophy, LSCD, epithelial defects, corneal erosion, SJS/TEN, Sjogren syndrome, filamentary keratitis, and HSV keratitis. When using the AM sheet, 0.12-mm forceps and smooth conjunctival forceps can be used to maneuver and affix the tissue to the cornea with fibrin glue, 10-0 nylon sutures, or 8-0 Vicryl sutures. Alternatively, self-retained AM in the form of PROKERA can be applied without sutures in the office, bedside, emergency room, intensive care unit, burn unit, or where it may not be amenable to bring the patient to the operating room due to medical reasons. With PROKERA, the epithelial healing process is generally complete within 1-3 weeks depending on the indication.

REFERENCES

1. de Rotth A. Plastic repair of conjunctival defects with fetal membrane. Arch Ophthalmol. 1940;23:522-5.
2. Sorsby A. Amniotic membrane grafts in burns. In: Sorsby A (Ed). Modern Trends in Ophthalmology. Vol. II ed. New York: Paul B. Hoeber, Inc., 1947, pp. 504-10.
3. Sorsby A, Symons H. Amniotic membrane grafts in caustic burns of the eye: (Burns of the second degree). Br J Ophthalmol. 1946;30:337.
4. Kim JC, Tseng SC. Transplantation of preserved human amniotic membrane for surface reconstruction in severely damaged rabbit corneas. Cornea. 1995;14:473-84.
5. Tighe S, Mead O, Lee A, Tseng S. Basic Science Review of Birth Tissue Uses in Ophthalmology. Taiwan J Ophthalmol. 2020;10.
6. Tseng SC, He H, Zhang S, Chen SY. Niche Regulation of Limbal Epithelial Stem Cells: Relationship between Inflammation and Regeneration. Ocul Surf. 2016;14:100-12.
7. Solomon A, Touhami A, Sandoval H, Tseng SCG. Neurotrophic keratopathy: basic concepts and therapeutic strategies. Comp Ophthalmol Update. 2000;3:165-74.
8. Solomon A, Meller D, Prabhasawat P, John T, Espana EM, Steuhl KP, et al. Amniotic membrane grafts for nontraumatic corneal perforations, descemetoceles, and deep ulcers. Ophthalmology. 2002;109:694-703.
9. Heinz C, Eckstein A, Steuhl KP, Meller D. Amniotic membrane transplantation for reconstruction of corneal ulcer in graves ophthalmopathy. Cornea. 2004;23:524-6.
10. Lee SH, Tseng SC. Amniotic membrane transplantation for persistent epithelial defects with ulceration. Am J Ophthalmol. 1997;123:303-12.
11. Kruse FE, Rohrschneider K, Völcker HE. Multilayer amniotic membrane transplantation for reconstruction of deep corneal ulcers. Ophthalmology. 1999;106:1504-11.
12. Azuara-Blanco A, Pillai CT, Dua HS. Amniotic membrane transplantation for ocular surface reconstruction. Br J Ophthalmol. 1999;8339:399-402.
13. Gabric N, Mravicic I, Dekaris I, Karaman Z, Mitrovic S. Human amniotic membrane in the reconstruction of the ocular surface. Doc Ophthalmol. 1999;98:273-83.
14. Chen HJ, Pires RTF, Tseng SCG. Amniotic membrane transplantation for severe neurotrophic corneal ulcers. Br J Ophthalmol. 2000;84:826-33.
15. Hanada K, Shimazaki J, Shimmura S, Tsubota K. Multilayered amniotic membrane transplantation for severe ulceration of the cornea and sclera. Am J Ophthalmol. 2001;131:324-31.
16. Letko E, Stechschulte SU, Kenyon KR, Sadeq N, Romero TR, Samson CM, et al. Amniotic membrane inlay and overlay grafting for corneal epithelial defects and stromal ulcers. Arch Ophthalmol. 2001;119:659-63.
17. Rodriguez-Ares MT, Tourino R, Lopez-Valladares MJ, Gude F. Multilayer amniotic membrane transplantation in the treatment of corneal perforations. Cornea. 2004;23:577-83.
18. Hick S, Data L, Brunette I, La C, Mabon M, Duchesne B. Amniotic membrane transplantation and fibrin glue in the management of corneal ulcers and perforations: a review of 33 cases. Cornea. 2005;24:369-77.
19. Seitz B, Das S, Sauer R, Mena D, Hofmann-Rummelt C. Amniotic membrane transplantation for persistent corneal epithelial defects in eyes after penetrating keratoplasty. Eye. 2009;23:840-8.
20. Nubile M, Dua HS, Lanzini M, Ciancaglini M, Calienno R, Said DG, et al. In vivo analysis of stromal integration of multilayer amniotic membrane transplantation in corneal ulcers. Am J Ophthalmol. 2011;151:809-22.e1.
21. Turkoglu E, Celik E, Alagoz G. A comparison of the efficacy of autologous serum eye drops with amniotic membrane transplantation in neurotrophic keratitis. Semin Ophthalmol. 2014;29:119-26.
22. Schuerch K, Baeriswyl A, Frueh BE, Tappeiner C. Efficacy of Amniotic Membrane Transplantation for the Treatment of Corneal Ulcers. Cornea. 2020;39:479-83.
23. Duchesne B, Tahi H, Galand A. Use of human fibrin glue and amniotic membrane transplant in corneal perforation. Cornea. 2001;20:230-2.
24. Ma DH-K, Wang SF, Su WY, Tsai RJF. Amniotic membrane graft for the management of scleral melting and corneal perforation in recalcitrant infectious scleral and corneoscleral ulcers. Cornea. 2002;21:275-83.
25. Prabhasawat P, Tesavibul N, Komolsuradej W. Single and multilayer amniotic membrane transplantation for persistent corneal epithelial defect with and without stromal thinning and perforation. Br J Ophthalmol. 2001;85:1455-63.
26. Peraka RP, Kalra P. Multilayered amniotic membrane transplantation in a case of chronic corneal fistula. BMJ Case Rep. 2020;13.
27. Chen JH, Ma DH, Tsai RJ. Amniotic membrane transplantation for pseudomonal keratitis with impending perforation. Chang Gung Med J. 2002;25:144-52.
28. Kim JS, Kim JC, Hahn TW, Park WC. Amniotic membrane transplantation in infectious corneal ulcer. Cornea. 2001;20:720-6.
29. Chen HC, Tan HY, Hsiao CH, Huang SC, Lin KK, Ma DH. Amniotic membrane transplantation for persistent corneal ulcers and perforations in acute fungal keratitis. Cornea. 2006;25:564-72.
30. Heiligenhaus A, Bauer D, Meller D, Steuhl KP, Tseng SC. Improvement of HSV-1 necrotizing keratitis with amniotic membrane transplantation. Invest Ophthalmol Vis Sci. 2001;42:1969-74.
31. Heiligenhaus A, Li H, Yang Y, Wasmuth S, Bauer D, Steuhl KP. [Amniotic membrane transplantation improves experimental herpetic keratitis. Modulation of matrix metalloproteinase-9]. Ophthalmologe. 2004;101:59-65.
32. Heiligenhaus A, Li H, Hernandez Galindo EE, Koch JM, Steuhl KP, Meller D. Management of acute ulcerative and necrotising herpes simplex and zoster keratitis with amniotic membrane transplantation. Br J Ophthalmol. 2003;87:1215-9.
33. Shi WY, Chen M, Wang FH, Zhao J, Ma L, Xie LX. [Multilayer amniotic membrane transplantation for treatment of necrotizing herpes simplex stromal keratitis]. Zhonghua YanKeZa Zhi. 2005;41:1107-11.
34. Mencucci R, Menchini U, Dei R. Antimicrobial activity of antibiotic-treated amniotic membrane: An in vitro study. Cornea. 2006;25:428-31.
35. Kim H-S, Sah W-J, Kim Y-J, Kim J-C, Hahn T-W. Amniotic membrane, tear film, corneal, and aqueous levels of ofloxacin in rabbit eyes after amniotic membrane transplantation. Cornea. 2001;20:628-34.

36. Resch MD, Resch BE, Csizmazia E, Imre L, Németh J, Szabó-Révész P, et al. Drug reservoir function of human amniotic membrane. J Ocul Pharmacol Ther. 2011;27:323-6.
37. Sara SH, Prajna NV, Senthilkumari S. Human amniotic membrane as a drug carrier - An in-vitro study using fortified cefazolin ophthalmic solution. Indian J Ophthalmol. 2019;67:472-5.
38. Pires RTF, Tseng SCG, Prabhasawat P, Puangsricharern V, Maskin SL, Kim JC, et al. Amniotic membrane transplantation for symptomatic bullous keratopathy. Arch Ophthalmol. 1999;117:1291-7.
39. Mrukwa-Kominek E, Gierek-Ciaciura S, Rokita-Wala I, Szymkowiak M. [Use of amniotic membrane transplantation for treating bullous keratopathy]. Klin Oczna. 2002;104:41-6.
40. Mejia LF, Santamaria JP, Acosta C. Symptomatic management of postoperative bullous keratopathy with nonpreserved human amniotic membrane. Cornea. 2002;21:342-5.
41. Espana EM, Grueterich M, Sandoval H, Solomon A, Alfonso E, Karp CL, et al. Amniotic membrane transplantation for bullous keratopathy in eyes with poor visual potential. J Cataract Refract Surg. 2003;29:279-84.
42. Sonmez B, Kim BT, Aldave AJ. Amniotic membrane transplantation with anterior stromal micropuncture for treatment of painful bullous keratopathy in eyes with poor visual potential. Cornea. 2007;26:227-9.
43. Shalabi N, Karp CL, Aziz H, Jeng BH, Galor A. Superficial epithelial keratectomy, cautery, and amniotic membrane transplant for the treatment of painful bullous keratopathy in eyes with poor visual potential. Cornea. 2014;33:755-9.
44. Chansanti O, Horatanaruang O. The results of amniotic membrane transplantation for symptomatic bullous keratopathy. J Med Assoc Thai. 2005;88 Suppl 9:S57-S62.
45. Anderson DF, Prabhasawat P, Alfonso E, Tseng SCG. Amniotic membrane transplantation after the primary surgical management of band keratopathy. Cornea. 2001;20:354-61.
46. Prabhasawat P, Kosrirukvongs P, Booranapong W, Vajaradul Y. Amniotic membrane transplantation for ocular surface reconstruction. J Med Assoc Thai. 2001;84:705-18.
47. Tosi GM, Traversi C, Schuerfeld K, Mittica V, Massaro-Giordano M, et al. Amniotic membrane graft: histopathological findings in five cases. J Cell Physiol. 2005;202:852-7.
48. Kwon YS, Song YS, Kim JC. New treatment for band keratopathy: superficial lamellar keratectomy, EDTA chelation and amniotic membrane transplantation. J Korean Med Sci. 2004;19:611-5.
49. Esquenazi S, Rand W, Velazquez G, Grunstein L. Novel therapeutic approach in the management of band keratopathy using amniotic membrane transplantation with fibrin glue. Ophthalmic Surg. Lasers Imaging. 2008;39:418-21.
50. Lavker RM, Tseng SC, Sun TT. Corneal epithelial stem cells at the limbus: looking at some old problems from a new angle. Exp Eye Res. 2004;78:433-46.
51. Puangsricharern V, Tseng SC. Cytologic evidence of corneal diseases with limbal stem cell deficiency. Ophthalmology. 1995;102:1476-85.
52. Tseng SC. Regulation and clinical implications of corneal epithelial stem cells. Mol Biol Rep. 1996;23:47-58.
53. Holland EJ, Schwartz GS. Changing concepts in the management of severe ocular surface disease over twenty-five years. Cornea. 2000;19:688-98.
54. Tseng SCG, Chen SY, Mead OG, Tighe S. Niche regulation of limbal epithelial stem cells: HC-HA/PTX3 as surrogate matrix niche. Exp Eye Res. 2020;199:108181.
55. Tseng SC, Prabhasawat P, Barton K, Gray T, Meller D. Amniotic membrane transplantation with or without limbal allografts for corneal surface reconstruction in patients with limbal stem cell deficiency. Arch Ophthalmol (Chicago, Ill: 1960). 1998;116:431-41.
56. Anderson DF, Ellies P, Pires RT, Tseng SC. Amniotic membrane transplantation for partial limbal stem cell deficiency. Br J Ophthalmol. 2001;85:567-75.
57. Gomes JA, dos Santos MS, Cunha MC, Mascaro VL, Barros JN, de Sousa LB. Amniotic membrane transplantation for partial and total limbal stem cell deficiency secondary to chemical burn. Ophthalmology. 2003;110:466-73.
58. Sangwan VS, Matalia HP, Vemuganti GK, Rao GN. Amniotic membrane transplantation for reconstruction of corneal epithelial surface in cases of partial limbal stem cell deficiency. Indian J Ophthalmol. 2004;52:281-5.
59. Kim JC, Tseng SCG. The effects on inhibition of corneal neovascularization after human amniotic membrane transplantation in severely damaged rabbit corneas. Korean J Ophthalmol. 1995;9:32-46.
60. Meallet MA, Espana EM, Grueterich M, Ti SE, Goto E, Tseng SC. Amniotic membrane transplantation with conjunctival limbal autograft for total limbal stem cell deficiency. Ophthalmology. 2003;110:1585-92.
61. Kheirkhah A, Raju VK, Tseng SC. Minimal conjunctival limbal autograft for total limbal stem cell deficiency. Cornea. 2008;27:730-3.
62. Sangwan VS, Basu S, MacNeil S, Balasubramanian D. Simple limbal epithelial transplantation (SLET): a novel surgical technique for the treatment of unilateral limbal stem cell deficiency. Br J Ophthalmol. 2012;96:931-4.
63. Amescua G, Atallah M, Nikpoor N, Galor A, Perez V. Modified Simple Limbal Epithelial Transplantation Using Cryopreserved Amniotic Membrane for Unilateral Limbal Stem Cell Deficiency. Am J Ophthalmol. 2014;158:469-75.
64. Tsubota K, Satake Y, Ohyama M, Toda I, Takano Y, Ono M, et al. Surgical reconstruction of the ocular surface in advanced ocular cicatricial pemphigoid and Stevens-Johnson syndrome. Am J Ophthalmol. 1996;122:38-52.
65. Pellegrini G, Traverso CE, Franzi AT, Zingirian M, Cancedda R, De Luca M. Long-term restoration of damaged corneal surface with autologous cultivated corneal epithelium. Lancet (London, England). 1997;349:990-3.
66. Koizumi N, Fullwood NJ, Bairaktaris G, Inatomi T, Kinoshita S, Quantock AJ. Cultivation of corneal epithelial cells on intact and denuded human amniotic membrane. Invest Ophthalmol Vis Sci. 2000;41:2506-13.
67. Meller D, Pires RT, Tseng SC. Ex vivo preservation and expansion of human limbal epithelial stem cells on amniotic membrane cultures. Br J Ophthalmol. 2002;86:463-71.
68. Wang DY, Hsueh YJ, Yang VC, Chen JK. Propagation and phenotypic preservation of rabbit limbal epithelial cells on amniotic membrane. Invest Ophthalmol Vis Sci. 2003;44: 4698-704.
69. Koizumi N, Inatomi T, Quantock AJ, Fullwood NJ, Dota A, Kinoshita S. Amniotic membrane as a substrate for cultivating limbal corneal epithelial cells for autologous transplantation in rabbits. Cornea. 2000;19:65-71.
70. Pan Z, Zhang W, Wu Y. [An experimental study on treatment of limbal alkali burn by allograft transplantation with cultured stem cells on amniotic membrane]. Zhonghua YanKeZa Zhi. 2000;36:32-5, 3.
71. Tsai RJ, Li LM, Chen JK. Reconstruction of damaged corneas by transplantation of autologous limbal epithelial cells. N Engl J Med. 2000;343:86-93.
72. Shimazaki J, Aiba M, Goto E, Kato N, Shimmura S, Tsubota K. Transplantation of human limbal epithelium cultivated on amniotic membrane for the treatment of severe ocular surface disorders. Ophthalmology. 2002;109:1285-90.
73. Nakamura T, Koizumi N, Tsuzuki M, Inoki K, Sano Y, Sotozono C, et al. Successful regrafting of cultivated corneal epithelium using

amniotic membrane as a carrier in severe ocular surface disease. Cornea. 2003;22:70-1.

74. Tseng SC, Chen SY, Shen YC, Chen WL, Hu FR. Critical appraisal of ex vivo expansion of human limbal epithelial stem cells. Curr Mol Med. 2010;10:841-50.
75. Kim JS, Kim JC, Na BK, Jeong JM, Song CY. Amniotic membrane patching promotes healing and inhibits proteinase activity on wound healing following acute corneal alkali burn. Exp Eye Res. 2000;70:329-37.
76. Meller D, Pires RTF, Mack RJS, Figueiredo F, Heiligenhaus A, Park WC, et al. Amniotic membrane transplantation for acute chemical or thermal burns. Ophthalmology. 2000;107:980-90.
77. Sridhar MS, Bansal AK, Sangwan VS, Rao GN. Amniotic membrane transplantation in acute chemical and thermal injury. Am J Ophthalmol. 2000;130:134-7.
78. Kobayashi A, Shirao Y, Yoshita T, Yagami K, Segawa Y, Kawasaki K, et al. Temporary amniotic membrane patching for acute chemical burns. Eye. 2003;17:149-58.
79. Pan DP, Li XX, Xu JF. [Therapeutic effect of amniotic membrane transplantation for ocular burn]. Zhongguo XiuFu ChongJianWai KeZa Zhi. 2003;17:318-20.
80. Arora R, Mehta D, Jain V. Amniotic membrane transplantation in acute chemical burns. Eye. 2005;19:273-8.
81. Katircioglu YA, Budak K, Salvarli S, Duman S. Amniotic membrane transplantation to reconstruct the conjunctival surface in cases of chemical burn. Jpn J Ophthalmol. 2003;47:519-22.
82. Tejwani S, Kolari RS, Sangwan VS, Rao GN. Role of amniotic membrane graft for ocular chemical and thermal injuries. Cornea. 2007;26:21-6.
83. Prabhasawat P, Tesavibul N, Prakairungthong N, Booranapong W. Efficacy of amniotic membrane patching for acute chemical and thermal ocular burns. J Med Assoc Thai. 2007;90:319-26.
84. John T, Foulks GN, John ME, Cheng K, Hu D. Amniotic membrane in the surgical management of acute toxic epidermal necrolysis. Ophthalmology. 2002;109:351-60.
85. Di Pascuale M. Correlation of corneal complications with eyelipid cicatricial pathologies in patients with Steven Johnson syndrome and toxic epidermal necrolysis syndrome. Ophthalmology. 2005.
86. Kobayashi A, Yoshita T, Sugiyama K, Miyashita K, Niida Y, Koizumi S, et al. Amniotic membrane transplantation in acute phase of toxic epidermal necrolysis with severe corneal involvement. Ophthalmology. 2006;113:126-32.
87. Kenyon KR. Amniotic membrane: mother's own remedy for ocular surface disease. Cornea. 2005;24:639-42.
88. Sridhar MS, Sangwan VS, Bansal AK, Rao GN. Amniotic membrane transplantation in the management of shield ulcers of vernal keratoconjunctivitis. Ophthalmology. 2001;108:1218-22.
89. Hong JW, Kang SM, Kim HJ, Kim HM. The effect of phototherapeutic keratectomy (PTK)-photorefractive keratectomy (PRK)-amniotic membrane transplantation (AMT) on myopic regression with corneal opacity after PRK in high myopia. Invest Ophthalmol Vis Sci. 1998;39:S354.
90. Kim JY, Wee WR, Choi YS, Lee JH. Clinical outcome of photorefractive keratectomy (PRK) retreatment using amniotic membrane. Ophthalmology. 1998:162.
91. Choi YS, Kim JY, Wee WR, Lee JH. Effect of the application of human amniotic membrane on rabbit corneal wound healing after excimer laser photorefractive keratectomy. Cornea. 1998;17:389-95.
92. Park WC, Tseng SC. Modulation of acute inflammation and keratocyte death by suturing, blood, and amniotic membrane in PRK. Invest Ophthalmol Vis Sci. 2000;41:2906-14.
93. Wang MX, Gray TB, Parks WC, Prabhasawat P, Culbertson W, Forster R, et al. Corneal haze and apoptosis is reduced by amniotic membrane matrix in excimer laser photoablation in rabbits. J Cat Refract Surg. 2001;27:310-9.
94. Kaminski SL, Lacombe E, Duchesne B, Fernandez V, Lamar P, Lee W, et al. Supradescemetic keratoprosthesis (SD-Kpro): A novel design. Invest Ophthalmol Vis Sci. 2002;43:2993.
95. Navas A, Hernandez-Camarena JC, Serna-Ojeda JC, Ramirez-Miranda A, Graue-Hernández EO. Boston type I Keratoprosthesis assisted with intraprosthetic amniotic membrane (AmniotiKPro sandwich technique). Acta Ophthalmologica. 2015;93:e87-e8.
96. Cooke M, Tan EK, Mandrycky C, He H, O'Connell J, Tseng SC. Comparison of cryopreserved amniotic membrane and umbilical cord tissue with dehydrated amniotic membrane/chorion tissue. J Wound Care. 2014;23:465-76.
97. Kruse FE, Joussen AM, Rohrschneider K, You L, Sinn B, Baumann J, et al. Cryopreserved human amniotic membrane for ocular surface reconstruction. Graefe's Arch Clin Exp Ophthalmol. 2000;238:68-75.
98. Kheirkhah A, Casas V, Blanco G, Li W, Hayashida Y, Chen YT, et al. Amniotic membrane transplantation with fibrin glue for conjunctivochalasis. Am J Ophthalmol. 2007;144:311-3.
99. Kheirkhah A, Casas V, Esquenazi S, Blanco G, Li W, Raju VK, et al. New surgical approach for superior conjunctivochalasis. Cornea. 2007;26:685-91.
100. Casas V, Kheirkhah A, Blanco G, Tseng SC. Surgical approach for scleral ischemia and melt. Cornea. 2008;27:196-201.
101. Shanbhag SS, Chodosh J, Saeed HN. Sutureless amniotic membrane transplantation with cyanoacrylate glue for acute Stevens-Johnson syndrome/toxic epidermal necrolysis. Ocul Surf. 2019.
102. Shanbhag SS, Rashad R, Chodosh J, Saeed HN. Long-term impact of a treatment protocol for acute ocular involvement in Stevens-Johnson syndrome/toxic epidermal necrolysis. Am J Ophthalmol. 2019.
103. Mead O, Tighe S, Tseng S. Amniotic Membrane Transplantation for Managing Dry Eye and Neurotrophic Keratitis. Taiwan J Ophthalmol. 2020.
104. Yin HY, Cheng AM, Tighe S, Kurochkin P, Nord J, Dhanireddy S, et al. Self-retained cryopreserved amniotic membrane for treating severe corneal ulcers: A comparative, retrospective control study. Sci Rep. 2020;10:1-5.
105. Brocks D, Mead OG, Tighe S, Tseng SCG. Self-retained Cryopreserved Amniotic Membrane for the Management of Corneal Ulcers. Clin ophthalmol. 2020;14:1437-43.
106. Nguyen P, Rue K, Heur M, Yiu SC. Ocular surface rehabilitation: Application of human amniotic membrane in high-risk penetrating keratoplasties. Saudi J Ophthalmol. 2014;28:198-202.
107. Kheirkhah A, Casas V, Raju VK, Tseng SC. Sutureless amniotic membrane transplantation for partial limbal stem cell deficiency. Am J Ophthalmol. 2008;145:787-94.
108. Shay E, Khadem JJ, Tseng SC. Efficacy and limitation of sutureless amniotic membrane transplantation for acute toxic epidermal necrolysis. Cornea. 2010;29:359-61.
109. Shammas MC, Lai EC, Sarkar JS, Yang J, Starr CE, Sippel KC. Management of acute Stevens-Johnson syndrome and toxic epidermal necrolysis utilizing amniotic membrane and topical corticosteroids. Am J Ophthalmol. 2010;149:203-13.e2.
110. Gregory DG. Treatment of acute Stevens-Johnson syndrome and toxic epidermal necrolysis using amniotic membrane: a review of 10 consecutive cases. Ophthalmology. 2011;118:908-14.
111. Hsu M, Jayaram A, Verner R, Lin A, Bouchard C. Indications and outcomes of amniotic membrane transplantation in the management of acute stevens-johnson syndrome and toxic epidermal necrolysis: a case-control study. Cornea. 2012;31:1394-402.
112. Ciralsky JB, Sippel KC. Prompt versus delayed amniotic membrane application in a patient with acute Stevens-Johnson syndrome. Clin Ophthalmol. 2013;7:1031-4.
113. Kolomeyer AM, Do BK, Tu Y, Chu DS. Placement of ProKera in the management of ocular manifestations of acute Stevens-Johnson syndrome in an outpatient. Eye Contact Lens. 2013;39:e7-11.

114. Tomlins PJ, Parulekar MV, Rauz S. "Triple-TEN" in the Treatment of Acute Ocular Complications From Toxic Epidermal Necrolysis. Cornea. 2013;32:365-9.
115. Hauswirth SG, Hom MM. Taking the Recurrence out of Recurrent Corneal Erosions: A Case Series. Invest Ophthalmol Vis Sci. 2017;58:2612.
116. Huang Y, Sheha H, Tseng SCG. Self-retained Amniotic Membrane Transplantation for Recurrent Corneal Erosion. J Clin Exp Ophthalmol. 2013;4:272.
117. Shafer B, Fuerst NM, Massaro-Giordano M, Palladino V, Givnish T, Macchi I, et al. The use of self-retained, cryopreserved amniotic membrane for the treatment of Sjogren syndrome: a case series. Digit J Ophthalmol. 2019;25:21-5.
118. Harthan J, Sicks L. Sutureless Amniotic Membranes (PROKERA) for filamentary keratitis: A case series. J Dry Eye Occ Surf Dis. 2019;2:e10-6.
119. Maharaj R. Cryopreserved Amniotic Membrane (ProKera) Treatment of Anterior Stromal Haze Secondary to HSV Keratitis. J Dry Eye Occ Surf Dis. 2019;2:e2-6.
120. Kheirkhah A, Johnson DA, Paranjpe DR, Raju VK, Casas V, Tseng SC. Temporary sutureless amniotic membrane patch for acute alkaline burns. Arch Ophthalmol. 2008;126:1059-66.
121. Kobayashi A, Ijiri S, Sugiyama K, Di Pascuale MA, Tseng SC. Detection of corneal epithelial defect through amniotic membrane patch by fluorescein. Cornea. 2005;24:359-60.
122. Yoshita T, Kobayashi A, Takahashi M, Sugiyama K. Reliability of intraocular pressure by Tono-Pen XL over amniotic membrane patch in human. J Glaucoma. 2004;13:413-6.
123. Marangon FB, Alfonso EC, Miller D, Remonda NM, Muallem MS, Tseng SC. Incidence of microbial infection after amniotic membrane transplantation. Cornea. 2004;23:264-9.

SECTION 6

Indication Specific Techniques of Corneal Transplantation

60 Pellucid Marginal Degeneration

Sohini Mandal, Somasheila I Murthy

INTRODUCTION

Pellucid marginal degeneration (PMD) is a noninflammatory, nonhereditary disorder, bilateral, often asymmetrical, characterized by peripheral thinning, and protuberance (ectasia) separated from the limbus by an area of 1–2 mm in width.[1] Predominantly this condition involves the inferior cornea, with peripheral thinning of 4 o'clock hours ranging from 4 to 8 o'clock position.[2] However, this disorder might also involve superior,[3,4] temporal,[5,6] and nasal[6] areas of cornea thus making itself a close differential of other conditions. The term was first coined by Schalaeppi in 1957 as "la dystrophie marginale inferieure pellucide de la cornee". The literal sense of "Pellucid" is clear and implies the intactness of corneal clarity with absence of scarring, lipid deposition, or vascularization.[7]

The exact data regarding incidence and prevalence of PMD is vaguely documented in literature as PMD remains a close differential to keratoconus with regards to their clinical presentation thus underestimated.[8,9] According to epidemiological studies, this is considered as the second most common corneal ectatic disorder after keratoconus. Other rare ectatic disorder includes keratoglobus and posterior keratoconus.[10]

ETIOLOGY

The etiology of pellucid marginal corneal degeneration (PMCD) is mostly unknown. One school of thought believes PMD, keratoconus and keratoglobus to belong to the same disease spectrum and represent different clinical presentations.[11,12] Systemic diseases such as obesity and related obstructive sleep apnea (OSA) have been reported to be accompanied with PMD in literature. The multiple episodes of hypoxia in patients with OSA have been theorized to result in anaerobic glycolysis and stromal acidosis. This would further lead to transcription of proinflammatory cytokines, tumor necrosis factor-alpha or interleukin-6, resulting in corneal thinning.[13] In addition, floppy eyelid syndrome is another common association in such obese patients that may lead to thinning and ectasia due to chronic mechanical rubbing.

The superior variant of PMD has been reported to be linked with vernal and atopic keratoconjunctivitis. Concurrent ocular and systemic pathologies such as retinitis pigmentosa, chronic open-angle glaucoma, scleroderma, and hyperthyroidism have been detected in few PMD cases, but direct causal relation could not be ascertained.[14-16]

Strong correlation exists between keratoconus and systemic disorders such as atopic disease, Down's syndrome, and connective tissue diseases (Sjögren syndrome, scleroderma). In the same vein, Pasztor et al.,[17] aimed to look for differences in chemical mediators from tear samples and could find a difference only in matrix metalloprotease-9 (MMP 9), while several other markers were similar. Studying these mediators in larger samples size may reveal differences or similarities to suggest different appearances of the same disorder.

EPIDEMIOLOGY

Several authors have proposed PMD to be just a peripheral form of keratoconus[18] that can affect all ethnicities and has more of a male preponderance.[19]

The most common affected age group is the second to fifth decade, but older individuals also seem to get affected. Rather than the onset truly being in older individual, it is more likely due to very slow progression of the condition, which tends to be unnoticed through-out life and only be diagnosed when an older patient seeks cataract surgery. Family members have been reported to have high astigmatism in few of these PMD patients,[20] however, genetic inheritance has not been reported yet. In 10% of patients with corneal ectasia, PMD, and keratoconus seems to coexist.

HISTOPATHOLOGY

Histopathological study on PMD corneas reveals an absent or uneven and discontinuous Bowman's membrane. Stroma shows an increased mucopolysaccharide content with thinning (**Fig. 1**). Electron microscopic studies are of particular significance as they show the irregular and random arrangement

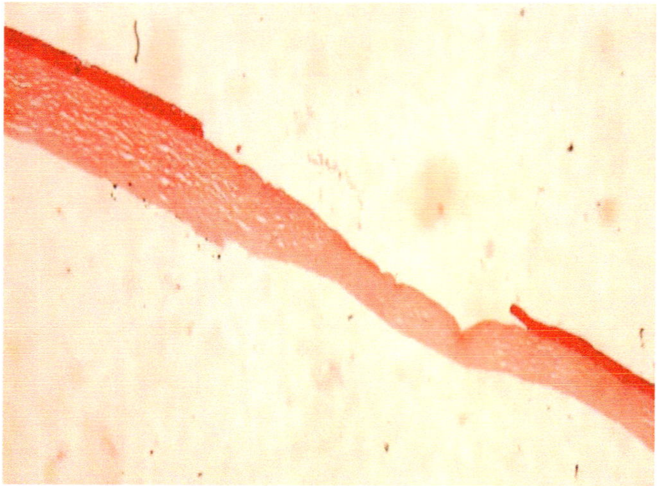

Fig. 1: Epithelial changes in patients with pellucid marginal degeneration showing elongation of superficial cells and the disruption of basement membrane.

of collagen fibrils with extracellular electron-dense deposits in the stroma. These electron-dense areas are islets of fibrous long-spacing collagen with 100–110 nm periodicity.

CLINICAL PRESENTATION

The patients usually present with gradual, progressive painless decline in vision or poor vision due to high astigmatism. Corrected distance visual acuity often declines in advanced stages of the disease and corneal topography reveals high irregular, against-the-rule astigmatism.[7] The vertical meridian is relatively flatter due to tissue loss and a thin stroma inferiorly. The steepening and ectasia occur at the intersection of the involved and uninvolved tissue, thereafter giving a typical high-cylindrical loop and high against-the-rule astigmatism. Rarely, they can present with an acute painful red eye with decline in vision with or without a history of minor trauma. On evaluation one can reach a diagnosis of acute hydrops and/or spontaneous corneal perforation.

Slit-lamp evaluation reveals crescent-shaped band of stromal thinning of the peripheral cornea, extending from 4 to 8 o'clock (**Fig. 2A**). When visualized sideways, advanced stages of PMD cornea gives an appearance of a beer belly as the zone of maximal ectasia lies above the thinnest location (**Figs. 2B and C**). Concentric Descemet's membrane folds have been noted in few cases as well.[21,22]

Although PMD is a bilateral condition, unilateral cases have also been stated.[23-25] Rarely, uncommon sites such as superior, nasal and temporal corneal involvement has also been recognized in literature.[26-30]

EVALUATION

Corneal tomography has been the gold-standard investigation for diagnosing and prognostication of PMD and other corneal ectasias. Topography machine-related technologies have advanced quite drastically from the old generation video keratography to recent technologies like slit-scanning (Orbscan) and Scheimpflug imaging (Pentacam) systems. These diagnostic modalities have made subclinical diagnosis of corneal ectatic disorders imaginable with a better evaluation of posterior corneal curvature. In the earliest stages, high against-the-rule astigmatism may be the only clue for development into PMD. In established cases, the topographical pattern is often confused with that of keratoconus. On a cursory glance, the topographical pattern is often confused with keratoconus due to the presence of inferior corneal steepening. However, the major difference is the presence of an island of flattening just below the midline within the steep area, which is pathognomonic for PMD. This gives rise to a characteristic "crab-claw", "butterfly", or "kissing doves" appearance on the curvature/keratometric map on topography[31,32] (**Figs. 3A and B**).

A typical hot-spot area or an area of elevation in the inferior periphery is pathognomonic on elevation maps. Greater emphasis must be given on the clinical and topographic relationship for a definitive diagnosis as sometimes, the elevation map change can also be observed in advanced keratoconus. The percentage thickness increase (PTI) on the Belin Ambrosio enhanced ectasia display (BAD) map of PMD patients shows the red curve moving upward, i.e., thinner pachymetry in the inferior periphery and thicker at the center.

The far peripheral changes cannot be picked up on topography as it is beyond the range of the corneal area sampled by the topography machine. To counteract this shortcoming, high-resolution anterior segment optical coherence tomography (ASOCT) and Scheimpflug imaging devices might guide in locating the thinnest corneal point (**Figs. 4A and B**).

DIFFERENTIAL DIAGNOSIS

As each ectatic disorder has its specific management, it becomes clinically very relevant to have a clear distinction between all the ectatic disorders.[33] The main differentiating points to differentiate PMD from rest of the ectatic disorders are elaborated in detail in this chapter.

Keratoconus versus Pellucid Marginal Degeneration

Keratoconus, which is far more common than PMD, is a progressive corneal thinning disorder with associated corneal protrusion leading to irregular astigmatism and decline in visual functions.[34-36] Topography reveals a well-delineated area of high-dioptric value, bounded by gradually reducing curvature zones that may be located centrally or somewhat displaced inferiorly (**Figs. 5A and B**).

"Crab-claw pattern" on topography is a classical topographic feature in cases of PMD however, few cases of keratoconus can also have such a characteristic pattern as noted in various case series as "pellucid-like keratoconus". In such cases of pellucid-like keratoconus the area of flattening beneath mid-line would be absent.[8] Scheimpflug devices provide information like elevation and pachymetry maps that

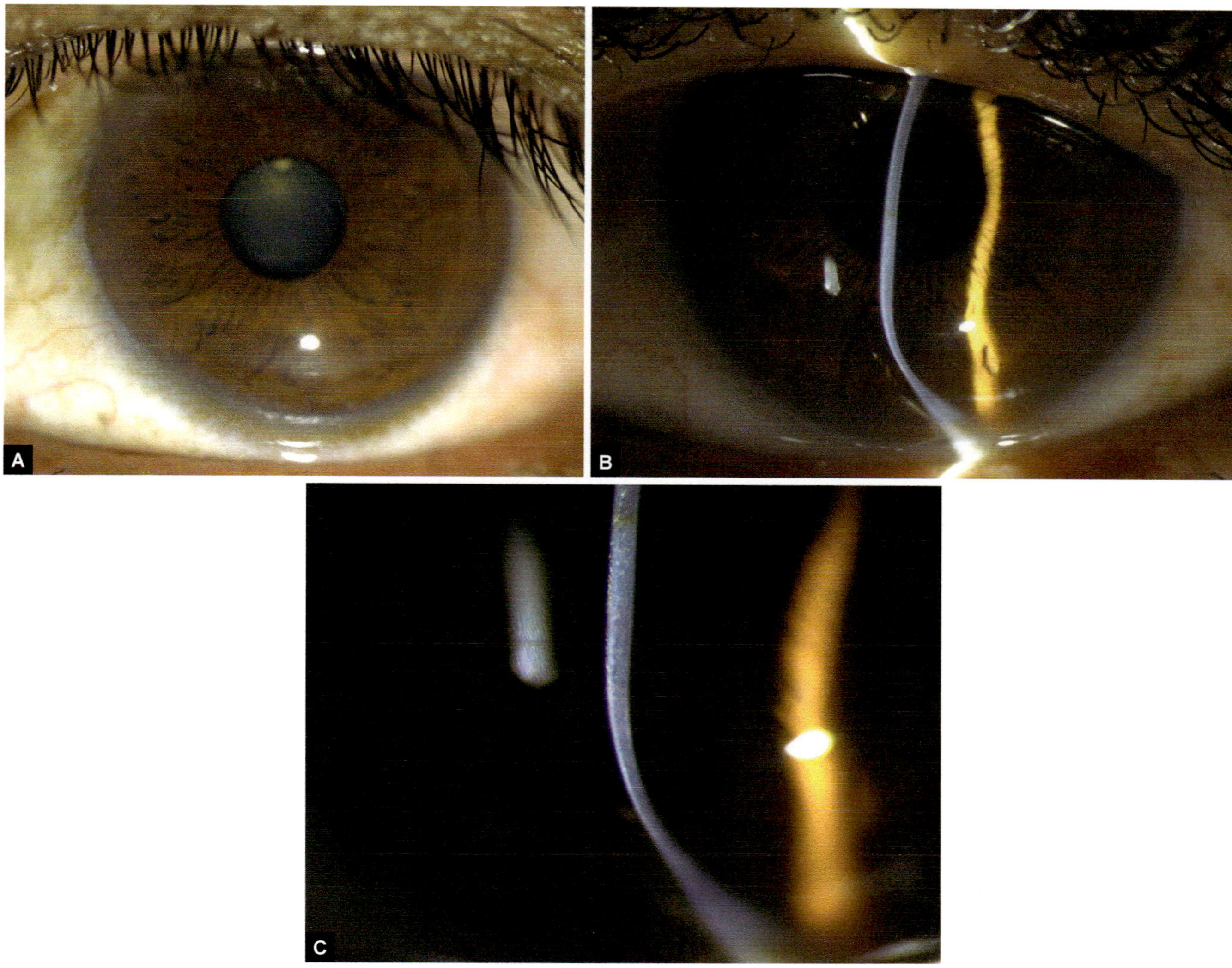

Figs. 2A to C: (A) Slit-lamp photograph in diffuse illumination examination reveals a crescentic band of corneal thinning that extends from 4 to 8 o' clock hours parted from limbus by a fairly healthy cornea of 1–2 mm in width with protuberance/ectasia; (B and C) Slit-lamp photography reveals localized inferior corneal thinning with ectasia just above it ("beer-belly appearance").

proves to be of great significance to come to a precise diagnosis of PMD.[37] In cases of PMD, the corneal thinning typically involves the peripheral cornea with a characteristic "bell" sign on topography that may be appreciated in advanced stage of the disease only.[8] Maximum thinning in the inferior cornea with a progressive increase in thickness through central and superior cornea explains the bell-sign very well. Sinjab et al.[8] have suggested pentacam map to be an important means to differentiate between keratoconus and PMD, especially as both maps reveal a "crab claw" pattern. The corneal hysteresis (CH) and corneal resistance factor (CRF) on Ocular Response Analyzer (ORA) are known to be reduced in keratoconus and PMD compared to normal eyes.[38-40] Therefore, neither of the parameters can be used as a diagnostic device to distinguish between keratoconus and PMD.

Keratoglobus versus Pellucid Marginal Degeneration

Keratoglobus is a rare, bilateral corneal ectatic disorder characterized by a globular protrusion of the cornea with diffuse limbus-to-limbus global thinning (**Fig. 6**). The maximal point of thinning is at the periphery that can reach up to about one-fifth of the central corneal thickness.[41] They generally present with clear corneas unless acute hydrops and associated scarring occur.[42] These corneas are thin enough making them prone to rupture spontaneously or with trivial trauma.[43] However, in cases of PMD corneal perforation is very rare. Karabatsas and Cook[44] have reported the association of frank keratoglobus in one eye with topographic features of PMD in the fellow eye. Therefore, they suggested keratoglobus to be occurring as a result of circumferential spread of the peripheral corneal thinning of PMD. Likewise, Rumelt and Rehany[45] also supported the hypothesis that both diseases are different phenotypic appearances of the same disorder. However, it is commonly believed that such coexisting keratoglobus and PMD are extremely rare. The significance of distinguishing the two conditions is that while keratoconus is not likely to progress beyond third decade of life progression of PMD is noted typically in thirties or later.

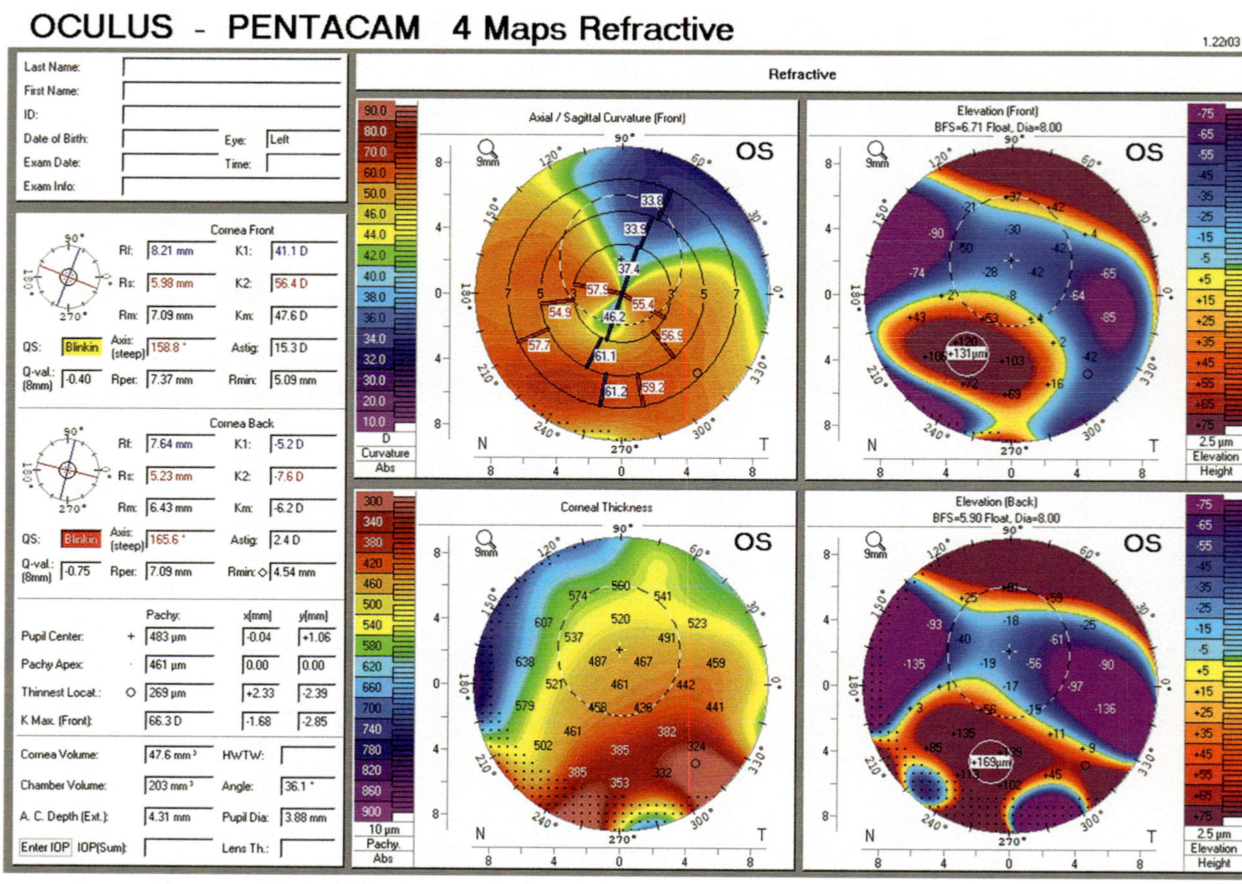

A

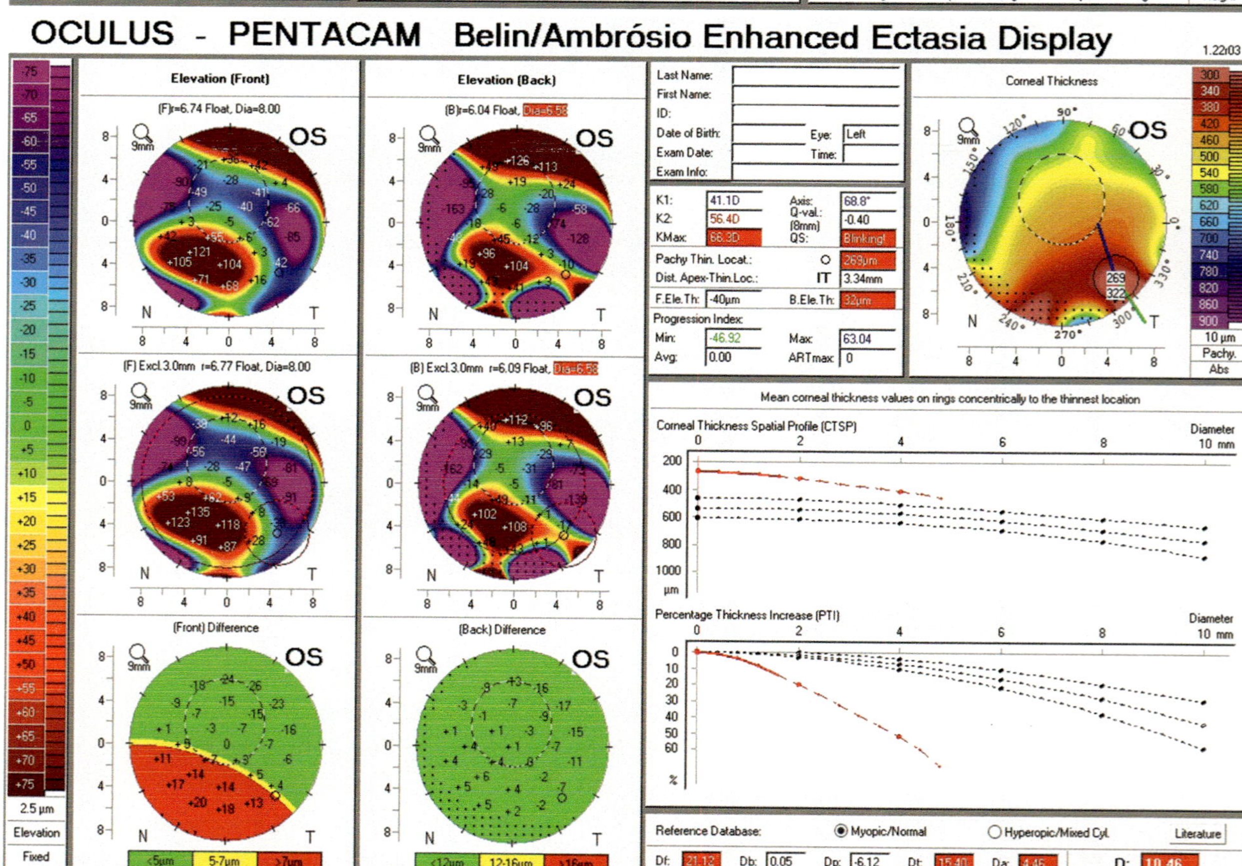

B

Figs. 3A and B: The axial curvature and Belin Ambrosio enhanced ectasia display of Pentacam topography maps that reveal the characteristic high against-the-rule astigmatism pattern seen in patients with pellucid marginal degeneration. Inferior steepening is also present, with the presence of the classic "crab claw" topographic appearance. There is presence of an island of flattening just below the midline within the steep area, which is pathognomonic for PMD.

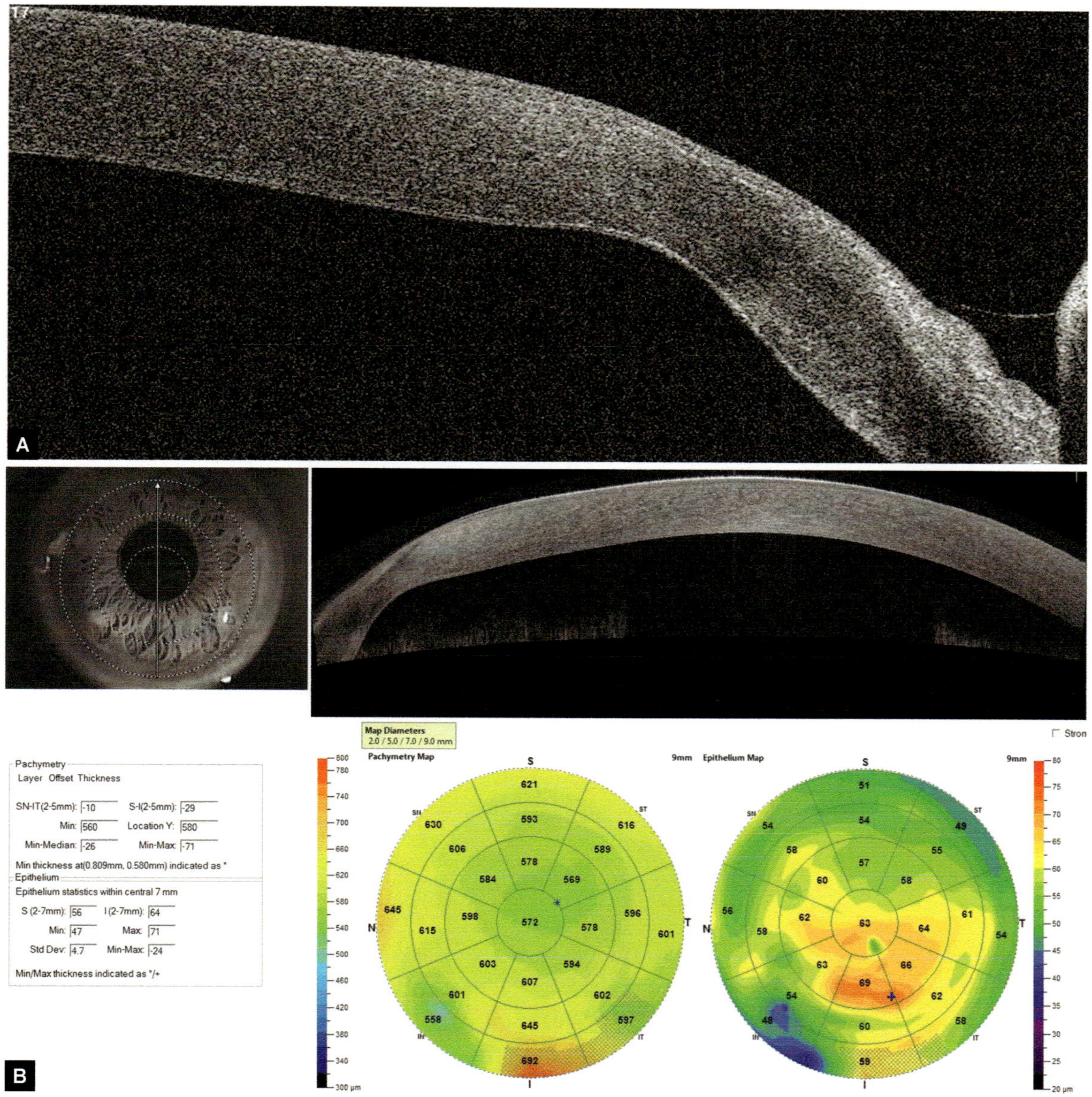

Figs. 4A and B: Anterior segment optical coherence tomography (ASOCT) image of a patient with pellucid marginal degeneration that reveals the exact location and extent of corneal thinning and the corresponding pachymetry and epithelial thickness map showing thinnest area of 48 microns in the inferonasal part of cornea.

Terrien Marginal Degeneration versus Pellucid Marginal Degeneration

Terrien marginal degeneration (TMD) is also a peripheral ectatic disorder mainly involving the superior cornea, and subsequently progress slowly and circumferentially.[46,47] The pathognomonic features of TMD includes a thinned-out band and furrowing of the peripheral cornea, lipid deposition at the anterior edge, and radial superficial vascularization (**Figs. 7A and B**).[48,49]

Mooren's Ulcer versus Pellucid Marginal Degeneration

Mooren's ulcer is a form of peripheral ulcerative keratitis of idiopathic origin characterized by unilateral or bilateral painful, inflammatory corneal thinning with ectasia in the absence of scleritis.[46] Slit-lamp examination reveals perilimbal corneal infiltrates, epithelial defect with overhanging anterior edges (**Figs. 8A and B**).[50] A classical Mooren's ulcer in its advanced stage cannot be misdiagnosed as PMD (**Fig. 9**). However, PMD may closely mimic early stages of Mooren's ulcer. Slit-lamp evaluation alone helps in differentiating the two, which lets the clinician assess the type of thinning process (inflammatory vs. noninflammatory) and evaluate the classical clinical signs.

Subclinical PMD

Advanced cases of PMD can be simply identified as the minimum corneal thickness (MCT) is located on the periphery and thinning can be easily appreciated on slit-lamp examination. In clinical practice, it is very difficult to detect cases with MCT in the central or paracentral zones. In such cases, pachymetric maps guide the clinician regarding

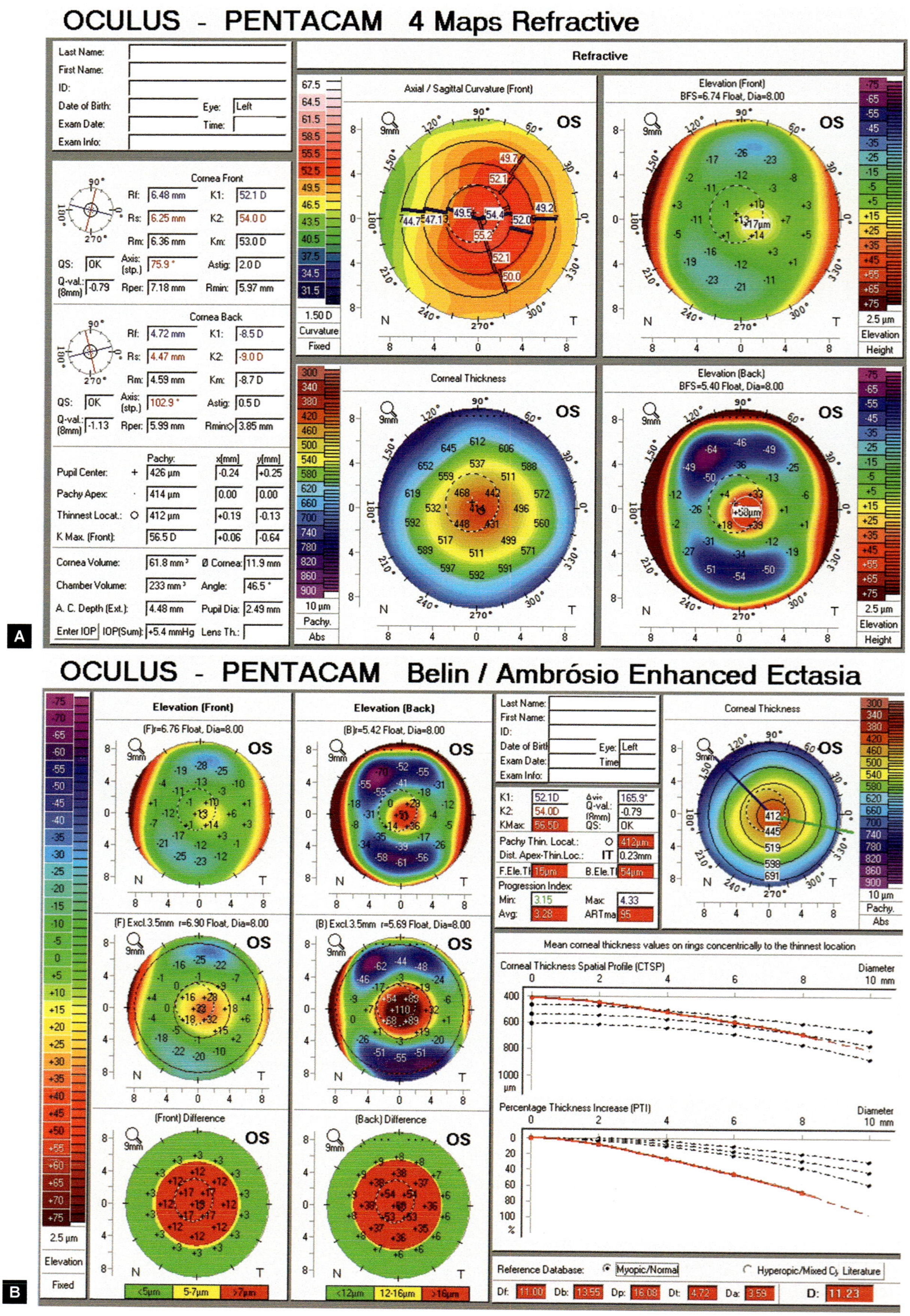

Figs. 5A and B: Pentacam map of a keratoconus patient showing (A) an asymmetric bow-tie pattern (inferior steepening) on the axial curvature map with corresponding corneal thinning; thinnest location of 412 µm with 0.19 mm and –0.13 mm displacement on the x- and y-axis, respectively; increased anterior and posterior elevation (maximum anterior elevation of 17 µm and maximum posterior elevation of 58 µm) at the location of maximum steepening (B) Belin-ambrosio-enhanced ectasia display map of the same patient showing hot colors in the elevation maps and difference map along with abnormal percentage thickness increase graph (steep dip from the 2 mm zone) and D value of 11.23.

the variations in corneal thickness as we go from periphery to center thus help in clinching the diagnosis aptly. Various studies[51-53] have reflected upon these cases as "subclinical PMD" due to the presence of peripheral thinning yet is not sufficient enough to be considered as frank PMD. However, there is no robust evidence in literature that supports the usage of this term of subclinical PMD. Some authors consider such cases as keratoconus or pellucid-like keratoconus as well.

MANAGEMENT

Patients with PMD can be managed either conservatively or surgically for optimal visual rehabilitation. Due to progressive corneal thinning with severe eccentric ectasia, the practicality of both these management options seems difficult. Still, majority of the PMD patients in early and moderate stage of the disease can be rehabilitated with optical aids such as spectacles or contact lenses (CLs). Contact lenses are more suitable for correction of irregular astigmatism.

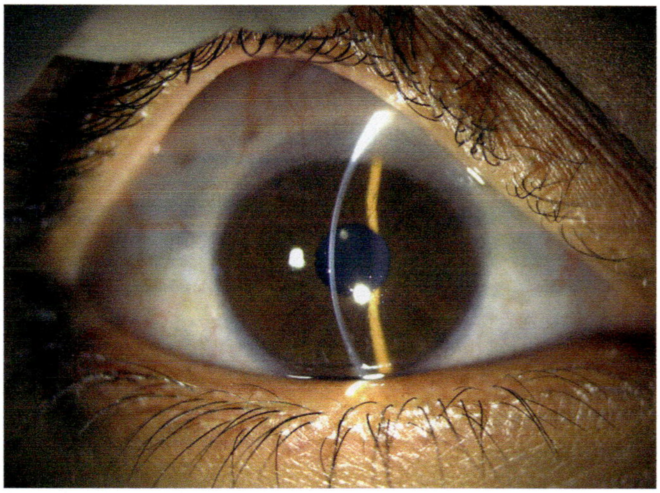

Fig. 6: Slit-lamp biomicroscopic examination reveals globular protrusion of the cornea associated with diffuse thinning from limbus-to-limbus with maximal thinning at the periphery.

Contact lens fitting in PMD remains more difficult because the ectasia involves a greater corneal area and often the CL is unable to cover the ectatic area completely. Routine rigid gas permeable (RGP) CLs are often associated with decentration. Other CLs such as large diameter RGP-CL, hybrid CL, semiscleral, miniscleral, and scleral CL [prosthetic replacement of ocular surface ecosystem (PROSE)] lenses are beneficial in such cases (**Figs. 10A to C**).[54,55]

Surgical treatment comprises collagen cross-linking (CXL), intracorneal ring segments (ICRS), and partial and total corneal replacement procedures.

Collagen cross-linking causes photopolymerization of disulfide covalent bonds that are both intra and intercollagen-linked within the corneal stroma. By the virtue of its principle, it is the only treatment modality known to halt the progression of corneal ectasia. However, there is significant paucity in literature regarding its role in PMD. The various challenges associated with its role in PMD are decentration of the UV-A rays to attain the desired outcome at the periphery and tendency of damage to the limbal stem cells due to decentered radiation.[56]

Intracorneal ring segments are basically polymethyl methacrylate (PMMA) segments that work on the principle of Hammock effect, i.e., redistribution of the biomechanical stress equally all throughout the corneal tissue, thereby steepening the corneal periphery and causing simultaneous central corneal flattening. However, there are few prerequisites for ICRS implantation like corneal thickness >450 μ with no scarring. Therefore, these segments are particularly efficacious in early to moderate stages of PMCD.

The various surgical options for visual rehabilitation in cases with PMD include lamellar or penetrating keratoplasty with a large diameter eccentric graft (**Figs. 11A and B**). The possible higher chances of graft rejection and limbal

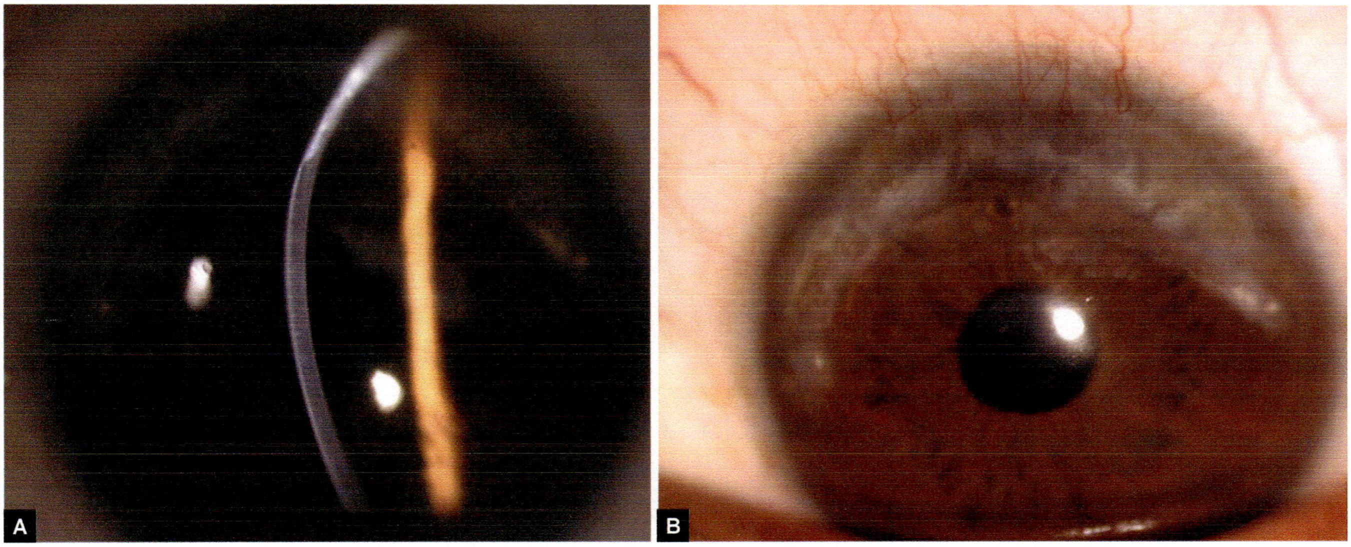

Figs. 7A and B: Patient with Terrien marginal degeneration displaying superior stromal thinning extending from 9 to 3 o'clock hours with intact epithelium, overlying pannus, and lipid at the leading edge.

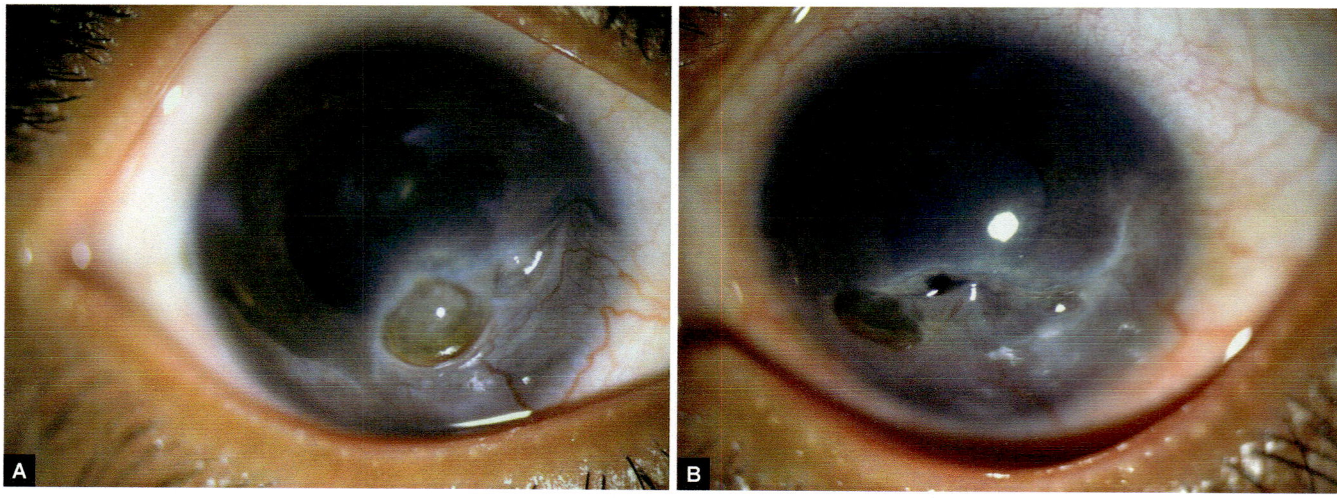

Figs. 8A and B: Slit-lamp photography in diffuse illumination reveals a peripheral corneal ulcer in a young male that ranged from 3 to 8 o'clock hours characterized by a grey, steep, overhanging leading edge with areas of stromal thinning, vascularization, and perforation.

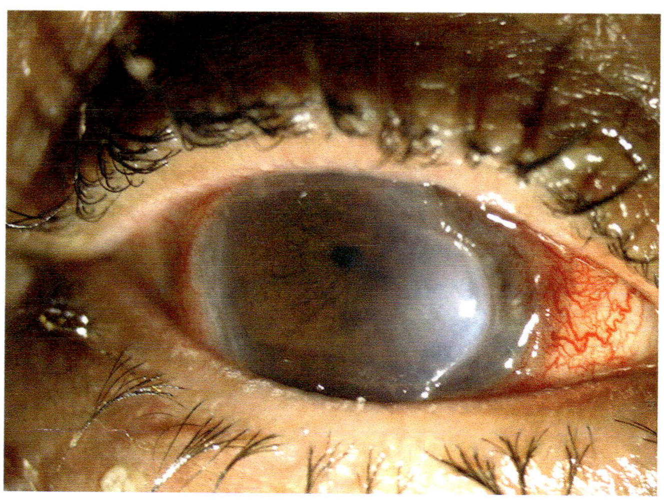

Fig. 9: Slit-lamp photography in diffuse illumination reveals a peripheral corneal ulcer of an elderly female patient ranging from 12 to 6 o'clock hours characterized by a grey, steep, overhanging leading edge with peripheral areas of stromal thinning, vascularization. There is no evidence of perforation.

stem cell damage make it a less feasible choice due to the proximity to the limbal vessels.[57]

"Tuck in" lamellar keratoplasty (TILK) is an exclusive category of lamellar keratoplasty introduced by Vajpayee et al., and is performed for advanced peripheral ectatic disorders such as PMD, keratoglobus, PMD combined with keratoconus, and post-PKP ectasia. It is comprised of a central donor corneal button obtained by lamellar dissection with an extra intrastromal tuck of the peripheral flange of the graft into the peripheral intrastromal pocket of the host (**Figs. 12 and 13**). TILK proved to be an effective surgical modality for the management of peripheral corneal thinning with very good results in patients with PMD.[58]

Other surgical procedures such as crescentic lamellar keratoplasty, combined central penetrating keratoplasty, intrastromal lamellar keratoplasty, lamellar, or full-thickness crescentic-wedge resection (**Figs. 14 and 15**), and epikeratoplasty have been tried successfully by various surgeons.[59-63] Some of these, such as crescentic-wedge resection have unpredictable and suboptimal visual results. There are several potential risks associated with lamellar procedures that include intraoperative DM macroperforation during lamellar dissection, double anterior chamber formation, graft dehiscence, stromal rejection, and interface problems like epithelial ingrowth.

PROGNOSIS

Since PMD is a slowly progressive disease, patients often seek medical care relatively late. Overall, there is a biphasic intervention in terms of age. Younger patients presenting in their late 20 or 30s usually do well with scleral contact lenses and collagen cross linking if progressive. Advanced PMD or CL failure required surgical intervention, usually DALK. In patients diagnosed for the first time in the fifth or sixth decade, cataract surgery with customized toric intraocular lens (IOL) works well.

The structural and functional outcomes following crosslinking and ICRS have been quite fruitful in mild to moderate cases of PMD. However, in literature the data remain inadequate to remark on the exact number of cases finally undergoing transplant procedure in the long run. In advanced cases of PMD, the structural and functional outcomes of TILK have particularly shown quite decent outcomes.

COMPLICATIONS

Although rare, complications can vary from extremely high-irregular astigmatism to development of acute corneal hydrops with or without subsequent corneal perforation (**Figs. 16A and B**). These cases need immediate surgical attention such as pneumatic descemetopexy, compression sutures or corneal perforation repair (**Figs. 17 and 18**). Few of them might eventually end up in visually impairing stromal opacity. Keratorefractive procedure remains an absolute contraindication in these patients due to increased risk of postoperative ectasia. Failure to recognize the pathology during refractive screening evaluation can have damaging consequences.

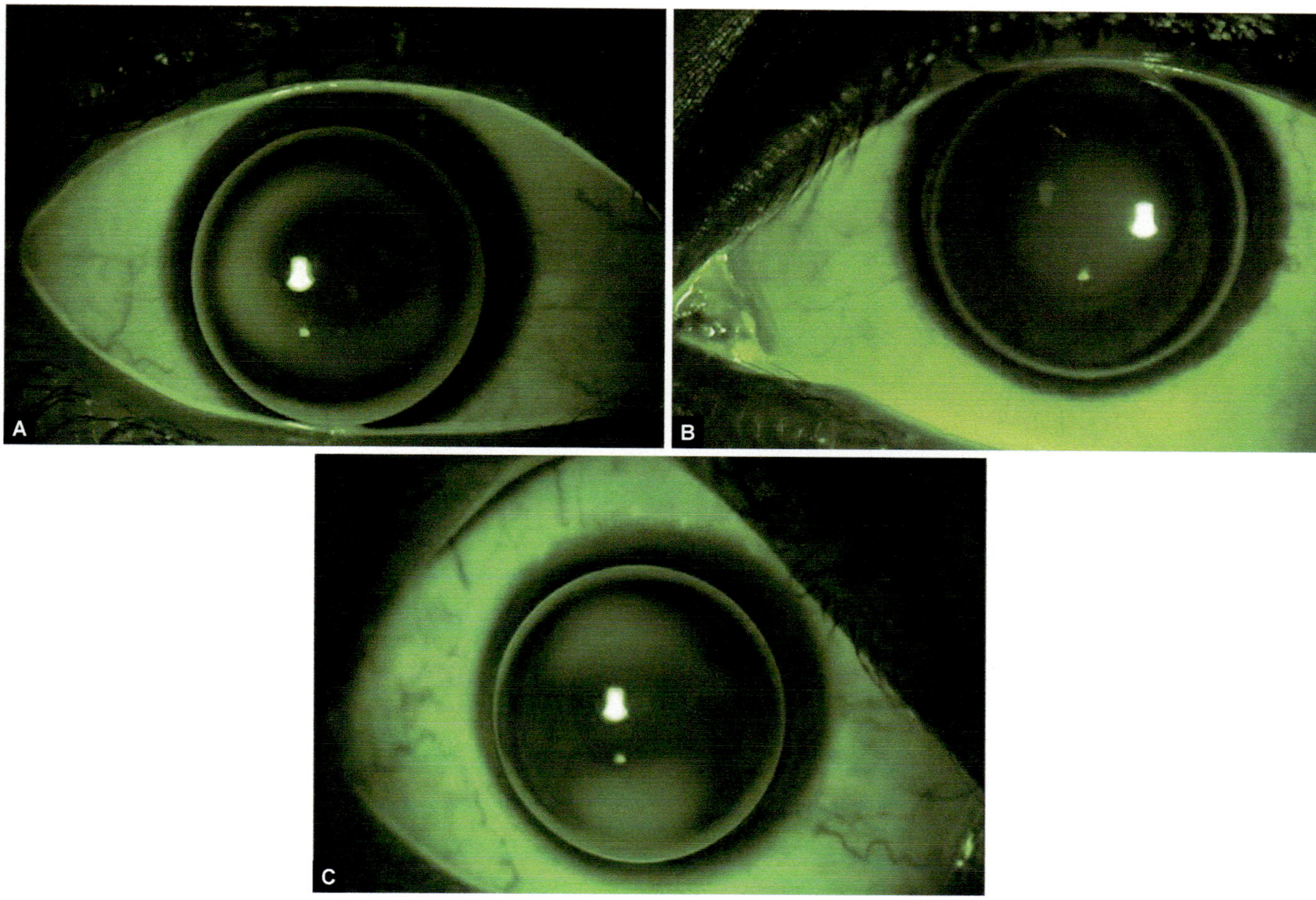

Figs. 10A to C: (A) Diffuse fluorescein in the center and midperiphery on either side depicting the divided touch or three-point touch; (B) Apical clearance—central fluorescein pooling and thin-edge clearance is visible; (C) Apical bearing—central bearing, seen as dark area because of lack of fluorescein in this area with thin-edge clearance at 3 o'clock position.

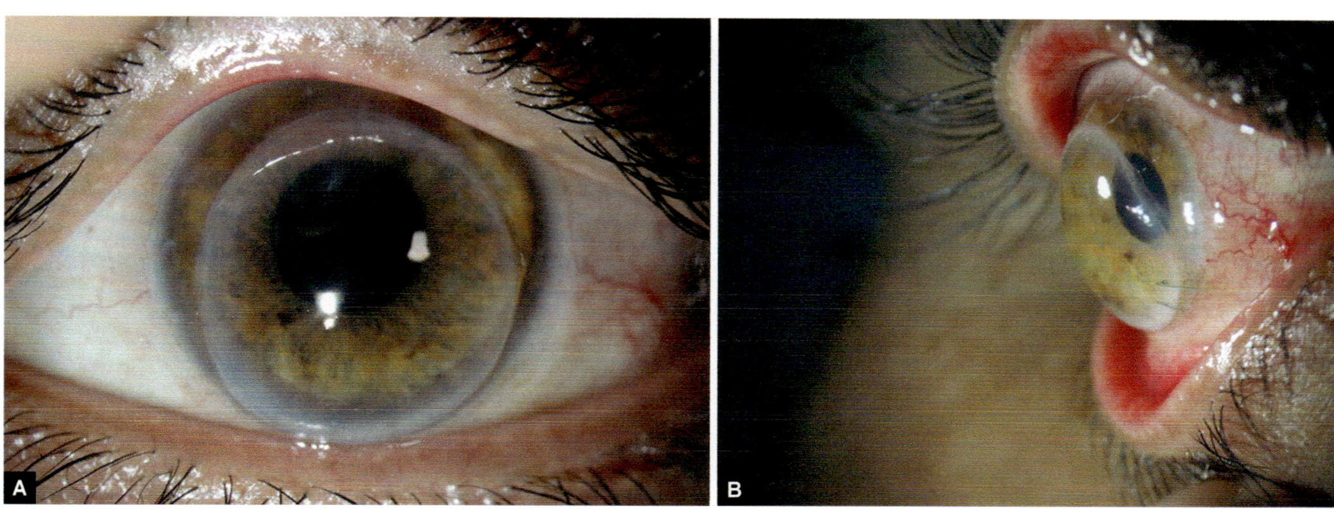

Figs. 11A and B: (A) Slit-lamp photography in diffuse illumination reveals clear graft following penetrating keratoplasty with a large diameter eccentric graft in the left eye; (B) Slit-lamp photography in diffuse illumination in side view reveals clear graft following penetrating keratoplasty with a large diameter eccentric graft in the left eye.

CATARACT SURGERY AND TORIC IOLs IN PELLUCID MARGINAL DEGENERATION

Toric IOLs can allow for the correction of refractive error and astigmatism independent of cornea alterations.[64] They can be implanted in anterior or posterior chamber with or without natural lens extraction (toric phakic IOLs). Stable PMD patients with cataract can be effectively managed by modern day phacoemulsification with toric IOL implantation. This approach helps in correcting high astigmatism, however this correction continues to be challenging. In preoperative work-up, it is important to know the BCVA that the patient has before cataract formation, the progression or stability

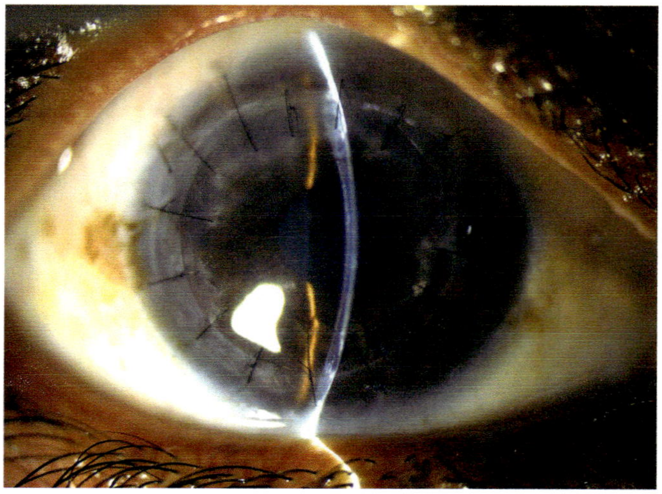

Fig. 12: Slit-lamp biomicroscopy reveals clear graft with minimal peripheral opacification at 6 months postoperative following tuck in lamellar keratoplasty. The graft host junction also shows the intrastromal tuck with well-integrated donor lamellar graft into the host corneal tissue.

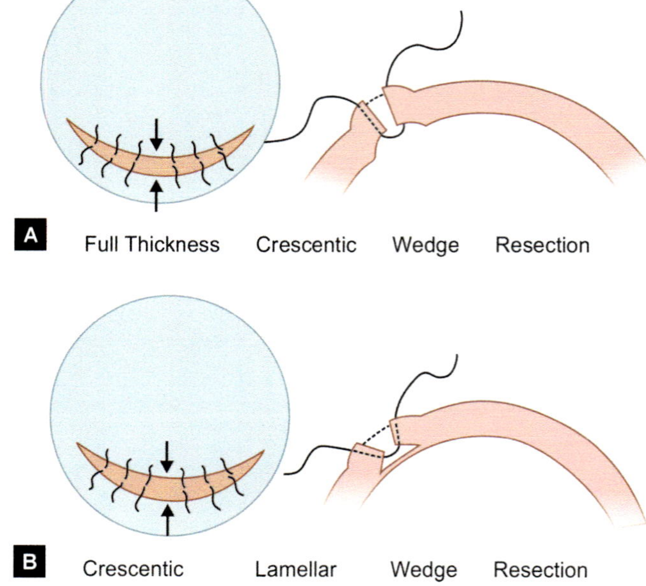

Figs. 14A and B: Schematic diagrams depicting full thickness and partial thickness crescentic-wedge resection in the area of peripheral corneal thinning followed by placement of interrupted 10-0 monofilament nylon sutures.

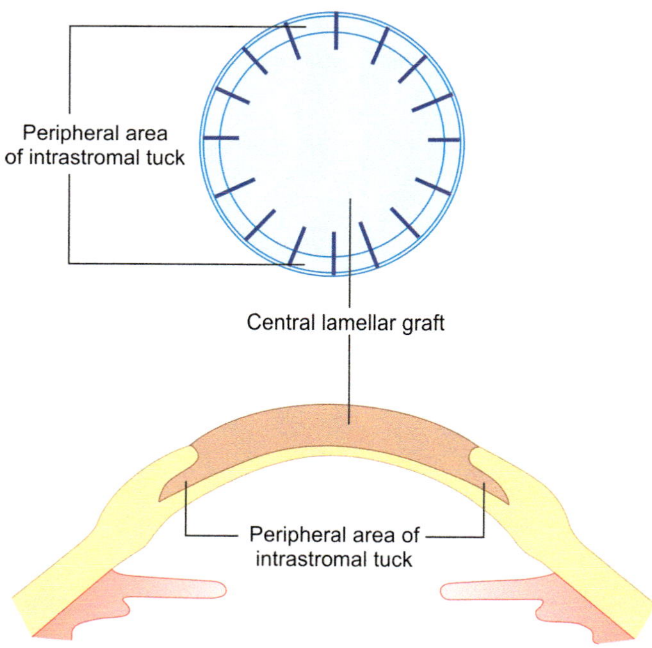

Fig. 13: Diagrammatic representation depicting central lamellar keratoplasty with peripheral tuck of the large graft into the intrastromal pocket of host corneal tissue.

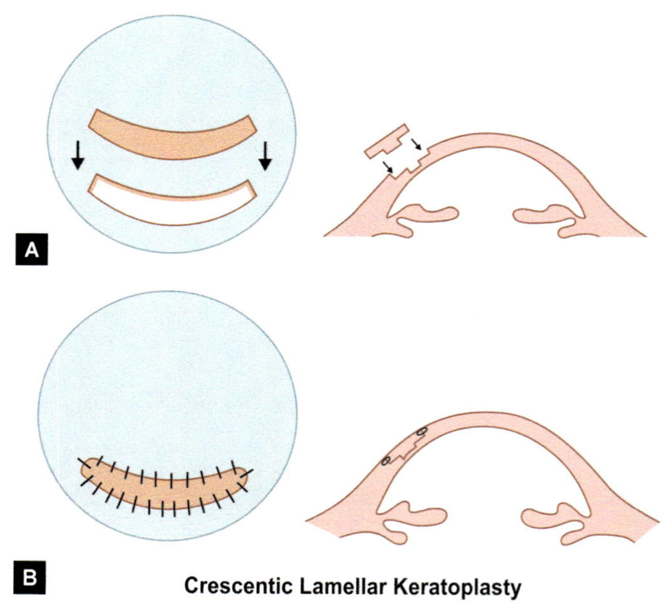

Figs. 15A and B: Schematic diagrams depicting crescentic lamellar keratoplasty that involves excision of the area of abnormally thinned stroma. A trimmed donor tissue stromal graft is fitted to the excised area (arrows). The donor tissue stromal graft is then sutured to the residual stromal edges.

of the disease and signs of ectasia progression should be well analyzed before implanting the toric IOL. An accurate biometry and IOL power calculation remain another grey area in cataract patients with PMD with high astigmatism and myopia.[65] PMD affects the keratometric readings to a lesser extent than keratoconus. Corneal tomography such as Scheimpflug imaging is a valuable diagnostic tool for diagnosing PMD. It also provides various data regarding ectasia progression, including the axial or sagittal curvature maps, anterior and posterior evaluation using the concept of enhanced best-fit sphere and corneal pachymetry. Orbscan is another such exceptional diagnostic device that provides us with keratometry values. The use of wavefront aberrometry in preoperative workup of cataract surgery and other procedures[66-68] has been described. AcrySof toric IOL is one of the most widely used toric IOL and has been confirmed to be effective in the reduction of refractive astigmatism by providing optimal visual outcomes.[65,69] Several concerns following implantation of toric IOLs in corneal ectasia are

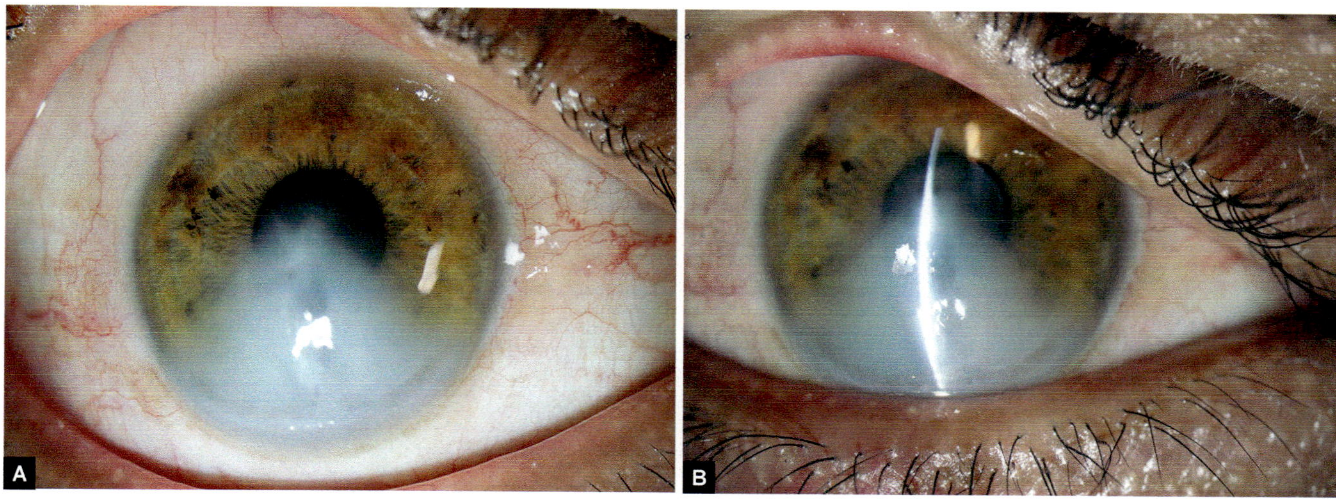

Figs. 16A and B: Slit-lamp biomicroscopy both in diffuse and slit illumination in the left eye reveals a dense inferior corneal edema encroaching the visual axis with large intrastromal fluid clefts in a patient with pellucid marginal degeneration.

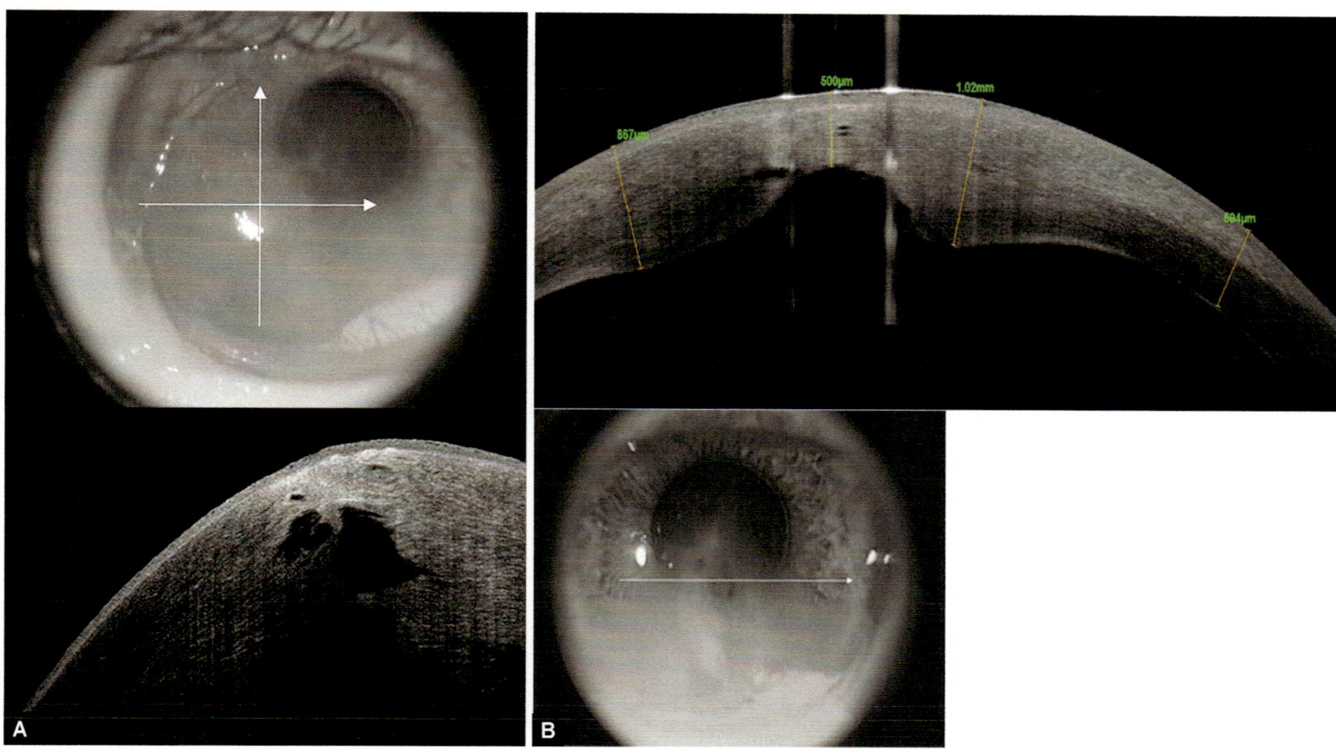

Figs. 17A and B: Anterior segment optical coherence tomography (AS-OCT) show (A) well-defined intrastromal fluid clefts, microcystic epithelial edema with increased corneal thickness; (B) Disappearance of intrastromal fluid clefts with scarring 1 month post intracameral C3F8 injection.

poor preoperative corrected distance visual acuity (CDVA), rotational stability of the IOL, and progression of the disease. Hence, careful and judicious case selection is necessary to achieve optimal visual outcomes. Corneal ectasia cases with poor BSCVA and/or irregular astigmatism are considered unfit for toric IOLs. This is because of high preexisting corneal higher order aberrations (HOAs) or corneal scarring. Ideally these cases should be taken up only by experienced hands as any intraoperative complications that may require extending of the incisions can higher the chances of astigmatism considerably.

The case series by Parikakis et al., have shown to attain optimal visual outcomes with toric IOL implantation in patients with stable KC or PMD with cataract.[70] Camoriano et al.,[71] in their study have recently reported regarding improvement in visual outcomes with toric IOL implantation for PMD in 10 eyes.[1]

Postoperative and Rehabilitation Care

Patients with PMD often will need lifelong follow-up. Suture loosening and graft rejection in the early postoperative period is a known complication following keratoplasty and

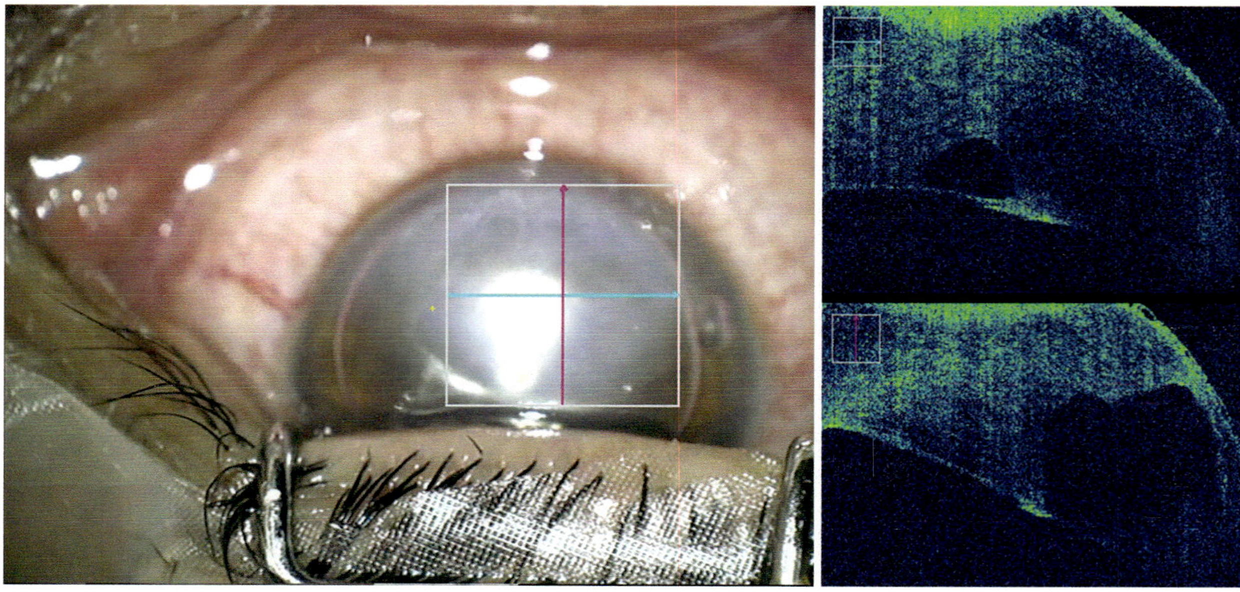

Fig. 18: The microscope integrated OCT (miOCT)-guided pneumodescemetopexy showing intracameral injection of isoexpansile perfluoropropane gas with residual intrastromal fluid cleft.

such cases require close follow-up. Spectacles and CLs are usually needed after keratoplasty for complete visual rehabilitation.

REFERENCES

1. Belin MW, Asota IM, Ambrosio R, Khachikian SS. What's in a name: keratoconus, pellucid marginal degeneration, and related thinning disorders. Am J Ophthalmol. 2011;152(2):157-62.
2. Sridhar MS, Mahesh S, Bansal AK, Nutheti R, Rao GN. Pellucid marginal corneal degeneration. Ophthalmology. 2004;111(6):1102-7.
3. Sridhar MS, Mahesh S, Bansal AK, Rao GN. Superior pellucid marginal corneal degeneration. Eye (Lond). 2004;18(4):393-9.
4. Dundar H, Kara N, Kaya V, Bozkurt E, Yazici AT, Hekimhan PK. Unilateral superior pellucid marginal degeneration in a case with ichthyosis. Cont Lens Anterior Eye. 2011;34(1):45-8.
5. Puy P, Stoica BT, Alejandre N, Toledano N. Temporal pellucid marginal degeneration displaying high "with-the-rule" astigmatism. Can J Ophthalmol. 2013;48(6):142-4.
6. Rao SK, Fogla R, Padmanabhan P, Sitalakshmi G. Corneal topography in atypical pellucid marginal degeneration. Cornea. 1999;18(3):265-72.
7. Krachmer JH. Pellucid marginal corneal degeneration. Arch Ophthalmol. 1978;96(7):1217-21.
8. Sinjab MM, Youssef LN, Pellucid-like keratoconus. F1000Res. 2012;1:48.
9. Tummanapalli SS, Maseedupally V, Mandathara P, Rathi VM, Sangwan VS. Evaluation of corneal elevation and thickness indices in pellucid marginal degeneration and keratoconus. J Cataract Refract Surg. 2013;39(1):56-65.
10. Jinabhai A, Radhakrishnan H, O'Donnell C. Pellucid corneal marginal degeneration: a review. Cont Lens Anterior Eye. 2011;34(2):56-63.
11. Krachmer JH, Feder RS, Belin MW. Keratoconus and related noninflammatory corneal thinning disorders. Surv Ophthalmol. 1984;28(4):293-322.
12. Rumelt S, Rehany U. Surgically induced keratoglobus in pellucid marginal degeneration. Eye (Lond). 1998;12(Pt 1):156-8.
13. Taylor CT. Interdependent roles for hypoxia inducible factor and nuclear factor-kappaB in hypoxic inflammation. J Physiol. 2008;586(17):4055-9.
14. Kompella VB, Aasuri MK, Rao GN. Management of pellucid marginal corneal degeneration with rigid gas permeable contact lenses. CLAO J. 2002;28(3):140-5.
15. Horodeński J. [Pellucid marginal corneal degeneration (author's transl)]. Klin Oczna. 1978;48(4):167-8.
16. Sii F, Lee GA, Sanfilippo P, Stephensen DC. Pellucid marginal degeneration and scleroderma. Clin Exp Optom. 2004;87(3):180-4.
17. Pásztor D, Kolozsvári BL, Csutak A, Berta A, Hassan Z, Ujhelyi B, et al. Tear mediators in corneal ectatic disorders. PLoS One. 2016;11(4).
18. Rodrigues MM, Newsome DA, Krachmer JH, Eiferman RA. Pellucid marginal corneal degeneration: A clinicopathologic study of two cases. Exp Eye Res. 1981;33(3):277-88.
19. Tzelikis PF, Cohen EJ, Rapuano CJ, Hammersmith K, Laibson PR. Management of pellucid marginal corneal degeneration. Cornea. 2005;24(5):555-60.
20. Taglia DP, Sugar J. Superior pellucid marginal corneal degeneration with hydrops. Arch Ophthalmol. 1997;115(2):274-5.
21. Robin JB, Schanzlin DJ, Verity SM, Barron BA, Arffa RC, Suarez E, et al. Peripheral corneal disorders. Surv Ophthalmol. 1986;31(1):1-36.
22. Golubović S, Parunović A. Acute pellucid marginal corneal degeneration. Cornea. 1988;7(4):290-4.
23. Kaushik S, Jain AK, Saini JS. Unilateral pellucid marginal degeneration. Eye (Lond). 2003;17(2):246-8.
24. Wagenhorst BB. Unilateral pellucid marginal degeneration in an elderly patient. Br J Ophthalmol. 1996;80(10):927-8.
25. Basak SK, Hazra TK, Bhattacharya D, Sinha TK. Unilateral pellucid marginal degeneration. Indian J Ophthalmol. 2000;48(3):233-4.
26. Rao SK, Fogla R, Padmanabhan P, et al. Corneal topography in atypical pellucid marginal degeneration. Cornea. 1999;18(3):265-72.
27. Ertan A, Bahadir M. Management of superior pellucid marginal degeneration with a single intracorneal ring segment using femtosecond laser. J Refract Surg. 2007;23(2):205-8.
28. Bower KS, Dhaliwal DK, Barnhorst DA, Warnicke J. Pellucid marginal degeneration with superior corneal thinning. Cornea. 1997;16(4):483-5.
29. Sridhar MS, Mahesh S, Bansal AK, et al. Superior pellucid marginal corneal degeneration. Eye (Lond). 2004;18(4):393-9.

30. Cameron JA, Mahmood MA. Superior corneal thinning with pellucid marginal corneal degeneration. Am J Ophthalmol. 1990;109(4):486-7.
31. Gruenauer-Kloevekorn C, Fischer U, Kloevekorn-Norgall K, Duncker GIW. Pellucid marginal corneal degeneration: evaluation of the corneal surface and contact lens fitting. Br J Ophthalmol. 2006;90(3):318-23.
32. Tang M, Shekhar R, Miranda D, Huang D. Characteristics of keratoconus and pellucid marginal degeneration in mean curvature maps. Am J Ophthalmol. 2005;140(6):993-1001.
33. Lee BW, Jurkunas UV, Harissi-Dagher M, Poothullil AM, Tobaigy FM, Azar DT. Ectatic disorders associated with a claw-shaped pattern on corneal topography. Am J Ophthalmol. 2007;144(1):154-6.
34. Martínez-Abad A, Piñero DP. New perspectives on the detection and progression of keratoconus. J Cataract Refract Surg. 2017;43(9):1213-27.
35. Imbornoni LM, McGhee CNJ, Belin MW. Evolution of keratoconus: From the diagnosis to therapeutics. Klin Monbl Augenheilkd. 2018;235(6):680-8.
36. Piñero DP, Nieto JC, Lopez-Miguel A. Characterization of corneal structure in keratoconus. J Cataract Refract Surg. 2012;38(12):2167-83.
37. Gokcinar NB, Yumusak E, Ornek N, Yorubulut S, Onaran Z. Agreement and repeatability of central corneal thickness measurements by four different optical devices and an ultrasound pachymeter. Int Ophthalmol. 2019;39(7):1589-98.
38. Ortiz D, Pinero D, Shabayek MH, Arnalich-Montiel F, Alió JL. Corneal biomechanical properties in normal, post-laser in situ keratomileusis, and keratoconic eyes. J Cataract Refract Surg. 2007;33(8):1371-5.
39. Piñero DP, Alio JL, Barraquer RI, Michael R, Jiménez R. Corneal biomechanics, refraction, and corneal aberrometry in keratoconus: an integrated study. Invest Ophthalmol Vis Sci. 2010;51(4):1948-55.
40. Sedaghat MR, Ostadi-Moghadam H, Jabbarvand M, Askarizadeh F, Momeni-Moghaddam H, Narooie-Noori F. Corneal hysteresis and corneal resistance factor in pellucid marginal degeneration. J Curr Ophthalmol. 2017;30(1):42-7.
41. Maharana PK, Dubey A, Jhanji V, Sharma N, Das S, Vajpayee RB. Management of advanced corneal ectasias. Br J Ophthalmol. 2016;100(1):34-40.
42. Wallang BS, Das S. Keratoglobus. Eye (Lond). 2013;27(9):1004-12.
43. Kiire C, Srinivasan S. Management of bilateral acute hydrops secondary to keratoglobus with perfluoroethane (C2F6) pneumodescemetopexy. Clin Exp Ophthalmol. 2009;37(9):892-4.
44. Karabatsas CH, Cook SD. Topographic analysis in pellucid marginal degeneration and keratoglobus. Eye (Lond). 1996;10(Pt 4):451-5.
45. Rumelt S, Rehany U. Surgically induced keratoglobus in pellucid marginal degeneration. Eye (Lond). 1998;12(Pt 1):156-8.
46. Robin JB, Schanzlin DJ, Verity SM, et al. Peripheral corneal disorders. Surv Ophthalmol. 1986;31(1):1-36.
47. Beauchamp GR. Terrien's marginal corneal degeneration J Pediatr Ophthalmol Strabismus. 1982;19(2):97-9.
48. Ceresara G, Migliavacca L, Orzalesi N, Rossetti L. In vivo confocal microscopy in terrien marginal corneal degeneration: a case report. Cornea. 2011;30(7):820-4.
49. Chan AT, Ulate R, Goldich Y, Rootman DS, Chan CC. Terrien marginal degeneration: Clinical characteristics and outcomes. Am J Ophthalmol. 2015;160(5):867-72.
50. Radhakrishnan H, O'Donnell C. Aberrometry in clinical practice: Case series. Cont Lens Anterior Eye. 2008;31(4):207-11.
51. Zhou X, Wang L, Chu R, Yu Z. Corneal thickness distribution and its relationship with corneal topography in ametropic population. Zhonghua Yan Ke Za Zhi. 2014;50(9):658-64.
52. Ueno Y, Hiraoka T, Miyazaki M, Ito M, Oshika T. Corneal thickness profile and posterior corneal astigmatism in normal corneas. Ophthalmology. 2015;122(6):1072-8.
53. Akhtar S, Kirat O, Alkatan H, Shu X, Almubrad T. Ultrastructural features of corneas with pellucid marginal degeneration. Microsc Res Tech. 2013;76(4):404-11.
54. Kamiya K, Hirohara Y, Mihashi T, Hiraoka T, Kaji Y, Oshika T. Progression of pellucid marginal degeneration and higher-order wavefront aberration of the cornea. Jpn J Ophthalmol. 2003;47(5):523-5.
55. Rathi VM, Dumpati S, Mandathara PS, Tanejac MM, Sangwanc VS. Scleral contact lenses in the management of pellucid marginal degeneration. Cont Lens Anterior Eye. 2016;39(3):217-20.
56. Hassan Z, Nemeth G, Modis L, Szalai E, Berta A. Collagen cross-linking in the treatment of pellucid marginal degeneration. Indian J Ophthalmol. 2014;62(3):367-70.
57. Varley GA, Macsai MS, Krachmer JH. The results of penetrating keratoplasty for pellucid marginal corneal degeneration. Am J Ophthalmol. 1990;110(2):149-52.
58. Kaushal S, Jhanji V, Sharma N, Tandon R, Titiyal JS, Vajpayee RB. "Tuck In" Lamellar Keratoplasty (TILK) for corneal ectasias involving corneal periphery. Br J Ophthalmol. 2008;92(2):286-90.
59. Kremer I, Sperber LT, Laibson PR. Pellucid marginal degeneration treated by lamellar and penetrating keratoplasty. Arch Ophthalmol. 1993;111(2):169-70.
60. Rasheed K, Rabinowitz YS. Surgical treatment of advanced pellucid marginal degeneration. Ophthalmology. 2000;107(10):1836-40.
61. Jabbarvand M, Hashemian H, Khodaparast M, Hassanpour N, Mohebbi M. Intrastromal lamellar keratoplasty in patients with pellucid marginal degeneration. J Cataract Refract Surg. 2015;41(1):2-8.
62. MacLean H, Robinson LP, Wechsler AW. Long-term results of corneal wedge excision for pellucid marginal degeneration. Eye (Lond). 1997;11 (Pt 5):613-7.
63. Fronterrè A, Portesani GP. Epikeratoplasty for pellucid marginal corneal degeneration. Cornea. 1991;10(5):450-3.
64. Moshirfar M, Edmonds JN, Behunin NL, Christiansen SM. Current options in the management of pellucid marginal degeneration. J Refract Surg. 2014;30:474-85.
65. Kersey JP, O'Donnell A, Illingworth CD: Cataract surgery with toric intraocular lenses can optimize uncorrected postoperative visual acuity in patients with marked corneal astigmatism. Cornea. 2007;26:133-5.
66. Maeda N. Clinical applications of wavefront aberrometry - a review. Clin Experiment Ophthalmol. 2009;37:118-29.
67. Cerviño A, Hosking SL, Montes-Mico R, Bates K. Clinical ocular wavefront analyzers. J Refract Surg. 2007;23:603-16.
68. Visser N, Berendschot TT, Verbakel F, Tan AN, de Brabander J, Rudy M. M. A. Nuijts RMMA. Evaluation of the comparability and repeatability of four wavefront aberrometers. Invest Ophthalmol Vis Sci. 2011;52:1302-11.
69. Visser N, Ruíz-Mesa R, Pastor F, Bauer NJ, Nuijts RM, Montés-Micó R. Cataract surgery with toric intraocular lens implantation in patients with high corneal astigmatism. J Cataract Refract Surg. 2011;37:1403-10.
70. Parikakis EA, Chatziralli IP, Peponis VG, David G, Chalkiadakis S, Mitropoulos PG. Toric intraocular lens implantation for correction of astigmatism in cataract patients with corneal ectasia. Case Rep Ophthalmol. 2013;4(3):219-28.
71. Camoriano GD, Aman-Ullah M, Purba MK, Sun J, Gimbel HV. Toric collagen copolymer phakic intraocular lens to correct myopic astigmatism in eyes with pellucid marginal degeneration. J Cataract Refract Surg. 2012;38:256-61.

61

Terrien's Marginal Degeneration

Sohini Mandal, Somasheila I Murthy

INTRODUCTION

Terrien marginal degeneration (TMD) is a rare, asymmetrically bilateral slowly progressive disease characterized by the following pathognomonic features: (1) a peripheral crescentic area of thin cornea with furrow formation, (2) superficial, radial, and tortuous or circumferential appearing blood vessels in the peripheral thinned area, (3) lipid deposition at the leading edge, and (4) undamaged corneal epithelium without apparent inflammatory signs or symptoms (**Figs. 1A and B**).[1]

ETIOLOGY

While the exact etiology is unknown, various authors have come up with different hypotheses behind the etiology of TMD. These assumptions are based on the histopathological results of the surgical specimens of TMD.

Degenerative Origin

The degenerative type of the disease is characterized by relatively slow progression with a long course, asymptomatic nature and lipid deposition at the leading edge. Iwamoto et al. had hypothesized the occurrence of fatty degeneration as a result of tissue hypoxia in the corneal stroma.[2]

Inflammatory Origin

In contrary to the previous theory, the inflammatory type of the disease is characterized by repeated episodes of pain, photophobia, watering, conjunctival injection, and/or epithelial defect. Iwamoto and Austin et al.[2,3] conjectured that immune responses incite this type of the disease. The degenerated basal epithelial cells secrete an immunogenic component to the basement membrane which results in hypersensitivity.[2]

Phagocytosis of Collagen by Histiocytes

Süveges proposed that stromal collagen lamellae are phagocytosed by histiocyte-like cells.[1] As reported by a recent study, an increased level of N-acetyl-β-D-glucosaminidase (lysosomal enzyme) has been detected in the tear film of

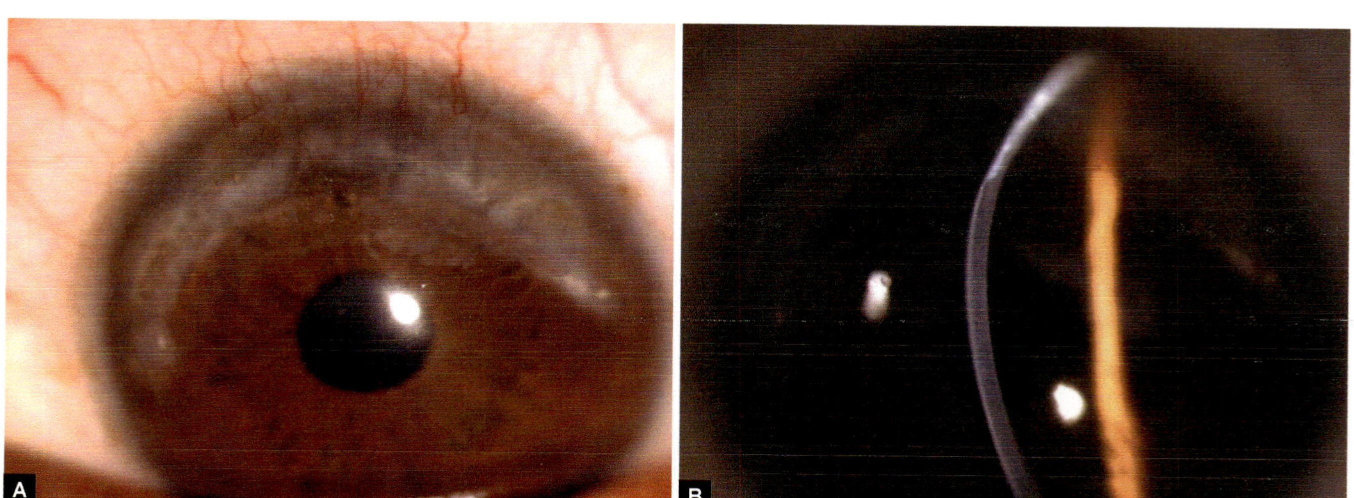

Figs. 1A and B: Slit-lamp examination, diffuse and slit illumination shows the presence of a fine, white-yellow peripheral opaque band with lipid deposition at the leading edge in the superior half of the cornea, as well as superficial vascularization in the transparent area between the limbus and the opaque band. The trajectory of the blood vessels is often radial with some tortuosity and circumferential extension.

TMD patients. This could be an indirect signal for histiocyte-like cell infiltration.[4]

In vivo confocal microscopy (IVCM) which is a recent addition to the existing literature, demonstrates clusters of lymphocytes and branched Langerhans cells in the early stage of the disease.[5] Langerhans cells are dendritic cells that process and present antigens to CD4+ and CD8+ cells. These cells secrete low-grade cytokines to induce corneal neovascularization as they steadily alter the morphology and function of stromal keratocytes.

Most common systemic and ocular associations reported with TMD are arthritis[6] and meibomian gland dysfunction,[7] respectively. However, these associations may only be a chance association as systemic disease might be absent in many TMD patients.

EPIDEMIOLOGY

There is no exact data on incidence and prevalence of TMD in literature, because of its rare occurrence. A recent case series has stated that the disease can occur at any ages, with a mean manifestation at 44 years and a slight male preponderance (54%).[7] In a similar study, 48.3% of TMD patients belonged to the age group between 40 and 59 years.

PATHOLOGY

Histochemical and electron microscopic studies aid in discovering the various ultrastructural changes in TMD.[1,2,8,9] Both in cases of degenerative as well as inflammatory variant of this disease, pyknotic nuclei and vacuole formation are observed in the corneal epithelium on light microscopy. Basement membrane appears thickened and fragmented with underlying collagen fibril degradation. Descemet membrane is also thickened with signs of previous breaking and healing. The endothelial cells can appear normal or degenerated. Inflammatory cells such as histiocytes, fibrocytes, lymphocytes, and plasma cells are distributed in various corneal layers with involvement of blood vessels as well.

Electron microscopic features of TMD reveal degenerated epithelial cells that contain dense cytoplasm with cytoplasmic projections, dilated interstitial spaces, intracellular vacuoles, and ill-defined organelles. Besides, fibrinoid collagen degeneration, which is typically seen in immune hypersensitivity, can also occur.[2,8] The pathognomonic hallmark of TMD is the presence of numerous intracellular and extracellular vacuoles.

Süveges et al. have classified these vacuoles into two types based on their composition.[10] One group consist of phagolysosomes comprising degraded collagen fibrils, while the other variety has phagolysosomes accumulating lipid-like materials. On the contrary, Iwamoto and Pouliquen et al. have reported only the lipid variant of vacuole formation.[2,8]

CLINICAL MANIFESTATIONS

Although, the disease is detected incidentally, TMD patients usually present with decline in visual acuity or mild foreign body sensation. It is a bilateral disease and progresses through five clinical stages.[1,2,11-14] TMD is characteristically associated with high against the rule astigmatism as the degenerative process typically originates from the superior or superonasal area of the cornea.[7] The peripheral corneal thinning leads to flattening in the vertical meridian, leading to relative steepening in the opposite meridian.[15]

Terrien marginal degeneration is a slowly progressive disorder reported, sometimes as late as over the course of 30 years.[3] A small number of cases of early TMD may be associated with atypical pterygia[12] that may be present outside the palpebral fissure. They have a broad, flat anterior edge, and often extending onto the cornea obliquely.

Complications include perforations which have been reported about 15%[3] cases in older literature, which is similar to the results reported by Chan et al.,[7] i.e., 11.6%. These can rarely happen spontaneously but more often are noted after trivial trauma such as finger nail injury. Descemet membrane detachments[16] and corneal hydrops[2,13] have also been described to occur very rarely. Hydrops in TMD appears as focal corneal edema with large intrastromal fluid caverna or clefts containing aqueous humor that can rarely spread underneath the conjunctiva, thus giving an appearance of a filtering bleb with subsequent danger of hypotony and associated maculopathy.[17]

The classical form of TMD encompasses to have intact epithelium in absence of any inflammatory signs or symptoms, however in the past decade, the debate about the latent existence of an inflammatory type of TMD has continued.

Iwamoto et al.[2] have classified the disease into two types: (1) inflammatory and (2) quiescent. Austin and Brown et al. have suggested the inflammatory variant of TMD to be a standard Terrien lesion with surrounding deep episcleritis. The associated episcleritis is the reason behind development of severe recurring ocular pain, conjunctival hyperemia, epiphora, and photophobia.

Terrien marginal degeneration is also reported to be associated with puberty and menstrual cycle.[3] TMD can be associated with various corneal and systemic diseases such as lattice stromal dystrophy,[18] posterior polymorphous corneal dystrophy,[19] vernal keratoconjunctivitis,[20] rheumatoid arthritis,[6] and erythema elevatum diutinum.[21]

DIFFERENTIAL DIAGNOSIS

The close differentials of TMD include: peripheral ulcerative keratitis (PUK), Mooren's ulcer, peripheral infectious keratitis, Fuchs superficial marginal keratitis, pellucid marginal degeneration (PMD), degenerative changes of peripheral cornea, and dellen. Therefore, these conditions need to be differentiated from each other.

Mooren's ulcer can be mistaken for TMD only in the early stages, where the patient may have a chronic indolent Mooren's ulcer with slow progression. In classical or full-blown Mooren's ulcer, the patient would have prominent symptoms such as redness and pain ranging from mild to severe and photophobia. There can often be rapid progression with high possibility of perforation.[22,23] Unlike classic form of TMD, Mooren's ulcer typically starts in the interpalpebral areas, with presence of epithelial defect, severe ocular pain, pathognomonic overhanging edge, and circulating immune complexes.[24]

Patients with PUK presents with pain, redness, and photophobia. Slit-lamp microscopic findings such as progressive stromal ulceration and epithelial loss as well as scleral involvement are not seen in TMD (**Figs. 2A and B**).[25] In case of granulomatosis with polyangiitis-associated PUK, patients would have additional systemic features that would help clinch the diagnosis. These would include respiratory associations such as chronic sinusitis, pneumonitis, nasopharyngeal ulceration, and urinary problem such as glomerulonephritis[26] which are absent in TMD. Similarly, patients with rheumatoid arthritis-associated PUK may present initially with constitutional symptoms such as fever, fatigue, anorexia, and typical joint pain.[27]

Fuchs superficial marginal keratitis is a very rare entity reported in literature. Slit-lamp microscopy reveals a well-defined gray band at the leading edge of the lesion.[28] There might be a possibility that Fuchs superficial marginal keratitis and TMD could be diverse appearances of the same disease spectrum.[29]

Marginal keratitis often presents secondary to blepharoconjunctivitis as a result of hypersensitivity reaction to *Staphylococcus* species.[23] Infective keratitis involving the corneal periphery is rapidly progressive in nature and is associated with purulent infiltrates often following trauma or contact lens wear.[22,23]

Pellucid marginal degeneration usually involves the inferior periphery of the cornea; however, rarely they can mimic TMD when superior cornea is affected.[30-32]

Very commonly, arcus senilis and senile marginal furrow degeneration can closely resemble TMD. They are physiological visually insignificant corneal degenerations.[23] Dellen are caused due to tear film instability manifested as local perilimbal elevation with desiccation of the adjacent cornea.[22]

USE OF RECENT INVESTIGATIVE MODALITIES IN TERRIEN MARGINAL DEGENERATION

The conventional topography map of TMD displays flattening over the areas of peripheral thinning and a consecutive steepening 90° away.

- *Orbscan II*: Scanning slit topography can pick up the disease in subclinical stage itself showing corneal elevation changes and increased astigmatism.[33]
- *Scheimpflug imaging*: It provides more detailed information about the cornea periphery compared to other diagnostic techniques.[34] Therefore, Scheimpflug imaging holds a significant place diagnosis and staging of TMD (**Figs. 3 to 6**).
- *Anterior segment optical coherence tomography (ASOCT)*: It is a noninvasive imaging modality that provides a high-definition in vivo cross-sectional image of the cornea.[35,36] It very well depicts the morphologic changes[37] and can help in surgical management by providing information about the thinnest corneal location, that may prevent intraoperative inadvertent perforation.[38]
  Wang et al. in their study have recently described a novel ASOCT-based staging system[39] with defining parameters

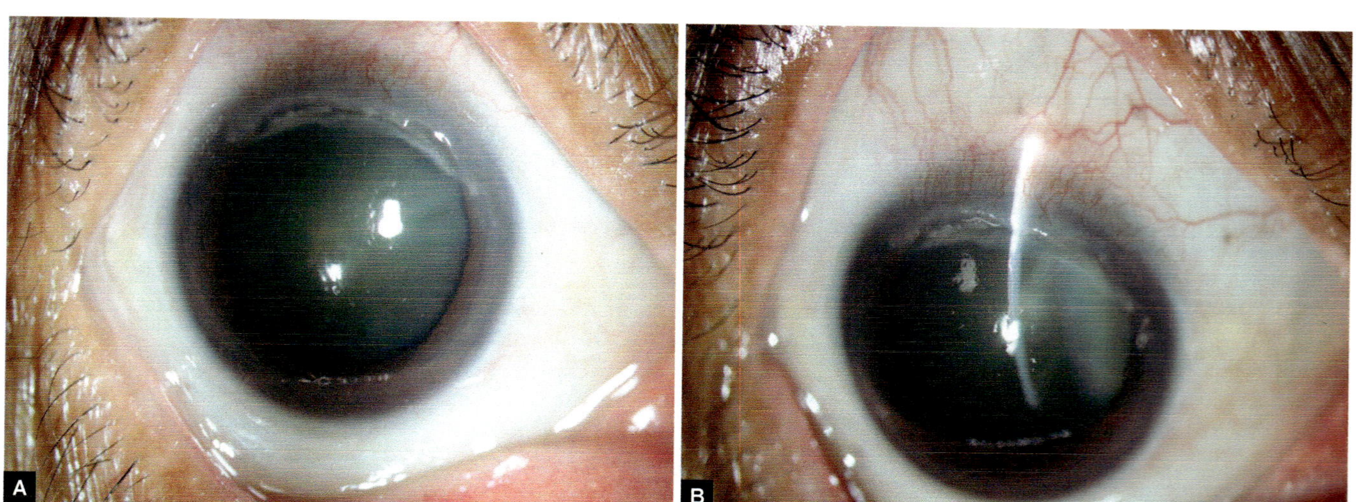

Figs. 2A and B: A case with superior peripheral ulcerative keratitis which was referred to as Terrien's marginal degeneration: Slit-lamp examination, diffuse and slit illumination shows a crescent-shaped narrow band of corneal stromal ulceration with epithelial defect in the superior cornea extending from 10 to 2 o' clock hours with adjacent sectoral conjunctival congestion.

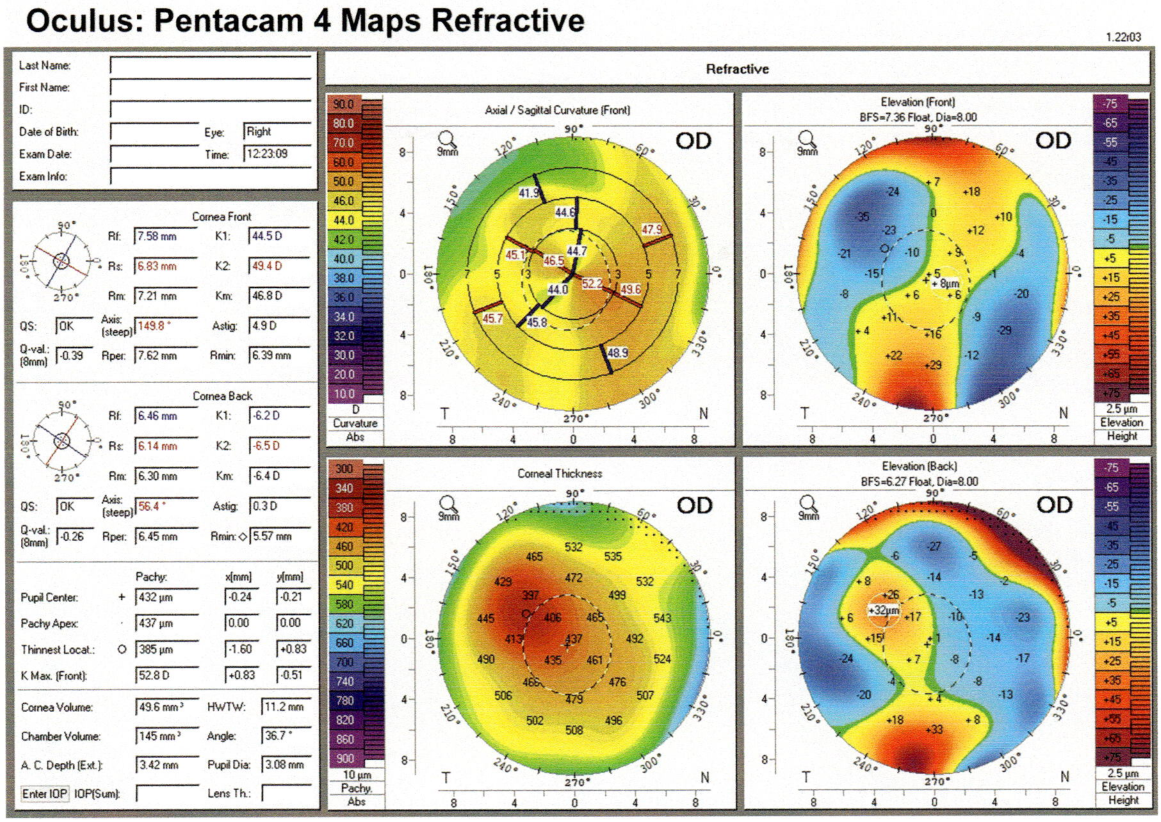

Fig. 3: Pentacam quad map of a patient of Terrien's marginal degeneration in right eye showing high against the rule astigmatism with flattening of the peripheral thinned cornea in the vertical meridian and relative steepening of the corneal 90° away on the axial sagittal curvature map. The thinnest point is located in the superotemporal quadrant.

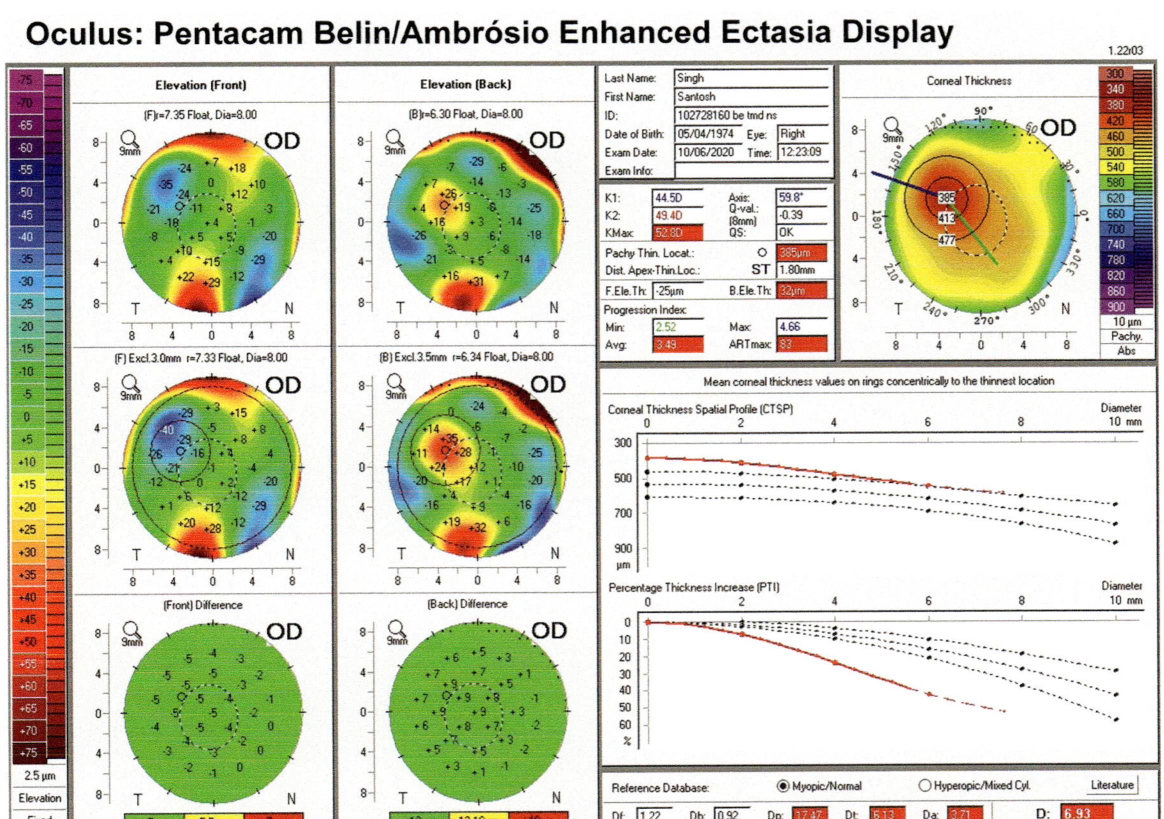

Fig. 4: The Pentacam Belin Ambrósio enhanced ectasia display of the same patient as shown in **Figure 3**, showing corneal graph lying outside 2 standard deviation with abnormal D value, pachymetry progression index and Ambrósio relational thickness.

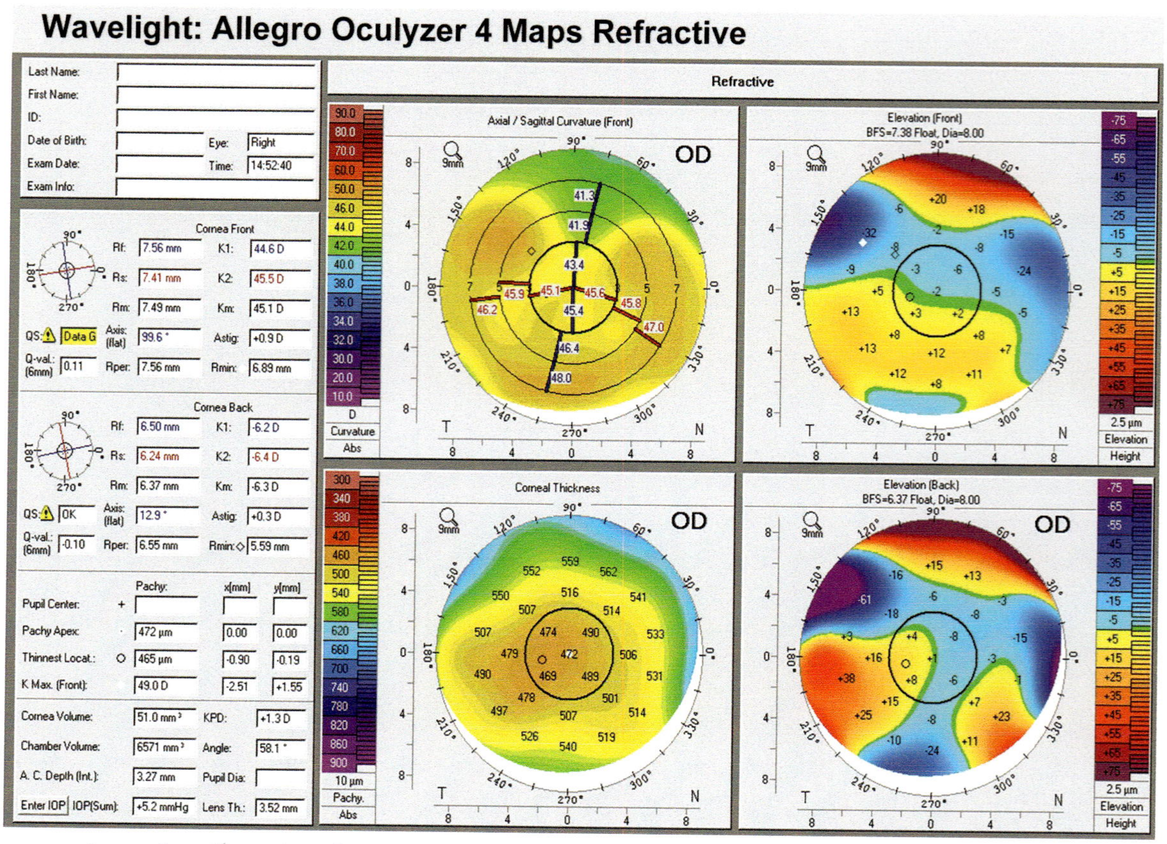

Fig. 5: Pentacam quad map of another patient of Terrien's marginal degeneration in right eye showing against the rule astigmatism with flattening of the peripheral thinned cornea in the vertical meridian and relative steepening in the opposite meridian on the anterior sagittal curvature map. There is also loss of the symmetric bow tie pattern with inferior steepening.

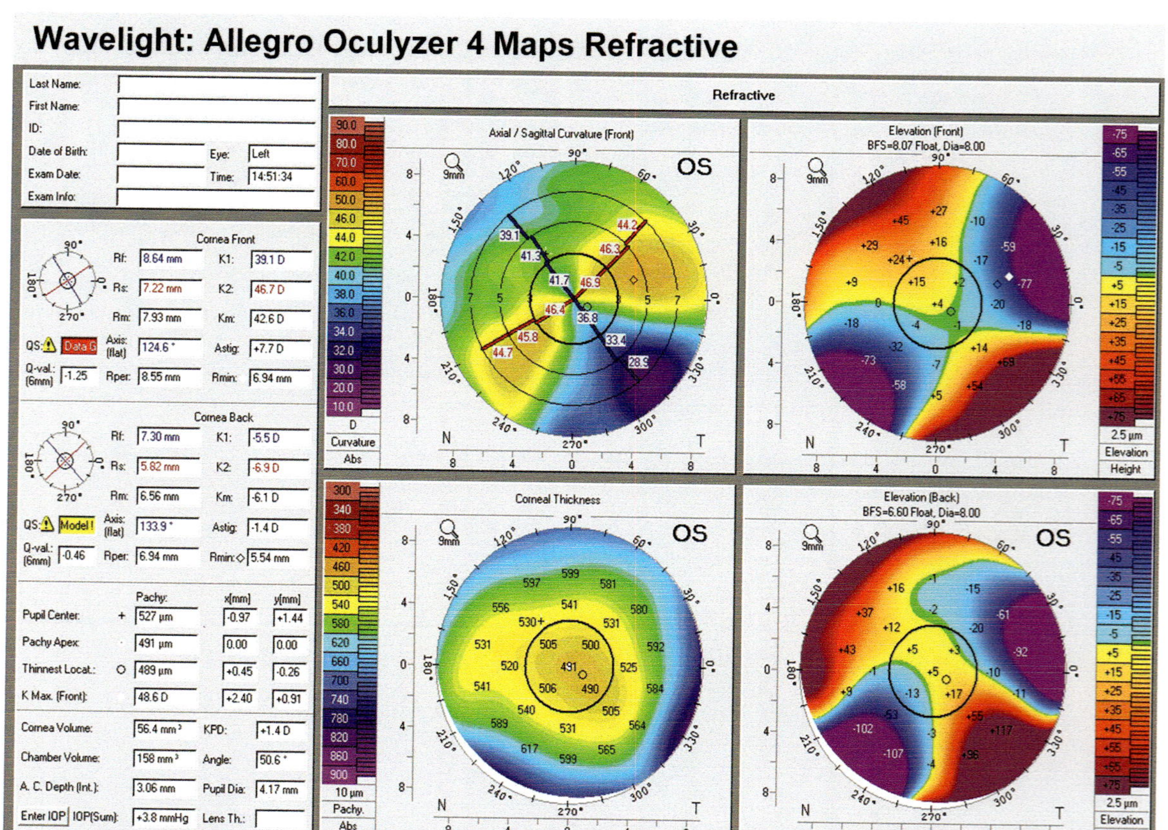

Fig. 6: Pentacam quad map of the same patient of Terrien's marginal degeneration in left eye showing high oblique astigmatism with marked flattening in the inferotemporal quadrant on the anterior sagittal curvature map.

as anterior curvature, posterior curvature, and the thinnest area of the cornea.

- *High-resolution ultrasound biomicroscopy (UBM)*: This modality very nicely demonstrates the morphological changes of the cornea in TMD.[40] On the contrary, IVCM provides more histological information on the disease.

TREATMENT

Nonsurgical Treatment

The progression of the disease cannot be halted with medical management. Symptomatic treatment for mild irritation experienced by a few patients can benefit with artificial tears and bandage contact lenses.

In early stage of the disease, spectacles alone can be used to visually rehabilitate the patient;[41] however, as the disease advances, high degree of against the rule and irregular astigmatism comes into play. Rigid gas permeable (RGP) or scleral contact lenses may be instituted in such cases. The prosthetic replacement of the ocular surface ecosystem (PROSE), is a customized scleral contact lens that vaults over the cornea and limbus.[42] An oxygenated tear pool rests between the contact lens and cornea, with presence of radial venting conduits to prevent suction.[43] Several studies have demonstrated the efficacy of PROSE contact lens in improving the visual acuity in such patients.[42-45] However, they come with several drawbacks such as accumulation of debris in tear film, haze, halo, and difficult manipulation.[46]

Surgical Treatment

Advanced cases of TMD often require surgical intervention which can be categorized into two groups: (1) tectonic and (2) vision enhancement surgeries.

1. Tectonic surgeries are primarily indicated for restoration of the globe integrity which include conjunctival flaps[47] and scleral autotransplantation[48] in cases of donor cornea paucity (**Figs. 7 and 8**). However, few shortcomings of this procedure are limited vision gain, cosmetic blemish, and difficulty for a second-stage penetrating keratoplasty.
2. Vision enhancement surgery intends to improve the visual acuity and restore globe integrity as well. These surgeries include ectatic tissue removal with suture apposition of the adjacent healthy cornea,[47] epikeratophakia,[49] partial or total full-thickness keratoplasty[50,51] or lamellar keratoplasty (LK).[10,38,52-57] LK using grafts with various shapes and depths (match and patch technique) is conventionally performed (**Fig. 9**). Femtosecond laser-assisted LK has an upper hand over conventional procedure in producing a smoother recipient bed, but endothelial damage remains a major setback.[58]

Surgical intervention is typically contraindicated in mild to moderate stages of TMD until there is a high risk of impending perforation.[7,52] There has been a major

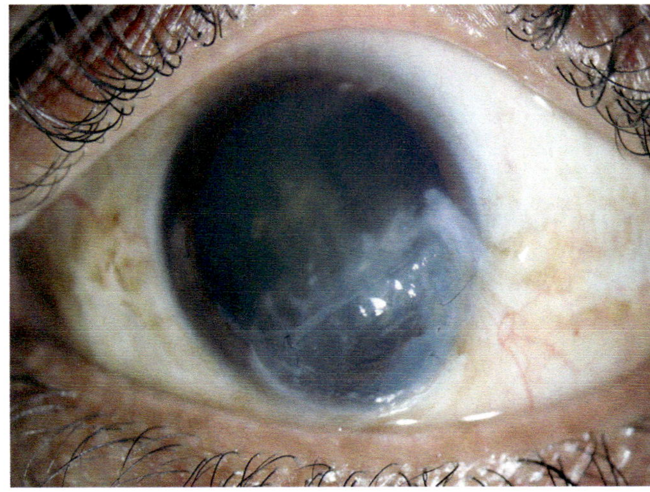

Fig. 7: Slit-lamp photograph (diffuse illumination) shows the left eye of a case of Terrien's marginal degeneration with operated crescentic patch graft for the repair of perforation following trivial trauma. The graft appears edematous, however, the chief purpose of restoring the integrity of the eye has been achieved.

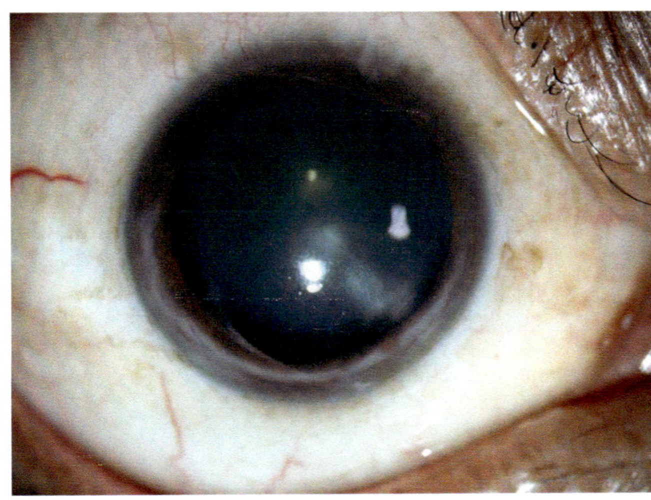

Fig. 8: Slit-lamp photograph (diffuse illumination) shows the right eye of the same case of Terrien's marginal degeneration with fine and white peripheral opaque band in the inferior half of the cornea without any evidence of lipid deposition and superficial vascularization.

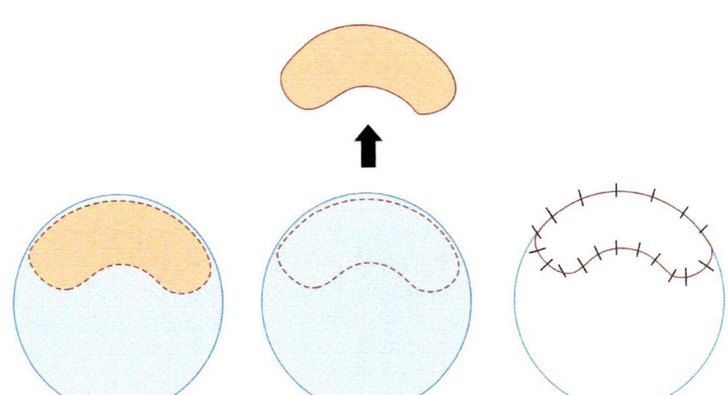

Fig. 9: Schematic representation of crescentic lamellar or full-thickness corneal patch graft anchored to the recipient bed using interrupted 10-0 monofilament nylon sutures.

conflict between two schools of thought; one that supports conservative management even in corneas below 150 µm thickness, and other that agrees with intervening when minimum corneal thickness reaches 150 µm.[54]

In a small scale study cohort, Hafezi et al. have successfully halted the progression of TMD through riboflavin-assisted corneal collagen cross-linking.[59] Therefore, large sample studies are required to authenticate the efficacy of cross-linking treatment.

Patients should be made aware regarding the prognosis, natural course, associated risk of perforation with trivial trauma, and respective treatment options according to various stages. Eye rubbing should be sternly evaded, and protective eyewear is recommended. Patients should be called on consistent follow-ups with serial ASOCT when the corneal thickness reaches 250 µm.

CONCLUSION

Although TMD has been familiar since the last century, the exact etiology remains unknown. Despite its ambiguous etiology, the management of TMD has evolved drastically with the target of enhancing the visual outcomes and corneal integrity. Preoperative assessment using ASOCT enables corneal surgeons to integrate manual or femtosecond-assisted LK in the treatment of the disease.

REFERENCES

1. Süveges I, Lévai G, Alberth B. Pathology of Terrien's disease: histochemical and electron microscopic study. Am J Ophthalmol. 1972;74(6):1191-200.
2. Ashenhurst M, Slomovic A. Corneal hydrops in Terrien's marginal degeneration: an unusual complication. Can J Ophthalmol. 1987;22(6):328-30.
3. Austin P, Brown SI. Inflammatory Terrien's marginal corneal disease. Am J Ophthalmol. 1981;92(2):189-92.
4. Hayasaka S, Tsuchiya M, Sekimoto M, Noda S, Shibuya Y, Setogawa T. Lysosomal enzymes in tear fluids from patients with Terrien's marginal corneal degeneration. Graefes Arch Clin Exp Ophthalmol. 1987;225(5):335-7.
5. Ceresara G, Migliavacca L, Orzalesi N, Rossetti L. In vivo confocal microscopy in Terrien marginal corneal degeneration: a case report. Cornea. 2011;30(7):820-4.
6. Zarei-Ghanavati S, Javadi MA, Yazdani S. Bilateral Terrien's marginal degeneration and posterior polymorphous dystrophy in a patient with rheumatoid arthritis. J Ophthalmic Vis Res. 2012;7(1):60-3.
7. Chan AT, Ulate R, Goldich Y, Rootman DS, Chan CC. Terrien marginal degeneration: clinical characteristics and outcomes. Am J Ophthalmol. 2015;160(5):867-72.e1.
8. Pouliquen Y, Dhermy P, Renard G, Goichot-Bonnat L, Foster G, Savoldelli M. Terrien's disease: clinical and ultrastructural studies, five case reports. Eye (Lond). 1989;3(Pt 6):791-802.
9. Guyer DR, Barraquer J, McDonnell PJ, Green WR. Terrien's marginal degeneration: clinicopathologic case reports. Graefes Arch Clin Exp Ophthalmol. 1987;225(1):19-27.
10. Pettit TH. Corneoscleral freehand lamellar keratoplasty in Terrien's marginal degeneration of the cornea—long-term results. Refract Corneal Surg. 1991;7(1):28-32.
11. Pesudovs K. Terrien's marginal degeneration: case reports and literature review. Clin Exp Optom. 1994;77(3):97-104.
12. Goldman KN, Kaufman HE. Atypical pterygium. A clinical feature of Terrien's marginal degeneration. Arch Ophthalmol. 1978;96(6):1027-9.
13. Soong HK, Fitzgerald J, Boruchoff SA, Sugar A, Meyer RF, Gabel MG. Corneal hydrops in Terrien's marginal degeneration. Ophthalmology. 1986;93(3):340-3.
14. Berrocal AM, Chen PC, Soukiasian SH. Ultrasound biomicroscopy of corneal hydrops in Terrien's marginal degeneration. Ophthalmic Surg Lasers. 2002;33(3):228-30.
15. Wilson SE, Lin DT, Klyce SD, Insler MS. Terrien's marginal degeneration: corneal topography. Refract Corneal Surg. 1990;6(1):15-20.
16. Vejdani A, Khakshoor H, McCaughey M, Moshirfar M. Partial and total Descemet's detachments in a patient with severe Terrien's marginal degeneration and juvenile idiopathic arthritis. Case Rep Ophthalmol Med. 2014;2014.279491.
17. Munro M, McWhae J, Romanchuk K, Crichton A, Carter G, Ball A. Two cases of spontaneous filtering blebs, one idiopathic and one associated with Terrien marginal degeneration. Cornea. 2014;33(7):752-4.
18. Zhang Y, Jia H. Terrien's marginal degeneration accompanied by latticed stromal opacities. Optom Vis Sci. 2014;91(5):110-6.
19. Wagoner MD, Teichmann KD. Terrien's marginal degeneration associated with posterior polymorphous dystrophy. Cornea. 1999;18(5):612-5.
20. Kremer I. Terrien's marginal degeneration associated with vernal conjunctivitis. Am J Ophthalmol. 2018;111(4):517-8.
21. Shimazaki J, Yang HY, Shimmura S, Tsubota K. Terrien's marginal degeneration associated with erythema elevatum diutinum. Cornea. 1998;17(3):342-4.
22. Mannis MJ, Holland EJ. Cornea, 4th edition. Philadelphia: Elsevier; 2017.
23. Robin JB, Schanzlin DJ, Verity SM, Barron BA, Arffa RC, Suarez E, et al. Peripheral corneal disorders. Surv Ophthalmol. 1986;31(1):1-36.
24. Berkowitz PJ, Arentsen JJ, Felberg NT, Laibson PR. Presence of circulating immune complexes in patients with peripheral corneal disease. Arch Ophthalmol. 1983;101(2):242-5.
25. Yagci A. Update on peripheral ulcerative keratitis. Clin Ophthalmol. 2012;6:747-54.
26. Greco A, Marinelli C, Fusconi M, Macri GF, Gallo A, De Virgilio A, et al. Clinic manifestations in granulomatosis with polyangiitis. Int J Immunopathol Pharmacol. 2016;29(2):151-9.
27. Grassi W, De Angelis R, Lamanna G, Cervini C. The clinical features of rheumatoid arthritis. Eur J Radiol. 1998;27 Suppl 1:S18-24.
28. Kotecha A, Raber IM. Superficial keratectomy and conjunctival autograft for Fuchs' superficial marginal keratitis. Cornea. 2001;20(2):214-6.
29. Keenan JD, Mandel MR, Margolis TP. Peripheral ulcerative keratitis associated with vasculitis manifesting asymmetrically as Fuchs superficial marginal keratitis and Terrien marginal degeneration. Cornea. 2011;30(7):825-7.
30. Bower KS, Dhaliwal DK, Barnhorst DA Jr, Warnicke J. Pellucid marginal degeneration with superior corneal thinning. Cornea. 1997;16(4):483-5.
31. Sridhar MS, Mahesh S, Bansal AK, Rao GN. Superior pellucid marginal corneal degeneration. Eye (Lond). 2004;18:393-9.
32. Maharana PK, Dubey A, Jhanji V, Sharma N, Das S, Vajpayee RB. Management of advanced corneal ectasias. Br J Ophthalmol. 2016;100(1):34-40.
33. Fernandes M. Scanning slit topography: Diagnostic boon in presumed unilateral Terrien's marginal degeneration. Contact Lens Anterior Eye. 2017;34(6):282-6.

34. Belin MW, Ambrósio R. Scheimpflug imaging for keratoconus and ectatic disease. Indian J Ophthalmol. 2013;61(8):401-6.
35. Chan TCY, Biswas S, Yu M, Jhanji V. Comparison of corneal measurements in keratoconus using swept-source optical coherence tomography and combined Placido-Scheimpflug imaging. Acta Ophthalmol. 2017;95(6):e486-94.
36. Jhanji V, Yang B, Yu M, Ye C, Leung CK. Corneal thickness and elevation measurements using swept-source optical coherence tomography and slit scanning topography in normal and keratoconic eyes. Clin Exp Ophthalmol. 2013;41(8):735-45.
37. Hattori T, Kumakura S, Mori H, Goto H. Depiction of cavity formation in Terrien marginal degeneration by anterior segment optical coherence tomography. Cornea. 2013;32(5):615-8.
38. Wang T, Shi W, Ding G, Li S, Liu M, Gao H. Ring-shaped corneoscleral lamellar keratoplasty guided by high-definition optical coherence tomography and Scheimpflug imaging for severe Terrien's marginal corneal degeneration. Graefes Arch Clin Exp Ophthalmol. 2012;250(12):1795-801.
39. Wang N, Wang CX, Lian XF, Duan SJ, Huang D, Zhou SY. Staging of development in Terrien's degeneration based on corneal curvatures detected by optical coherence tomography. Graefes Arch Clin Exp Ophthalmol. 2015;253(10):1757-64.
40. Skribek A, Sohár N, Gyetvai T, Nógrádi A, Kolozsvári L. Role of ultrasound biomicroscopy in diagnosis and treatment of Terrien Disease. Cornea. 2008;27(4):427-33.
41. Thurschwell LM. Terrien's marginal degeneration. J Am Optom Assoc. 1983;54(5):441-6.
42. Stason WB, Razavi M, Jacobs DS, Shepard DS, Suaya JA, Johns L, et al. Clinical benefits of the Boston ocular surface prosthesis. Am J Ophthalmol. 2010;149(1):54-61.
43. Rosenthal P, Croteau A. Fluid-ventilated, gas-permeable scleral contact lens is an effective option for managing severe ocular surface disease and many corneal disorders that would otherwise require penetrating keratoplasty. Eye Contact Lens. 2005;31(3):130-4.
44. Lee JC, Chiu GB, Bach D, Bababeygy SR, Irvine J, Heur M. Functional and visual improvement with prosthetic replacement of the ocular surface ecosystem scleral lenses for irregular corneas. Cornea. 2013;32(12):1540-3.
45. Rathi VM, Mandathara PS, Dumpati S, Vaddavalli PK, Sangwan VS. Boston ocular surface prosthesis: an Indian experience. Indian J Ophthalmol. 2011;59(4):279-81.
46. Pecego M, Barnett M, Mannis MJ, Durbin-Johnson B. Jupiter Scleral Lenses: the UC Davis eye center experience. Eye Contact Lens. 2012;38(3):179-82.
47. Caldwell DR, Insler MS, Boutros G, Hawk T. Primary surgical repair of severe peripheral marginal ectasia in Terrien's marginal degeneration. Am J Ophthalmol. 1984;97(3):332-6.
48. MV H. Marginal degeneration of the cornea: Report of a case treated with a scleral autograft. Arch Ophthalmol. 1964;72(1):29-31.
49. Chen L, Chen J, Yang B, Liu Z, Feng C, Lin Y, et al. [A preliminary report of epikeratophakia for the treatment of Terrien's degeneration]. Yan Ke Xue Bao. 1997;13(2):79-81.
50. Brown AC, Rao GN, Aquavella JV. Peripheral corneal grafts in Terrien's marginal degeneration. Ophthalmic Surg. 1983;14(11):931-4.
51. Mohammadi H, Morton RL, Wetterholm D. Total keratoplasty in peripheral corneal degeneration. Ophthalmic Surg. 1982; 13(5):400-2.
52. Huang D, Qiu W, Zhang B, Wang BH, Yao YF. Peripheral deep anterior lamellar keratoplasty using a cryopreserved donor cornea for Terrien's marginal degeneration. J Zhejiang Univ Sci B. 2014;15(12):1055-63.
53. Gao H, Wang X, Echegaray JJ, Li S, Wang T, Shi W. Partial lamellar keratoplasty for peripheral corneal disease using a graft from the glycerin-preserved corneoscleral rim. Graefes Arch Clin Exp Ophthalmol. 2014;252(6):963-8.
54. Li L, Zhai H, Xie L, Cheng J, Liu W. Therapeutic effects of lamellar keratoplasty on Terrien marginal degeneration. Cornea. 2018;37(3):318-25.
55. Hahn TW, Kim JH. Two-step annular tectonic lamellar keratoplasty in severe Terrien's marginal degeneration. Ophthalmic Surg. 1993;24(12):831-4.
56. Cheng CL, Theng JT, Tan DT. Compressive C-shaped lamellar keratoplasty: a surgical alternative for the management of severe astigmatism from peripheral corneal degeneration. Ophthalmology. 2005;112(3):425-30.
57. Fernandes M, Vira D. Patch graft for corneal perforation following trivial trauma in bilateral Terrien's marginal degeneration. Middle East Afr J Ophthalmol. 2015;22(2):255-7.
58. Arenas E, Esquenazi S, Anwar M, Terry M. Lamellar corneal transplantation. Surv Ophthalmol. 2012;57(6):510-29.
59. Hafezi F, Gatzioufas Z, Seiler TG, Seiler T. Corneal collagen cross-linking for Terrien marginal degeneration. J Refract Surg. 2014;30(7):498-500.

62

Keratoglobus

Priyadarshini K, Ritu Nagpal, Namrata Sharma, Rasik B Vajpayee

INTRODUCTION

Keratoglobus is a nonprogressive, noninflammatory bilateral, ectatic disorder of the cornea, involving thinning from limbus to limbus with globular protrusion. It can be congenital or acquired.

Congenital keratoglobus usually affects and is present bilaterally since birth. Although no definitive inheritance pattern has been described, autosomal recessive inheritance is the most common. It is seen in association with other ocular and systemic syndromes including the Marfan's syndrome, Rubinstein–Taybi syndrome, blue sclera syndromes such as Ehlers–Danlos type VI and osteogenesis imperfecta and Leber's congenital amaurosis.[1]

Acquired keratoglobus occurs later in life usually secondary to other preexisting ocular disorders. It has been reported to be associated with vernal keratoconjunctivitis, chronic marginal blepharitis, dysthyroid ophthalmopathy, posterior polymorphous dystrophy, idiopathic orbital inflammation, and syphilis.[2]

Brittle cornea syndrome is an autosomal recessive generalized connective tissue disorder involving mutations in the genes *ZNF469* and *PRDM5*.[3] Patients with this disorder are prone to corneal thinning and rupture. Systemic manifestations of this disorder include deafness, developmental dysplasia of the hip, scoliosis, arachnodactyly, joint hypermobility, and hyperelasticity of skin with abnormal scarring. The ocular manifestations are progressive and may lead to the development of keratoconus or keratoglobus, blue sclera, and retinal detachment.

ETIOLOGY

No definitive etiology has been attributed to the disease, nor is any specific inheritance pattern documented in the literature. However, it is seen in association with collagen vascular disorders such as Ehlers–Danlos syndrome, Marfan's syndrome, and blue sclera. Keratoconus is also commonly seen in family members of those with keratoglobus.

PATHOGENESIS

Though it is associated with defects in collagen synthesis and degradation, the exact pathogenesis of keratoglobus remains to be elucidated.

HISTOPATHOLOGY

Histopathologically, it shows diffuse stromal thinning with scarring and disruptions or complete absence of Bowman's membrane. Despite its global thinning, it exhibits normal configuration of stromal lamellar collagen organization. In addition to it, disruption and thickening of Descemet's membrane, scarring and neovascularization of stroma, and central epithelial hyperplasia may also be seen.[4]

IMMUNOHISTOCHEMISTRY

Decreased levels of alpha1-proteinase inhibitor (A1PI) are found in the corneal stroma of patients with keratoglobus. Correspondingly, increased levels of the transcription factor Sp1, which suppress A1PI promoter activity has also been noted.[4] The levels of matrix metalloproteinases (MMP1, MMP2, and MMP3) are also increased in eyes with keratoglobus. Thus alterations in stromal degradation could also be contributory to corneal thinning seen in noninflammatory corneal ectasias.

DIAGNOSIS

Clinical Diagnosis

Suboptimal vision with spectacle and contact lens correction, episodes of pain followed by resolution or decreased visual acuity are the usual presenting complaints.

Clinical signs include high myopia with or without irregular astigmatism, irregular retinoscopic reflex, diffuse corneal thinning that is more pronounced peripherally, globular protrusion of the cornea, Descemet's membrane abnormalities (folds, breaks, thickening, or rupture), acute hydrops, and scarring or neovascularization of the stroma. The typical slit-lamp finding indicating early presentation in an asymptomatic

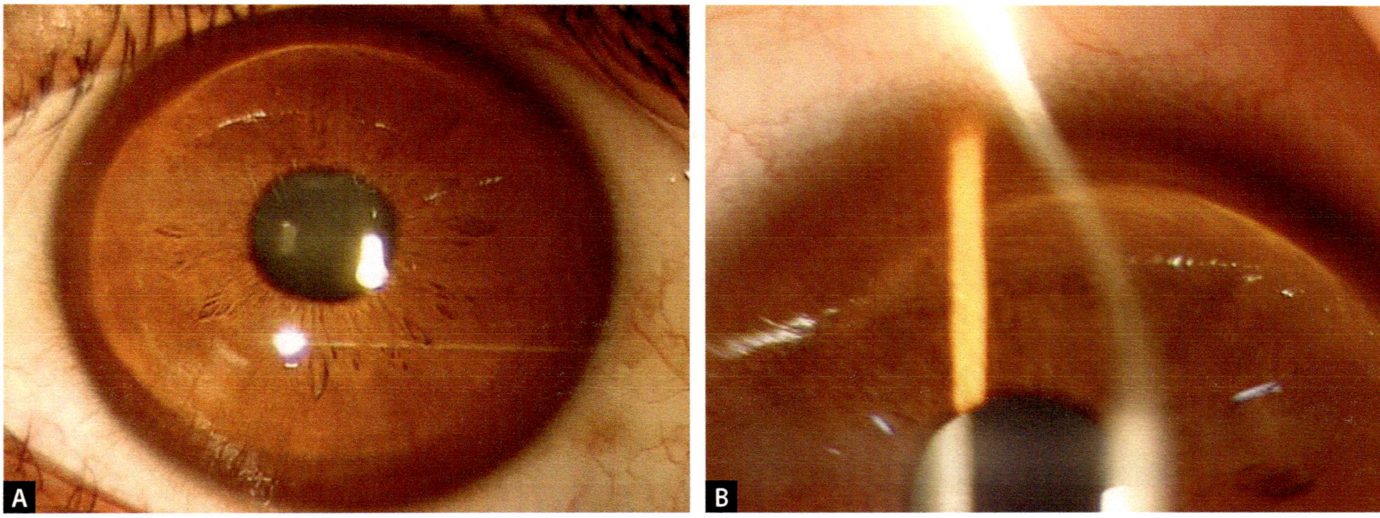

Figs. 1A and B: (A) Slit-lamp photograph of a patient with keratoglobus under diffuse illumination; (B) Clinical photograph of the same eye examined with a slit beam showing pronounced peripheral corneal thinning.

Table 1: Differentiating features between various corneal ectasias.[7]

	Keratoconus	*Pellucid marginal degeneration*	*Keratoglobus*	*Posterior keratoconus*
Frequency	Most common	Less common than keratoconus and keratoglobus	Less common than keratoconus	Least common
Laterality	Usually bilateral	Bilateral	Bilateral	Usually unilateral
Age at onset	Puberty	20–40 years	Usually at birth	Birth
Thinning	Inferior paracentral	Inferior band 1–2 mm wide	Global; Most at periphery	Paracentral posterior excavation
Protrusion	Thinnest at apex	Superior to band of thinning	Generalized	Usually none
Fleischer's ring	Seen	Not present	Not present	Sometimes
Scarring	Common	Only after hydrops	Mild	Common
Vogt's striae	Common	Sometimes	Sometimes	None
Progression	Seen	Seen	Seen	Does not progress
Anterior curve	Steep	Steep in periphery	Flat above and steep below	Normal usually
Posterior curve	Steep	Steep in periphery	Flat above and steep below	Steep

patient shows globular protrusion of the cornea with diffuse thinning (**Figs. 1A and B**).

While acute hydrops is not as common as in keratoconus, patients with keratoglobus are more prone to corneal rupture after a relatively mild trauma. Poole et al. postulated the theory behind keratoglobus eyes being more prone to rupture with minimal trauma.[5] According to Laplace law,

$$\text{Stress} = pr/2t$$

where, p is the intraocular pressure, r is the radius of curvature, and t the corneal thickness. Thus, reduced corneal thickness increases the corneal stress, making it susceptible to breakdown following a trivial trauma. Both spontaneous corneal ruptures and ruptures to trivial trauma have been reported in eyes with keratoglobus. It was found that most patients had poor visual prognosis postoperatively after episodes of corneal rupture.[6]

The differentiating features of keratoglobus from other corneal ectasias such as keratoconus, pellucid marginal degeneration and posterior keratoconus are tabulated in **Table 1**.[7]

Investigations

Investigations which aid in diagnosis include ultrasound pachymetry, corneal topography and tomography, ideally using Scheimpflug imaging and anterior segment optical coherence tomography (**Figs. 2A and B**). Ultrasound pachymetry shows decreased thickness of the cornea. Corneal tomography shows central and paracentral steepening associated with generalized thinning of the cornea. Generalized thinning can also be documented through ASOCT, which can also aid intraoperatively in surgical maneuvers.

Differential Diagnosis

Differential diagnosis of keratoglobus apart from other ectatic corneal disorders include megalocornea and congenital glaucoma.

Megalocornea presents with corneal diameters above 12.5 mm at birth, wherein the corneal diameters are usually normal in keratoglobus. Keratoglobus shows marked

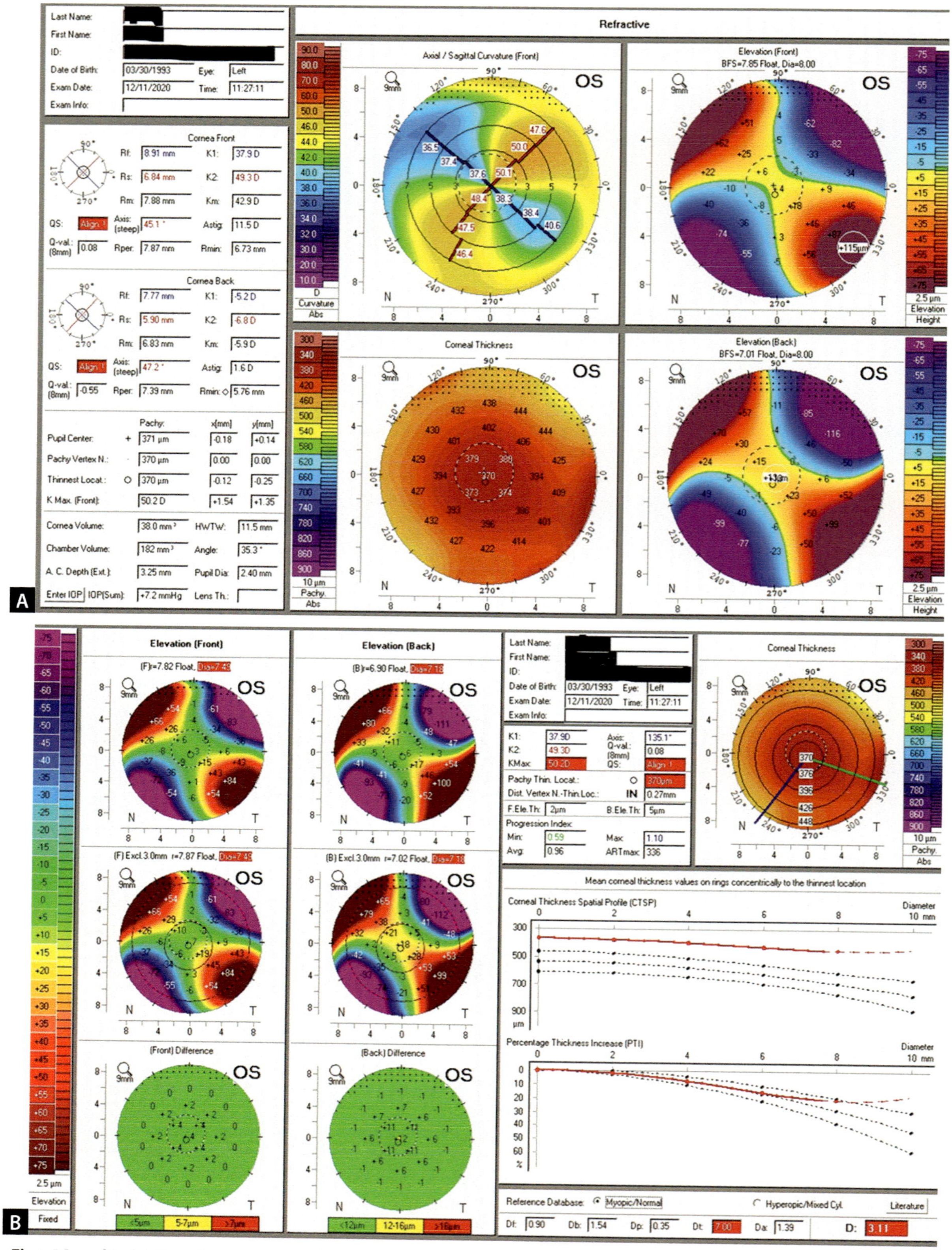

Figs. 2A and B: (A) The 4 Maps Refractive Pentacam scan of a keratoglobus eye illustrating diffuse corneal thinning and steepening; (B) The Belin/Ambrosio' Enhanced Ectatic display map of the same patient.

thinning and protrusion of the cornea resulting in moderate to marked astigmatism, whereas these features are not seen in megalocornea. Hydrops, scarring, and corneal rupture can occur in later stages of keratoglobus, which are never a spectrum of megalocornea.

Congenital glaucoma presents with increased corneal diameters and elevated intraocular pressures with edematous cornea in contrast to keratoglobus, which does not show any of these features. Corneal scarring in the form of Haab's striae may also be seen in congenital glaucoma.

MANAGEMENT

Conservative Management

Initially spectacle correction can be given for optimizing visual acuity. It plays an important role in initial stages, especially in children, to prevent amblyopia. Spectacle correction is preferred with polycarbonate lenses which help in protecting the cornea from trivial trauma, thus preventing corneal rupture, since they have higher tendency to flex and deform rather than shatter.[8]

Use of contact lens for correction of visual acuity is controversial in patients with keratoglobus. As with other ectatic disorders, contact lens trial is started with soft contact lenses and then shifted toward rigid gas permeable, hybrid, or scleral contact lenses as per patient's requirement.[9] Excessively flat rigid contact lenses can cause thinning at corneal apex or epitheliopathy, whereas excessively steep lenses can worsen preexisting ectasia.[10] The risk of corneal rupture in keratoglobus with trivial trauma should also be taken into consideration while opting for contact lenses. Though it is difficult to provide a stable fit due to changing corneal contour, prosthetic replacement of the ocular surface ecosystem (PROSE) scleral contact lenses may provide a good fit in cases of keratoglobus.

Thus, it is better to consider the corneal thickness, patient's comfort and fit of contact lenses before prescribing them in keratoglobus patients.

Surgical Management

Surgery is indicated when conservative measures fail to provide desired visual correction or in cases of contact lens intolerance or hesitancy in prescribing contact lenses due to severe corneal thinning. Various surgical techniques of keratoplasty have evolved over time for the management of keratoglobus. Following are the surgical procedures described so far in cases of keratoglobus:

- Penetrating keratoplasty
- Large diameter penetrating keratoplasty
- Eccentric penetrating keratoplasty
- Tuck in lamellar keratoplasty (TILK)

The advantages and disadvantages of the above mentioned techniques with respect to keratoglobus are briefly discussed below.

Penetrating Keratoplasty

The advantage of this procedure is that it is technically less challenging. However, since a normal thickness graft had to be approximated to a thin host rim, the graft-host disparity results in higher astigmatism, leading to poor visual outcomes.[11]

Large Diameter Penetrating Keratoplasty

Larger diameter grafts >9 mm were then incorporated to circumvent the challenges of regular penetrating keratoplasty in keratoglobus. The complications associated with larger grafts are increased risk of graft rejection, delayed re-epithelialization and higher risk of postoperative glaucoma. However, the initial case report with 9.5 mm graft documented a postoperative visual acuity of 20/60 with just an aqueous leak as a postoperative complication.[12]

Eccentric Penetrating Keratoplasty

This technique was described to overcome the disadvantages of a regular penetrating keratoplasty and large diameter keratoplasty. In the initial case report of the procedure described, the graft was decentered inferiorly over the thinnest pachymetry of the cornea noted on tomography. The report documented a postoperative visual acuity of 20/50.[11]

Tuck in Lamellar Keratoplasty

First described by Vajpayee et al., it has been widely used for the management of keratoglobus.[13] Following host trephination, lamellar dissection is extended centrifugally into the sclera to create a plane to tuck in the donor corneal tissue flange. Thus, the procedure provides graft-host junction stability, decreases postoperative astigmatism, avoids risk of endothelial rejection by being an extraocular procedure, and preserves the limbal stem cells. **Figures 3A to F** shows the difference between a standard deep anterior lamellar keratoplasty and the tuck-in keratoplasty procedure. Various modifications of the procedure have been described. In case of cornea involving deeper opacities, a two-step procedure in which penetrating keratoplasty is followed by TILK has also been described.[14] Femtosecond (FS)-assisted tuck in penetrating keratoplasty has also been described for keratoglobus, wherein the host and graft dissection is done using 60 kHz FS-laser in patients with endothelial damage.[15]

Management of Acute Hydrops

Acute hydrops, though rare, can occur in patients with keratoglobus. It is usually treated conservatively with topical hypertonic saline, cycloplegics, and bandage contact lenses. Stromal uptake of fluid has also been found to reduce with aqueous suppressants.[16]

Nonexpansile concentration of intracameral perfluoropropane gas (14%) has also been used for the management of acute hydrops in keratoglobus.[17] However, it was not found to be significantly useful as in cases of acute hydrops with keratoconus, which may be due to the relatively larger size of tears in keratoglobus. Another novel procedure using a combination of intracameral injection of sulfur hexafluoride and full-thickness corneal sutures has also been described and has been found to be quite successful in the management of acute hydrops occurring in association with all forms of corneal ectasias.[18] In cases of such large tears, conservative management

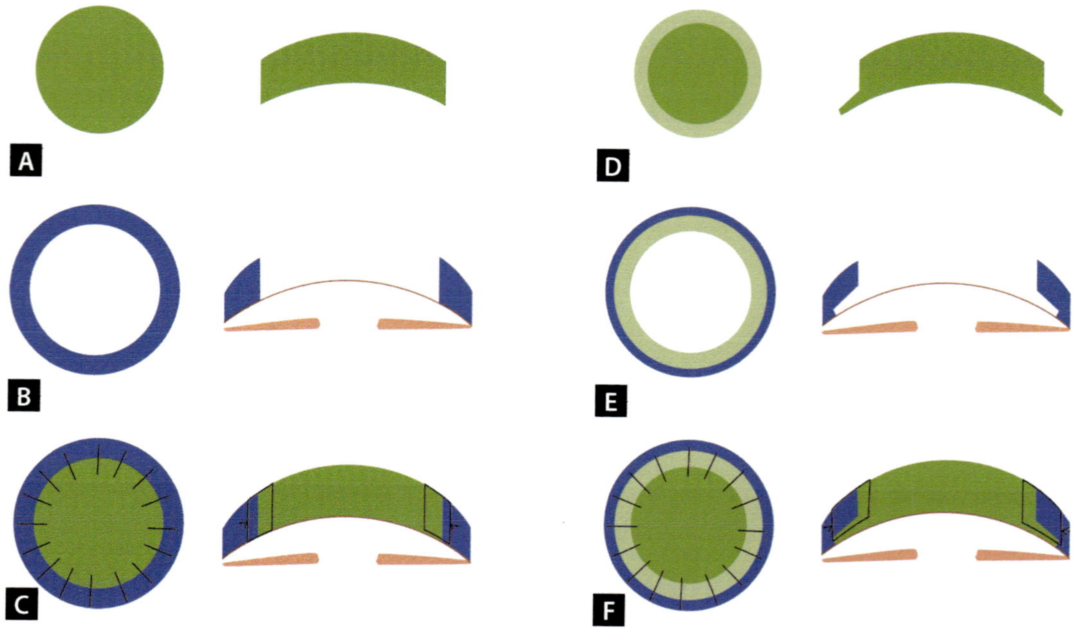

Figs. 3A to F: The difference between a standard deep anterior lamellar keratoplasty (DALK) technique and the tuck-in DALK procedure. (A to C) Cross-sectional view of the donor button (A), post-dissection host bed (B) and apposition between donor and host (C) for a standard DALK procedure. (D to F) Cross-sectional view of the mushroom shaped donor button (D), host bed (E) and apposition between donor and host tissue (F) for tuck-in DALK technique.

followed by Descemet's stripping automated endothelial keratoplasty (DSAEK) has also proven to be useful for visual rehabilitation.[19]

Management of Cataract in Keratoglobus

In patients with keratoglobus on conservative management with spectacles or contact lenses, cataract surgery can pose multiple challenges. There have been case reports of cataract surgery performed in patients keratoglobus and posterior subcapsular cataract and intumescent cataract.[20,21]

The intraocular lens (IOL) power calculation can be quite challenging in eyes with keratoglobus. None of the IOL power calculation formulae accept K-readings of >60 D, which can be quite challenging in advanced cases. In addition to that, the optical biometry formulae tend to overestimate IOL power in ectatic corneas, which can lead to a postoperative hyperopic shift. Thus, the final IOL power should be calculated, after taking into consideration, all these discrepancies. The K-readings taken from Scheimpflug imaging are most reliable. In cases of dense cataracts, ultrasound pachymetry might be useful for determining axial length, in case it is not assessed by optical biometry.

Intraoperatively, the surgical technique should ideally be modified to accommodate for the corneal thinning and a deep anterior chamber. The procedures described in literature use a superior scleral tunnel incision 2.5 mm from the limbus, to avoid traumatizing the peripheral thin cornea. The incisions can also be customized as per the steep axis on Scheimpflug imaging. The side ports are also made toward the scleral limbus avoiding the thin cornea. After capsulorhexis, the nucleus can be prolapsed into the anterior chamber with viscoelastic to compensate for the deep anterior chamber in these eyes, facilitating ease of phacoemulsification. An IOL of appropriate power is then inserted into the bag and the incisions are sutured.

CONCLUSION

The management of keratoglobus is quite challenging. Most patients do not respond to conservative measures of visual rehabilitation and hence require surgical correction. Currently described surgical procedures requires expertise and have, a steep learning curve time. The choice of treatment needs to be individualized, depending upon the age of presentation, the severity of clinical presentation and patient's requirements.

REFERENCES

1. Rumelt S, Rehany U. Surgically induced keratoglobus in pellucid marginal degeneration. Eye (Lond). 1998;12(Pt 1):156-8.
2. James AC. Keratoglobus. Cornea. 1993;12(2):124-30.
3. Burkitt Wright EMM, Spencer HL, Daly SB, Manson FDC, Zeef LAH, Urquhart J, et al. Mutations in PRDM5 in brittle cornea syndrome identify a pathway regulating extracellular matrix development and maintenance. Am J Hum Genet. 2011;88:767-77.
4. Meghpara B, Nakamura H, Vemuganti GK, Murthy SI, Sugar J, Yue BY, et al. Histopathologic and immunohistochemical studies of keratoglobus. Arch Ophthalmol. 2009;127(8):1029-35.
5. Poole TA. Calculation of stress distribution in keratoconus. N Y State J Med. 1973;73:1284-8.
6. Rathi VM, Murthy SI, Bagga B, Taneja M, Chaurasia S, Sangwan VS. Keratoglobus: An experience at a tertiary eye care center in India. Indian J Ophthalmol. 2015;63(3):233-8.
7. Feder RS, Gan TG. Non-inflammatory ectatic disorders. In: Krachmer JH, Mannis MJ, Holland EJ (Eds). Cornea:

Fundamentals, Diagnosis, and Management, 3rd edition. St. Louis, MO: Mosby; 2011. p. 879.

8. Diallo ML, Simonet P, Frenette B, Sanschagrin B. Resistance of plastic ophthalmic lenses: the effect of base curve on different materials during static load testing. Optom Vis Sci. 2001;78(7):518-24.
9. Krachmer JH, Feder RS, Belin MW. Keratoconus and related noninflammatory corneal thinning disorders. Surv Ophthalmol. 1984;28(4):293-322.
10. McMonnies CW. The biomechanics of keratoconus and rigid contact lenses. Eye Contact Lens. 2005;31(2):80-92.
11. Kodjikian L, Baillif S, Burillon C, Grange JD, Garweg JG. Keratoglobus surgery: Penetrating keratoplasty redux. Acta Ophthalmol Scand. 2004;82(5):625-7.
12. Papaioannou L, Papathanassiou M. Large penetrating keratoplasty in the management of keratoglobus: A case report. Open J Ophthalmol. 2016;6(1):51-5.
13. Vajpayee RB, Bhartiya P, Sharma N. Central lamellar keratoplasty with peripheral intralamellar tuck: A new surgical technique for keratoglobus. Cornea. 2002;21(7):657-60.
14. Jones DH, Kirkness CM. A new surgical technique for keratoglobus-tectonic lamellar keratoplasty followed by secondary penetrating keratoplasty. Cornea. 2001;20(8):885-7.
15. Del Barrio JL, Al-Shymali O, Alió JL. Femtosecond laser-assisted Tuck-In penetrating keratoplasty for advanced keratoglobus with endothelial damage. Cornea. 2017;36(9):1145-9.
16. American Academy of Ophthalmology. External Disease and Cornea. Basic and Clinical Science Course, Section 8. San Francisco: AAO; 2011. pp. 302-3.
17. Basu S, Vaddavalli PK, Ramappa M, Shah S, Murthy SI, Sangwan VS. Intracameral perfluoropropane gas in the treatment of acute corneal hydrops. Ophthalmology. 2011;118(5):934-9.
18. Mohebbi M, Pilafkan H, Nabavi A, Mirghorbani M, Naderan M. Treatment of acute corneal hydrops with combined intracameral gas and approximation sutures in patients with corneal ectasia. Cornea. 2020;39(2):258-62.
19. Palioura S, Chodosh J, Pineda R. A novel approach to the management of a progressive Descemet membrane Tear in a patient with keratoglobus and acute hydrops Cornea. 2013;32(3):355-8.
20. Singh B, Sharma S, Bharti N, Ranjan R, Bharti S. Hypermature intumescent cataract in advanced keratoglobus. Int Med Case Rep J. 2020;13:507-11.
21. Ku JY, Grupcheva CN, Fisk MJ, McGhee CN. Keratoglobus and posterior subcapsular cataract: Surgical considerations and in vivo microstructural analysis. J Cataract Refract Surg. 2004;30(1):237-42.

63 Severe Corneoiridic Scars

Priyadarshini K, Ritu Nagpal, Namrata Sharma

INTRODUCTION

The burden of corneal diseases in our country is on a rise and accounts for the second leading cause for blindness. Ninety percent of ocular trauma and corneal ulcer cases are prevalent in developing countries like ours.[1] Corneal scars account for 28.1% cases of corneal blindness in adults residing in less-developed countries.[2] In pediatric population, nontraumatic corneal scars account for 71.32% of corneal blindness in the developing nations.[3]

Corneal scars can be graded either as nebular, macular or leukomatous depending on the density of opacity and transparency of the cornea. Leukomatous corneal opacities are dense opacities involving almost the entire thickness of corneal stroma, causing total loss of transparency. Corneoiridic scars result if the iris tissue is incarcerated or incorporated in a leukomatous corneal opacity.

ETIOLOGY

Corneoiridic scars can occur as a sequel of various corneal pathologies such as:

- Infective keratitis
- Perforated corneal ulcers
- Corneal perforations
- Keratomalacia
- Congenital
- Postuveitic

Infective keratitis tends to heal with corneal scarring and vascularization. When there is severe inflammation associated with an active ulcer, it may eventually heal with peripheral anterior synechiae formation resulting in a corneoiridic scar.

Perforated corneal ulcers when left untreated get plugged by the iris tissue. The wound eventually heals with pseudocornea formation and scarring resulting in adherent leukoma (**Fig. 1**).

Post-traumatic corneal perforations are usually repaired by primary closure. Extensive iris tissue manipulation and a shallow anterior chamber lead to corneoiridic scar formation (**Fig. 2**).

Nutritional deficiencies such as vitamin A deficiency can cause keratin plaques, stromal punched out ulcers, and diffuse or focal corneal melting. Congenital corneal opacities associated with anterior segment dysgenesis, Peter's

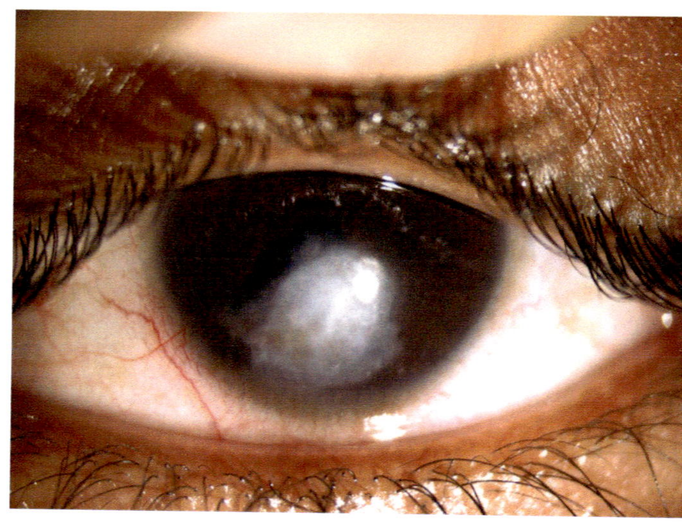

Fig. 1: Slit-lamp image of a patient with an adherent leukoma formed as a sequelae of a perforated corneal ulcer.

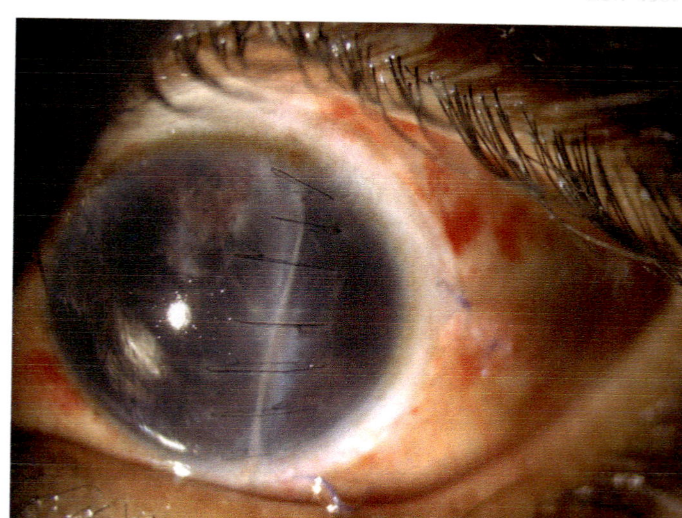

Fig. 2: Postoperative slit-lamp image of the left eye of a patient with severe corneoiridic scar formation following repair of a corneal perforation subsequent to an open globe injury.

anomaly, and anterior staphyloma also present with severe corneoiridic adhesions. These cases carry a suboptimal visual prognosiss due to the presence of other associated ocular comorbidities such as glaucoma.

Recurrent cases of uveitis can sometimes lead to extensive anterior and posterior synechiae formation associated with iris bombe and secondary glaucoma.

CLINICAL PRESENTATION

Patients usually present with diminution of vision which may be associated with complaints of glare. There is usually a preceding history of trauma, keratitis, or uveitis. The extent and depth of corneal opacity, extent of anterior synechiae, presence of vascularization (superficial or deep) and extent of vascularization in clock hours should be documented. Intraocular pressures should be recorded wherever possible (**Fig. 3**).

MANAGEMENT

The depth of corneal scarring and the extent of anterior synechiae should be assessed using ultrasound biomicroscopy (UBM) and anterior segment optical coherence tomography (AS-OCT). B-mode ultrasonography should be done to assess the status of posterior segment. Electrophysiological examination with visually evoked responses (VERs) should be recorded to assess the visual potential before planning any kind of surgical intervention. Coexisting glaucoma should be managed using various methods such as topical antiglaucoma drugs, YAG-peripheral iridotomy (YAG-PI), micropulse diode laser photocoagulation and diode laser cyclophotocoagulation (DLCP).

In cases of nil visual prognosis, corneal tattooing or cosmetic contact lens can be used to improve cosmesis.

Penetrating keratoplasty is the definitive management in cases with severe corneoiridic scars. The integrity of the iris might get compromised, leading to intraoperative difficulties in preserving the lens, forming the anterior chamber and facilitating implantation of intraocular lens during the keratoplasty procedure. Hence, some improvisations in the technique of keratoplasty have been described.

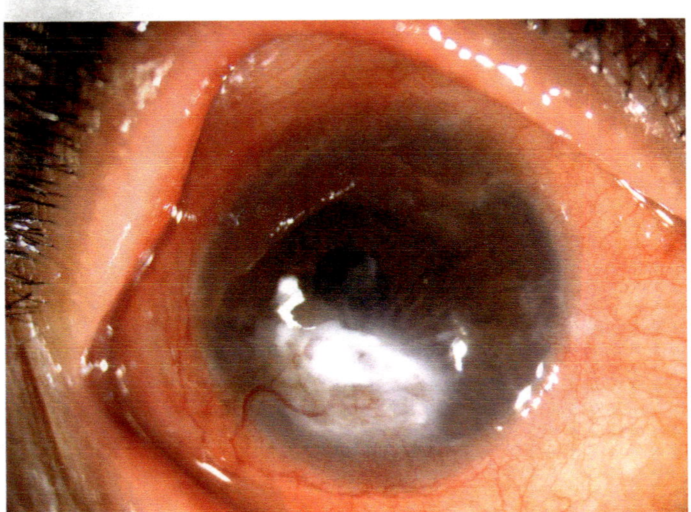

Fig. 3: Slit-lamp image of an inferonasal corneoiridic scar with superficial vascularization developing following an episode of keratitis.

In cases of localized corneoiridic scars, an optical iridectomy (OI) can be planned after assessing the optimal site by using cycloplegic refraction under stenopic slit. It is a simple and safe procedure that can be used as an alternative to penetrating keratoplasty in selective cases.

The management options available for severe corneoiridic scars have been described below in brief, with emphasis to special precautions taken during penetrating keratoplasty, which is the mainstay of management.

Optical Iridectomy

The two important prerequisites of this surgical procedure are the presence of a sector of clear cornea and lens. According to a study done by Aasuri et al, penetrating keratoplasty is likely to fail in children below 5 years of age and thus an optical iridectomy (OI) should be preferred.[4] It can also be done as an intermediary procedure in patients, who can later be planned for penetrating keratoplasty, especially in developing nations, where there are constraints of tissue availability. Doing an OI in pediatric patients can thus reduce chances of graft rejection and delay the onset of amblyopia. It can also be used in patients with multiple graft rejections and in whom there is high risk of graft rejection. In a study by Miller et al., it was proven that patients with clear peripheral cornea can gain visual acuity of ≥20/30 with an OI.[5]

In this procedure, the anterior chamber is formed after making a limbal incision followed by synechiae release as much as possible. Care should be taken not to damage the lens. Optical iridectomy is done in the quadrant with clear lens and cornea. If there is coexisting cataractous lens, lens aspiration with intraocular lens fixation can be done along with OI.[6]

Complications such as graft rejection and secondary glaucoma associated with penetrating keratoplasty can be avoided by performing an OI. Visual rehabilitation can be ensured by correction of residual refractive error on follow-up and prescription of glasses or contact lens.

Penetrating Keratoplasty

Penetrating keratoplasty should be performed with utmost care to preserve the integrity of iris tissue and lens matter as much as possible. Vajpayee et al., described the modified technique of corneal debulking while performing keratoplasty in perforated corneal ulcers with pseudocornea in order to preserve the iris tissue.[7] This can also be adopted in severe corneoiridic scars to preserve the iris anatomy. In this technique, host cornea is initially trephined up to a depth of 75%, following which the corneal button is removed in two layers. The dissection is carried out from periphery towards the center at the level of posterior stroma using a lamellar dissector. An intraoperative optical coherence tomography (iOCT) can also aid in this process of debulking, avoiding any perforation at the sites of corneal thinning and corneoiridic adhesions, similar to performing a lamellar keratoplasty.[8] After bulk of corneal stroma is removed, an anterior chamber entry is made in the area devoid of any underlying adhesions and viscoelastic is injected. The deeper parts of the cornea and the fibrous membranes present between the iris and the cornea are then gently dissected and peeled away, taking care not to damage the friable iris tissue beneath. The iOCT serves as a great tool in aiding visualization of the retrocorneal membranes thus helping in retaining the iris anatomy[9] (**Fig. 4**).

Additional procedures such as cataract extraction, anterior vitrectomy and pupilloplasty can be performed wherever needed. The graft is oversized by 1 mm and sutured to the host with interrupted 10-0 nylon sutures. Oversizing the corneal grafts by 1 mm in cases of corneoiridic adhesions and, in pediatric cases, was found to increase the morphologic success rates.[10,11]

The outcome of penetrating keratoplasty has been seen to be better in cases of post-traumatic and postinfectious corneal scars in comparison to eyes with adherent leukoma and congenital corneoiridic scars.[12] It was also found that eyes with scars associated with ≥2 quadrants vascularization had lower survival rate than those that were nonvascularized.[12] The causes of graft failure include immunological rejection, secondary glaucoma, persistent epithelial defect, and graft infection. The graft survival rates are better in adult patients compared to pediatric population. In pediatric population, the probability of obtaining a clear graft at the end of 1 year has been reported to be 60% in cases of congenital opacities and 70% for acquired opacities.[13] In cases of healed keratomalacia, the success rate of penetrating keratoplasty was found to be 57.14%.[14] Poor visual outcomes of pediatric keratoplasty are attributed to amblyopia, astigmatism, and higher chances of graft failures.[15]

The major complications associated with penetrating keratoplasty performed in eyes with corneoiridic scars include secondary glaucoma, cataract, graft rejection, and graft infection. The most dreaded complications are expulsive suprachoroidal hemorrhage and endophthalmitis which can lead to total loss of vision.

Autorotational penetrating keratoplasty requires special mention in relation to the management of localized corneoiridic scars. In this technique, the clear peripheral cornea of the ipsilateral eye is rotated toward the area of corneal scarring and vice versa thus facilitating optical clarity in the visual axis. It has the advantage of lesser chances of immunological rejection in compared to an allogenic transplant. It is also useful in areas with scarcity of donor tissue. However, in comparison to penetrating keratoplasty, it was found to have poor visual outcomes due to high postoperative corneal astigmatism and endothelial cell loss.[16]

Corneal Tattooing

It is a commonly used technique for improving the cosmetic outcome in eyes with unsightly corneal scars. Commercially available drawing ink (Rotring GmbH; Hamburg, Germany) in black, brown, or blue shades are used for corneal tattooing. In cases with associated degenerative changes such as band-shaped keratopathy, simultaneous ethylenediaminetetraacetic acid (EDTA) chelation is performed after epithelial debridement. The details of the surgical technique of corneal tattooing have been covered in chapter number 69.

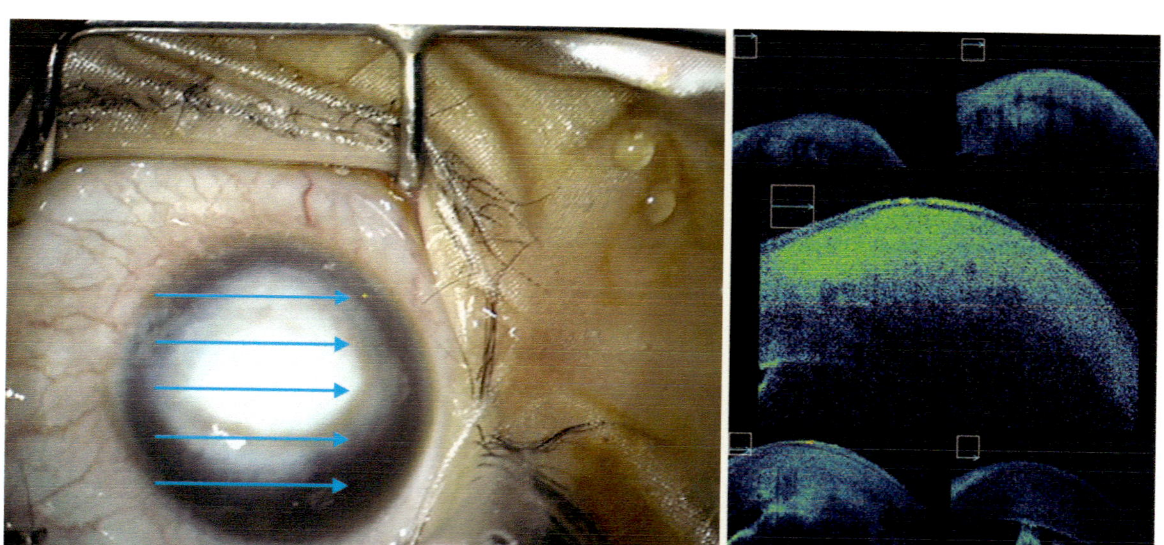

Fig. 4: Intraoperative optical coherence tomography image of a patient with healed keratitis showing corneoiridic adhesions at various levels.

Cosmetic contact lenses are an another alternative option for managing patients with unsightly corneal scars.

CONCLUSION

The primary management of cases of keratitis, trauma, keratomalacia, and uveitis plays a major role in preventing the sequel of severe scarring. Penetrating keratoplasty should be considered in cases, wherein an optical iridectomy is either not feasible or is unlikely to yield adequate results. Optical iridectomy is a useful surgical modality especially for pediatric eyes wherein a full thickness keratoplasty carries a high risk of graft rejection.

REFERENCES

1. Kumar A, Vashist P. Indian community eye care in 2020: Achievements and challenges. Indian J Ophthalmol. 2020;68(2): 291-3.
2. Garg P, Krishna PV, Stratis AK, Gopinathan U. The value of corneal transplantation in reducing blindness. Eye. 2005;19(10):1106-14.
3. Dada T, Sharma N, Vajpayee RB. Indications for pediatric keratoplasty in India. Cornea. 1999;18(3):296-8.
4. Aasuri MK, Garg P, Gokhle N, Gupta S. Penetrating keratoplasty in children. Cornea 2000;19:140-4.
5. Miller D, Atebara N, Stegmann R. The role of the limbal cornea in vision. Eye. 1989;3:128-31.
6. Foster J. Optical iridectomy, indications, method, and value. Br J Ophthalmol. 1932;16(8):476-84.
7. Vajpayee RB, Singhvi A, Sharma N, Sinha R. Penetrating keratoplasty for perforated corneal ulcers: preservation of iris by corneal debulking. Cornea. 2006;25(1):44-6.
8. Titiyal JS, Kaur M, Nair S, Sharma N. Intraoperative optical coherence tomography in anterior segment surgery. Surv Ophthalmol. 2021;66(2):308-26.
9. Sharma N, Priyadarshini K, Agarwal R, Bafna RK, Nagpal R, Sinha R, et al. Role of microscope-intraoperative optical coherence tomography in pediatric keratoplasty: A comparative study. Am J Ophthalmol. 2021;221:190-8.
10. Vajpayee RB, Ramu M, Panda A, Sharma N, Tabin GC, Anand JR. Oversized grafts in children. Ophthalmology. 1999;106(4): 829-32.
11. Vajpayee RB, Dada T, Ray M, Tandon R, Sethi A, Turaka K. Oversized corneal grafts for corneal opacities with iridocorneal adhesions. Ophthalmology. 2001;108(11):2026-8.
12. Joshi SA, Jagdale SS, More PD, Deshpande M. Outcome of optical penetrating keratoplasties at a tertiary care eye institute in Western India. Indian J Ophthalmol. 2012;60(1):15-21.
13. Stulting RD, Sumers KD, Cavanagh HD, Waring III GO, Gammon JA. Penetrating keratoplasty in children. Ophthalmology. 1984; 91(10):1222-30.
14. Vajpayee RB, Vanathi M, Tandon R, Sharma N, Titiyal JS. Keratoplasty for keratomalacia in preschool children. Br J Ophthalmol. 2003;87(5):538-42.
15. Limaiem R, Chebil A, Baba A, Ben Youssef N, Mghaieth F, El Matri L. Pediatric penetrating keratoplasty: indications and outcomes. Transplant Proc. 2011;43(2):649-51.
16. Jonas JB, Rank RM, Budde WM. Autologous ipsilateral rotating penetrating keratoplasty. Am J Ophthalmol. 2001;131(4): 427-30.

64 Anterior Staphyloma

Priyadarshini K, Ritu Nagpal, Namrata Sharma

INTRODUCTION

Staphyloma is defined as an abnormal protrusion of the uveal tissue through a weak area in the eyeball. Anterior staphyloma is the protrusion of an enlarged, opaque, and ectatic cornea, lined posteriorly by uveal pigments, through the interpalpebral fissure. It can occur congenitally or may be acquired later in life as a sequel of perforated corneal ulcers. A rare case of an untreated cocaine-associated corneal ulcer has also been reported as a cause of acquired anterior staphyloma.[1]

The incidence of congenital corneal opacities range from 3/100,000 to 6/100,000 in newborns.[2] Congenital anterior staphyloma accounts for about 11% of congenital corneal opacities.[3] In 1827, FA von Ammon reported the first clinical case of congenital anterior staphyloma.[4] The first extensive pathological description was, presented by Hirschberg and Birnbacher.[5] Congenital anterior staphyloma presents with an enlarged, ectatic and vascularized cornea with thinning and ectasia of the surrounding anterior segment structures. It may be associated with other anterior segment anomalies such as corneoiridic adhesions and partial aniridia. Crystalline lens may also be found adherent to the cornea and iris as in cases of Peter's anomaly. It may also be associated with subluxation of lens, aphakia, or cataractous changes.

ETIOPATHOGENESIS

As per G Coats' concepts, there are two hypotheses ascribed to the occurrence of congenital anterior staphylomas: (1) ulcerative hypothesis and (2) malformation/non-differentiation hypothesis.[6]

Congenital Anterior Staphyloma

Ulcerative Hypothesis

This theory postulates infection to be the origin of the inflammatory process that ends up in the formation of staphyloma. The source of infection can be either endogenous acquired through the fetal circulation or exogenous acquired through the amniotic fluid. Endogenous infections may present as deep-seated keratitis resulting in sloughing of cornea causing pseudocornea formation as in cases of perforated corneal ulcers. However, cornea being a relatively avascular structure, this hypothesis remains questionable.

Exogenous infections can cause antepartum ophthalmia via organisms which travel upward through the vaginal canal, thus damaging the fetal membranes and gaining entry into the liquor amnii. Any infection of the placenta which has a similar effect as endometritis can break into the amniotic fluid and cause an infection of the fetal cornea. However, fetal eyelids that are normally fused from the 2nd month until shortly around 6–7th months of gestation would not permit infection to take place during this period. In that case, if there is a small defect in the fusion of eyelids, an infection might enter due to the toxic properties of amniotic fluid and cause keratitis.

Malformation or Nondifferentiation Hypothesis

The anterior chamber is initially formed as a cleft between the cornea and pupillary membranes which is later followed by the ingrowth of the iris. The paraxial mesoderm forms substantia propria of the cornea, Descemet's membrane, endothelium, and the anterior fibrovascular sheath of lens which is composed of uniform cells. They, then get separated to the anterior and posterior part of cornea with Descemet's membrane in between. Lack of differentiation of cells during this process would hence lead to severe malformations, causing the mesoblast to remain adherent, thus resulting in maldevelopment of the iris and cornea. It would also cause disturbances in aqueous drainage resulting in increased intraocular pressure. Hence, a fused iris and pseudocornea may bulge through the interpalpebral fissure resulting in anterior staphyloma.

The familial incidence supporting this hypothesis is also quite remarkable. Steinheim[7] reported familial incidence in which children of the same family presented with following features: a boy aged 6 years in whom both eyes had anterior staphyloma; a girl aged 4 years with anterior staphyloma in one eye and cystic ectasia in the other; a girl aged 3 years with total staphyloma in both eyes; and a boy aged 2 months in which both eyes were shrunken. This supports various stages of developmental malformations resulting in congenital anterior staphyloma in different members of the same family.

Acquired Anterior Staphyloma

The most common cause of acquired anterior staphylomas is untreated/perforated corneal ulcers, usually following fungal, pseudomonas, or acanthamoeba keratitis.[8] In literature, there are some reports of narcotic abuse causing epithelial defect and ulceration progressing into anterior staphyloma.[9-11] Fulminant keratitis which results in corneal thinning leads to corneal perforation. The iris then plugs over the wound with pseudocornea formation. However, the pseudocornea formed is unable to withstand the normal intraocuar pressure resulting in the formation of an anterior staphyloma (**Figs. 1 and 2**).

HISTOPATHOLOGY

In congenital anterior staphyloma the epithelium is usually thickened and intact with keratinization due to exposure.[12] Bowman's membrane may be absent or fragmented, thin and atrophic with hypercellular, disorganized, and vascularized stroma. The irregular cellularity and presence of fibrovascular tissue in the stroma indicates a preceding inflammatory or an ulcerative process. Descemet's membrane and endothelium are absent with posterior aspect of cornea being lined by an atrophic iris.[12,13] Peter's anomaly may also present with absence of Descemet's membrane and endothelium, without corneal ectasia and hence represents an earlier stage of mesenchymal dysgenesis in comparison to congenital anterior staphyloma. However, posterior segment appears normal except for changes attributed to concomitant glaucoma. Acquired staphyloma also has a similar histopathological picture.

DIFFERENTIAL DIAGNOSIS

Cases of congenital anterior staphyloma need to be differentiated from other causes of congenital anomalies such as Peter's anomaly and other anterior segment dysgenesis, keratectasia, sclerocornea, and buphthalmos.

MANAGEMENT

In cases of congenital anterior staphylomas, the child needs to be assessed clinically to know the presenting visual acuity and expected visual potential. An examination under anesthesia is be required in most cases to plan further treatment.

Under anesthesia, the corneal diameter, intraocular pressure, and pupillary status are assessed. Anterior segment assessment under ultrasound biomicroscopy (UBM) and intraoperative optical coherence tomography (iOCT) is done, whenever possible to understand the anatomy of anterior segment and know the extent of iridocorneal adhesions as well as the lens status. The posterior segment is evaluated using a B scan ultrasonography. Most of these cases do not have a good visual prognosis. However, keratoplasty can be attempted as a last resort for restoring visual acuity, especially in bilateral cases. In most cases of acquired anterior staphylomas, visual potential tends to be poor and surgical management is performed with the aim of improving overall cosmesis.

Medical Management

Patients can be medically treated with lubricants, wherein the visual potential is poor. Concomitant secondary glaucoma is managed using antiglaucoma medications in patients planned for penetrating keratoplasty. Cyclodestructive procedures like diode laser cyclophotocoagulation (DLCP) may be required in patients with intractable glaucoma and painful blind eye.

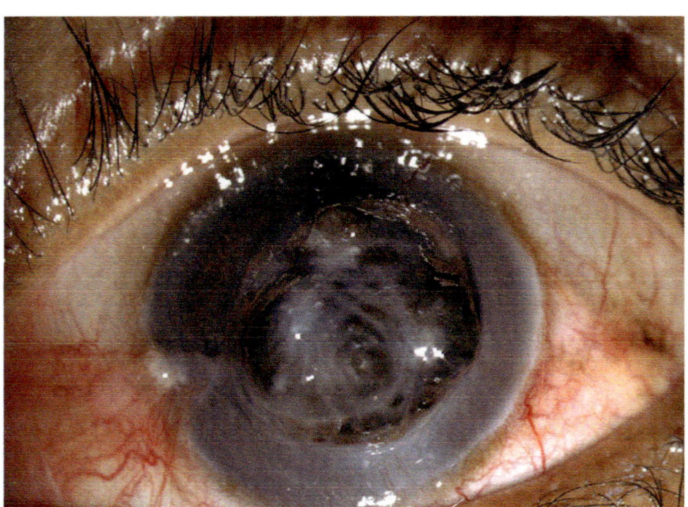

Fig. 1: Diffuse slit-lamp image of a case of anterior staphyloma as a sequel of a perforated corneal ulcer.

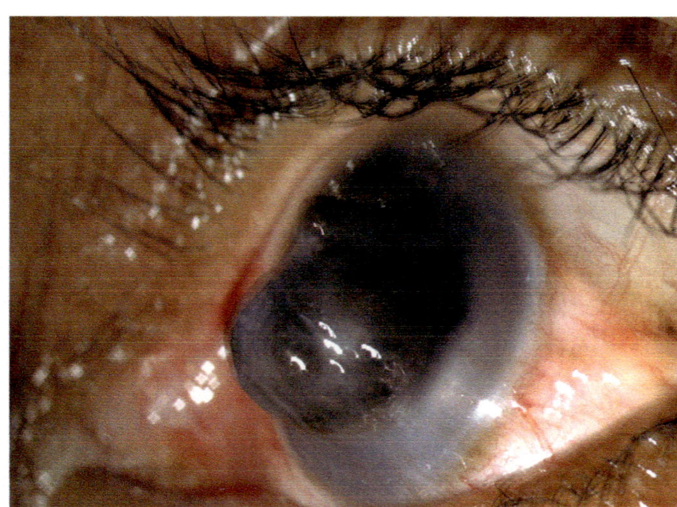

Fig. 2: Side view of the slit-lamp image of the same patient with acquired anterior staphyloma as shown in **Figure 1**.

Surgical Management

Initially enucleation and evisceration were the preferred surgical practices in cases of congenital anterior staphylomas. However, due to the extreme psychological trauma and physical disability induced by these procedures, they are no longer preferred.

Sclerokeratoplasty or a large full-thickness keratoplasty is the procedure of choice to restore cosmesis and visual potential. Sclerokeratoplasty was found to have better postoperative visual prognosis and good cosmetic results due to absence of suture marks in comparison to penetrating keratoplasty in cases of anterior staphylomas.[14] Panda et al. also reported a lower risk of reinfection and secondary glaucoma as a result of avoiding direct trauma to the trabecular meshwork in sclerokeratoplasty.[14] A successful attempt at a staged procedure in which penetrating keratoplasty was performed after sclerokeratoplasty has also been described in literature in an acquired case of anterior staphyloma.[15]

Sclerokeratoplasty

In this procedure both the donor and recipient tissues are prepared freehand. A 360° peritomy is performed on the recipient eye with relaxing conjunctival incisions. The circumference of the required scleral excision margin is marked, ideally extending 1 mm beyond the diseased area. Then a circumferential incision 50% beveled into sclera is made until the peripheral cornea is reached followed by a 360° sclerokeratectomy.

Donor graft is harvested with a graft-host disparity of 1 mm. The scleral margin is beveled such that a large mushroom-shaped pattern is created. The harvested donor sclerocorneal graft is then sutured to the beveled recipient bed using 10-0 nylon interrupted sutures. In a sclerokeratoplasty nearly 22–24 interrupted sutures might be needed to suture the graft adequately to the host bed in comparison to 16 sutures usually required in penetrating keratoplasty, due to the large graft size. Concurrent procedures, such as, synechiolysis, iridectomy, pupilloplasty, lensectomy/cataract extraction and anterior vitrectomy are done wherever required. The graft is tucked into the host bed and the overlying conjunctival peritomy is sutured using 8-0 Vicryl sutures (**Fig. 3**).

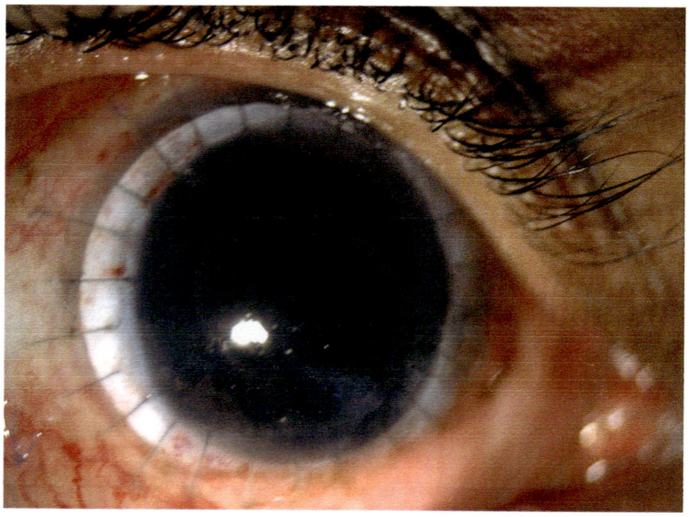

Fig. 3: Postoperative slit-lamp image of a case of anterior staphyloma following sclerokeratoplasty with a large graft in situ.

Penetrating Keratoplasty

A large corneal graft is required for penetrating keratoplasties in cases of anterior staphyloma. The lesion should be removed completely with 1 mm margin of normal cornea. After removing the diseased cornea, additional procedures such as iridectomy, synechiolysis, anterior vitrectomy, lensectomy, and pupilloplasty are done wherever required to restore the normal anterior segment anatomy as much as possible. A layer-by-layer lamellar dissection of the host cornea is done to avoid any inadvertent injury to the iris tissue. Goniosynechialysis and gonioplasty can be done if required such as in cases of concurrent anterior segment dysgenesis associated with angle anomalies.

The harvested graft tissue is sutured to the host bed with a graft host disparity of 1.0 mm using interrupted 10-0 nylon sutures. The graft tissue is tucked in after creating a ledge in the host and all sutures are buried.

The host specimen in both sclerokeratoplasty and penetrating keratoplasty should be sent for histopathological examination.

Surgical Complications

Intraoperative Complication

The most dreaded, though rare, intraoperative complication of any open-sky procedure is expulsive suprachoroidal hemorrhage. Preoperative control of intraocular pressure is an important prerequisite in order to avoid this dreaded complication.

Postoperative Complications

Ocular hypotony is more frequently associated with sclerokeratoplasty. Other postoperative complications, especially in pediatric eyes are loose sutures and graft failure, which may require frequent follow-ups and interventions. Persistent epithelial defects, secondary glaucoma, graft infection, endophthalmitis, and late retinal detachments are other complications that have been reported following penetrating keratoplasty in these eyes.

Postoperative Management

Postoperatively, the patients should be treated with topical antibiotics, corticosteroids, and preservative-free lubricants.

System immunosuppressants can also be started in high-risk cases. Frequent postoperative examinations under anesthesia (EUAs) may be required, especially in pediatric patients. Pediatric patients also require management of concurrent issues such as glaucoma and amblyopia. Thus, the parents should be counseled regarding the requirement of a long-term follow-up and compliance to obtain the best possible results.

CONCLUSION

Congenital cases of anterior staphyloma tend to have a dismal prognosis. Hence, any patient with even a little hope of visual prognosis should be treated as early as possible to salvage vision. Penetrating keratoplasty with a large graft or sclerokeratoplasty is the definitive treatment option in these cases. However, in cases with no visual potential, an anterior staphylectomy, or an evisceration can be performed followed by prosthesis fitting for cosmetic reasons.

REFERENCES

1. Vasconcelos SB, Guerra FM, Morato GM, Neves NT, Tzelikis PF. Acquired anterior staphyloma after corneal ulcer associated with the use of crack. Arq Bras Oftalmol. 2016;79(4):268-9.
2. Ciralsky J, Colby K. Congenital corneal opacities: A review with a focus on genetics. Semin Ophthalmol. 2007;22:241-6.
3. Shigeyasu C, Yamada M, Mizuno Y, Yokoi T, Nishina S, Azuma N. Clinical features of anterior segment dysgenesis associated with congenital corneal opacities. Cornea. 2012;31(3):293-8.
4. Schoen. Handbuch d. path. Anat. d. menschlich. Aug, 1828, p. 68.
5. Hirschberg J, Birnbacer. Dentralbi. f. prakt. Augenh., 1886, x, p. 225.
6. De Long P. Congenital anterior staphyloma. Trans Am Ophthalmol Soc. 1933;31:315-328.
7. Steinheim. Centralbl. f. prakt. Auge 1897, xxi, p. 353.
8. Grieser EJ, Tuli SS, Chabi A, Schultz S, Downer D. Blueberry eye: Acquired total anterior staphyloma after a fungal corneal ulcer. Cornea. 2009;28(2):231-2.
9. Ghosheh FR, Ehlers JP, Ayres BD, Hammersmith KM, Rapuano CJ, Cohen EJ. Corneal ulcers associated with aerosolized crack cocaine use. Cornea. 2007;26(8):966-9.
10. Sachs R, Zagelbaum BM, Hersh PS. Corneal complications associated with the use of crack cocaine. Ophthalmology. 1993;100(2):187-91.
11. Pilon AF, Scheiffle J. Ulcerative keratitis associated with crack-cocaine abuse. Cont Lens Anterior Eye. 2006;29(5):263-7.
12. Schanzlin DJ, Robin JB, Erickson G, Lingua R, Minckler D, Pickford M. Histopathologic and ultrastructural analysis of congenital corneal staphyloma. Am J Ophthalmol. 1983;95:506-14.
13. Weizenblatt S. Congenital malformations of cornea associated with embryonic arrest of ectodermal and mesodermal structures. Arch Ophthalmol. 1954;52:415-25.
14. Panda A, Sharma N, Angra SK, Singh R. Sclerokeratoplasty versus penetrating keratoplasty in anterior staphyloma. Ophthalmic Surg Lasers. 1999;30(1):31-6.
15. De la Torre-Gonzalez E, de León Ascencio CP. Staged penetrating sclerokeratoplasty and penetrating keratoplasty for management of advanced acquired anterior staphyloma. J Ophthalmic Vis Res. 2011;6(2):147-50.

65

Descemetocele

Rinky Agarwal, Prerna Agarwal, Ritu Nagpal, Namrata Sharma

INTRODUCTION

A descemetocele is commonly defined as a cystic protrusion of Descemet's membrane (DM) on the anterior surface of the cornea.[1] Normally, the tectonic strength of the cornea is majorly contributed by its stromal layer and the DM is 8–10 μm thick, transparent, elastic acellular membrane that protects the endothelium from various destructive stromal processes. In descemetocele, corneal stroma is thinned out to such an extent that DM is the only anatomical layer maintaining the integrity of the eyeball.[2,3]

PATHOGENESIS

Any infectious or inflammatory ocular trauma can lead to localized or diffuse destruction of corneal stroma from loss of keratocytes and structural framework of collagen (**Figs. 1A and B**). Relentless progression of this process can expose the bare DM to the external environment that may give way to even trivial external trauma or rise of intraocular pressure (IOP). Two well-known theories related to the pathogenesis of descemetoceles are summarized as follows:[4,5]

Law of Laplace

According to the law of Laplace, the tension in a spherical wall is directly proportional to its pressure and inversely proportional to its radius of curvature. This law explains the ability of a 5–10 μm thin DM to resist changes in IOP and also proposes the three stages of descemetocele formation.

First stage involves building of a relatively large tension in DM as the protruded DM is less than a hemisphere and has a relatively large radius of curvature. The second stage involves minimal tension in DM as the diameter of curvature of DM is equal to the diameter of the stromal defect. However, as the DM distends further, and its radius of curvature increases, the risk of perforation increases from a blowout in the third stage. The law of Laplace also explains that the tension in the wall of descemetocele is directly proportional to the IOP and lays a basis for administering antiglaucoma medications in this condition.

Role of Proteolytic Enzymes

Proteases are enzymatic structures that cleave the protein molecules to yield active chemotactic peptides in the corneal layers. Twinning et al. suggested that proteases

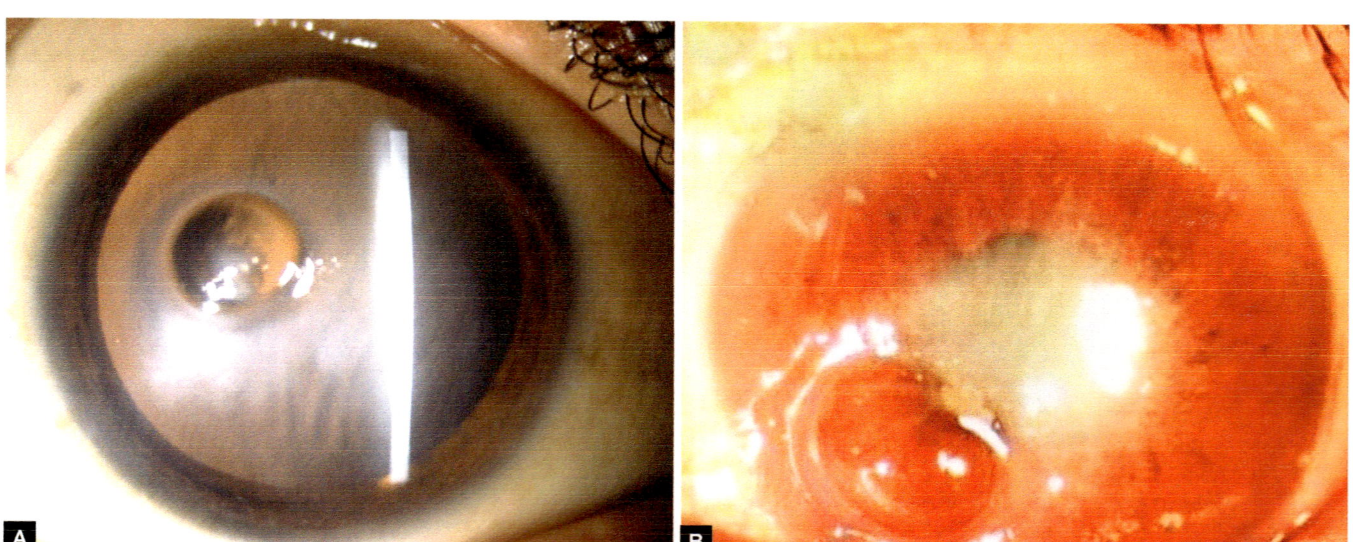

Figs. 1A and B: Descemetocele in sterile melt (A) and in presence of active infection (B).

(alkaline protease, total protease, and elastase activity) play an important role in the genesis of a descemetocele. In an experimental rabbit eye model, the authors demonstrated that certain strains of *Pseudomonas* (102, 115, 118) with higher production of protease, presence of added Ca^{+} and Mg^{++} and fewer inflammatory cells induced massive destruction of the stromal matrix, rapid descemetocele formation, and perforation when compared to others (107, 111, 113).

ETIOLOGY

As mentioned before, descemetoceles are an end-point of corneal tissue degradation. Microbial keratitis remains the most common cause of descemetocele formation and various ocular and systemic conditions that can cause descemetocele are mentioned in **Box 1**.[1,2,6]

DIFFERENTIAL DIAGNOSIS

Predescemetocele and dellen are two important differential diagnoses of a descemetocele. Various differences between all three lesions are mentioned in **Table 1**[7] and **Figures 2A to C**.

Box 1: Etiology of descemetocele.

Microbial keratitis:
- Herpetic
- Bacterial (particularly *Pseudomonas*)
- Fungal (*Carpoligna pleurothecii, Rhodotorula rubra, and Colletotrichum Corda*)
- Acanthamoebal
- Oropharyngeal commensals such as (*Rothia dentocariosa*)

Neurotrophic keratitis:
- *Neuroparalytic keratitis-associated lagophthalmos and exposure keratopathy*
- *Complete corneal anesthesia*:
  - Postsurgical excision of parotid carcinoma
  - High-dose radiation therapy
  - Topical anesthetic abuse
- *Immune-mediated corneal melt*:
  - Mooren's ulcer
  - Rheumatoid arthritis
  - Systemic lupus erythematosus
- *Cicatrizing dry eye*:
  - Stevens–Johnson syndrome
  - Ocular cicatricial pemphigoid
- *Post-traumatic descemetocele*:
  - Alkali burns
- *Iatrogenic*:
  - Pterygium excision
  - Radial keratotomy
  - Excimer laser phototherapeutic keratectomy
  - Collagen cross-linking
  - Cataract removal
- *Miscellaneous*:
  - Corneal dellen
  - Fuchs' superficial marginal keratitis
  - Ocular rosacea
  - Advanced keratomalacia
  - Protein-calorie malnutrition
  - Common variable immunodeficiency-associated hypogammaglobulinemia
  - Alpha-1 antitrypsin
  - Intravesical bacille Calmette–Guérin injection

INVESTIGATIONS

Different ocular and systemic investigations required for descemetocele are mentioned in **Box 2** and **Figure 3**.[8]

Table 1: Differences between descemetocele, predescemetocele, and dellen.

Finding	*Descemetocele*	*Predescemetocele*	*Dellen*
Corneal ectasia	Present	Present	Absent
Corneal thickness	8–10 µm	28–36 µm	Decreased up to one-third thickness
Integrity of epithelium	Compromised unless epithelialized	Compromised	Variable, usually intact
Stromal destruction	Present	Present	Absent to minimal
Residual layers	DM	PDL, DM	Stroma, PDL, DM
Pathogenesis	Stromal destruction	Stromal destruction	Stromal dehydration
Disruption of tear film	May or may not be present	May or may not be present	Usually disrupted
Surrounding elevation	Absent	Absent	Present
Timing of treatment	Urgent	Can monitor	Within a day or two of onset
Management	Medical or surgical	Keratoplasty	Lubricants, topical antibiotic-steroids
Prognosis	Poor	Poor	Good

(DM: Descemet's membrane; PDL: predescemetic layer)

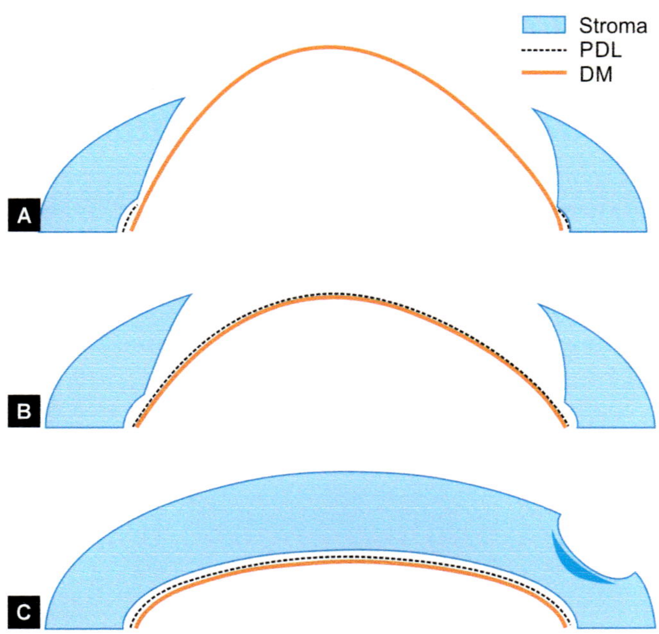

Figs. 2A to C: Pictorial representation of descemetocele (A), pre-descemetocele (B), and dellen (C).

MANAGEMENT

Urgent intervention is mandatory in descemetoceles due to risk of imminent perforation.[9] The main aim of management remains maintaining corneal integrity by providing tectonic support to the DM along with suppression of coexisting ocular and systemic inflammation.

Box 2: Investigations for descemetoceles.

Ophthalmic

Visual acuity
- *Slit-lamp examination*:
  - Ulcer size, site, depth, and margins, surrounding infiltrates
  - Epithelial defect
  - Size and site of descemetocele
  - Descemet membrane folds
  - Presence of perforation by Seidel's test
  - Corneal sensations and ocular surface
  - Anterior chamber depth, reaction
  - Lens—cataract, position, and stability of intraocular lens, should also be noted
  - Intraocular pressure by noncontact procedures
- *Microbiological work-up*: Staining and culture sensitivity and rarely, histopathological examination:
  - Surrounding infiltrates
  - Mucoid discharge
  - Contact lens samples
- *Anterior segment optical coherence tomography*:
  - Helpful when clinical visualization is limited due to overlying debris and mucoid discharge
  - Helps in differentiating descemetocele form predescemetocele and dellen
  - Helps in serial monitoring
- *Ultrasonography*:
  - Gentle B-scan ultrasonography to rule out endophthalmitis

Systemic

- *Suspected Sjogren syndrome*:
  - Immunology referral
  - Rheumatoid factor
  - Immune complexes
  - C-reactive protein
  - Antineutrophilic cytoplasmic antibodies
  - Erythrocyte sedimentation rate
- *Diabetes mellitus*:
  - Blood sugar levels

The choice of therapy is majorly determined by the size and location of descemetocele, presence of perforation, and various options available and their cost. Large descemetoceles, severe/deep/rapidly progressing ulcers, children, functionally one-eyed and noncompliant patients can be considered for hospital admission, while all others can be managed on an out-patient basis.

Medical Management

Topical Therapy

For descemetoceles associated with infectious keratitis, broad-spectrum antibiotics should be started immediately and specific antibiotics can be added later based on culture sensitivity results. Topical lubricants, mydriatics, cycloplegics, steroids, and antiglaucoma medications can be added to the regime as and when required.

Topical steroids should be prescribed cautiously for descemetocele. While they are absolutely contraindicated for fungal keratitis, they are beneficial for ocular rosacea.[10] They are known to exacerbate collagenase-induced stromal necrosis in alkali-burned corneas.

Hydrophilic bandage contact lens provides temporary structural reinforcement to the DM and protects it from lid-margin trauma during blinking. However, these are not free of complications and should be used cautiously in already thinned out corneas.

Systemic Agents

Steroids and/or steroid-sparing agents should be administered to reduce inflammation-induced ocular surface damage in immune-mediated disorders. For descemetoceles secondary to herpetic and fungal infections, appropriate therapeutic dose of oral acyclovir/valacyclovir and systemic antifungals should be started respectively, along with the topical therapy. Oral doxycycline and carbonic anhydrase inhibitors can be administered for impending perforations secondary to ocular rosacea and for aqueous humor suppression respectively.

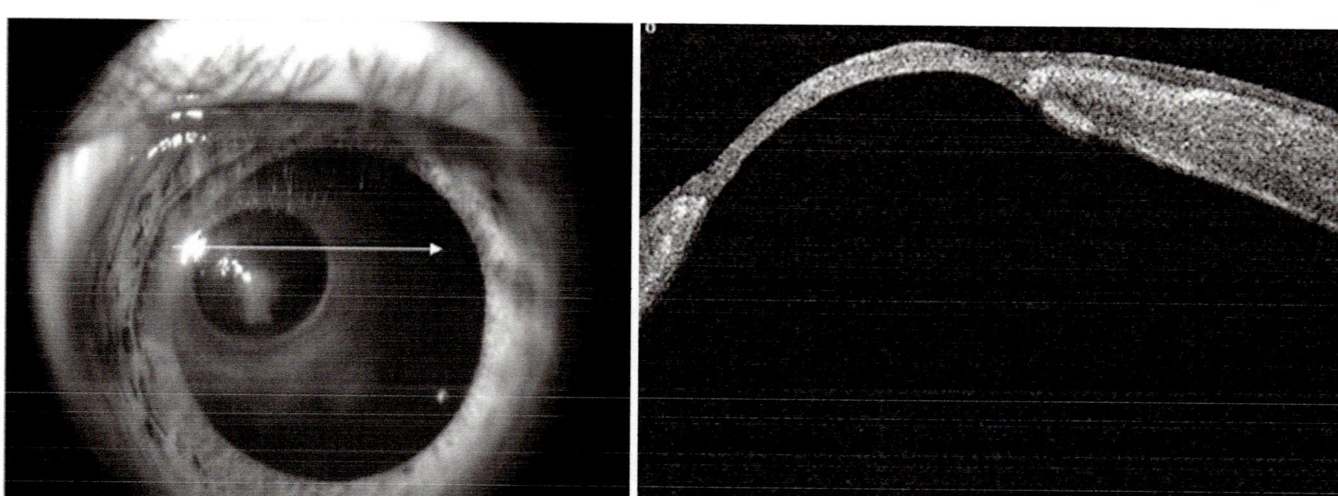

Fig. 3: Anterior segment optical coherence tomography imaging of descemetocele.

Vitamin A supplements (oral or intramuscular) should be administered to children with keratomalacia.

Surgical Management

Commonly, surgical intervention is required to provide tectonic support to the cornea in descemetoceles. Most cases can be usually dealt with local anesthesia with general anesthesia being reserved for children and uncooperative adults. Extreme caution should be maintained and minimal pressure must be applied to prevent inadvertent perforation during eyeball prepping (cleaning, draping, and placing eye speculum). The indications and complications of each of these techniques are mentioned in **Table 2**.

Table 2: Indications and complications of different surgical techniques for descemetocele.

	Indications	*Complications*
Tissue adhesives	• Small-sized descemetoceles • Wound dehiscence postkeratoplasty	• Progressive corneal melting in immune-mediated disorders or neurotrophic keratopathy • Dislodgment of the tissue adhesive necessitating repeat applications • Irritation of eyelids • Inflammation of iris, endothelium, and the lens • Cautious use in microbial keratitis and in hypogammaglobulinemia
Amniotic membrane grafting (AMG)	• Small (<2 mm) descemetoceles if tissue adhesives fail repeatedly • Ulcers with active infection or inflammation, those refractory to medical therapy and those secondary to ocular rosacea and exposure keratopathy	• Not suitable for traumatic cases and perforated corneas • Dislocation • Persistent leakage in perforated cornea • Prolonged time for dissolution • Hazy neocorneal stroma formation • Barrier to antibiotic penetration
Platelet-rich fibrin (PRF) membrane	• Central descemetoceles • For preventing corneal perforation while waiting for a donor graft • For failed single-layer AMG	• Leukocytes present in the PRF membrane may cause excessive inflammatory response • Postoperative corneal opacification
Umbilical cord patch-amniotic membrane	Deep ulcers and perforations	• Requires strict criteria and specialized equipment for preparation • Carries a risk of transmitting infections
Patch graft	• Peripheral corneal perforations and descemetoceles which are too small for full-sized penetrating keratoplasty and too large for tissue adhesives • Nonresolving dellen • Cases with failed tissue adhesives	• Wound dehiscence, rejection • Graft melt • Graft infection • Suture-related complications • Encroachment of graft edge or sutures into visual axis • Interface haze, infection and vascularization and late perforation with lamellar grafts
Deep anterior lamellar keratoplasty	• Small as well as large descemetoceles • Leaking descemetoceles, and perforations >2 mm • Descemetoceles with microbial keratitis, RA, neurotrophic keratitis, Mooren's ulcer, alkali burns and postpterygium avulsion • Leaking descemetoceles	*Intraoperative*: • Descemet membrane perforations may require a back-up approach or shift to another approach of stromal dissection • Continuous aqueous sweating in the area of descemetocele *Postoperative*: • Sequestration of infection in the interface • Double chamber formation • Graft melt
Penetrating keratoplasty	• Perforated descemetoceles when other approaches have failed • Extensive infections	• Graft melt • Endothelial rejection • Graft failure • Synechiae • Glaucoma • Uveitis • Endophthalmitis • Suboptimal visual gain
Conjunctival flaps	• Descemetoceles with poor visual potential • Perforated descemetoceles after failed AMG • Smaller flaps for peripheral descemetoceles	• Persistence of infection under the flap • Cystic flap formation • Graft retraction and dissolution • Poor cosmetic result • Hinder visualization of intraocular structures • Damage to conjunctiva

Tissue Adhesives

Cyanoacrylate glue (CG) is an ophthalmic sealant composed of esters of cyanoacrylic acid and provides good tectonic support and is bacteriostatic and halts corneal melting with minimal effect on stromal healing.[11] Fibrin glue is a biological tissue adhesive derived from blood. It is made of a fibrinogen component and a thrombin component and dissolves on itself. Both CG and fibrin glue can be employed as either primary treatment modality or as an interim tectonic measure for descemetoceles. However, poor tensile strength of fibrin glue makes it suitable for sealing small descemetoceles only.

Amniotic Membrane Graft

Amniotic membrane graft (AMG) is a biological membrane prepared under sterile conditions from human placentas obtained immediately after elective cesarean section.[12-14] It contains various forms of protease inhibitors and a high content of nerve growth factors that help in suppressing inflammation, promoting epithelialization and improving ocular surface in deep neurotrophic ulcers. Depending on the size, depth, and localization of descemetocele, AMG can be applied as a monolayer or a multilayer and secured to the cornea either with the help of 10-0 nylon sutures (interrupted or continuous) or fibrin glue. Injection bevacizumab can be given in eyes with neovascularization.

Platelet-rich Fibrin Membrane Grafting

Platelet-rich fibrin (PRF) membrane is a second-generation platelet concentrate, composed of three-dimensional polymerized autologous fibrin matrix.[15] It is prepared from autologous blood immediately before surgery and is double-layered and thicker than AMG. Concentrated platelets, growth factors, matrix proteins, cytokines, circulating stem cells, and few leukocytes are found in this membrane and provide both mechanical and chemotactic support for ocular surface reconstruction. The method of application is similar to AMG.

Umbilical Cord Patch Transplantation

The cryopreserved umbilical cord patch (UCP) is a biological graft derived from AM-UC and exerts therapeutic actions similar to AMG.[16] Similar to PRF membrane, UCP is thicker and more compact than AMG. The cryopreserved UC possesses anti-inflammatory, antiscarring, and antiangiogenic effects due to numerous biological signals incorporated in it. The membrane is prepared from the placental tissues by separating AM from chorion by blunt dissection and applied in a manner similar to that of AMG.

Keratoplasty

Keratoplasty is usually considered for descemetoceles when aforementioned approaches have failed. Also, keratoplasty overcomes the limitations of above methods such as temporary support to the cornea with limited increase in inherent tensile strength or visual rehabilitation. Besides, keratoplasty also rids the cornea of necrotic tissue, which is a source of destructive proteolytic enzymes and also provides samples for microbiological and histopathological analysis.

- *Patch graft*: A full-thickness or a lamellar patch graft can be employed as a temporary or definitive method of stabilizing the eyeball. These grafts can be round, crescentic, or customized depending on the size and shape of the ulcer. The donor corneal button is usually oversized by 0.25–0.50 mm and sutured to host with interrupted 10-0 nylon sutures.
- *Lamellar keratoplasty*: Lamellar keratoplasty (LK) involves transplanting a partial thickness donor tissue. Although LK is technically more difficult to perform than PKP, it reduces the risk of postoperative endophthalmitis, allograft rejection, and endothelial failure. Also, preserved host DM forms an effective barrier to deeper microbial invasion.

  Various techniques of deep anterior lamellar keratoplasty (DALK) have been described in eyes with descemetocele. These include Gabison's air-assisted DALK, Sharma's viscoelastic-assisted DALK, and Tong's hydrodissection DALK.[17-19] The donor tissue, stripped of DM, is commonly sutured to the recipient with interrupted 10/0 nylon sutures. Other types of LK inclusive of manual, automated, or femtosecond laser-assisted dissection may also be undertaken for these cases. Infrequently, a sandwich technique of Descemet stripping automated endothelial keratoplasty succeeded by an AMG has also been tried for a case with descemetocele >2 mm.[20]
- *Penetrating keratoplasty*: Penetrating keratoplasty (PKP) is technically easier to perform than LK procedure and also carries a lower risk of donor tissue injuries, such as DM perforation. The surgical steps are similar to any routine full-thickness keratoplasty except for a gentle trephination to decrease the risk of perforation. A 4-mm customized polymethylmethacrylate hard contact lens can also be temporarily applied to the cornea for easy trephination. The donor button is usually kept 0.25–0.50 mm larger than the host and similar to patch graft and DALK, secured with intermittent 10-0 nylon sutures.

  Tectonic epikeratoplasty, where a corneal button is directly sutured to the cornea, was once used as an alternative to PKP for preserving globe integrity in descemetoceles.[21] However, this is rarely practiced now-a-days due to refinements in LK and PKP techniques, increased risk of vascularization, and need for repeat surgeries or urgent PKP. **Figures 4A to H** shows a collage of preoperative and postoperative clinical photographs representing descemetocele managed by different surgical treatment options.

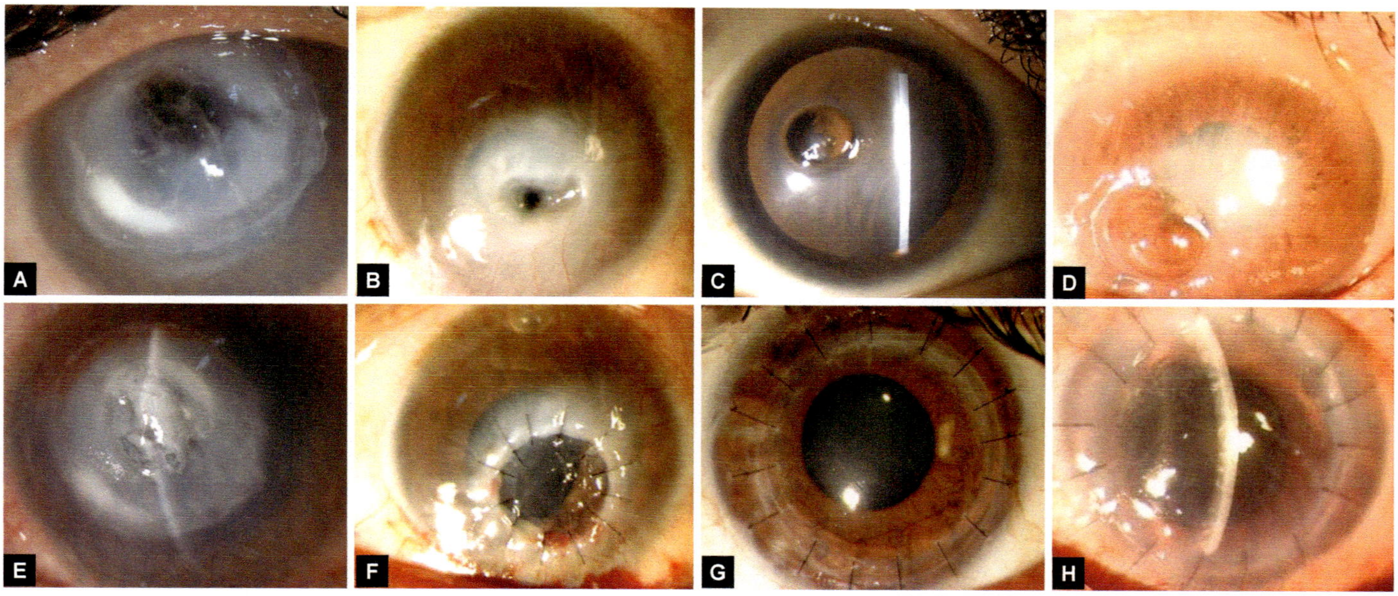

Figs. 4A to H: Preoperative (A to D) and postoperative (E to H) clinical photographs representing descemetocele managed by cyanoacrylate glue application, patch graft, deep anterior lamellar keratoplasty and full thickness keratoplasty respectively.

Flowchart 1: Management algorithm for the treatment for descemetocele, based on the underlying etiology and its size.

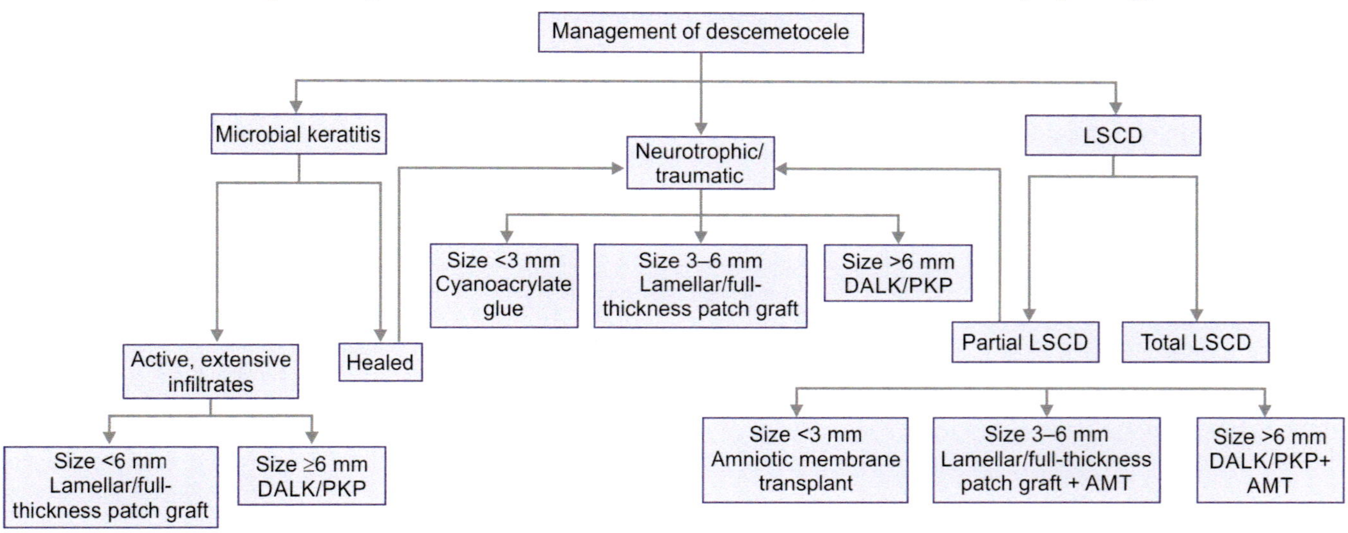

(LSCD: limbal stem cell disorder; DALK: deep anterior lamellar keratoplasty; PKP: penetrating keraplasty; AMT: amniotic membrane transplantation)

Conjunctival Flaps

Conjunctival flaps are usually considered for stabilizing globe integrity in refractory corneal ulcers, corneal perforations, and ocular surface disorders. In Gundersen's procedure, a thin flap of conjunctiva is harvested either from the limbus or from the superior fornix. The flap is repositioned over the cornea and sutured to the sclera just posterior to the limbus with absorbable sutures. Although conjunctival flaps are a time-honored method of ocular surface rehabilitation, they have largely been replaced by alternative methods.

Other reconstructive procedures such as partial thickness scleral patch grafts, Tenon's patch graft, and bioengineered corneas can also be tried in the future for less dependency on donor tissues. **Flowchart 1** representing the management algorithm for a patient presenting with descemetocele, based on the underlying etiology and its size.

POSTOPERATIVE CARE

In general, it is important to continue preoperative medications in the postoperative phase as surgical therapy without an added medical therapy is bound to fail. A common postoperative regime consists of topical antibiotics, lubricants, and steroids (unless contraindicated), with mydriatics, cycloplegics, and antiglaucoma agents added depending on the situation. All patients should be followed-up regularly, preferably bimonthly, for assessing ocular integrity and control of inflammation.

PROGNOSIS

The primary outcome measure of any surgical intervention undertaken for a descemetocele remains the restoration of ocular integrity. The functional and the visual success are secondary to anatomical outcomes.

Anatomical Outcomes

Solomon and colleagues reported 85% success rates with AMG with an epithelialization time of 2–8 weeks.[14] Xie and colleagues showed a marked decrease in ocular surface inflammation with complete epithelialization within 1 month post UCP grafting. Can and colleagues also reported reduction in pain, irritation, and lacrimation after PRF membrane application. While AMG and PKP have similar anatomical outcomes, PKP is reported to be more surgically successful than AMG with a lower rate of perforation.

Functional Outcomes

The visual outcomes of AMG and PRF membrane remain poor and these surgeries may require a second keratoplasty in the future for visual rehabilitation as corneal transplantation provides a transparent medium for achieving better visual results. Krysik and colleagues, demonstrated 13.7%, 57%, and 27.6% improvement in visual acuity after corneoscleral patch grafts, anterior LK, and PKP, respectively.[22] The postoperative visual acuity may worsen in some patients due to cystoid macular edema or visual axis opacification.[23]

Factors Affecting Postoperative Outcome

The prognosis of a descemetocele is dependent on its size, site, cause, and presence of perforation.

Although the location of the descemetocele can affect the visual outcome, Özdemir and colleagues reported no significant effect of site of the descemetocele on visual acuity and the success of surgery in both AMG and PKP group. Immune-mediated disorders carry grim visual prognosis as they respond poorly to conventional medical and surgical interventions. Previous studies have shown that emergent PKPs in perforated eyes have higher rates of graft failure than those performed several weeks to months later. In a recent study by Ozdemir and colleagues, the surgical success was 94.1% in AMG group and 100% in PKP group, respectively if the size of perforation was <1 mm, and it was 90.9% for AMG group and 82.3% for PKP group if the size of perforation was 1–2 mm.[24]

PREVENTION

The best way of managing a descemetocele is to prevent progression of any corneal ulcer to extreme stromal thinning by their early diagnosis and timely management of all corneal infections and inflammations.

Most cases of epithelial defects due to exposure and neurotrophic keratopathy can be prevented from progression to descemetocele by the timely administration of lubricating eye drops/ointment, pressure padding and evasion of the triggering factors. Sometimes, even autologous serum, prophylactic tarsorrhaphy/botulinum toxin-induced ptosis, and punctal occlusion may be required in presence of persistent epithelial defect, lagophthalmos/poor Bells' phenomenon and dry eyes respectively.

SUMMARY

Descemetocele is rare but serious complication of progressive stromal destruction due to various ocular and systemic disorders. The stromal thinning is so severe that the DM is the only layer maintaining the ocular integrity. This condition mandates urgent intervention to restore corneal stability due to the risk of imminent perforation. While medical therapy is preliminary in its management, surgical intervention forms the major requirement. Although anatomical outcomes are usually convincing, the visual prognosis varies with the size and site of descemetocele, presence of perforation, and the underlying cause. With the presently evolving role of microscope-integrated optical coherence tomography in improving outcomes of various corneal surgeries, further studies exploring its effect on management of descemetocele are awaited.[25-26]

REFERENCES

1. Agarwal R, Nagpal R, Todi V, Sharma N. Descemetocele. Surv Ophthalmol. 2021;66(1):2-19.
2. Bafna RK, Agarwal R, Beniwal A, Bhandari A, Sharma N, Titiyal JS. Emulsion polymer isocyanate-gluing: Autologous epithelial transplant with cyanoacrylate glue application for small corneal perforations. Indian J Ophthalmol. 2020;68:1636-9.
3. Ozdemir ES, Burcu A, Akkaya ZY, Ornek F. Surgical outcomes of perforated and unperforated corneal descemetocele. Int Ophthalmol. 2018;38(1):327-35.
4. Can ME, Dereli Can G, Cagil N, Cakmak HB, Sungu N. Urgent therapeutic grafting of platelet-rich fibrin membrane in descemetocele. Cornea. 2016;35(9):1245-9.
5. Gabison EE, Doan S, Catanese M, Chastang P, Ben M'hamed M, Cochereau I. Modified deep anterior lamellar keratoplasty in the management of small and large epithelialized descemetoceles. Cornea. 2011;30(10):1179-82.
6. Gelender H. Descemetocele after intraocular lens implantation. Arch Ophthalmol. 1982;100:72-6.
7. Arentsen JJ, Laibson PR, Cohen EJ. Management of corneal descemetoceles and perforations. Trans Am Ophthalmol Soc. 1984;82:92-105.
8. Berguiga M, Mameletzi E, Nicolas M, Rivier D, Majo F. Long-term follow-up of multilayer amniotic membrane transplantation (MLAMT) for non-traumatic corneal perforations or deep ulcers with descemetocele. Klin Monbl Augenheilkd. 2013;230(4):413-8.
9. Carmichael TR, Gelfand Y, Welsh NH. Topical steroids in the treatment of central and paracentral corneal ulcers. Br J Ophthalmol. 1990;74(9):528-31.
10. Davanger M. Descemetocele and the law of Laplace. Acta Ophthalmol (Copenh). 1971;49(5):715-8.
11. Dua HS, Faraj LA, Said DG, Gray T, Lowe J. Human corneal anatomy redefined: A novel pre-Descemet's layer (Dua's layer). Ophthalmology. 2013;120(9):1778-85.

12. Graue-Hernandez EO, Zuñiga-Gonzalez I, Hernandez-Camarena JC, Jaimes M, Chirinos-Saldaña P, Navas A, et al. Tectonic DSAEK for the management of impending corneal perforation. Case Rep Ophthalmol Med. 2012;2012:916528.
13. Krachmer JH, Mannis MJ, Holland EJ. Cornea. China: Mosby/Elsevier; 2011. p. 1967.
14. Krysik K, Dobrowolski D, Lyssek-Boron A, Jankowska-Szmul J, Wylegala EA. Differences in surgical management of corneal perforations, measured over six years. J Ophthalmol. 2017;2017:1582532.
15. Lifshitz T, Oshry T. Tectonic epikeratoplasty: a surgical procedure for corneal melting. Ophthalmic Surg Lasers. 2001;32(4):305-7.
16. Mohammadpour M, Sabet FA. Long-term Outcomes of amniotic membrane transplantation in contact lens-induced pseudomonas keratitis with impending corneal perforation. J Ophthalmic Vis Res. 2016;11(1):37-41.
17. Medsinge A, Gajdosova E, Moore W, Nischal KK. Management of inflammatory corneal melt leading to central perforation in children: A retrospective study and review of literature. Eye (Lond). 2016;30(4):593-601.
18. Narang P, Agarwal A, Kumar DA. Predescemetocele: A distinct clinical entity. Indian J Ophthalmol. 2017;65(11):1224-6.
19. Sharma N, Kumar C, Mannan R, Titiyal JS, Vajpayee RB. Surgical technique of deep anterior lamellar keratoplasty in descemetoceles. Cornea. 2010;29(12):1448-51.
20. Solomon A, Meller D, Prabhasawat P, John T, Espana EM, Steuhl KP, et al. Amniotic membrane grafts for nontraumatic corneal perforations, descemetoceles, and deep ulcers. Ophthalmology. 2002;109:694-703.
21. Sultana N, Chaurasia S, Ramappa M. High-resolution optical coherence tomography in a case of descemetocele managed with amniotic membrane transplantation. Indian J Ophthalmol 2018;66:315-7.
22. Tong L, Tan DT, Abańo JM, Lim L. Deep anterior lamellar keratoplasty in a patient with descemetocele following gonococcal keratitis. Am J Ophthalmol. 2004;138(3):506-7.
23. Twining SS, Davis SD, Hyndiuk RA. Relationship between proteases and descemetocele formation in experimental Pseudomonas keratitis. Curr Eye Res. 1986;5(7):503-10.
24. Xie HT, Zhao D, Liu Y, Zhang MC. Umbilical cord patch transplantation for corneal perforations and descemetoceles. J Ophthalmol. 2017;2017:2767053.
25. Agarwal R, Sidhu N, Sinha R, Sharma N. Real-time optical coherence tomography-guided scleral flap creation for intrascleral haptic fixation of posterior chamber intraocular lens. Clin Exp Ophthalmol. 2020;48(9):1310-12.
26. Sharma N, Priyadarshini K, Agarwal R, Bafna R, Nagpal R, Sinha R, et al. Role of microscope-intraoperative optical coherence tomography in paediatric keratoplasty: A comparative study. Am J Ophthalmol. 2021;221:190-8.

66 Sclerokeratoplasty

Shreya Thatte, Ankita B Dube, Trupti Dubey

INTRODUCTION

Corneal pathologies caused by a wide variety of infectious and inflammatory insults can lead to severe vision loss and blindness. According to World Health Organization (WHO), corneal pathologies stand as the 4th leading cause of blindness (5.1%) and the second major cause of preventable blindness, worldwide.[1] For pathologies involving all layers of cornea, penetrating keratoplasty is the answer and if the pathology involves the adjoining sclera as well, it warrants a penetrating sclerokeratoplasty.[2]

The first successful penetrating keratoplasty was performed by Edward Conrad Zirm in 1906.[3] Since then various modifications have been introduced in the technique of keratoplasty to address various corneal as well as corneoscleral pathologies. Penetrating sclerokeratoplasty was first introduced by Girard in 1956, and was defined as, the transplantation of full-thickness cornea including the adjacent scleral rim.[4] The surgical technique involves transplantation of relatively large-sized grafts in order to provide structural support to the globe.[4]

Compared to a routine performed optical penetrating keratoplasty, the technique is more risky as well as more challenging.[5] It is usually kept as a last resort while managing patients with advanced corneal pathologies. The severity or chronicity of the primary disease, along with concurrent distortion of the anterior segment anatomy and the use of a large size graft, all these factors serve to increase the likelihood of serious complications such as recurrence of the primary pathology, immune-mediated graft rejection, graft failure, and secondary glaucoma. It requires a great deal from the surgeon to obtain better tectonic as well as optical results.

INDICATIONS

There are multiple etiologies comprising both ocular as well as systemic diseases which mandate the use of sclerokeratoplasty procedure so as to salvage the eye. These indications can be broadly classified into two groups:

1. Infective etiologies
2. Noninfective etiologies

Infective Etiologies

These include eyes with rapidly progressive, necrotizing sclerokeratitis (**Fig. 1**), and cases with large corneal perforation.[6-8]

This is one of the most common indications especially encountered in developing countries. The etiology is most commonly due to mixed pathogens and is usually refractory to all forms of medical therapies.[9,10] The most severe forms of corneal ulceration or abscess are encountered with *Pseudomonas, Staphylococcal, Aspergillus,* or *Fusarium* species.[2,11,12] Such eyes require urgent therapeutic or tectonic sclerokeratoplasty.

Noninfective Etiologies

These include a broad spectrum of diseases which can be further subdivided into autoimmune, neoplastic, or traumatic causes.

Autoimmune causes include eyes with sterile sclerocorneal melts, seen in patients with rheumatoid arthritis, Wegener's granulomatosis, and relapsing polychondritis. Similarly, corneal melts associated with advanced, late stages of Mooren's ulcer also need this procedure.[13,14]

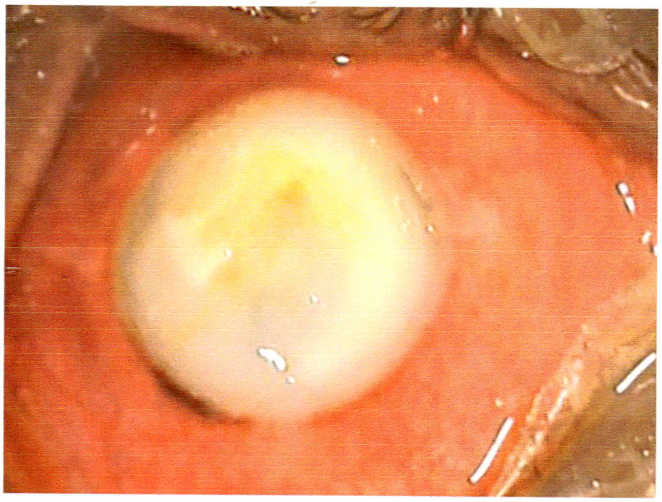

Fig. 1: Slit-lamp photograph showing corneal abscess with adjacent scleral involvement.

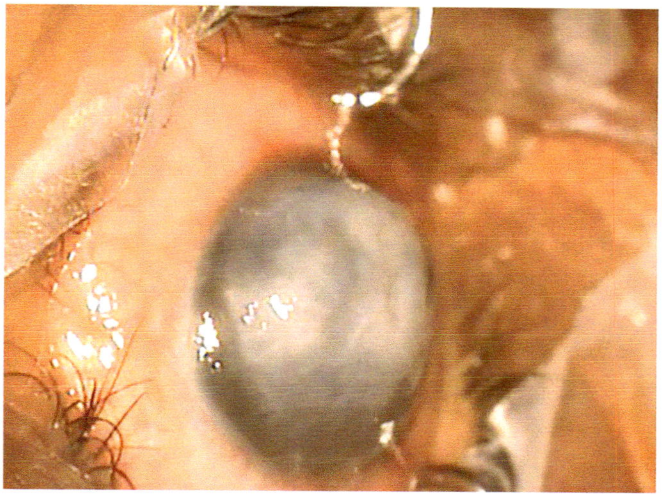

Fig. 2: Slit lamp showing large anterior staphyloma in an eye resulting from a prior corneoscleral infection.

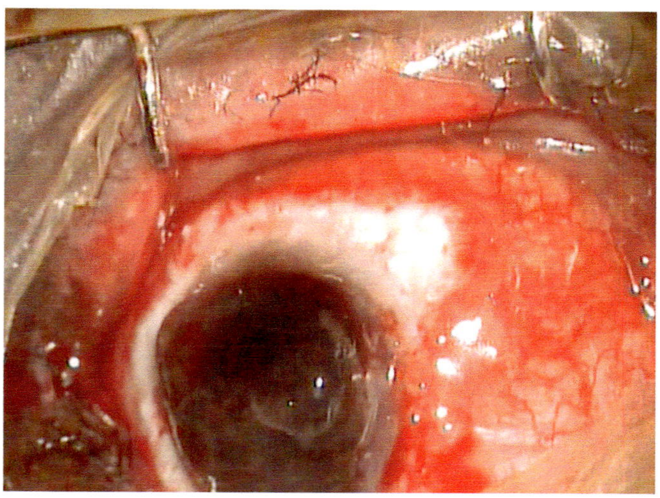

Fig. 3: Slit-lamp photograph of an eye with extensive tissue loss following a chemical burn.

- *Eyes with anterior staphyloma* resulting from a long standing poorly healed corneoscleral infection (**Fig. 2**) and noninflammatory ectatic disorders such as advanced keratoconus, keratoglobus, and pellucid marginal degeneration also need sclerokeratoplasty.[14-18]
- Sclerokeratoplasty is also indicated as a first-line treatment in eyes which have suffered extensive mechanical trauma with resulting tissue loss and as a last resort procedure in eyes with chemical injuries, not responding to alternative tissue-preserving treatment strategies (**Fig. 3**).[13,19,20]
- Extensive tumors such as large congenital limbal dermoids and cases of widespread infiltrating conjunctival squamous cell carcinoma also require sclerokeratoplasty.[21]

PENETRATING/LAMELLAR KERATOPLASTY VERSUS SCLEROKERATOPLASTY

Penetrating/lamellar keratoplasty, which is most commonly performed as an elective procedure, is quite different from sclerokeratoplasty. In sclerokeratoplasty, there is disturbance in the limbal, scleral as well as conjunctival anatomy. Therefore, these eyes are more prone for both nonimmunological as well as immune-mediated graft failure. Distorted anterior segment anatomy in the form of anterior iris synechiae, vitreous adhesions, deep stromal vascularization, large-sized graft, proximity to limbal vessels, and host immune cells, and presence of preexisting lymphocytotoxic antibodies[22-26] are more frequently encountered in eyes undergoing sclerokeratoplasty.

Compression or distortion of the anterior chamber angle either due to preexisting pathology, surgical trauma associated with use of large graft, and suturing technique account for a higher incidence of glaucoma in eyes undergoing sclerokeratoplasty.[27,28] Performing trephination and dissection during full-thickness sclerokeratoplasty is more angle-threatening as opposed to sclerokeratoplasty done with lamellar scleral dissection and with other special precautions to safeguard the angle structures.[29-32]

Hence, this high-risk nature of sclerokeratoplasty demands a meticulous and detailed approach to such challenging cases in order to achieve a desired outcome.

PREOPERATIVE CONSIDERATIONS

It is prudent to perform a comprehensive preoperative workup of patients so as to have a clue about the etiology and thus to provide appropriate postoperative care. It encompasses the following:

- *History*: Detailed history pertaining to the actual pathology and related systemic disease needs to be elicited.
- *Anterior segment evaluation*: A thorough slit-lamp examination is necessary to evaluate anterior segment-associated pathologies. As these cases involve a larger part of the cornea, it is difficult to examine the anterior segment in detail. Therefore, a procedure which can reveal anterior segment details is needed. There are many techniques to visualize the anterior segment based on principle of penetration of light and ultrasonic rays. The opaque media in these eyes obscures the light rays to penetrate deeply. Since the ultrasonic waves penetrate deeply, ultrasound biomicroscopy (UBM) is thus a helpful investigative modality in these cases (**Fig. 4**).

  Another important investigation is the assessment of intraocular pressure (IOP). Methods such as applanation tonometry and Schiotz tonometry are not accurate in view of extensive corneal involvement, digital assessment of IOP is therefore the preferred option.
- *Posterior segment evaluation*: Retinal evaluation by direct and indirect ophthalmoscope may not be possible due to extensive corneal involvement. B-scan is therefore useful to detect gross posterior segment pathologies.
- *Special Investigations*: Corneal scraping and culture and sensitivity testing is recommended in infective cases. Blood cultures should be obtained in cases with

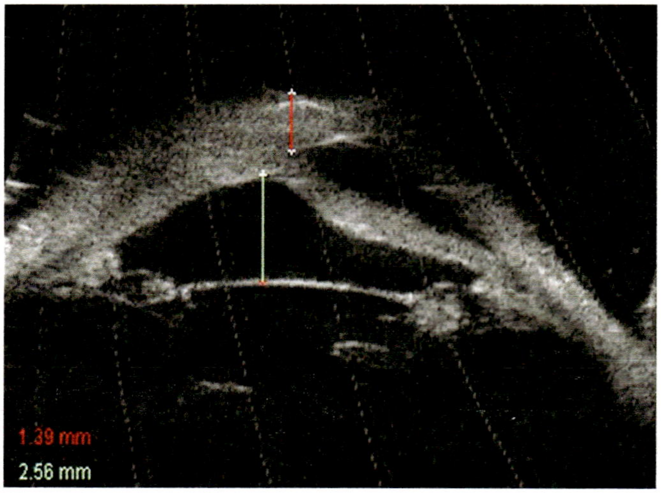

Fig. 4: Ultrasound biomicroscopy image showing dense iridocorneal adhesions on the nasal side with shallow temporal anterior chamber.

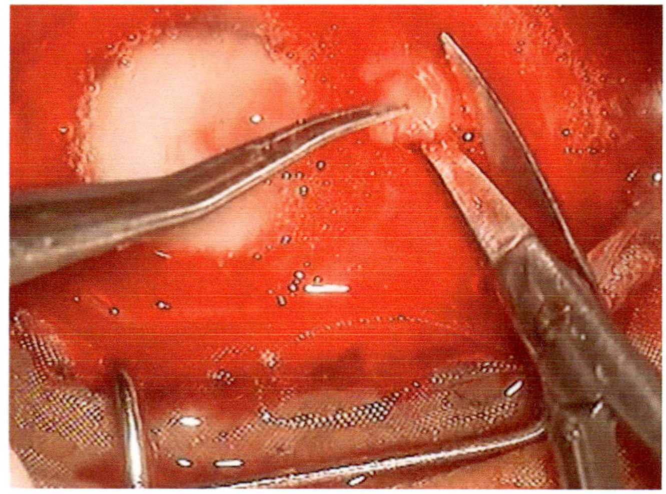

Fig. 5: Conjunctival peritomy to delineate the areas of underlying scleral involvement.

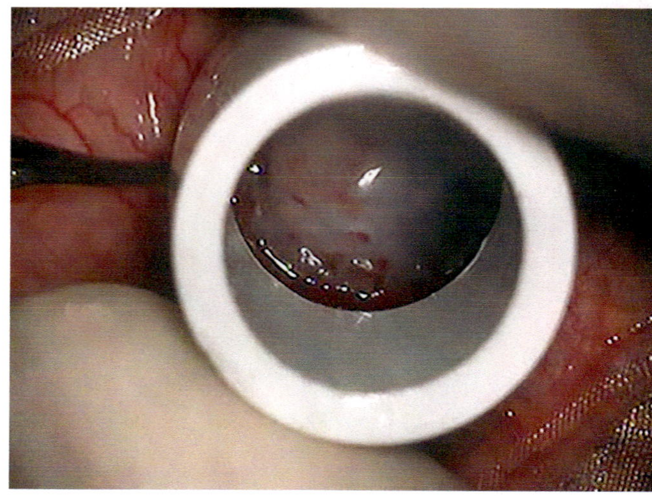

Fig. 6: Host marking using a handheld trephine.

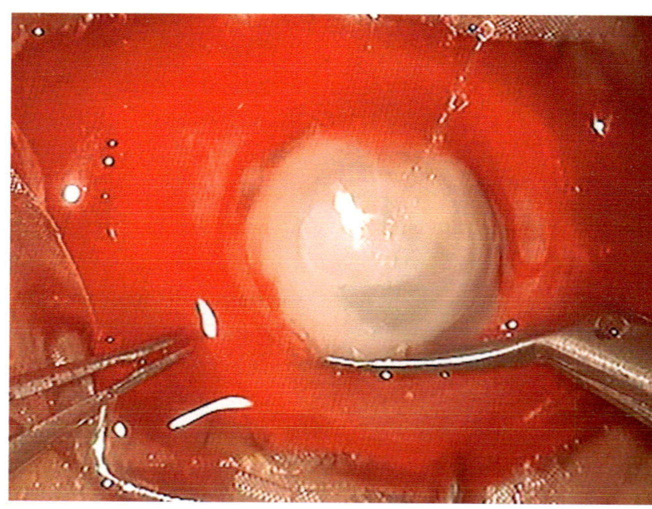

Fig. 7: Manual dissection of the host tissue using scissors.

extensive scleral involvement to rule out any systemic foci of sepsis.

Patients with underlying autoimmune disorders need a comprehensive autoimmune work-up to determine the disease activity in conjunction with a physician and rheumatologist.

- *Counseling and consent*: The most crucial step before preparing for surgery is counseling of the patient and close relatives about the procedure and its complications, its guarded prognosis, requirement for subsequent procedures as well as compulsion to maintain compliance, and regular follow-up.

PATIENT PREPARATION BEFORE SURGERY

Approximately 30–45 minutes prior to surgery, intravenous mannitol 20%, 1 g per kg body weight should be administered. It is logical to perform the surgery under general anesthesia in patients with large perforations or the ones wherein administering a peribulbar block is cumbersome due to the disturbed anatomy of the globe.

SURGICAL TECHNIQUE

It is advised to use a light weight wire speculum or even lid everting sutures in perforated eyes in order to avoid spontaneous extrusion of lens and vitreous intraoperatively. Conjunctival peritomy is performed, starting at the site of corneoscleral involvement, which may extend to complete 360° in cases with total limbal involvement (**Fig. 5**). It is important to vigorously remove the diseased conjunctiva and underneath devitalized tissue, wherever present so as to obtain a healthy graft-host junction, void of all nonviable tissue.

The diseased corneoscleral host tissue is then gently marked using hand held trephine (**Fig. 6**) or a Vernier caliper and then excision is carried out with using a trephine or manually with Castroviejo's scissors (**Fig. 7**). Corresponding to the host defect, the donor graft size and shape are customized. The graft diameter chosen is 1 mm larger than the area of host dissection.

The donor graft can be procured either using a corneal punch or by freehand dissection depending on its size and shape (**Fig. 8**). The edges of host defect are excised

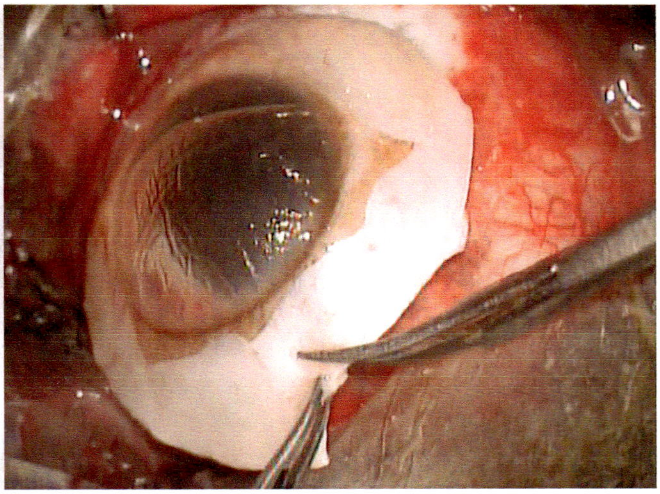

Fig. 8: Manual preparation of the donor corneal button.

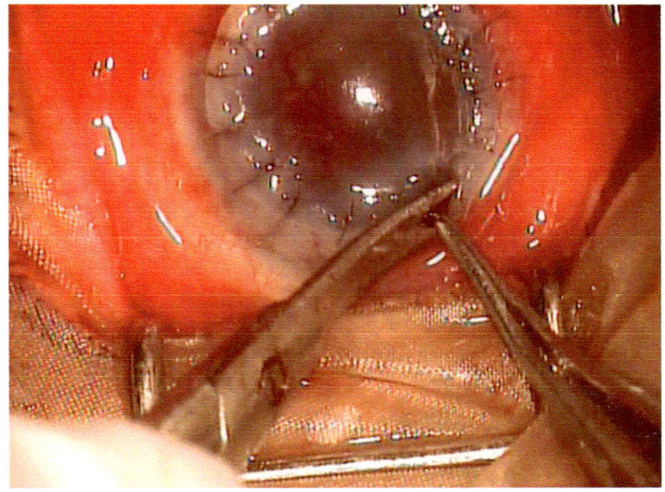

Fig. 10: Peripheral buttonhole iridectomy.

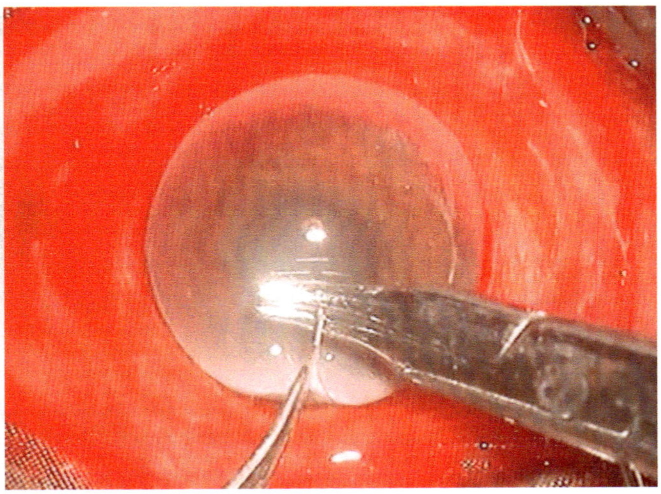

Fig. 9: The relatively thicker and denser scleral tissue where the suturing is being initiated.

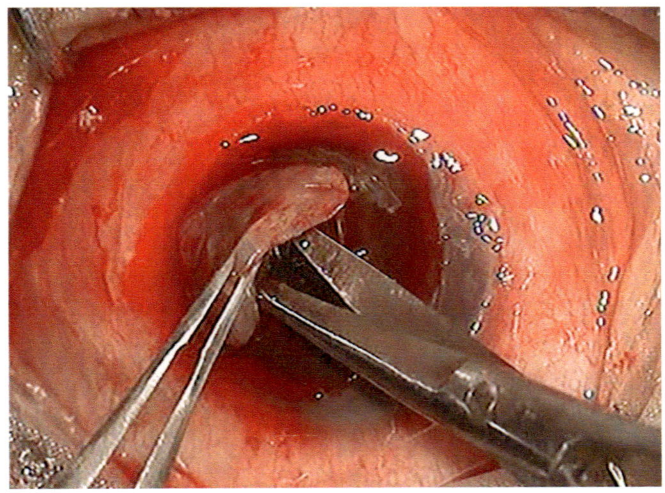

Fig. 11: Release of anterior iris synechia using Vannas scissors.

obliquely keeping the base toward sclera and slope toward iris. Similarly, donor tissue is also excised obliquely but in reverse manner with thinner part toward sclera and base toward iris for proper fitting of graft over the recipient bed.

Suturing in these eyes requires special mention. Obtaining a perfectly apposed graft-host junction is difficult due to variable thickness and uneven surfaces of corneal and scleral tissue and the differences in corneal and scleral tissue rigidity (**Fig. 9**). Continuous suturing is not advocated in these high-risk cases.

Peripheral iridectomy has to be performed in all eyes to avoid postoperative glaucoma (**Fig. 10**).[2,7] Lateral tarsorrhaphy is to be routinely done in eyes with extensive tissue damage especially to the limbal stem cells to promote epithelial healing postoperatively.[8,31]

Although the main purpose of sclerokeratoplasty is to help in maintaining the globe integrity, salvaging as much viable host tissue as possible and restoring near-normal anterior segment anatomy is equally important in order to obtain favorable postoperative results.

Thus, it is wise to implement few modifications or additional procedures as per the case scenario. These include:

- *Releasing anterior synechiae*: In staphylomatous eyes with broad anterior synechiae and a strongly adhered iris, gentle superficial separation of the iris tissue from the cornea is advised using either a swab stick, an iris repositor or using a fine scissors (**Fig. 11**). In cases with gross iris and pupillary distortion, iris reconstruction/pupilloplasty is also recommended.[33]
- *Removal of dense fibrinous membranes*: In infected cases, the fibrinous exudative membrane should be gently peeled off using nontraumatizing fine forceps taking care not to cause any further damage to the underlying iris tissue and the lens capsule (**Fig. 12**). Subsequently, a thorough wash of the anterior chamber is done using broad-spectrum antibiotics (preservative-free moxifloxacin)[34] or antifungal drugs (amphotericin B 5 μg/0.1 mL[35] and voriconazole 50 μg/0.1 mL[36]) depending upon the nature of the causative organism.

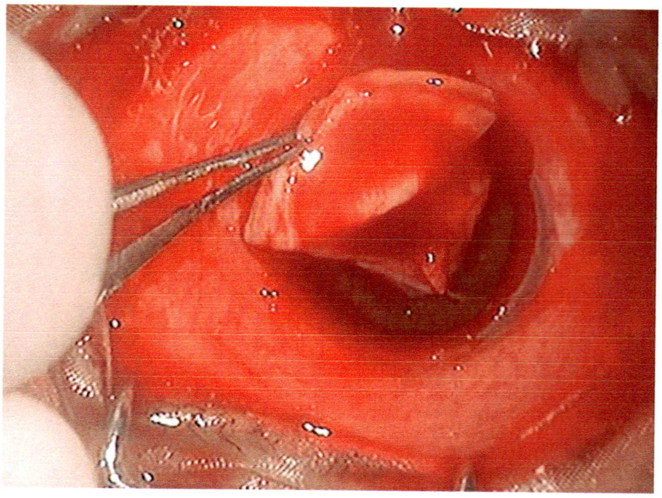

Fig. 12: Thick fibrous membrane removed from the anterior chamber.

- It is critical to perform a meticulous anterior vitrectomy in cases where spontaneous lens extrusion is encountered.[14,17,37]

Modifications to Protect the Angle

Many techniques have been introduced to curb damage to the angle during surgery. The most commonly followed method is lamellar preparation of the host scleral bed extending almost 1 mm into the peripheral cornea followed by a penetrating excision of the remaining host cornea described by many authors.[7,14,21] Studies have also described use of angle support sutures and interrupted, horizontal, running mattress sutures.[31] Another technique is to use fibrin glue instead of sutures to secure the donor tissue after lamellar preparation, so as to safeguard the angle structures.[38]

POSTOPERATIVE MANAGEMENT

In eyes with an infective etiology corticosteroids in any form are not to be administered for a minimum of 10 days postoperatively. Systemic and topical antibiotics are employed depending upon the culture-sensitivity report. These patients require frequent follow up to pick up any early signs of recurrence of infection. In case of no signs of reinfection for a period of 10 days, corticosteroids may be initiated under a close follow-up.[39]

In cases with noninfective etiology, topical corticosteroids should be started immediately following surgery supplemented by systemic steroids at the rate of 1 mg/kg body along with topical broad-spectrum antibiotics and lubricating eye drops.[16,17]

During follow-up visual acuity, graft clarity, IOP, occurrence of any signs of suture-related complications, graft rejection, recurrence of preexisting corneal pathology, and other complications should be assessed and treated accordingly.

POSTOPERATIVE COMPLICATIONS AND MANAGEMENT

The complications encountered after sclerokeratoplasty can be attributed either to the preexisting pathology or the complications associated with the surgical procedure.

- *Reinfection*: Studies have reported a lower incidence of reinfection following sclerokeratoplasty compared to therapeutic keratoplasty.[6] Subjecting the surgically excised host tissue to culture sensitivity, isolating the offending microorganism and accordingly administering intraocular as well as systemic antibiotics is of utmost importance. Treatment includes regrafting in most of cases. In highly resistant cases, enucleation or evisceration might be warranted.
- *Epithelial defect*: This is seen in almost every patient undergoing sclerokeratoplasty. In conventional penetrating keratoplasty the graft re-epithelialization is carried out only by the host limbal stem cells unlike sclerokeratoplasty wherein the donor limbal cells are presumed to be responsible for regenerating the graft epithelium. Thus, a healthy population of donor stem cells is required to prevent recurrent epithelial breakdowns and to maintain the structural integrity of the graft. Long-term use of intensive lubricants, vitamin A ointment, bandage contact lens, and ultimately tarsorrhaphy facilitate in rehabilitating the ocular surface.
- *Graft rejection*: As discussed earlier, use of a large graft and close proximity to host blood vessels account for higher chances of graft rejection. Apart from this, another mechanism thought to be responsible for triggering graft rejection is the delayed epithelial rejuvenation especially in eyes with chemical injury and neurotrophic keratopathy.[15,40] Systemic steroids (1 mg/kg/day) are to be included in the routine treatment regime as a prophylactic measure. However, if the rejection episode is noticed, the treatment has to be intensified by increasing the dose of oral prednisolone (1.5 mg/kg/day) and adding oral cyclosporine A (200 mg/day). Blood cyclosporine levels should be monitored and maintained within the therapeutic range (0.14–0.13 mg/dL).[14,41,42] Routine blood investigations are frequently advised to monitor the adverse effects of cyclosporine A. The oral immunosuppressive treatment other than steroids should be continued for a minimum of 6 months to one year. Topical corticosteroid medications should be instilled every half hourly for the initial 24–48 hours followed by gradual tapering.
- *Secondary glaucoma*: The surgical dissection close to the angle, frequent episodes of immunological graft rejection, use of high-dose corticosteroids and preoperative inflammatory status of the eye altogether contribute to the development of secondary glaucoma. Absolute glaucoma seems to be a possibility due to the

disturbed anatomy of angle structures.[43] The surgical technique described previously to safeguard the angle also reduces the incidence of secondary glaucoma. IOP reduction is achieved using oral as well as topical antiglaucoma drugs. Surgical intervention in the form of trabeculectomy, glaucoma drainage device or even cyclocryotherapy is recommended in highly recalcitrant cases.[8,13,14]

- *Graft failure*: Recurrence of disease, repeated graft rejection episodes, persistent epithelial defect causing stromal melting, secondary glaucoma, secondary infections, and autoimmune nature of the underlying disease, all these factors may lead to graft failure.
- *Suture-related complications*: Suture-related complications such as sterile or infective infiltrates and loose sutures are commonly expected in the postoperative period, loosening is expected to be more common and may be encountered quite early in the postoperative period following sclerokeratoplasty. This needs to be addressed immediately in order to avoid immune-mediated graft rejection. Early suture removal is advisable in such situations, even before 6 weeks following sclerokeratoplasty.[21] It is important to differentiate between sterile and infective infiltrates in order to address the situation appropriately.
- *Hypotony*: This may occur due to extensive physical or chemical trauma, infectious etiology, frequent episodes of graft rejection or postoperative uveitis, and repeated need for cyclocryotherapy.
- Other complications such as hyphema, shallow anterior chamber, and postoperative uveitis may be noted as early as on postoperative day one, requiring immediate medical or surgical intervention.

OUTCOMES OF SCLEROKERATOPLASTY

Sclerokeratoplasty is considered as a viable treatment option in eyes with extensive corneoscleral lesions. With the complications well managed, it helps to preserve the structural integrity of eyeball. Corneoscleral grafts of 12–14 mm diameter, function well with good anatomic success rates.[14,21] Sclerokeratoplasty alone however does not suffice in restoring vision and a subsequent central optical penetrating keratoplasty may be required as a second stage procedure which needs to be incorporated in the treatment paradigm.

REFERENCES

1. Whitcher JP, Srinivasan M, Upadhyay MP. Corneal blindness: A global perspective. Bull World Health Organ. 2001;79:214-21.
2. Krysik K, Wroblewska-Czajka E, Lyssek-Boron A, Wylegala EA, Dobrowolski D. Total penetrating keratoplasty: Indications, therapeutic approach, and long-term follow-up. J Ophthalmol. 2018;2018:9580292.
3. Zirm EK. Eine erfolgreiche totale Keratoplastik (A successful total keratoplasty). 1906. Refract Corneal Surg. 1989;5(4):258-61.
4. Krachmer JH, Mannis MJ, Holland EJ. Cornea: Fundamentals, Diagnosis and Management. New York: Elsevier Inc.; 2011.
5. Tourkmani AK, Sánchez-Huerta V, De Wit G, Martínez JD, Mingo D, Mahillo-Fernández I, et al. Weighing of risk factors for penetrating keratoplasty graft failure: Application of risk score system. Int J Ophthalmol. 2017;10(3):372-7.
6. Panda A, Sharma N, Angra SK, Singh R. Therapeutic sclerokeratoplasty versus therapeutic penetrating keratoplasty in refractory corneal ulcers. Aust N Z J Ophthalmol. 1999;27:15-9.
7. Jonas JB, Rank RM, Budde WM. Tectonic sclerokeratoplasty and tectonic penetrating keratoplasty as treatment for perforated or predescemetal corneal ulcers. Am J Ophthalmol. 2001;132(1):14-8.
8. Hirst LW, Lee GA. Corneoscleral transplantation for end stage corneal disease. Br J Ophthalmol. 1998;82(11):1276-9.
9. Sony P, Sharma N, Vajpayee RB, Ray M. Therapeutic keratoplasty for infectious keratitis: A review of the literature. CLAO J. 2002;28(3):111-8.
10. Cristol SM, Alfonso EC, Guildford JH, Roussel TJ, Culbertson WW. Results of large penetrating keratoplasty in microbial keratitis. Cornea. 1996;15(6):571-6.
11. Koçluk Y, Sukgen EA. Results of therapeutic penetrating keratoplasty for bacterial and fungal keratitis. Int Ophthalmol. 2017;37(5):1085-93.
12. Rush SW, Rush RB. Outcomes of infectious versus sterile perforated corneal ulcers after therapeutic penetrating keratoplasty in the United States. J Ophthalmol. 2016;2016:6284595.
13. Taylor DM, Stern AL. Reconstructive keratoplasty in the management of conditions leading to corneal destruction. Ophthalmology. 1980;87(9):892-904.
14. Burk RO, Joussen AM. Corneoscleroplasty with maintenance of the angle in two cases of extensive corneoscleral disease. Eye (Lond). 2000;14(Pt 2):196-200.
15. Rozycki R, Nowak-Gospodarowicz I, Bialas D, Pawlik R, Rekas M. Sclerokeratoplasty as the therapy for corneal perforation due to exposure and neurotrophic keratopathy. Case Rep Ophthalmol Med. 2014;2014:467249.
16. Panda A, Sharma N, Angra SK, Singh R. Sclerokeratoplasty versus penetrating keratoplasty in anterior staphyloma. Ophthalmic Surg Lasers. 1999;30:31-6.
17. de la Torre-Gonzalez E, de León Ascencio CP. Staged penetrating sclerokeratoplasty and penetrating keratoplasty for management of advanced acquired anterior staphyloma. J Ophthalmic Vis Res. 2011;6(2):147-50.
18. Esquenazi S, Shihadeh WA, Abderkader A, Kaufman HE. A new surgical technique for anterior segment ectasia: Tectonic lamellar sclerokeratoplasty. Ophthalmic Surg Lasers Imaging. 2006;37:434-6.
19. Iyer G, Srinivasan B, Rishi E, Rishi P, Agarwal S, Subramanian N. Large lamellar corneoscleral grafts: tectonic role in initial management of severe ocular chemical injuries. Eur J Ophthalmol. 2016;26(1):12-7.
20. Viestenz A, Seitz B, Struck HG, Viestenz A Sclerocorneal graft and sequential removal of melted cornea after severe corneal burn with perforation. Clin Anat. 2018;31(1):39-42.
21. Panda A. Lamellolamellar sclerokeratoplasty. Where do we stand today? Eye (Lond). 1999;13(Pt 2):221-5.
22. Maguire MG, Stark WJ, Gottsch JD, Stulting RD, Sugar A, Fink NE, et al. Risk factors for corneal graft failure and rejection in the collaborative corneal transplantation studies. Ophthalmology. 1994;101:1536-47.
23. Völker-Dieben HJ, D'Amaro J, Kok-van Alphen CC. Hierarchy of prognostic factors for corneal allograft survival. Aust N Z J Ophthalmol. 1987;15:11-18.
24. Boisjoly HM, Bernanrd PM, Dube I, Laughera PA, Bazin R, Bermier J. Effect of factors unrelated to tissue matching on

corneal transplant endothelial rejection. Am J Ophthalmol. 1989;107:647-54.
25. Des Marchais B, Bazin R, Boisjoyly HM, Laughera PA, Dube I, Lille S, et al. Role of presensitization and donor-recipient crossmatching in corneal graft outcome. Cornea. 1998;17:141-5.
26. Khodadoust AA. The allograft rejection reaction: the leading cause of late failure of clinical allografts. In: Porter R, Knight J, (Eds). Corneal Graft Failure. Amsterdam: Elsevier; 1973. pp. 151-67.
27. Kirkness CM, Moshegov C. Post-keratoplasty glaucoma. Eye (Lond). 1988;2 Suppl:S19-26.
28. Lass JH, Pavan-Langston D. Timolol therapy in secondary angle closure glaucoma post penetrating keratoplasty. Ophthalmology. 1979;86:54-9.
29. Karesh JW, Nirankari VS. Factors associated with glaucoma after penetrating keratoplasty. Am J Ophthalmol. 1983;96:160-4.
30. Kirkness CM, Ficker LA. Risk factors for the development of post PK glaucoma. Cornea. 1992;11:427-32.
31. Cobo M, Ortiz JR, Safran SG. Sclerokeratoplasty with maintenance of the angle. Am J Ophthalmol. 1992;113:533-7.
32. Panda A. Sclerokeratoplasty vs PK. Visiscan. 1994; DOS 2:22-4.
33. Cohen EJ, Kenyon KR, Dohlmam CH. Iridoplasty for prevention of post keratoplasty angle closure glaucoma. Ophthalmic Surg. 1982;13:994-6.
34. Arshinoff SA, Modabber M. Dose and administration of intracameral moxifloxacin for prophylaxis of postoperative endophthalmitis. J Cataract Refract Surg. 2016;42(12):1730-41.
35. Kuriakose T, Kothari M, Paul P, Jacob P, Thomas R. Intracameral amphotericin B injection in the management of deep keratomycosis. Cornea. 2002;21(7):653-6.
36. Shen YC, Wang CY, Tsai HY, Lee HN. Intracameral voriconazole injection in the treatment of fungal endophthalmitis resulting from keratitis. Am J Ophthalmol. 2010;149(6):916-21.
37. Parwez H, Tourkmani AK, Kazakos D, Jones M, Anderson D; NHS blood and transplant ocular tissue advisory group and contributing ophthalmologists. Emergency corneal grafting in the UK: A 6-year analysis of the UK transplant registry. Br J Ophthalmol. 2018;102:26-30.
38. Kumar S, Panda A. Fibrin Glue aided sutureless sclerokeratoplasty with maintenance of chamber angle. Cornea. 2011;30(5):588-90.
39. Skeens HM, Holland EJ. Large-diameter penetrating keratoplasty: indications and outcomes. Cornea. 2010;29(3):296-301.
40. Redbrake C, Buchal V. Keratoplasty with scleral rim after the most severe chemical eye burns of the anterior eye segment. Klin Monbl Augenheilkd. 1996;208:145-51.
41. Reinhard T, Sundmacher R, Heering P. Systemic cyclosporine A in high-risk keratoplasties. Graefes Arch Clin Exp Ophthalmol. 1996;234 Suppl 1:S115-21.
42. Sundmacher R, Reinhard T. Central corneolimbal transplantation under systemic cyclosporin A cover for severe limbal stem cell insufficiency. Graefes Arch Clin Exp Ophthalmol. 1996;234 (Suppl 1):S122-5.
43. Lustbader JM, Barraquer J, Green WR. Corneoscleral autotransplant. Arch Ophthalmol. 1988;106:953-7.

SECTION

7

Alternatives to Corneal Transplantation

67

Keratoprosthesis: A Broad Overview

Hiren Matai, Shweta Agarwal, Bhaskar Srinivasan, Geetha Iyer

INTRODUCTION

Keratoprosthesis form the last resort for bilateral end stage corneal and ocular surface disorders. The Kpros are classified based on the type of eye they cater to. As important as it is to choose a patient for keratoprosthesis, equally important is the process of selecting the correct Kpro for the patient. The indications, perioperative care, nuances of the surgical technique, identifying and managing complications are all crucial in determining the outcome and have been outlined in the chapter in detail.

Along with the revolution in corneal transplants over the past 2 decades, modifications and refinements in techniques have also been witnessed in the field of keratoprosthesis. Kpros are not an alternative to corneal transplants and are reserved for end stage bilateral corneal/ocular surface disorders. In these eyes, Kpros reserve a special place in rehabilitating these patients. Keratoprosthesis are broadly divided into two categories—Type 1 and 2 based on the eye on which they are transplanted. The decision on the choice of Kpro is made depending on the underlying etiology, the ocular surface anatomy, and the status of the tear film.

At the Sankara Nethralaya Ocular Surface Clinic, Kpro procedures are being performed since 2003, with the initiation of the modified osteo-odonto Kpro (MOOKP) procedure for the first time in India under the guidance of the father of OOKP, Professor Giancarlo Falcinelli from Italy. This was followed by initiation of the Type 1 Kpro in January 2008, followed subsequently by the Boston Type 2 Kpro in January 2013 and the osteo-Kpro in January 2014, thus in all probability making it the only center currently that actively performs and offers all types of Kpros.

This chapter details the guidelines regarding the choice of Kpro with the corresponding surgical techniques, the author's experience with the various Kpro types thereby providing an insight into understanding the virtues of the different Kpro types as well as their shortcomings. It also highlights the result of the several types of Kpro procedures performed at our institute, comparing the same with the results from large single-center studies of distinct types of Kpros. Multicenter studies as well as etiology- and complication-specific studies have been excluded due to an overlap with patients from the single-center studies.

The success of a Kpro procedure depends not just on the appropriate patient but also on the correct choice of Kpro. Patients with normal lid anatomy, blink, and tear film sans an underlying immunological disorder merit a Type 1 Kpro, the prototype of which is the Boston Type 1 keratoprosthesis. Patients having a severely dry or even worse, a keratinized ocular surface with an underlying autoimmune disease and associated lid abnormalities are candidates for Type 2 Kpros.

Most of the series reported thus far from a single center cater to only one type of Kpro predominantly and its outcomes. Boston Type 1 Kpro has gained popularity in many centers worldwide chiefly because of its ready availability, straightforward technique, and a lesser dependence on ancillary disciplines. Contrarily, the 'biological' Kpros as well as the Boston Type 2 Kpro are presently performed only at a few centers globally. Both the biological and the Boston Type 2 Kpros are mutually exclusive.

DESIGN AND TYPES OF KERATOPROSTHESIS

The design of a Kpro consists of an optic and a haptic, like the design of an intraocular lens. The optic, is the central part of the Kpro which creates an optically clear window, thus allowing the patient to see,

It is a cylinder, mostly made of polymethyl methacrylate (PMMA) the haptic of the Kpro determines the type of the prosthesis which could be classified as:

- Biocompatible—consists of usually a PMMA skirt with the corneal graft as in the Boston Type 1 and 2 Kpro.
- Biointegrated—as in the Pintucci Kpro with the Dacron mesh forming the skirt around the PMMA optic.
- Biological—as in the osteoodonto—and the osteo-Kpro where the tooth or the bone respectively form an autologous biological tissue that supports the optical cylinder.

Apart from the haptic and the optic, the supporting cover tissue also adds to the Kpro complex. In Type 1 Kpro, it is the bandage contact lens which prevents the carrier graft desiccation whereas in Type 2 Kpros, the supporting cover is the skin in the Boston Type 2 and the buccal mucosa for the osteo and the osteo-odonto and Pintucci Kpros, respectively.

INDICATIONS

Kpro procedures are carried out for bilateral corneal disorders that are intractable with conventional penetrating keratoplasty. The indications for the Type 1 and the Type 2 Kpros are discussed *vide infra*.

Indications for Type 1 Kpro

With better outcomes, the indications for Type 1 Kpro have fanned out over the past decade. But there is always an increased risk of developing complications in eyes with guarded prognosis which makes it best to enlist the indications based on prognostic hierarchy.

Good Prognosis

1. Multiple failed grafts
2. Aniridia
3. Herpetic keratitis
4. Silicon oil-filled eyes

Guarded Prognosis

1. Pediatric corneal conditions
2. Chemical injuries

Very Guarded Prognosis

1. Underlying auto-immune disorders such as Stevens–Johnson syndrome (SJS)/ocular cicatricial pemphigoid (OCP)
2. Severe chemical injuries with severe forniceal shortening and lid abnormalities

Indications for Type 2 Kpros

Considering the long-term anatomical and functional outcomes, the MOOKP is the preferred choice of Kpro in severe end-stage ocular surface disorders. If MOOKP is not an option, the other Type 2 Kpros are resorted to for the following conditions:

1. Stevens-Johnson syndrome
2. OCP/Mucous membrane pemphigoid (MMP)
3. Severe chemical injuries
4. Severely keratinized surface

Box 1 enlists the exclusion criteria for Kpros. Kpro in the pediatric population a separate entity.

The Type 1 Kpro is performed in children to visually rehabilitate those with congenital bilateral corneal disorders where conventional PK forms a poor management choice.

Type 2 Kpros are rarely if ever performed in the pediatric age group.

Box 1: Exclusion criteria for keratoprosthesis surgery.

Exclusion criteria
- Nil perception of light
- Unrealistic expectations
- Advanced glaucoma/retinal conditions
- Unwilling or unable to report for regular follow-ups
- Unwilling to follow postoperative care and restrictions
- Dense amblyopia

Specific for Boston Type 2
- Absent eye lids

Specific for MOOKP
- <18 years of age
- Edentulous
- Poor oral hygiene
- Unfit for general anesthesia

(MOOKP: modified osteo-odonto keratoprosthesis)

PREOPERATIVE EVALUATION

1. The importance of a detailed history taking to determine etiology, onset (to gauge extent of amblyopia—loss of vision prior to 5 years of age is considered as a poor visual prognostic factor) and previous intraocular surgeries cannot be overemphasized.
2. A detailed ophthalmic evaluation including a B scan with axial length measurement is mandatory in all patients.
3. Assessment of perception of light and accurate projection of rays.
4. Intraocular pressure (IOP) is estimated by digital tonometry.
5. In cases of scarred opaque corneas, ultrasound biomicroscopy (UBM)/anterior segment optical coherence tomography (ASOCT) helps assess the anterior segment details.
6. Adequacy of blink is confirmed for Type 1 Kpros.
7. Schirmer's I wetting is assessed for adequacy of tears (Type 1).
8. Patency of the nasolacrimal duct is confirmed by syringing to rule out focus of infection (for Type 1, if puncta open for Type 2).
9. If an MOOKP is planned for a patient, then he/she should undergo a detailed dental and oral mucosal evaluation with a spiral computed tomography scan to evaluate the canines preoperatively. Also, fitness should be obtained for general anesthesia.
10. The most important aspect which should never be disregarded preoperatively is counseling. Counseling of the patient and his/her caretakers/family with respect to reasonable and grounded expectations, the need for compliance with postoperative care and follow-ups, the anticipated cosmesis and the need to report back or to the nearest ophthalmologist immediately in case of unexplained drop in vision or pain, should be done while giving enough time to clear doubts or queries to make the decision.
11. A detailed checklist is verified prior to every procedure/stage to ensure a complete preoperative evaluation.

SURGICAL TECHNIQUE AND POSTOPERATIVE CARE

Boston Type 1 Kpro

1. The type of Kpro is to be decided and ordered based on pseudophakic or aphakic status; also, the diameter of the backplate is mentioned while ordering—adult (8.5 mm backplate)/pediatric (7.0 mm backplate).
2 Axial length also needs to be specified for aphakic Kpro
3. An extra Kpro is also ordered as a standby
4. Local or general anesthesia is mentioned as indicated for the case
5. The host cornea is marked with the trephine as necessary
6. The Kpro is then assembled prior to trephining the recipient cornea. The backplate of the Kpro measures 8.5 mm and hence, the minimum donor graft size must be 8.5 mm. The donor cornea is oversized by 0.5 mm.
7. For the stem of the Kpro optic, the central 3 mm opening in the donor corneal graft is subsequently trephined.
8. Fresh therapeutic grade donor cornea is preferably opted for to assemble the Kpro.
9. The donor corneal graft is then slid down the stem of the optic, which is placed on an adhesive strip upside down, into its slot using a wrench. Subsequently, backplate is slid in place. Lastly the titanium ring then locks the Kpro assembly which is then checked for a snug fit.
10. The recipient corneal trephination is completed and excised. Any intraocular procedure is performed, as planned.
11. The assembled Kpro is then sutured like in a conventional penetrating keratoplasty using 16 interrupted 9-0 nylon sutures, with the knots preferably buried.
12. Lastly, a bandage contact lens is placed on the Kpro.

Postoperative Regimen

1. A fourth generation fluoroquinolone is instilled four times a day for a month, and then continued twice daily indefinitely
2. For high-risk eyes, it is preferable to use topical vancomycin (14 mg/mL) four times daily for a month, and continued once daily indefinitely
3. Topical corticosteroids are tapered to 2 times/day, indefinitely or are discontinued after 6 months
4. Topical lubricants prescribed as required
5. BCL should be changed once in 3 months, with instillation of 5% povidone iodine in clinic at the time of BCL replacement
6. Regular follow-ups every 3 monthly, is recommended.

Examination at the Time of Each Follow-up Visit

1. *Refractive change*: A hyperopic shift could point towards an early leak, while a myopic shift could indicate raised intraocular pressure.
2. Deposits on BCL, if any, are preferably subjected to routine microbiological evaluation.
3. Air bubbles under the optic flange as well as immobile bubbles beneath the BCL should always be looked for as these could indicate early ectasia of the carrier graft.
4. The graft surrounding the optic should be inspected for any infiltrates.
5. A proper slit beam examination should be done to assess for any irregularity in the carrier graft.
6. Presence of a retroprosthetic membrane (RPM) should be looked for as well as loose sutures which, if any, should be removed with proper aseptic precautions.
7. Intraocular pressure is assessed and monitored by digital tonometry.
8. A central fundus examination with a 90D lens should always be done to document the optic disk and posterior pole findings.
9. Whenever the BCL is to be replaced, the graft should always be inspected for the presence of any epithelial defect or leak by staining it with sterile fluorescein.
10. As already discussed, 5% povidone iodine is to be instilled in the eye at the time of BCL replacement.
11. It is always good to document the status of the eye with slit-lamp phtotography.
12. Visual field analysis with perimetry is recommended once in 6 months.
13. An ASOCT to identify early graft thinning, periprosthetic tissue loss, retroprosthetic membrane, and anterior chamber angle details once in 6 months is preferable.
14. B-scan ultrasonography should be performed at least once in a year or as and when necessary.

Boston Type 2 Kpro

The surgical technique bears a large resemblance to the Boston Type 1 Kpro in terms of Kpro assembly and suturing with the following differences:

1. The anterior nub of the Kpro protrudes by 2 mm to accommodate the skin around it.
2. The backplate itself is made up of titanium which snaps on to the Kpro complex. This obviates the need for a separate titanium ring.
3. In the recipient eye, the conjunctival mucosa is removed in totality from lid margin.
4. Sphincterotomy is performed to keep the pupil in a mid-dilated state.
5. After the Kpro is sutured, pars plana vitrectomy is performed along with Ahmed glaucoma valve implantation in all eyes.
6. The lid margins are excised to completely get rid of hair follicles. A meticulous suturing of the lid margins is essential and in two layers is done around the optic.

Postoperative Regimen

1. Systemic and topical corticosteroids to be tapered and stopped over a month's.
2. A fourth generation topical fluoroquinolone is to be instilled for 2 weeks.
3. A topical antibiotic ointment at bedtime to be continued indefinitely.
4. To prevent skin overgrowth, meticulous cleaning over the Kpro is done for the first postoperative week.
5. Lid sutures are removed on 10th postoperative day.
6. A follow-up once every 3 months is recommended.

MODIFIED OSTEO-ODONTO KERATOPROSTHESIS (MOOKP)

It is done as a three-staged procedure, as per the Rome-Vienna Protocol. The 1st stage consists of prepping the eye for the procedure by removing the iris, performing a cryo lens extraction with a limited anterior vitrectomy. This stage is called Stage 1 A of the 1st stage of the procedure. A tectonic PK is undertaken at this stage only if any corneal thinning is noted.

The next stage, Stage 1B + C is performed a month later. This involves harvesting the chosen canine tooth, preferably a maxillary canine and fashioning it into an osteo-odonto alveolar lamina with the optical cylinder fixed. The lamina is then placed in the subcutaneous pouch of the contralateral cheek so that it develops its fibrovascular covering over the next 2–3 months. Along with this, buccal mucosa measuring 3 cm in diameter is harvested and draped over the ocular surface securing it to the four recti muscles.

The next stage, Stage 2 of the procedure is performed 3 months later. The osteo-odonto alveolar lamina is removed from the subcutaneous pouch of the cheek and prepared. The ocular surface mucosa is reflected with an inferior hinge. After trephination of the central cornea according to the posterior diameter of the optical cylinder, the lamina is placed in the eye and the mucosa is then reflected over the lamina and sutured. A central aperture is fashioned in the mucosa for the cylinder to protrude through.

Postoperative Regimen

1. Systemic as well as topical corticosteroids and antibiotics are administered after every stage as necessary.
2. Topical antibiotic ointment is continued once daily along with topical lubricants for an indefinite period.
3. A follow-up visit once every 6 months is mandatory. The health of the oral mucosa and the lamina is also assessed.

OSTEO-KERATOPROSTHESIS

The major difference between the osteo Kpro (OKP) and the MOOKP is that in the former, the tibia is harvested and fashioned into an osteo-lamina instead of a tooth. The optical cylinder is fixed into this osteo-lamina.

Figures 1A to C illustrates the final appearance of the eyes following each of the Kpro procedures.

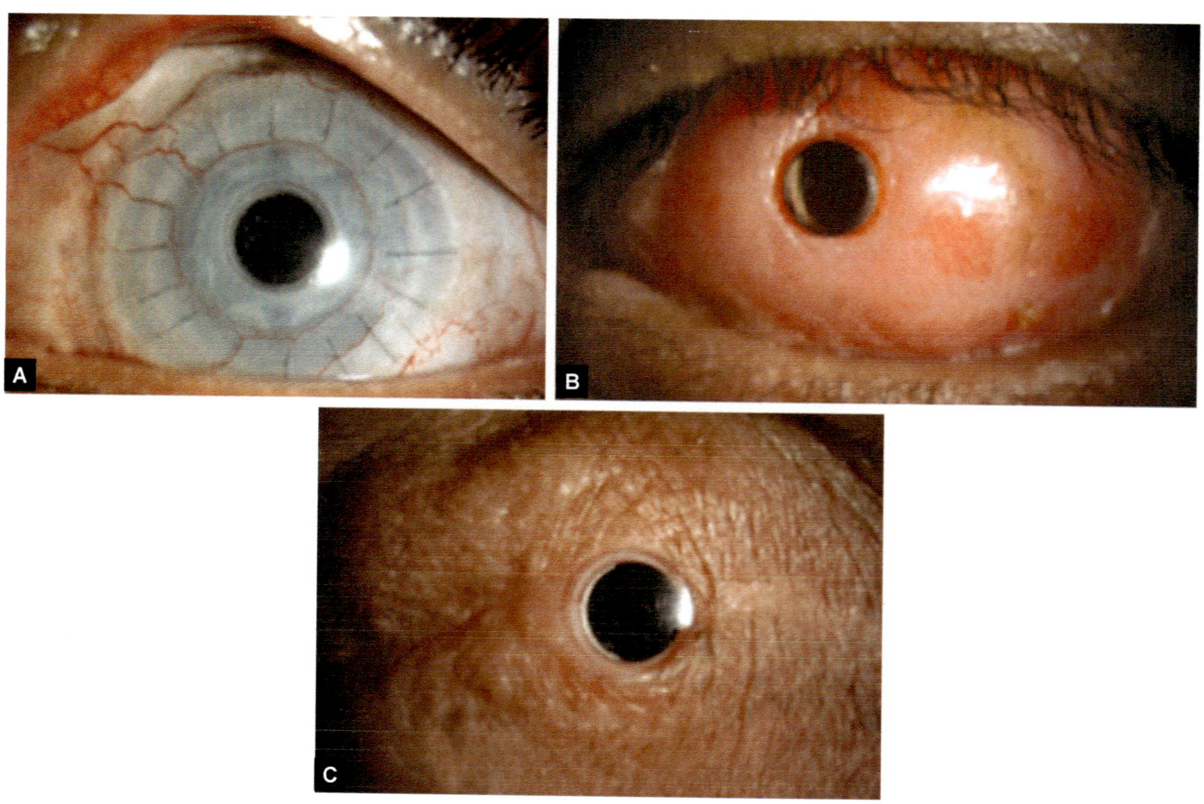

Figs. 1A to C: (A) 13 years following Boston type 1 Kpro in silicon oil filled eye, patient maintaining BCVA of 20/120, with a regular 3 monthly change of BCL; (B) 15 years following MOOKP in eye following Stevens–Johnson syndrome, patient maintaining BCVA of 20/20; (C) 6 years following Boston type 2 Kpro for Stevens–Johnson syndrome, patient maintaining BCVA of 20/20.

Box 2: General guidelines and practical pearls regarding keratoprosthesis procedures

1. Recommend Kpro only in cases with bilateral corneal blindness
2. Kpro is not an alternate to penetrating keratoplasty
3. It benefits neither the visual field nor the stereoacuity, and hence, these should not be advised in patients with one normal eye
4. Improving cosmesis is not an indication for performing Kpro
5. All options to attempt visual recovery should be exhausted before considering Kpro
6. Multiple prior intraocular procedures can impact the outcome of Kpro, hence, a judicious decision needs to be taken regarding Kpro versus multiple grafts in eyes amenable to penetrating keratoplasty. Conversely, Kpro is usually considered as the last resort, since complications related to Kpro can be globe threatening
7. Patients have to be willing to be compliant with medications and follow-up
8. Type 1 Kpro is a viable alternative in eyes with chronic hypotony with silicon oil in the eye. 5,000 centistokes oil is the preferred choice for long-term retention of oil
9. Type 1 Kpro is not primarily recommended in patients with underlying immunological conditions such as SJS or MMP, even if the tear film is adequate
10. Bilateral Kpro is contraindicated

(Kpro: keratoprosthesis; MMP: matrix metalloproteinases; SJS: Stevens–Johnson syndrome)

Certain general guidelines concerning the Kpros must be followed at all costs beyond the surgical technique and postoperative care. The same has been highlighted in **Box 2**.

KERATOPROSTHESIS SETUP

Significant planning and execution go into establishing a keratoprosthesis unit. A resolute and committed team forms the backbone of a Kpro unit. The team should comprise subspecialists from glaucoma, vitreoretinal, and oculoplasty along with anesthetists, and nursing staff.

Type 2 Kpros demand a more elaborate setup. General anesthesia is required besides coordination with an oral maxillofacial surgeon and a radiologist. Availability of appropriate instruments must be ensured for the dental or bone graft procedures.

While ordering for Type 1 aphakic Kpros the axial length of the eye needs to be provided. It is always a good practice to keep a second Kpro ready as a back-up in case of an inadvertent loss or breakage of the Kpro during the procedure.

An eye bank affiliation is mandatory to procure the corneal tissue for Kpros that requires carrier graft and as a standby tissue for the others that need a tectonic PK intraoperatively.

Consent forms and checklists must be elaborate and should be duly cross-checked prior to every stage of the surgery. The services of a psychologist can be sought for a smooth transition of the patient in the perioperative period. The importance of a mentor and formal training in the procedure cannot be overemphasized keeping in mind the nuances involved of the procedures.

OUTCOMES

the outcomes of the Type 1 Kpro especially, have improved dramatically in the current times. The indication affects the visual outcome and is found to be the best among patients operated for multiple-failed corneal grafts. The most common complications encountered include sterile melts, glaucoma, and retroprosthetic membrane.

These are discussed further in detail *vide infra*.

Sterile Melts

As noted in various series, sterile corneal graft melts have been noted to occur in up to 26% of eyes (**Fig. 2A**). It is important to take note of the early signs described earlier.

The extent of melt is first assessed and managed accordingly. In mild cases, cyanoacrylate glue application to the area of thinning mostly suffices. In moderate cases involving more clock hours, a crescentic or an annular lamellar graft is required to address the issue. In cases of extensive melts, associated with aqueous leak, it is prudent to replace the Kpro with a new one altogether, unless the area of leak is small enough to be addressed by the above-mentioned options. Adjuvant medical measures include topical medroxyprogesterone and systemic doxycycline with copious lubrication and a tarsorrhaphy in cases with frequent BCL displacements leading to graft desiccation.

Sterile melt was noted in close to 50% of the cases in our series, primarily in patients with chemical injuries. A similar finding has also been reported by Chan et al. with chemical injuries accounting for 35% of sterile melts in their series. Acknowledging the fact that the Type 1 Kpro is performed in a larger number (27% compared to 7%) of patients with chemical injuries in India, Kpro surgeons in India should be aware of this complication and hence, attempt to pick up early signs of melt to salvage the Kpro. This can occur at any period following the Kpro procedure.

Periprosthetic tissue loss has been cited as one of the associations with idiopathic sterile vitritis and the same nomenclature can be broadened to the melts which involve the haptic in other types of Kpro. A related process in the MOOKP/OKP is called as laminar resorption (**Fig. 3**). Due to proximity, a sterile inflammatory process which initiates the keratolysis could involve the vitreous also, especially in aphakic eyes leading to a sterile vitritis. Sterile vitritis leads to a decrease in vision which was the most common presenting symptom of laminar resorption in our MOOKP series. In most instances, it resolved completely with systemic steroid-antibiotic management.

Retroprosthetic Membrane

Retroprosthetic membrane (RPM) with a reported occurrence of greater than 50% in most of the studies, is the most common complication in the literature published so far. However, in our series, only 25% of the eyes, especially silicone oil-filled eyes, were complicated by RPM. Although

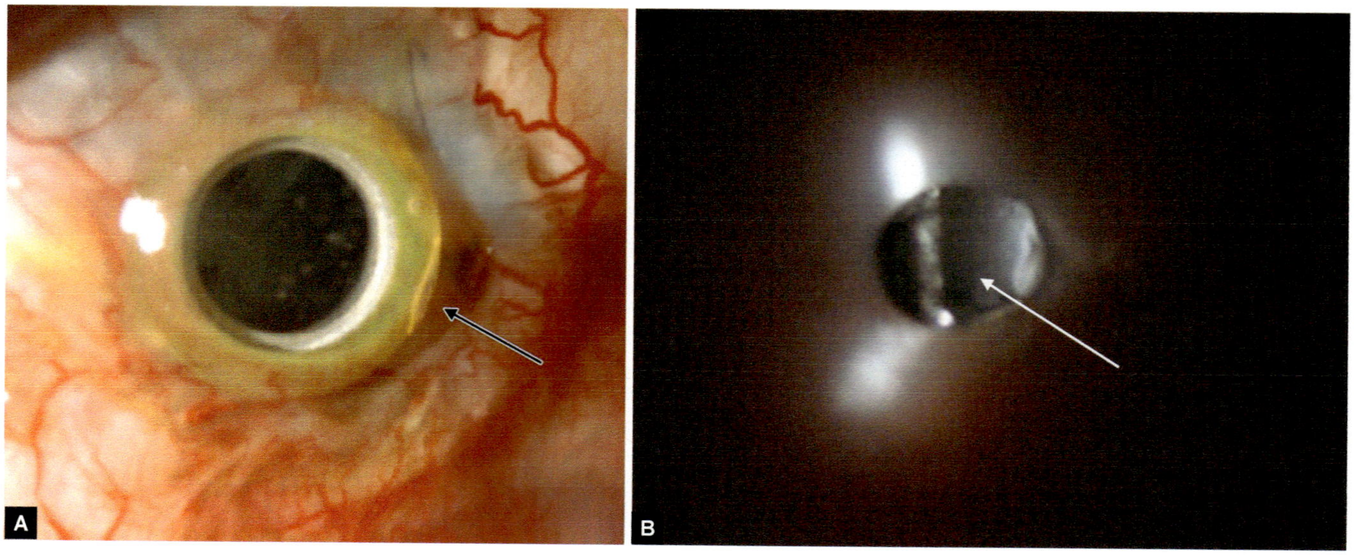

Figs. 2A and B: (A) Perioptic melt noted 4 years following a type 1 Kpro for chemical injury; (B) Retroprosthetic membrane noted 8 years following MOOKP for Stevens–Johnson syndrome.

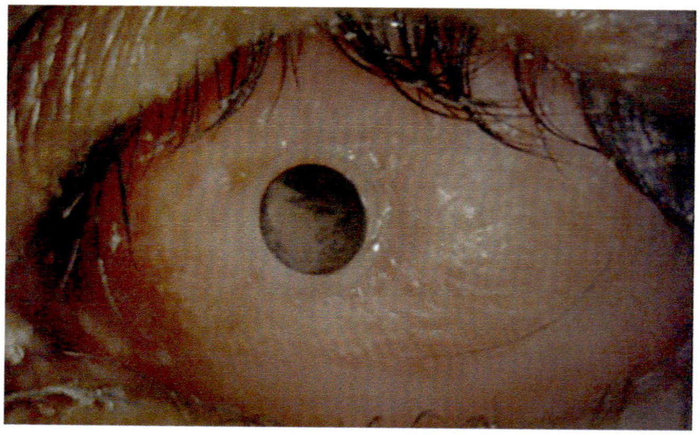

Fig. 3: Aqueous leak around the optic indicating laminar resorption, 8 years after MOOKP.

RPM (**Fig. 2B**) was reported to be the most common complication in the group performed outside of the United States, it was noticed in only 26.7% of the eyes at a mean follow-up of 14.2 months. RPM has also been victimized for one of the causes of sterile corneal melts as it prevents the access of aqueous to the carrier graft. As shown by a recent study, there is no advantage of a titanium back-plate over a PMMA backplate in the formation of RPM, with parallel rates of RPM noted in both. A total pars plana vitrectomy appears to be protective against the formation of RPM. The details regarding the Kpro (whether aphakic or pseudophakic) were unavailable for all the series but the International arm of the multicenter study, of which Indian centers formed an important group, had aphakic Kpros implanted in 62% of the eyes. In our series, all the Type 1 Kpros in were aphakic Kpros.

Whether the aphakic or the pseudophakic state of the operated eye contributes to the formation of RPM or not needs to be studied further. Theoretically an aphakic eye sans the posterior capsule and the iris in certain instances does not provide any scaffold for the formation of RPM, quite like what is seen in the MOOKP eyes where the rate of primary RPM formation is very minimal.

Visually insignificant RPMs do not need any intervention and can be monitored. Those affecting the vision can be managed by means of either neodymium: yttrium-aluminum-garnet laser membranotomy or a surgical membranectomy.

Glaucoma

Glaucoma is the most common comorbid factor with progressive diminution of vision post-Kpro occurring mostly secondary to continued progression of glaucoma. Of note is the fact that no de novo glaucoma was noted in the MOOKP eyes in our series. In patients with coexistent glaucoma and planned for a Kpro procedure, glaucoma requires to be managed proactively and aggressively. It is best to simultaneously place a drainage device in eyes undergoing the Type 1 Kpro while the timing of placing a valve in eyes undergoing the MOOKP procedure is based on the stage of surgery.

Endophthalmitis

Our series of Type 1 Kpros noted endophthalmitis in 15.4% of the eyes and is more as compared to the other single-center studies over a mean follow-up of 38 months (9% in the international study group at 14.2 months mean follow-up).

Further, endophthalmitis was noted in 10% of the eyes with the MOOKP as well as the Boston Type 2 Kpro in our series. Fungal endophthalmitis was noted in almost the same number of eyes as those with bacterial endophthalmitis.

CONCLUSION

India has a subtropical climate with an agrarian population primarily, which accounts for the substantial risk of infection vis-a-vis that quoted in the literature from the West. Also, in developing countries, a major proportion of the patients which undergo Type 1 Kpro fall into the guarded and the very guarded prognostic categories. Hence, it might not be apt to make head-on comparisons of the outcomes and complications between different geographical zones. In a single-center series from Thailand by Lekhanont et al., infective keratitis was reported in 21.4% of the eyes and endophthalmitis in 11.9% at a mean follow-up period of 64.9 months.

Even among the MOOKP subset of patients, SJS forms a major proportion of cases, unlike other studies wherein chemical injuries predominate. Eyes with SJS are more prone to specific complications like laminar resorption and its consequences and, therefore have led to suboptimal outcomes in India when compared to reported outcomes in the non-SJS category of patients. However, if followed up for a longer period in a similar SJS group of patients, the results with the MOOKP appear to be superior to the Boston Type 2 Kpro, making MOOKP the procedure of choice in these eyes.

As a word of caution, novice Kpro surgeons should avoid deviating from the existing techniques of Kpro procedures. Variations and modifications from the current procedures in a bid to improvise or simplify techniques and outcomes is best attempted in a controlled manner, comparing the outcomes with the present benchmarks.

The most important aspect of being a Kpro surgeon is knowing when to operate and when not to and counseling the patient. The necessity of following strict postoperative compliance with medications, regular follow-ups and restrictions cannot be overemphasized.

ACKNOWLEDGMENT

Professor James Chodosh, Boston Kpro Foundation.

FURTHER READING

1. Iyer G, Srinivasan B, Agarwal S, Talele D, Rishi E, Rishi P, et al. Keratoprosthesis: Current global scenario and a broad Indian perspective. Indian J Ophthalmol. 2018;66(5):620-9.
2. Khan B, Dudenhoefer EJ, Dohlman CH. Keratoprosthesis: an update. Curr Opin Ophthalmol. 2001;12(4):282-7.
3. Saeed HN, Shanbhag S, Chodosh J. The Boston keratoprosthesis. Curr Opin Ophthalmol. 2017;28(4):390-6.
4. Yaghouti F, Nouri M, Abad JC, Power WJ, Doane MG, Dohlman CH. Keratoprosthesis: preoperative prognostic categories. Cornea. 2001;20(1):19-23.
5. Dohlman CH, Harissi-Dagher M, Graney J. The Boston keratoprosthesis: a new threadless design. Digit J Ophthalmol. 2007;13(3):1-6.
6. Hille K, Grabner G, Liu C, Colliardo P, Falcinelli G, Taloni M, et al. Standards for modified osteoodontokeratoprosthesis (OOKP) surgery according to Strampelli and Falcinelli: the Rome-Vienna Protocol. Cornea. 2005;24(8):895-908.
7. Chan CC, LoVerde L, Qiang J, Nordlund ML, Holland EJ. Incidence, risk factors, and surgical management of boston type 1 keratoprothesis corneal melts, leaks, and extrusions. Cornea. 2016;35(8):1049-56.
8. Bouhout S, Robert MC, Deli S, Harissi-Dagher M. Corneal melt after Boston keratoprosthesis: clinical presentation, management, outcomes and risk factor analysis. Ocul Immunol Inflamm. 2018;26(5):693-9.
9. Goins KM, Kitzmann AS, Greiner MA, Kwon YH, Alward WL, Ledolter J, et al. Boston type 1 keratoprosthesis: visual outcomes, device retention, and complications. Cornea. 2016;35(9):1165-74.
10. de la Paz MF, Stoiber J, de Rezende Couto Nascimento V, de Toledo JA, Seyeddain O, Hitzl W, et al. Anatomical survival and visual prognosis of Boston type I keratoprosthesis in challenging cases. Graefes Arch Clin Exp Ophthalmol. 2014;252(1):83-90.
11. Aravena C, Yu F, Aldave AJ. Long-term visual outcomes, complications, and retention of the Boston type I keratoprosthesis. Cornea. 2018;37(1):3-10.
12. Patel AP, Wu EI, Ritterband DC, Seedor JA. Boston type 1 keratoprosthesis: the New York eye and ear experience. Eye (Lond). 2012;26(3):418-25.
13. Güell JL, Arcos E, Gris O, Aristizabal D, Pacheco M, Sanchez CL, et al. Outcomes with the Boston type 1 keratoprosthesis at Instituto de Microcirugía Ocular IMO. Saudi J Ophthalmol. 2011;25(3):281-4.
14. Lekhanont K, Thaweesit P, Muntham D, Chuckpaiwong V, Vongthongsri A. Medium-term outcomes of Boston type 1 keratoprosthesis implantation in Bangkok, Thailand. Cornea. 2014;33(12):1312-9.
15. Greiner MA, Li JY, Mannis MJ. Longer-term vision outcomes and complications with the Boston type 1 keratoprosthesis at the University of California, Davis. Ophthalmology. 2011;118(8):1543-50.
16. Chew HF, Ayres BD, Hammersmith KM, Rapuano CJ, Laibson PR, Myers JS, et al. Boston keratoprosthesis outcomes and complications. Cornea. 2009;28(9):989-96.
17. de Oliveira LA, Pedreira Magalhães F, Hirai FE, de Sousa LB. Experience with Boston keratoprosthesis type 1 in the developing world. Can J Ophthalmol. 2014;49(4):351-7.
18. Duignan ES, Ní Dhubhghaill S, Malone C, Power W. Long-term visual acuity, retention and complications observed with the type-I and type-II Boston keratoprostheses in an Irish population. Br J Ophthalmol. 2016;100(8):1093-7.
19. Shihadeh WA, Mohidat HM. Outcomes of the Boston keratoprosthesis in Jordan. Middle East Afr J Ophthalmol. 2012;19(1):97-100.
20. Al Arfaj K, Hantera M. Short-term visual outcomes of Boston keratoprosthesis type I in Saudi Arabia. Middle East Afr J Ophthalmol. 2012;19(1):88-92.
21. Falcinelli G, Falsini B, Taloni M, Colliardo P, Falcinelli G. Modified osteo-odonto-keratoprosthesis for treatment of corneal blindness: long-term anatomical and functional outcomes in 181 cases. Arch Ophthalmol. 2005;123(10):1319-29.
22. Liu C, Okera S, Tandon R, Herold J, Hull C, Thorp S. Visual rehabilitation in end-stage inflammatory ocular surface disease with the osteo-odonto-keratoprosthesis: results from the UK. Br J Ophthalmol. 2008;92(9):1211-7.
23. Charoenrook V, Michael R, de la Paz MF, Ding A, Barraquer RI, Temprano J. Osteokeratoprosthesis using tibial bone: surgical technique and outcomes. Ocul Surf. 2016;14(4):495-506.
24. Lee R, Khoueir Z, Tsikata E, Chodosh J, Dohlman CH, Chen TC. Long-term Visual outcomes and complications of Boston keratoprosthesis type II implantation. Ophthalmology. 2017;124(1):27-35.
25. Aldave AJ, Sangwan VS, Basu S, Basak SK, Hovakimyan A, Gevorgyan O, et al. International results with the Boston type I keratoprosthesis. Ophthalmology. 2012;119(8):1530-8.
26. Iyer G, Pillai VS, Srinivasan B, Falcinelli G, Padmanabhan P, Guruswami S, et al. Modified osteo-odonto keratoprosthesis—the Indian experience—results of the first 50 cases. Cornea. 2010;29(7):771-6.

27. Iyer G, Srinivasan B, Gupta J, Rishi P, Sen PR, Bhende P, et al. Boston keratoprosthesis for keratopathy in eyes with retained silicone oil: a new indication. Cornea. 2011;30(10):1083-7.
28. Grassi CM, Cruzat A, Taniguchi EV, Crnej A, Colby KA, Dohlman CH, et al. Periprosthetic tissue loss in patients with idiopathic vitreous inflammation after the Boston keratoprosthesis. Cornea. 2015;34(11):1378-82.
29. Iyer G, Srinivasan B, Agarwal S, Rachapalle SR. Laminar resorption in modified osteo-odonto-keratoprosthesis procedure: a cause for concern. Am J Ophthalmol. 2014;158(2):263-9.e2.
30. Talati RK, Hallak JA, Karas FI, de la Cruz J, Cortina MS Retroprosthetic membrane formation in Boston keratoprosthesis: a case-control-matched comparison of titanium versus PMMA backplate. Cornea. 2018;37(2):145-50.
31. Perez VL, Leung EH, Berrocal AM, Albini TA, Parel JM, Amescua G, et al. Impact of total pars plana vitrectomy on postoperative complications in aphakic, snap-on, type 1 Boston keratoprosthesis. Ophthalmology. 2017;124(10):1504-9.
32. Iyer G, Srinivasan B, Agarwal S, Shetty R, Krishnamoorthy S, Balekudaru S, et al. Glaucoma in modified osteo-odonto-keratoprosthesis eyes: role of additional stage 1A and Ahmed glaucoma drainage device-technique and timing. Am J Ophthalmol. 2015;159(3):482-9.e2.
33. Iyer G, Srinivasan B, Gupta N, Padmanabhan P. Outcome of Boston keratoprosthesis in a developing country-importance of patient selection, education, and perioperative care: the Indian experience. Asia Pac J Ophthalmol (Phila). 2012;1(4): 202-7.
34. Iyer G, Srinivasan B, Agarwal S, Pillai VS, Ahuja A. Treatment modalities and clinical outcomes in ocular sequelae of Stevens-Johnson syndrome over 25 years—a paradigm shift. Cornea. 2016;35(1):46-50.

68

The Boston Type II Keratoprosthesis

Shaunak K Bakshi, James Chodosh

INTRODUCTION

The Boston keratoprosthesis (BK) was originally developed by Dr Claes H Dohlman (Massachusetts Eye and Ear, Boston, USA), to manage patients with severe corneal disease in whom a standard penetrating keratoplasty carries a poor prognosis. Since its initial development, the BK has risen to become the most commonly used keratoprosthesis, with over 16,000 units implanted worldwide (J Chodosh, personal communication). The most commonly used BK, the "type 1" (BK1), is composed of a poly(methyl methacrylate) (PMMA), mushroom-shaped front plate/optic, and a PMMA or titanium back plate, and assembled in "nut and bolt" fashion in a donor cornea and sutured in place as with standard keratoplasty (**Fig. 1**). The BK1 is designed for patients with a normal tear film and blink, and is not appropriate for patients with severe, cicatrizing ocular surface disease. For these patients, the BK "type 2" (BK2) was developed. The design of the BK2 is similar to that of the BK1 except for an anterior extension of the front plate/optic to be positioned through surgically closed eyelids, thus permitting vision with complete and permanent eye closure (**Fig. 2**). To date, around 450 BK2 devices have been implanted.

INDICATIONS

The BK2 is indicated in select patients with severe dry eye, ocular surface keratinization, and/or ankyloblepharon, as can occur due to end-stage Sjögren's syndrome, Stevens-Johnson syndrome/toxic epidermal necrolysis (SJS/TEN), mucous membrane pemphigoid (MMP), and severe chemical and thermal burns. Patients with end-stage glaucoma or an irreparable retinal detachment are not candidates. Also, some patients with burn injuries lack sufficient eyelid excursion, due to cicatricial skin changes, to permit the tension-free medial and lateral tarsorrhaphies essential to retention of the device.

BOSTON KERATOPROSTHESIS TYPE II SURGERY

Preoperative Considerations

Before implantation of the BK2, it is imperative to inform the patient of the associated risks of this procedure, the cosmetic changes induced by the surgery, and the frequent postoperative visits required, the latter necessary to maintain the implanted device. The significant alteration in cosmetic appearance after eyelid closure and device insertion should

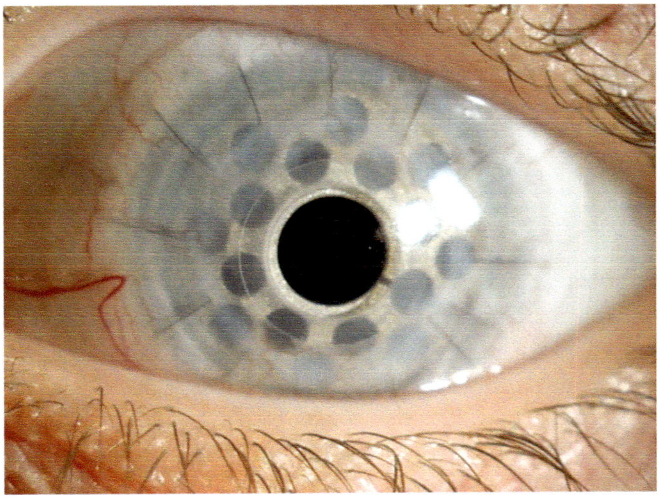

Fig. 1: Postoperative appearance of the Boston keratoprosthesis type 1 (BK1).

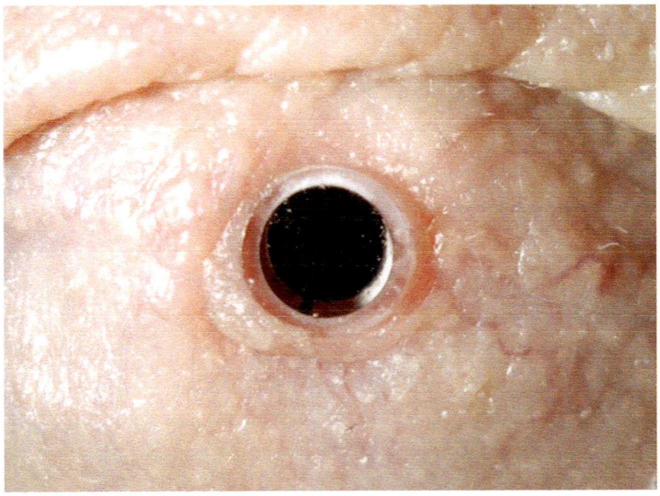

Fig. 2: Postoperative appearance of the Boston keratoprosthesis type 2 (BK2).

be described, along with communication of the limited options (i.e., use of tinted glasses) to improve cosmesis after the procedure. Postoperatively, lifelong and regular eye care with a corneal specialist trained in management of the device is vital. Daily adherence to topical antibiotics and regularly scheduled examinations with the operating surgeon are critical to monitor for and treat serious complications, including infection and glaucoma, either of which can cause total loss of vision, leaving the BK2 recipient worse off than prior to implantation. If a BK2 candidate is unable or unwilling to return for lifelong postoperative care, they should not undergo the surgery.

Occult infection of the lacrimal drainage system can contaminate surgical implantation of the BK2 or infect the cornea beneath surgically closed eyelids after surgery. If there is even one patent lacrimal puncta, occult lacrimal drainage system infection must be considered and ruled out. Chronic retinal detachment is not an absolute contraindication to BK2 surgery, if the macula is attached and repair is feasible. On the other hand, glaucoma limits the vision of many otherwise successful BK2 recipients. Candidates for BK2 should be asked about a history of elevated intraocular pressure and/or treatment with glaucoma medications. All candidates must have a preoperative B-scan ultrasound to look for evidence of retinal detachment, and also to identify optic nerve cupping that might preclude a successful outcome. In cases where the optic nerve status is uncertain, but there is a definite history of glaucoma, it may be advisable to perform endoscopy prior to BK2 surgery to visualize the optic nerve head. If the retina is attached and there is no history of glaucoma or evidence of optic nerve head cupping on ultrasound, but the candidate lacks the capacity to correctly project light from the nasal side, the prognosis for visual recovery is guarded. Even the densest corneal opacity should still permit projection of the direction of light if the posterior segment is intact and healthy. Although it is difficult to project light through a closed eyelid, and absence of nasal light projection can be discounted in patients with ankyloblepharon, in patients in whom the cornea is not covered by eyelid skin, failure to correctly distinguish a light source as nasally projected suggests the patient will not recover vision with surgery.

As part of preoperative assessment, an A-scan ultrasound is critical to determine the specific power of the keratoprosthesis to be implanted. If the patient is phakic, lens removal and aphakia are planned. If the patient is pseudophakic, then the opposite eye can be measured. If the opposite eye has been enucleated or is phthisical, then the average axial length for BK recipients is adopted for the operative eye (23.5 mm, personal communication, James Chodosh), adjusted accordingly if the intended recipient eye appears prephthisical or has a known history of axial myopia. Although a pseudophakic model of the BK2 is available and can be considered for patients with a stable posterior chamber intraocular lens, it should be reserved for those in whom for medical reasons, it is judged important to shorten the anesthesia by avoiding posterior segment procedures. Otherwise, as discussed below, planned aphakia is the goal. Typical concomitant procedures with a BK2 include a pars plana vitrectomy and pars plana Ahmed valve placement. Therefore, preoperative consultation should also include a vitreoretinal and a glaucoma surgeon.

Operative Technique

The BK2 procedure, when inclusive of pars plana vitrectomy and Ahmed valve placement as described below, can take 5 hours to complete, and therefore is typically performed under general anesthesia.

Preparation of Ocular Surface and Eyelid

All ocular surface epithelium is removed from the tarsal, forniceal, bulbar, and limbal surfaces, to prevent formation of a fistula or delayed epithelial cyst beneath the fully closed eyelids. Tenon's capsule is left in place, but any fibrous tissue restricting full movement of the globe is divided. The upper and lower eyelid margins are infiltrated with 1% lidocaine supplemented with epinephrine for hemostasis, followed by excision of the anterior eyelid margins to remove all eyelash follicles and avoid lash ingrowth after closure of the eyelids. The corneal diameter and thickness are assessed and the optimal host cornea trephination diameter is chosen.

Assembly of the Boston Keratoprosthesis Type II

Prior to assembly of the BK2, it is necessary to decide on the trephination diameters of the donor and host corneas, which should differ by 0.5 mm (donor size > host size). The donor cornea trephination diameter should be at least 7 mm in order to allow for suturing to the host—at least 1 mm corneal tissue peripheral to the 4.5 mm diameter front plate is the minimum needed to pass sutures. However, this assumes near perfect centration of the inner trephination (discussed below), and if decentered, suturing can be difficult or impossible. In general, larger trephinations make for easier implantation. If a temporary keratoprosthesis is planned to facilitate visualization for pars plana vitrectomy, then the trephination size is chosen to accommodate the fixed diameter of the temporary keratoprosthesis, and the donor cornea intended for assembly with the BK2 is sized accordingly. In general, unless otherwise restricted by a small corneal diameter in the recipient eye, a donor size of at least 8.5 mm diameter is recommended (with corresponding host trephination diameter 0.5 mm less—many temporary keratoprosthesis designs can be used with a 8 mm host trephination). For thin corneas, the chosen trephination of the host cornea should be large enough to enable suturing to the limbus.

Following a choice of trephines, each component of the device should be visually inspected. The supplied components include the 3 mm skin biopsy punch, the PMMA front plate/optic, the 8.5 mm diameter "click-on" titanium back plate, the assembly tool, and the adhesive patch. The donor cornea is prepared with two trephinations, an inner trephination using the 3.0 mm skin biopsy punch, and the outer trephination with a standard corneal donor trephine, in the order preferred by the operating surgeon. If both trephinations are done free-hand, it is easier to perform the outer trephination first. If the outer trephination is performed with a sized punch, the inner trephination can be performed first and then the donor centered on the trephination block for the outer trephination.

Once the corneal trephinations are complete, the coverings on the enclosed double-sided adhesive patch are removed and the patch is placed on a smooth sterile surface. The PMMA component is placed front side down on the adhesive patch. The donor cornea is slide down the PMMA stem, with the endothelial side up. The back plate is then positioned above the donor cornea with the concave side up, and locked into place, applying downward pressure with the assembly tool. The device should then be carefully inspected, best done under the operating microscope, to assure proper assembly. Specifically, an equal length of PMMA should be visible behind the back plate while the device is turned 360°, and the slitted sides of the back plate should be parallel and close together. The assembled device is then placed in a sterile container with corneal preservation medium and covered until needed.

Implantation

After device assembly, the patient's cornea is marked with the selected trephine, and any corneal and limbal epithelium peripheral to the mark is removed. The host cornea is trephined and removed. If phakic, the lens is extracted. Total iridectomy, lens capsule removal, pars plana vitrectomy, and pars plana Ahmed valve implantation are performed as per the surgeon's judgment to reduce the risk of postoperative glaucoma and retinal detachment. These concomitant procedures may be conducted in collaboration with a vitreoretinal and glaucoma specialist. The intraocular lens, if stable, can be left in place, assuming the surgeon has chosen a BK2 powered for pseudophakia. Finally, the assembled keratoprosthesis is implanted using either 12 interrupted 9-0 or 16 interrupted 10-0 nylon sutures. Rotation of the resulting knots to the host side is recommended, but it is not necessary to bury them. Injections of broad-spectrum antibiotics and a corticosteroid are performed in peribulbar fashion.

Management of the Eyelids

To ensure long-term retention of the BK2, the eyelid skin must be closed to securely surround the BK2 optic and protect the globe from desiccation and infection. No epithelium can be allowed to persist or invade beneath the eyelids. The method employed to create medial and lateral tarsorrhaphies around the BK2 optic is up to the surgeon's preference. In general, a two layer closure is recommended, for example with use of interrupted 6-0 Vicryl sutures to oppose the upper and lower tarsal plates, followed by bolster-supported sutures of the eyelid skin to properly evert the skin edges for optimal healing. This will leave the optical component of the BK2 covered by skin, and the final step of surgery is to create an opening in the upper eyelid margin for the device. This is most easily performed with curved Vannas scissors. It is important that the opening be placed to align with the eye in primary gaze. At the conclusion of the procedure, injection of a peribulbar anesthetic can reduce postoperative pain, before general anesthesia is reversed. Antibiotic ointment is placed over the eyelid margins and eyelid notch followed by a patch and Fox shield.

POSTOPERATIVE CARE

No data exist to support any particular postoperative regimen after BK2 implantation, although antibiotic ointment is indicated until the skin has healed. Penetration of topical medications to the underlying cornea is limited by the eyelid closure. However, topical antibiotic drops are recommended on the theoretical basis that they may reduce colonization of the skin adjacent to the optic and prevent infection of the underlying and presumably vulnerable donor cornea. If the intraocular pressure is elevated, oral acetazolamide or methazolamide is mandatory—topical antiglaucoma medications will not be effective. Daily or every other day debridement of blood and exudate from the optical surface by the surgeon is essential to prevent skin overgrowth. At 10 days postoperatively, the skin sutures and bolsters are removed, and the ointment is discontinued. The patient is taught to clean the optical surface, for example with a cellulose sponge, on a daily basis. Intraocular pressure must be assessed at every visit (see later).

OUTCOMES, COMPLICATIONS, AND MANAGEMENT

Published series with the BK2 are limited as compared to those with the BK1, given the smaller population of patients managed with the BK2. A study by Sayegh et al.,[1] published in 2008, reviewed outcomes of patients with a diagnosis of SJS/TEN, implanted with either a BK1 or BK2 between January 2000 and December 2005. Sayegh reported 16 eyes of 15 patients, with mean follow-up of 3.6 years (range 10.2 months–5.6 years). 10 of 16 eyes received the BK2. 75% (12 of 16 eyes) reached at least 20/200 acuity after implantation, and 50% (8 of 16 eyes) measured at least 20/40. At last follow-up, vision of at least 20/70 was found in 43.8% (7 of 16 eyes), while 31.2% (5 of 16 eyes), after originally experiencing improvement in acuity after implantation, dropped to under 20/200. As indicated, these findings represent a compilation of outcomes of both BK1 and BK2 devices, and particularly given the small sample size, should be interpreted with caution.

A retrospective review in 2011 by Pujari et al.[2] examined outcomes specific to the BK2, for the 9 years inclusive of January 2000 to December 2009, with analysis of 29 eyes of 26 patients operated on at the Massachusetts Eye and Ear. Preoperative diagnoses included MMP (51.7%), SJS/TEN (41.4%), and other conditions (6.9%), including one chemical burn and one treatment-associated radiation keratopathy for lymphoma. Prior to device implantation, 96.6% of eyes had acuity of 20/200 or worse. 26.9% of patients with MMP and 11.5% with SJS/TEN were on an immunosuppressive regimen when implanted with the BK2. After implantation, among individuals with follow-up of 1 year, 57.1% (12 eyes) maintained acuity of 20/200 or better. Among 13 eyes with follow-up of at least 5 years, 46.2% (6 eyes) maintained 20/200 or better acuity. 6 of 29 eyes (20.7%) did not reach 20/200 acuity or better at any time after surgery due to underlying conditions: in the case of 4 eyes with SJS/TEN, this included 1 with end-stage glaucoma, 1 with occult retinal detachment, and 2 with age-related macular degeneration; in the case of 2 eyes with MMP, 1 with occult retinal detachment and 1 with unknown cause. For a total of 12 of 29 eyes (41.4%), reimplantation of the BK2 was performed. Overall follow-up amounted to 107.9 person-years, with a hazard rate of 0.11 per person-year.

The largest retrospective study of BK2 outcomes was conducted by Lee et al.,[3] who analyzed outcomes of 48 eyes in 44 patients treated at the Massachusetts Eye and Ear, with mean follow-up length of 70.2 months (range 6 months to 19.8 years). Surgical indications for implanted patients included SJS (41.7%), MMP (41.7%), chemical injury (8.3%), neurotrophic keratopathy (4.2%), Sjögren's syndrome (2.1%), and Kearns–Sayre syndrome (2.1%). Prior to surgery, 95.8% (46 of 48 eyes) presented with acuity of 20/200 or worse. Acuity of 20/200 or better was achieved in 37.5% (18 of 48 eyes), and 20/100 or better in 33.3% (16 of 48 eyes), at last follow-up, with the initially placed device retained in 50%. Notably, patients included in the study were treated between January 1992 and April 2015—thus, the earliest cases were initially managed nearly 3 decades in the past, and many of these with older versions of the device. The currently used BK2 with a titanium back plate was approved for use by the United States Food and Drug Administration (USFDA) only in 2013. In addition, recognition of the most frequently encountered complications has led to iterative progress, particularly in the last 10 years, in preoperative selection, intraoperative decision-making, and postoperative care.

Among BK2-associated postoperative complications, retroprosthetic membrane (RPM) has emerged as perhaps the most common, occurring in 60.4% of eyes in the study by Lee et al.[3] and 48.3% in the series reported by Pujari et al.[2] Not all of these were visually significant, but if so, neodymium-doped yttrium aluminum garnet (Nd:YAG) laser may be used for treatment, or if more severe, surgical membranectomy may be performed. In Lee et al., 45.8% (22 of 48 eyes) were managed with a laser procedure, and 8.3% (4 of 48 eyes) required surgical membranectomy.[3] In Pujari et al., 48.3% (14 of 29 eyes) required laser membranectomy and 3.4% (1 of 29 eyes) were treated with a surgical membranectomy.[2] Other notable complications reported by Lee et al. included retinal detachment in 18.8% (9 of 48 eyes), choroidal detachment or hemorrhage in 8.3% (4 of 48 eyes), and infectious endophthalmitis in 6.3% (3 of 48 eyes).[3] Pujari et al. reported loss of better than 20/200 visual acuity due to retinal detachment in 17.4% (4 of 23 eyes), choroidal detachment in 8.7% (2 of 23 eyes), and endophthalmitis in 4.3% (1 of 23 eyes).[2]

Postoperative complications with glaucoma, either progression of prior disease or de novo occurrence, have been encountered frequently with both BK designs, and are nonspecific to BK2. Lee et al. reported glaucoma progression in 27.1% (13 of 48 eyes), and de novo disease in 8.3% (4 of 48 eyes) after implantation.[3] Pujari et al. noted eventual loss of visual acuity in 2 eyes that had initially reached at least 20/200 vision after surgery, in the setting of glaucoma progression.[2] This occurred despite a prior history of tube placement, or concurrent drainage device insertion at the time of BK2 implantation, which was the case in 69% (20 of 29 eyes). Accurate measurement of intraocular pressure after BK2 implantation is not possible, and clinical judgment relies on palpation of the globe through the upper eyelid. Therefore, regular examination of the optic nerve and performance of formal visual field testing are essential. Topical antiglaucoma medications do not penetrate the eyelid skin and are useless after BK2 implantation, limiting therapeutic options to oral agents and surgery, with Ahmed valve implantation and endoscopic cyclophotocoagulation,[4] the two most commonly employed options. Thus, it is strongly recommended to consider placement of an Ahmed valve at the time of initial BK2 implantation, unless a glaucoma drainage device is already in place and working. Typically, the Ahmed tube is inserted through the inferotemporal pars plana incision utilized by the vitreoretinal surgeon for vitrectomy, leaving the superior globe available for later surgery should it become necessary. For example, in patients with elevated intraocular pressure after BK2, endoscopic cyclophotocoagulation can then be performed through a single arcuate incision in the upper eyelid, fashioned at 9 mm from the center of the keratoprosthesis to approximate a distance from the limbus of 3 mm.[4] This method obviates the necessity of fully opening the eyelids, a sometimes challenging task because of fusion of the tarsal plate to Tenon's capsule.

Other postoperative challenges associated with BK2 implantation include retraction of the skin surrounding the optic (**Fig. 3**), which exposes the underlying cornea to desiccation, keratolysis, and infection. Alternatively, if the optic is not cleaned daily, there is the potential for overgrowth of skin (**Fig. 4**), which then requires excision. In the first decade of BK2 implantation, eyelid closure included removal of the tarsal plate, but this led to significant retraction of the skin adjacent to the stem (personal communication, Dr Claes H Dohlman). Today, careful preservation of the tarsus during removal of mucosal epithelium, and then suture closure of the upper and lower tarsal plates are considered critical steps to ensure stable medial and lateral tarsorrhaphies and long-term device retention. In the earlier study by Sayegh et al.,[1] 4 of 10 eyes (40%) implanted with a BK2 were impacted by skin retraction around the stem, first observed at mean 18.6 months (range 10–33 months) postoperatively.[1] These were managed with multiple skin revisions, and in one case, device replacement. In Lee et al., tarsorrhaphy/skin revision was noted in 52.1% (25 of 48 eyes).[3] In the study by Pujari et al., skin revisions were required in 34.5% (10 of 29 eyes), but were most commonly for treatment of overgrowth.[2] Reported approaches to management of skin retraction after BK2 implantation include two cases with retraction treated with forehead pericranial flaps,[5] and use of a porous polyethylene implant incorporated as a lid spacer around the stem during repair.[6]

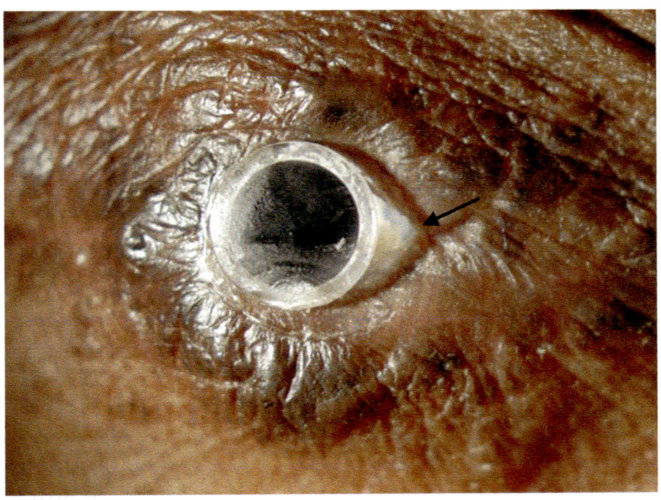

Fig. 3: Postoperative appearance of skin retraction (arrow) following implantation of the Boston keratoprosthesis type 2 (BK2).

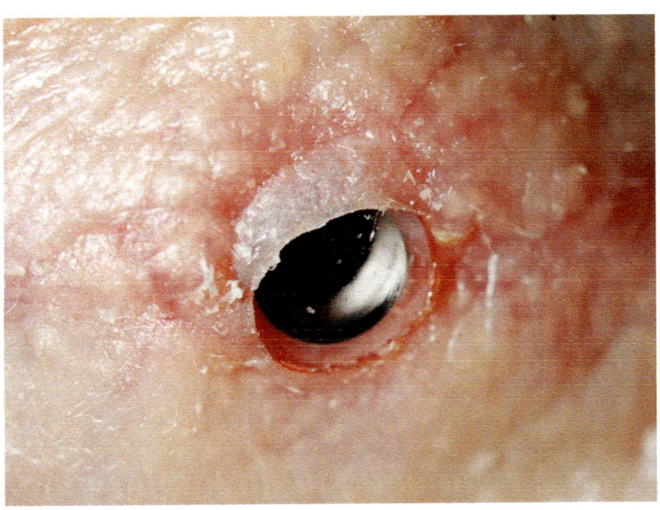

Fig. 4: Postoperative appearance of the Boston keratoprosthesis type 2 (BK2) with early overgrowth of skin onto optic.

Epithelial inclusion cysts involving the eyelid have been reported in BK2 recipients, and may involve the meibomian glands and on histopathology, these appear similar to a chalazion with lipogranulomatous inflammation.[7] In one report, a patient with a history of chemical burns treated with a BK2 presented with gradual cyst-like enlargement beneath the lower eyelid that on histopathology was shown to be a dacryops.[8]

Very few surgeons/centers outside of those at the Massachusetts Eye and Ear currently implant the BK2. However, given the heavy burden of corneal disease associated with SJS and chemical injuries seen specifically in ocular surface centers in India, surgeons at the world-famous Sankara Nethralaya, a tertiary eye care center in Chennai, India, recently reported their results with the BK2, which they first began to implant in January 2013,[9] with results first reported 5 years later.[10] 10 eyes of 10 patients were implanted with the BK2, with mean follow-up of 2.75 (range 0.5–5 years). Indications for surgery included SJS (80%), MMP (10%), and chemical injury (10%). Visual acuity of better than 20/200 was achieved in 70%, and 20/30 or better in 50% at last follow-up, with device retention in 90%. Complications were infrequent, with RPM, retinal detachment, endophthalmitis, and sterile keratolysis requiring device replacement occurring in 1 eye (10%) each. No glaucoma-associated complications were noted. 20% required skin revision within 2 weeks after initial BK2 implantation, and 10% required excision due to skin overgrowth. This is the only published case series describing BK2 outcomes from a center other than the Massachusetts Eye and Ear, and demonstrates that BK2 implantation can be an effective treatment modality in other centers dedicated to severe corneal disorders. Further, in a review of 5-year outcomes in 11 patients implanted with a BK2, the cost utility of the device was estimated at $ 63,196/quality-adjusted life year (QALY), which qualifies the procedure as a moderately cost-effective measure.[11]

CONCLUSION

Implantation of the BK2 is a viable option to restore vision in the most severe corneal pathologies, in particular for those patients with significant ocular dryness and conjunctival cicatrix in which neither a corneal allograft nor a BK1 would be successful. BK2 implantation is a high-risk, high-reward intervention, and although the procedure can be associated with significant complications, it can also provide a dramatic and life-altering improvement in visual function. Additional advances in device design, intraoperative decision-making, and postoperative management are needed to further improve the long-term prognosis for BK2 recipients.

REFERENCES

1. Sayegh RR, Ang LP, Foster CS, Dohlman CH. The Boston keratoprosthesis in Stevens-Johnson syndrome. Am J Ophthalmol. 2008;145:438-44.
2. Pujari S, Siddique SS, Dohlman CH, Chodosh J. The Boston keratoprosthesis type II: The Massachusetts Eye and Ear Infirmary experience. Cornea. 2011;30:1298-303.
3. Lee R, Khoueir Z, Tsikata E, Chodosh J, Dohlman CH, Chen TC. Long-term visual outcomes and complications of Boston keratoprosthesis type II implantation. Ophthalmology. 2017; 124:27-35.
4. Poon LY, Chodosh J, Vavvas DG, Dohlman CH, Chen TC. Endoscopic cyclophotocoagulation for the treatment of glaucoma in Boston keratoprosthesis type II patient. J Glaucoma. 2017;26:e146-e149.
5. Nanavaty MA, Avisar I, Lake DB, Daya SM, Malhotra R. Management of skin retraction associated with Boston type II keratoprosthesis. Eye. 2012;26:1384-6.
6. Sivaraman KR, Aakalu VK, Sajja K, Cortina MS, de la Cruz J, Setabutr P. Use of a porous polyethylene lid spacer for management of eyelid retraction in patients with Boston type II keratoprosthesis. Orbit. 2013;32:247-9.
7. Choi CJ, Stagner AM, Jakobiec FA, Chodosh J, Yoon MK. Eyelid mass in Boston keratoprosthesis type 2. Ophthalmic Plast Reconstr Surg. 2017;33:e39-e41.
8. Gonzalez-Saldivar G, Lee NG, Chodosh J, Freitag SK, Stacy RC. Dacryops in the setting of a Boston type II keratoprosthesis. Ophthalmic Plast Reconstr Surg. 2014;30:e73-5.
9. Iyer G, Srinivasan B, Agarwal S, Talele D, Rishi E, Rishi P, et al. Keratoprosthesis: Current global scenario and a broad Indian perspective. Indian J Ophthalmol. 2018;66:620-9.
10. Iyer G, Srinivasan B, Agarwal S, Ravindran R, Rishi E, Rishi P, et al. Boston type 2 keratoprosthesis—mid term outcomes from a tertiary eye care centre in India. Ocul Surf. 2019;17:50-4.
11. Ament JD, Stryjewski TP, Pujari S, Siddique S, Papaliodis GN, Chodosh J, et al. Cost effectiveness of the type II Boston keratoprosthesis. Eye (Lond). 2011;25:342-9.

69

Phototherapeutic Keratectomy

Ritu Nagpal, Somasheila I Murthy, Christopher J Rapuano, Namrata Sharma

INTRODUCTION

Phototherapeutic keratectomy (PTK) is a technique in which excimer laser is used to ablate the corneal tissue in order to treat epithelial and stromal pathologies limited to the anterior one third of the cornea. By uniformly ablating the corneal stroma, it not only helps in improving the corneal clarity but also helps to attain a smooth optical surface. The procedure was first approved by the United States Food and Drug Administration (FDA) in the year 1995, for treating anterior corneal stromal pathologies. The excimer laser uses 193 nm ultraviolet rays to disrupt intermolecular bonds in the cornea by a process called "photoablative decomposition".[1] This process is athermal and works with submicroscopic precision with minimal collateral damage.[2]

AIMS AND INDICATIONS

The goal of the surgery is to remove the anterior stromal pathology whilst maintaining a minimum residual stromal bed thickness (RSBT) of 250 µm, in order to maintain the structural as well as functional integrity of the cornea.[3]

Phototherapeutic keratectomy has been most commonly employed to treat elevated corneal lesions, anterior corneal stromal lesions, and recurrent erosions.[4] The primary aim of PTK in eyes with elevated corneal lesions is to smoothen and regularize the corneal surface thereby causing improvement in visual acuity and reduction of symptoms of foreign body sensation, tearing, and photophobia. In keratoconic eyes with nodules, smoothening of corneal surface helps in improving the contact lens tolerance of patients by providing a stable tear film. In eyes with progressive keratoconus, PTK can be combined with other procedures such as intracorneal ring segment (ICRS) implantation and collagen cross-linking to arrest the ectatic process, besides improving visual outcome. Eyes with anterior corneal dystrophies are benefitted by reduction of symptoms of recurrent corneal erosions and improved visual outcome due to reduction of corneal stromal opacities. PTK can also be employed as an interim procedure to delay the need for an invasive surgical procedure such as deep anterior lamellar or full thickness keratoplasty.

This is of special utility in those dystrophies that rapidly recur or have an onset at an early age, such as gelatinous drop-like dystrophy (GDLD). Eyes with recurrent corneal erosions; either dystrophic or nondystrophic in origin are benefitted by the formation of a stable epithelium with strong adhesion complexes.

Other less commonly employed indications include eyes with bullous keratopathy,[5] band keratopathy,[6] primary and recurrent pterygium,[7] postrefractive surgery complications,[8,9] and certain miscellaneous situations.[10-12] Ablation of sub-epithelial nerve plexus in eyes with bullous keratopathy helps in alleviation of pain by reducing corneal sensations in addition to reducing the osmotic load. Certain complications that develop as a result of laser in situ keratomileusis (LASIK) and photorefractive keratectomy (PRK), which are not amenable to medical therapy, have been seen to respond to excimer laser ablation. Eyes with recurring episodes of diffuse lamellar keratitis (DLK) are benefitted by PTK since it helps to remove the residual foci of inflammatory cells, responsible for recurrent attacks of inflammation.[9] Persistent folds in the LASIK flap respond to excimer laser ablation since the mechanical memory of the Bowman layer is reduced due to its reduced thickness.[13] Other situations include large decentrations, central islands persisting beyond 6–12 months of initial surgery,[14] post-PRK corneal haze,[15] and eyes with post-LASIK keratitis, nonresponsive to medical therapy.[16]

Phototherapeutic keratectomy has also been performed in eyes post-Descemet stripping automated endothelial keratoplasty (DSAEK) to address anterior surface irregularities developing as a result of long-standing corneal edema.[17] Various indications of PTK have been briefly summarized in **Box 1**.

GUIDELINES FOR PATIENT SELECTION

- *Depth of opacity < 100 µm*: In order to achieve good clarity of the cornea, the depth of opacity should be <100 µm, after accounting for the first 50 µm of epithelium.

Box 1: Indications of phototherapeutic keratectomy.

- *Elevated corneal lesions*:
  - Salzmann nodular degeneration
  - Spheroidal degeneration
  - Keratoconus nodules
- *Anterior corneal stromal dystrophies*:
  - Epithelial basement membrane dystrophy
  - *Bowman layer dystrophies*:
    - Reis–Bücklers corneal dystrophy
    - Thiel–Behnke corneal dystrophy
  - *Stromal dystrophies*:
    - Granular corneal dystrophy (GCD)
    - Lattice corneal dystrophy (LCD)
    - Macular corneal dystrophy (MCD)
    - Schnyder corneal dystrophy
- Recurrent corneal erosions
- Symptomatic bullous keratopathy
- *Postrefractive surgery complications*:
  - Diffuse lamellar keratitis
  - Flap folds and striae
  - Decentered ablations and central islands
  - Post-PRK corneal haze
  - Post-LASIK keratitis
- Primary and recurrent pterygium
- Band keratopathy
- Keratitis
- Postkeratoplasty
- *Miscellaneous*:
  - Primary amyloidosis
  - Trachomatous scarring
  - Subepithelial cryoglobulin deposits
  - Dye migration following corneal tattooing
  - Recurrent intraepithelial corneoconjunctival carcinoma

(LASIK: laser in situ keratomileusis; PRK: photorefractive keratectomy)

- *Minimum residual stromal bed thickness*: Ablation of corneal stroma should be limited to anterior one-third of stroma, leaving behind a RSBT of 250 µm in order to the withstand the normal intraocular pressure and prevent postoperative corneal ectasia.
- Superficial, homogeneous, and diffuse opacities are easier to treat than focal and deep scars.
- *Realistic expectations*: Postoperative visual outcome should be explained to the patient in accordance with the underlying corneal pathology and other ocular co-morbidities. Need for glasses or contact lenses should also be explained as a hyperopic shift is expected.

METHODS

Preoperative Evaluation

A comprehensive preoperative evaluation is important to achieve optimal anatomical as well as functional outcome and avoid any sort of patient dissatisfaction. This includes accurate estimation of corneal thickness and the depth of lesion in order to decide the depth of ablation. The other important parameter which should be evaluated preoperatively is the health of ocular surface. Presence of dry eye and corneal neurotrophicity should be ruled out since they interfere with postoperative corneal epithelial healing.

The preoperative checklist includes following points:

- Detailed history
- Uncorrected and best-corrected visual acuity (BCVA)
- Detailed slit-lamp biomicroscopic evaluation
- Posterior segment evaluation by indirect ophthalmoscopy
- Ultrasonography, if posterior segment not visible
- Anterior segment optical coherence tomography (AS-OCT)
- Corneal topography
- Nine point pachymetry, if possible
- Refraction, if possible.

Anesthesia

The surgical procedure is usually performed under topical anesthesia except in children and in patients who are not able to cooperate well during the surgical procedure. Topical proparacaine 0.5% is instilled every 5 minutes three times before the start of the procedure. A written and informed consent should be obtained after explaining the nature and possible outcome of the surgical procedure.

Preparation of Eye

The procedure is performed with the patient lying in supine position. The eye and periocular area are cleaned with povidone iodine 5% solution. The eye is draped and a wire speculum is placed to retract the eyelids and adequately expose the cornea and ocular surface.

SURGICAL TECHNIQUE

Step 1: Removal of Corneal Epithelium

Central 9 mm epithelium is usually removed manually using a blunt instrument such as a hockey stick spatula (**Figs. 1A to I**). Eyes with superficial stromal scarring tend to have a tightly adherent epithelium making manual removal difficult and time consuming. Chemical agents such as 20% alcohol can be used in these eyes to loosen the attachments between epithelium and the underlying stromal bed, allowing easy peeling. This method is also preferred in post-LASIK cases, where too much of epithelial manipulation might dislodge the flap. The excimer laser itself can be used for epithelial removal especially in eyes with a smooth surface and presence of subepithelial opacities. In eyes with Salzmann nodular degeneration, or spheroidal degeneration with dense deposits, the nodules are also manually removed along with the epithelium either using a hockey stick spatula or with a lamellar dissector, followed by ablation of the underlying stroma.

Step 2: Ablation of Corneal Stroma

After removal of the corneal epithelium, the corneal surface is subjected to ablation by excimer laser (*see* **Figs. 1A to I**). The ablation zone diameter can vary from 6.0 to 7.0 mm in

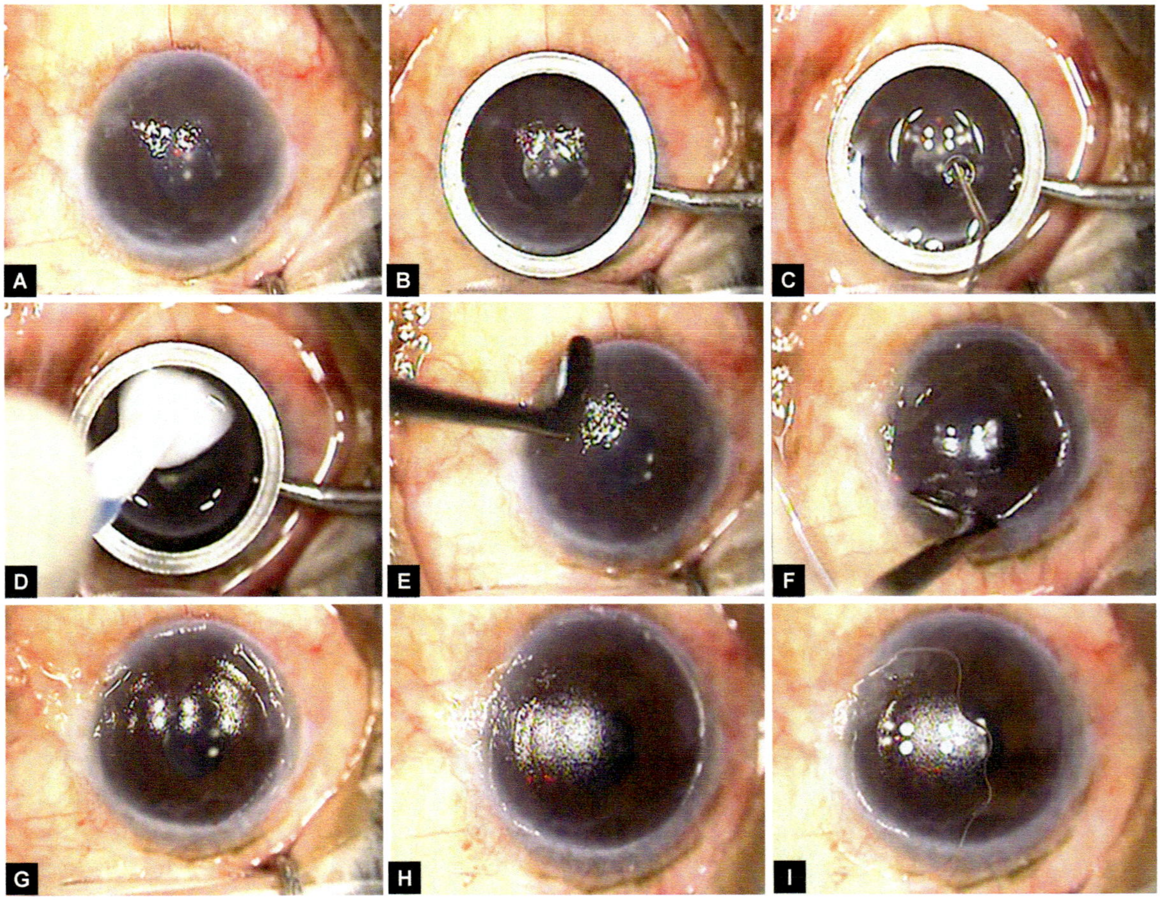

Figs. 1A to I: The collage shows various steps of a PTK procedure performed in an eye with bullous keratopathy. (A) Adequate exposure of the eye to be treated is ensured by proper draping and application of a wire speculum; (B) A well is placed over the corneal surface; (C) 20% alcohol is instilled to facilitate epithelial loosening; (D) Using a cellulose sponge the excess alcohol is removed; (E and F) central 9 mm epithelium is manually debrided using a hockey stick spatula; (G and H) Excimer laser ablation is then performed; (I) A therapeutic bandage contact lens is applied at the end of the procedure.

diameter. The amount of ablation depends upon the depth of the corneal opacity. It is usually kept between 50 and 100 µm. Less than 50 µm ablation does not produce the desired effect in most cases and >100 µm ablation can lead to subepithelial haze in the postoperative period. In eyes with irregular surface, a coupling fluid may be used to spare the depressions and ablate the elevations to achieve an even distribution of excimer laser over the area being treated.

Using the slit-lamp attachment of the microscope, the corneal surface is inspected for clarity and adequate removal of the diseased tissue. If this is not satisfactory, additional tissue can be ablated as retreatment. However, care must be taken not to ablate beyond 100 µm so as to prevent the occurrence of subepithelial haze. Another option is application of Mitomicin C, over the bare stroma if a deeper ablation is performed.

During the process of stromal ablation, patients are asked to fixate on coaxial red and green target lights within the delivery system, positioned above the patient's head and the eye-tracking system is kept on. However, if the opacity is too dense, and the patient is unable to maintain appropriate fixation, the eye-tracker is turned off.

Step 3: Placement of Bandage Contact Lens

Once, the ablation is complete, a therapeutic bandage contact lens is placed on the eye and one drop of moxifloxacin 0.5% eye drops is instilled in the conjunctival sac. During placement of the BCL, care should be taken to avoid contamination of the lens or of the bare stroma with the eye lashes, and patient should be discouraged against squeezing the eye on removal of the speculum to avoid dislodgement of the BCL.

Transepithelial Phototherapeutic Keratectomy

Herein, the corneal epithelium acts as a natural masking agent, facilitating smoothening of surface irregularities. The surgical technique has been employed mainly for the management of recurrent corneal erosions, postrefractive surgery complications, epithelial debridement in eyes undergoing PRK, and in eyes with irregular corneal surface.[18-20]

Excimer laser ablation through the epithelium removes a homogeneous layer of epithelial cells, stimulating the basal cells to regenerate with stronger underlying adhesions thereby preventing further erosions. Studies comparing pain scores between alcohol-assisted epithelial debridement and transepithelial PTK have shown significantly lower pain scores following transepithelial ablation with comparable epithelial healing.

Adjuncts to Phototherapeutic Keratectomy

Various adjuvants have been described and used in combination with PTK in an attempt to promote postoperative epithelial healing, limit corneal scarring and reduce recurrences of the original corneal pathology. These include:

- Mitomycin C (MMC)
- Autologous serum
- Amniotic membrane transplantation (AMT)

Mitomycin C

Mitomycin C decreases cellular proliferation by inhibiting the synthesis of nucleic acids and proteins in rapidly growing cells. This property of MMC has been employed to limit and modulate wound healing response at various sites. As far as corneal wound healing is concerned, by decreasing the number as well as the activity of keratocytes, it helps to limit stromal haze and scarring.[21] In eyes with anterior corneal dystrophies, it helps to prevent postoperative recurrences thereby delaying the need for keratoplasty.[22-25] 0.02–0.04% is the usual concentration used for a duration of 1–2 minutes.

Autologous Serum

Autologous serum contains various epithelial-friendly growth factors and cytokines which help to promote its migration and closure. The presence of transforming growth factor beta additionally aids in stromal repair process. These eye drops are superior to the commercially available tear drops by being autologous in nature and by having additional growth factors and cytokines, which are absent in the later.[26]

Amniotic Membrane Transplantation

Amniotic membrane by virtue of its antiangiogenic, anti-inflammatory, and antifibroblastic activities helps in stromal repair process and prevents scar formation, besides providing a cover for the bare ocular surface.[27]

POSTOPERATIVE MANAGEMENT

Patients are evaluated immediately following the surgical procedure, on day 1, day 3, at 1 week, after 4–6 weeks of surgical treatment, and then depending upon the underlying pathology and the response to initial treatment. Medical management includes prophylactic topical antibiotics (0.5% moxifloxacin) and lubricants to prevent secondary infection and promote early epithelial closure. Once the epithelial cover is re-established, bandage contact lens is removed and topical corticosteroids are initiated in tapering doses over a period of 4–6 weeks to limit postoperative corneal haze and scarring. Unlike post-PRK where the BCL is typically removed within three to five days of surgery, the BCL should be removed relatively later as recurrent epithelial breakdown can be noted.

OUTCOMES OF PHOTOTHERAPEUTIC KERATECTOMY

Phototherapeutic keratectomy has been used for the management of many clinical entities and has been reported to be a safe and effective procedure in selected superficial corneal pathologies that might otherwise need keratoplasty.[28-31] The efficacy of PTK is evaluated by improvement in BCVA comparable with the results of a full-thickness or lamellar keratoplasty in a similar clinical situation.[32] Studies have shown 47–78% improvement in BCVA following PTK.[32] In a series of 26 patients with anterior corneal pathology, Hersh et al. reported improvement in uncorrected and best corrected visual acuity in 20 eyes following PTK. Loss of two lines of BCVA occurred in two eyes and another two required penetrating keratoplasty. The average refractive shift in this series was +1.4 D.[33] The Summit PTK Study group has reported results of PTK in 232 eyes with corneal pathologies limited to the anterior 100 μm of stroma. BCVA improved by a mean of in 1.6 Snellen with a mean hyperopic shift of 0.87D.[34] Treatment was found to be most effective in eyes with hereditary corneal dystrophies, SND and corneal scars and least effective in eyes with calcific band keratopathy.

Phototherapeutic keratectomy has been shown to be effective and safe in improving visual acuity in clinical entities such as SND[35] (**Figs. 2A to C**), any superficial corneal opacity,[36] Reis-Bücklers dystrophy[37] (**Figs. 3A and B**), granular dystrophy (**Figs. 4A to C**) and recurrence of a granular dystrophy in a corneal graft,[38] residual corneal opacity after pterygium surgery, band-shaped keratopathy lattice corneal dystrophy in naive cornea (**Figs. 5 and 6**), and those recurring after a prior keratoplasty (**Figs. 7A to D**), macular corneal dystrophy (**Figs. 8A and B**) and for post traumatic corneal scars.[39,40]

It has been shown to be an effective procedure for delaying or avoiding the requirement of penetrating or lamellar keratoplasty.[41,42] It is a minimally invasive technique that results in improvement of visual acuity significantly in many clinical entities. Hence, the patient may not require a keratoplasty which is quite invasive and also carries the risk of rejection and failure due to causes other than rejection as well. However, in some situations, the visual improvement may not be as good as a keratoplasty. In such conditions, a keratoplasty may be done at a later date as a definitive procedure for visual gain. In these cases, the PTK may act as an interim procedure to provide some visual improvement. In condition like band-shaped keratopathy following a vitreoretinal surgery, the procedure makes the cornea clearer so that a retinal evaluation can be performed properly.

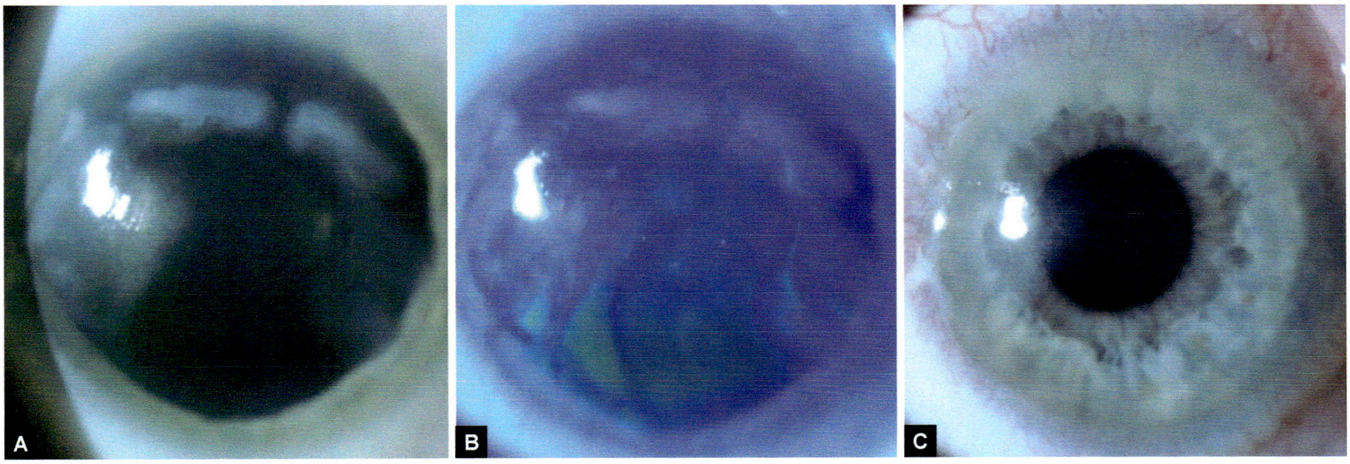

Figs. 2A to C: Slit-lamp photographs of a patient who underwent PTK for Salzmann nodular degeneration. (A) Preoperative photograph of the right eye of a patient showing well demarcated dense white nodules in the superior half of cornea with nearly 270-degree limbal stem cell deficiency; (B) Fluorescein-stained photograph of the same eye clearly delineating the extent of LSCD; (C) Day 1 postoperative photograph, following PTK with mitomycin-C showing complete disappearance of nodules, with residual some anterior haze.

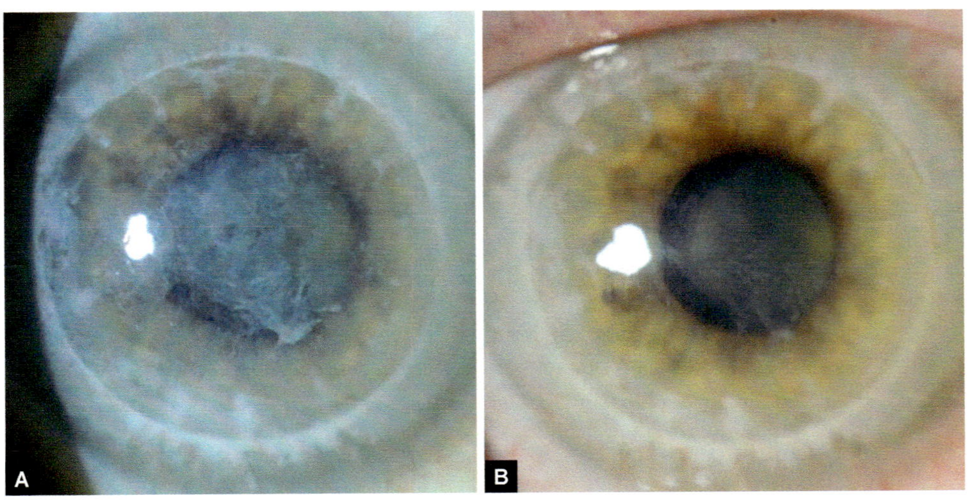

Figs. 3A and B: Slit-lamp photographs of a patient with Reis-Bücklers corneal dystrophy, who underwent PTK. (A) Preoperative, diffuse illumination photograph of the right eye of a patient showing confluent, irregular opacities predominantly involving the central part of a full thickness graft obscuring pupillary details; (B) Day 5 postoperative photograph of the same eye following PTK with mitomycin-C, showing significant clearing of the graft with improved visibility of anterior segment details.

Elevated Corneal Lesions

Das et al. reported significant reduction in median surface irregularity values and regularization of surface following PTK performed in eyes with SND.[35]

Ward et al.[43] in their series of patients with keratoconic nodules observed improvement in contact lens tolerance in all cases following 2–4 months of PTK. Similar results of successful removal of nodules followed by resumption of contact lens wear have also been reported by Steinert et al.[30] and Elsahn et al.[44] Transepithelial PTK (TE-PTK) has also been performed in combination with corneal cross-linking (CXL) in eyes with progressive keratoconus. In a study by Kymionis et al.,[45] 38 eyes with progressive keratoconus underwent TE-PTK with CXL superior outcomes were observed in eyes where TE-PTK was used for epithelial removal, compared to eyes where the epithelium was manually removed. This was attributed to customized epithelial removal and stromal smoothening during TE-PTK. Yeung et al. noticed significant improvement in visual acuity in keratoconic eyes by combining implantation of intrastromal ring segment (ICRS) with TE-PTK and CXL at 6-month follow-up.

Anterior Corneal Dystrophies

Phototherapeutic keratectomy has been used in both naïve as well in grafted eyes for the management of corneal dystrophies. In a study by Ellies et al., 42 eyes with recurrent TGFBI dystrophies following full-thickness keratoplasty underwent PTK with optimal visual results. Das et al.[46] observed improvement in visual acuity along with regularization of keratometric mires in eyes with granular corneal dystrophy (GCD) and lattice corneal dystrophy (LCD) with predominantly superficially located opacities. A significant improvement in surface regularity was seen in eyes with GCD as evident by reduction of SRI/SRA values. Kamiya et al.[47] reported significant reduction in cornea hysteresis and corneal resistance factor in eyes with GCD undergoing PTK. Hafner et al.[48] observed significant improvement in visual acuity in eyes with macular corneal dystrophy (MCD) with corneal surface regularization. 90% eye however experienced recurrence after a mean follow-up of 3 years, with two-thirds requiring keratoplasty after a period of 5 years. Wagoner et al. performed PTK in one eye and keratoplasty in the second of patients with MCD. Eyes undergoing PTK experienced gain in visual acuity, while it deteriorated in eyes undergoing keratoplasty due to irregular astigmatism. Postoperative recurrences were however higher in eyes undergoing PTK.

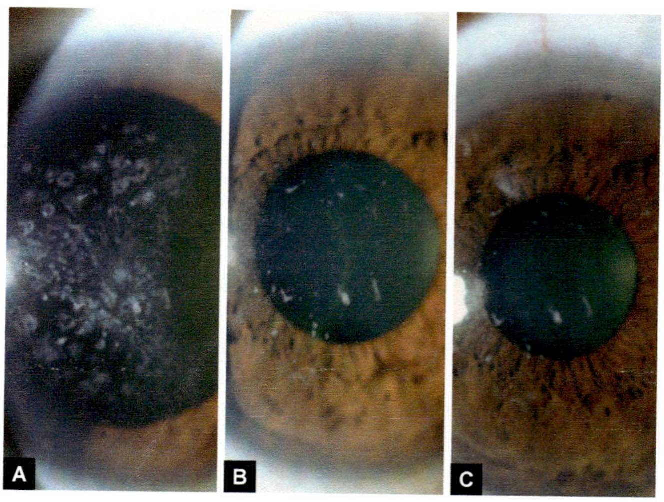

Figs. 4A to C: Pre- and postoperative slit-lamp photographs of the right eye of a patient who underwent PTK for granular corneal dystrophy. (A) Preoperative photograph showing bread crumb like opacities, tightly clustered in the central cornea; (B) 6 weeks postoperative photograph of the same eye, showing significant reduction in the number of opacities with clearing of central cornea; (C) 3.5 months postoperative photograph, showing further clearing of the cornea.

Recurrent Corneal Erosions

Eyes with recurrent corneal erosions respond well to PTK in terms of reduction of both symptoms as well as postoperative recurrences. Complications such as stromal haze and refractive shifts are less commonly observed due to limited amount of stroma ablated. Ablation depths usually range from 5 to 7 µm. In a study by Chan E et al., the efficacy of PTK was randomly compared with alcohol delamination in eyes with recurrent corneal erosions. The outcomes of both procedures were favorable in terms of resolution of symptoms, subepithelial haze formation, and mean time for recurrences.[49]

Bullous Keratopathy

Phototherapeutic keratectomy is primarily indicated for symptomatic improvement in patients with bullous keratopathy, either waiting for a keratoplasty for with poor visual potential. Sharma et al.[50] in their study of 203 eyes performed PTK in eyes with bullous keratopathy and other superficial corneal pathologies. The results were optimal in terms of alleviation of symptoms due to smoothening of corneal surface supporting the formation of a stable tear film. The epithelial closure time was found to be

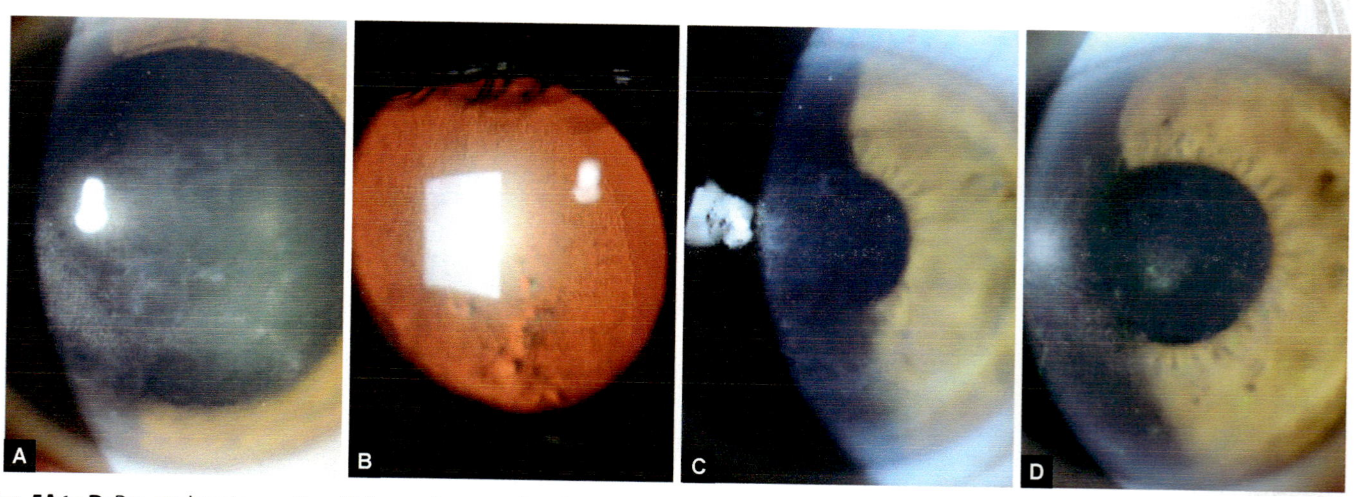

Figs. 5A to D: Pre- and postoperative slit-lamp photographs of a patient who underwent PTK for lattice corneal dystrophy that worsened after LASIK. (A) Preoperative photograph of the left eye of a patient who developed central linear, branched deposits in the central cornea following LASIK. Margins of the LASIK flap can be made out. The opacities are limited to the flap area; (B) Retro illumination image of the same eye showing a network of very fine, branching opacities limited to the area of the LASIK flap; (C) Day 1 postoperative photograph of the same eye, following PTK with mitomycin-C application, showing clearing of the central cornea; (D) 1-year postoperative photograph, showing only residual opacities.

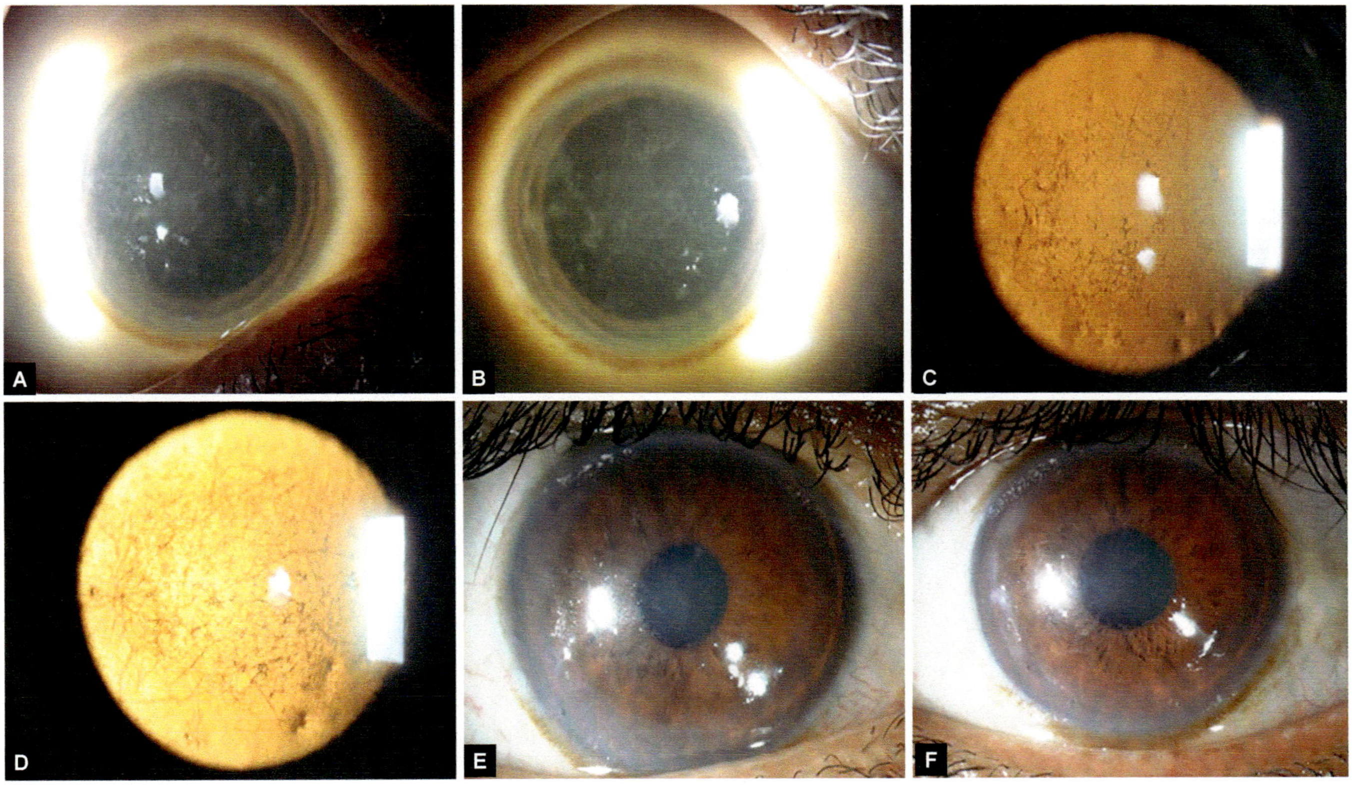

Figs. 6A to F: 47-year-old diabetic male presented with bilateral lattice corneal dystrophy and bilateral severe non-proliferative diabetic retinopathy. Preoperative vision was 20/400 and 20/600 in his right and left eye respectively. (A and B) Preoperative slit-lamp photograph with multiple diffuse gelatinous deposits at anterior to mid-stromal level, with lattice lines noted prominently on retro-illumination (C and D). PTK was done to improve the view for planning pan-retinal photocoagulation (PRP). Post-PTK there was significantly clearing of the opacities in the right (E) as well as the left eye (F) and the patient could successfully undergo PRP due to the improved retinal view.
Courtesy: Dr Pratik Gogri; Consultant, Cataract and Refractive Services. The Cornea Institute, LV Prasad Eye Institute, Hyderabad, India.

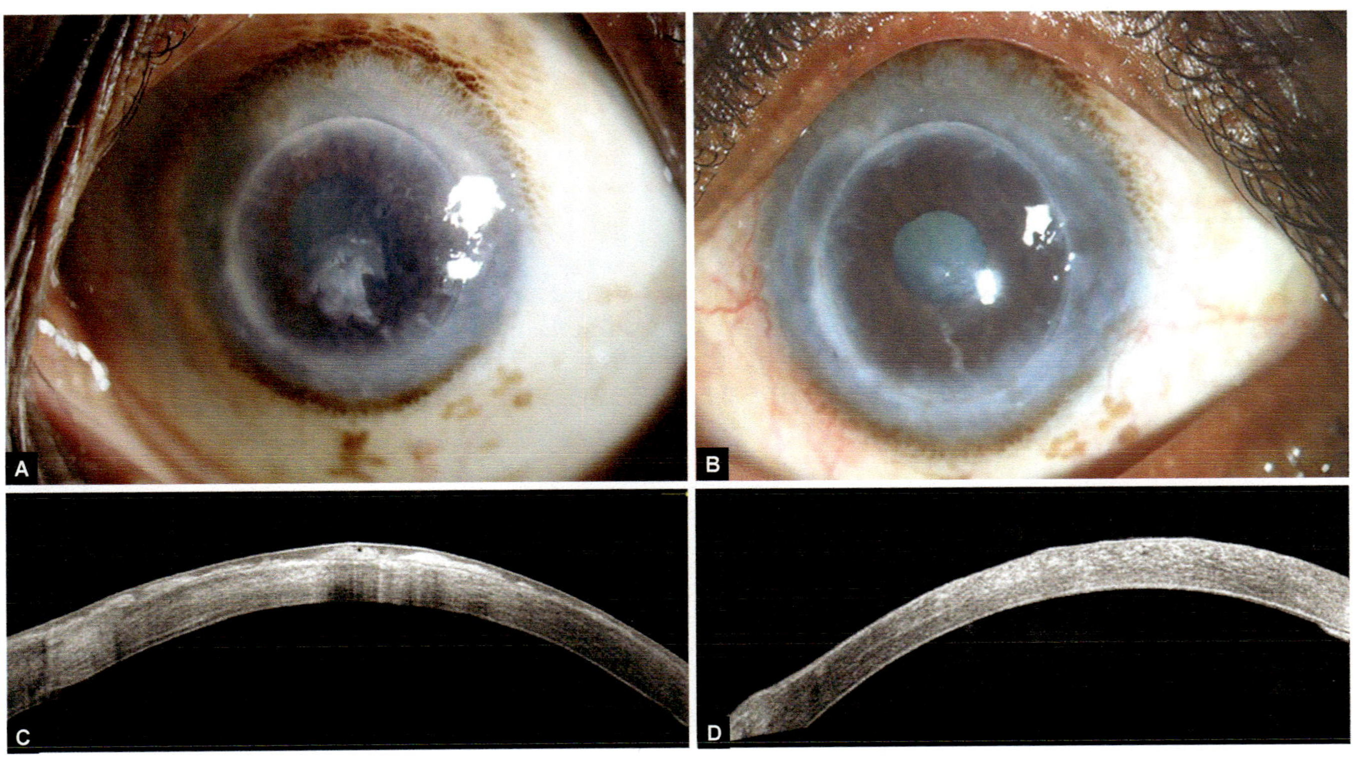

Figs. 7A to D: A 57-year-old male had undergone bilateral penetrating keratoplasty, 10 years ago for lattice corneal dystrophy. He presented with decreased vision due to advanced cataracts and recurrence of the dystrophy (A). The preoperative OCT (B) shows an uneven anterior corneal surface with deposits located predominantly in the anterior stroma. He underwent PTK following which he could also undergo cataract surgery. Postoperative image shows an optically clearer surface (C), and the corresponding OCT shows absence of these deposits.
Courtesy: Dr Sunita Chaurasia; Consultant, Cornea and Refractive Services. The Cornea Institute, LV Prasad Eye Institute, Hyderabad, India.

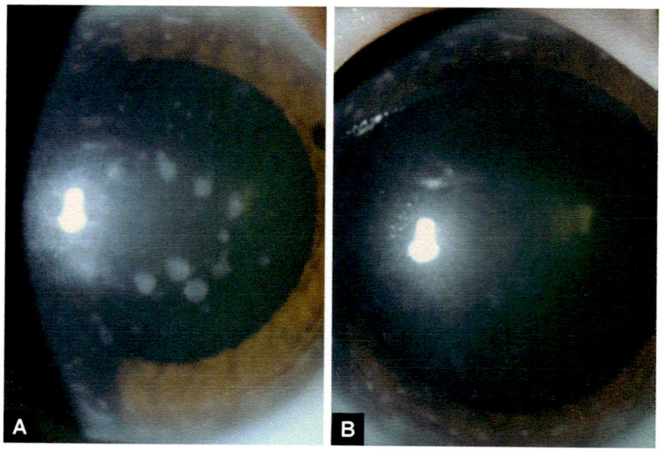

Figs. 8A and B: Pre- and postoperative slit-lamp photograph of a patient who underwent PTK for macular corneal dystrophy. (A) Preoperative, diffuse illumination photograph of the right eye of a patient showing well demarcated round to oval dense creamy white opacities involving the central as well as peripheral cornea with clearer intervening areas. The central cornea also shows anterior stromal haze; (B) 7 weeks postoperative photograph of the same eye, showing significant reduction in the number of central opacities with improvement in corneal clarity.

higher in eyes with a comparatively higher preoperative pachymetry.

Band Keratopathy

Excimer laser ablation effectively helps to smoothen the stromal surface in eyes with consequent improvement in visual acuity in eyes with both rough as well as smooth bands.[51] Im et al. combined PTK with ethylenediaminetetraacetic acid (EDTA) chelation and AMT in 11 eyes with band keratopathy and noticed symptomatic improvement in 100% eyes with no recurrences over a period of 11 months.[6]

Pterygium

Phototherapeutic keratectomy has been used in eyes with both primary as well as recurrent pterygia to reduce the recurrence rates. Combining excimer laser ablation with surgical excision serves to smoothen the corneal surface by removing the residual fibrous tissue, which is not visible clinically. Talu et al. observed regularization of keratometry mires following bare sclera excision combined with PTK in eyes with recurrent pterygium. Out of the 22 eyes, only one eye experienced postoperative recurrence. Promesberger et al., retrospectively analyzed the outcomes of conjunctival autograft (CAG) with and without PTK, in 81 eyes with primary and recurrent pterygium. The study found significantly reduced recurrence rates in eyes with primary pterygium which received additional PTK procedure in combination with CAG. This could be attributed to the difference in the distribution of gene expression between primary and recurrent pterygium, as observed on immunohistochemical studies.[52]

Post-Descemet Stripping Endothelial Keratoplasty

Eyes undergoing DSAEK with anterior stromal scarring respond well to excimer laser ablation of anterior corneal surface. PTK serves to improve visual acuity by clearing the visual axis and by reducing the higher order aberrations.[53,54]

Postrefractive Surgery Complications

Leu et al. reported successful resolution of recalcitrant DLK following PTK, performed on the undersurface of flap as well as the stromal bed.[9] TE-PTK has been observed to successfully address refractive changes occurring due to flap striae following LASIK.[12] In a study of 47 eyes with post-LASIK flap striae, TE-PTK was performed with stable visual and refractive outcomes, till 2-year follow-up. 40% eyes developed trace to 1+ haze with a mean hyperopic shift of 0.80 D.[55] Rachid et al. in another retrospective study reported reduction in spherical equivalent values with improvement in visual acuity following PTK performed for the treatment of decentration and central islands developing after PRK.[14]

The outcomes of PTK in various corneal stromal pathologies have been summarized in **Table 1**.

COMPLICATIONS OF PHOTOTHERAPEUTIC KERATECTOMY

- *Hyperopic shift*: Induced hyperopia is the most common refractive error seen following PTK, although all types of refractive errors may occur. This occurs due to central corneal thinning and flattening.[56] The amount of actual hyperopic shift developing per the amount of tissue ablated is not exactly known. The Munnerlyn formula, developed initially for myopic excimer laser treatments has been used by some surgeons for the estimation of refractive shift following PTK, but the correlation is not that strong. A shallow ablation depth (<100 μm), large diameter ablation zones, and use of masking agents significantly helps to decrease the amount of hyperopic shift.
- *Corneal haze*: Subepithelial corneal haze following excimer laser ablation occurs due to a process of wound remodeling involving corneal basal epithelial cells as well as keratocytes.[57] It is more commonly encountered in association with deep stromal ablations and in eyes with delayed epithelial healing. Laser-induced haze is usually subepithelial in location, stays confined to the ablation zone and has a gray reticulated appearance in contrast to the residual opacification which is deep-seated in location, has a ground glass appearance and extends beyond the area of laser ablation.
- *Glare*: Night time glare and photic phenomenon may be seen in some cases as seen in any other excimer laser refractive procedure.

Table 1: Outcomes of PTK in various corneal stromal pathologies.

S. No.	Author/Year	Study type	N	Indication	Intervention	Outcome
1.	Kymionis GD et al./2014	P	23	Progressive keratoconus	TE-PTK + CXL	UDVA and CDVA improved significantly with reduction in flat and steep keratometry and corneal astigmatism
2.	Elsahn F et al./2009	R	15	Keratoconic nodules	PTK	Contact lens tolerance improved in majority of eyes. (73%) three eyes experienced recurrence of nodule formation
3.	Yeung SN et al./2013	R	16	Progressive keratoconus	TE-PTK + ICRS implantation	UDVA and CDVA improved significantly with reduction corneal astigmatism
4.	Das S et al./2005	R	22	SND	PTK + pannus tissue removal	Visual acuity improved in 86% eyes. four eyes experienced recurrence of nodules requiring repeat PTK
5.	Hieda O et al./2013	R	10	TBCD	PTK	100% eyes experienced two line improvement in visual acuity with 50% experiencing recurrences
6.	Germundsson J et al./	C	52	EBMD	PTK	Overall 46% eyes experienced recurrences, of which 40% had morphologic recurrence and 13% had symptomatic recurrence
7.	Hafner A et al./2005	R	10	MCD	PTK	Visual acuity improved in 100% eyes, 90% however experienced postoperative recurrence
8.	Das S et al./2005	P	62	GCD (n = 50) LCD (n = 12)	PTK	10/50 eyes with granular dystrophy while two eyes with lattice dystrophy experienced postoperative recurrence of deposits
9.	Maclean H et al./1996	P	3	Recurrent GCD, postkeratoplasty	PTK	All eyes experienced improvement in visual acuity with recurrence seen in one eye
10.	Heinz P et al./1995	P	3	Recurrent GCD, postkeratoplasty	PTK	100% eyes experienced improved cornea clearing with no further recurrences till 1-year follow-up
11.	Dedes W et al./2015	P	89	Dystrophic and nondystrophic refractory RCEs	PTK	25 eyes experienced postoperative recurrence. The dystrophic eyes had a higher rate of recurrence compared to the nondystrophic ones
12.	Suri K et al./2013	R	272	Dystrophic and nondystrophic RCEs	a. Conservative management b. Epithelial debridement c. PTK d. Diamond burr polishing	Eyes treated with conservatively had highest rate of recurrence followed by PTK. Least recurrence rates observed in eyes managed by diamond burr polishing
13.	Sridhar MS et al./2002	R	43	RCEs in eyes with EBMD	a. PTK b. Diamond burr polishing	Eyes in both groups were comparable in terms of visual outcomes, occurrence of corneal haze and recurrences
14.	Jain S et al./1999	R	77	Dystrophic and nondystrophic refractory RCEs	a. PTK 71/77 b. PTK + PRK 6/77	Overall, 68.8% eyes achieved complete resolution of symptoms
15.	Reddy JC et al./2014	P	13	SND	PTK+ MMC	All eyes had significant improvement in visual quality in terms of improvement in contrast sensitivity and reduction of corneal higher order aberrations
16.	Vyas S et al./2009	R	18	Symptomatic bullous keratopathy	PTK + AMT	91.67% eyes achieved complete resolution of symptoms

(AMT: amniotic membrane transplantation; CDVA: corrected distance visual acuity; CXL: corneal cross-linking; EBMD: epithelial basement membrane dystrophy; GCD: granular corneal dystrophy; ICRS: intracorneal ring segment; LCD: lattice corneal dystrophy; MMC: Mitomycin C; N: number of eyes; P: prospective; PRK: photorefractive keratectomy; R: retrospective; RCE: recurrent corneal erosions; SND: Salzmann nodular degeneration; TBCD: Thiel-Behnke corneal dystrophy; TE-PTK: transepithelial phototherapeutic keratectomy; UDVA: uncorrected distance visual acuity)

- *Myopic shift*: Myopic shift after PTK is usually rare and it may be due to accumulation of plume in the central part of the cornea and in some situations where the ablation is done in the peripheral part of the cornea in order to remove a peripheral corneal opacity.
- *Infection*: Infectious keratitis may be seen rarely. The eye is predisposed to infection by the ocular commensals due to presence of a large epithelial defect and use of therapeutic bandage contact lens in the immediate postoperative period.

- *Recurrence of the original corneal pathology*: Recurrence of a corneal dystrophy such as Reis-Bücklers or a granular dystrophy may be seen. This may be treated by a re-ablation; and can be repeated several times. However, some cases may require a keratoplasty. The recurrence patterns following PTK vary depending upon the underlying corneal pathology. Dinh et al. observed eyes with epithelial basement membrane dystrophy to experience recurrence much earlier after an average interval of 6–9 months, compared to other dystrophies. This was attributed to the involvement of epithelial basement membrane as opposed to stromal involvement in eyes with other dystrophies.[58] Sorour et al. observed 100% recurrence rates in their study involving eyes with Thiel-Behnke corneal dystrophy, after a mean follow-up period of 9.7 ± 7.97 years.[59] Hafner et al. in their largest study of eyes with MCD, observed 90% recurrence rates after a mean follow-up period of 3.4 ± 0.4 years. Almost two-thirds eyes required a subsequent keratoplasty, all grafts remaining clear over a follow-up period of 4 years. Post-PTK recurrences are seen early in eyes with MCD compared to eyes with GCD, and at a higher rate. This is in contrast to the recurrence pattern observed following keratoplasty, where they develop early on and at a higher rate, in eyes with GCD.[48]
- *Reactivation of viral keratitis*: Excimer laser ablation is known to reactivate herpetic disease by stimulating viral shedding in tears and reactivation of the virus. Corneal trauma and corticosteroid-induced local immunosuppression are the other predisposing factors.[60]
- *Graft rejection*: In eyes with a prior graft, the inflammatory anterior segment reaction induced by the excimer laser might compromise survival of the graft.[61]
- *Corneal edema*: Persistent corneal edema has been described to occur following PTK in eyes receiving continued administration of MMC, as a consequence of endothelial dysfunction.[62]
- *Keratolysis*: This is a rare complication, encountered in cases where the epithelium fails to heal. Progressive keratolysis due to exposed stromal surface might progress to descemetocele formation, requiring emergent keratoplasty.[63]

CONCLUSION

Phototherapeutic keratectomy is a useful and satisfying procedure provided its limitations are understood. It may provide visual improvement in many superficial corneal disorders. This may reduce the requirement of keratoplasty in some cases, thereby reducing the load on the eye bank. This is specifically advantageous in countries where the availability of donor corneal tissue is a limiting factor. However, the visual improvement in some conditions may not be optimal. Use of PTK as an interim procedure helps to buy time for keratoplasty in such cases. The procedure being repeatable and can be performed in both naïve as well as in grafted corneas without significantly altering the outcomes of a subsequently performed keratoplasty.

ACKNOWLEDGMENTS

The authors would like to acknowledge Dr Pratik Gogri and Dr Sunita Chaurasia for providing pre- and postoperative clinical photographs and anterior segment OCT images of their patients undergoing PTK. Dr Pratik Gogri: Consultant, Cataract and Refractive surgery services, LV Prasad Eye Institute, Hyderabad, India. Dr Sunita Chaurasia: Consultant, Cornea Services, The Cornea Institute, LV Prasad Eye Institute, Hyderabad, India.

REFERENCES

1. Wu WC, Stark WJ, Green WR. Corneal wound healing after 193-nm excimer laser keratectomy. Arch Ophthalmol. 1991;109:1426-32.
2. Marshall J, Trokel SJ, Rothery S, Krueger RR. Long-term healing of the central cornea after photorefractive keratectomy using an excimer laser. Ophthalmology. 1988;95:1411-21.
3. Stasi K, Chuck RS. Update on phototherapeutic keratectomy. Curr Opin Ophthalmol. 2009;20(4):272-5.
4. Ayres BD, Rapuano CJ. Excimer laser phototherapeutic keratectomy. Ocul Surf. 2006;4(4):196-206.
5. Lin PY, Wu CC, Lee SM. Combined phototherapeutic keratectomy and therapeutic contact lens for recurrent erosions in bullous keratopathy. Br J Ophthalmol. 2001;85(8):908-11.
6. Im SK, Lee KH, Yoon KC. Combined ethylenediaminetetraacetic acid chelation, phototherapeutic keratectomy and amniotic membrane transplantation for treatment of band keratopathy. Korean J Ophthalmol. 2010;24(2):73-7.
7. Talu H, Taşindi E, Ciftci F, Yildiz TF. Excimer laser phototherapeutic keratectomy for recurrent pterygium. J Cataract Refract Surg. 1998;24(10):1326-32.
8. Kymionis G, Ide T, Yoo S. Flap amputation with phototherapeutic keratectomy (PTK) and adjuvant mitomycin C for severe post-LASIK epithelial ingrowth. Eur J Ophthalmol. 2009;19(2):301-3.
9. Leu G, Hersh PS. Phototherapeutic keratectomy for the treatment of diffuse lamellar keratitis. J Cataract Refract Surg. 2002;28(8):1471-4.
10. John ME, Martines E, Cvintal T, Ballew C. Excimer laser photoablation of primary familial amyloidosis of the cornea. Refract Corneal Surg. 1993;9(2 Suppl):S138-41.
11. Kremer I, Blumenthal M. Excimer phototherapeutic keratectomy for corneal subepithelial cryoglobulin deposits. J Cataract Refract Surg. 1997;23(7):1119-21.
12. Steinert RF, Ashrafzadeh A, Hersh PS. Results of phototherapeutic keratectomy in the management of flap striae after LASIK. Ophthalmology. 2004;111(4):740-6.
13. Hernandez-Matamoros J, Iradier MT, Moreno E. Treating folds and striae after laser in situ keratomileusis. J Cataract Refract Surg. 2001;27(3):350-2.
14. Rachid MD, Yoo SH, Azar DT. Phototherapeutic keratectomy for decentration and central islands after photorefractive keratectomy. Ophthalmology. 2001;108(3):545-52.
15. Choi H, Ju L, Kim J, Choi S, Lee D. Successful treatment with combined PTK/PRK guided by intraoperative skiascopy of

patients with corneal haze after surface ablation. Korean J Ophthalmol. 2015;29(1):74-6.

16. Lindbohm N, Moilanen JA, Vesaluoma MH, Tervo TM. Acinetobacter and Staphylococcus aureus ulcerative keratitis after laser in situ keratomileusis treated with antibiotics and phototherapeutic keratectomy. J Refract Surg. 2005;21(4):404-6.
17. Awdeh RM, Abbey AM, Vroman DT, Ying MS, Goldman D, Kymionis G, et al. Phototherapeutic keratectomy for the treatment of subepithelial fibrosis and anterior corneal scarring after descemet stripping automated endothelial keratoplasty. Cornea. 2012;31(7):761-3.
18. Muller LT, Candal EM, Epstein RJ, Dennis RF, Majmudar PA. Transepithelial phototherapeutic keratectomy/photorefractive keratectomy with adjunctive mitomycin-C for complicated LASIK flaps. J Cataract Refract Surg. 2005;31(2):291-6.
19. Ibarz Barberá M, García González M, Teus Guezala M. Transepithelial phototherapeutic keratectomy to treat chronic laser in situ keratomileusis-flap macrostriae. A case review. Arch Soc Esp Oftalmol. 2012;87(12):407-10.
20. Holzer MP, Auffarth GU, Specht H, Kruse FE. Combination of transepithelial phototherapeutic keratectomy and autologous serum eyedrops for treatment of recurrent corneal erosions. J Cataract Refract Surg. 2005;31(8):1603-6.
21. Rajan MS, O'Brart DP, Patmore A, Marshall J. Cellular effects of mitomycin-C on human corneas after photorefractive keratectomy. J Cataract Refract Surg. 2006;32(10):1741-7.
22. Kim T, Pak JH, Chae J, Kim EK, Tchah H. Mitomycin C inhibits recurrent Avellino dystrophy after phototherapeutic keratectomy. Cornea. 2006;25(2):220-3.
23. Sykakis E, Papadopoulos R, Lake D. Phototherapeutic keratectomy with mitomycin C for recurrent granular corneal dystrophy under femtosecond-assisted anterior lamellar keratoplasty. Cornea. 2015;34(6):e17-8.
24. Khaireddin R, Katz T, Baile RB, Richard G, Linke SJ. Superficial keratectomy, PTK, and mitomycin C as a combined treatment option for Salzmann's nodular degeneration: a follow-up of eight eyes. Graefes Arch Clin Exp Ophthalmol. 2011;249(8):1211-5.
25. Reddy JC, Rapuano CJ, Felipe AF, Nagra PK, Hammersmith KM. Quality of vision after excimer laser phototherapeutic keratectomy with intraoperative mitomycin-C for Salzmann nodular degeneration. Eye Contact Lens. 2014;40(4):213-9.
26. Akcam HT, Unlu M, Karaca EE, Yazici H, Aydin B, Hondur AM. Autologous serum eye-drops and enhanced epithelial healing time after photorefractive keratectomy. Clin Exp Optom. 2018; 101(1):34-7.
27. Vyas S, Rathi V. Combined phototherapeutic keratectomy and amniotic membrane grafts for symptomatic bullous keratopathy. Cornea. 2009;28(9):1028-31.
28. Starr M, Donnenfeld E, Newton M, Tostanoski J, Muller J, Odrich M. Excimer laser phototherapeutic keratectomy. Cornea. 1996;15:557-65.
29. Gaster RN, Binder PS, Coalwell K, Berns M, McCord RL, Burstein NL. Corneal surface ablation by 193 nm excimer laser and wound healing in rabbits. Invest Ophthalmol Vis Sci. 1989;30:90-8.
30. Steinert RF, Puliafito CA. Excimer laser phototherapeutic keratectomy for a corneal nodule. Refract Corneal Surg. 1990;6:352.
31. Saini JS, Reddy MK, Jain AK, Ravindra MS, Jhaveria S, Raghuram L. Perspectives in eye banking. Indian J Ophthalmol. 1996;44:47-55.
32. Stark WJ, Charmon W, Kamp MT, Enger CL, Rencs EV, Gottsch JD. Clinical follow-up of 193-nm ArF excimer laser phototherapeutic keratectomy. Ophthalmology. 1992:99:805-12.
33. Hersh PS, Burnstein Y, Carr J, Etwane G, Mayers M. Excimer laser phototherapeutic keratectomy. Surgical strategies and clinical outcomes. Ophthalmology. 1996;103:1210-22.
34. Maloney RK, Thompson V, Ghiselli G, Durrie D, Waring GO 3rd, O'Connell M. A prospective multicenter trial of excimer laser phototherapeutic keratectomy for corneal vision loss. The Summit Phototherapeutic Keratectomy Study Group. Am J Ophthalmol. 1996;122:149-60.
35. Das S, Langenbucher A, Pogorelov P, Link B, Seitz B. Long- term outcome of excimer laser phototherapeutic keratectomy for treatment of Salzmann's nodular degeneration. J Cataract Refract Surg. 2005;31:1386-91.
36. Amano S, Oshika T, Tazawa Y, Tsuru T. Long-term follow-up of excimer laser phototherapeutic keratectomy. Jpn J Ophthalmol. 1999;43:513-6.
37. el Aouni A, Briat B, Mayer F, Saragoussi JJ, Abenhaim A, Assouline M, et al. [Reis-Buckler dystrophy: therapeutic photo-ablation with the excimer laser]. J Fr Ophtalmol. 1998;21:23-7.
38. Heinz P, Wiegand W, Kroll P. [Phototherapeutic keratectomy in recurrences of granular corneal dystrophy after keratoplasty]. Klin Monbl Augenheilkd. 1995;206:184-7.
39. Förster W, Atzler U, Ratkay I, Busse H. Therapeutic use of the 193-nm excimer laser in corneal pathologies. Graefes Arch Clin Exp Ophthalmol. 1997;235:296-305.
40. Kozobolis VP, Siganos DS, Meladakis GS, Pallikaris IG. Excimer laser phototherapeutic keratectomy for corneal opacities and recurrent erosion. J Refract Surg. 1996;12:S288-90.
41. Nagy ZZ, Süveges I, Németh J, Füst A. [Phototherapeutic use of excimer laser]. Orv Hetil. 1996;14:137:75-8.
42. Förster W, Grewe S, Busse H. [Clinical use of the excimer laser in treatment of surface corneal opacities—therapeutic strategy and case reports]. Klin Monbl Augenheilkd. 1993;202:126-9.
43. Ward MA, Artunduaga G, Thompson KP, Wilson LA, Stulting RD. Phototherapeutic keratectomy for the treatment of nodular subepithelial corneal scars in patients with keratoconus who are contact lens intolerant. CLAO J. 1995;21(2):130-2.
44. Elsahn AF, Rapuano CJ, Antunes VA, Abdalla YF, Cohen EJ. Excimer laser phototherapeutic keratectomy for keratoconus nodules. Cornea. 2009;28(2):144-7.
45. Kymionis GD, Grentzelos MA, Kounis GA, Diakonis VF, Limnopoulou AN, Panagopoulou SI. Combined transepithelial phototherapeutic keratectomy and corneal collagen cross-linking for progressive keratoconus. Ophthalmology. 2012; 119(9):1777-84.
46. Das S, Langenbucher A, Seitz B. Excimer laser phototherapeutic keratectomy for granular and lattice corneal dystrophy: A comparative study. J Refract Surg. 2005;21(6):727-31.
47. Kamiya K, Shimizu K, Ohmoto F. The changes in corneal biomechanical parameters after phototherapeutic keratectomy in eyes with granular corneal dystrophy. Eye (Lond). 2009; 23(9):1790-5.
48. Hafner A, Langenbucher A, Seitz B. Long-term results of phototherapeutic keratectomy with 193-nm excimer laser for macular corneal dystrophy. Am J Ophthalmol. 2005;140(3):392-6.
49. Chan E, Jhanji V, Constantinou M, Amiel H, Snibson GR, Vajpayee RB. A randomised 1 controlled trial of alcohol delamination and phototherapeutic keratectomy for the treatment of recurrent corneal erosion syndrome. Br J Ophthalmol. 2014;98(2):166-71.
50. Sharma N, Prakash G, Sinha R, Tandon R, Titiyal JS, Vajpayee RB. Indications and outcomes of phototherapeutic keratectomy in the developing world. Cornea. 2008;27(1):44-9.
51. O'Brart DP, Gartry DS, Lohmann CP, Patmore AL, Kerr Muir MG, Marshall J. Treatment of band keratopathy by excimer laser phototherapeutic keratectomy: Surgical techniques and long term follow up. Br J Ophthalmol. 1993;77(11):702-8.
52. Promesberger J, Kohli S, Busse H, Uhlig CE. Pterygium recurrence, astigmatism and visual acuity following bare-sclera excision and conjunctival autograft with or without additional phototherapeutic keratectomy. Ophthalmic Res. 2014;51(1):52-8.
53. Lee BS, Hardten DR. Visual and subjective outcomes of phototherapeutic 1 keratectomy after Descemet's stripping endothelial keratoplasty. Clin Ophthalmol. 2014;8:1011-5.

54. Hongyok T, Kim A, Jun AS, Ladas JG, Chuck RS. Phototherapeutic keratectomy with mitomycin C after Descemet stripping automated endothelial keratoplasty. Br J Ophthalmol. 2010;94(3):377-8.
55. Ashrafzadeh A, Steinert RF. Results of phototherapeutic keratectomy in the management of flap striae after LASIK before and after developing a standardized protocol: Long-term follow up of an expanded patient population. Ophthalmology. 2007;114(6):1118-23.
56. Dogru M, Katakami C, Yamanaka A. Refractive changes after excimer laser phototherapeutic keratectomy. J Cataract Refract Surg. 2001;27:686-92.
57. Lee YC, Wang IJ, Hu FR, Kao WW. Immunohistochemical study of subepithelial haze after phototherapeutic keratectomy. J Refract Surg. 2001;17(3):334-41.
58. Dinh R, Rapuano CJ, Cohen EJ, Laibson PR. Recurrence of corneal dystrophy after excimer laser phototherapeutic keratectomy. Ophthalmology. 1999;106(8):1490-7.
59. Sorour HM, Yee SB, Peterson NJ, Li FT, Macsai MS, Zhao XC, et al. Recurrence of chromosome 10 Thiel-Behnke corneal dystrophy (CDB2) after excimer laser phototherapeutic keratectomy or penetrating keratoplasty. Cornea. 2005;24(1):45-50.
60. Deai T, Fukuda M, Tomoda Y, Higaki S, Hayashi K, Shimomura Y. Excimer laser photokeratectomy reactivates latent herpes simplex virus. Jpn J Ophthalmol. 2004;48(6):570-2.
61. Pisella PJ, Albou-Ganem C, Bourges JL, Debbasch C, Limon S. Evaluation of anterior chamber inflammation after corneal refractive surgery. Cornea. 1999;18(3):302-5.
62. Pfister RR. Permanent corneal edema resulting from the treatment of PTK corneal haze with mitomycin: A case report. Cornea. 2004;23(7):744-7.
63. Lahners WJ, Russell B, Grossniklaus HE, Stulting RD. Keratolysis following excimer laser phototherapeutic keratectomy in a patient with keratoconus. J Refract Surg. 2001;17(5):555-8.

70

Optical Sector Iridectomy

M Vanathi, Sarath S, Rasik B Vajpayee, Namrata Sharma

INTRODUCTION

Corneal opacities account for 37.5% of blindness in less than 50 years age group and 8.2% of blindness in the age group 50 years and above, in India.[1] More than half of these cases are treatable and curable. Penetrating keratoplasty is the procedure of choice for full-thickness opacities involving the central cornea. The procedure demands a good quality donor material, surgical expertise, and long-term follow-up to achieve optimal visual results. In developing countries, there is a paucity of good quality donor material and therefore patients have to wait for a long period of time to undergo corneal transplantation. Also, a paucity of trained corneal specialists at the peripheral healthcare centers precludes proper long-term care of grafted patients resulting in failure of many successfully performed transplantation surgeries. Moreover in developing countries poor socioeconomic status and lack of adequate transport facilities in remote areas preclude a regular follow-up. All these factors do significantly reduce the chances of survival of a corneal graft. In such patients if one graft fails, chances of a second graft being successful are even more remote. Such a situation is particularly disastrous for one-eyed patients.

If the opacity does not occupy the entire circumference and leaves some area of the cornea still transparent, an optical iridectomy may help in providing a good ambulatory vision.[2,3] This vision may not be equal to the vision achieved initially after a corneal transplantation surgery, but it may last lifelong and enable these patients to carry out their routine activities.

The surgical procedure being simple and safe compared to penetrating keratoplasty, is particularly advantageous for children with central leukomas such as in Peters anomaly. Obtaining a clear visual axis early on is of utmost importance for visual development in these eyes. Full thickness keratoplasty performed in children has limitations in the form of high failure rate, difficult postoperative follow-ups, need for repeated examinations under anesthesia and the complications of long-term corticosteroid use. A simple surgical technique that helps to re-establish visual axis clarity with minimal postoperative complications and reduced duration of follow up is specifically suited for pediatric eyes.

MECHANISM OF ACTION

Understanding mechanism of action of optical iridectomy is vital, if optimal results are to be achieved.[4] Although the peripheral part of the human optical system does not form as sharp an image as the central part does optical iridectomy helps to add a peripheral bundle of rays so that a relatively clear vision is produced by the superimposition of a clear peripheral and a blurred central image. One may not attain a visual acuity of 6/6, but a significant improvement of vision does happen.

The best site for optical sector iridectomy is debated. The part of peripheral cornea, which is maximally clear, should be chosen as the site of iridectomy. A superiorly placed iridectomy gets covered by the upper lid and therefore will not serve its purpose. Hence, iridectomy should be placed in the lower nasal and lower temporal quadrant.

INDICATIONS OF OPTICAL IRIDECTOMY

An optical sector iridectomy is ideally indicated in those cases where the corneal opacity is off center and encroaches on to the pupillary area.[5-7] It has also been advocated in cases in which the scar is central and sufficient part of the peripheral cornea is clear (**Fig. 1**).[8] Optical iridectomy is especially indicated in one eyed patients, patients with corneal scars where the chances of graft failure are very high such as with ocular surface disorders and in cases of bilaterally blind patients awaiting for keratoplasty.

Optical iridectomy is an ideal alternative in cases of partial opacification of cornea, where penetrating keratoplasty is contraindicated or cannot be performed.[9,10]

PREOPERATIVE EVALUATION

Patient selection for iridectomy is of utmost importance to achieve optimal results. The prerequisites for performing an optical sector iridectomy are the presence of an area of

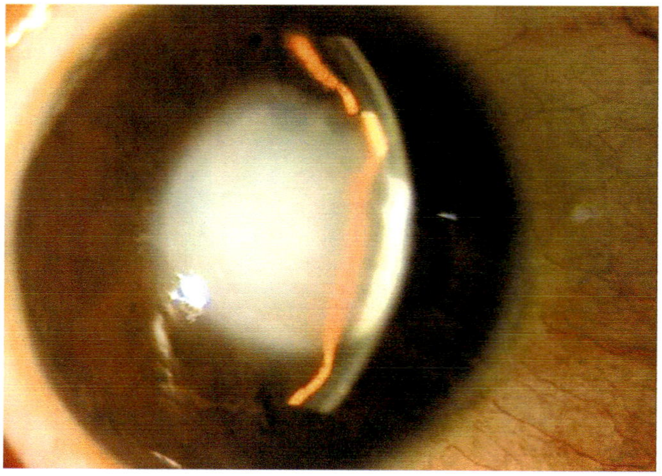

Fig. 1: Preoperative slit-lamp photograph of the right eye of a patient with central corneal opacity and clear periphery.

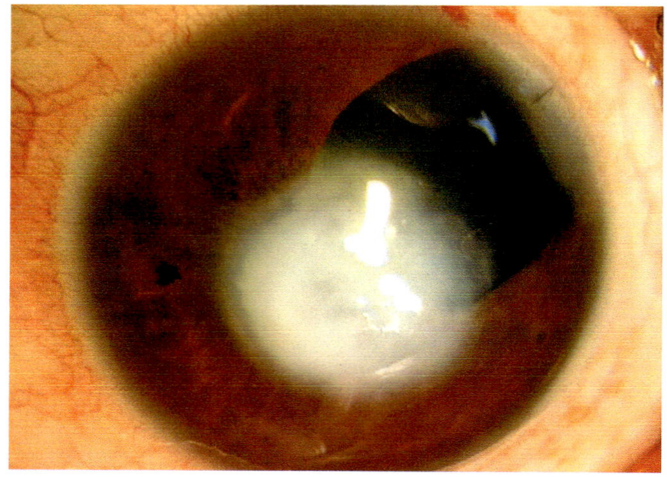

Fig. 2: Postoperative slit-lamp photograph of the same patient as shown in **Figure 1**, following optical sector iridectomy.

clear cornea, a clear peripheral lens and a successful possible estimation of achievable visual acuity based on the clarity of fundus, as viewed through the area of proposed iridectomy. Patients with additional ocular problems such as nystagmus, macular degeneration or optic atrophy should be expected to achieve subnormal level of visual acuity and are not the ideal candidates. An estimation of best-corrected visual acuity with a stenopic slit, aids in optimal placement of iridectomy.[11] Further, if the media is hazy an indirect ophthalmoscopy or ultrasound for posterior segment evaluation should be done to rule out any posterior segment pathology.

SURGICAL TECHNIQUE

A small fornix-based conjunctival flap is made at the previously selected location with a conjunctival scissors and undermined. Mild cautery of the bleeding vessels is done. A 3.2 mm groove incision is made at the posterior limbus. A corneolimbal tunnel is dissected 0.5 mm into the clear cornea. The 3.2 mm keratome blade is inserted into the tunnel and advanced horizontally parallel to the iris causing a linear horizontal cut through the Descemet's membrane into the anterior chamber. Care is taken to avoid injury to the iris tissue. A small amount of viscoelastic is injected to deepen the anterior chamber. Subsequently, the midperiphery of the iris is caught with the forceps and pulled out of the incision gently and a complete iridectomy is facilitated using an iris forceps. Care is taken to avoid inadvertent injury to the lens. The anterior chamber is cleared of viscoelastic and formed with balanced salt solution (BSS). The wound is sutured (**Fig. 2**).

Alternatively, another method can be used to perform optical iridectomy, especially in cases of adherent leukomas.[11,12] An automated vitrector can be used to release the adherent leukoma and create an optical iridectomy. Release of iris adhesions with creation of an optical iridectomy improves visualization and also aid in performing phacoemulsification in case of coexisting cataract. A radial 1.2 mm incision is made at the limbus, opposite to the site of adherent leucoma. An additional side port is made 2 to 3 clock hours away on the clear cornea. Viscoelastic is injected below the iris in order to lift it away from the crystalline lens. A 20-gauge vitrectomy probe is then inserted into the anterior chamber keeping the aspiration setting at 100 mm Hg and cutter-setting at 700 cpm. The adherent leucoma is released by occluding the iris stroma with the aspiration port and cutting in a controlled manner under direct visualization, taking care not to disturb the angle structures. A customized iridectomy is thus made in the desired quadrant, leaving rest of the iris tissue undisturbed. The anterior chamber is then irrigated with balanced salt solution followed by hydration of side ports. Postoperatively, topical antibiotic corticosteroids and cylcoplegics are prescribed.

RESULTS AND OUTCOMES

Optical sector iridectomy has been used for clearing of visual axis in cases of congenital corneal opacities, specifically for Peters anomaly.[6,7] Visual outcomes following optical iridectomy for Peters anomaly have been reported to be equivalent to that of keratoplasty.[6,13]

We evaluated visual outcomes after optical sector iridectomy in 17 patients with corneal opacities.[8] In this study, an optical iridectomy was performed in the inferior quadrant with 94% eyes achieving a visual acuity of 6/60 or better.

In the largest study of optical iridectomy performed in 29 eyes with Peters anomaly, visual improvement was seen in 72.4% eyes.[14] In another 17.2% eyes, it remained stable while in 10.3% eyes a deterioration was noted. The visual improvement was significant in patients with bilateral disease. No intraoperative complications were reported. Over a mean follow-up period of 41 months 5 eyes were diagnosed with glaucoma and one patient required additional sector iridectomy. Overall the surgical technique was found to be a safe and a noninferior alternative to penetrating keratoplasty.

The complications, which can occur during optical sector iridectomy, include postoperative hyphema, secondary glaucoma, and injury to the lens causing cataract formation.

REFERENCES

1. Murthy GVS, Jose R, Vashist P, John N. Rapid Assessment of Avoidable Blindness - India Report. National Program for Control of Blindness Directorate General of Health Services, Ministry of Health and Family Welfare, Government of India.
2. Summers CG, Holland EJ. Neodymium: YAG pupilloplasty in pediatric aphakia. J Pediatr Ophthalmol Strabismus. 1991; 28:155-6.
3. Weber SW, Crawford JS, Arndt JH, Parker JS. Visual acuity after iridectomy or aspiration for congenital cataracts: Experimental and clinical studies. Can J Ophthalmol. 1978;13:229-36.
4. Drews LC, Drews RC. Optical iridectomy. Am J Ophthalmol. 1964;58:789-96.
5. Costenbader FD, Albert DG. Conservatism in the management of congenital cataract. Arch Ophthalmol. 1957;58:426-30.
6. Jünemann A, Gusek GC, Naumann GO. Optical sector iridectomy: an alternative to perforating keratoplasty in Peter's anomaly. Klin Monbl Augenheilkd. 1996;209:117-24.
7. Zaidman GW, Rabinowitz Y, Forstot SL. Optical iridectomy for corneal opacities in Peter's anomaly. J Cataract Refract Surg. 1998;24:719-22.
8. Vajpayee RB, Sharma N, Dada T, Pushker N. Optical sector iridectomy in corneal opacities. Cornea. 1999;18:262-4.
9. Sundaresh K, Jethani J, Vijayalakshmi P. Optical iridectomy in children with corneal opacities. J AAPOS. 2008;12:163-5.
10. Vajpayee RB, Vanathi M, Tandon R, Sharma N, Titiyal JS. Keratoplasty for keratomalacia in preschool children. Br J Ophthalmol. 2003;87:538-42.
11. Agarwal T, Jhanji V, Dutta P, Tandon R, Sharma N, Titiyal JS, Vajpayee RB. Automated vitrector-assisted optical iridectomy: Customized iridectomy. J Cataract Refract Surg. 2007;33(6): 959-61.
12. Agarwal T, Jhanji V, Dutta P, Titiyal JS. Automated vitrector-assisted optical iridectomy and phacoemulsification in eyes with coexisting cataract and adherent leucomas. Eye (Lond). 2009;23:1345-8.
13. Zaidman GW. Optical sector iridectomy in corneal opacities. Cornea. 2000;19:870.
14. Spierer O, Cavuoto KM, Suwannaraj S, McKeown CA, Chang TC. Outcome of optical iridectomy in Peters anomaly. Graefes Arch Clin Exp Ophthalmol. 2018;256:1679-83.

71

Corneal Tattooing

Nikhil S Gokhale

INTRODUCTION

Tattooing is an age-old procedure done to improve cosmesis in a corneal opacity. It was described way back by Galen using copper sulfate.[1] Despite advances in treatment of corneal disorders, tattooing continues to have a role in patients with corneal opacities.

BASIC PRINCIPLE

Corneal tattooing involves impregnation of colored substances into the corneal stroma to imitate the patient's iris and a central pupil. It not only enhances the cosmesis of the eye, but it may also be used for optical purposes by converting a diffuse semitransparent nebula with irregular edges into an opaque plaque with well-defined margins.[2] This eliminates the undesirable effect of irregular scattering of the light. In such cases, the light is refracted regularly by the surrounding clear cornea into the macula, thus giving an undistorted image. Although, this image has the disadvantage of small positive scotomata and a diminution of the intensity, it causes fewer disturbances to the patient as compared to an irregular distorted image due to a nebulomacular corneal opacity. This principle has also been used to treat the significant glare and monocular diplopia associated with traumatic iris defects and aniridia.[3]

INDICATIONS AND CONTRAINDICATIONS

Corneal tattooing is done for improving cosmesis in corneal opacities and mature white cataracts when there is a high chance of failures with other surgical methods. For cosmetic improvement, it may be undertaken for old, firm, and flat scars in quiet blind eyes, especially in cases where iris print contact lens is either not accepted by the patient or is uncomfortable. In selected cases with corneal opacity an optical iridectomy may be used in addition to tattooing as this confers an optical advantage especially when tattooed area covers a major part of the pupillary aperture (**Fig. 1**).[4] It has also been done to reduce glare or diplopia in eyes with large iris defects due to trauma or surgery.[3] It is contraindicated in cases of corneal ectasia and thin corneas due to the risk of intraoperative perforation, however, it can be done if combined with a lamellar tectonic keratoplasty. It can incite an iridocyclitis in eyes with adherent leukoma, anterior staphyloma, phthisis bulbi, and glaucoma.[4]

METHODS OF TATTOOING

The methods used to accomplish tattooing use two principles—(1) the chemical reduction method and (2) the direct method.

Chemical Reduction Methods

Colored pigments are deposited in the cornea through a chemical reaction using salts and reagents.[5] Different pigments are used to give different colors to match the other eye color. These techniques however have the disadvantage of the colors fading over time. However, being easy and quick the procedure can be repeated.[6]

Gold chloride, reduced by epinephrine or tannic acid gives a golden brown color while platinum chloride gives a jet black color.[6-8]

Platinum chloride is the preferred salt for corneal tattooing even today. The technique involves the removal

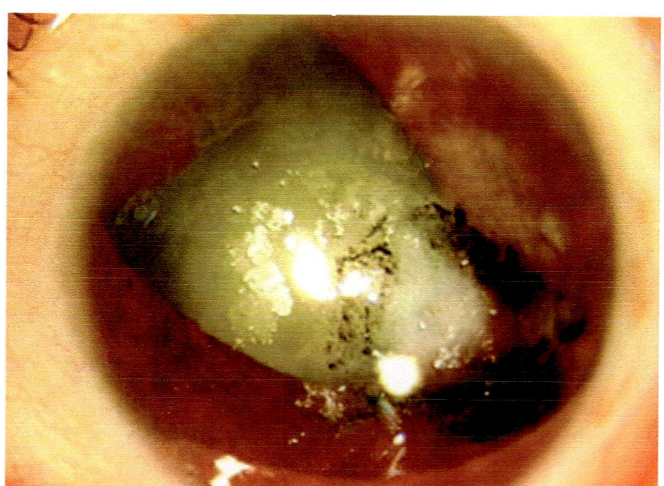

Fig. 1: Corneal tattooing with optical iridectomy.

of corneal epithelium over the opacified area and a piece of blotting paper of same size, soaked in fresh 2% solution of platinum chloride, is applied for 2 minutes to impregnate the subjacent tissues. On removal of the blotting paper, a few drops of fresh hydrazine hydrate 2% solution are poured for 25–30 seconds to reduce the platinum chloride. This causes precipitation of platinum black in situ making this area appears black in color. The eye is irrigated with saline, and a drop of parolein is instilled. Pad and bandage is applied over the eye. The epithelium grows over the black deposit of platinum black in 4–5 days. However, with the passage of time, the epithelium may breakdown.[9]

Tattooing with Gold Chloride

The procedure is done under topical anesthesia. The scar area to be tattooed is marked on the cornea and the surface is de-epithelialized. A freshly prepared solution of 2% gold chloride is used. pH is adjusted to a point of faint acidity with soda bicarbonate, so that litmus paper turns only slightly pink. The solution is then applied to the de-epithelialized corneal surface for 3–7 minutes. The duration of application determines the color obtained. Shorter applications give a lighter brown shade and longer ones give a darker shade. Two percent tannic acid solution (freshly prepared) is then applied to reduce the gold chloride. Alternatively, a solution of epinephrine 1:1,000 can be used. The treated area turns brown to black in about 2 minutes. The eye is patched with an antibiotic ointment and a cycloplegic. Patients are observed till corneal re-epithelialization is complete. In most cases, there is no significant inflammatory reaction.

Corneal Tattooing with Palladium Oxide

Vabutta and Toth reported a new method of the corneal tattooing by using palladium oxide, which is reduced by vitamin C solution. This is simpler than other methods and is said to give the best cosmetic results. It produces a deep black color, which lasts for many years.[10]

Proper demarcation of the pupillary area and the colored area corresponding to the iris is essential for a good cosmetic result. Anastas (1995) used excimer laser to create a perfectly circular corneal bed for the pupil.[11] Holth (1928) used a variety of solutions to achieve different colors of the corneal tattoo. About 5% $FeSO_4$ gives a black color, silver salts a brown color, cobalt tannate a bluish color, and burnt sienna a greenish color.[12]

Direct Inoculation Methods

Direct introduction of the coloring agent into the corneal stroma is an older and a crude method of corneal tattooing. It is technically more difficult, more time consuming, and requires experienced handling of the needles. However, it produces more permanent results as compared to the chemical reduction methods.[13] This is due to the fact that these dyes tend to be phagocytosed by the keratocytes thus preventing leaching of the dyes. When chemical reduction method is used, the metallic compounds are mainly deposited in the extracellular matrix of cornea thus allowing early fading of the color.[14]

The dye may be inoculated into the corneal stroma with the help of various instruments such as 10/0 suture needle, hollow needle, bundle of thin needles, and blepharopigment needle. A 26-gauge hypodermic needle bent as a capsulotomy needle can also be used for the same purpose. This has the advantage of easy availability and prevents inadvertent full-thickness corneal perforation. Tattooing with needles is a longer and more tedious procedure, which may require two or more sittings for completion. The dye may also be inserted into a lamellar pocket made in the cornea in the area of opacity.[15] This can be used in cases where the superficial stroma is clear.

With this method also there is corneal reaction but is comparatively less as compared to the chemical methods. Other complications include under and over coloring, change in color over time, migration of pigment, corneal perforation, uveitis, and infection. Various coloring agents, which directly stain the cornea, are Indian ink, combination of Chinese ink and gold dust, uveal pigment from animal eyes, lamp black candle soot, animal charcoal, titanium dioxide (blue and white), ferric oxide (Fe_2O_3 brown), iron oxide (Fe_3O_4 black). Use of iron compounds carries a theoretical risk of toxicity though the compound used contain ferric form which is nontoxic for ocular tissues.[14]

Corneal Needle Tattooing with Pigments

Lampblack or India ink may be used to produce a black pupil. Stored powders or inks can be autoclaved for sterilizing them. Lampblack can be freshly prepared in the operation theater using a burner and a small bowl to collect the soot. In this technique, the surface is not de-epithelialized after marking the area of treatment. A thick paste of black pigment is prepared by adding a few drops of sterile saline to the powder. A small amount of this paste is placed on the area to be treated. A multiple tattoo needle is held slanting at about 45° and multiple superficial punctures are made into the corneal stroma. This drives the pigment into the subepithelium and anterior stroma underneath. The pigment is washed off to check the color obtained and the process is repeated till satisfactory coloration is achieved. It is better to achieve a darker color than desired to compensate for the slight reduction of color with time. Postoperative care is similar to chemical methods. Being a simple technique, it can be repeated if necessary. Breaks in the conjunctival mucosa should be avoided to prevent inadvertent staining of the conjunctival surface. A three-edged spatula needle (CSA-48°C) available with a conventional 10-0 nylon suture can also be used for this technique. Commercially available tattoo machines (**Fig. 2**) with micropuncture needles, which have puncture depth setting are now available and give very good results (**Fig. 3**). They are definitely better than manual micropuncture with a 26-gauge needle.

Corneal Tattooing with Pigments (Lamellar Pocket Method)

This method is beneficial for cases with a clear superficial cornea. A partial thickness incision is made in the peripheral cornea which is extended to a lamellar intracorneal pocket in a plane anterior to the opacity. The pigment is made into a thick paste after mixing with a few drops of saline and inserted into the pocket. This technique has the advantage of requiring only single sitting with more permanent results (**Fig. 4**).[16]

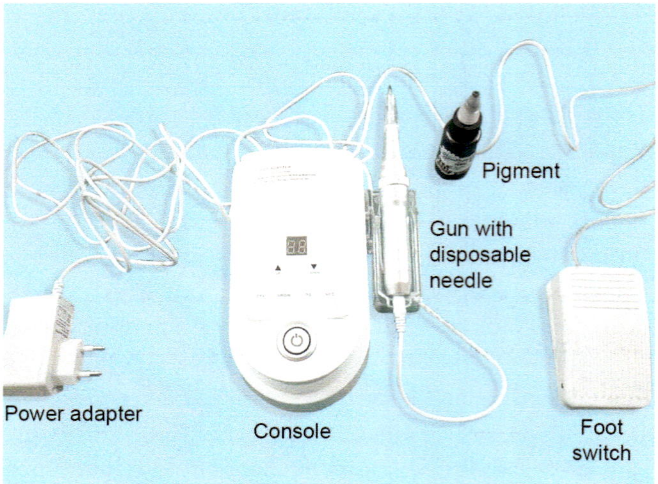

Fig. 2: Commercially available tattoo machine.
Courtesy: Dr Aditya Pradhan, Disha Eye Hospital.

Use of femtosecond laser has also been described as a tool to create lamellar flaps and pockets for corneal tattooing.[16,17] A free flap can be created with femtosecond laser which can be dipped in tattooing pigment and then repositioned on the corneal bed.[16] The versatility of the femtosecond laser can also be used to create a lamellar pocket where the pigment can be injected as a paste.[17] The limitation of the femtosecond laser-based techniques include the high cost and the inability of the laser to penetrate opaque cornea. This prevents the use of this technique for most of the patients especially where, the opacity also involves the subepithelial stroma.

Lamellar Keratoplasty with Interface Tattoo

This technique is useful for patients with dense full-thickness scarring with an irregular anterior surface profile scars following multiple failed surgeries, trauma, ectatic scars, scars with calcific or degenerative changes, etc. can all be managed with this technique. A large trephine mark is made and with the help of lamellar dissectors a superficial dissection is done to raise a free flap, which is then excised. Care needs to be taken to avoid perforation. A preoperative

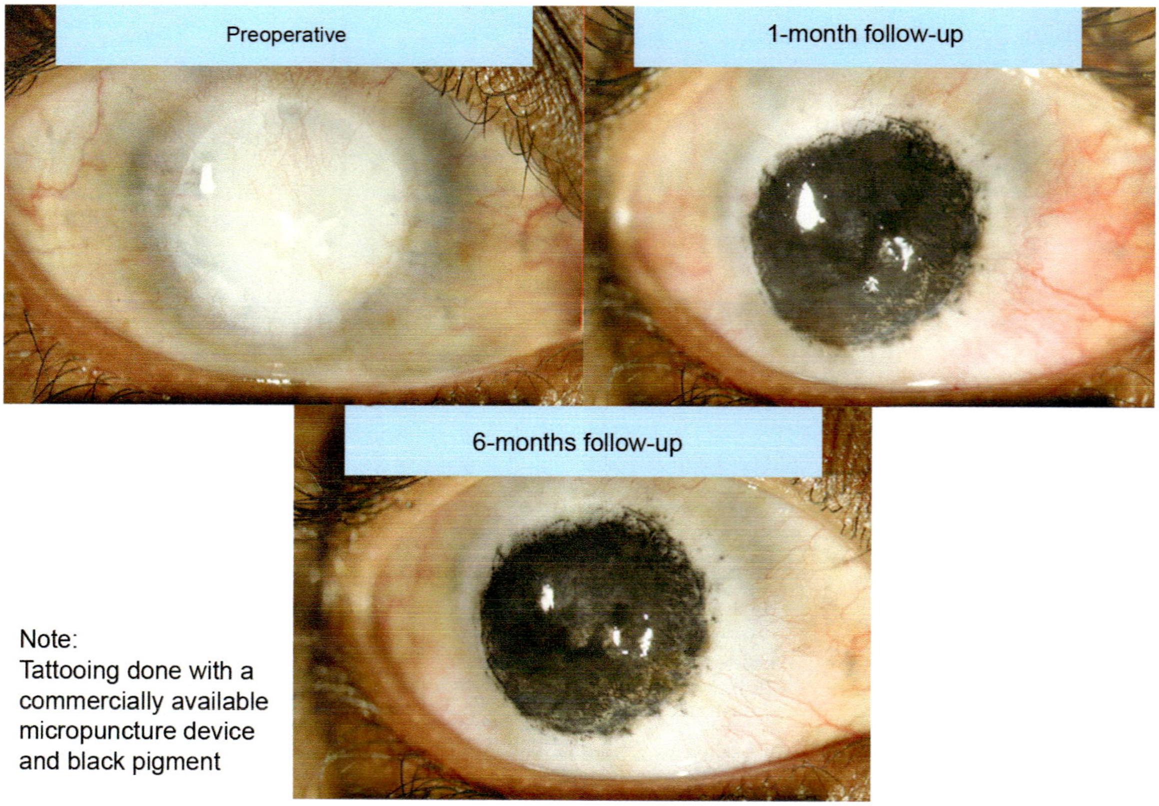

Fig. 3: Preoperative and postoperative pictures of tattooing with micropuncture device.
Courtesy: Dr Aditya Pradhan, Disha Eye Hospital.

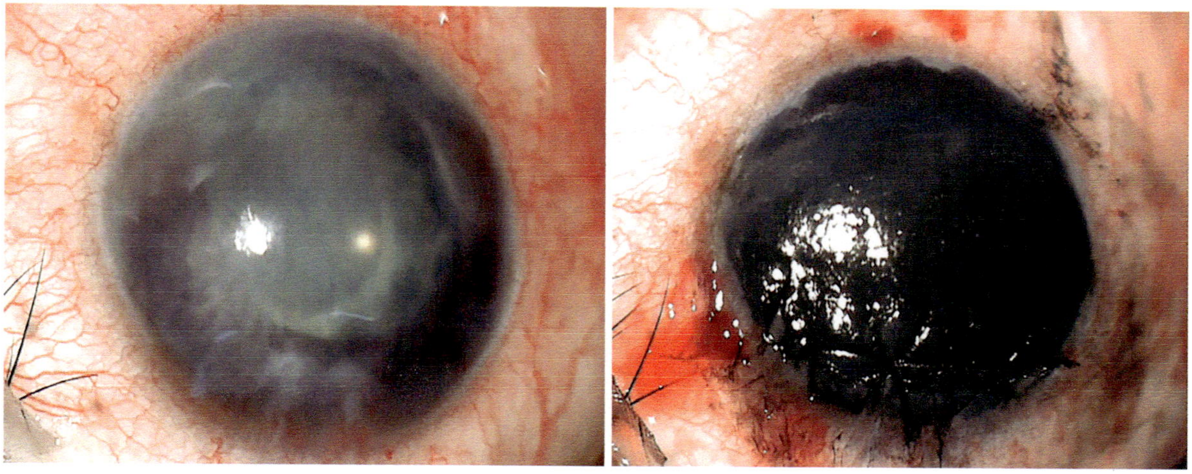

Fig. 4: Lamellar pocket with tattoo.
Courtesy: Dr Aditya Pradhan, Disha Eye Hospital.

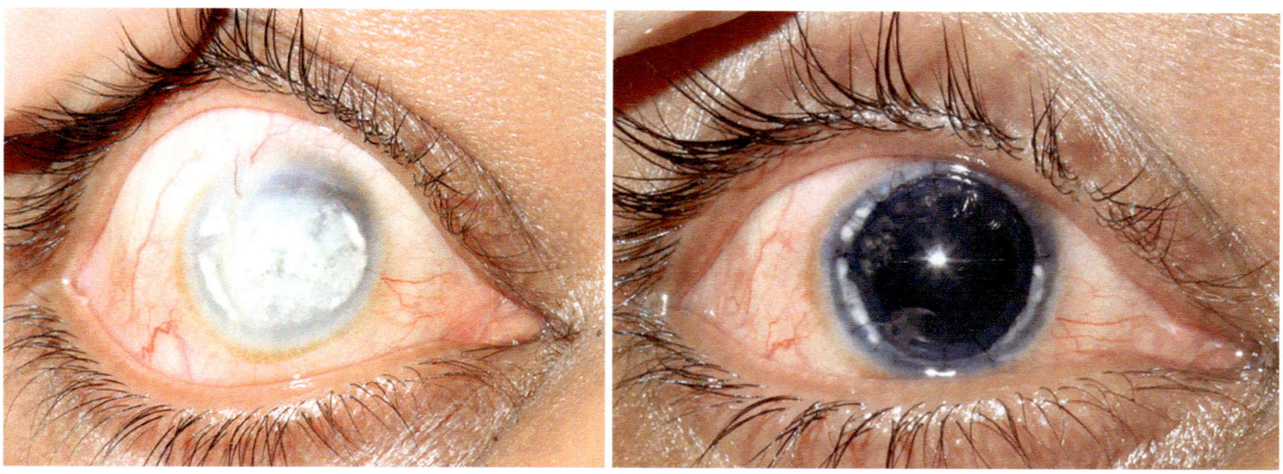

Fig. 5: Corneal opacification with extensive calcareous degeneration. Postlamellar graft with interface tattoo.

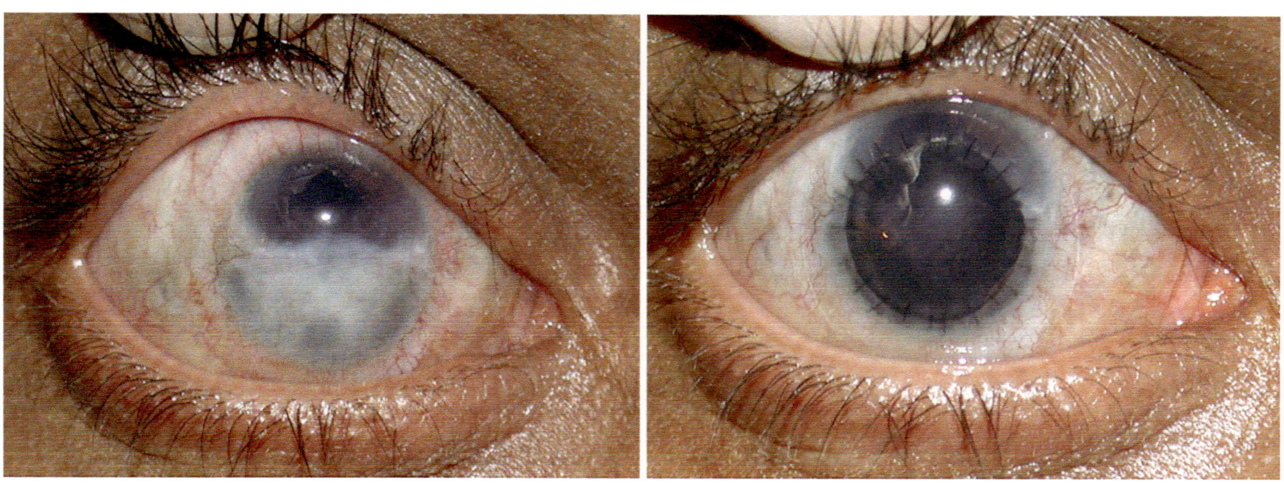

Fig. 6: Post-trauma and multiple failed surgeries with dense scarring following an interface tattoo with lamellar graft.

AS-OCT can be helpful in planning these surgeries. The peripheral host rim is undermined with a lamellar dissector till the limbus. Pigment is directly applied to the bed and also pushed into the peripheral rim pocket till the limbus all around. A 0.25-mm oversized corneal lamellar graft is dissected from a donor cornea fixed onto a King's clamp or an artificial anterior chamber. The graft is sutured with interrupted sutures. This provides tectonic support, a smooth anterior surface, and traps the pigment in the interface. The long-term results of this technique are excellent, though follow-up care is needed till all sutures are removed (**Figs. 5 and 6**).

PRESENT STATUS

The practice of corneal tattooing to conceal cosmetically bad corneal opacities is still actively practiced. Though cosmetic contact lenses may give superior cosmesis than tattooing, it is still a very good alternative for patients with intolerance to contact lenses due to irregular corneal curvature or ocular surface problems.

Tattooing may also serve as a cheaper and safer alternative to cosmetic contact lenses for patients living in tropical climates and for those with poor socioeconomic and hygienic status.

REFERENCES

1. Duke-Elder S. Disease of the outer eye. London: Henry Krimptom Publishers/Mosby; 1977.
2. Duggan JN, Nanavati BP. Tattooing of corneal opacity with gold and platinum chloride. Br J Ophthalmol. 1936;20:419-2.
3. Beekhuis WH, Drost BH, van der Velden/Samderubun EM. A new treatment for photophobia in post-traumatic aniridia: A case report. Cornea. 1998;17:338-41.
4. Knapp AA. Corneal graft or tattooing with iridectomy? With a brief report on corneal studies after electrocution. Nav Med Bull Wash. 1944;42:1366-70.
5. Forbes SB. New pigment for corneal tattooing. Am J Ophthalmol. 1960;50:325.
6. Gifford SR, Steinberg A. Gold and silver impregnation of the cornea for cosmetic purposes. Am J Ophthalmol. 1927;10:240-7.
7. Levis RJ. The new operation for coloring corneal opacities. Phil Med Times. 1946;3:1872-3.
8. Pischel DK. Tattooing the cornea with gold and platinum chloride. Arch Ophthalmol. 1930;3:176.
9. Taylor CB. The art of tinting opacities of the cornea. Br Med J. 1872;2:214.
10. Vebutta A, Toth I. New operative method for corneal tattooing. Szemeszet. 1960;97:78-81.
11. Anastas CN, McGhee CN, Webber SK, Bryce IG. Corneal tattooing revisited: Excimer laser in the treatment of unsightly leucomata. Aust N Z J Ophthalmol. 1995;23:227-30.
12. Miller SJH. Parson's diseases of the eye (Eighteenth edition). London: Churchill Livingstone; 1990.
13. Pitz S, Jahn R, Frisch L, Duis A, Pfeiffer N. Corneal tattooing: An alternative treatment for disfiguring corneal scars. Br J Ophthalmol. 2002;86:397-9.
14. Mannis MJ, Eghbali K, Schwab IR. Keratopigmentation: A review of corneal tattooing. Cornea. 1999;18:633-7.
15. Burris TE, Holmes-Higgin DK, Silvestrini TA. Lamellar intrastromal corneal tattoo for treating iris defects (artificial iris). Cornea. 1998;17:169-73.
16. Kymionis GD, Ide T, Galor A, Yoo SH. Femtosecond-assisted anterior lamellar corneal staining-tattooing in a blind eye with leukocoria. Cornea. 2009;28:211-3.
17. Kim JH, Lee D, Hahn TW, Choi SK. New surgical strategy for corneal tattooing using a femtosecond laser. Cornea. 2009;28:80-4.

72 Prosthetic Contact Lenses

Monica Chaudhry

INTRODUCTION

Failed grafts may lead to dense corneal scars and prosthetic contact lenses support as an important beneficial tool in the management of diseased and disfigured eyes. This article discusses general clinical fitting considerations of prosthetic soft contact lenses and highlights the use of an opaque hydrogel prosthetic lens with a decompensated cornea secondary to failed keratoplasties.[1]

A blind or disfigured eye which is not enucleated but has maintained its shape is ideal indication for this kind of lenses. Acceptance for enucleation is a mental trauma and this lens offers respite as it is noninvasive and a good substitute to cover the opaque corneas. The look may not be as instinctive but much more cosmetically appealing compared to the eye without it.

One of the major benefits is upturn in mental well-being. The disfigured scarred eye inhibits one from socializing and interacting. Loneliness, depression, and inferiority complex are frequently observed in these patients. Enhancing the cosmetic appearance brings in a change in quality of life of such individuals. Their social interaction improves, and confidence builds up.[2]

The soft contact lens with iris painted on the front surface hides the corneal scars. These are like regular soft contact lens material with customized iris and pupil painted over it. To fit them the eyeball should be complete. If the eye is enucleated or shrunken, a prosthetic scleral shell is the option proposed and it is referred to an ocularist for management.[3]

PROSTHETIC LENS OPTIONS

Prosthetic contact lens is available in soft lens material and can be customized to range diameters from 13 to even 18 mm size. The standard options are available in 14 mm size soft lens, hydrogel material with 11 mm iris paint zone, and about 4.5 mm pupil size. The standard parameters usually fit most of the eyes. However, one-fourth of the patients may require further customization.

Tints and shades of brown iris color typical to Indian iris color are available as light, medium, and dark tint. These can further be customized to make the tint shade lighter or darker to match the good eye by the local laboratory. Silicone hydrogel material is also an option available globally but not in our country. Indian iris shades are predictable and straightforwardly matchable compared to light colored irises. Iris colors other than brown or black are available across some global brands.

Prosthetic soft lenses are broadly classified into two main designs:

1. Iris painted (**Fig. 3**) center clear (**Fig. 1**)
2. Iris painted center black/opaque (**Fig. 2**)

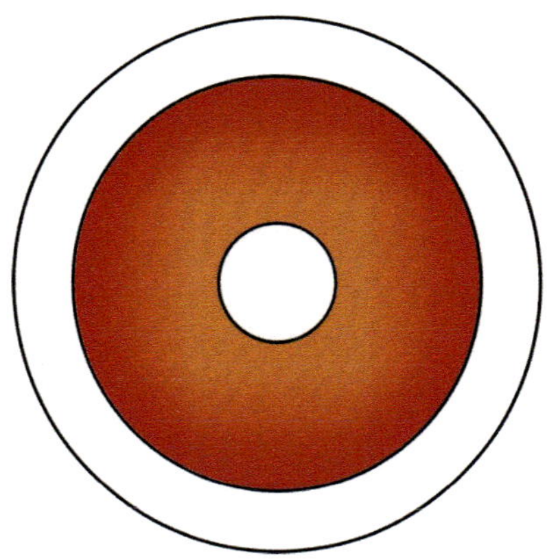

Fig. 1: Iris painted clear pupil.

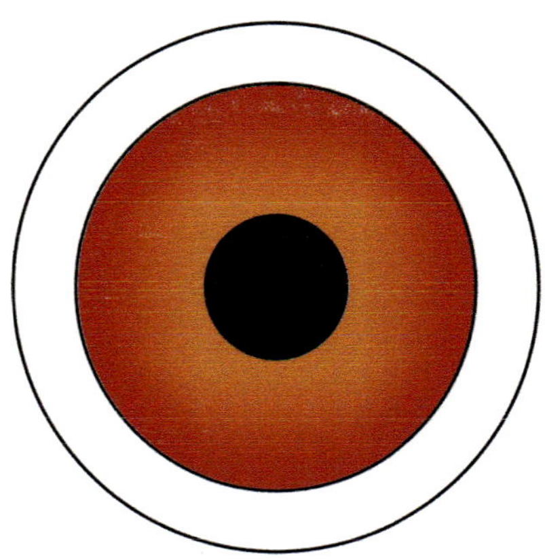

Fig. 2: Iris painted black pupil.

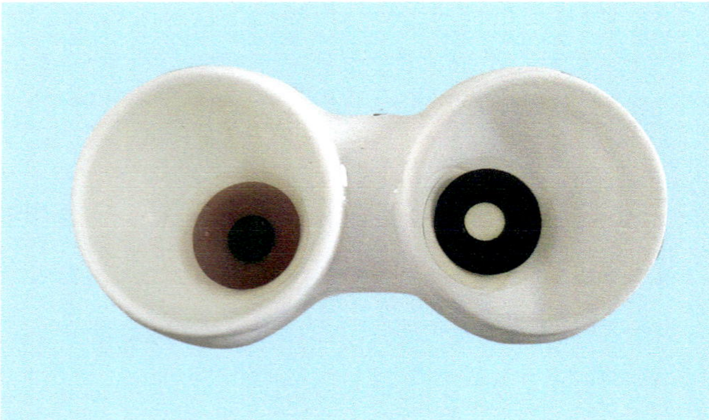

Fig. 3: Center dark and center clear iris painted prosthetic lens.

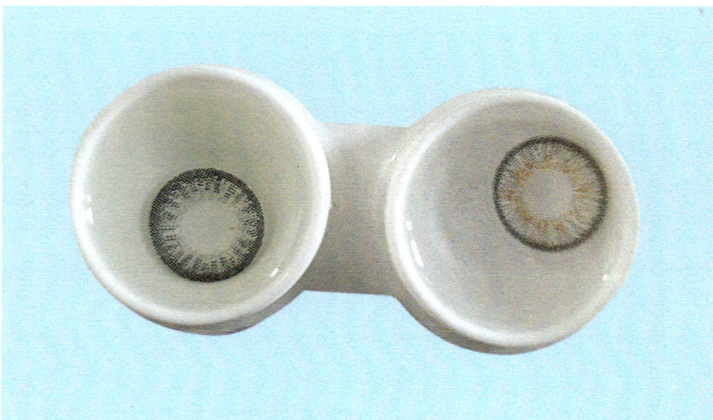

Fig. 4: Transparent tinting.

Indications of center clear pupil are in conditions such as albinism, aniridia, coloboma, microphthalmos which has some practical residual vision.

With a nonseeing eye, one has the possibility of using a black opaque pupil. If there is nothing to hide in the pupil area then there is no need to use an opaque pupil in the lens.

The iris painting can be of three types:

1. Transparent tinting—which enhances the natural tones of the iris. It is like making brown iris more enhanced or mixed with shades of blue, green or grey (**Fig. 4**).
2. Standard tint—these are standard tones of iris in light, medium, dark iris tones, and are customized lathe cut soft lenses. Most of Indian eyes would match the standard shades and are less expensive and easily reproducible (**Fig. 5**).
3. *Customized tinting*: It is hand painted or customized matching of the iris.

Iris rim enhancer—where the zone of iris is only added to increase the size of the cornea like in case of microcornea or microphthalmos or shrunken eye (**Fig. 6**).

The use of prosthetic contact lenses is:

- Reducing glare and photophobia in conditions by using a clear pupil design.
- Enhancing contrast—by adding contrast enhancing color tint in the pupil area. These are typical yellow-colored tints which augment the contrast acuity. This is less prescribed in postgraft eye.

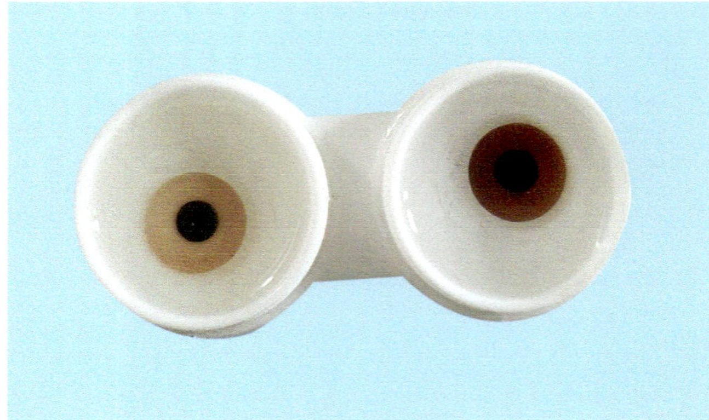

Fig. 5: Standard tint.

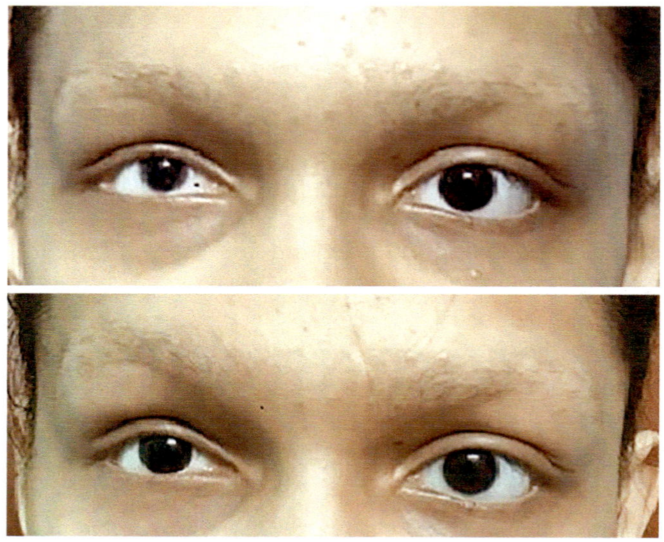

Fig. 6: Iris rim enhancer prosthetic lens.

- Occluder lens—by using the dark opaque center dark pupil to prevent diplopia, and mostly used for occlusion therapy.

PREFIT EXAMINATION

- Prefitting evaluation of eye begins with assessment to rule out contraindication of contact lenses.
- Lose sutures, severe dryness, neovascularization, active abrasion, papillae, etc., are few contraindications specific to these corneas.
- *Assess the visual acuity status*: Blind eyes with disfigurement or scar in the center, select the center. For patients who have residual vision, the best-corrected visual acuity and refraction needs to be incorporated in the contact lens, optic zone and the pupil area needs to be kept clear, so select center clear design.
- *Corneal curvature and topography measurements*: These may or may not be attainable in the scarred eye. The corneal curvature measurement and diameter of the fellow eye are then taken as the reference.
- Images or simple digital smart phone pictures of eyes both healthy and unhealthy are taken in the beginning. This is done for documentation and even reference guide shared with laboratory in case customization has to be done.

The essential measurements of the affected and the fellow eye are:

- Horizontal visible iris diameter (HVID)
- Pupil diameter in bright, average, and dim light conditions
- Visual acuity and refraction with best-corrected visual acuity in each eye
- *Observe and note the following*:
  - Iris color
  - Any hyperemia of the conjunctiva/sclera
  - Careful examination of the tears, cornea, limbus, conjunctivas, and lids using the slit-lamp microscope
  - Position and nature of scar tissue
- Custom hand-painted contact lenses are selected from the catalog. Although there is a limited range of iris colors available with shades, yet corresponding Indian iris colors with diameters are available which is expected to fit nearly all eyes. By small alterations and customization almost all eyes can attain the desired cosmetic and anatomic result.

PROSTHETIC FITTING PROCEDURE

Prosthetic matching process: The first step is to liaise with the local laboratory, who shall generate the lens and same trial lens set should be used. For Indian eyes the shades of light, medium, and dark brown tint with standard base curve should be kept ready at hand. The trial set with standard base curve, diameter, iris size, and pupil size is put as trial on the eye and variations to customize based on this trial. Select a shade darker than the healthy eye as the whiteness of the corneal scar at the back of the prosthetic lens also varies the color of the lens.

The laboratory needs to be sent descriptions and estimated parameters to customize for the patient. Like the HVID of the healthy eye should match the HVID of scarred eye. Photograph taken in room light and natural light helps a lot in matching and guides the local laboratory too.

Expectations of the patients can be handled by using these trial lenses. The match is never comparable to the normal eye and the observer can identify the non-natural look of the eye from a closer view. There is a constraint to the wearing hours since they are usually hydrogel material soft lens and the eye itself is not a healthy cornea. The recommendation is to use it for average 8 hours a day or even less if the cornea is compromised. Most of the patients would use it while going outdoors or only during social interactions. Long-term hypoxia complications are a possibility if worn for longer hours and worse if used for extended wear that is during sleep. Additionally, the dye used in tinting itself adds to poor oxygen transmission. Nevertheless, the rewards are still many that patients are willing to curb its own expectations.

The trial lens method is advisable as the patient can then appreciate the difference and have an idea of the outcome. Response to the lens wear and fitting assessment can also be done on the eye. In case the trial set is not available then the local laboratory can be sent the corneal curvatures, HVID, pupil size of the healthy eye and refraction and pictures of the unhealthy eye. Based on these measurements, the laboratory can make an empirical lens and the fine-tuning can be done with this lens on the patient's eye.

To summarize the steps are:

- History and indication for the lens assessment
- Rule out contraindication of contact lens wear if any and ensure eye condition is healthy. Manage that before lens wear.
- Record corneal curvature of both healthy and unhealthy eye with the help of keratometer. It is usually the healthy eye taken as reference for base curve calculation.
- Other measurements are HVID, that is the white-to-white diameter of the healthy eye to determine the painted iris dimensions. The pupil size is also measured to determine the pupil size such that it matches the good eye.
- Use a diagnostic lens. Local brands usually give standard base curve and diameter in three shades—(1) dark, (2) medium, and (3) light brown, select a hue which you feel is best match and match the one closest by picking various hues from the trial set. This match should be done in both indoor and natural light outdoors. Patient expectations on matching the hue should be set as the painted lens may still have some synthetic look when observed from very close distance.
- Wait for the lens to settle on the eye and then do the slit-lamp biomicroscopic assessment of the fit. Normal fitting criteria apply for aspects such as push-up test, lens movement between blinks, excursion movements, etc. The eye is kept under observation over time in order to assess if these compromises are adversely affecting the ocular tissues (**Figs. 7 and 8**). The bottom line is that the lens should be comfortable, stable, and allow sufficient tear exchange.
- Generally, such lenses fit slightly larger (0.5 mm) than normal to get the best centration. If some sector of the underlying cornea is showing, larger iris portion in 0.5 mm steps can be ordered.

PROBLEMS IN FITTING

Sometimes fitting this soft lens may lead the issue of lens centration. If there have been any severe changes in the corneal topography, perilimbal scarring or chemosis; there is a chance that the lens may not center well. Additionally, the fit of the lens periphery and edge may well be compromised. However, this may not mean that fitting is impossible—one needs to advise the patient that wearing time might be limited and/or the white of the eye may become a little pink with lens wear. One must accept some compromises in fitting compared to normal lenses on normal eyes. If centration is

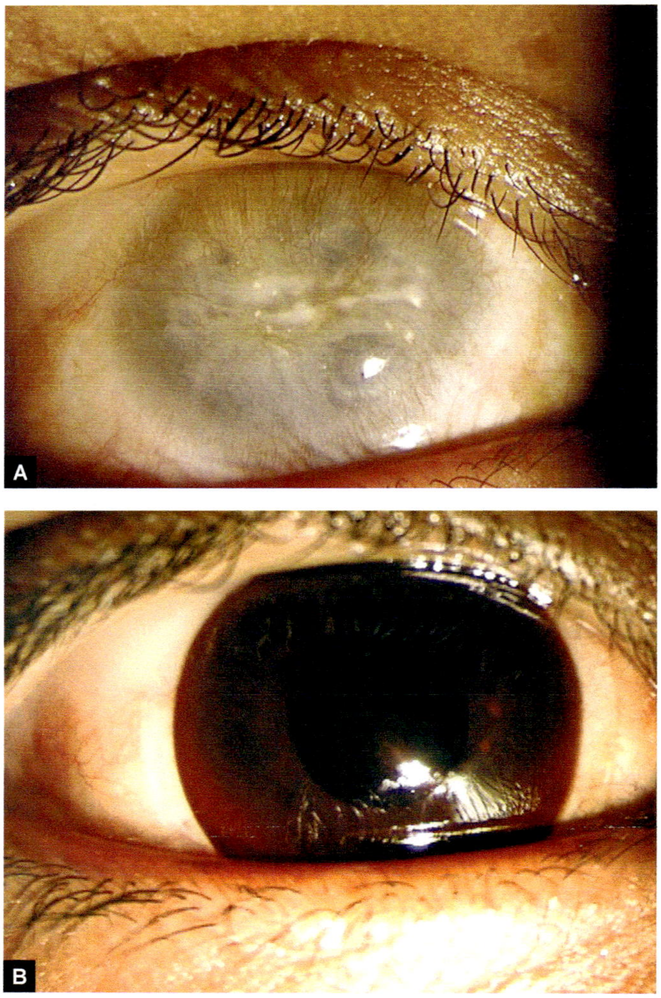

Figs. 7A and B: (A) Corneal opacity; (B) Prosthetic contact lens with iris painted center dark pupil covering the white opaque cornea.

poor, trying a larger total diameter could help. To assess the tolerance in terms of comfort a clear soft lens with customized base curve can first be ordered and later refinement over the first lens may be done. Shades or sunglasses can be worn over them to overcome mild variations in the shades. They also protect the healthy eye which is a vital recommendation.

Pupil size problems: This is always a difficult decision because the pupil size will not be correct when the fellow pupil is noticeably smaller or larger. Sometimes, this difference in pupil size can be noticeable and is of concern to the patient. One should try to aim for a size in average photopic conditions so that in bright light the lens' pupil is slightly bigger and in dull conditions the lens' pupil is slightly smaller. If you have some trial lenses with different size pupils, this is useful. The patient can take a mirror and look at the effects in different light conditions while ignoring the color of the trial lenses. If in doubt err toward the larger size as in dull conditions any difference will be less obvious. Indian eyes with dark brown irides are easily compromised in terms of pupil size and color, as there is less contrast between the pupil and iris colors.

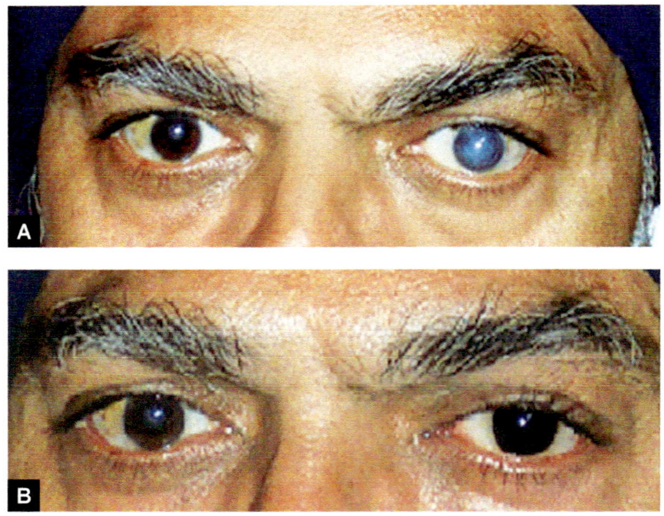

Figs. 8A and B: (A) Unilateral corneal opacity; (B) Prosthetic contact lens.

In case of pale iris, pay attention to the limbal ring, because otherwise the lens will look artificial. It is easier again to fit Indian eyes as the texture is more homogeneous compared to lighter eyes.

FOLLOW-UP

The lens schedule is built gradually from 2 hours first day to increasing 1 hour daily reaching maximum of 8 hours in a week. The first follow-up is done after 1 week, where the patient is instructed to wear the lens for 4 hours at least and visit the clinic.

The aftercare includes assessment of lens on the eye first followed by removal of lens and evaluating the eye and cornea with fluorescein. Any staining indicates an intervention and management should be accordingly done. The lenses available in our country are hydrogel material and one has to follow-up the patients and ensure no hypoxia signs arise. These signs can be corneal edema, neovascularization, limbal hyperemia, etc. The follow-up should ideally be done every 3 months and lenses should be replaced frequently. The usual replacement schedule is quarterly disposability.

PROSTHETIC LENS CARE

The care and maintenance are similar to clear soft lenses. Since they are lathe cut lenses with quarterly disposability, protein removal regimen can be recommended. Peroxide-based solutions are usually avoided as it leads to discoloration. Solution compatibility can be an issue and if any such toxicity is seen, combination of different preservative based solution should be used. Regular replacement of such lenses is also important and shorter is better. Set of four lenses as frequent planned replacement is provided to the patient as an annual supply.

Prosthetic lens fitting encompasses the disfigurement of the eye in many cases thus avoiding enucleation. These lenses are an appealing option for patients postgraft disfigurements and corneal scars. The enhancement of cosmetic appearance and retaining the integrity of the orbit improves the mental health of the patient.[4-6]

REFERENCES

1. Kanemoto M, Toshida H, Takahiro I, Murakami A. Prosthetic soft contact lenses in Japan. Eye Contact Lens. 2007;33:300-3.
2. Yildirim N, Basmak H, Sahin A. Prosthetic contact lenses: Adventure or miracle. Eye Contact Lens. 2006;32:102-3.
3. Bator KK, Salituro SM. Prosthetic soft contact lenses and you. Eye Contact Lens. 2005;31:215-8.
4. Yildirim N, Basmak H, Sahin A. Prosthetic contact lenses: Adventure or miracle. Eye Contact Lens. 2006;32(2):102-3.
5. Barron C, Dishman A, Garofalo R, Akerman D, Bekritsky G. Opaque hydrogel prosthetic contact lens correction for the disfigured eye. Int Contact Lens Clin. 1992;19(5):125-9.
6. Kamble VB, Kumar M, Panigrahi D. An ocular prosthesis for a geriatric patient: A case report. J Clin Diagn Res. 2013; 7(6):1236-8.

73 Gundersen Flap

Prakash Chand Agarwal, Sarath S, Ritu Nagpal, Namrata Sharma, Rasik B Vajpayee

INTRODUCTION

Schoeler in Berlin described a conjunctival flap in 1877, which was later popularized by Kuhnt in 1884. Byers described flaps in cataract surgery, eviscerations, and corneoscleral lacerations in 1912. In 1927, Green advocated wound healing by conjunctivalization to be beneficial for corneal ulcerations, Mooren's ulcer and for corneal perforations.

In 1958, Gunderson described a technique for creating a thin conjunctival flap, devoid of the underlying tenon's fascia.[1] Such thin flaps allow permanent coverage of the diseased cornea. Gundersen flaps may be performed as a temporary procedure in acute cases, later on to be followed up by a suitable optical rehabilitation procedure such as a penetrating keratoplasty. These can also be performed as a permanent procedure in eyes with chronic non-healing pathologies.

In addition to the total conjunctival flaps described by Gundersen, partial flaps may be used to cover a particular sector of the diseased cornea. Racquet flaps are created by rotating or swinging a flap of limbal conjunctiva onto the cornea. Thick flaps including the Tenon's fascia are beneficial in eyes with stromal melting and thinning (**Fig. 1**). Gunderson advocated the use of thick flaps in eyes with bullous keratopathy.

The exact mechanism for the success of conjunctival flaps remains unclear. In general prompt relief of pain is felt after flap placement. Inflammation subsides and refractory ulcers and necrotic areas heal with scar formation. Gunderson in his original description, hypothesized that a thin flap provides protection from tears and various irritants besides providing blood-borne factors from the conjunctival vessels (**Fig. 2**). These blood borne factors help to reduce the inflammation, allowing early healing and wound repair. Placement of a conjunctival flap also helps to provide tectonic support, especially if the underlying Tenon's fascia is included within the flap. Flaps help in the restoration of an epithelized ocular surface, thereby improving tear film stability, reducing patient's symptoms and the risk of phthisis bulbi. In eyes with bullous keratopathy, flaps help in alleviation of pain by covering the exposed nerve endings. In severe cases of herpetic stromal necrosis unresponsive

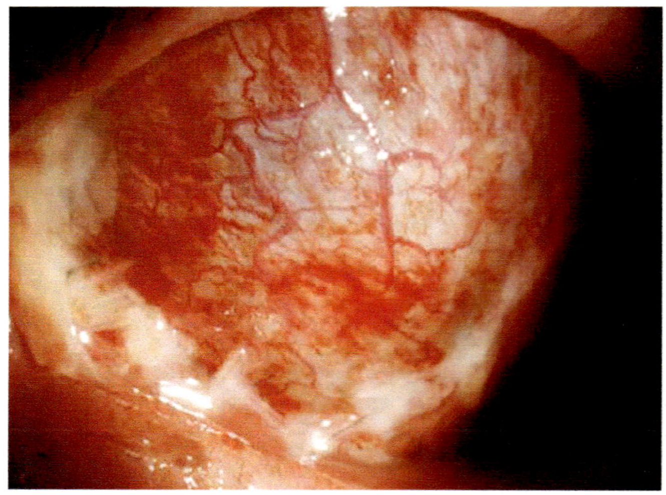

Fig. 1: Slit-lamp photograph of an eye with a thick conjunctival flap including the underlying Tenon's fascia.
Courtesy: Medical Photographic Imaging Centre, Royal Victorian Eye and Ear Hospital.

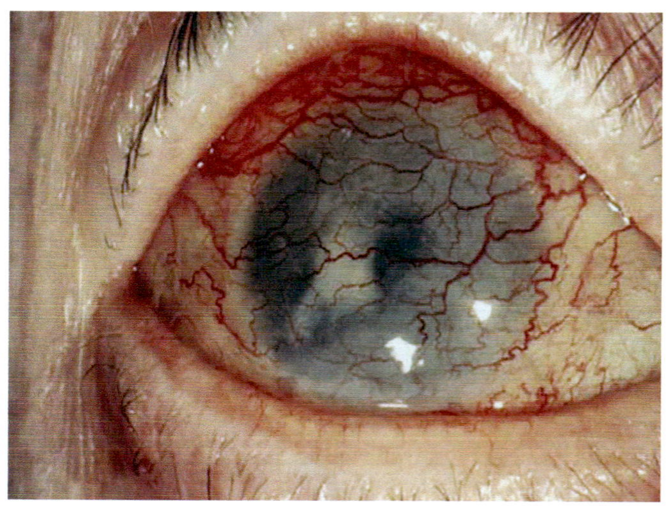

Fig. 2: Slit-lamp photograph of an eye with a thin vascularized flap.
Courtesy: Medical Photographic Imaging Centre, Royal Victorian Eye and Ear Hospital.

to topical and systemic antivirals, a conjunctival flap may often be the only effective means for arresting the inflammatory disease process. By providing a stable epithelial surface and introducing anti-inflammatory cytokines to the stromal bed, flaps helps to limit the active infective or inflammatory and stromal lysis.[2] In eyes with non-infective pathologies, such as neuroparalytic keratopathy, neutrophil recruitment and subsequent liberation of collagenases are the key factors responsible for the disease pathogenesis.[2] Introduction of vascularized structures at such sites helps to contain the process of tissue destruction, by bringing various anti-collagenolytic factors from the circulation.[3] Once the active infective or inflammatory process has settled down, flaps may be removed and replaced by a full thickness or a lamellar corneal graft combined with limbal stem cell transplantation in order to maintain the stability of the ocular surface.[4]

The Gundersen flap does have some disadvantages such as impairment of vision and inability to visualize the details of the anterior segment. This is more pronounced in eyes with thicker flaps. Monitoring the course of an infective pathology beneath the flap, might be difficult. This is more pronounced in eyes with thicker flaps. Persistence of infection with subsequent perforation under the flap has also been reported in case with herpetic stromal keratitis.[5]

Requirement of a relatively large area of healthy conjunctiva is another limiting factor, limiting its use in ocular surface diseases with significant conjunctival involvement and in eyes with a history of previous retinal or glaucoma surgery. Last but not the least, removal of the limbal epithelium results in limbal stem cell deficiency, necessitating a future limbal stem cell transplant in order to maintain the stability of the ocular surface.

SURGICAL TECHNIQUE

- Local anesthesia is achieved using a peribulbar block.
- The corneal epithelium is scraped off with the help of a blade or using a repositor. Any necrotic tissue is also removed. A superficial keratectomy may be performed if required. Areas of dystrophic calcification as well as any surface deposits or infiltrates should also be debrided.
- A 360° peritomy is done and hemostasis is achieved using a bipolar cautery.
- Either a superior rectus hook or a superior corneal traction suture may be secured.
- The area to be dissected is marked. The vertical height of the flap is marked at 15–18 mm above the superior limbus and the horizontal extent is kept around 18–20 mm.
- Conjunctiva is separated from the underlying Tenon's fascia by injecting lignocaine (2%) admixed with 1:100,000 epinephrine (1:100,000) in the subconjunctival space.
- The superior edge of the flap is incised horizontally.
- Blunt dissection is carried out using either a scissors or by using a moist cotton tip applicator. The flap is then pulled down to cover the cornea.
- The inferior edge of the flap is secured to the inferior limbus with 10-0 monofilament nylon sutures. The superior edge is secured to either with the superior limbus or the episcleral tissue.
- Antibiotic ointment is instilled and a pressure dressing is applied.

Sutures are removed at 1 month postoperatively.

Modifications and Evolution of Surgical Technique

Gundersen originally advocated performing lamellar keratectomy at the time of initial surgery, as being one of the essential steps for the success of a Gundersen flap.[6] Various reports later on however showed that lamellar keratectomy may not be necessary.[4,7] The original technique described by Gundersen in 1958, involved the use of thinner flaps, which were devoid of Tenon's fascia. However, later on modifications were done and surgeons used thicker flaps in eyes with corneal melting to prevent underlying tissue lysis. This has several advantages over the traditional Gundersen conjunctival flap, in terms of lower rates of flap retraction, and more resistance against tissue lysis. Gundersen flaps have also been combined with oral mucous membrane grafting in eyes with corneal melting following ocular burns.[8]

The use of Gundersen flap has considerably declined in the developed countries with the advent of other treatment options such as therapeutic penetrating keratoplasty, amniotic membrane transplants (AMTs),[9,10] therapeutic extended wear bandage contact lenses (BCLs),[11] and cultured epithelial transplantation techniques for ocular surface reconstruction.[12,13] These techniques represent significant technological advancements, but have their limitations in the form of limited availability of corneal donor tissue and laboratory equipment. The Gundersen flap is thus still a relevant but often overlooked procedure today. Gundersen flaps are mainly performed in cases with poor visual potential. In selected cases, conjunctival flaps also have the potential to improve visual acuity. Insler and Pechous[14] reported visual improvement in 8 of 33 patients (24%) with conjunctival flaps performed as the only procedure. In acutely inflamed eyes, conjunctival flaps may also be used as a temporizing measure and on an emergent basis to maintain the structural integrity of eye ball.[4]

Fibrin glue can be used as an alternative to suturing for securing the conjunctival flaps with optimal results.[15]

Microsurgical approach offers an appropriate option to the method developed by Gunderson without its deficiencies. The steps to an efficient pedicle conjunctival flap include choosing the proper site and size, movement of the flap without traction, conserving the flap's blood supply, avoiding cautery and conjunctival or corneal epithelial entrapment, debridement, application of povidone-iodine to infected ulcers, securing the flap over the denuded area with running 10-0 monofilament nylon sutures, and avoiding excessive traction on sutures.[16] The pedicle conjunctival flap can also supply further support in the healing of a corneal ulcer. Depending on the depth of the ulcer, it can be thin (without Tenon's capsule) in cases of superficial ulcers or thick (with Tenon's capsule) in eyes with deeper lesions.

Complications of Conjunctival Flap

Both intraoperative and postoperative complications can occur but most of these are avoidable by a careful case selection, preoperative evaluation and meticulous care with regards to instrumentation and surgical technique.[17] Suturing is one of the most essential steps for the success of this procedure. The flap over the cornea should not be too tight or too loose. Sutures that are too tight may cut through a tight flap and a loose conjunctival flap may not heal and get detached in the postoperative period.[18,19] The most frequently reported complications include:[20]

- Flap retraction
- Conjunctival buttonholes and erosions
- Epithelial inclusion cysts
- Persistence of infection and corneal perforations
- Ptosis
- Recurrence of the original pathology (**Fig. 3**).

Therapeutic keratoplasty, AMT, BCLs, and cultured ocular surface epithelial transplants have supplanted conjunctival flaps in many cases. These newer procedures are not without their complications and limitations. Donor corneal tissue is usually not freely available. AMT harvesting and preparation requires specialized equipment and technical expertise, with a small but definite risk of infectious or prion disease transmission. Extended wear BCLs are expensive, usually do not eliminate medication requirements, and are associated with an increased risk of microbial keratitis. The transplantation of cultured epithelial equivalents is perhaps the most promising modality, but it is technically difficult. For these reasons, and particularly in developing countries where the burden of disease frequently exceeds the capacity of the healthcare delivery system, Gundersen flap is still an important procedure and should be considered as a means of stabilizing globe integrity while managing cases with severe ocular surface diseases.

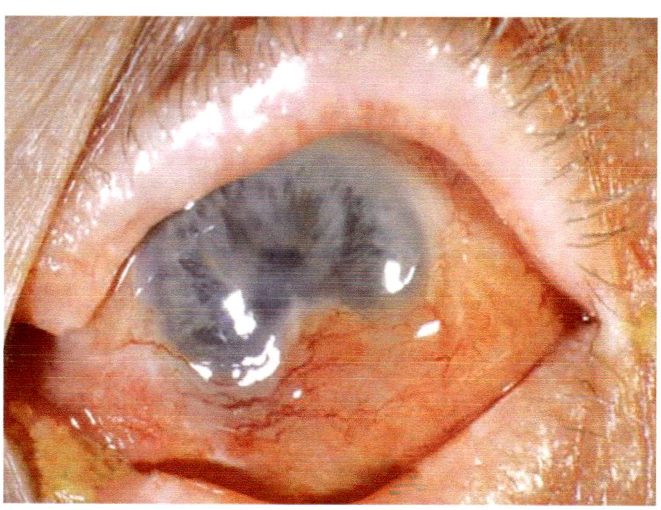

Fig. 3: Recurrence of original pathology following a Gundersen flap.
Courtesy: Medical Photographic Imaging Centre, Royal Victorian Eye and Ear Hospital.

REFERENCES

1. Gundersen T. Conjunctival flaps in the treatment of corneal disease with reference to a new technique of application. AMA Arch Ophthalmol. 1958;60:880-8.
2. Gundersen T, Pearlson HR. Conjunctival flaps for corneal disease: Their usefulness and complications. Trans Am Ophthalmol Soc. 1969;67:78-95.
3. Berman MB. The role of alpha-macroglobulins in corneal ulceration. Prog Clin Biol Res. 1976;5:225-59.
4. Geria RC, Zarate J, Geria MA. Penetrating keratoplasty in eyes treated with conjunctival flaps. Cornea. 2001;20:345-9.
5. Lesher MP, Lohman LE, Yeakley W, Lass J. Recurrence of herpetic stromal keratitis after a conjunctival flap surgical procedure. Am J Ophthalmol. 1992;114:231-3.
6. Gundersen T. Surgical treatment of bullous keratopathy. Arch Ophthalmol. 1960;64:260-7.
7. Gokhale NS. Penetrating keratoplasty after a total conjunctival flap. Indian J Ophthalmol. 2004;52:341-2.
8. Cheng KC, Chang CH. Modified Gunderson conjunctival flap combined with an oral mucosal graft to treat an intractable corneal lysis after chemical burn: A case report. Kaohsiung J Med Sci. 2006;22:247-51.
9. Sippel KC, Ma JJ, Foster CS. Amniotic membrane surgery. Curr Opin Ophthalmol. 2001;12:269-81.
10. Fernandes M, Sridhar MS, Sangwan VS, Rao GN. Amniotic membrane transplantation for ocular surface reconstruction. Cornea. 2005;24:643-53.
11. Arora R, Jain S, Monga S, Narayanan R, Raina UK, Mehta DK. Efficacy of continuous wear PureVision contact lenses for therapeutic use. Cont Lens Anterior Eye. 2004;27:39-43.
12. Kinoshita S, Koizumi N, Sotozono C, Yamada J, Nakamura T, Inatomi T. Concept and clinical application of cultivated epithelial transplantation for ocular surface disorders. Ocul Surf. 2004;2:21-33.
13. Ang LP, Nakamura T, Inatomi T, Sotozono C, Koizumi N, Yokoi N, et al. Autologous serum-derived cultivated oral epithelial transplants for severe ocular surface disease. Arch Ophthalmol. 2006;124:1543-51.
14. Insler MS, Pechous B. Conjunctival flaps revisited. Ophthalmic Surg. 1987;18:455-8.
15. Chung HW, Mehta JS. Fibrin glue for Gundersen flap surgery. Clin Ophthalmol. 2013;7:479-84.
16. Khodadoust A, Quinter AP. Microsurgical approach to the conjunctival flap. Arch Ophthalmol. 2003;121:1189-93.
17. Mannis MJ. Conjunctival flaps. Int Ophthalmol Clin. 1988;28: 165-8.
18. Cremona G, Carrasco MA, Tytiun A, Cosentino MJ. Treatment of advanced acanthamoeba keratitis with deep lamellar keratectomy and conjunctival flap. Cornea. 2002;21:705-8.
19. Grange JD, Duquesne N, Roubeyrol F, Branisteanu D, Sandon K, Fleury J, et al. Double irradiation for macroscopic radioresistance or recurrence of melanomas of the posterior uvea: Clinical, ballistic, therapeutic and prognostic aspects. Series of 19 cases among 462 patients. J Fr Ophtalmol. 1999;22:1054-63.
20. Lim LS, How AC, Ang LP, Tan DT. Gundersen flaps in the management of ocular surface disease in an Asian population. Cornea. 2009;28:747-51.

74

Future Developments

Vishal Jhanji, Karl David Brown, Ritu Nagpal, Sarath S, Hugh R Taylor

INTRODUCTION

Corneal surgery has come a long way since Dr Edward Zirm performed the first successful corneal transplantation in 1905. In the succeeding 30 years, corneal transplants were rare, and used only from tissues obtained from the living donors. In those days, cornea was removed from the donor, who was often in the same operating room as the person receiving the donated tissue. We are fortunate to have been practicing in an era with a well-established eye banking system, better transport media, binocular microscopes, and novel surgical instruments. Despite these significant advances in the field of corneal transplantation, issues like management of high-risk keratoplasty and prevention of graft failure remain major concerns. This is especially relevant for high-risk cases such as chemical injury, chronic inflammatory conditions, and repeated grafts.[1,2] In this chapter we will briefly discuss ongoing developments in the field of corneal diseases with an emphasis on treatment options that aim to increase the sucess rates and provide for improved utilization of existing resources, particularly the donor tissues. The main focus areas for the development of corneal treatments include:

- Component surgery of the cornea
- Development of artificial cornea
- Novel surgical techniques
- Cultured corneal endothelial cells
- Regenerative medicine and gene therapy

COMPONENT SURGERY OF THE CORNEA

The cornea consists of three cellular layers: (1) epithelium, (2) corneal stroma (comprising most of the corneal thickness), and (3) the single-layered endothelium. Each layer of the cornea is prone to disease or injury that can cause irreversible opacification and decreased visual acuity.[3]

Although penetrating keratoplasty (PKP) has long been the standard procedure for transplanting corneal tissue, all three layers of the cornea may not be needed in cases where, disease is limited to a specific layer only.[3] For example, PKP may not be required in every case of bullous keratopathy. Similarly, a full-thickness corneal transplantation may increase the risk of endothelial graft rejection in a patient with keratoconus who could otherwise benefit from an anterior lamellar keratoplasty. The ideal corneal transplant surgery should replace only the diseased part or "components" in these situations.[3]

Recent innovations in component surgery of the cornea include Descemet's stripping automated endothelial keratoplasty[4] (DSAEK) and Descemet's membrane endothelial keratoplasty[4] (DMEK) for cases with endothelial dysfunction, automated anterior lamellar keratoplasty for anterior stromal diseases and Deep anterior lamellar keratoplasty (DALK) for the management of corneal stromal dystrophies as well as keratoconus. Epithelial tissue transplantation can be successfully used in the treatment of cicatrizing ocular surface diseases like Stevens–Johnson syndrome, chemical injury, and ocular cicatricial pemphigoid.[3,5] All these surgical techniques have certain advantages over the conventional full-thickness corneal transplantation which may represent "overkill therapeutics" in these diseased states.[6] Furthermore, the new techniques allow for effective utilization of the donor tissue so that one donor cornea can be used for more than one recipient. This is especially useful in countries with shortage of donor corneal tissues.[6]

DEVELOPMENT OF ARTIFICIAL CORNEA

Keratoprosthesis

Artificial materials are used to recreate the injured or damaged cornea as an alternative procedure to high risk corneal transplantations.[7-10] When multiple corneal transplants fail, these materials can be used as a last resort to restore functional vision rather than attempting a regraft. Most prosthesis are made up of plastic polymers consisting of a central transparent zone [acrylic, polymethyl methacrylate (PMMA), hydroxyethyl methacrylate (HEMA), etc.], with a surrounding skirt which becomes integrated with the host tissue. The challenges in making a keratoprosthesis (KPro) are its biocompatibility, need for long-term integration with host cornea, and the permanent exposure of the outer component with the host tissue. Several modifications have been made to circumvent these issues, such as creating an intrastromal pocket for resting the implant (AlphaCor, KeraKlear), integrating the implant with human bone [osteo-odonto keratoprosthesis (OOKP) and modified OOKP (MOOKP)], and implanting a clear cylinder in the center of the corneal graft with front and back plates that snap together with corneal tissue sandwiched in-between (Boston K-Pro).[11-16] The modified KPro designs have an anterior surface that promotes epithelialization, and inhibits the downgrowth of epithelial cells into the stroma/implant interface.[17-20]

Tridimensional Cornea Scaffold Models

With improvements in tissue engineering and cell printing have enabled, various 3D scaffolds that partially replicate the human corneal structure have been manufactured from materials including aligned collagen fibrins, silk, chitin, collagen-chitosan hydrogels, fibrin-agarose hydrogels, and synthetic polymer hydrogels.[21-23]

Tissue-engineered Cornea

Tissue-engineered corneas are structured to provide the basic anatomic and functional characteristics of a natural cornea.[24] Bioengineering has many benefits over KPro but has its own limitations and hence hybrid materials which have features of both biologic and artificial materials may come into future research.[3] These are mostly prepared by combining human cells with synthetic biomaterials to imitate human cornea. Histopathological similarity as well as expression of extracellular matrix components and integrins are demonstrated in 3D models made by growing human corneal epithelial cells on a stroma synthesized by human corneal fibroblasts. Type 1 collagen accounts for the majority of extracellular matrix protein in the cornea and has been tried to recreate artificial cornea. These have also been used for in vitro cultivation of stromal fibroblasts. The mechanical properties as well as permeability of collagen gels undergoes changes via cell scaffold interactions in these cultures. The University of Ottawa model is a hydrogel corneal substitute that has successfully been implanted into a variety of animal models.[24] These kinds of hydrated gels can be moulded into different sizes and curvatures that can easily transmit 90% or more of white light. Trials have been conducted in pigs by using recombinant human collagen fibrils type 1 (RHCI) and type 3 (RHCIII) for replacing corneal stromal matrix.[25] Since these are obtained from yeast cells, the risk of transmission of diseases and immune reactions are eliminated unlike in cases of collagens of animal origin. Phase 1 trials are ongoing in Sweden using RHCIII as materials for deep anterior lamellar grafts.[25] However long-term trials with larger sample size are required to determine the usefulness of these materials as substitutes for human cornea. Also, more enhancements are required to make them amenable for use in a variety of clinical scenarios.

NOVEL SURGICAL TECHNIQUES

Corneal surgeons around the world have been performing and publishing novel techniques for corneal transplantation. These techniques are aimed at management of challenging cases, reducing intraoperative problems, as well as increasing the chances of achieving a successful overall outcome. Many of these surgical endeavors include fashioning of the corneal wound to provide good integrity of the graft-host junction and to induce rapid visual recovery.[26,27]

More recently, the femtosecond laser is being tested for performing lamellar as well as full-thickness corneal transplantation procedures. Use of the femtosecond laser to create complex keratoplasty wound designs is a novel technological advancement. The femtosecond laser-assisted penetrating grafts utilize stepped incisions, with "top hat" or "mushroom" shapes, and Z-shaped "zig-zag" incisions. These incisions have more wound surface area to better resist rupture, plus the laser seems to induce a fibrotic healing response along the vertical portion of the corneal incision. All these features contribute to faster as well as better visual recovery.[28-32] Introduction of anterior segment intraoperative optical coherence tomography (OCT) has led to tremendous improvement in lamellar corneal transplantation surgery by helping in continuous monitoring of intraoperative surgical maneuvers. Intraoperative OCT is helpful for the measurement of host and donor corneal thickness, which are the key parameters in choosing the size of microkeratome head. During DALK, intraoperative OCT helps in guiding the exact depth of trephination, assessment of plane of formation of a big bubble, identify the areas of stromal thinning, and assessment of graft-host junction apposition.[33] Even a small perforation could be easily detected and appropriate precautions may then be taken to avoid conversion into a full-thickness keratoplasty. In cases of DSAEK,[34] it helps in deciding the adequate thickness of donor tissue, ensuring complete scoring of host Descemet's membrane in eyes with hazy cornea, identifying the correct graft orientation, and to confirm the graft host apposition, on table at the end of surgery. Complications such as small peripheral detachments,[35] fluid pockets,[35] reverse orientation of graft,[35] and interface debris[35] are easily identified with the help of intraoperative OCT, which can otherwise be missed in hazy corneas.[35] Even, in DMEK, the correct orientation of DMEK scroll[35] can be identified using an intraoperative OCT.

CULTURED CORNEAL ENDOTHELIAL CELLS

The proposed use of cultured corneal endothelial cells[36,37] in cases with endothelial dysfunction has been a topic of discussion for a few years.[37] Only the endothelial layer is affected in cases of bullous keratopathy and corneal endotheliopathy and hence requires only endothelial cell replacement.[36] With the increasing demand for donor corneas many researchers have investigated cultivating human endothelial cells and transplanting them alone on to Descemet's membrane.

Normal human corneal endothelial cells do not proliferate and are arrested in the G1 phase of cell cycle, in vivo. Even though the endothelial cells of older donors show ability to proliferate in vitro they enter very slowly into the cell cycle compared to young donors. To circumvent this issue many growth promoting agents such as fibroblast growth factor, epidermal growth factor, and endothelial cell growth supplements have been used to promote endothelial cell proliferation (**Figs. 1A and B**). Alternative solutions include producing corneal endothelial cells from the stem cells[38] rather than cadaveric donors or direct reprogramming of more numerous somatic cells,[39] though the latter approach is in its infancy. Multiple models have been trialled by transplanting cultivated animal or human endothelial cells in the past.[40-44] Recently Chen et al. proposed a model which has healthy monolayer of endothelium without the help of immortalized cells. Early data suggest the successful maintenance of host stromal dehydration by the transplanted cultured endothelial cells.[36] Future studies will determine whether any of these gigantic efforts will be successful at the clinical level. The ongoing studies will open the horizons of future in vivo endothelial transplants with better methods and long-term outcomes.

REGENERATIVE MEDICINE APPROACH TO ENDOTHELIAL REPLACEMENT

Rho-associated kinases (ROCK) belong to the AGC (cAMP-dependent protein kinase/protein kinase G/protein kinase C) family of serine-threonine protein kinases.[45-47] ROCK kinase inhibitors act by promoting cell cycle proliferation, migration,[48] enhances cell adhesions, and inhibition of apoptosis of corneal endothelial cells.[49,50] When ROCK gets activated, it phosphorylates the downstream targets which in turn controls the contraction of smooth muscle by sensitizing calcium ions. Thus, cyclin D levels increase and suppress phosphorylation of cyclin-dependent kinase inhibitors 1B, p27/kip1 that regulates endothelial cell cycle. They regulate signal transductions for stress fiber contraction, cell adhesion, cellular motility, cell proliferation, and apoptosis.[51] The effect of ROCK inhibitors varies in different tissues and they are currently used in treatment of open-angle glaucoma and endothelial regeneration in cornea. It achieved FDA approval for use in glaucoma in 2017 and was recently approved in Japan and few other countries for Fuchs corneal dystrophy.[49,50,52-55] They can also be used for in vitro cultivation and proliferation of endothelial cells also which can be used in cell-based therapy.[56] Cultivated corneal endothelial cells along with ROCK inhibitors are injected into the anterior chamber and patient is kept prone.[53,55] In Japan, injection of cultivated corneal endothelial cells to treat corneal endothelial failure is in clinical trial.[57] ROCK inhibitors have also been tried for preventing allograft rejection by their effect on preventing angiogenesis and lymph angiogenesis and improving graft survival by maintaining endothelial cell viability.[58]

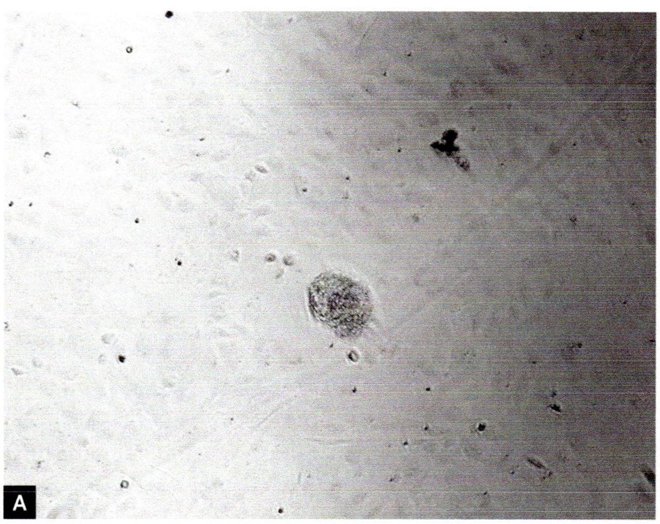

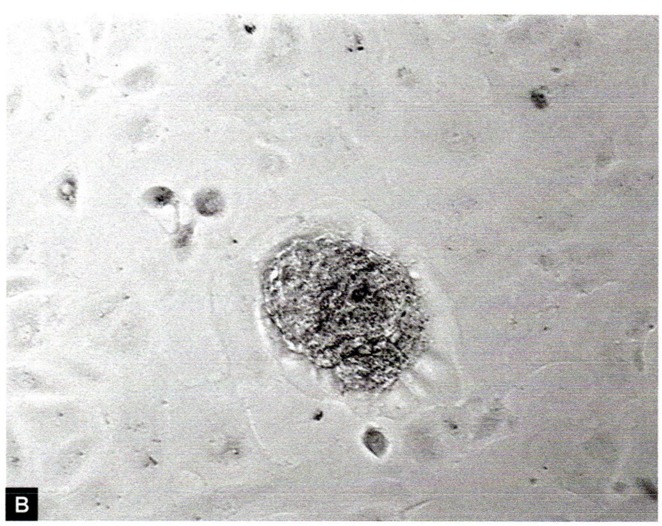

Figs. 1A and B: Human corneal endothelial cells in vitro. Human corneal endothelial cells cultured from a primary cell suspension. Cells shown at day 33 of culture. (A) Endothelial cell sheet and (B) Central mass has morphology consistent with being a holoclone (a colony descended from a single stem cell).

GENE THERAPY

Advancement in gene therapy has created a new technique, known as the *clustered regularly interspaced short palindromic repeats* (CRISPR)-*associated protein 9* (CRISPR-Cas9). This technique is simple and very efficient compared to older technologies for gene editing like zinc-finger proteins.[59] It uses an RNA-guided DNA endonuclease with enzymatic activity of Cas9 nuclease derived from bacteria *Streptococcus pyogenes* which has the ability to create double-stranded breaks at targeted locations of DNA sequence. *Cas9* gene knockout occurs by nonhomologous end joining (NHEJ) repairing of DNA that results in production of nonfunctional proteins.[60] The greatest advantage of this technology is that it can alter the gene to express positively (gene activation) or negatively (repression). In such cases, the Cas9 enzyme is deactivated (dCas9) and coupled with enhancers (such as VP16)[61] or repressors of chromatin compaction such as the Krüppel associated-box (KRAB) domain.[62] Many in vitro studies with CRISPR-Cas9 are underway for the treatment of corneal dystrophies such as TGFβ1-related corneal dystrophies,[63] Schnyder corneal dystrophy[64] and other corneal diseases by targeting human herpes viruses.[65]

The cornea is also ideal for CRISPR-Cas9 use[20] because of its immune privilege status and the absence of vascularity.[66] This helps in reducing the immunological response against the plasmids which are used in gene therapy[67] as well as limits the components to inside the cornea and prevents systemic spread to other organs.[20] Gene therapy was tried initially in vitro on human tissue-engineered cornea (hTEC) as it shares features with native cornea. Since the hTEC can be maintained at the air–liquid interface for many days, the CRISPR-Cas9 components can be deposited directly on the humid upper surface of the hTEC without dilution by culture media and quantitative measurement of components in contact can be done easily.[20] The CRISPR-Cas9-targeted gene alteration can then be passed to the daughter cells of the superficial epithelial layers by simply raising the hTEC to the air–liquid interface. CRISPR-Cas9 can be combined with cell culture by transfecting the 3D models of cornea with them as a monolayer and then producing a 3D model from this.[20] However, to produce quality cornea models using such methods, the edited genes should not interfere with the cell proliferation and maturation of cells to produce tissue cultured corneas with well-differentiated epithelium.[20]

SUMMARY

With all these exciting and novel strategies being developed to combat various problems associated with corneal transplantation, the future seems promising. The era of penetrating keratoplasty as the solution to all severe corneal disease cases is over and emerging technologies are poised to progressively replace keratoplasty.

REFERENCES

1. Birnbaum F, Mayweg S, Reis A, Böhringer D, Seitz B, Engelmann K, et al. Mycophenolate mofetil (MMF) following penetrating high-risk keratoplasty: Long-term results of a prospective, randomised, multicentre study. Eye (Lond). 2009;23(11):2063-70.
2. Unal M, Yücel I. Evaluation of topical ciclosporin 0.05 percent for prevention of rejection in high-risk corneal grafts. Br J Ophthalmol. 2008;92:1411-4.
3. Shimmura S. Component surgery of the cornea. Cornea. 2004; 23:S31-5.
4. Ong HS, Ang M, Mehta J. Evolution of therapies for the corneal endothelium: past, present and future approaches. Br J Ophthalmol. 2021;105(4):454-67.
5. Sangwan et al. Simple limbal epithelial transplantation (SLET): A novel surgical technique for the treatment of unilateral limbal stem cell deficiency. Br J Ophthalmol. 2012;96(7):931-4.
6. Vajpayee RB, Sharma N, Jhanji V, Titiyal JS, Tandon R. One donor cornea for 3 recipients: A new concept for corneal transplantation surgery. Arch Ophthalmol. 2007;125:552-4.
7. Chew HF, Ayres BD, Hammersmith KM, Rapuano CJ, Laibson PR, Myers JS, et al. Boston keratoprosthesis outcomes and complications. Cornea. 2009;28(9):989-96.
8. Khan BF, Harissi-Dagher M, Pavan-Langston D, Aquavella JV, Dohlman CH. The Boston keratoprosthesis in herpetic keratitis. Arch Ophthalmol. 2007;125:745-9.
9. Holak SA, Holak HM, Bleckmann H. AlphaCor keratoprosthesis: postoperative development of six patients. Graefes Arch Clin Exp Ophthalmol. 2009;247:535-9.
10. Bradley JC, Hernandez EG, Schwab IR, Mannis MJ. Boston type 1 keratoprosthesis: The university of california davis experience. Cornea. 2009;28:321-7.
11. Schrage N, Hille K, Cursiefen C. Current treatment options with artificial corneas: Boston Kpro, Osteo-odontokeratoprosthesis, Miro Cornea® and KeraKlear®. Ophthalmologe. 2014;111: 1010-8.
12. Jiraskova N, Rozsival P, Burova M, Kalfertova M. AlphaCor artificial cornea: Clinical outcome. Eye (Lond). 2011;25:1138-46.
13. Studeny P, Krizova D, Kuchynka P. Use of pocketmaker microkeratome for creation of corneal pocket for foldable keratoprosthesis keraklear implantation—case series. Open Ophthalmol J. 2015;9:126-30.
14. Casey TA. Osteo-odonto-keratoprosthesis. Proc R Soc Med. 1966;59:530-1.
15. Zerbe BL, Belin MW, Ciolino JB; Boston Type 1 Keratoprosthesis Study Group. Results from the multicenter Boston type 1 keratoprosthesis study. Ophthalmology. 2006;113:1779.e1-7.
16. Falcinelli G, Falsini B, Taloni M, Colliardo P, Falcinelli G. Modified osteo-odonto-keratoprosthesis for treatment of corneal blindness: Long-term anatomical and functional outcomes in 181 cases. Arch Ophthalmol. 2005;123:1319-29.
17. Aldave AJ, Kamal KM, Vo RC, Yu F. The Boston type I keratoprosthesis: Improving outcomes and expanding indications. Ophthalmology. 2009;116:640-51.
18. Ciolino JB, Dohlman CH. Biologic keratoprosthesis materials. Int Ophthalmol Clin. 2009;49:1-9.
19. Liu C, Hille K, Tan D, Hicks C, Herold J. Keratoprosthesis surgery. Dev Ophthalmol. 2008;41:171-86.
20. Campillo-Fernandez AJ, Pastor S, Abad-Collado M, Bataille L, Gomez-Ribelles JL, Meseguer-Dueñas JM, et al. Future design of a new keratoprosthesis. Physical and biological analysis of polymeric substrates for epithelial cell growth. Biomacromolecules. 2007;8:2429-36.
21. Guérin LP, Le-Bel G, Desjardins P, Couture C, Gillard E, Boisselier E, et al. The human tissue-engineered cornea (hTEC): Recent progress. Int J Mol Sci. 2021;22(3):1291.

22. Ozcelik B, Brown KD, Blencowe A, Ladewig K, Stevens GW, Abberton K, et al. Biodegradable and biocompatible poly(ethylene glycol)-based hydrogel films for the regeneration of corneal endothelium. Adv Healthc Mater. 2014;3(9):1496-507.
23. Chen Z, Liu X, You JJ, Song Y, Tomascovik-Crook E, Sutton G, et al. Biomimetic corneal stroma using electro-compacted collagen. Acta Biomater. 2020;113:360-71.
24. Griffith M, Jackson WB, Lagali N, Merrett K, Li F, Fagerholm P. Artificial corneas: A regenerative medicine approach. Eye (Lond). 2009;23(10):1985-9.
25. Fagerholm P, Lagali N, Carlsson DJ, Merret K, Griffith M. Corneal regeneration following implantation of a biomimetic tissue-engineered substitute. Clin Transl Sci. 2009;2(2):162-4.
26. Kaushal S, Jhanji V, Sharma N, Tandon R, Titiyal JS, Vajpayee RB. "Tuck in" lamellar keratoplasty (TILK) for corneal ectasias involving corneal periphery. Br J Ophthalmol. 2008;92:286-90.
27. Lee J, Winokur J, Hallak J, Azar DT. Femtosecond dovetail penetrating keratoplasty: Surgical technique and case report. Br J Ophthalmol. 2009;93:861-3.
28. Farid M, Steinert RF, Gaster RN, Chamberlain W, Lin A. Comparison of penetrating keratoplasty performed with a femtosecond laser zig-zag incision versus conventional blade trephination. Ophthalmology. 2009;116:1638-43.
29. Farid M, Steinert RF. Deep anterior lamellar keratoplasty performed with the femtosecond laser zigzag incision for the treatment of stromal corneal pathology and ectatic disease. J Cataract Refract Surg. 2009;35:809-13.
30. Soong HK, Malta JB. Femtosecond lasers in ophthalmology. Am J Ophthalmol. 2009;147:189-97.
31. Bahar I, Kaiserman I, Lange AP, Levinger E, Sansanayudh W, Singal N, et al. Femtosecond laser versus manual dissection for top hat penetrating keratoplasty. Br J Ophthalmol. 2009;93:73-8.
32. Cheng YY, Hendrikse F, Pels E, Wijdh RJ, van Cleynenbreugel H, Eggink CA, et al. Preliminary results of femtosecond laser-assisted descemet stripping endothelial keratoplasty. Arch Ophthalmol. 2008;126:1351-6.
33. Steven P, Le Blanc C, Lankenau E, Krug M, Oelckers S, Heindl LM, et al. Optimising deep anterior lamellar keratoplasty (DALK) using intraoperative online optical coherence tomography (iOCT). Br J Ophthalmol. 2014;98:900-4.
34. Pasricha ND, Shieh C, Carrasco-Zevallos OM, Keller B, Izatt JA, Toth CA, et al. Real-time microscope-integrated OCT to improve visualization in DSAEK for advanced bullous keratopathy. Cornea. 2015;34:1606-10.
35. Juthani VV, Goshe JM, Srivastava SK, Ehlers JP. Association between transient interface fluid on intraoperative OCT and textural interface opacity after DSAEK surgery in the PIONEER study. Cornea. 2014;33:887-92.
36. Chen KH, Azar D, Joyce NC. Transplantation of adult human corneal endothelium ex vivo: A morphologic study. Cornea. 2001;20:731-7.
37. Engelmann K, Friedl P. Optimization of culture conditions for human corneal endothelial cells. Invest Ophthalmol Vis Sci. 1989;25:1065-72.
38. McCabe KL, Kunzevitzky NJ, Chiswel BP, Xia X, Goldberg JL, Lanza R. Efficient generation of human embryonic stem cell-derived corneal endothelial cells by directed differentiation. PLoS One. 2015;10(12):e0145266. doi: 10.1371/journal.pone.0145266.
39. Pan SH, Zhao N, Feng X, Jie Y, Jin ZB. Conversion of mouse embryonic fibroblasts into neural crest cells and functional corneal endothelia by defined small molecules. Sci Adv. 2021;7(23):eabg5749.
40. Engelmann K, Friedl P. Growth of human corneal endothelial cells in a serum-reduced medium. Cornea. 1995;14:62-70.
41. Bohnke M, Eggli P, Engelmann K. Transplantation of adult human or porcine corneal endothelial cells onto human recipients in vitro. Part II: evaluation in the scanning electron microscope. Cornea. 1999;18:207-13.
42. Gospodarowicz D, Greenburg G, Alvarado J. Transplantation of cultured bovine corneal endothelial cells to species with nonregenerative endothelium. The cat as an experimental model. Arch Ophthalmol. 1979;97:2163-9.
43. Jumblatt NM, Maurice DM, McCulley JP. Transplantation of tissue-cultured corneal endothelium. Invest Ophthalmol Vis Sci. 1978;17:1135-41.
44. Aboalchamat B, Engelmann K, Böhnke M, Eggli P, Bednarz J. Morphological and functional analysis of immortalized human corneal endothelial cells after transplantation. Exp Eye Res. 1999;69:547-53.
45. Leung T, Manser E, Tan L, Lim L. A novel serine/threonine kinase binding the Ras-related RhoA GTPase which translocates the kinase to peripheral membranes. J Biol Chem. 1995;270:29051-4.
46. Matsui T, Amano M, Yamamoto T, Chihara K, Nakafuku M, Ito M, et al. Rho-associated kinase, a novel serine/threonine kinase, as a putative target for small GTP binding protein Rho. EMBO J. 1996;15:2208-16.
47. Ishizaki T, Maekawa M, Fujisawa K, Okawa K, Iwamatsu A, Fujita A, et al. The small GTP-binding protein Rho binds to and activates a 160 kDa Ser/Thr protein kinase homologous to myotonic dystrophy kinase. EMBO J. 1996;15:1885-93.
48. Biro M, Munoz MA, Weninger W. Targeting Rho-GTPases in immune cell migration and inflammation. Br J Pharmacol. 2014;171:5491-506.
49. Okumura N, Nakano S, Kay EP, Numata R, Ota A, Sowa Y, et al. Involvement of cyclin D and p27 in cell proliferation mediated by ROCK inhibitors Y-27632 and Y-39983 during corneal endothelium wound healing. Invest Ophthalmol Vis Sci. 2014;55:318-29.
50. Okumura N, Ueno M, Koizumi N, Sakamoto Y, Hirata K, Hamuro J, et al. Enhancement on primate corneal endothelial cell survival in vitro by a ROCK inhibitor. Invest Ophthalmol Vis Sci. 2009;50:3680-7.
51. Liao JK, Seto M, Noma K. Rho kinase (ROCK) inhibitors. J Cardiovasc Pharmacol. 2007;50:17-24.
52. Feng Y, LoGrasso PV, Defert O, Li R. Rho Kinase (ROCK) inhibitors and their therapeutic potential. J Med Chem. 2016; 59:2269-300.
53. Okumura N, Koizumi N, Kay EP, Ueno M, Sakamoto Y, Nakamura S, et al. The ROCK inhibitor eye drop accelerates corneal endothelium wound healing. Invest Ophthalmol Vis Sci. 2013;54:2493-502.
54. Okumura N, Okazaki Y, Inoue R, Kakutani K, Nakano S, Kinoshita S, et al. Effect of the Rho-associated kinase inhibitor eye drop (Ripasudil) on corneal endothelial wound healing. Invest Ophthalmol Vis Sci. 2016;57:1284-92.
55. Koizumi N, Okumura N, Ueno M, Nakagawa H, Hamuro J, Kinoshita S. Rho-associated kinase inhibitor eye drop treatment as a possible medical treatment for Fuchs corneal dystrophy. Cornea. 2013;32:1167-70.
56. Peh GS, Adnan K, George BL, Ang HP, Seah XY, Tan DT, et al. The effects of Rho-associated kinase inhibitor Y-27632 on primary human corneal endothelial cells propagated using a dual media approach. Sci Rep. 2015;5:9167.
57. Ong HS, Peh G, Neo DJH, Ang HP, Adnan K, Nyein CL, et al. A novel approach of harvesting viable single cells from donor corneal endothelium for cell-injection therapy. Cells. 2020;9(6):1428. Published 2020 Jun 9.
58. Inomata T, Fujimoto K, Okumura Y, Zhu J, Fujio K, Shokirova H, et al. Novel immunotherapeutic effects of topically administered ripasudil (K-115) on corneal allograft survival. Sci Rep. 2020; 10(1):19817.

59. Barrangou R, Birmingham A, Wiemann S, Beijersbergen RL, Hornung V, Smith A. Advances in CRISPR-Cas9 genome engineering: Lessons learned from RNA interference. Nucleic Acids Res. 2015;43:3407-19.
60. Jasin M, Haber JE. The democratization of gene editing: Insights from site-specific cleavage and double-strand break repair. DNA Repair (Amst). 2016;44:6-16.
61. Xu X, Gao J, Dai W, Wang D, Wu J, Wang J. Gene activation by a CRISPR-assisted trans enhancer. Elife. 2019;8:e45973.
62. Thakore PI, D'Ippolito AM, Song L, Safi A, Shivakumar NK, Kabadi AM, et al. Highly specific epigenome editing by CRISPR-Cas9 repressors for silencing of distal regulatory elements. Nat Methods. 2015;12:1143-9.
63. Usui T. To protect corneal transparency against diseases. Nippon Ganka Gakkai Zasshi. 2016;120:246-62; discussion 263.
64. Dong F, Jin X, Boettler MA, Sciulli H, Abu-Asab M, Del Greco C, et al. A mouse model of schnyder corneal dystrophy with the N100S point mutation. Sci Rep. 2018;8:10219.
65. van Diemen FR, Lebbink RJ. CRISPR/Cas9, a powerful tool to target human herpesviruses. Cell Microbial. 2017;19(2).
66. Cursiefen C. Immune privilege and angiogenic privilege of the cornea. Chem Immunol Allergy. 2007;92:50-7.
67. Charlesworth CT, Deshpande PS, Dever DP, Camarena J, Lemgart VT, Cromer MK, et al. Identification of preexisting adaptive immunity to Cas9 proteins in humans. Nat Med. 2019;25:249-54.

Index

Page numbers followed by *b* refer to box, *f* refer to figure, *fc* refer to flowchart, and *t* refer to table

I

K

L

M

N

O